AIDS - ACQUIRED IMMUNE DEFICIENCY SYNDROME - AND OTHER MANIFESTATIONS OF HIV INFECTION

AIDS

—

Acquired Immune Deficiency Syndrome

—

and Other Manifestations of HIV Infection

Epidemiology, Etiology, Immunology, Clinical Manifestations, Pathology, Control, Treatment and Prevention

Edited by

Gary P. Wormser, M.D.

Division of Infectious Diseases
New York Medical College
Valhalla, New York

Associate Editors

Rosalyn E. Stahl, M.D.

Department of Pathology
New York Medical College
Valhalla, New York

Edward J. Bottone, Ph.D.

Departments of Microbiology
and Pathology
Mount Sinai School of Medicine
New York, New York

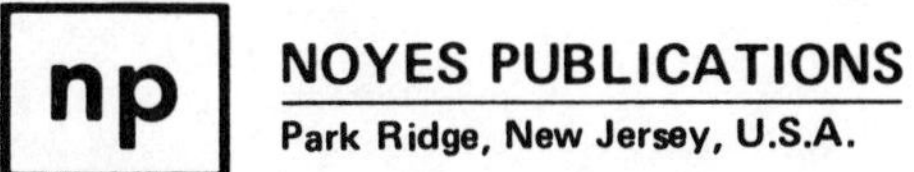
NOYES PUBLICATIONS
Park Ridge, New Jersey, U.S.A.

Library of Congress Catalog Card Number: 86-33308
ISBN: 0-8155-1108-6
Printed in the United States

Published in the United States of America by
Noyes Publications
Mill Road, Park Ridge, New Jersey 07656

10 9 8 7 6 5 4 3 2 1

Library of Congress Cataloging-in-Publication Data

AIDS, acquired immune deficiency syndrome, and other manifestations of HIV infection.

Includes bibliographies and index.
1. AIDS (Disease) 2. Human immunodeficiency viruses.
I. Wormser, Gary P. II. Stahl, Rosalyn. III. Bottone, Edward J. [DNLM: 1. Acquired Immunodeficiency Syndrome. 2. HTLV-III. WD 308 A2877]
RC607.A26A3453 1987 616.97'92 86-33308
ISBN 0-8155-1108-6

This book is dedicated to the health care workers throughout the world engaged in the management of victims of HIV infection—that they may render, with compassion, the highest level of care possible.

Foreword

Human history has been marked by episodic plagues and AIDS is only a recent virulent expression of one of these natural phenomena. AIDS has, however, the potential to be the greatest natural tragedy in human history. This book provides an interim report on Acquired Immune Deficiency Syndrome and other manifestations of HIV infection.

The thought that the great infectious diseases of mankind are under control has made us complacent and optimistic about human health and we have scientific accomplishments and health care to thank for this. Preventive medicine is now coming into its own in attempting to maintain the status quo.

In recent times we have experienced the influenza epidemic, a viral disease that mowed down twenty million people. In this century, viruses have increasingly come to our attention through technological and conceptual developments that have revealed this fascinating microcosmos of miniscule pathogens. Many of these are still in search of diseases and most of them are, as yet, untreatable, although a few are preventable with vaccines. The elusive nature of viruses is no doubt associated with their unique life-style, best characterized by the intimacy with their host. They are obligate parasites, depending, for their procreation and survival, on the biosynthetic mechanisms of the host cell. The intimate cell-virus relationship makes it difficult to sort out viral molecules from cellular molecules, both being of the same fundamental nature, nucleic acids, proteins and lipids and sharing basic properties. Consequently, attempts to target viral molecules therapeutically have yielded few successes. The discovery of Interferons, which are natural broad-spectrum antivirals *in vitro,* initially raised hopes of a universal viral inhibitor but its application to human viral diseases is, as yet, replete with frustation. The most consistently successful approach to dealing with viral diseases has been with vaccines which take advantage of our exquisitely specific immune system to ferret out and neutralize viral molecules.

The human AIDS virus, HIV, like the earlier human retroviruses (HTLV-I and II), is an example of a super-intimate virus. It has the capacity to transform itself into and become integrated with cellular genes. As such, the virus becomes occult and capable of the ultimate degree of parasitism. This makes it all the more difficult to deal with. The capacity of all retroviruses to do this is all the more remarkable considering the fact that their genome is RNA, a molecule that is unable to integrate with cellular DNA. These viruses accomplish this feat by means of a unique enzyme, reverse transcriptase, that makes DNA, the provirus, from the viral genomic RNA. The provirus then can integrate with cellular genes and become cryptic. This accounts for the unpredictable and frequently long latent period between infection with HIV and disease manifestations.

Reverse transcriptase and the process of reverse transcription are common to the family of viruses, the Retroviruses, which have been known by the name RNA tumor viruses for three quarters of a century and have been associated with viral-induced cancers in various species, most recently also in man. The first human retroviruses (HTLV-I and HTLV-II) that were discovered nearly ten years ago and the study of these viruses, made possible by the earlier discovery of Interleukin-2 or TCGF (1976), provided the background information and technical know-how for the discovery, growth, and study of the AIDS virus (1983–84) and the development of a successful screening test (1985). Research achievements in the short time since then have been rapid and have made enormous inroads in the understanding of the biology, epidemiology and clinical aspects of AIDS.

HIV, the virus that causes the human immunodeficiency syndrome also has the capacity to destroy the functioning of the very system the body uses in its defense, the immune system. Latent intracellular HIV can be induced by activation of the virus carrier cell by antigenic stimulation, lysing its host cell and spreading to other cells. This compounds the already difficult task of dealing with this disease. The cytopathic effect on immune cells, particularly the T-helper cells, central to the regulation of the immune system, depletes this cell population and progressively leads to an array of immune system dysfunctions and many opportunistic infections. The disease is also associated with frequent development of certain tumors and with impairment of the central nervous system.

It is clear that such a complicated viral strategy and the resulting manifestations of this fatal disease offer a great challenge to virologists, immunoologists, and clinicians and it is more than obvious that a concerted effort is essential to the understanding of this enigma. Luckily, we are now helped by the abundant knowledge stemming from animal and human retrovirology and from the many significant advances in immunology and molecular biology. The unique enzyme, reverse transcriptase, has provided one specific target of attack and this has recently yielded a first generation anti-HIV drug, AZT. Other similar drugs are on trial. Molecular biology studies of the viral genes and their products will no doubt reveal other potential targets and also address the problem of the heterogeneity of the virus by which the virus can escape the immune system and which seems to anticipate the need for a cocktail of immunogens as an effective vaccine. The immunologists will identify the *in vivo* immune responses that protect against HIV, determine how to protect against both free virus and cells infected with the virus, try to modify and restore certain immune responses, discover ways to prevent the occult virus from being activated and evaluate the use of animal models for testing vaccine candidates for safety and efficacy. Clinicians will design clinical trials, determine which groups of people should receive test vaccines and how to measure vaccine efficacy in humans. Recently, a clinical trial with a candidate vaccine has been initiated in Zaire and similar trials in the U.S. are imminent.

The war on AIDS requires a global effort on the part of governments, multinational organizations, industry, scientists, public health workers and educators. The virus is transmitted sexually and no one is immune. It is not confined to certain minorities of life style (drug addicts), sexual preference (homosexuals), or color, as the power and lability of human sexuality makes most of us susceptible and spread of the virus is an exponential process, giving the disease its relentless character and making the fight against it a race against time. If we can make rapid and fundamental changes in our sexual behavior, we can, at least, slow its spread and buy time for the development of more effective drugs and a vaccine.

Evolution cares little for its agents, viruses or humans, but we care for humans. If we use the unique human features of imagination, focus and effort and, if these features are supported by means and by cooperation, there is optimism that the AIDS epidemic is only a temporary problem of nature's tinkering, and that it will be overcome and then have beneficial effects on the greater issues, the quality of life, human relationships and perhaps even a return to romanticism. In an era in which we have witnessed nuclear war, the holocaust and now the AIDS pandemic, it appears that mind and technology are not omnipotent, that progress through technology is not the solution to all human problems and certainly is not a potion for human happiness. But for now we must use mind and technology to unravel the mechanism of AIDS and its many complications described and discussed in this book. If we can dream it, we can do it. By addressing ourselves to the biological problem of the intimacy of the cell-virus relationship in AIDS, we can hope to restore the intimacy of human relationships.

Bethesda, Maryland
April, 1987

Robert C. Gallo, M.D.
Emmanuel Heller, Ph.D.
National Cancer Institute
Laboratory of Tumor Cell Biology

Foreword

The first cases of *Pneumocystis carinii* pneumonia were reported among young immunocompromised men in the United States in 1981, nearly six years ago. Since that time, the scientific progress in understanding AIDS, and its etiologic agent, the human immunodeficiency virus (HIV) has been nearly incredible. In parallel with this scientific understanding of AIDS has come increased recognition of the significance of AIDS as a worldwide public health problem. During the first six years, AIDS has been reported from citizens of most nations. Societies throughout the world are grappling with solutions to minimize transmission of HIV. Discovery of HIV and development of diagnostic tests have provided fundamental tools for prevention, but further advances are urgently needed, particularly in therapy and vaccines.

Provision of accurate up-to-date information on HIV infection and AIDS forms the basis of current prevention efforts. Today, those of us in health care must have a fundamental knowledge of the clinical and social aspects of HIV infection. *AIDS - Acquired Immune Deficiency Syndrome - and Other Manifestations of HIV Infection* edited by Dr. Wormser and his colleagues provides comprehensive and up-to-date information on the subject. This text should greatly assist health care workers in fulfilling their dual roles as providers of care and sources of accurate information to patients.

Atlanta, Georgia
April, 1987

James W. Curran, M.D., M.P.H.
Director
AIDS Program
Center for Infectious Diseases
Centers for Disease Control

Preface

Up to March of 1987, two landmark events have occurred in the history of our understanding of AIDS: one is the recognition of the entity as a distinct clinical syndrome; the other is the discovery of the etiologic agent. The clinical syndrome was first described in 1981, and many fundamental concepts of its epidemiology were worked out in the ensuing two years. In 1983-1984, the etiologic viral agent was discovered. In the next several years numerous aspects of its molecular and pathobiology were elucidated, although there is clearly still much to be learned. Already a number of antiviral agents have been tested and at least one has shown some clinical efficacy. Hopefully, the third epoch in this historical process will be the development of an effective vaccine and/or curative antiviral medication. Alternatively, discovery of a means for permanent restoration of the immunologic system, even without eradication of the causative virus, would be an immensely important achievement.

With these considerations in mind, this book was written to provide as comprehensive an overview as possible of the biologic properties of the etiologic viral agent, its clinico-pathological manifestations including AIDS, the epidemiology of its infection, and present or future therapeutic and preventive options. In the same manner as for other infectious diseases when they have become better understood, AIDS is approached from the perspective of the etiologic agent. Consequently, AIDS is seen as a complex manifestation of an even more complex array of clinical and laboratory findings in the biologic expression of this viral infection of man.

As more and more patients seek health care for complications of HIV infection, it is clear that a rapidly enlarging number and scope of health care practitioners must become comfortable with, and facile in, the care of these patients. First entering into this field may be an intimidating experience for the health care professional for several reasons, including unfamiliarity with retroviral diseases, personal concerns over potential communicability, lack of experience with unusual opportunistic infections or tumors, and uncertainty with issues related to death and dying for a young adult population. A formidable amount of medical literature has amassed on the subject of AIDS. For example, over 5,600 citations are listed in the NLM/MEDLARS data base. Consequently, it is doubtful that the busy health care practitioner would have the time to learn about this illness through an extensive survey of this literature.

Thus, it is our hope and intention that this book will provide a reference source for the essential information needed by most practitioners and specialists. Further, interested readers may avail themselves of the extensive bibliographical material provided on each topic.

In this volume, the etiologic retrovirus is referred to as "human immunodeficiency virus" (HIV) except on those occasions when attention is called to a specific isolate. In such situations, the virus is referred to by the name designated by the laboratory in which it was originally isolated. In some chapters, the authors have preferred, however, to continue to use the name, "human T-lymphotropic virus type III" (HTLV-III). Also, in places the term "lymphadenopathy-associated virus" (LAV) is used.

Special thanks go to Ann Marie Everett Fiore, without whose tireless efforts, and consummate secretarial skill, this volume could not have been published. Also, I would like to acknowledge Richard D. Levere, Soldano Ferrone, and George Narita for their helpful advice, generous understanding and never-ending support during this endeavor.

We hope this book has contributed not only to a better understanding of AIDS and HIV infections, but also to helping health care workers render the highest level of medical care possible.

Valhalla, New York
April, 1987

Gary P. Wormser, M.D.
Editor

Contributors

Gerard Agius, M.D.
International AIDS Epidemiology
National Cancer Institute
Bethesda, Maryland

Tauseef Ahmed, M.D.
Department of Medicine
New York Medical College
Valhalla, New York

Rosemary Ancelle, M.D.
WHO Collaborating Center on AIDS
Paris, France

Rudolph Bedford, M.D.
Sloan-Kettering Institute for Cancer Research
New York, New York

Robert J. Biggar, M.D.
International AIDS Epidemiology
National Cancer Institute
Bethesda, Maryland

Edward J. Bottone, Ph.D.
Departments of Microbiology and Pathology
Mount Sinai School of Medicine
New York, New York

John F. Brundage, M.D., M.P.H.
Division of Preventive Medicine
Walter Reed Army Institute of Research
Washington, D.C.

J.B. Brunet, M.D.
WHO Collaborating Center on AIDS
Paris, France

Kenneth G. Castro, M.D.
AIDS Program
Centers for Disease Control
Atlanta, Georgia

Tran C. Chanh, Ph.D.
Department of Virology and Immunology
Southwest Foundation for Biomedical Research
San Antonio, Texas

Peggy Clarke, M.P.H.
Assistant Commissioner for AIDS
New York City Department of Health
New York, New York

Clay J. Cockerell, M.D.
Department of Dermatology
New York University Medical Center
New York, New York

John M. Coffin, Ph.D.
Department of Molecular Biology and Microbiology
Tufts University School of Medicine
Boston, Massachusetts

Mary Ann Adler Cohen, M.D.
Department of Psychiatry
Metropolitan Hospital Center
New York, New York

Beca Damsker, M.D.
Department of Clinical Microbiology
The Mount Sinai School of Medicine
New York, New York

Don C. Des Jarlais, Ph.D.
New York State
Division of Substance Abuse Services
New York, New York

Gordon R. Dressman, Ph.D.
Department of Virology and Immunology
Southwest Foundation for Biomedical Research
San Antonio, Texas

D. Peter Drotman, M.D., M.P.H.
AIDS Program
Centers for Disease Control
Atlanta, Georgia

Frederick P. Duncanson, M.D.
Division of Infectious Diseases
Metropolitan Hospital Medical Center
New York, New York

Brad M. Dworkin, M.D.
Department of Medicine
New York Medical College
Valhalla, New York

Jorg Eichberg, D.V.M., Ph.D.
Dept. of Virology and Immunology
Southwest Foundation for Biomedical Research
San Antonio, Texas

Wafaa El-Sadr, M.D.
New York Veterans Administration Medical Center
New York University School of Medicine
New York, New York

Myron Essex, D.V.M., Ph.D.
Department of Cancer Biology
Harvard School of Public Health
Boston, Massachusetts

Ann Giudici Fettner
Writer Journalist
Washington, DC

Samuel R. Friedman, Ph.D.
Narcotics and Drug Research, Inc.
New York, New York

Patricia N. Fultz, M.D.
AIDS Program
Centers for Disease Control
Atlanta, Georgia

Dana H. Gabuzda, M.D.
Massachusetts General Hospital
Harvard Medical School
Boston, Massachusetts

Stuart M. Garay, M.D.
Department of Medicine
New York University School of Medicine
New York, New York

Johanna Goldfarb, M.D.
Division of Pediatric Pharmacology and Critical Care
Rainbow Babies and Childrens Hospital
Cleveland, Ohio

Asha Gupta, M.D.
Department of Pediatrics
Westchester County Medical Center
Valhalla, New York

John W. Hadden, M.D.
Program of Immunopharmacology
University of South Florida
Medical College
Tampa, Florida

Keith Haffer, Ph.D.
Research and Development Dept.
Norden Laboratories
Lincoln, Nebraska

Ann M. Hardy, Dr. P.H.
AIDS Program
Centers for Disease Control
Atlanta, Georgia

Harry W. Haverkos, M.D.
AIDS Program
National Institute of Allergy and
Infectious Diseases
Bethesda, Maryland

Anne K. Hennig, M.S.
Division of Clinical Pathology
State University of New York
Health Science Center
Syracuse, New York

John R. Herbold, D.V.M., M.P.H., Ph.D.
Office of the Assistant Secretary of
Defense
Health Affairs
Washington, DC

David D. Ho, M.D.
Massachusetts General Hospital
Harvard Medical School
Boston, Massachusetts

Kenneth B. Hymes, M.D.
Department of Medicine
New York University School of
Medicine
New York, New York

Patricia A. John, M.S.
Division of Clinical Pathology
State University of New York
Health Science Center
Syracuse, New York

Carol Joline R.N. B.A. C.I.C.
Westchester County Medical Center
Valhalla, New York

Vijay V. Joshi, M.D., FRC Path
United Hospitals Medical Center
The College of Medicine and
Dentistry of New Jersey
Newark, New Jersey

Patrick Kanda, Ph.D.
Dept. of Virology and Immunology
Southwest Foundation for
Biomedical Research
San Antonio, Texas

Phyllis J. Kanki, D.V.M. D.Sc.
Department of Cancer Biology
Harvard School of Public Health
Boston, Massachusetts

Joan C. Kaplan, Ph.D.
Department of Neurology
Massachusetts General Hospital
Harvard Medical School
Boston, Massachusetts

Patrick W. Kelley, M.D., M.P.H.
Division of Preventive Medicine
Walter Reed Army Institute of
Research
Washington, DC

Ronald C. Kennedy, Ph.D.
Dept. of Virology and Immunology
Southwest Foundation for
Biomedical Research
San Antonio, Texas

Natalie C. Klein, M.D., Ph.D.
Department of Medicine
Metropolitan Hospital Medical Center
New York, New York

Bruce E. Kloster, M.D.
Division of Clinical Pathology
State University of New York
Health Science Center
Syracuse, New York

Barbara S. Koppel, M.D.
Department of Neurology
Metropolitan Hospital Center
New York, New York

Lauren B. Krupp, M.D.
Neuroimmunology Branch of NINCDS
National Institutes of Health
Bethesda, Maryland

Louis J. Lafrado, Ph.D.
Department of Veterinary Pathobiology
Ohio State University
Columbus, Ohio

Patrick K. Lai, Ph.D.
Molecular Biology Laboratory
University of Nebraska Medical Center
Omaha, Nebraska

Edward Lebovics, M.D.
Department of Medicine
New York Medical College
Valhalla, New York

Theodore H. Lenox, M.D.
Department of Medicine
Metropolitan Hospital Medical Center
New York, New York

Mark G. Lewis, Ph.D.
Department of Veterinary Pathobiology
Ohio State University
Columbus, Ohio

Alan R. Lifson, M.D., M.P.H.
AIDS Program
Centers for Disease Control
Atlanta, Georgia

Richard B. Lipton, M.D.
Department of Neurology
Albert Einstein College of Medicine
Bronx, New York

Phillip D. Markham, Ph.D.
Department of Cell Biology
Bionetics Research, Inc.
Rockville, Maryland

William J. Martone, M.D.
Hospital Infections Program
Centers for Disease Control
Atlanta, Georgia

Joseph R. Masci, M.D.
City Hospital Center at Elmhurst
Mount Sinai School of Medicine
Elmhurst, New York

Henry Masur, M.D.
Critical Care Medicine Department
National Institutes of Health
Bethesda, Maryland

Lawrence E. Mathes, Ph.D.
Comprehensive Cancer Center
Ohio State University
Columbus, Ohio

Usha Mathur-Wagh, M.D.
Beth Israel Medical Center
Mount Sinai School of Medicine
New York, New York

Eugene McCray, M.D.
Hospital Infections Program
Centers for Disease Control
Atlanta, Georgia

Craig E. Metroka, M.D., Ph.D.
St. Luke's–Roosevelt Hospital Center
Dept. of Hematology/Oncology
New York, New York

Donna Mildvan, M.D.
Beth Israel Medical Center
Mount Sinai School of Medicine
New York, New York

Linda E. Miller, Ph.D.
Division of Clinical Pathology
State University of New York
Health Science Center
Syracuse, New York

Richard N. Miller, M.D., M.P.H.
Walter Reed Army Institute of Research
Washington, DC

Cliff Morrison, M.S., R.N., C.S., C.N.A.
California Nurses Association
AIDS Education and Training Project
San Francisco, California

W. John W. Morrow, Ph.D.
Cancer Research Institute
University of California
San Francisco, California

James M. Oleske, M.D., M.P.H.
United Hospitals Medical Center
The College of Medicine and
Dentistry of New Jersey
Newark, New Jersey

Richard G. Olsen, Ph.D.
Comprehensive Cancer Center
Ohio State University
Columbus, Ohio

Robert R. Redfield, M.D.
Division of Communicable Disease
and Immunology
Walter Reed Army Institute of Research
Washington, DC

Martha F. Rogers, M.D.
AIDS Program
Centers for Disease Control
Atlanta, Georgia

Susanna Cunningham-Rundles, Ph.D.
Division of Pediatric Hematology/
Oncology
The New York Hospital-Cornell
Medical Center
New York, New York

Mangalasseril G. Sarngadharan, Ph.D.
Department of Cell Biology
Bionetics Research, Inc.
Rockville, Maryland

Steve Savona, M.D.
Department of Medicine
New York Medical College
Valhalla, New York

Robert T. Schooley, M.D.
Massachusetts General Hospital
Harvard Medical School
Boston, Massachusetts

David J. Sencer, M.D., M.P.H.
Management Sciences for Health
Boston, Massachusetts

Richard Sharpee, Ph.D.
Research and Development
Department
Norden Laboratories
Lincoln, Nebraska

Paul S. Shneidman, M.D.
Molecular Genetics Branch of
NINCDS
National Institutes of Health
Bethesda, Maryland

Gurdip S. Sidhu, M.D.
New York Veterans Administration
Medical Center
New York University School of
Medicine
New York, New York

Frederick P. Siegal, M.D.
Department of Medicine
Long Island Jewish Medical Center
New Hyde Park, New York

Michael S. Simberkoff, M.D.
Department of Medicine
New York University School of
Medicine
New York, New York

Steven L. Sivak, M.D.
Westchester County Medical Center
New York Medical College
Valhalla, New York

Rosemary Soave, M.D.
Departments of Medicine and Public Health
The New York Hospital-Cornell Medical Center
New York, New York

Rosalyn E. Stahl, M.D.
Department of Pathology
New York Medical College
Valhalla, New York

Anthony F. Suffredini, M.D.
Critical Care Medicine Department
National Institutes of Health
Bethesda, Maryland

Ernest T. Takafuji, M.D., M.P.H.
Office of the Surgeon General
Department of the Army
Falls Church, Virginia

Russell H. Tomar, M.D.
Division of Clinical Pathology
State University of New York Health Science Center
Syracuse, New York

Edmund C. Tramont, M.D.
Division of Communicable Disease and Immunology
Walter Reed Army Institute of Research
Washington, DC

Susan Tross, Ph.D.
Psychiatry Services
Memorial Sloan-Kettering Cancer Center
New York, New York

Marius P. Valsamis, M.D.
Bird S. Coler Hospital
New York Medical College
New York, New York

Markus W. Vogt, M.D.
Massachusetts General Hospital
Harvard Medical School
Boston, Massachusetts

David J. Volsky, Ph.D.
Molecular Biology Laboratory
University of Nebraska Medical Center
Omaha, Nebraska

Christina Walsh, M.D.
Division of Oncology
New York University School of Medicine
New York, New York

John W. Ward, M.D.
AIDS Program
Centers for Disease Control
Atlanta, Georgia

Stanley H. Weiss, M.D.
Environmental Epidemiology Branch
National Cancer Institute
Bethesda, Maryland

Gary S. Wood, M.D.
Veterans Administration Medical Center
Stanford University Medical Center
Palo Alto, California

Gary P. Wormser, M.D.
Department of Medicine
New York Medical College
Valhalla, New York

Robert L. Yarrish, M.D.
Department of Medicine
New York Medical College
Valhalla, New York

Abigail Zuger, M.D.
New York Veterans Administration Medical Center
New York University School of Medicine
New York, New York

NOTICE

In this work, the Editors and Contributors have synthesized their experiences and research, to bring together fundamental information regarding AIDS. The information contained herein is intended as a guide to assist in the understanding of the etiology, epidemiology, clinical manifestations, treatment and management of AIDS. But, the facts regarding AIDS are changing almost daily, as new information is uncovered. Future research could reveal facts contrary to those now found in this book, or information that materially alters the significance of particular facts or theories advanced herein. To the best of our knowledge, the information in the book is accurate at the time of publication. However, neither the Publisher nor the Editors or Contributors will be responsible or liable for the use of any information contained herein.

This work is not intended to describe the scope of risks incurred or avoided by those seeking to prevent infections from AIDS. Avoidance of AIDS can result only from the exercise of great personal prudence and careful attention to the most recent social and scientific information obtainable. This book does not, and cannot serve as a substitute for such prudence and attention.

hool District
R HIGH SCHOOL
RAPH ROAD
SOURI 63129

338

FLOYD J. LAHAY
Assistant Principal

Send two
who from 19th
Dec.

Add ethereal visits to Carmin
Odd - references to amin.

Contents

PART IV
CLINICAL MANIFESTATIONS

PART VI
INFECTION CONTROL CONSIDERATIONS

Part I
Background and Epidemiology

1
The Discovery of AIDS: Perspectives from a Medical Journalist

Ann Giudici Fettner

The scientific accomplishments of this century had led us into complacently thinking along with Dr. Lewis Thomas that "the great infectious diseases of humankind were completely under control and would soon, maybe in my own lifetime, vanish as threats to human health" (1). That viral infection accounts for 85 percent of such illness in the developed world seemed merely a sign of our success in dealing with those caused by other pathogens. The attention of biomedical researchers had gradually turned to areas such as birth defects, cancer, chronic cardiac disease, while preventionists focused on smoking, obesity and alcoholism. But complacency has evaporated in the presence of a novel agent whose apparent ability to target a single type of lymphocyte has thrust on modern medicine a presently untreatable infectious disease.

Medical historians likely will express envy of those who had the unique opportunity to participate in the genesis of an important new disease. But for those struggling to make sense of the elegant and mysterious mechanisms by which the immune system is literally destroyed, for those attempting to treat the mostly young victims of the acquired immunodeficiency syndrome (AIDS), the present is too pressing for thoughts of the historical event in which they are playing a role. AIDS has and will tax the endurance of society in countless ways. Emotionally, physicians are burdened by unexpected impotence, researchers frustrated by their inability to make sense of a plethora of tantalizing clues. Society and the health care delivery system are struggling to accept the new burdens imposed on them by AIDS; and compounding everything is the identification of little-loved segments of the population as the initial and principal victims of the new disease in this country.

Uncertainty is everywhere. As yet, the natural history of AIDS is unknown, and estimates of latency, of the probable numbers of those infected, of the number infected who will progress to active disease, are constantly being rethought. For the first time, the general population mistrusts scientific assurance and goes its own way, some demanding quarantine of victims, others deeming AIDS "God's punishment." The frustrated press views even esoteric molecular discoveries as worthy of front page play and public perception swings back and forth between disinterest and panic. Few aspects of society will escape this change-by-AIDS, from sexual mores to industry, from the military to the political arena.

Doubtless, in time, the mysteries will be resolved, and an effective treatment, perhaps a cure and a vaccine, will be found. In tandem with these discoveries will be heightened knowledge of the immune system, of dealing with those elusive strands of genetic material that cause much of man's disease, the viruses. Then we will be able to look back and evaluate that rare event, the moment in time when a truly new disease made its appearance, as all must have, unremarked except by its first victim.

"SOME NEW FACTOR"

The June 5, 1981 issue of the *Mortality and Morbidity Weekly Report* (MMWR) (2) carried a small report by Michael Gottlieb of UCLA's School of Medicine of five cases of *Pneumocystis carinii* pneumonia (PCP) in homosexual men. Taking second place to that week's cover story of dengue fever in travellers to the Caribbean, that a few previously healthy young men were suffering from an opportunistic infection was of little more than passing interest to most readers. But the manuscript fit in with an on-going survey being conducted by James Curran and Harold Jaffe of the Centers for Disease Control (CDC) in Atlanta.

"That report hit us right between the eyes," Curran recalls. "We had just been working with two other diseases that are very common in homosexual men and that are sexually transmitted--hepatitis B and gonorrhea. So our first thought was that the occurrence of pneumocystis pneumonia in homosexual men might involve sexual transmission." The timing was good: Curran and Jaffe were in the middle of a series of national seminars for public health officials and the week after the Gottlieb report appeared, held a sexually transmitted disease seminar in San Diego. Robert Bolan of Presbyterian Medical Center attended from San Francisco and while talking with Curran, mentioned that he'd also seen a few cases of PCP in gay men.

Back in New York City, Frederick Siegal of the Mount Sinai Hospital was puzzling over the recent referral of a 29 year-old man with a perianal ulcer unresponsive to treatment. Uncontrollable diarrhea and fevers of 104°F seemed the culprits of the patient's severe weight loss. A colostomy had been performed to see if the passage of feces might be keeping the growing ulcer infected, but it did nothing to improve his condition. Experimental drugs affected the man's nervous system; interferon had no effect. Then he developed pneumonia and Siegal was called in. "I found his immune system was strangely, severely depressed. When all the hypotheses we knew to make, when all rational treatment was exhausted, we had to stand around and watch him die," Siegal recalled

Unaware of what was happening in New York, Curran and Jaffe returned to Atlanta from the West Coast and with other CDC workers formed an ad hoc working group to see if they were indeed facing a novel outbreak of illness in California. Their first activity: telephone calls around the country to determine whether other institutions were experiencing unusual illness in gay men. The calls turned up no PCP, but physicians in two New York City hospitals had patients with severe perianal herpes infections. In addition to the one seen by Siegal, there were four others. At Memorial Sloan-Kettering Cancer Center, Jon Gold recalls these early patients: saying that he hadn't known what to make of the ulcers in their first patient, "then we had a few other patients with similar features -- young men with uncontrollable ulcers who later developed infections of the central nervous system with an unusual parasite called toxoplasma, or else got PCP -- and we realized that we had probably seen the first case of this type in 1979."

In common with some of the California patients, many in New York were infected with *Candida albicans* (3),(4) and cytomegalovirus (CMV) (5), and as well were experiencing debilitating fevers, extreme weight loss and swollen lymph nodes (6). The publication by Siegal and others in December 1981, in the *New England Journal of Medicine* (7), described the cases as "part of a nationwide epidemic of immunodeficiency among male homosexuals." Through 1980 and 1981, there had been as many as 40 independent observations of one or two patients by physicians in their private practices, but until the *NEJM* and *MMWR* described the groupings, these remained merely curiosities.

As quickly as cases accumulated, so would reports of rare opportunistic infections (8). There would be *Mycobacterium avium-intracellulare* which, prior to the new illness, had been reported only rarely in adults worldwide. Cryptococcus and toxoplasmosis were shortly to be found in the brains of some men. And several were infected with cryptosporidium, so rare in man that only six cases were known to have occurred between 1976 and 1981: in 1981 and 1982, Pearl Ma of St. Vincent's Hospital in New York diagnosed it in fourteen. Donald Armstrong, head of Infectious Diseases at Sloan-Kettering Cancer Center, said to Jim Curran, "I've been here for twenty years and I've never seen anything like this before."

The same surprise was being felt by Alvin Friedman-Kien at New York University when, in March of 1981, a young man with an unconfirmed Hodgkin's lymphoma "mentioned that he had these funny spots on his legs" which were spreading to his chest and abdomen: his internist sent him to dermatologist Friedman-Kien. Within a week, another patient with these lesions was referred by the same physician. "They turned out to have very similar backgrounds. Both were in their late 30's, both had been extremely promiscuous--and into a lot of what is called "kinky" sex. And both men had a multiplicity of sexual partners over an extended period of time as well as a habit of using a variety of recreational drugs--cocaine, marijuana, LSD,... and amyl nitrite, a drug I'd never heard of except for treating cardiac conditions," recalls Friedman-Kien. In his years of practice, Friedman-Kien had seen around thirty cases of Kaposi's sarcoma (KS), all in elderly men. The Cancer Registry at New York University for the previous nine years recorded no cases of KS in men younger than fifty.

Again the telephone served as the initial epidemiological tool: calls by Friedman-Kien turned up six cases from private practices, and another half dozen from Memorial Sloan-Kettering, where the head of the dermatology department, Dr. Bijan Safai's special area of study was the rare tumor. "We had already been doing immune-function tests on transplant patients with KS, so when these young men started coming in, we did the same tests on them. We found profound immune depression," said Safai (9). His puzzlement was felt by all physicians who came early to the disease: "The KS was recognized, but it took a while to connect it to their being gay."

Continuing his investigation, Friedman-Kien discovered that in his own institution, Linda Laubenstein had several sick men with KS and a call to a friend in Oakland, California, within a week resulted in reports of three more. A common thread, the presence of amebiasis, led the New York University researcher to telephone Dennis Juranek, chief of the CDC's parasitology unit. With Curran, Juranek flew to New York to review the charts of the KS patients, which by late spring of 1981 totalled nineteen. Shortly after the *MMWR* reported the outbreak of PCP in gay men, Friedman-Kien's paper on KS in a similar population was published in the *Journal of the American Academy of Dermatology* (10).

At the CDC during 1981 it was obvious that something peculiar was happening. One tantalizing lead was the discovery in New York that most of those with KS had the HLA marker DR5 (11), which is known to confer a special predisposition in the classic cases in elderly Italian and Jewish men. An interesting early observation made by Rosalyn Stahl and others at New York University (12) was that patients with KS had seriously deranged cellular immune functions. But because 90 percent of the sick men had used amyl (or butyl) nitrite, "our best clue to the cause of the disease was 'poppers'", recalls Curran (13). This tentative lead was confounded by a spate of activities and infections among gay men that suggested there might be a multiplicity of initiating events. But there were problems with life-style speculations: though there was something new about, as Dave Durack of Duke University commented, "homosexuality is at least as old as humanity." Later, however, some correlation between certain sexual practices and the likelihood of developing immune dysfunction was identified (14).

T-CELL RATIOS EXPLORED

After initial disbelief, others began tracking the mysterious illness: said Anthony Fauci, now Director of the National Institute for Allergy and Infectious Disease, "When I first read about the California cases in the June 1981 *MMWR*, I thought, 'Fluke! They probably have ingested some bad drugs.' and I just forgot about it. Then the July issue came out: pneumocystis had been joined by Kaposi's and I thought, 'Oops! This is strange!' Then I started hearing things from my colleagues in New York and, knowing the sexual exposure of gay men, I became vaguely anxious that it might be a new disease--and that it would spread".

When immunologist Fauci started looking at the immune functions of two patients admitted to the National Institute's Clinical Center, he noted two novel aspects: "The first was that while opportunistic infections usually affect people with across-the-board immune suppression, this one was very selective. The second was absolutely new to me: certain lymphocytes, the T-4 cells, that should have been there, were simply gone, absent." Also, though hyperactively churning-out immunoglobulins, the B-cells in these patients had lost the ability to make antibody against new foreign substances. In addition, there was massive destruction of platelets, and circulating immune complexes were found in many of the patients: immune regulatory functions seemed to be in a state of total anarchy.

The most intriguing aspect of the dysregulation was the reversed ratio of T-4 and T-8 cells, though as Robert Biggar of the National Cancer Institute said, "There is a dearth of information about the general public in terms of helper/suppressor ratios. The T4/T8 ratio is a brand new entity that's been around only since 1980, so there's a whole lot of data tumbling out now relating this to every conceivable disease". Many suffering from KS alone had T-cell ratios well within normal parameters; those with PCP often had virtually no T-4 cells left to measure. In the new syndrome, instead of there being increased numbers of T-8 cells, as is usual in immunocompromised persons, the ratio was unbalanced by the disappearance of the T-4's. Studies of healthy gay men used as controls showed that up to 80 percent had some degree of ratio reversal (12),(13). Said Bijan Safai, "It all shows us how ignorant we are about these very important things."

AN EARLY PAIR OF THEORIES

The early hope that what Jim Curran called "a quick and dirty study" would produce an answer to the geometrically increasing illness was destined to be unfulfilled. Nitrites were impossible to implicate because their hoped-for contamination couldn't be found and, though widely used, were not universal. Another theory suggested that contamination of some aspect of the "baths", clubs used by some gay men for socializing and anonymous sexual encounters, might be implicated; again, no evidence of this could be found. Two biologic possibilities were put forward and each immediately attracted adherents. One was that antigenic overload of infection was responsible (16). After all, virtually all of the sick men had a combination of venereal disease (5), intestinal parasites and hepatitis: most were also infected with cytomegalovirus and many recalled having had Epstein-Barr virus-caused mononucleosis. In addition, sperm on the fragile rectal mucosa was proposed as itself being immunosuppressive (17).

Others demurred: none of this was new and Gottlieb insisted that "people in third-world countries, and some in the U.S., are constantly being challenged with antigens, by repeated infections through their lives. Yet no failure of the immune system of this dimension has been documented previously, which is a good argument for a new infectious agent as the cause of this new disease". But what agent? A virus or perhaps a bacteriophage? A mutation of cytomegalovirus or Epstein-Barr virus, both known previously to cause abnormalities in immune function? No, said James Goedert, "not unless they've changed so much they're no longer still the same viruses."

"...AND TWO CLUSTERS"

Early in the burgeoning epidemic of what would come to be called AIDS, in an atmosphere some perceived as desperate, physicians were trying to make sense of the entirely peculiar illnesses afflicting young homosexual men. At New York University, Linda Laubenstein and Friedman-Kien were attempting to track the sexual contacts of a man whose pseudonym became "Erik." Erik had worked for a Canadian airline, had been diagnosed much earlier with KS, and was found to have had sex with another gay man who had died at NYU. "Someone else also knew that Erik had stayed in a house on Fire Island where three men had died," remembers Friedman-Kien, but no one could locate him. As an expert in KS, Friedman-Kien was invited to attend a meeting of gay physicians in San Francisco. At the meeting, "a doctor came over to me and said, "I have a date tonight with a Canadian who has Kaposi's sarcoma. Do you think it's okay for me to go to bed with him?" relates Friedman-Kien. "I just stared at him and then said, "Is it a man named Erik?" "Yes," he said, "do you know him?" Friedman-Kien said, "I almost fell off my seat."

Through this lucky accident, Erik was found and his co-operation proved the first firm evidence of sexual transmission. During the previous three years, Erik had had approximately 250 sexual contacts and was able to provide medical anthropologist, William Darrow of the CDC, with names and addresses of 72. Contacted by Darrow, four biopsy-confirmed cases of KS, and many men with lymphadenopathy and reversed T cells were identified among Erik's contacts.

In the Los Angeles area, sexual histories were being taken from the surviving 13 of 19 cases. Joel Weisman, from whose practice many of the first patients had come, reported to Epidemic Intelligence Service (EIS) officer David Auerbach that in discussing the growing epidemic, a VD patient had told him about eight men who had attended a party where there had been "a lot of sex": all eight subsequently came down with the disease. When this was confirmed by Auerbach, there were two clusters linked by sexual contact and Erik was involved in both. Recalled Auerbach, "We have now identified about forty cases in ten cities that we can put on a schematic map that are linked by sexual contact." Harold Jaffe said "our statistician tells us that the probability of all of these contacts among men with the same rare disease occurring by random chance not only approaches zero--it _is_ zero. And that's an unusual statement for a statistician." Mini-clusters began turning up here and there and theories of substances, sperm and antigenic overload paled.

As information accumulated several probabilities became evident: a specific, infectious agent seemed the likely culprit; one did not have to have a great number of sexual contacts to be at risk; many men appeared to have been exposed to the illness but remained healthy: were they able to infect others? But it was evidence for a new viral entity that became the game after which most investigators began tracking in earnest (18).

HAITIANS CONFOUND THE EARLY THEORIES

George Hensley, chief pathologist at Jackson Memorial Hospital in Miami, kept looking at the frozen sections of brain. Although the young Haitian had died from a particularly vicious case of tuberculosis, "it just didn't look right," recalled Hensley. This wasn't the first such slide the pathology lab people had worried over in the spring of 1981 soon after straggling boatloads of Haitians began to appear in the southern metropolis. As he had before, Hensley froze and filed the latest specimens. These were soon joined by other equally puzzling sections as Haitian patients died of tuberculosis with neurological manifestations such as seizures, disorientation and confusion. Finally, a section covered with the distinctive protozoan *Toxoplasma gondii* came into focus and, "Bang!" says Hensley; "We had an epidemic." (19)

The CDC telephone survey inquiring about immunosuppressed gay men was received just after Hensley's diagnosis of toxoplasmosis. "We don't have anything like that," Hensley answered, "but we do have several Haitians who've died with toxoplasmosis and cytomegalovirus in their brains." By the middle of 1982, gay men in Miami were joining what had become a steady flow of Haitians who were starting to be seen in Brooklyn, New Jersey and Montreal, as well as in Florida. The social aspects of the new illness, still thought of by most as a "gay" disease, were doubly confusing in Haitians who, in most respects, are of a completely foreign culture. Questioned about homosexuality, the Haitians categorically denied such practices. Exotica briefly became a focus, with voodoo practices and ritual scarring mentioned frequently in the press. Among other problems raised by this new group of AIDS patients, the first cases in women would appear.

THE AFRICAN CONNECTION

There were numerous indications that AIDS had begun in Haiti at approximately the same time as in the U.S. But epidemiologic studies on the island were patently flawed and many contended that the true incidence was being concealed by the government of then President-for-Life, "Baby Doc" Duvalier. Despite official Haitian attempts to relate AIDS to homosexual activities exclusively in the tourist city of Port-au-Prince, where American gay men had been going since the early 1970's, there were hints that Haitians might have brought the disease from Zaire in central Africa.

When the Belgian government relinquished their colonial oversight of the vast, poverty-stricken nation in the early 1960's, Zaire was left without trained citizens to run the state. At once, French-speaking Haitians were signed to long- and short-term technical assistance and teaching contracts and a regular traffic between the island and the former Belgian Congo commenced. Early speculation that AIDS may have arisen in Africa was partly predicated on similarities between the virulent Kaposi's sarcoma known to afflict African's, and the KS in AIDS. Soon, however, more substantial evidence of Africa's involvement occurred in Europe: in France and Belgium prior to 1981, more than a dozen cases in both Africans and Europeans who had lived or travelled on the African continent were seen (20). None had had contact with Americans or Haitians, and many were women.

The question that immediately arose was, was this an old illness in central and west Africa? "No," stated Charles Olweny, formerly of Makerere University Medical School in Kampala, Uganda, who insisted that he had never before seen such an illness complex. Other physicians with similar experience agreed. Later, researchers examining African sera frozen in Europe would suggest that the putative virus had been present in Uganda since the late 1970's (21); but like much seroepidemiology in Africa, this may have been confounded by poorly stored blood or by malaria (22). Despite such questions, AIDS has spread rapidly across central Africa infecting women as frequently as men. Questions of transmission there, initially cast in the homosexual mode, have yielded to acceptance that heterosexual spread is obviously taking place. The incidence of venereal disease, parasites and marginal nutrition in these populations, added to poor sanitation and inadequate sterilization of syringes in health facilities and among traditional healers, probably accounts for the 1:1 male-female ratio in most areas.

BLOOD AND BABIES

While the new illness in gay men was caught relatively early in the burgeoning epidemic, New York City's intravenous (IV) drug abusers with opportunistic pneumonias largely were overlooked or, according to Harold Jaffe, "we thought, well maybe there is a common drug usage between the homosexuals and IV drug users." The possibility of blood transmission (23) wasn't considered until interviews with the drug users revealed that they didn't use nitrites and had moderate sexual activity. Many of the first female cases were IV drug abusers (24).

In January of 1982, the CDC learned of a hemophiliac who had died of pneumocystis in Florida. All they could do was tag the pentamidine file: "If this is real, there will be another case and another," said William Foege, then head of CDC. That summer, hemophiliacs in Ohio and Colorado joined the growing list (25),(26).

During late 1980 at St. Michael's Hospital in Newark, New Jersey and at Albert Einstein Medical Center in the Bronx, New York, babies were dying with a puzzling immune-deficiency illness. Slowly and cautiously, the pediatric immunologists managing these children tried to sort out from the range of possible pediatric immune deficiencies something that could be classified. "These symptoms didn't fit into any known congenital immune deficiency," recalls Ayre Rubinstein of Einstein; then "we thought of congenital infections that might have affected the immune system--Epstein-Barr virus, cytomegalovirus, rubella--but couldn't find any evidence of them."

In Newark, James Oleske was having identical problems with critically and mysteriously ill infants, when a series of fortuitous coincidences inclined him towards the possibility that the newly identified disease in gay men might also be affecting children. Recognizing the father of one of the dead babies in a hospital corridor, Oleske found the man had come for immune function tests, which showed reversed T-cell ratios. The father, an IV drug user, also had many AIDS-related opportunistic infections and severe weight loss. Then, identical twins--one ill, the other healthy--convinced Oleske that he was not seeing an heritable condition. Of Oleske's babies, Jim Curran said, "Unfortunately, he realized there was a pattern only after some of the kids had died, so there was not an adequate clinical or laboratory workup to make a diagnosis of AIDS."

A major problem in diagnosing AIDS in children was the apparent dissimilarity of disease manifestations. Where adults were infected primarily with viral and fungal entities, the babies were succumbing to bacterial agents. Their failure-to-thrive was seen by Oleske as analogous to the weight loss in adults. Still, it was not until the May 1983 issue of *JAMA* that AIDS in children was presented to the scientific community. In an editorial in *JAMA* (27) accompanying articles by Oleske and Rubinstein (28),(29), Anthony Fauci wrote, "The evidence for a transmissible agent being the cause of AIDS is about as strong as it could be, despite the fact that, up to this point, no agent has been identified or isolated."

A PUTATIVE AGENT IDENTIFIED

In May 1983, four research reports appeared in *Science* (30)-(33) describing an apparent relationship between AIDS and the new retroviral family called HTLV--human T-cell leukemia virus. Robert Gallo of the National Cancer Institute, who earlier had identified the first in this family as the cause of a type of leukemia, had isolated HTLV from a number of AIDS patients, as had Luc Montagnier of the Pasteur Institute in France. The American papers described HTLV-I and the newly identified HTLV-II (which is thought to be a precipitator of hairy-cell leukemia). The French virus, though apparently different from those described in the Gallo articles, was tentatively identified by Montagnier as another HTLV: it had been isolated from an American patient with AIDS.

Almost exactly one year later, Secretary of Health and Human Services, Margaret Heckler, called a hurried press conference in Washington. Introduced by then-Assistant Secretary Edward Brandt, Heckler announced that "the arrow of funds has hit the target," and that the cause of AIDS had been identified by Gallo's people as a new variant of the retrovirus, which they were calling HTLV-III. The Gallo virus was almost identical to the one described earlier by Montagnier, and which he had designated LAV--lymphadenopathy-associated virus.

Ms. Heckler introduced Dr. Gallo, whose group had also devised a culture technique for the virus that was to be made available to other researchers, and said that a test to detect antibodies for HTLV-III would be available "within six months" to screen blood donations. Heckler also claimed that a vaccine would be "ready for testing" within two years. Controversy of many kinds was kicked-off by this announcement, much of which continues to this day. Although most accept HTLV-III/LAV as the prime agent, many researchers remain convinced that without one or more co-factors, as yet unidentified, AIDS does not result. Most available research funding immediately found its way into proposals designed to investigate various aspects of this new pathogen, leaving those with alternative ideas to scramble for other funding sources. But most have experienced difficulty in gaining adequate funding, particularly for clinical research and education, and Congress has had to push a reluctant Administration into allocating even what many perceive as a paltry response to the nation's "No. 1 health priority."

In 1984, Jay Levy and others from the University of California, San Francisco published a report (34) describing a retroviral isolate which was identified as being "similar to LAV." Making a clear distinction between the type C morphology of the HTLV-I and II types and that of the new isolate, Levy named the type D retrovirus, ARV, or AIDS-associated retrovirus. The three claims on the nomenclature of the virus implicated in AIDS have led to confusion in the lay public, as well as often ascerbic disagreements between professionals. Many questioned the designation of the identified agent as properly belonging to the HTL family of viruses, stating that its closer homology with visna, a viral infection of sheep and goats which produces a similar disease course, is a more natural association (35).

A serious on-going lack of cooperation between government agencies was revealed when the report by the Office of Technical Assessment (36), a Congressional watch-dog group, was published in February 1985. The report delineated the controversy regarding whether Gallo or Montagnier was the first to identify the implicated retrovirus, explored the lack of federal funding available for the new epidemic and set out many of the problems concerning the ELISA antibody test. The test was patented by Dr. Gallo and the US Department of Health and Human Services on April 23, 1984 and soon thereafter, five firms were awarded licenses to produce the test which was approved by the Food and Drug Administration for protecting the national blood supply. In the summer of 1985, testing of all blood donations was put into effect (37).

THE BLOOD TEST

Questions of legality concerning using the antibody test other than for screening blood donations arose immediately. Many groups were concerned with civil rights and job discrimination. A lengthy article in *The New England Journal of Medicine* (38) in May of 1985 suggested that "as donors become better informed about the likelihood of a reactive test, they may begin to view a donation as a major risk to their well-being", meaning their peace of mind. The article also questioned the accuracy of the blood test, despite manufacturers' claims of near-99 percent accuracy (39). Questions also remained about false-negatives, and James Goedert of the National Cancer Institute cautioned that there are probably antibody-negative persons who are carriers. Self-excluded from the donation pool, those in designated risk-groups were joined by many in the general population who either unrealistically feared contracting AIDS from giving blood, or were apprehensive that their names would appear on lists of those infected. In the winter of 1985, the Armed Forces decided to test all new recruits and soon followed this with a plan to test all military personnel. Robert Redfield's group at Walter Reed Hospital in Washington also came up with a Staging Classification for HTLV-III/LAV infection (40).

FEARS OF TRANSMISSION AND PREVENTION EFFORTS

In the minds of most persons concerned with AIDS, many critical questions affecting the public have been less than well-managed and many certainly are not yet resolved. From wide-spread early refusal to care for patients with the disease, most hospital staffs have gradually learned that AIDS is indeed difficult to contract in ways other than sexual contact or relatively large inoculations of infected blood. Thousands of accidental needle sticks in medical settings have resulted in virtually no infection of personnel (41),(42). Reports from areas where sick children have been cared for at home have demonstrated that casual household contact also does not transmit the virus (43). But such evidence has done little to reassure the public, and disputes over allowing HTLV-III/LAV positive children to attend public school, over infected prison inmates, over AIDS in the workplace, continue unabated. International travel to and from areas with high incidences of AIDS may someday require special clearance from immigration health officials.

The "dis-ease" of the public is understandable: with little funding, educational efforts have fallen far short of convincing most people that AIDS cannot be contracted casually. Despite medical assurances to the contrary, uncertainties over latency and projections that two to three million Americans may unknowingly be able to transmit the deadly virus, have caused considerable fear. Presently, the only prevention method available is the practice of "safe sex" for those not in monogamous relationships, but this has little meaning to the majority of Americans, most of whom do not perceive themselves to be at risk. And while most gay men have changed their sexual practices -- as evidenced by a dramatic fall-off in the incidence of other sexually transmitted diseases, IV drug abusers remain inaccessible. That the majority of female cases in America and Europe have connections to IV drug abuse is of major concern (44).

In Africa, Latin America, and throughout the Caribbean, few governments have come to grips with AIDS in their populations and the disease can be expected to follow the geometric six-to-nine-month rate of doubling experienced in this country in the early days of the epidemic. Many novel compounds are being tested in an effort to break the infectious cycle of the AIDS virus, among which azidothymidine (AZT) (45) to date is viewed as the most promising. A vaccine is still "iffy" against this virus because of its ability to change its surface coat and because of other concerns. While it is true that science has never moved so rapidly as in these past few years, it still is unable to offer more than supportive care and treatment for specific opportunistic infections to those experiencing any part of the spectrum of AIDS-related illness.

Socially and politically, the picture has been and remains even less optimistic, as subtle but significant changes begin to insinuate themselves into every aspect of life. AIDS is now a major cause of death in young males and a major burden for the already hard-pressed health care delivery system which, Edward Brandt remarked in 1983, could not "support additional thousands of chronically sick people suffering from recurrent infections for which they must be hospitalized again and again." At that time, it was inconceivable that AIDS would not soon yield to scientific innovation, but we still stand at the gate, working against time to circumvent the terror of a world described by poet W. B. Yeats:

> "Things fall apart; the center cannot hold.
> Mere anarchy is loosed upon the world."

REFERENCES

1. Thomas L., On the AIDS Problem. Discover 42:103 (1983)

2. CDC., Pneumocystis pneumonia-Los Angeles. MMWR 30:250-252 (1981)

3. Gottleib, M.S., Schroff, R,, Schanker, H.M., et al., *Pneumocystis carinii* pneumonia and mucosal candidiasis in previously healthy homosexual men. N Engl J Med, 305:1425-31 (1981)

4. Klein, R.S., Harris, C.A., Butkus-Small, C., et al., Oral candidiasis in high-risk patients as the original manifestation of the acquired immune deficiency syndrome. N Engl J Med 311:354-58 (1984)

5. Drew, W.L., Mintz, L., Miner, R.C., et al, Prevalence of cytomegalovirus infection in homosexuals. J Infect Dis 143:1888-1892 (1981)

6. Metroka, C.E., Cunningham-Rundles, S., Pollack, M., et al., Generalized lymphadenopathy in homosexual men. Ann Intern Med 99:585-591 (1983)

7. Siegal, F.P., Lopez, C., Hammer, G.S., et al., Severe acquired immunodeficiency in male homosexuals, manifested by chronic perianal ulcerative *Herpes simplex* lesions. N Engl J Med 305:1439-44 (1981)

8. Mildvan, D., Mathur, U., Enlow, R.W., et al., Opportunistic infections and immune deficiency in homosexual men. Ann Intern Med 96:700-704 (1982)

9. Safai, B., Good, R.A., Kaposi's sarcoma: a review and recent developments. Cancer 31:1-12 (1981)

10. Friedman-Kien, A., Disseminated Kaposi's sarcoma syndrome in young homosexual men. J Am Acad Derm 5:468-471 (1981)

11. Friedman-Kien, A., Laubenstein, L., Rubinstein, P., et al., Disseminated Kaposi's sarcoma in homosexual men. Ann Intern Med 96:693-700 (1982)

12. Stahl, R.E., Friedman-Kien, A., Dubin, R., et al., Immunologic abnormalities in homosexual men: relationship to Kaposi's sarcoma. Am J Med 73:171-178 (1982)

13. Goedert J.J., Nouland, C.Y., Wallen, W.C., et al., Amyl nitrite may alter T-lymphocytes in homosexual men. Lancet 1:412-416 (1982)

14. Detels, R., Fahey, J.L., Schwartz, K., et al., Relationship between sexual practices and T-cell subsets in homosexually active men. Lancet 1:609-11 (1983)

15. Kornfeld, H., Stouwe, R.A.V., Lange, M., et al., T-lymphocyte subpopulations in homosexual men. N Engl J Med 307:729-731 (1982)

16. Sonnabend J., Witkin, S.S., Purtilo, D.T., Acquired immunodeficiency syndrome, opportunistic infections, and malignancies in male homosexuals. JAMA 249:2370-2374 (1983)

17. Hertenbach, U., Shearer, G.M., Germ-cell induced immune suppression in mice. J Exp Med 155:1719-1729 (1982)

18. CDC., Epidemiologic aspects of the current outbreak of Kaposi's sarcoma and opportunistic infections. N Engl J Med 306:240-252 (1982)

19. Moskowitz L.B., Kory, P., Chan, J.C., et al., Unusual causes of death in Haitians residing in Miami. JAMA 250:1187-1190 (1983)

20. Clumeck, N., Mascart-Lemone, F., DeMaubeuge, F., et al., Acquired immune deficiency syndrome in black Africans. Lancet 1:642 (1983)

21. Saxinger, W.C., Levine, P.H., Lange-Wantzin, G., et al., Evidence for exposure to HTLV-III in Uganda before 1973. Science 227:1036-1038 (1985)

22. Norman, C., Africa as the origin of AIDS. Science 230: 1140-1141 (1985)

23. CDC., Possible transfusion-associated acquired immune deficiency syndrome (AIDS)--California. MMWR 321:652-654 (1982)

24. Masur, H., Michelis, M.A., Wormser, G.P., et al., Opportunistic infection in previously healthy women: initial manifestation of a community acquired cellular immunodeficiency. Ann Intern Med 97:533-539 (1982)

25. Poon, M., Landay, A., Prasthofer, E.F., et al., Acquired immunodeficiency syndrome with *Pneumocystis carinii* and pneumonia and *Mycobacterium avium-intracellulare* in a previously healthy patient with classic hemophilia: clinical, immunologic, and virologic findings. Ann Intern Med 98:287-290 (1983)

26. CDC., *Pneumocystis carinii* pneumonia among persons with hemophilia A. MMWR 31:365-367 (1982)

27. Fauci, A., The acquired immune deficiency syndrome: The ever broadening clinical spectrum. JAMA 249:2375-2376 (1983)

28. Oleske, J., Minnefor, A., Cooper, R., et al., Immunodeficiency syndrome in children. JAMA 249:2345-2349 (1983)

29. Rubinstein, A., Sicklick, M., Gupta, A., et al., Acquired immunodeficiency with reversed T4/T8 ratios in infants born to promiscuous and drug-addicted mothers. JAMA 249:2350-2356 (1983)

30. Gallo, R.C., Sarin, P., Gelmann, E.P., et al., Isolation of human T-cell leukemia virus in acquired immune deficiency syndrome (AIDS). Science 220:865-867 (1983)

31. Barre-Sinoussi, F., Chermann, J.C., Rey, F., et al., Isolation of a T-lymphotrophic retrovirus from a patient at risk for acquired immune deficiency syndrome (AIDS). Science 220: 868- 871 (1983)

32. Gelmann, E.P., Popovic, M., Blayney, D., et al., Proviral DNA of a retrovirus, human T-cell leukemia virus, in two patients with AIDS. Science 220:862-865 (1983)

33. Essex, M., McLane, M.F., Lee, T.H., et al., Antibodies to cell membrane antigens associated with human T-cell leukemia virus patients with AIDS. Science 220:859-862 (1983)

34. Levy, J., Hoffman, A.D., Kramer, S.A., et al., Isolation of lymphocytopathic retroviruses from San Francisco patients with AIDS. Science 225:840-842 (1984)

35. Gonda, M., Wong-Staal, F., Gallo, R.C., et al., Sequence homology and morphologic similarity of HTLV-III and visna virus, a pathogenic lentivirus. Science 227:173-177 (1985)

36. Review of the Public Health Service to AIDS, Office of Technical Assessment, Washington, D.C., February 1985

37. Culliton, B., Five firms with the right stuff. Science 225: 1129 (1984)

38. Osterholm, M.T., Bowman, R.J., Chopek, M.W., et al., Screening donated blood and plasma for HTLV-III antibody. Facing more than one crisis? N Engl J Med 312:1185-1190 (1985)

39. CDC., Update: Public Health Service workshop on human T-lymphotropic virus type III antibody testing -- United States. MMWR 34:477-478 (1985)

40. Redfield, R.R., Wright, D.C., Tramont, E., et al., The Walter Reed staging classification for HTLV-III/LAV infection. N Engl J Med 314:131-132 (1986)

41. Hirsch, M.S., Wormser, G.P., Schooley, R.T., et al., Risk of nosocomial infection with human T-cell lymphotrophic virus III (HTLV-III). N Engl J Med 312:1-4 (1985)

42. McCray, E. Occupational risk of the acquired immunodeficiency syndrome among health care workers. N Engl J Med 314:1127-1132 (1986)

43. Curran, J.W., Morgan, W.M., Hardy, A.M., et al., The epidemiology of AIDS: current status and future prospects. Science 229:344-350 (1985)

44. CDC., Immunodeficiency among female sexual partners of males with acquired immune deficiency syndrome (AIDS) - New York. MMWR 31:697-698 (1983)

45. Yarchoan, R., Klecker, R.W., Weinhold, K.J., et al., Administration of 3'-azido-3'deoxythymidine, an inhibitor of HTLV-III/LAV replication, to patients with AIDS or AIDS-related complex. Lancet 1:575-580 (1986)

2
AIDS in the United States

John W. Ward, Ann M. Hardy, D. Peter Drotman

The first cases of what was later termed the acquired immunodeficiency syndrome (AIDS) were reported to the Centers for Disease Control in the spring of 1981 (1),(2). The patients were all young, previously healthy homosexual men with similar patterns of opportunistic illnesses due to an unexplained suppression of the immune system. In 1982, this pattern of illness was recognized in intravenous (IV) drug abusers, persons with hemophilia, and blood-transfusion recipients (3), and epidemiologists postulated that a transmissible agent was responsible for the syndrome. During 1983 and 1984, several reports documented the isolation of a retrovirus from persons with AIDS (4)-(6). This virus, variously termed lymphadenopathy-associated virus (LAV), human T-lymphotropic virus type III (HTLV-III), and AIDS-associated retrovirus (ARV) is now recognized as the cause of AIDS. The International Committee on the Taxonomy of Viruses has recommended that human immunodeficiency virus (HIV) be used to supplant the three existing names (7).

In 1981, well before the discovery of the AIDS virus, CDC developed a surveillance case definition for AIDS (8). This definition was based on the early observation that patients with AIDS developed certain opportunistic illnesses secondary to a specific defect in the cell-mediated component of the immune system (9). If no other cause for the cellular immune dysfunction was present, the diagnosis of one of 12 opportunistic illnesses was considered indicative of AIDS (Table 1). Following the discovery of the virus that causes AIDS and the development of serologic tests to detect antibodies specific for it, the case definition was modified to include other diseases as part of the spectrum of AIDS, if antibody to HIV is also found (10).

Following the initial case reports, CDC set out to determine the magnitude of the problem by actively seeking other cases meeting the surveillance definition. Physicians in 18 metropolitan areas were contacted and tumor registries were surveyed to identify persons with unexplained cases of opportunistic illnesses. Investigators found an additional 125 cases, with the earliest occurring in the late 1970s. This provided evidence that AIDS was a larger problem than initially suspected and that it was a relatively new disease in the United States and not a previously present but unreported one.

Table 1. Opportunistic Diseases in the CDC Surveillance Case Definition for AIDS in Adults

Diseases Indicative of AIDS

- Atypical mycobacteriosis--disseminated
- Candidiasis--esophageal
- Cytomegalovirus infection--pulmonary, gastrointestinal or central nervous system
- Cryptococcosis--meningitis or disseminated
- Cryptosporidiosis--chronic enteritis
- *Herpes simplex* virus infection--chronic mucocutaneous or disseminated
- Kaposi's sarcoma--in patients less than 60 years of age
- Papovavirus infection--progressive multifocal leukoencephalopathy
- *Pneumocystis carinii* pneumonia
- Primary lymphoma--limited to the brain
- Strongyloidiasis--pulmonary, central nervous system or disseminated
- Toxoplasmosis--encephalitis or disseminated

Diseases Indicative of AIDS--but Requiring Serologic or Virologic Evidence of HIV* Infection

- Candidiasis--bronchial or pulmonary
- Histoplasmosis--disseminated
- Isosporiasis--chronic diarrhea
- Kaposi's sarcoma--in patients 60 years of age or older
- Non-Hodgkin's lymphoma--diffuse, undifferentiated

* HIV = Human immunodeficiency virus

THE AIDS EPIDEMIC

The number of AIDS cases has increased rapidly. Between June 1, 1981 and December 1, 1986, 28,246 (27,843 adult, 403 pediatric) AIDS cases were reported in the United States. The first 1,000 cases were reported over a 21-month period. In contrast, 1,000 cases were reported over a four-week period in early 1986 (11). At the present rate, the number of AIDS cases is expected to double by December, 1987 (12).

Based on an empirical mathematical model that extrapolates from the cases reported by June 1986, approximately 16,000 AIDS cases are expected to be reported during 1986 and 24,000 cases are projected in 1987 (13) (Table 2). Approximately 74,000 AIDS cases will be diagnosed in 1991 and 54,000 (73%) of these patients will die by 1992. The cumulative total of AIDS cases will reach an estimated 270,000 by the end of 1991.

Table 2. Projections of AIDS Cases and Deaths by Year - United States

Year	Cases	Deaths
1978-1985	19,000	9,000
1986	16,000	9,000
1987	24,000	14,000
1988	33,000	22,000
1989	45,000	30,000
1990	59,000	41,000
1991	74,000	54,000
Cumulative:	270,000	179,000
Range:	(201,000-311,000)	(141,000-201,000)

Data from Reference 13.

The case fatality rate from AIDS is high. Over 55% of all adult and adolescent patients are known to have died and the rate increases sharply with time: over 76% of reported AIDS patients died within three years of diagnosis. Because of incomplete reporting of patient deaths, this rate may underestimate the true impact of AIDS.

The large number of AIDS cases and the high fatality for AIDS has had a significant impact on premature mortality rates in areas with large numbers of AIDS cases. By 1984, AIDS had become the fourth leading cause of death for single, never-married males aged 25-50 years in New York City (14). In 1986, AIDS became the leading cause of death in New York City for men aged 30-39 years, and 33% of all deaths of single males in areas of the city with large homosexual populations were due to AIDS (15). Other studies have shown a similar effect on mortality patterns among homosexual men in San Francisco (14).

AIDS TRANSMISSION GROUPS

AIDS cases in adults and adolescents have occurred in six transmission groups (Table 3). These groups are arranged in a hierarchy so that patients with multiple risks are placed in only one group. The distribution of AIDS patients by groups has been remarkably stable over the course of the epidemic in the United States. Seventy-two percent of reported AIDS cases are homosexual/bisexual men. Approximately 17% of cases occur in persons who have abused illicit intravenous drugs. These two groups overlap; about 9% of the homosexual/bisexual men with AIDS report using intravenous drugs. Another 1% of AIDS patients have hemophilia, and 2% have received transfusions. About 3% of AIDS patients have reported heterosexual contact with persons who have AIDS or with members of one of the other risk groups. This last category includes persons born in countries (primarily Haiti) where heterosexual contact is believed to be the major mode of transmission. The remaining 3-4% are persons for whom a risk could not be identified because of severe illness or early death, refusal to cooperate with interviews, or lack of information. A proportion of these patients with no identified risk are probably persons acquiring the infection through heterosexual contact but did not know their partner was at risk for AIDS. In addition, a small number of persons who do not have AIDS but whose illnesses meet the criteria of the case definition may be counted in this group.

Most of the AIDS cases through 1991 are expected to continue to occur in homosexual/bisexual men (70% of cases) and IV drug abusers (16%) (Table 3). However, several small but important changes in the distribution of cases among the transmission groups have been noted and will continue in the coming years.

First, the proportion of AIDS cases associated with transfusion increased from 1.4% in 1983 to 2% in 1986 and is expected to represent 2.5% of cases by the end of 1991 (13),(16). Patients in this group were transfused before 1985. The interval from the date of transfusion to the development of AIDS is long; AIDS develops a mean of 29 months after the infecting transfusion (range 5 to 62 months) (17). The mean incubation period for this group is probably longer because the reported cases are those diagnosed earlier after infection and bias this estimate. Serologic screening of blood donations (begun in 1985) and the self-deferral of those at increased risk (begun in 1983) can be expected to have their greatest impact on the occurrence of transfusion-associated AIDS cases after the mean incubation period has passed (1990 or later).

Second, the proportion of American AIDS patients born outside the United States decreased from 3.7% in 1983 to 1.3% in 1986; this risk group is projected to represent less than 1% of cases

Table 3. Projected Distribution of Adult AIDS Cases by Transmission Group - United States, 1983, 1986, and 1991

Transmission Group	1983		1986		1991	
	No.	%	No.	%	No.	%
Homosexual/bisexual men	1929	72.1	11300	72.6	51100	70.0
Heterosexual IV drug abusers	486	18.2	2700	17.3	12000	16.4
Persons with hemophilia	12	0.4	200	0.9	1000	1.4
Transfusion recipients	37	1.4	300	2.0	1800	2.5
Heterosexual men & women	123	4.6	500	3.3	3900	5.3
(Heterosexual contact)	(25	0.9)	(300	2.0)	(3700	5.0)
(Born outside U.S.)*	(98	3.7)	(200	1.3)	(200	0.3)
Other	89	3.3	600	3.7	3200	4.5
Total	2676	100.0	15600	100.0	73000	100.0

* Includes persons born in countries (primarily Haiti) where heterosexual contact is believed to be the major mode of transmission. Data from Reference 13.

by 1991 (13),(16). The cause of this decline is not known; but may be due to a decrease in the number of HIV infected immigrants from these countries or the overall spread of the disease in U.S. residents.

The fraction of cases attributed to heterosexual exposures has inceased slightly compared with the other transmission modes (Table 3). The proportion of AIDS cases in this group is expected to rise from 2% of cases in 1986 to approximately 5% in 1991 (13),(16). This increase is due to an increase in the number of persons who have had heterosexual contact with persons infected with HIV and to better recognition of these cases among persons previously reported as having no identified risks (11).

DEMOGRAPHIC CHARACTERISTICS OF AIDS PATIENTS

Age

The mean age of all AIDS patients is 36.6 years, and over 90%

of all cases occur in persons 20-49 years of age. The age distribution of AIDS patients varies for the various transmission groups (Table 4). Patients with transfusion-associated AIDS are older than patients in the other groups, probably because of the older age of transfusion recipients in general.

Sex

Over 93% of adult and adolescent AIDS patients are men. Of these men with AIDS, 79% are homosexual/bisexual, and another 15% are heterosexual IV drug abusers. Men in the other transmission groups account for less than 7% of total cases. Of the women patients, over one-half (52%) are IV drug abusers, and 30% have histories of sexual contact with men at high risk for AIDS or who were born in countries where heterosexual contact is believed to be the major mode of transmission. Nine percent of women with AIDS are blood transfusion recipients.

Race

A striking feature of the AIDS epidemic is the large number of patients in minority groups. Overall, 60% of AIDS cases occur in whites, 25% in blacks, and 14% in Hispanics (Table 4). This racial distribution varies greatly by transmission group. Seventy-four percent of homosexual/bisexual men with AIDS are white, 15% are black, and 10% are Hispanic. For non-homosexual IV drug abusers, 51% are black, and 30% are Hispanic. Only 18% of IV drug abusers with AIDS are white. Gay/bisexual men who also abuse IV drugs are racially distributed between these two (Table 4).

The racial distribution of AIDS patients who report heterosexual contact with persons at risk for AIDS (82% are women) is similar to that of IV drug abusers; 52% of these patients are black, and 26% are Hispanic. For women in this group, 60% of the blacks and 77% of the Hispanics reported their male sexual contacts were IV drug abusers. This high proportion of blacks and Hispanics among heterosexual patients and IV drug abusers has resulted in a similar racial distribution of AIDS in children --over 80% of all pediatric AIDS cases occur in black and Hispanic children.

Geographic Distribution

All 50 states, the District of Columbia, and three U.S. territories have reported at least one AIDS case. Two states, New York and California, accounted for 55% of all AIDS cases reported through 1986. Florida (6%), New Jersey (6%), and Texas (5%) have also reported substantial proportions of the U.S. AIDS cases. Some of the transmission groups cluster in certain geographic areas. Over 75% of persons with histories of IV drug abuse who have developed AIDS live in New York and New Jersey. Almost 78% of persons with AIDS born in countries where heterosexual transmission is believed to be the major mode of transmission live in New York and Florida. Seventy-one percent of transfusion-associated AIDS cases occur in areas outside New York and California.

The two metropolitan areas with the highest incidence of AIDS cases have been New York City and San Francisco, which accounted for 35% of all reported cases through 1986 (Table 5). This proportion decreased from 47% of all cases at the end of 1983. The decrease in New York City has been concomitant with the decline in the percentage of AIDS cases in homosexual or bisexual men (11).

Table 4. Age and Racial Distribution of AIDS Cases by Transmission Group, United States, 1986

Transmission Group	Mean Age (years)	Racial Group - % White	Black	Hispanic	Other
Homosexual/bisexual men	37.1	74	15	10	1
Homosexual/bisexual men and IV drug abusers	33.9	64	22	14	1
Heterosexual IV drug abusers	34.8	18	51	30	1
Persons with hemophilia	36.8	83	6	8	2
Transfusion recipients	53.9	79	13	6	2
Heterosexual men and women	33.1	10	76	13	1
(Heterosexual contact)	33.6	21	52	26	1
(Born outside U.S.*)	32.7		99		1
Other	36.5	35	43	20	2
Total	36.6	60	25	14	1

* Includes persons born in countries (primarily Haiti) where heterosexual contact is believe to be the major mode of transmission.

The declining proportion of cases from these areas (despite the continued exponential increase in the absolute numbers of cases) is clearly due to the even more rapid increase in the number of cases being reported from the rest of the country. The number of AIDS cases reported by mid-1986 from other states had doubled in 10.5 months. In contrast, the number of AIDS cases in

Table 5. Projected Distribution of AIDS Cases By Geographic Area - United States, 1983, 1986, and 1991

Area	1983		1986		1991	
	No.	%	No.	%	No.	%
New York City	985	36.0	3900	24.9	8700	11.9
San Francisco	306	11.2	1600	10.1	5900	8.1
Other	1448	52.8	10100	65.0	58400	80.0
Total	2739	100.0	15600	100.0	73000	100.0

New York and California had doubled in 13.6 months. By 1991, only about 20% of all cases will be reported from New York City and San Francisco (13).

Since the first reports from the United States, AIDS has been reported from other countries throughout the world. Two other countries in North America and the Caribbean have reported a substantial number of AIDS cases: Canada (638 cases) and Haiti (377 cases) (18). By July 31, 1986, the World Health Organization Collaborating Centre on AIDS had received reports of 2,856 cases in Europe (18). Most of these were reported from France (707), the Federal Republic of Germany (539), and the United Kingdom (465). AIDS has also been reported from countries of Central (144 cases) and South America (634 cases) and from Australia (256 cases). Most of the cases in countries other than Haiti have occurred in homosexual/bisexual men or IV drug abusers. The proportion of AIDS cases in these transmission groups may differ from one country to another. The largest porportion of AIDS cases in Spain, Italy and Greece are IV drug abusers (19). In Haiti, AIDS appears to be transmitted by heterosexual contact, or parenterally, through injections given by nonmedical personnel (20). The AIDS problem in Africa is probably great, but it has not been well documented. Published studies suggest that AIDS is not rare and that infection with HIV may be common (21),(22). Asia has been underrepresented, but Asian nations have reported numbers of cases. Few Asian Americans living in the United States have developed AIDS.

DISEASE PRESENTATIONS

Of all the opportunistic diseases seen in adult patients with AIDS, the two most commonly reported are *Pneumocystis carinii* pneumonia (PCP) (63% of patients) and Kaposi's sarcoma (KS) (23%). The proportion of AIDS adult patients with KS has decreased from 24% of those reported before December 1984 to 13% in 1985 and 1986. This decrease may be due to a reporting artifact or an actual unexplained decline in the number of these cases.

The other opportunistic illnesses associated with AIDS are seen less frequently. Of these, esophageal candidiasis is the most common initial diagnosis (14% of cases). Less commonly reported initial diagnoses include cytomegalovirus infection (7%), cryptococcosis (7%), atypical mycobacteriosis (5%), chronic *Herpes simplex* (4%), cryptosporidiosis (3%), and toxoplasmosis (3%) (11).

The type of opportunistic disease has a great impact on outcome. Patients with KS alone have had a lower case-fatality rate (38%) than those with other diseases (52%-63%). Patients with KS have tended to live longer after diagnosis; for patients with KS diagnosed in 1983 or earlier, approximately 40% were still living in 1986. In contrast, only 16% of patients with PCP and 21% of patients with the other opportunistic illnesses survived from 1983 to 1986. Other studies have shown the median survival period for persons with KS alone ranges from 14 to 30 months after diagnosis, compared with a 9 to 15 month median survival time for patients with KS and another opportunistic illness and a 4 to 10 months survival interval for patients with an opportunistic illness without KS (23),(24).

The rates of opportunistic infection vary by transmission group. KS has been reported in 29% of homosexual/bisexual males but in only 6% of patients in all other groups at risk for AIDS. The reason for this excess in homosexual/bisexual men is not known; both nitrite inhalents and cytomegalovirus infection have been suggested as possible cofactors for KS in AIDS patients (25),(26).

Forty-four percent of AIDS patients born in Haiti have developed opportunistic illnesses other than KS and PCP. Of these, toxoplasmosis (39%), cryptococcosis (27%), and cytomegalovirus infections (12%) are the most common initial diagnoses. The different disease presentation in Haiti is probably not due to chance and deserves further study.

MODES OF TRANSMISSION

HIV is transmitted in limited ways: through sexual contact, through sharing contaminated IV needles, through transfusion of infected blood components and clotting factor concentrates, and perinatally. HIV has been isolated from a variety of body fluids, including blood, saliva, semen, and tears (27)-(31). The virus preferentially infects T-helper lymphocytes and conceivably could be recovered from any site where such cells are found. However, such findings do not necessarily have public health importance. There is no evidence that contact with saliva or tears results in infection with HIV.

Several studies have examined risk factors for AIDS and HIV infection in homosexual/bisexual men. The most consistent risk factor identified was a large number of male sexual partners

(32),(33). Receptive anal intercourse and other potentially traumatic sexual activities have been associated with HIV infection (32),(34).

Needlesharing and frequent injection are risk factors for AIDS in IV drug abusers (35). Most cases in IV drug abusers (71%) have been reported in New York City and northern New Jersey. This geographic clustering may be related to the more frequent use of "shooting galleries" where sharing of "rented" needles and syringes ("works") is common.

AIDS in persons with hemophilia and in blood-transfusion recipients was reported in 1982 and led to the recognition that AIDS could be transmitted by contaminated blood. Persons with hemophilia acquired the infection through pooled plasma products, especially clotting factor concentrates, which are derived from 2,500 to 22,500 individual donations. The prevalence of HIV antibody is greater in persons with severe hemophilia (36). The use of cryoprecipitate also has been implicated in HIV transmission. AIDS has also occurred in recipients of blood or blood components derived from a single donation. The highest incidence rates occur among those receiving large numbers of transfusions (usually more than 10 units) and children (37). Investigation of donors of blood given to patients with transfusion-associated AIDS has nearly always identified a person at high risk for AIDS; often these donors can be demonstrated to be infected with HIV (27). Most of such infected donors were asymptomatic at the time of the investigation years after the implicated donation. Blood components that presumably have transmitted HIV include whole blood, red cells, platelets, and plasma (14). One study has shown that virtually all recipients of blood from HIV infected donors will become infected (38).

The epidemiology of AIDS and HIV infection is consistent with the routes of transmission listed above and fails to support concerns about transmission of HIV from occupational contact with infected persons (14). Health-care workers who have contact with AIDS patients have not themselves had an increased incidence of AIDS. At least five studies in the United States involving more than 1,498 persons have provided information on health-care workers exposed to HIV-infected persons (39). This total included 666 persons who had needlestick injuries or direct mucosal exposures to persons with AIDS or HIV infection or their specimens. Of the health-care workers in these studies, only three without risk factors were positive for HIV antibody. Two of these workers were investigated, and their infections were termed due to "probable" occupational exposures even though neither worker had a preexposure or early postexposure serum sample tested to document the onset of infection (40). The risk of HIV infection following needlestick injury to health-care workers in these studies has been estimated to be less than 1% (41). Since these reports, another health-care worker seroconverted within six months after being injured with a needle contaminated with blood from an AIDS patient (42). A similar, well-documented case of HIV transmission following an injury with a contaminated needle had previously been reported from England (43). However, these needlestick injuries were unusual; in at least one case, the needlestick injury involved direct inoculation of about 2cc of HIV-contaminated blood.

The collective evidence strongly suggests that the risk to health-care workers of occupational transmission of HIV is low and can be most effectively reduced by following recommended guidelines for the care of HIV-infected persons and the handling of their specimens (39).

There is no convincing evidence that AIDS or HIV can be transmitted through air, food, water, or fomites or by arthropods or casual contact (14).

MANIFESTATIONS OF HIV INFECTION

So far, the number of persons infected with HIV is much greater than the number who have developed AIDS. Between 1 and 1.5 million Americans were estimated to be infected with HIV in 1986 (13),(14). Seroprevalence studies of frozen sera collected periodically since 1978 from a cohort of asymptomatic bisexual men in San Francisco showed an increasing prevalence of infection, from 5% in 1978 to 73% in 1985 (44). In New York City, 75 (87%) of 86 recent IV drug abusers enrolled in a drug detoxification center had antibody to HIV (45). For persons with hemophilia who use factor VIII concentrate, one study identified 18 (72%) of 25 as having HIV specific antibody (45).

Clinical Spectrum of HIV Infection

The AIDS epidemic is a small part of a much larger epidemic of HIV infection. Other symptoms and signs may be seen in some infected persons and some may remain healthy for a number of years. CDC has proposed the adoption of a standard classification system for HIV infection (46). The system includes four mutually exclusive groups (Table 6) ranging from acute and asymptomatic HIV infection (Groups I and II) to persistent generalized lymphadenopathy (Group III) to constitutional symptoms, secondary infections and cancers, and other conditions (Group IV) (47), (48). Patients in Group IV may have one or more of the secondary conditions, and the severity of illness may vary over time. The full clinical spectrum of diseases associated with HIV infection continues to unfold. As more is learned, the classification system can be revised to accomodate additional information.

Recently HIV infection has been associated with neurologic disease, and the virus has been isolated from central nervous system tissue of AIDS patients (49),(50). HIV infection has been associated with aseptic meningitis in otherwise asymptomatic HIV-infected persons recently infected with the virus and has been related to a decrease in intellectual functioning in persons who have aleady developed AIDS (49),(50). The proportion of HIV-infected persons that may ultimately develop HIV-related neurologic illness remains to be determined.

The natural history of HIV infection has been the subject of

Table 6. Summary of Classification System for Human Immunodeficiency Virus Infection

Group I	Acute Infection
Group II	Asymptomatic infection*
Group III	Persistent generalized lymphadenopathy*
Group IV	Other disease
Subgroup A.	Constitutional disease
Subgroup B.	Neurologic disease
Subgroup C.	Secondary infectious diseases
Category C-1.	Specified secondary infectious diseases listed in the CDC surveillance definition for AIDS**
Category C-2	Other specified secondary infectious diseases
Subgroup D.	Secondary cancers**
Subgroup E.	Other conditions

* Patients in Groups II and III may be subclassified on the basis of a laboratory evaluation.

** Includes those patients whose clinical presentation fulfills the definition of AIDS used by CDC for national reporting.

intensive study. Not all HIV-infected persons have progressed to Group IV or developed AIDS. In a longitudinal study of homosexual/bisexual men in San Francisco, 57 men were followed for an average of 44 months after their initial seropositive specimen. Of these, 10 (18%) developed AIDS, and 27 (47%) developed illnesses related to HIV infection (51) (Table 7). The proportion who developed AIDS has increased steadily, and a larger number ultimately may develop AIDS. Approximately 30% of this group are expected to develop AIDS within 72 months of the first evidence of HIV infection. In other studies, a similar proportion developed AIDS, although over a shorter period after infection (52). In longitudinal studies of HIV-infected homosexual/bisexual men, no infectious or pharmacologic cofactors have been identified as increasing the risk of developing AIDS, although such cofactors may exist. So far, the most important risk factor for developing AIDS is duration of infection with HIV (24).

Table 7. Clinical Outcomes for 57 Men with Long-Term HIV Infection

Outcomes	Number of Cases	Percent of Cases	95% Confidence Interval
AIDS	10	17.5	7.6 - 27.4
HIV-related conditions:			
generalized lymphadenopathy;	16	28.1	16.4 - 39.8
other signs or symptoms*;	3	5.3	0 - 11.1
hematologic abnormalities**	8	14.0	5.0 - 23.0
Subtotal	27	47.4	34.4 - 60.4
Asymptomatic	20	35.1	22.7 - 47.5

* Oral candidiasis, weight loss, or persistent idiopathic fever or diarrhea.

** Anemia, neutropenia, or lymphopenia

SUMMARY

The number of persons with AIDS has increased dramatically since the first case reports in 1981. AIDS is the most severe manifestation of HIV infection, and the full clinical spectrum of diseases resulting from this viral infection continues to be defined. This virus has been shown to be transmitted almost exclusively by sexual contact, exposure to contaminated blood, infected needles shared by IV drug abusers, or perinatally.

REFERENCES

1. CDC., Pneumocystis pneumonia - Los Angeles. MMWR 30:250-252 (1981)

2. CDC., Kaposi's sarcoma and Pneumocystis pneumonia among homosexual men, New York City and California. MMWR 30:305-308 (1981)

3. CDC., Acquired immunodeficiency syndrome (AIDS) update, United States. MMWR 33:309-311 (1983)

4. Barre-Sinoussi, F., Chermann, C., Rey, F., et al., Isolation of a T-lymphotropic retrovirus from a patient at risk for acquired immunodeficiency syndrome (AIDS). Science, 220:868-871 (1983)

5. Gallo, R.C., Salahuddin, S.E., Popovic, M., et al., Frequent detection and isolation of cytopathic retroviruses (HTLV-III) from patients with AIDS and at risk for AIDS. Science 224:500-503 (1984)

6. Levy, J.A., Hoffman, A.D., Kramer, A.D., et al., Isolation of lymphocytopathic retroviruses from San Francisco patients with AIDS. Science 225:840-842 (1984)

7. Coffin, J., Haase, A., Levy, J.A., et al., Human immunodeficiency viruses. Science 223:697 (1986)

8. CDC., Update on the acquired immune deficiency syndrome (AIDS) - United States. MMWR 31:507-514 (1982)

9. Masur, H., Michelis, M.A., Greene, J.B., et al., An outbreak of community-acquired *Pneumocystis carinii* pneumonia: Initial manifestation of cellular immune dysfunction. N Engl J Med 305:1431-1438 (1981)

10. CDC., Revision of the case definition of acquired immunodeficiency syndrome for national reporting - United States, MMWR 34:373-375 (1985)

11. Hardy, A.M., Allen, J.R., Starcher, E.T., et al., AIDS trends in the United States: Analysis of the first 15,000 cases in adults and adolescents. International Conference on Acquired Immunodeficiency Syndrome (AIDS), Paris, June, (1986)

12. Morgan, W.M., Selik, R.M., Hardy, A.M., et al., Current trends of AIDS in the United States. International Conference on Acquired Immunodeficiency Syndrome (AIDS), Atlanta, April, (1985)

13. Coolfont Report. A PHS plan for prevention and control of AIDS and the AIDS virus. Public Health Rep 101:341-347 (1986)

14. Curran, J.W., Morgan, W.M., Hardy, A.M., et al., The epidemiology of AIDS: Current status and future prospects. Science 229:1352-1357 (1985)

15. Kristal, A.R., The impact of the acquired immunodeficiency syndrome in New York City. JAMA 255:2306-2310 (1986)

16. CDC., Update: Acquired immunodeficiency syndrome (AIDS) - United States. MMWR 35:17-21 (1986)

17. Peterman, T.A., Jaffe, H.W., Feorino, P.M., et al., Transfusion associated acquired immunodeficiency syndrome in the United States. JAMA 254:2913-2917 (1985)

18. AIDS report. World Health Organization, September 1, 1986

19. CDC., Update: Acquired immunodeficiency syndrome - Europe, MMWR 35:25-38, 43-46 (1986)

20. Pape, J., Lieutaud, B., Thomas, F., et al., AIDS: Risk factors in Haiti. Twenty-fourth Interscience Conference on Antimicrobial Agents and Chemotherapy. Washington, D.C., October (1984)

21. Kreiss, K., Koech, D., Plummer, F., et al., AIDS virus infection in Nairobi prostitutes: Spread of the epidemic to East Africa. N Engl J Med 314:414-418 (1986)

22. Clumeck, N., Guroff, M., Van De Perre, P., et al., Seroepidemiological studies of HTLV-III antibody prevalence among selected groups of heterosexual Africans. JAMA 254:2599-2602 (1985)

23. Riven, B.E., Monroe, J.M., Habschman, B.P., et al., AIDS outcome: A first follow-up. N Engl J Med 311:857 (1984)

24. Moss, A.R., McCallum, G., Volberding, P.A., et al., Mortality associated with mode of presentation in the acquired immune deficiency syndrome. J Natl Can Inst 73:1281-1284 (1984)

25. Haverkos, H.W., Pinsky, P.F., Drotman, D.P., et al., Disease manifestation among homosexual men with the acquired immunodeficiency syndrome (AIDS): A possible role of nitrites in Kaposi's sarcoma. Sex Transm Dis 12:203-208 (1985)

26. Marmor, M., DesJarlais, D., Spira, T., et al., AIDS and cytomegalovirus exposure in New York City drug abusers. International Conference on Acquired Immunodeficiency Syndrome (AIDS), Atlanta, April (1985)

27. Feorino, P.M., Jaffe, H.W., Palmer, E., et al., Transfusion-associated acquired immunodeficiency syndrome: Evidence for persistent infection in blood donors. N Engl J Med 312: 1293-1296 (1985)

28. Groopman J.E., Salahuddin S.Z., Sarngadharan M.G., et al., HTLV-III/LAV in saliva of people with AIDS related complex and healthy homosexual men at risk for AIDS. Science 226: 447-449 (1984)

29. Zagury D., Bernard J., Leibowitch J., et al., HTLV-III in cells cultured from semen of two patients with AIDS. Science 226:449-451 (1984)

30. Jaffe H.W., Feorino P.M., Darrow W.W., et al., Persistent infection with human T-lymphotropic virus type III/lymphadenopathy-associated virus in apparently healthy homosexual men. Ann Intern Med 102:627-628 (1985)

31. Goedert J.J., Sarngadharan M.G., Biggar R.J., et al., Determinants of retrovirus (HTLV-III) antibody and immunodeficiency conditions in homosexual men. Lancet 2:711-716 (1984)

32. Jaffe, H.W., Choi, K., Thomas, P.A., et al., National case-control study of Kaposi's sarcoma and *Pneumocystis carinii* pneumonia in homosexual men: Part 1, epidemiologic results. Ann Intern Med 99:145-151 (1983)

33. Marmor, M., Friedman-Kien, A.E., Zolla-Pazner S., et al., Kaposi's sarcoma in homosexual men: A seroepidemiologic case-control study. Ann Intern Med 100:809-815 (1984)

34. Darrow, W.W., Byers, R.H., Jaffe, H.J., et al., Cofactors in the development of AIDS and AIDS-related conditions. International Conference on AIDS, Paris, June, (1986)

35. Harris, C.A., Small, C.B., Klein, R.S., et al., Needle sharing as a route of transmission of the acquired immune deficiency syndrome. Twenty-Third Interscience Conference on Antimicrobial Agents and Chemotherapy. Las Vegas, October, (1983)

36. McGrady, G., Gjerset, G., Kennedy, S., Risk of exposure to HTLV-III/LAV and type of clotting factor used in hemophilia. International Conference on Acquired Immunodeficiency Syndrome (AIDS) Atlanta, April, (1985)

37. Hardy, A.M., Allen, J.R., Morgan, W.M., et al., The incidence rate of acquired immunodeficiency syndrome in selected populations. JAMA 253:215-220 (1985)

38. Ward, J.W., Deppe, D.A., Sampson, S., et al., The risk of HIV infection for recipients of blood from donors who later developed the acquired immunodeficiency syndrome (In press)

39. CDC., Recommendations for preventing transmission of infection with human T-lymphotropic virus type III/lymphadenopathy-associated virus in the workplace. MMWR 34:681-686, 691-695 (1985)

40. CDC., Update: Evaluation of human T-lymphotropic virus type III/lymphadenopathy-associated virus infection in health-care personnel - United States, MMWR 34:575-578 (1985)

41. McCray, E., et al., Occupational risk of the acquired immunodeficiency syndrome among health care workers, N Engl J Med 314:1127-1132 (1986)

42. Stricoff, R.L., Morse, D.L., HTLV-III/LAV seroconversion following a deep intramuscular needlestick injury [letter]. N Engl J Med 314:1115 (1986)

43. Needlestick transmission of HTLV-III from a patient infected in Africa. Lancet 2:1376-1377 (1984)

44. CDC., Update: Acquired immunodeficiency syndrome in the San Francisco cohort study. MMWR 34:573-575 (1985)

45. CDC., Antibodies to a retrovirus etiologically associated with acquired immunodeficiency syndrome (AIDS) in populations with increased incidences of the syndrome. MMWR 33:377-379 (1984)

46. CDC., Classification system for human T-lymphotropic virus type III/lymphadenopathy-associated virus infections. MMWR 35:334-339 (1986)

47. Metroka, C.E., Cunningham-Rundles, S., Pollack, M.W., et al., Generalized lymphadenopathy in homosexual men. Ann Intern Med 99:585-591 (1983)

48. Mathur-Waugh, U., Spigland, I., Sacks, H.W., et al., Longitudinal study of persistent generalized lymphadenopathy in homosexual men: relation to the acquired immunodeficiency syndrome. Lancet 1:1033-1038 (1984)

49. Resnick, L., diMarzo-Veronese, F., Schubpach, J., et al., Intra-blood-brain synthesis of HTLV-III specific IgG in patients with neurologic symptoms associated with AIDS or AIDS-related complex. N Engl J Med 313:498-504 (1985)

50. Ho, D.D., Rota, T.R., Schooley, R.T., et al., Isolation of HTLV-III from cerebrospinal fluid and neural tissue of patients with neurologic symptoms related to the acquired immunodeficiency syndrome. N Engl J Med 313:1493-1497 (1985)

51. Rutherford, G.W., Echenberg, D.F., O'Malley, P.M, et al., The natural history of HTLV-III/LAV infection and viremia in homosexual and bisexual men in a 6-year follow up study. International Conference on Acquired Immunodeficiency Syndrome (AIDS), Paris, June, (1986)

52. Goedart, J.J, Biggar, R.J., Weiss, S.H., et al., Three year incidence of AIDS in five cohorts of HTLV-III infected risk group members. Science 231:992-995 (1986)

3

The Epidemiology of Pediatric HIV Infections

Martha F. Rogers

Since the Centers for Disease Control (CDC) began surveillance for the acquired immunodeficiency syndrome (AIDS) in 1981, reports of over 20,000 cases of AIDS in the United States have been received. As of April 1986, 281 of these cases have occurred in children under 13 years of age, and another 83 cases have occurred in adolescents aged 13-19 years. Through CDC's national surveillance for AIDS, the epidemiologic characteristics of the most severe form of human immunodeficiency virus (HIV) infection have been well defined. This chapter will summarize the epidemiologic characteristics of children with AIDS, describe transmission patterns of HIV in the pediatric population, and give recommendations on how the spread of infection can be reduced.

SURVEILLANCE FOR AIDS IN CHILDREN

Under CDC's national surveillance system practicing physicians and hospital personnel voluntarily report cases of AIDS to state or local health departments. For reporting purposes, the CDC case definition of AIDS requires that an opportunistic disease or malignancy indicating an underlying cellular immune deficiency be present (Table 1). Therefore, not all cases of HIV infection are reported, and reported cases represent the most severe form of the infection. The case definition for pediatric AIDS was revised in June of 1985 to include biopsy-proven lymphoid interstitial pneumonitis (1). Pediatric cases are defined as cases in children under 13 years

Table 1. Diseases Considered by CDC at Least Moderately Predictive of Underlying Cellular Immunodeficiency Associated with AIDS

Protozoal and Helminthic Infections

Intestinal cryptosporidiosis causing diarrhea > 1 month
Pneumocystis carinii pneumonia
Strongyloides infection of the lungs, CNS, disseminated infection
Disseminated toxoplasmosis infection of internal organs other than liver, spleen, or lymph nodes
Isosporiasis causing chronic diarrhea*

Fungal Infections

Candida esophagitis
Bronchial or pulmonary candidiasis*
Disseminated or meningeal cryptococcosis
Disseminated histoplasmosis*

Bacterial Infections

Disseminated nontuberculous mycobacterial infections

Viral Infections

Cytomegalovirus infection of internal organs other than liver, spleen, or lymph nodes
Chronic mucocutaneous *Herpes simplex* virus infection or infection of the lungs or gastrointestinal tract beyond the mouth, throat, or rectum
Progressive multifocal leukoencephalopathy

Cancer

Kaposi's sarcoma
Brain lymphoma
Non-Hodgkin's lymphoma*

Idiopathic

Chronic lymphoid interstitial pneumonitis*

* Must also have a positive test for HIV

of age at the time of diagnosis.

CDC has conducted surveillance for AIDS since June 1981, a few months after recognition of the first cases in adults. The initial case of AIDS in a child was reported to CDC in 1982. Since that time, the number of reported cases has increased each year (Figure 1).

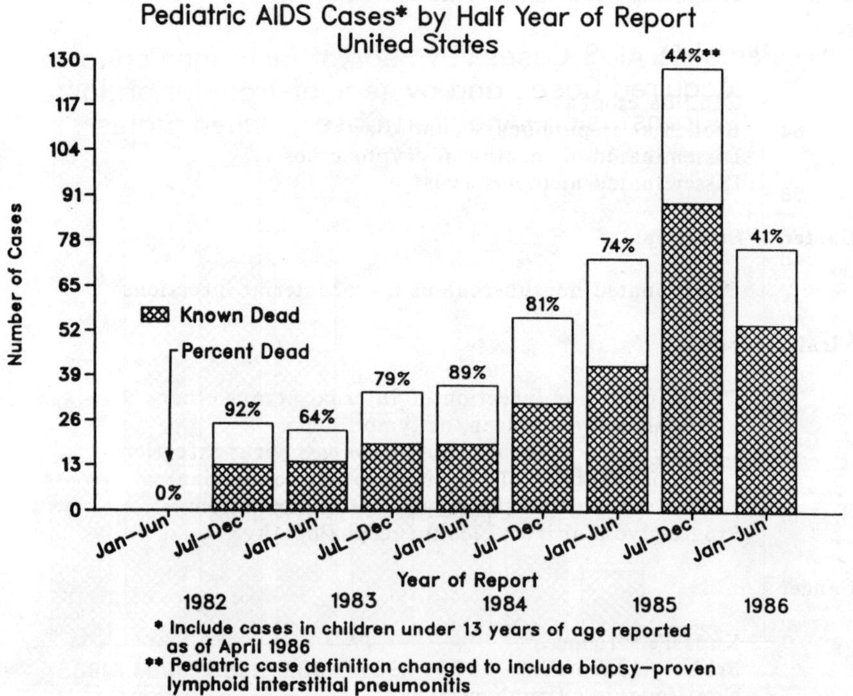

Figure 1.

The time at which the virus was transmitted to children who developed AIDS can be estimated by the year of birth for those children who acquired the virus perinatally and the year of transfusion for those acquiring the virus through blood transfusion (Figure 2). For the perinatally acquired cases, the earliest year of birth is 1977. The first blood transfusion that transmitted HIV to a child was given in 1978.

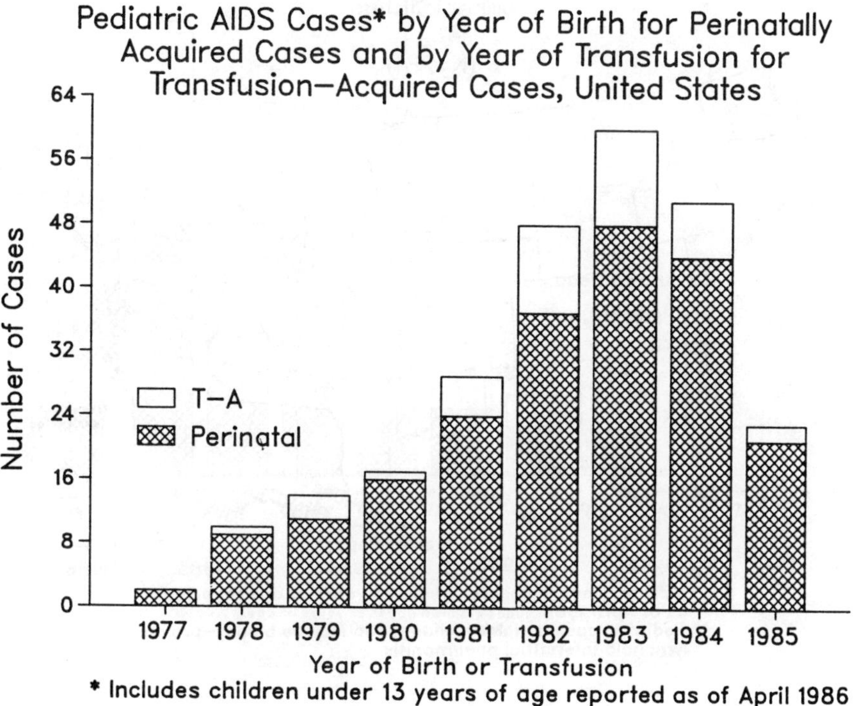

Figure 2.

Children with AIDS have been reported from 22 states, Washington, D.C., and Puerto Rico (Figure 3). Seventy-five percent of cases were reported from New York, New Jersey, Florida, or California, with 40% reported from New York State alone.

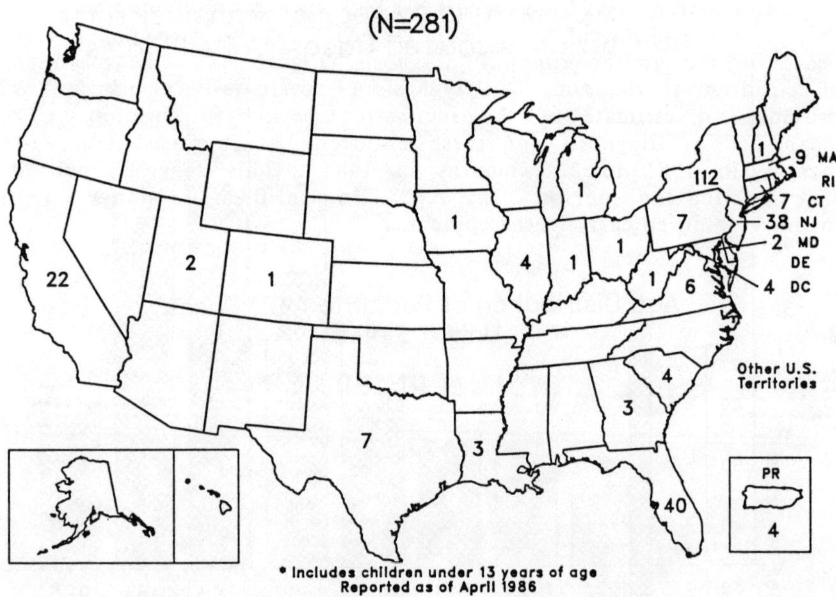

Figure 3.

The demographic characteristics of pediatric AIDS patients differ from those of adult patients and vary by risk factor. Fifty-four percent of children are male compared with 93% of adults, most of whom are gay men. Eighty-one percent of pediatric cases occur in blacks and Hispanics, compared with 39% in adults. The racial characteristics of the children are, however, similar to those of adults who use intravenous drugs (51%, black and 30%, Hispanic).

The male:female ratio of children with perinatally acquired AIDS is 1:1.1, indicating that both sexes are equally affected by this means of transmission. However, there is a marked male predominance (68%) among children with transfusion-acquired AIDS, even when children with hemophilia are excluded. The reason for this distribution is unclear, but a similar observation has been made in Zaire where there is a marked male predominance among children who presumably acquired the infection from transfusions or medical injections, since their mothers were seronegative (personal communication, Jon Mann, M.D., Project SIDA, Zaire).

In children, AIDS is a disease of infants and toddlers. Of the reported children with pediatric AIDS, 80% were under three years of age at the time of diagnosis (Figure 4). The mean age of children at the time of diagnosis of perinatally acquired AIDS provides an estimate of the incubation period in children. The mean age at diagnosis for these children has increased from 10.4 months in 1981 to 22.3 months in 1985. This suggests that the true incubation period for AIDS in children is longer than initially observed early in the epidemic.

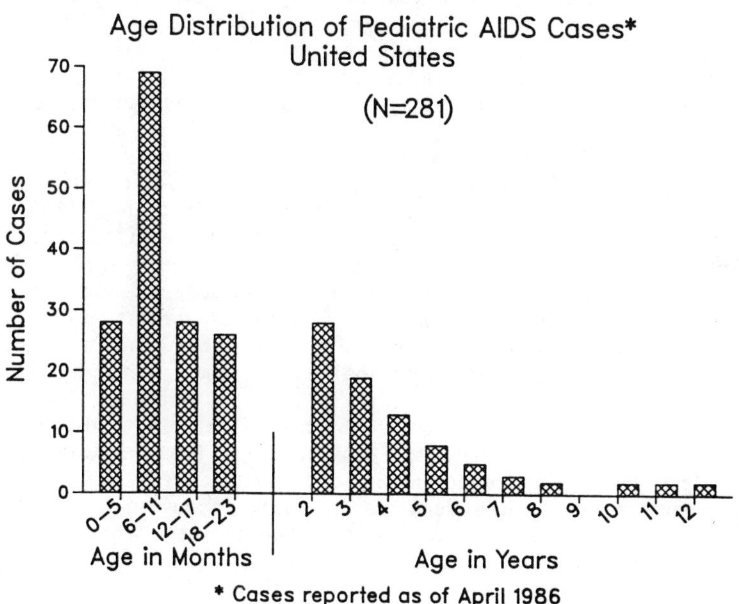

Figure 4.

The prognosis for children with AIDS is poor. Overall, 61% of the children reported are dead (Figure 1). Of children diagnosed before 1984, 74% are dead. These case fatality rates are probably underestimates since not all deaths are reported to CDC.

Risk factors associated with AIDS in children are: 1) perinatal exposure to infected mothers (75% of reported cases); 2) hemophilia (4%); 3) transfusion of blood or blood products (16%); and 4) unknown or indeterminate factors (5%). The 212 mothers of the perinatally exposed children were: 1) intravenous drug users (61%); 2) born in Haiti (19%); 3) sexual partners of men who are intravenous drug users (12%); 4) sexual partners of bisexual men (3%); 5) recipients of infected blood transfusions (2%); 6) women with HIV infection but no reported risk factors (2%); and 7) women with sexual exposure to HIV-infected partners whose risk factors were unknown (1%).

TRANSMISSION

As the risk factors for children indicate, HIV is transmitted in two ways -- through perinatal exposure to infected mothers and through parenteral exposure to infected blood or blood products. Of 43 children with transfusion-associated AIDS, 40 received their transfusion in the neonatal period. Although infants receive only about 2% of red cell transfusions, they account for about 10% of all transfusion-associated AIDS cases reported in both adults and children.

There are several possible explanations for the higher attack rate in infants. First, neonates may be more susceptible to AIDS, perhaps because of their immature immune systems. Second, transfused neonates may receive a larger inoculum of virus relative to their body size. Third, infants may appear to have a higher attack rate than adults because of the shorter incubation period in children.

Both cellular and plasma products derived from infected whole blood can transmit the virus. In one study, factor VIII concentrate recipients had the highest seropositivity rate (74%), compared with factor IX recipients (39%) and persons receiving multiple transfusions of packed red cells (4%) (3).

Perinatal transmission may occur prenatally, during delivery, and possibly postnatally through ingestion of breast milk. Transmission of the virus during pregnancy or labor and delivery has been demonstrated by two reported AIDS cases occurring in children who had no contact with their infected mothers after birth. One was delivered by cesarean section (4),(5). In addition, virus has been isolated from fetal tissues (6). Transmission of the virus after birth was suggested in one case of HIV infection in a child born to a mother reported to have acquired the infection from a postpartum blood transfusion. The mother, who reported no other risk factors for AIDS, breastfed the child for six weeks. The authors of the report describing this case suggested breast-feeding as the most likely mode of transmission. HIV has been isolated from the breast milk of infected women (8).

The frequency of transmission from mothers to infants is unknown. In one study of 20 infants born to infected mothers who had already delivered one infant with AIDS, 13 infants (65%) had serologic and/or clinical evidence of infection with HIV several months after birth (9). Since these woman were selected because they had previously transmitted HIV perinatally, this study may overestimate the average risk of transmission for all infected pregnant women. Other retrospective studies have found transmission rates ranging from 0% to 22% (10)-(13).

It is not known whether pregnancy increases an infected woman's risk of developing AIDS or related conditions. Pregnancy is associated with suppression of cell-mediated immunity and increased susceptibility to some infections (14). In a study of mothers of infants with AIDS or related conditions, 15 infected women who were well at the time of delivery were followed an average of 30 months after the births of their children (9). Five (33%) subsequently developed AIDS, seven (47%) developed AIDS-related conditions, and only three (20%) remained asymptomatic. These results may not apply to all infected pregnant women, but they do suggest an increased likelihood of developing symptomatic disease when HIV infection occurs in association with pregnancy.

HIV has not been transmitted through casual exposure to infected persons, including young children with behaviors that might be expected to increase the likelihood of transmission (e.g., incontinence, drooling, biting, etc.). Studies of household members have not revealed transmission within the family setting even in families of young children with AIDS (10),(13), (15)-(20).

There has been only one instance of transmission from a child to another person. This instance involved a mother who sero-converted 13 to 17 months after her baby had acquired HIV infection from a contaminated blood transfusion (21). The child had a congenital intestinal abnormality which required colonic and ileal resections. The mother had prolonged and extensive contact with blood and body fluids of the child while providing nursing care, including drawing blood through the child's indwelling catheter, removing peripheral intravenous lines, emptying and changing ostomy bags, inserting rectal tubes, changing diapers and surgical dressings, and changing nasogastric tubes. The mother did not always observe the recommended precautions for preventing such transmission (22).

PREVENTION

Prevention of HIV infection in children requires prevention of the infection in women, prevention of pregnancy in infected women, screening blood and blood products, and the use of heat-treated factor products for children with coagulation defects. The latter two prevention strategies are already in place. The number of infected cases attributable to transfusions of blood and blood products is expected to decrease markedly over the next few years. Although routine screening procedures cannot detect units of blood from recently infected blood donors who may be viremic but seronegative, such units will be rare.

To assist in preventing perinatally transmitted cases of HIV infection, the U.S. Public Health Service has recommended that counselling services and testing for antibody to the virus be offered to women who are members of groups at increased risk for acquiring HIV who are pregnant or may become pregnant (23). For women who are seronegative, prevention of infection is key. Transmission through intravenous drug use indirectly accounts for 72% of perinatally acquired cases and 54% of all pediatric cases. Efforts to prevent transmission among drug users should prevent cases in children.

Women who are already infected should be advised to consider delaying pregnancy until more is known about perinatal transmission of the virus. Infants born to these women should be followed closely for signs and symptoms of HIV infection. Breast-feeding is not recommended for infants of infected mothers.

Since HIV transmission in casual settings appears extremely unlikely, the U.S. Public Health Service has recommended that most infected school-age children can safely attend school without fear of transmission to other students or staff (24). These recommendations stress the need to evaluate each child individually, considering the risk of HIV transmission in the school setting, the risks of acquiring potentially harmful infections in the school setting for the immunodeficient child, and the need for confidentiality.

The risk of transmission in the school setting is thought to be minimal to non-existent in general, but the guidelines advise caution in placing very young children, or those who are neurologically handicapped and lack control of their body secretions or who display behavior such as biting, and those children who have uncoverable oozing lesions. Because other infections in addition to HIV can be present in blood or body fluids, the recommendations stress the need for all schools and daycare/nursery facilities, regardless of whether HIV-infected children are attending, to adopt routine procedures for handling blood or body fluids in the school setting.

The guidelines do not recommend mandatory screening for anti-HIV in school children, but suggest that adoption and foster care agencies consider adding such screening to their routine medical evaluations of children at increased risk of infection before placement, since adoptive and foster parents must make decisions regarding the medical care of the child and must consider the possible social and psychological effects on their family.

Finally, these recommendations stress the need to provide information and education regarding HIV and its transmission for parents, school officials, and others to alleviate the fear and hysteria surrounding the AIDS epidemic.

CONCLUSION

In summary, the problem of HIV infection and AIDS in children is increasing as more children become infected each year. Without effective vaccines, our only means of prevention of AIDS in children is through counselling and education. Geographic areas with an increased incidence of perinatally acquired infection need to establish such prevention programs immediately.

Continued national surveillance for AIDS and monitoring of infection rates in certain populations at increased risk is mandatory for establishing effective prevention programs to control the spread of the disease. Physicians and other health care personnel are strongly encouraged to report patients with AIDS to their local health department and to provide for prevention counselling of their patients who may be at increased risk for infection.

REFERENCES

1. CDC., Revision of the case definition of acquired immunodeficiency syndrome for national reporting--United States. MMWR 34:373- 375 (1985)

2. Peterman, T.A., Jaffee, H.W., Feorino, P.M., et al., Transfusion-associated acquired immunodeficiency syndrome in the United States. JAMA 254:2913-2917 (1985)

3. Jason, J., McDougal, S., Holman, R.C., et al., Human T-lymphotropic retrovirus type III/lymphadenopathy-associated virus antibody. JAMA 253:3409-3415 (1985)

4. Cowan, M.J., Hellmann, D., Chudwin, D., et al., Maternal transmission of acquired immune deficiency syndrome. Pediatrics 73:382-386 (1984)

5. Lapointe, N., Michaud, J., Pekovic, D., et al., Transplacental transmission of HTLV-III virus. (Letter) N Engl J Med 312:1325-1326 (1985)

6. Jovaisas, E., Koch, M.A., Schafer, A., et al., LAV/HTLV-III in 20-week fetus. Lancet 2:1129 (1985)

7. Ziegler, J.B., Cooper, D.A., Johnson, R.O., et al., Postnatal transmission of AIDS-associated retrovirus from mother to infant. Lancet 1:896-897 (1985)

8. Thiry, L., Sprecher-Goldberger, S., Jonckheer, T., et al., Isolation of AIDS virus from cell-free breast milk of three healthy virus carriers. Lancet 2:891-892 (1985)

9. Scott, G.B., Fischl, M.A., Klimas, N., et al., Mothers of infants with the acquired immunodeficiency syndrome. International Conference on Acquired Immunodeficiency Syndrome (AIDS), Atlanta, GA, April 1985

10. Friedland, G.H., Saltzman, B.R., Rogers, M.F., et al., Lack of household transmission of HTLV-III infection. N Engl J Med 314:344-349 (1986)

11. Stewart, G.J., Tyler, J.P.P., Cunningham, A.L., et al., Transmission of HTLV-III virus by artificial insemination by donor. Lancet 2:581-584 (1985)

12. Rogers, M.F., Ewing, E.P., Warfield, D., et al., Virologic studies of HTLV-III/LAV in pregnancy: case report of a woman with AIDS. Obstet Gynecol (in press)

13. Thomas, P.A., Lubin, K., Enlow, R.W., et al., Comparison of HTLV-III serology, T cell levels, and general health status of children whose mothers have AIDS with children of healthy

inner city mothers in New York. International Conference on Acquired Immunodeficiency Syndrome (AIDS), Atlanta, GA, April 1985

14. Weinberg, E.D., Pregnancy-associated depression of cell mediated immunity. Rev Infect Dis 6:814-831 (1984)

15. Jason, J.M., McDougal, J.S., Lawrence, D.N., et al., Lymphadenopathy-associated virus (LAV) antibody and immune status of household contacts and sexual partners of persons with hemophilia. JAMA 255:212-215 (1986)

16. Kaplan, J.E., Oleske, J.M., Getchell, J.P., et al., Evidence against transmission of HTLV-III/LAV in families of children with AIDS. Ped Infect Dis 4:468-471 (1985)

17. Lewin, E.B., Zack, R., Ayodele, A., Communicability of AIDS in a foster care setting. International Conference on Acquired Immunodeficiency Syndrome (AIDS), Atlanta, GA, April 1985.

18. Lawrence, D.N., Jason, J.M., Bouhasin, J.D., et al., HTLV-III/LAV antibody status of spouses and household contacts assisting in home infusion of hemophilia patients. Blood 66:703-705 (1985)

19. Fischl, M.A., Dickinson, G., Scott, G., et al., Evaluation of household contacts of adult patients with the acquired immuno deficiency syndrome. International Conference on Acquired Immunodeficiency Syndrome (AIDS), Atlanta, GA, April, 1985.

20. Redfield, R.R., Markham, P.D., Salahuddin, S.Z., et al., Frequent transmission of HTLV-III among spouses of patients with AIDS-related complex and AIDS. JAMA 253:1571-1573 (1985)

21. CDC., Apparent transmission of HTLV-III/LAV from a child to a mother providing health care. MMWR 35:76-79 (1986)

22. CDC., Recommendations for preventing transmission of infection with human T-lymphotropic virus type III/lymphadenopathy-associated virus in the workplace. MMWR 34:681-695 (1985)

23. CDC., Recommendations for assisting in the prevention of perinatal transmission of human T-lymphotropic virus type III/lymphadenopathy-associated virus and acquired immunodeficiency syndrome. MMWR 34:722-732 (1985)

24. CDC., Education and foster care of children infected with human T-lymphotropic virus type III/lymphadenopathy-associated virus. MMWR 34:517-521 (1985)

4
AIDS in Prisons

Gary P. Wormser

Prison inmates are a growing population whose complex medical and social needs seriously challenge the health care profession. Figure 1 depicts the steady increase in the number of prisoners incarcerated in state and federal correctional facilities throughout the United States from 1970 through 1985 (1), (2). At the end of 1985 there were over 500,000 prisoners in these institutions. In addition, another 250,000 or more inmates are imprisoned in local jails outside of the state or federal systems. Therefore, in the United States a total of 750,000 persons are incarcerated, or one out of every 320 Americans (2)-(3).

In this chapter, the clinical and epidemiologic characteristics of prisoners with the acquired immunodeficiency syndrome (AIDS) are discussed. How certain features unique to prisoners in New York State contributed to an improved understanding of the AIDS epidemic is described. Finally, data regarding the risk of spread of human immunodeficiency virus (HIV) infection in prison, as well as the special problems faced by correctional systems in dealing with the AIDS epidemic, are reviewed.

CHARACTERISTICS OF PRISONERS PERTINENT TO THE DEVELOPMENT OF AIDS

Prisoners as a group differ from the general population in regard to several important demographic features pertinent to the AIDS epidemic. First, the vast majority of prisoners are young men. For example, in 1981 when AIDS was first described, the median age of inmates in prisons in the New York State correctional system was 27.8 years and 96 percent were male (4). Secondly, a background of illicit drug use is very common. A survey in 1978 by the U.S. Department of Justice found that 61 percent of inmates had used either heroin, methadone, cocaine, marijuana, amphetamines or barbituates without medical sanction (5). In a 1975 study of more than 1400 detainees of New York City prisons, 41 percent were found to have used illicit drugs and more than 80 percent of those inmates abused heroin (6). Specifically among New York State prisoners, it has been estimated that more than 50% used intravenous drugs before incarceration (7). Thirdly, male homosexual activity during confinement is known to take place and may well occur with greater frequency than it does among civilians. In one study in which inmates from 17 different federal facilities were surveyed, 30 percent of prisoners admitted to homosexual activity in prison (8). In many cases the homosexual activities that occur in prison represent the first such experiences for the inmate. According to a recent report of prisoners in Tennessee, 7% of prisoners interviewed admitted to homosexual activity before entering prison, but more than double this number, 18%, admitted to such experiences after incarceration (9).

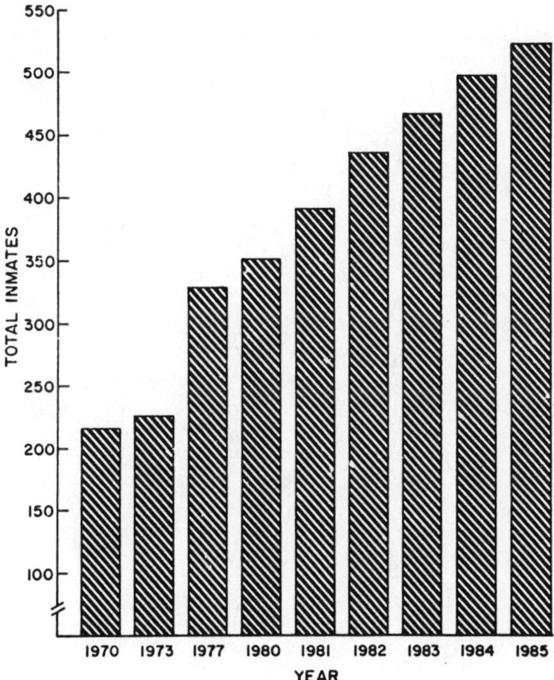

Figure 1. The total number of inmates incarcerated in federal and state correctional facilities (in thousands) is shown by year for selected years from 1970 to 1985.

Table 1. Comparison of Prisoners in the New York State Correctional System with AIDS Patients Diagnosed in the United States (Refs. 10, 11)

	Prisoners*	AIDS Patients
Median Age	28 years	34 years
Percent Male	96%	94%
History of Intravenous Drug Abuse	50%	24%**
Homosexuality	Not Known	73%

* All figures are approximations.
** Includes both heterosexual and homosexual intravenous drug abusers.

The similarity of these characteristics of prisoners to those of AIDS patients throughout the United States (Table 1) (10), (11), is so striking as to suggest that prisoners are likely to be a high risk group for AIDS. Evidence to support this conjecture came in late 1981 when the first prisoner with the syndrome was identified. The first report of this event appeared in the medical literature in 1982 (12). In 1983, Wormser and colleagues (13) described in detail seven previously healthy male inmates from the New York State correctional system who were diagnosed to have AIDS and *Pneumocystis carinii* pneumonia between September 1981 and June 1982. The seven prisoners had a mean age of 29 years and had been incarcerated for 18 months on average prior to the diagnosis of AIDS. All of these inmates were heterosexual before incarceration and vehemently denied homosexual contact while in prison. However, all readily admitted to use of intravenous narcotics prior to incarceration with a mean reported duration of use of 12 years (range, 7 to 25 years). Like other AIDS patients, these prisoners had profound defects in cellular immune function as indicated by cutaneous anergy, lymphopenia, and inversion of the normal ratio of helper to suppressor T-cell lymphocyte populations. Since this report, an escalating number of cases of AIDS have been diagnosed among New York State prisoners, and AIDS has been diagnosed in prisoners in other states and in other countries as well.

Table 2. Risk Groups for 292 New York State Prisoners with AIDS

Group	Number	Percent
Heterosexual IVDA	205	(70.2)
IVDA, sex-orientation unknown	48	(16.4)
IVDA, homosexual/bisexual	26	(8.9)
Homosexual/Bisexual, not IVDA	5	(1.7)
Homosexual/Bisexual, IV drug use unknown	3	(1.0)
Under investigation	5	(1.7)
Total IVDA	279	(95.5)
Total homosexual/bisexual	34	(11.6)
Total all groups	292	(99.9)

IVDA = Intravenous drug abuser
(Adapted from reference 15)

CHARACTERISTICS OF PRISONERS WITH AIDS IN THE NEW YORK STATE CORRECTIONAL SYSTEM

The New York State correctional system is the third largest correctional system in the country with 35,845 inmates as of February 20, 1986 (14). AIDS has been diagnosed in over 300 prisoners from this system, 96.5% of which were men. The typical prisoner with AIDS is in his early 30's, and over 80% of inmate cases are non-white, similar to the overall ethnic composition of the New York State prison population (14). Risk groups for AIDS for 292 New York State prisoners are shown in Table 2 (15). In contrast to the general experience with AIDS in the United States in which homosexual/bisexual men are the leading risk group, intravenous drug abuse is overwhelmingly the most significant risk factor among prisoners, accounting for over 95% of cases. The accuracy of this figure is borne out by the infrequent occurrence in prisoners of Kaposi's sarcoma, a complication of AIDS principally seen among gay men (16). Review of the primary diagnosis for AIDS of the first 292 New York State inmates with the syndrome, showed that prisoners had a significantly lower prevalence of Kaposi's sarcoma (2.7% vs. 21.9%) and a significantly higher prevalence of *Pneumocystis carinii* pneumonia (76.4% vs. 64%) than was observed among the first 25,650 U.S. patients with AIDS ($P < .01$) (Table 3) (15). It is of interest that intravenous drug abuse, not homosexual behavior, has also been the primary identified risk factor for hepatitis B among prisoners (9).

Table 3. Primary Diagnosis in AIDS Patients

Diagnosis	Prisoners	All USA Cases	Significance*
	No. 292	No. 25,650	
Pneumocystis carinii pneumonia	76.4%	64%	P < .01
Kaposi's sarcoma	2.7%	21.9%	P < .01

* By chi-square analysis
(Adapted from reference 15)

In regard to other clinical manifestations of AIDS, prisoners are quite similar to non-prisoners, although clinically symptomatic cytomegalovirus infection and chronic *Herpes simplex* infection in the perianal location specifically, are infrequent manifestations in prisoners. These differences also likely reflect the absence of homosexuality as an important risk factor for AIDS among prisoners. Paralleling recent experience with intravenous drug abusers outside of prison (17)-(19), tuberculosis is emerging as a common problem in New York State prisoners with AIDS. Among 319 prisoners with AIDS, 19 (6%) have had tuberculosis, and conversely, of 120 prisoners with tuberculosis, 19 (16%) have also had AIDS (20). Furthermore, of the 14 state prisoners diagnosed to have tuberculosis at our medical center between May 1985 and September 1986, at least 10 (71%) were positive for HIV antibody (G. Wormser, S. Offutt, unpublished data).

INCIDENCE AND MORTALITY OF AIDS IN THE NEW YORK STATE CORRECTIONAL SYSTEM

Since 1981, a progressive increase in incidence of AIDS among New York State prisoners has been documented (Figure 2) (21). The incidence rate for 1985 was 328.6 per 100,000, which is approximately equal to the annual incidence rate for all cancers in the U.S. population, which was 331.5 per 100,000 for the years 1973-1977 (22). However, the incidence of AIDS among New York State prisoners, although high, is comparable to other established high risk groups for AIDS such as hemophiliacs and intravenous drug abusers (Table 4) (22).

AIDS is a highly lethal disease in prisoners (Table 5). The cumulative mortality among New York State prisoners with AIDS was at least 63% as of the end of 1985 (21). Even this high figure, however, must be considered a minimum estimate since it does not take into consideration the fate of approximately 16% of inmates with AIDS who were released from the correctional system and not

Table 4. Incidence Rate of AIDS in Selected Populations per 100,000

Population		Year	Rate
New York State Prisoners		1985	- 328.6
		1984	- 213.0
Single Men	- NYC	1984	- 263.2
IVDA	- USA	1984	- 167.7
	- NYC	1984	- 261.1
Hemophilia Type A		1984	- 345.7

IVDA = Intravenous drug abuser
(Adapted from references 21, 22)

further evaluated. Since 1982, the average survival of prisoners from time of diagnosis of AIDS to death has consistently been between five and six months (14).

The average age of AIDS inmates at time of death was 34 years (range 19-59) (14). Fifty-six percent of inmates who died had been in the state correctional system for 1-18 months at the time of their death. Another 28% had completed 19-36 months, 12% had served 37-54 months, 4% had been in the system 4.6 - 6 years and one individual had been in continuous custody for seven years.

Table 5. Mortality Due to AIDS - New York State Correctional System

Year	AIDS Deaths/Total AIDS Cases (%)	AIDS Deaths/Total Deaths Percent
1982	4/15 (27%)	5%
1983	26/64 (41%)	35%
1984	79/133 (59%)	51%
1985	155/248 (63%)	58%

(Adapted from references 14, 21)

Pneumocystis carinii pneumonia, found in 41% of cases, was the predominant opportunistic infection at post-mortem examination in a study of 27 consecutive prisoners who died (Table 6) (23). In contrast to the results of autopsy studies of homosexual men with AIDS, Kaposi's sarcoma and cytomegalovirus infection were less frequently diagnosed in prisoners (14),(24).

Table 6. Opportunistic Infections and Neoplasms Found on Post-Mortem Examination of 27 Prisoners with AIDS (Ref. 23)

Condition	Percentage
Pneumocystis carinii pneumonia	41%
Cytomegalovirus infection	37%
Disseminated fungal infection	30%
Primary brain lymphoma	11%
Disseminated mycobacterial infection	4%
Kaposi's sarcoma	4%

AIDS has had a major impact on the overall mortality rate of prisoners and is now the most common cause of death in the New York State correctional system, accounting for over 50% of prisoner deaths since 1984 (Table 5) (14),(21). Between 1980 and 1985 the average mortality rate for AIDS in state prisoners was 568/100,000 compared to the much lower rate of 17.6/100,000 for overall AIDS mortality in the state of New York.

AIDS IN CORRECTIONAL FACILITIES OUTSIDE OF NEW YORK STATE

According to a recent joint report by the National Institute of Justice of the U.S. Department of Justice, and the American Correctional Association, as of the end of 1985 a total of 766 AIDS cases (meeting the CDC surveillance definition) were recognized among inmates. These inmates were incarcerated in 24 (48%) of 50 state prison systems, 20 large city and county jail systems or in the Federal Bureau of Corrections. Fifty-two percent of the state systems had no reported cases (25). The geographic distribution of cases was uneven. Among state and federal systems, 80% of the systems accounted for only 5% of the total AIDS cases, while 4% of the systems contributed 72% of the cases. Among participating city and county systems, 69% accounted for only 5% of the total AIDS cases, while 6% accounted for 77% of the cases. Of note, 70% of AIDS cases occurring in state, city or county jail systems have occurred in New York, New Jersey or Pennsylvania (25).

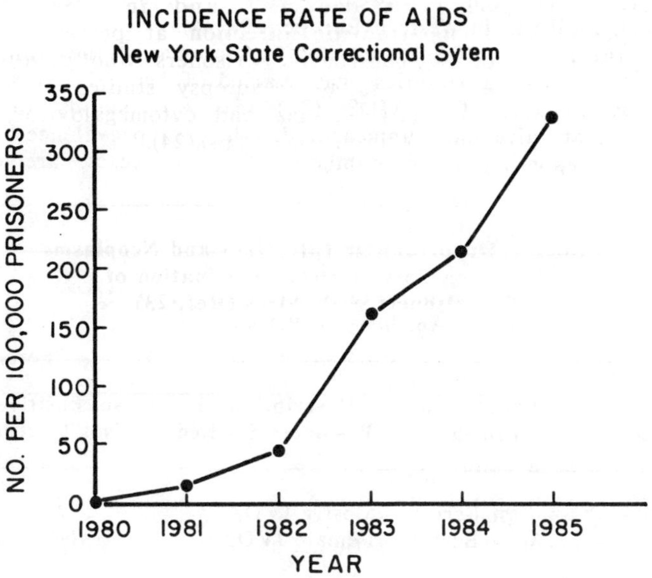

Figure 2. Incidence of AIDS per 100,000 for New York State prisoners is plotted for the years 1981 - 1985.

In jurisdictions with large numbers of AIDS cases among inmates, the majority have occurred among persons with histories of intravenous drug abuse. This observation would appear to explain the skewed geographic distribution of prisoners with AIDS, since the prevalence of HIV infection and AIDS among intravenous drug abusers is closely tied to geographical location. For example, New York and New Jersey have reported 62% of all U.S. AIDS cases associated with histories of intravenous drug abuse (25). In addition, the proportion of intravenous drug abusers with HIV antibody is higher in New York City and Northern New Jersey than in other parts of the country (26)-(28).

PREVALENCE OF HIV INFECTION AMONG INMATES

Comparatively little information is known on prevalence of antibody to HIV among prisoners, especially in the states where the majority of inmates with AIDS have been diagnosed. Available data are summarized in Table 7 (29)-(34). In one study conducted in 1983-1984 among American military prisoners, 1.0% of 913 incoming inmates were positive for antibody to HIV (30). In a more recent investigation in 1985 in prisons in Maryland, 7% of 748 incoming male inmates and 17% of 35 incoming female prisoners were seropositive (31). Among selected subsegments of the prisoner population (especially intravenous drug abusers), seroprevalence rates as high as 44-50% have been recorded in certain correctional facilities in Western Europe (29),(34).

The ratio of AIDS cases to asymptomatic individuals seropositive for HIV antibodies has varied from 1:28 to 1:825 in populations at risk for AIDS (22),(35). It stands to reason, therefore, that although unmeasured, the seroprevalence rates in the prisons reporting large numbers of AIDS cases, are considerable.

Table 7. Studies of Seroprevalence of HIV Antibody in Prisoners

Ref.	Date	Location of Prison	Description of Prisoners Studied	No. Positive/ No. Tested	Percentag[e] Positive
29	1980-1981	West Berlin	Mostly IVDA	0/760	0%
	1985	West Berlin	Female IVDA	NG	50%
30	1983-1984	Military Prison, USA	Incoming inmates	9/913	1.0%
31	1985	Maryland	Incoming males	52/748	7%
			Incoming females	6/35	17%
			Long-term (≥ 7 yrs) inmates	2/137	1.5%
32	?1985	San Remo, Italy	All inmates (30% IVDA)	11/92	12%
33	1985	Los Angeles, CA	Female prostitutes (50% IVDA)	5/89	6%
34	?1985	Austrian Tyrol	IVDA	15/34	44%

IVDA = Intravenous drug abuser; NG = Not given

FEATURES ASSOCIATED WITH INCARCERATION PERTINENT TO RESEARCH ON AIDS

Certain features peculiar to the New York State prison system make prisoners unique and permit studies not possible in other populations with AIDS (Table 8).

Inclusion of New York State prisoners in the AIDS epidemic helped to clarify an early controversy of whether or not AIDS was a new illness or one that had been merely overlooked by the medical community. Unlike most other patient groups with AIDS, New York State prisoners who die are required by law to undergo a postmortem examination. If undiagnosed cases of AIDS had been commonly occurring in the general population prior to recognition of the syndrome, it is reasonable to assume some prisoners would have been affected and very likely would have died because of it. However, review of postmortem records on all 168 prisoners who died from non-traumatic causes during an approximately five year period preceding the first recognized case of AIDS in a New York State prisoner, failed to show a single case with findings suggestive of AIDS (13). Additionally, even for the three prisoners who had an unexplained respiratory death, there was no evidence of *Pneumocystis carinii* pneumonia on subsequent re-examination of lung tissue using special stains for this organism. These observations, along with other data, helped to establish that AIDS was genuinely a new illness in the United States (36).

Table 8. Features Associated with Incarceration in the New York State Correctional System Pertinent to the Study of AIDS

Size of Population Precisely Known
Laboratory Studies and Medical Examination Routinely Performed on Entry
Date of Discontinuation (or Reduction) of Intravenous Drug Use Known
Postmortem Examinations Required by Law
Limited Environmental Exposures

Other characteristics of prisoners proved useful in helping to address some difficult issues well before the discovery of the etiologic agent of AIDS. One important feature of the prison setting is that laboratory studies and medical examinations are routinely performed on entry. Prisoners with AIDS may well be the only group of AIDS patients for whom systematic retrospective reviews can be done of medical records from an earlier time period when these patients may have been completely asymptomatic. This characteristic helped to clarify whether or not AIDS was usually acquired in prison, i.e., did inmates already have evidence of illness prior to incarceration? Another issue concerned the incubation period of AIDS in intravenous drug abusers, a group particularly hard to evaluate since most addicts regularly and continuously engage in high risk behaviors up to the time symptoms of AIDS begin. In contrast, intravenous drug abusers who are imprisoned have an interrupted exposure history, stopping or drastically reducing intravenous drug use at the time of incarceration.

It was reasoned that if AIDS actually predated entry into the state corrections system, that some laboratory abnormality might be discovered through retrospective inspection of the routine blood tests done on all prisoners when they enter the system. To this end, Hanrahan et al. studied entrance total leukocyte counts on 19 prisoners who were diagnosed with AIDS between November 1981 and January 1983 (37). Leukocyte counts were chosen for study since anecdotal experience had suggested that these counts were usually depressed in AIDS patients. Five prisoners were excluded, three because symptoms were present on entry, one because no leukocyte count was done, and one because of the absence of an identifiable risk factor for AIDS (this prisoner was subsequently shown not to have either AIDS or HIV infection). The 14 remaining prisoners were all heterosexual intravenous drug abusers prior to incarceration.

Each prisoner with AIDS was matched with three control prisoners of the same age (within three years), sex, race, and with a similar date of entry into the New York State correctional system, as well as a history of intravenous drug use prior to imprisonment. The three control prisoners chosen were those with an identification number closest to that of an index case and who met each of the five matching criteria.

The 14 inmates with AIDS first developed symptoms of the disease 12.4 $\pm$ 7.6 months (mean $\pm$ SD) after the leukocyte counts were done. Nevertheless, 12 (86%) had entrance leukocyte counts of <5000 cells/mm^3 vs. only six (14%) of the 42 controls ($p < .00001$ by Fisher's exact test). The mean leukocyte count for the AIDS inmates was 4430 cells/mm^3 compared to 6320 cells/mm^3 for the controls ($p<.005$ by F test for matched samples).

These findings were consistent with the premise that the inmates had been infected prior to the entrance laboratory test. They also suggested that leukopenia is a typical (but non-diagnostic) laboratory abnormality associated with the incubation period of AIDS. Since all but three of the prisoners denied participation in high risk activities (intravenous drug use or homosexual activities) following incarceration, it was deduced that they were most likely infected prior to entering prison. Since the mean interval from time of incarceration to onset of AIDS was 22.6 months (4-36 months) for these 14 prisoners, it was reasonable to conclude that the incubation period in intravenous drug abusers with AIDS may be in excess of two years, a figure consistent with the results of other studies done on recipients of contaminated blood transfusions (38). Furthermore, most of these prisoners had been incarcerated between 1979 and 1981, around the time of, or shortly after, entry of HIV into the United States. This information, coupled with the study findings, suggests that the mean incubation period from onset of HIV infection to development of AIDS for this specific group of intravenous drug abusers was between two and four years.

An additional feature of the prison population is that it is a well defined group for whom population sizes are known and incidence figures can be calculated. This information helped to strengthen the association of lymphoma and AIDS. Lymphomas, especially non-Hodgkin's lymphomas, had been suspected to be an important clinical manifestation of AIDS based on their occurrence in homosexual men at risk for AIDS (39),(40). However, the total number of homosexual men is unknown, and consequently, it is impossible to compute exact incidence or prevalence figures for lymphoma in this group. Thus, it has never been conclusively established that homosexual men have a greater frequency of this neoplasm than does the general population.

Ahmed and co-workers (41) determined the incidence rate of non-Hodgkin's lymphoma among New York State prisoners based on patients seen at one medical center. Among the general population aged 20-49 years, the incidence of non-Hodgkin's lymphoma is approximately 3.8 per 100,000. In contrast, among the prisoners studied of the same age group, the incidence rate was 21.5 to 67.2 per 100,000, representing a relative risk 5.7 to 17.7 times higher than in the general population. Similar to the experience with AIDS in prisoners, non-Hodgkin's lymphoma occurred almost exclusively in the prisoner subpopulation who were former intravenous drug abusers. Indeed, in this group the relative risk of non-Hodgkin's lymphoma may have been as high as 164 fold greater than in the general population. These data added support to the theory that non-Hodgkin's lymphoma may be a manifestation of AIDS.

Restricted environmental exposure is an essential feature of prison life. This characteristic is helping to address the question of whether or not *Mycobacterium avium-intracellulare* infection is also a regional disease in AIDS patients, as it has been in other patient populations prior to the AIDS epidemic (42). To determine if regional differences may exist in frequency of *Mycobacterium avium-intracellulare* infection in AIDS patients, we compared the rate of isolation of this organism from patients at two medical centers in the Northeast. The centers (Westchester County Medical Center, Valhalla, NY and St. Francis Hospital, Trenton, NJ) were selected because the majority of AIDS patients seen there are prisoners from area prisons, with well-defined environmental exposures. Also, *Mycobacterium avium-intracellulare* is known to be highly endemic in soil and water in Westchester County. Preliminary results from this study have shown striking differences. At Westchester County Medical Center, 26 (43%) of 61 AIDS patients who had mycobacterial cultures submitted (an average of seven cultures per patient) had at least one positive culture. In contrast, none of 27 patients from St. Francis Hospital had even a single positive culture (an average of six cultures were done per patient) ($p<.01$ by chi square) (43). These results support the premise that *Mycobacterium avium-intracellulare* infection/colonization in AIDS patients is greatly influenced by environmental exposure.

HIV TRANSMISSION IN PRISONS

Although prior studies have suggested that prisoners with AIDS were most likely infected with HIV prior to incarceration (37), there is no reason to doubt that transmission within confinement might occur. In addition to needle sharing for illicit drug use and male homosexual activities, intra-prison tattooing and sharing of razors may also pose some measure of risk (44). Transmission of hepatitis B is well documented in prisons occurring with an incidence rate of 800 to 1300 per 100,000 per year (45), (46).

Despite the potential for HIV transmission, there has still not been a well documented case of HIV infection or AIDS where intra-prison transmission was proven, but too few studies have been done to address this question specifically. In one investigation, conducted from April through July 1985, serologic testing for HIV was offered to all 360 inmates who had been incarcerated for seven years or longer at a correctional facility in Maryland. Of the 137 inmates who participated, two (1%), both of whom had been in custody for nine years, were seropositive (25). Similarly, the question of HIV transmission in prison was raised for six inmates with AIDS who died in the New York State correctional system because they had been continuously incarcerated for over 4.6 years before the onset of symptoms of AIDS (14). Although all these cases must be regarded as suspicious due to the long periods of incarceration before illness, they do not represent conclusive evidence of HIV transmission within prison, since the upper time limit for the incubation period of AIDS is undefined.

In the only serosurvey on prisoners reported to date in which serial specimens were collected for HIV antibody testing, no seroconversion was documented over a combined 1326 patient-year experience (30). This study, however, was done in a military prison with a low baseline prevalence of seropositivity (1%).

Since the late 1970's there has been a progressive increase in the HIV seropositivity rate among drug addicts in New York City, with recent figures showing an overall rate of approximately 50% (26),(47). Since intravenous drug use in prison is highly likely to be less than that which would have taken place outside of prison, the ironic conclusion that arises is that incarceration may have actually benefited seronegative intravenous drug users by protecting them from AIDS and HIV infection. In other words, the risk of HIV infection seems likely to have been far greater outside of prison than within. Direct evidence, however, to support this conjecture is unavailable.

PRISON RESPONSE TO AIDS

Not withstanding a recent publication by the American Public Health Association (48) which provided guidelines for management of prisoners with HIV infection, actual practice is diverse and varies from prison to prison. For example, according to a recent survey, HIV antibody testing is done routinely in approximately 12% of state and federal systems, done only for diagnosis, incident response, or epidemiologic studies in 76% and not done at all in 5% (25). Housing policies range from segregation of all infected inmates (16%), to selective segregation (65%), to no segregation (4%), to no policy at all (16%) (25).

One rational that is often given for segregation, and which is perhaps unique to correctional institutions, is to protect prisoners with AIDS from possible physical injury or death inflicted by their fellow prisoners (49). In general, however, there are few convincing arguments that can be made for segregation on the bases of individual or public health concerns (48).

A clearly recognized priority for prisons is educating staff and inmates on AIDS. In 1985, 93% of prisons surveyed were currently providing or were developing AIDS training or educational material for staff, and 83% claimed the same for inmates (25). Such programs have been considered effective in reducing fears of staff and inmates; timely and effective educational efforts have prevented threatened job actions by correctional staff unions and generally forestalled hysteria over AIDS within several correctional systems.

Other potentially important AIDS risk reduction measures, such as the provision of condoms or sterile needles are unlikely to be adopted by correctional systems, as the activities surrounding their use are never condoned. Additionally, the availability of needles would pose a clear security risk. Nevertheless, education about sterilization techniques and/or the provision of disinfectant solutions might serve the same purpose as sterile needles with less controversy or danger. Furthermore, condoms might be made available through a mechanism devised to insure anonymity.

CONCLUSION

Prisoners, especially those with a history of intravenous drug abuse from New York and New Jersey, are a high risk group for AIDS. So far, the principal explanation for the high incidence of AIDS in this population is HIV infection before incarceration. Future studies need to address the risk of seroconversion in prisons with identification of behavioral factors pertinent to this event.

Because New York State prisoners with AIDS are different from other risk groups in regard to several important epidemiologic features associated with incarceration (Table 8), certain studies of this patient population were done that would have been difficult, it not impossible, to do in other risk groups. Results of these investigations have given insight into the date of onset of AIDS in the United States, the incubation period of AIDS, the association of leukopenia with prodromal AIDS, the association of non-Hodgkin's lymphoma outside of the central nervous system with AIDS, and, possibly, the regional nature of *Mycobacterium avium-intracellulare* infections in AIDS patients.

Proper management of the AIDS epidemic by correctional systems should include a vigorous educational campaign in an attempt to decrease unnecessary fears and anxiety and to diminish known or presumed high risk behaviors.

ACKNOWLEDGMENTS

The author gratefully thanks the following for their many contributions to the research efforts described in the manuscript: Drs' J. Hanrahan, L. Krupp, E. Gelberg, S. Cunningham-Rundles, E. Allen, G. Gavis, M. Hyland, R.E. Stahl, R. Yarrish, F. Duncanson, R. Broaddus and Ms' B. Maguire and S. Gamble.

REFERENCES

1. Department of Justice, Personal Communication, (1986)

2. Bureau of Justice, Personal Communication, (1986)

3. U.S. Census Bureau, Personal Communication, (1986)

4. Krupp, L.B., Gelberg, E.A., Wormser, G.P., Prisoners as medical patients. (Manuscript submitted)

5. Barton, W.I., Drug histories and criminality of inmates of local jails in the United States: Implication for treatment and rehabilitation of the drug abuser in a jail setting. Int J Addict 17:417-444 (1982)

6. Novick, L.F., Dello Penna, R., Schwartz, M.S., Health status of the New York City prison population. Med Care 15:205-216 (1977)

7. Gustave Gavis, M.D., Health Services, New York State Department of Corrections, Personal Communication (1986)

8. Nacci, P.L., Pane, T.R., Sex and Sexual Aggression in Federal Prisons: Progress Report U.S. Department of Justice Washington, D.C. (1982)

9. Decker, M.D., Vaughn, W.K., Brodice, J.S. et al., Seroepidemiology of hepatitis B in Tennessee prisoners. J Infect Dis 150:450-459 (1984)

10. Jaffe, H.W. Bregman, D.J., Selik, R.M. Acquired immunodeficiency syndrome in the United States: the first 1000 cases. J Infect Dis 148:339-345 (1983)

11. Wormser, G.P., Prisoners with AIDS, In: The Acquired Immune Deficiency Syndrome and Infections of Homosexual Men (Ma, P., Armstrong, D., eds), Second Edition, York Medical Books, New York (In press)

12. Hanrahan, J.P., Wormser, G.P., Maguire, G.P., et al., Opportunistic infections in prisoners. N Engl J Med 307:498 (1982)

13. Wormser, G.P., Krupp, L.B., Hanrahan, J.P., et al., Acquired immunodeficiency syndrome in male prisoners. New Insights into an emerging syndrome. Ann Intern Med 98:297-303 (1983)

14. Gaunay, W., Gido, R.L., Acquired Immune Deficiency Syndrome. A Demographic Profile of New York State Inmate Mortalities 1981-1985, New York State Commission of Corrections. (1986)

15. Bureau of Communicable Disease Control, New York State Department of Health. AIDS Surveillance Monthly Update, September (1986)

16. Haverkos, H., Drotman, D.P., Morgan, M., Prevalence of Kaposi's sarcoma among patients with AIDS. N Engl J Med 312:1518 (1985)

17. Maayan, S., Wormser, G.P., Hewlett, D., et al., Acquired immunodeficiency syndrome (AIDS) in an economically disadvantaged population. Arch Intern Med 145:1607-1612 (1985)

18. Duncanson, F.P. Hewlett, D., Maayan, S., et al., *Mycobacterium tuberculosis* infection in the acquired immunodeficiency syndrome. A review of 14 patients. Tubercle (In press)

19. Hewlett, D., Duncanson, F.P., Lieberman, J., et al., Lymphadenopathy in intravenous drug users with suspected AIDS. Interscience Conference on Antimicrobial Agents Chemotherapy. Minneapolis, MN (1985)

20. Braun, M.M., Truman, B.I., Morse, D.L., et al., Tuberculosis and AIDS in prisoners (Manuscript submitted)

21. Barbara Maguire, RN, Director of Health Services, New York State Department of Corrections, Personal Communication (1986)

22. Curran, J.W., Morgan, W.M., Hardy, A.M., et al., The epidemiology of AIDS: Current status and future prospects. Science 229:1352-1357 (1985)

23. Stahl, R.E. Wormser, G.P., Fiore, A.R., et al., Autopsy findings in 27 consecutive prisoners with AIDS. (Manuscript in preparation)

24. Macher, A.M., Reichert, C.M., Straus, S.E., et al., Death of the AIDS patient: role of cytomegalovirus. N Engl J Med 23:1454 (1983)

25. Hammett, T.M., Acquired immunodeficiency syndrome in correctional facilities: A report of the National Institute of Justice and the American Correctional Association. MMWR 35:195-199 (1986)

26. Maayan, S., Backenroth, R., Rieber, E., et al., Antibody to lymphadenopathy-associated virus/human T lymphotropic virus type III in various groups of illicit drug users in New York City. J Infect Dis 152:843 (1985)

27. Weiss, S.H., Ginzburg, H.M., Goedert, J.J. et al., Risk factors for HTLV-III infection among parenteral drug abusers. Proc Am Soc Clin Oncol (Abstract) 5:11 (1986)

28. Levy, N., Carlson, J.R., Hinrichs, S., et al., The prevalence of HTLV-III/LAV antibodies among intravenous drug users attending treatment programs in California: A preliminary report. N Engl J Med 314:446 (1986)

29. Kohler, H., Lange, W., Rex, W., et al., Antibodies to LAV/HTLV-III in Berlin prison inmates with risk factors for hepatitis B from 1980-1985. International Conference on Acquired Immunodeficiency Syndrome (AIDS), Paris, France (1986)

30. Kelley, P.W., Redfield, R.R., Ward, D.L., et al., Prevalence and incidence of HTLV-III in a prison. JAMA 256:2197-2198 (1986)

31. Polk, B.F., Brewer, F., Britz, J., et al., Serologic evidence of infection with HTLV-III/LAV in prison inmates in Maryland, USA., International Conference on Acquired Immunodeficiency Syndrome (AIDS), Paris, France (1986)

32. Crovari, P., Cassini, U., Infante, D., et al., Prevalence of infections caused by AIDS and hepatitis B virus in jailed people. Boll Ist Sieroter Milan 64:367-370 (1985)

33. Gill, P.S., Levine, A.M., Ross, R., et al., Prevalance of antibody to HTLV-III in female prostitutes from Los Angeles. International Conference on the Acquired Immunodeficiency Syndrome (AIDS), Paris, France (1986)

34. Fuchs, D., Blecha, H.G., Deinhardt, F., et al., High frequency of HTLV-III antibodies among heterosexual intravenous drug abusers in the Austrian Tyrol. Lancet 1:1506 (1985)

35. Sivack, S., Wormser, G.P., How common is HTLV-III infection in the United States? N Engl J Med 313:1352 (1985)

36. Auerbach, D.M., Bennett, J.V., Brachman, P.S., et al., Report of the Centers for Disease Control task force on Kaposi's sarcoma and opportunistic infections: Epidemiological aspects of the current outbreak of Kaposi's sarcoma and opportunistic infections. N Engl J Med 306:248-52 (1982)

37. Hanrahan, J.P., Wormser, G.P., Reilly, A.A., et al., Prolonged incubation period of AIDS in intravenous drug abusers: Epidemiologic evidence in prison inmates. J Infect Dis 150:263-266 (1984)

38. Curran, J.W., Lawrence, D.N., Jaffe, H., et al., Acquired immunodeficiency syndrome (AIDS) associated with transfusions. N Engl J Med 310:69-75 (1984)

39. Levine, A.M., Meyer, P.R., Begandy, M.K., et al., Development of B-cell lymphoma in homosexual men: clinical and immunologic findings. Ann Intern Med 100:7-13 (1984)

40. Ziegler, J., Beckstead, J.A., Volberding, P.A., et al., Non-Hodgkin's lymphadenopathy and the acquired immunodeficiency syndrome. N Engl J Med 311:565-570 (1984)

41. Ahmed, T., Wormser, G.P., Stahl, R.E., et al., Increased risk for Hodgkin's disease and non-Hodgkin's lymphomas in a population at risk for AIDS. International Conference on Acquired Immunodeficiency Syndrome (AIDS), Atlanta, Georgia (1985)

42. Edwards, L.B., Palmer, C.E., Epidemiological studies of tuberculin sensitivity. I. Preliminary studies with purified protein derivatives prepared from atypical acid-fast organisms. Am J Hyg 68:213-229 (1985)

43. Wormser, G.P., Porwancher, R., Dupree, M., et al., (Unpublished data)

44. Peyton, H.J., Paleo, L., AIDS education in federal, state and local prisons: model programs for administrative, medical and custodial staff and inmate populations. International Conference on Acquired Immunodeficiency Syndrome (AIDS) Paris, France (1986)

45. Hull, H.F., Lyons, L.H., Mann, J.M., et al., Incidence of hepatitis B in the penitentiary of New Mexico. Am J Public Health 75:1213-1214 (1985)

46. Decker, M.D., Vaughn, W.K., Brodie, J.S., et al., Incidence of hepatitis B in Tennessee prisoners. J Infect Dis 152: 214-217 (1985)

47. Des Jarlas, D.C., Friedman, S.R., Hodgkins, W., Risk reduction for the acquired immunodeficiency syndrome among intravenous drug users. Ann Intern Med 103:755-759 (1985)

48. Dubler, N. N., Standards for Health Services in Correctional Institutions. Second edition American Public Health Association, Washington, D.C., p 117-119 (1986)

49. Guerro, I.C., Koenigsfest, A., AIDS in prisons - an update of a continuing saga. International Conference on Acquired Immunodeficiency Syndrome (AIDS), Paris, France (1986)

5 The Importance of HIV Infection for the Military

Patrick W. Kelley, Ernest T. Takafuji, Edmund C. Tramont, Robert R. Redfield, John F. Brundage, John R. Herbold, Richard N. Miller

The recent epidemic spread of human immunodeficiency virus (HIV) infection in predominantly young sexually active populations, concern over factors inherent in a military career that may jeopardize the health of HIV infected individuals, and specific requirements for a safe blood supply in the military operational setting, led the Department of Defense in the summer of 1985 to embark upon a comprehensive program to reduce the threat of this infection to military readiness (1). An immediate program goal is to control the prevalence of HIV infection in military populations. A number of measures were instituted including recruit applicant and phased total force serologic testing, serologic testing of select high risk groups such as sexually transmitted disease patients, and targeted health education programs. Secondarily, the program has provided and will continue to provide to the scientific community unique opportunities for expanding current understanding of the epidemiology, pathogenesis, prevention, and treatment of HIV infection.

The organizational structure of the military medical care system lends itself to the efficient conduct of natural history studies, preventive and therapeutic clinical trials, and other epidemiologic studies. Except for the national blood donor screening program, military HIV control programs provide the only HIV seroprevalence data on large cross-sections of the U.S. population. Military accession, active duty, reserve, and National Guard populations are especially valuable because they are probably a more representative cross-section of young adult members of the U.S. population than are blood donors; however, both blood donors and military populations may represent somewhat biased samples of the U.S. population since homosexuals and intravenous drug abusers are underrepresented in both groups. Infected active duty military populations, unlike blood donors, also lend themselves to the relatively efficient collection of follow-up information due to the worldwide centrally administered military health care systems used for the care of these individuals.

In this country, HIV disease is largely confined to a young male segment of the population. As of August 25, 1986, 88% of the reported 24,189 cases of the acquired immunodeficiency syndrome (AIDS) reported to the Centers for Disease Control (CDC) occurred in individuals between the ages of 20 and 49, and 92% were adult males (2).

Because 81.1% of the active duty servicemembers in the U.S. Armed Forces are males in this age range, and in light of an increasing appreciation for potentially significant levels of heterosexual HIV transmission, this infection is of particular interest to the military (3)-(7). This chapter discusses the background for the military's HIV control program, outlines the procedures in place to limit the prevalence of infection and maximize force readiness, and describes the epidemiology of this infection in selected military populations.

BACKGROUND FOR THE MILITARY HIV PROGRAM

It is the mission of this country's Armed Forces to maintain a force capable of initiating and sustaining timely and effective military operations in any environment throughout the world. The successful accomplishment of this mission is predicated on the maintenance of a force that is physically, psychologically, and intellectually fit to fight. Though clearly many servicemembers do not have primary duties in a combat specialty, it is imperative to maximize the number of individuals on active duty capable of coping with the physical, mental, and emotional demands of combat anywhere in the world.

During deployments, servicemembers not only must cope with the opposing military forces, but they must also be prepared to face the threat of climatic and infectious disease hazards. In addition to concerns of combat, however, are issues relevant to international policy and the maintenance of a peacetime force in specific overseas areas. The rationale for the military HIV programs was developed after consideration of these issues.

Military Blood Supply

In recent conflicts involving U.S. or British forces, such as actions in Vietnam and the Falklands, medical doctrine for accomplishing necessary fresh blood replacement under battlefield conditions required use of servicemembers in the field as blood donors (8),(9). This "walking blood bank" concept was also employed after the Beirut bombing in 1983 (LTC A. Polk, Department of Defense Armed Services Blood Program Office, personal communication). Contingency planning on board U.S. Navy ships calls for direct transfusion in the event of fires, explosions, and other mass casualties. For example, in 1983 during operations in the Mediterranean, a pilot from the U.S.S. Kennedy crashed into the water. His injuries necessitated transfusions with 14 units of blood from the "walking blood bank." Though the use of frozen blood supplies is incorporated into U.S. military contingency plans, such supplies would not be sufficient to meet the demand in all cases nor would the reduced concentration of clotting factors in frozen blood always be sufficient to achieve hemostasis. Even with current medical technology, it is doubtful that blood obtained and transfused under field conditions could always be screened for HIV antibody. To limit the obvious medical and morale concerns associated with maintaining a doctrine that may not always permit HIV testing of battlefield collections, it is imperative that the HIV status of soldiers eligible for donating under such circumstances be known with as much certainty as possible. Similarly, identified hepatitis B surface antigen carriers are precluded from donating blood for transfusions.

Projected Military Service

Personnel acquisition and management in the military has the goal of selecting and training physically and mentally fit individuals so that they are ready for military action. Standards of fitness have been established to define factors existing prior to service that identify individuals who either are at unusual risk of becoming disabled before the end of their tour of military service, or for whom necessary modifications to usual procedures or equipment would be unacceptably expensive (10). For example, the ergonomic requirements of various pieces of military hardware and other cost considerations implicit in outfitting a military force, have necessitated setting height minimums and maximums for new recruits. Similarly, because of the increased probability of certain medical conditions being associated with future health problems, e.g., an undescended testicle predisposing to testicular cancer, individuals have also historically been denied entry into the service for various pre-existing medical conditions.

A significant percentage of persons identified with HIV infection as a result of the presence of antibody to HIV have been shown to progress to advanced stages of immunodeficiency. Although follow-up of a male homosexual cohort in San Francisco indicated that 10 of 31 infected men developed AIDS or related conditions over a median of 61 months of follow-up, the actual proportion of infected individuals showing progression may be higher, given a longer follow-up period (11),(12). The probability of an HIV antibody-positive recruit completing his/her military career without becoming disabled seems to be less than desirable.

Economic Considerations

Disability retirements prior to 20 years of service are expensive and will become even more costly as the proportion of servicemembers holding technologically sophisticated military specialties increases. To replace disabled soldiers, new recruits need to be trained, again often at substantial expense depending on the occupational specialty. The cost of providing care for patients with HIV disease is high. The Centers for Disease Control estimates that costs for care of the first 10,000 U.S. AIDS patients exceeded $140,000 per patient (13). As of the summer of 1986, the three services had already identified nearly 1000 infected members; it is estimated that as many as 3000-4000 people will be identified with HIV infections among the 2.1 million members of the active duty force. Considering the likelihood of disease progression, the cost of providing care for HIV infected patients, and the potential for expensive disability retirement payments, it is clear that an ever increasing HIV infected patient load would consume a significant amount of the already limited resources available.

Peacetime Travel

Even during peacetime, U.S. servicemembers are deployed throughout the world for prolonged assignment or limited training. Large contingents of troops are currently stationed in Central America, Korea, Japan, the Phillipines, Europe, and the Middle East. Moreover, large populations of sailors and Marines regularly take shore leave in ports throughout the world. At present, HIV infection is unevenly distributed among the countries of the world (14)-(16). Some U.S. troops perform duty overseas in geographical areas with a relatively high HIV prevalence and others serve in regions of extremely low prevalence. Concerns arise over whether U.S. forces could import HIV infections into the U.S., since overseas they commonly acquire at high rates other sexually transmitted diseases such as hepatitis B and penicillinase-producing *Neisseria gonorrhoeae* (17),(18). Studies have reported relatively high prevalence rates of HIV infection among prostitutes, not only in some U.S. cities, but also in Europe and Africa (19)-(21). The solicitation of prostitutes by soldiers is not an infrequent occurrence. Although data suggest that intravenous drug abuse is a major HIV risk factor for prostitutes, a high degree of sexual activity with multiple sexual partners is also a likely factor. Observations of military and civilian AIDS cases suggest that prostitutes may represent a noteworthy source of infection for heterosexual men (7).

In contrast to the concern over HIV acquisition by soldiers stationed in highly endemic areas overseas, countries with low HIV prevalence wish to avoid having their burden of infection increased. Either possibility, whether real or hypothetical, has obvious geopolitical ramifications which must be addressed (22).

Tactical Considerations

Combat is commonly characterized by physical, mental, and emotional stress and confusion. Lines of communication, transportation, and access to medical facilities are often compromised. Scenarios for future conflicts suggest that the battlefields will be fluid and rapidly evolving, further complicating logistic support and evacuation arrangements (23). Combat soldiers with psychological, medical, or other needs due to evolving HIV disease could not be assured necessary care under such circumstances. The concept of "buddy first aid" for combat injuries could also be difficult to implement if infected soldiers were assigned to deployed units.

A growing body of literature details the potential psychologic and neurologic complications of HIV infection (24),(25). Progressive dementia in the absence of immunodeficiency poses a special concern (26). Performance in combat requires self-confidence and trust in one's peers and leaders. Problems with impaired judgement, memory, and affect secondary to progressive HIV infection could compromise mission success, as can similar deficits secondary to alcoholism and drug abuse, two other conditions of current importance to the military leadership. More needs to be learned about this potential problem area.

Immunologic Issues

A cornerstone of military preventive medicine is the use of vaccines for the prevention of infections among basic trainees and servicemembers deployed worldwide. Army recruits routinely receive a total of at least 17 live and inactivated immunogens during basic training. These incude oral trivalent polio, tetanus, diphtheria, adenovirus 4 and 7, smallpox, trivalent influenza, measles, rubella, and tetravalent meningococcal vaccines (27). Troops assigned to rapid deployment units also commonly receive yellow fever, plague, and typhoid vaccines. Soldiers permanently assigned to Korea are administered the hepatitis B vaccine (27). Military health care providers are also encouraged to voluntarily receive this vaccine. In addition to the above mentioned immunizations, servicemembers may be required to receive specific vaccines based on anticipated exposures during a deployment, e.g., Rift Valley fever, Venezuelan equine encephalitis, and Japanese B encephalitis vaccines. Passive immunization with immune globulin is commonly used for military members deployed to areas where there is an increased risk of hepatitis A transmission.

One of the first indications that HIV might cause special concerns for the military surfaced in 1982 when a basic trainee developed disseminated vaccinia after vaccination against smallpox. Smallpox, though classified by the World Health Organization as having been eradicated from the world, remains a potential biological warfare and terrorist threat to U.S. troops. This recruit, who was confirmed shortly after receiving his entrance immunizations to have AIDS associated with cryptococcal meningitis, required such a large amount of vaccinia immune globulin (VIG) that the military's supply of VIG was compromised. The temporary VIG shortage resulted in suspension of the military smallpox vaccination requirement for over 15 months. Resumption of smallpox vaccination only occurred after VIG stocks were replenished and an HIV screening program was in place. The occurrence of this uncommon vaccine complication in the context of underlying HIV-induced immunodeficiency raised concerns that similar life-threatening outcomes might be seen with continued administration of live virus vaccines to recruits with unrecognized HIV infections.

Activation of T-lymphocytes through vaccination may be a hazard for the asymptomatic HIV-infected individual. In vitro evidence suggests that T-cell activation promotes HIV expression and release; consequently, T-cell activation may increase the probability of other T4 cells becoming secondarily infected (28). Thus, immunization may be associated with a deleterious effect on those in the early stages of the infection. Relative T-helper cell deficiencies and other immune system defects seen in HIV infection may also result in poor or inappropriate responses to vaccines. Evidence to support a reduced ability of AIDS patients to respond to polysaccharide (pneumococcal) and soluble tetanus toxoid protein antigens has been documented (29),(30).

Servicemembers deployed to distant locales are likely to have exposures not only to vaccine-preventable infections but also to exotic diseases such as malaria, leishmaniasis, dengue, amebiasis, hepatitis A, leptospirosis, tuberculosis, etc. Concerns over decreased immunocompetence and T-cell activation secondary to antigenic stimulation by infectious agents, make worldwide deployability of HIV infected individuals problematic (28). For example, Salata and Ravdin have reported that the lectin responsible for the invasiveness of pathogenic amebae is mitogenic for human peripheral-blood lymphocytes (31). Theoretically, mitogens such as these may activate lymphocytes, leading to accelerated virus expression, cell death, and progression of HIV infection (28), (32).

In light of these issues, the Department of Defense, after consultation with distinguished civilian scientists from academia and other governmental agencies who serve on the Armed Forces Epidemiological Board (AFEB), developed the following HIV control program to select, train, and maintain a healthy and effective combat force.

THE MILITARY HIV CONTROL PROGRAM

The military's HIV control program is multifaceted and includes screening of recruit applicants; phased serologic testing of the active and reserve components; screening of blood donors; testing of high risk groups, such as sexually transmitted disease patients and selected recipients of blood or blood products; troop and community health education; contact tracing and testing; clinical staging of infection; periodic follow-up of infected individuals; and research into the virology, epidemiology, pathogenesis, and clinical aspects of this infection.

Procedures adopted by the military for all HIV screening and clinical programs include Western blot testing of all specimens that are repeatedly ELISA positive. A Western blot positive result is defined by Department of Defense policy to be a blot containing at a minimum a gp41 glycoprotein band or both p24 and p55 protein bands (33). A specimen with a p24 band alone is considered negative, but repeat follow-up testing with secondary confirmatory assays is indicated. Individuals are not classified as confirmed HIV positive patients until two independently collected and tested specimens are shown to have one of the defined Western blot patterns. This is done to reduce the chance of misclassification due to administrative or laboratory errors. Pending receipt of the second Western blot result, the potential need for interim counseling and other support services is recognized.

A rigorous quality-assurance program for all contract laboratories performing ELISA and Western blot testing for the Army is conducted by the Department of Virus Diseases at the Walter Reed Army Institute of Research (WRAIR), Washington, DC. This detailed program is characterized by on-site inspections and specific performance criteria including successful analysis of both in-house controls and blind and unblinded panels supplied by the WRAIR (33). Analysis of quality assurance panels and inspections are repeated each month. By contract, failure to correctly identify at least 95% of the panel specimens in a given month would necessitate that the contractor repeat all tests performed that month. All contractor performed Western blots are interpreted by researchers at the WRAIR.

Recruit Applicant Testing

On August 30, 1985 the Deputy Secretary of Defense directed that HIV serologic testing (by an FDA approved ELISA method) be started on all new enlisted and officer accessions into the military. Confirmatory testing of all ELISA positive sera by Western blot was also directed. Accession screening began in October 1985 with serologic services supplied by a single contract laboratory.

Based on considerations delineated above, military policy calls for Western blot positive recruit candidates to be declared ineligible for military service. By directive from the Military Entrance Processing Command (MEPCOM), an HIV antibody-positive applicant is requested by registered letter to report with his/her recruiter to the processing station to discuss the results of the entrance physical examination. At the processing station, antibody-positive applicants are informed by a physician of the abnormal serologic test and are advised to see a civilian medical care provider for further evaluation and counseling. A list of civilian referral agencies is also provided. Again, to ensure accuracy, a second blood specimen for a repeat ELISA and Western blot is obtained at the notification meeting. Final determination of an applicant's status is not made until the second specimen result is available.

Analysis of data derived from screening 308,076 recruit applicants between October 1, 1985 and March 31, 1986, showed an overall antibody prevalence of 1.5 per 1,000. Among the 265,361 men, the rate was 1.6 per 1,000; among 42,715 females the rate was 0.6 per 1,000. Prevalence by race showed striking differences, with a prevalence rate among whites of 0.9/1,000, a rate of 3.9/1,000 in blacks, and a rate for the remaining applicants of 2.6/1,000. Antibody positivity correlated with age. The rate among the 17 year old applicants was 0.2/1000. Thereafter, there was a steady progression from a rate of 1.1/1000 in the 20 year olds, to 2.5/1000 in those 21-25 years, and to a level of 4.4/1000 for those greater than 25 years. The relationship of seroprevalence rates to sex and race persisted after age adjustment. Seroprevalence rates were highest in the coastal regions of the country other than New England. Recruits from urban areas had higher positivity rates than those from non-urban backgrounds (34).

Force Testing

On October 24, 1985, the Secretary of Defense directed that all active duty and reserve component servicemembers undergo HIV antibody screening. The directive with subsequent modifications in general gave highest priority for testing to individuals serving in, or subject to deployment on short notice to areas of the world with a high risk of endemic infectious diseases or with minimal existing medical capability. Servicemembers assigned overseas, awaiting assignment overseas, or in units subject to overseas deployment, were given the next highest priority. Persons in military schools or seeking entrance to such schools and ROTC students were also to be tested. Timetables for screening the various priority groups were developed by each service. Timetables for repeat screens to identify incident infections within the Armed Forces are to be determined.

Blood Bank Screening

In March 1985, the Department of Defense Armed Services Blood Program Office directed that routine testing of all donated blood be implemented by June 30, 1985. In July, the Assistant Secretary of Defense for Health Affairs directed that all potential donors be informed prior to blood donation that HIV antibody testing would be done. Blood that is initially ELISA-positive is retested, and if found to be repeatedly ELISA-positive, is sent for Western blot confirmation. It is current military policy to discard all units of blood that are singly or repeatedly ELISA-positive. Civilian donors with positive HIV antibody results are notified in accordance with local and state laws and regulations.

In August 1985, civilian blood collection agencies collecting blood on military installations were required to notify appropriate medical authorities of active duty donors with serologic tests indicating the presence of hepatitis B surface antigen or antibodies to either HIV or syphilis. This federal requirement, which takes precedence over any state laws that regulate the disclosure of blood-test results or other medical information, was issued to insure medical follow-up of infected servicemembers.

Every year, approximately 200,000 units of blood are collected by the military. An additional 500,000 units are collected on military posts by civilian agencies. The prevalence of HIV antibody (Western blot confirmed) in military donations is approximately 0.5-0.6/1000 (LTC A. Polk, Department of Defense Armed Services Blood Program Office, personal communication). This compares with reported civilian rates of approximately 0.3/1000 (35). A retrospective program to screen certain past blood transfusion recipients for HIV infection is under development.

High Risk Groups

In March 1986, the U.S. Public Health Service defined high risk groups to include: homosexual and bisexual men, present or past intravenous drug abusers, persons with clinical or laboratory evidence of HIV infection, persons born in countries where heterosexual transmission is thought to play a major role, male or female prostitutes and their sex partners, sex partners of infected persons or persons at increased risk, all persons with hemophilia who have received clotting factor products, and newborn infants of high-risk or infected mothers (36). Earlier recommendations of the U.S.P.H.S. also included persons who had received transfusions of contaminated blood (37). The Armed Forces have included these categories as high risk categories. In addition, the Army has further defined high risk categories to include sexually transmitted disease patients and inmates of selected long-term correctional facilities; screening of these two populations has also begun.

Existing data on the prevalence of HIV infection among Army sexually transmitted disease patients indicates significant risk. James et al. documented an HIV antibody prevalence of 5.3% among 75 patients seen in an Army sexually transmitted disease clinic in Berlin (4). Other locations have reported rates ranging from 1-30/1000 (E. Takafuji, OTSG, and M. Benenson, 7th Medical Command, personal communications).

In the civilian sector, long-term confinement facility inmates have been identified as possible high risk populations for HIV infection, based on the relatively high prevalence of other risk factors such as drug abuse and intraprison homosexual behaviors (38),(39). Studies recently completed at the United States Disciplinary Barracks (USDB), Fort Leavenworth, KS, showed that nine of 913 (1.0%) inprocessing inmates screened during 1983-1984 had Western blot confirmed HIV antibody (40). This prevalence rate was approximately seven-fold greater than that seen in active duty Army troops based on the first 63,000 serologic test results reported in 1985-1986 (P. Kelley, unpublished data). Follow-up blood collected in July 1985 from 549 of the prisoners who provided an inprocessing specimen showed that none of those originally negative by ELISA seroconverted during the interval. In addition 199 specimens collected in May 1982 were paired with July 1985 specimens, again without evidence of seroconversion in the three year period. Therefore, the combined annual seroconversion rate assuming both a potential risk for all 1326 person-years of observation and sufficient time for any infections to result in seroconversions was 0.0% (95% confidence interval 0.0 to 0.2%). Currently both inprocessing and outprocessing inmates are screened for HIV antibody. Data from these screens should allow more definitive assessments of the risk of intraprison transmission at the USDB.

In order to determine their immune status, confirmed antibody positive inmates undergo a medical evaluation similar to that in place for infected soldiers identified through force screening. Provided that the inmate shows no signs of advanced disease, he is returned to the prison. If, after several days of close psychological observation in the prison, the inmate appears to be adjusting satisfactorily to the diagnosis, he is returned to his usual pre-diagnosis prison routine provided that the level of supervision is felt by the Director of Custody to be sufficient to preclude participation in high risk behaviors and to avoid being the target of violence (40). As a matter of policy, knowledge of a prisoner's antibody status is limited to the prison commandant, his senior staff, and appropriate medical representatives.

In addition to the screening programs outlined above, there are opportunities for military health care beneficiaries to receive HIV screening at their initiation.

Medical Evaluation and Staging

Each branch of the service has some flexibility in defining policies for periodic evaluation procedures, epidemiologic data collection and analysis, and personnel management. As an illustration of the comprehensive approach to HIV infections taken by the military, the following is the Army's program for evaluation and counseling of those identified as HIV antibody positive.

To assist in the application of standardized criteria for use in evaluating the immune status of infected adults in both the military and the civilian sectors, the Walter Reed Staging Classification for HIV Infection was developed by the Army and adopted by the Department of Defense (Figure 1) (41). This system, which is composed of seven major stages, moves from antibody-negative high-risk contacts (WR0), through stages characterized by the development of HIV antibody positivity (WR1), chronic adenopathy (WR2), a T-helper cell deficiency (WR3), partial cutaneous anergy (WR4), complete cutaneous anergy and/or thrush (WR5), and opportunistic infection (WR6). Suffix codes are added for various constitutional or diarrheal symptoms (coded B), Kaposi's sarcoma (K), other neoplasms (N), or central nervous system disease (CNS). Assignment to a stage is based on the persistence of stage-specific findings for at least three months.

Infected active-duty soldiers are initially evaluated at their local Army community hospital. Prior to evaluation, the patient is individually notified of his/her antibody status by a physician, and the individual's commander is also personally notified.

Customarily, the patient also undergoes a contact interview prior to, or during admission, to identify potential sources of infection and possible secondary cases. Extensive and repeated counseling by physicians and other trained professionals is provided to educate the individual about the infection, about mechanisms to prevent its spread, and about the need to inform others who may have been exposed. Family counseling is also an essential feature of the program. Respect for privacy and compassion from health care providers, commanders, and family members are emphasized as part of the evaluation and counseling process. Formal psychiatric help is arranged if needed.

Walter Reed Staging Classification of HIV Infection

Stage	HIV Antibody	Chronic Lymphadenopathy	T Helper Cells/mm^3	Delayed Hypersens.	Thrush	Opportunistic Infections
WR 0	-	-	>400	Normal	-	-
WR 1	+	-	>400	Normal	-	-
WR 2	+	+	>400	Normal	-	-
WR 3	+	+/-	<400	Normal	-	-
WR 4	+	+/-	<400	P	-	-
WR 5	+	+/-	<400	C and/or Thrush		-
WR 6	+	+/-	<400	P/C	+/-	+

P = Partial C = Complete

Figure 1.

The medical evaluation undertaken for all HIV infected Army personnel usually includes a thorough history and physical; chest roentgenograms; routine and special chemical, serologic, and hematologic studies including absolute T4 and T8 lymphocyte levels; and skin tests for anergy to mumps, trichophyton, candida, and tetanus. Other specialized exams may be done at the discretion of the attending physician. HIV infected patients under evaluation are also provided with additional education including guidance on warning signs of potential disease progression. Current policy calls for annual (or sooner should symptoms develop) reappraisals of disease progression.

To ensure an orderly movement of HIV patients and information between local hospitals, referral hospitals, and other organizations, each Army hospital has a designated physician point-of-contact who serves as the hospital's clinical and administrative HIV program coordinator.

The Department of Defense has adopted a policy to retain HIV antibody-positive individuals who manifest no evidence of clinical illness or other indication of immunologic or neurologic impairment related to HIV infection, and are determined to be fit for duty. Pending additional medical and administrative experience in managing such individuals, they are not considered to be disabled and appear to be capable of making worthwhile contributions in a military capacity. It is current policy for all infected soldiers stationed overseas to be returned to the United States for permanent reassignment as soon as possible. Except for being barred from overseas or deployable assignments, HIV infected soldiers are permitted to work in their military occupational specialty. Due to regulations which require Army aviators to meet more stringent accession fitness standards rather than the usual retention standards, these servicemen represent the only current exception to the Army policy of no occupational restriction. Regulatory alteration of this occupational restriction is under consideration.

Soldiers who demonstrate advanced infections undergo a medical board action to determine their fitness for retention on active duty. Those separated as a result of such action are eligible for a disability pension and for medical care through either the military or the Veterans Administration medical care system, depending on the nature of their retirement classification.

HIV-infected individuals who demonstrate advanced infection are considered for a fitness-for-duty determination under Title 10 United States Code Section 1201, et seq. Individuals infected with HIV who are found not to have complied with preventive medicine counseling are subject to appropriate administrative and disciplinary action.

To assist in the orderly management of HIV patient-care requirements within the Army Medical Department and for policy development purposes, the Army Surgeon General has organized a secure, centralized, automated data system. The system is designed to maintain demographic, epidemiologic, clinical, and laboratory data on all Western blot positive soldiers. Data are updated periodically as re-evaluations are completed. The system provides tracking information to clinicians on individual patients and information to hospital commanders to document in summary fashion the distribution and staging status of infected soldiers within their areas of responsibility. This data system compliments the Defense Medical Support System Center's Reportable Disease Database that was established to provide Department-wide information on the distribution of infection within the total force. These systems have patient care and personnel management functions; in addition, they serve as repositories for data critical to answering questions concerning the prevalence, incidence, and natural history of HIV infection.

Health Education and Contact Tracing

Another critical element in the military's HIV control program is education. Along with the requirements for education of cases and high/moderate risk contacts, extensive programs have been developed for various segments of the military community. These have included production by the military of audience specific videotapes, pamphlets, and slide sets, and the procurement of commercially available films and videotapes. Health education on the prevention of HIV infection is included in classes on sexually transmitted diseases. The overall health education effort is designed to reach all segments of the military community to include dependents, health care providers, commanders, and servicemembers. Adolescents are a special concern.

A key element of the Army's HIV control program is case-contact notification and counseling. Evaluation and education are offered to high-risk contacts, including those potentially infected through having received certain blood or blood products, through transmission from an infected mother, through participation in sexual acts with possibly infected individuals, or through other high risk behaviors. Health care providers who may be at some increased risk (such as those with percutaneous needle sticks or other exposures to infected body fluids) are also evaluated. Usually these individuals are identified through contact tracing or self-referral.

The Army contact-evaluation program includes a preventive medicine interview, counseling, and a clinical evaluation for contacts entitled to care under the military medical care system. The program calls for HIV-infected persons with a history of donating blood to be identified, and information for tracing the ultimate recipient of the blood to be transmitted to the appropriate blood bank office. Counseling includes discussion of pertinent Public Health Service recommendations for preventing further spread of the infection (36),(37),(42)-(47). Contacts who are initially seronegative are followed up with additional tests at least every 12 months. Seropositive Army active-duty contacts receive a medical evaluation as described previously. Other beneficiary contacts are urged to undergo a similar staging evaluation.

Information on high/moderate risk non-beneficiary civilian contacts is shared with local health departments if requested by the civilian authorities.

Medical-Legal Considerations

The implementation of HIV force testing poses not only obvious logistic challenges but also a variety of medical and legal questions related to patient confidentiality. Military physicians legally do not retain the level of doctor-patient privilege found in the civilian sector. Line commanders have a special and legitimate interest in this infection, since, by regulation, they are responsible for the health and welfare of their command and must know about major individual health events to assess their impact on unit readiness. Under routine circumstances, military physicians can be required by regulation to inform a servicemember's commander of information obtained concerning an individual's participation in the abuse of drugs or in homosexual activity. Special concern is directed toward individuals holding extremely sensitive national security responsibilities, such as those serving in a nuclear weapons specialty. Servicemembers convicted of participating in homosexual acts or drug abuse are subject to punishment under the Uniform Code of Military Justice. Clearly a conflict is posed between the restrictions on confidentiality inherent to the military doctor-patient relationship and the mandate to conduct epidemiological assessments to develop scientifically based information regarding the natural history and transmission pattern of HIV infections. Recognizing this problem, the Department of Defense has directed that information disclosed by a Service member as part of or as a result of an HIV epidemiological assessment may not be used against the Service member in a court martial; non-judicial punishment; involuntary separation (other than for medical reasons); administrative or punitive reduction in grade; denial of promotion; an unfavorable entry in a personnel record; a bar to reenlistment; and any other action considered by the Secretary of Defense to be an adverse personnel action. HIV serologic test results may not be used as the basis for separation except for a separation based upon physical disability. The limitations on the use of epidemiologic information do not apply to the introduction of evidence for impeachment or rebuttal purposes in any proceeding in which the evidence for drug abuse or relevant sexual activity (or lack thereof) has been first introduced by the servicemember; disciplinary or other action based on independently derived evidence; reassignment; disqualification from a personnel reliability program; removal from flight status; denial, suspension, or revocation of a security clearance; and suspensions or terminations of access to classified information.

Medical Research Efforts

The military provides an ideal environment in which to learn about HIV infection. Ready access to at-risk sexually active populations coupled with an integrated worldwide medical care and research system are just two assets. The screening of several million asymptomatic servicemembers will generate thousands of individuals who are infected in the relatively recent past and who still have an intact immune system. These people should prove to be of particular value in studying the pathogenesis of the disease and in trials of chemotherapy and immunotherapy. Military medical research and development organizations have been traditional leaders in the development of vaccines for control of diseases incuding meningococcal infections, adenoviral infections, typhoid, shigella, malaria, dengue, gonorrhea, and viral hemorrhagic fevers. Considerable expertise from these vaccine endeavors can be brought to bear on this aspect of AIDS prevention.

Servicemembers early in their HIV infection also constitute a valuable population for documenting the natural history of this infection, since, for operational reasons, these patients will be receiving at least annual assessments of disease status until they have progressed to the point where they can not be retained on active duty. Following separation they would usually still be eligible for care under the military or Veterans Administration health care systems and presumably accessible for follow-up data collection. Though studying risk factors for transmission of HIV infection in the military does present some difficulties, there are ample opportunities to gather solid data on heterosexual transmission of this infection, especially between regular sexual partners. As illustrated above, seroprevalence data ascertained from recruit applicants, active duty members, and members of the reserve component can shed considerable light on the evolving epidemiology of HIV infections in this country. Specifically, the size and dispersion of various screened populations provide opportunities to examine the relationship between current prevalence of infection and subsequent incidence. There are numerous opportunities to evaluate the effectiveness of various educational approaches in modifying behavior and reducing the incidence of infection. The military has already worked both independently and in collaborative relationships to undertake many of these epidemiologic and clinical studies.

Through a vigorous HIV management and research program, the Department of Defense is committed to finding answers to many questions concerning this rapidly spreading epidemic in order to develop appropriate policies on military readiness and to provide invaluable information on which to base sound public health policies. Program objectives have been defined; responsibilities have been assigned; and necessary funds have been appropriated to carry out ambitious serologic case identification and educational programs to limit the incidence of this infection among those in uniform and their dependents. This commitment was established on the belief that the only practical mechanisms available today to curtail transmission of this tragic disease are based on aggressive identification of those infected and appropriate effective education programs for all. Anything less will lead to unnecessary anxiety, continued viral transmission and more deaths.

REFERENCES

1. Herbold J.R., AIDS Policy Development within the Department of Defense. Military Med 151:623-630 (1986)

2. CDC., Acquired Immunodeficiency Syndrome (AIDS) Weekly Surveillance Report - United States. August 25 Issue (1986)

3. Redfield, W.R., Markham, P.D., Salahuddin, S.Z., et al., Frequent transmission of HTLV-III among spouses of patients with AIDS-related complex and the acquired immunodeficiency syndrome. JAMA 253:1571-1573 (1985)

4. James, J.J., Hatten, J.A., Morgenstern, M., et al., HTLV-III and hepatitis A and B serological markers among U.S. military venereal disease patients. Milit Med 151:193-198 (1986)

5. Harris, C., Butkus Small, C., Klein, R.S., et al., Immunodeficiency in female sexual partners of men with the acquired immunodeficiency syndrome. N Engl J Med 308:1181-1184 (1983)

6. Piot, P., Taelman, H., Minlangu, K.B., et al., Acquired immunodeficiency syndrome in heterosexual population in Zaire. Lancet 2:65-69 (1984)

7. Redfield, R., Markham, P., Salahuddin, S., et al., Heterosexual acquired HTLV-III/LAV disease (AIDS-related complex and AIDS): epidemiologic evidence for female-to-male transmission. JAMA 254:2094-2096 (1985)

8. Barrett, O., "U.S. Medicine in Vietnam: The Early Years" In: Internal Medicine in Vietnam, Vol II - General Medicine and Infectious Diseases. Office of the Surgeon General and Center of Military History, United States Army, p 21-38 (1982)

9. Harmon, J.W., Llewllyn, C., Lessons of the Falklands. Medical Bulletin of the U.S. Army, Europe 41:11-13 (1984)

10. Headquarters, Department of the Army. Medical Services Standards of Fitness. Army Regulation 40-501. Interim Change 104 (July 1986)

11. Jaffe, H.W., Darrow, W.W., Echenberg, D.F., et al., The acquired immunodeficiency syndrome in a cohort of homosexual men: a six-year follow-up study. Ann Intern Med 103:210-214 (1985)

12. Association of State and Territorial Health Officials Foundation. Guide to Public Health Practice: HTLV-III Antibody Testing and Community Approaches. Publication No. 85, (1985)

13. Hardy, A.M., Rauch, K., Echenberg, D., et al., The economic impact of the first 10,000 cases of acquired immunodeficiency syndrome in the United States. JAMA 255:209-211 (1986)

14. Mann, J.M., Francis, H., Quinn, T., et al., Surveillance for AIDS in a Central African City: Kinshasa, Zaire. JAMA 255:3255-3259 (1986)

15. CDC., Update: acquired immunodeficiency syndrome - Europe. MMWR 35:43-46 (1986)

16. Chang, R.S., French, G.L., Leong, S., et al., HTLV-III antibody testing in Hong Kong. JAMA 256:41 (1986)

17. Lemon, S.M., Lednar, W.M., Bancroft, W.H., et al., Etiology of viral hepatitis in American soldiers. Am J Epidem 116:438-450 (1982)

18. Berg, S.W., Sexually transmitted diseases in the military. In: Sexually Transmitted Diseases, (Holmes, K.K., Mardh, P.A., Sparling, P.F., Wiesner, P.J., eds), McGraw-Hill Book Company, New York (1984)

19. Haseltine, W.A., HTLV-III/LAV-antibody-positive soldiers in Berlin. N Engl J Med 314:55-56 (1986)

20. Tirelli, U., Vaccher, E., Sorio, R., et al., HTLV-III antibodies in drug-addicted prostitutes used by U.S. soldiers in Italy. JAMA 256:711-712 (1986)

21. Kreiss, J.K., Koech, D., Plummer, F.A., et al., AIDS virus infection in Nairobi prostitutes: spread of the epidemic to East Africa. N Engl J Med 314:414-418 (1986)

22. Franceschi, S., Tirelli, U., Vaccher, E., et al., Increased prevalence of HTLV-III antibody among drug addicts from Italian province with U.S. military base. Lancet 1:804 (1986)

23. Headquarters, Department of the Army. Field Manual (FM) 100-5, Operations, (1982)

24. Navia, B.A., Jordan, B.D., Price, R.W., et al., The AIDS dementia complex: I. Clinical features. Ann Neurol 19:517-524 (1986)

25. Ho, D.D., Rota, T.R., Schooley, R.T., et al., Isolation of HTLV-III from cerebrospinal fluid and neural tissues of patients with neurologic syndromes related to the acquired immunodeficiency syndrome. N Engl J Med 313:1493-1497 (1985)

26. Mirra, S.S., Anand, R., Spira, T.J., HTLV-III/LAV infection of the central nervous system in a 57 year-old man with progressive dementia of unknown cause. N Engl J Med 314:1191-1192 (1986)

27. Headquarters, Department of the Army. Army Regulation 40-562. (In press)

28. Zagury, D., Bernard, J., Leonard, R., et al., Long-term cultures of HTLV-III-infected T cells: a model of cytopathology of T-cell depletion in AIDS. Science 231:850-853 (1986)

29. Ammann, A.J., Schiffman, G., Abrams, D., et al., B-cell immunodeficiency in acquired immune deficiency syndrome. JAMA 251:1447-1449 (1984)

30. Lane, H.C., Depper, J.M., Greene, W.C., et al., Qualitative analysis of immune function in patients with the acquired immunodeficiency syndrome: evidence for a selective defect in soluble antigen recognition. N Engl J Med 313:79-84 (1985)

31. Salata, R.A., Ravdin, J.I., N-acetyl-D-galactosamine-inhibitable adherence lectin of *Entamoeba histolytica*. II. Mitogenic activity for human lymphocytes. J Infect Dis 151:816-822 (1985)

32. Petri, W.A., Ravdin, J.I., Treatment of homosexual men infected with *Entamoeba histolytica*. N Engl J Med 315:393 (1986)

33. Burke, D.S., Redfield, R.R., False-positive Western blot tests for antibodies to HTLV-III. JAMA 256:347 (1986)

34. CDC., Human T-lymphotropic virus type III/lymphadenopathy-associated virus antibody prevalence in U.S. military recruit applicants. MMWR 35:421-424 (1986)

35. Sandler, S.G., Testing Blood Donors for HTLV-III antibodies: the American Red Cross experience. Abstract. NIH Consensus Development Conference: Impact of Routine HTLV-III Antibody Testing on Public Health. Bethesda, MD, p 26-27 (1986)

36. CDC., Additional recommendations to reduce sexual and drug-abuse-related transmission of human T-lymphotrophic virus type III/lymphadenopathy-associated virus. MMWR 35:152-155 (1986)

37. CDC., Recommendations for preventing transmission of infection with human T-lymphotrophic virus type III/lymphadenopathy-associated virus in the workplace. MMWR 34:681-686 (1985)

38. Marini, J.L., Bridges, C.I., Sheard, M.H., Multiple drug abuse: examination of drug-abuse patterns in male prisoners. Int J Addict 13:493-502 (1978)

39. Nacci, P.L., Kane, T.R., The incidence of sex and sexual aggression in federal prisons. Federal Probation 47:31-36 (1983)

40. Kelley, P.W., Redfield, R.R., Ward, D.L., et al., Intraprison transmission of HTLV-III. JAMA 256:2197-2198 (1986)

41. Redfield, R.R., Wright, D.C., Tramont, E.C., The Walter Reed staging classification for HTLV-III/LAV infection. N Engl J Med 314:131-132 (1986)

42. CDC., Prevention of acquired immune deficiency syndrome (AIDS): report of inter-agency recommendations. MMWR 32: 101-103 (1983)

43. CDC., Provisional Public Health Service inter-agency recommendations for screening donated blood and plasma for antibody to the virus causing acquired immunodeficiency syndrome. MMWR 34:1-5 (1985)

44. CDC., Testing donors of organs, tissues, and semen for antibody to human T-lymphotrophic virus type III/lymphadenopathy-associated virus. MMWR 34:294 (1985)

45. CDC., Education and foster care of children infected with human T-lymphotrophic virus type III/lymphadenopathy-associated virus. MMWR 30:517-521 (1985)

46. CDC., Update: revised Public Health Service definition of persons who should refrain from donating blood and plasma - United States. MMWR 34:547-548 (1985)

47. CDC., Recommendations for assisting in the prevention of perinatal transmission of human T-lymphotrophic virus type III/ lymphadenopathy-associated virus and acquired immunodeficiency syndrome. MMWR 34:721-726, 731-732 (1985)

Footnote

The military HIV control program is subject to periodic review by Congress and various offices within the Department of Defense. The interpretations of current and imminent policies and procedures described in the chapter are believed accurate as of November 26, 1986.

6
AIDS Cases with "No Identified Risk"

Alan R. Lifson, Kenneth G. Castro

The Centers for Disease Control (CDC) receives reports of patients with acquired immunodeficiency syndrome (AIDS) on a standard case report form. Based on the information contained in this report, patients are classified into various groups that suggest a possible means of disease acquisition. Ninety-seven percent of all reported adults are known to belong to groups at increased risk for AIDS (Table 1). The remaining 3% are classified as persons with unknown, or "no identified" risk (NIR). The proportion of all AIDS patients with NIR has not significantly changed over time.

All AIDS patients with NIR are referred for further investigation by state or local public health personnel. This investigation includes an in-depth interview and, if possible, serologic testing for human immunodeficiency virus ([HIV], also referred to as human T-lymphotropic virus type III [HTLV-III] and lymphadenopathy-associated virus [LAV]). This chapter will present reasons for classification of an AIDS patient as NIR, and discuss whether investigation of these patients reveals new modes of HIV transmission.

OUTCOME OF INVESTIGATIONS

Of 22,964 adults with AIDS reported to CDC as of August 1, 1986, 1,133 (5%) were initially classified as NIR on the basis of the case report form (1) (Table 2). Of these cases, 346 have not yet been investigated or are currently under investigation. Further information with respect to risk history was unobtainable on 196 because of the patients' death, refusal to be interviewed, or loss to follow-up. Interviews or other follow-up information were available on the remaining 591 patients. Risk factors were ultimately identified for 68% of these patients. An additional 5% of these patients were considered not to have AIDS based on normal serologic and immunologic studies, the presence of another reason for immunocompromise or failure to meet the criteria of the case definition for other reasons.

TABLE 1. Cases of AIDS in U.S. Adults by Risk Groups* and Year of Diagnosis (through August 1, 1986)

	Before Jan 1983	1983	1984	1985	1986	Total
Homosexual/ Bisexual	939(73%)	1944(72%)	4018(74%)	6650(74%)	3343(73%)	16894(74%)
IV Drug Abuser	202(16%)	489(18%)	916(17%)	1536(17%)	804(18%)	3947(17%)
Hemophiliac	8(1%)	12(1%)	46(1%)	88(1%)	34(1%)	188(1%)
Heterosexual cases:						
Heterosexual contact,high risk person**	14(1%)	27(1%)	72(1%)	160(2%)	102(2%)	375(2%)
Born outside U.S.***	75(6%)	98(4%)	125(2%)	130(1%)	58(1%)	486(2%)
Transfusion recipient	8(1%)	36(1%)	79(1%)	171(2%)	95(2%)	389(2%)
None of the above (NIR)	43(3%)	84(3%)	149(3%)	267(3%)	142(3%)	685(3%)
	1289	2690	5405	9002	4578	22,964

* Risk groups are ordered hierarchically.

** Persons who have had heterosexual contact with a person with AIDS or a person at risk for AIDS.

*** Persons born in countries where heterosexual transmission is believed to play a major role.

TABLE 2. Outcome of NIR Investigations as of August 1, 1986

1,133 patients initially classified as NIR based on case report form:

346 cases: Not yet investigated, currently under investigation

196 cases: Further information unobtainable

157 patients died, no further information from family
30 patients refused interview
9 patients lost to follow-up

591 cases: Interviews or other follow-up information obtained

431 patients reclassified

401 reclassified into high risk groups
30 did not meet criteria of case definition for AIDS

160 patients remained NIR

REASONS FOR CLASSIFICATION OUTSIDE OF RISK GROUPS

Evaluation of surveillance data and in-depth interviews suggest that there are four major reasons for classification of an AIDS patient as NIR. First, for some individuals incomplete information exists regarding risk history. CDC surveillance data indicate that the majority of persons initially classified as "no identified risk" are reclassified when additional information becomes available.

Second, risk factors may not be identified because the patient with AIDS may be reluctant to disclose personal information such as sexual preference or drug use for personal, social or economic reasons. In a study of the first 201 "no identified risk" AIDS cases, investigators found that many of these patients were demographically similar to populations recognized to be at increased risk for AIDS, such as IV drug users and sexual contacts of high risk persons, suggesting that risk factors may have been present but not reported (2).

Third, some patients may be incorrectly classified as cases of AIDS. Patients with opportunistic infections may have other unrecognized causes for immunodeficiency. Also, diseases such as Kaposi's sarcoma may occur in the immunocompetent individual not infected with HIV (3). These patients represent background, sporadic cases of these diseases. According to the revised case definition, patients are excluded as AIDS cases if they have a negative test for HIV antibody, have no other HIV test with a positive result, and have normal immunologic studies (4). If such testing is not available or is not done, a patient who does not have AIDS may be inappropriately classified as an AIDS case.

Fourth, heterosexual transmission may account for many cases in patients not belonging to recognized risk groups. For example, a person may have acquired infection through sexual contact with someone he or she did not know was infected with HIV or belonged to a high risk group. This may be particularly true for individuals who report multiple or "anonymous" sexual partners, prostitution or contact with prostitutes. Such individuals are at increased risk for acquiring other sexually transmitted diseases. Data from 133 in-depth interviews indicate that 50 (38%) NIR patients with AIDS had a history of other sexually transmitted diseases, such as gonorrhea (27%) and syphilis (14%) (1). Although the efficiency of male-to-female and female-to-male transmission of HIV continues to be studied, preliminary data from the United States and other countries suggest that bidirectional transmission occurs (5),(6),(7)-(11).

SPREAD OF INFECTION BY PROSTITUTES

Because of evidence suggesting that HIV may be transmitted from infected females to their heterosexual partners, CDC is studying the potential role of female prostitutes in such transmission. Nineteen (29%) of 66 NIR men interviewed reported a history of sexual contact with a female prostitute within the preceding five years (1). Not all of these men necessarily became infected through this contact. Some investigators have suggested that a report of contact with prostitutes may be offered by some persons belonging to high-risk groups for HIV infection to prevent further risk factor investigation (12). However, reports suggesting female-to-male HIV transmission, the isolation of this virus from cervical and vaginal secretions (13),(14), and preliminary data indicating that 5%-40% of female prostitutes have antibody to HIV (7), suggest that such transmission may occur. Studies of AIDS in persons from Haiti and central Africa also suggest that female prostitutes might play a role in HIV transmission (6),(15),(16). Because of the possibility of bidirectional heterosexual transmission, the U.S. Public Health Service has included male and female prostitutes and their sex partners among those persons at increased risk of HIV infection (17).

ALTERNATE ROUTES OF TRANSMISSION

Concern has been raised regarding the safety of products derived from human blood or plasma, such as therapeutic immune globulin preparations and the hepatitis B vaccine. There is no laboratory or epidemiologic evidence to suggest that HIV is transmitted by receipt of any of these products (18),(19). Patients with no identified risk are not more likely to have received immune globulins than are members of high risk groups

(18). Several studies have shown that recipients of hepatitis B immune globulin and other immune globulin preparations, including lots known to be positive for antibody to HIV, have not seroconverted or developed other evidence of HIV infection (18),(20). Patients with no identified risk are also not more likely to have received the hepatitis B vaccine than are members of high risk groups (1). Laboratory data evaluating the processes for preparing immune globulins and the hepatitis B vaccine also support the safety of these products (18),(19).

Of all health care workers reported to CDC as of August 1, 1986, 95% were known to belong to high risk groups for AIDS (21). Specific occupational exposures which could be implicated as the source of HIV infection (such as needlesticks from infected persons) have not been identified for any health care worker with AIDS reported to CDC. However, several reports from the United States and England have indicated that HIV may, on rare occasions, be transmitted from infected persons to health care workers through parenteral exposures (22)-(24), although the risk associated with such exposures is extremely low (25)-(28). Adherence to recommended guidelines for health care workers should further decrease this risk (29)-(32).

To date, there remains no evidence that HIV is spread by casual contact. Such transmission, if it occurs, might be evident in the household or family setting. One study evaluated this possibility in 101 household contacts (68 adults and 33 children) of AIDS or ARC patients who had close personal interaction with these patients (excluding sexual contact) and shared household items and facilities (33). Of these contacts, only one young child had evidence of HIV infection, which was most likely acquired perinatally; none of the other household contacts had evidence of HIV infection. Other studies evaluating the possibility of HIV transmission through casual contact in the family setting have also not found serologic or virologic evidence of such transmission within families (34)-(37).

Although HIV has been isolated from saliva (38) and tears (39), there have been no AIDS cases in which contact with these fluids is known to have transmitted HIV infection. In one study, HIV was only infrequently isolated from the saliva of seropositive individuals (one of 83 persons tested), much less commonly than it was isolated from blood (28 of 50 persons tested) (40), suggesting that contact with saliva carries even lower risk than the small risk associated with parenteral contact with blood.

There is also no evidence that HIV is transmitted by contact with mosquitoes or other insects (41),(42). For example, the relative absence of NIR AIDS cases in populations which might have heavy mosquito exposure, such as preadolescent children and adolescents, suggests that such transmission does not play an important role. Studies from one community in south Florida evaluated the prevalence of antibody to nine arboviruses endemic in that region as a measure of exposure to mosquito vectors (43). Antibodies to one or more of these viruses did not correlate significantly with HIV infection. No arthropod transmission has ever been documented for hepatitis B, which is more readily transmitted than HIV after needlestick injury in health care settings (42).

CHILDREN OUTSIDE OF RISK GROUPS

CDC also receives reports of children with AIDS on a standard case report form. Based on the information contained in this form, children are also classified into groups that suggest a possible means of disease acquisition. Of all children with AIDS, 79% had a parent with HIV infection or a parent at increased risk for HIV infection; 4% of children were hemophiliacs, and 15% had been transfused with blood or blood products.

Of 324 children with AIDS reported to CDC as of August 1, 1986, 25 were initially classified as NIR on the basis of the case report form (44). Three cases are currently under investigation. Further information was unobtainable on six patients. Of the 16 cases on whom some follow-up information was obtained, 15 were reclassified. Information on the sixteenth case was felt to be incomplete because the parents were not interviewed in their native language. These data suggest that the major reason for classification of a child with AIDS as NIR is incomplete information with respect to risk history.

In summary, both surveillance data and studies considered in this chapter support previously described modes of HIV transmission: sexual contact, contact with infected blood or blood products, and perinatal transmission from an infected mother to her neonate. Evaluation of NIR cases does not support the existence of major alternate modes of transmission which to date have gone undetected.

REFERENCES

1. Lifson A.R., Castro, K.G., White, C.R., et al., "No identified risk" cases of AIDS. Twenty-sixth Interscience Conference on Antimicrobial Agents and Chemotherapy, New Orleans, Louisiana (1986)

2. Chamberland, M.E., Castro, K.G., Haverkos, H.W., et al., Acquired immunodeficiency syndrome in the United States: An analysis of cases outside high risk groups. Ann Intern Med 101: 617-623 (1984)

3. Biggar, R.J., Horm, J., Fraumeni, J.F., et al., Incidence of Kaposi's sarcoma and mycosis fungoides in the United States including Puerto Rico, 1973-1981. J Nat Can Inst 73:89-94 (1984)

4. CDC., Revision of the case definition of acquired immunodeficiency syndrome for national reporting -- United States. MMWR 34:373-375 (1985)

5. Piot P., Quinn T., Taelman, H. et al., Acquired immunodeficiency syndrome in a heterosexual population in Zaire. Lancet 2: 65-69 (1984)

6. Van de Perre P., Rouvroy D., Lepage, P., et al., Acquired immunodeficiency syndrome in Rwanda. Lancet 2: 62-65 (1984)

7. CDC., Heterosexual transmission of human T-cell lymphotropic virus type III/lymphadenopathy associated virus. MMWR 34:561-562 (1985)

8. Redfield, R.R., Markham, P.D., Salahuddin, S.Z., et al., Heterosexually acquired HTLV-III/LAV disease (AIDS related complex and AIDS): Epidemiologic evidence for female to male transmission. JAMA 254:2094-2096 (1985)

9. Calabrese, L.H., Gopalakrishna, K.V. Transmission of HTLV-III infection from man to woman to man. N Engl J Med 314:987 (1986)

10. Peterman, T.A., Stoneburner, R.L., Allen, J.R. Risk of transmission of human T-lymphotropic virus type III/ lymphadenopathy associated virus in households. Epidemic Intelligence Service 35th Annual Conference, Atlanta, Georgia, April 14-18 (1986)

11. Johnson, W., Liautaud, B., Thomas, F., et al., Heterosexual transmission of HTLV-III/LAV in Haiti. Twenty-fifth Interscience Conference on Antimicrobial Agents and Chemotherapy. Minneapolis, Minnesota. (1985)

12. Schultz, S., Milberg, J.A., Kristal, A.R., et al., Female to male transmission of HTLV-III. JAMA 255:1703-1704 (1986)

13. Vogt, M.W., Witt, D.J., Craven, D.E., et al., Isolation of HTLV-III/LAV from cervical secretions of women at risk for AIDS. Lancet 1:525-527 (1986)

14. Wofsy, C.B., Cohen, J.B., Hauer, L.B., et al., Isolation of AIDS associated retrovirus from genital secretions of women with antibodies to the virus. Lancet 1:527-529 (1986)

15. Castro, K.G., Fischl, M., Landesman, S., et al., Risk factors for AIDS among Haitians in the United States. International Conference on the Acquired Immunodeficiency Syndrome, Atlanta, Georgia, April (1985)

16. Kreiss, J.K., Koech, D., Plummer, F.A., et al., AIDS virus infection in Nairobi prostitutes. N Engl J Med 314:414-418 (1986)

17. CDC., Additional recommendations to reduce sexual and drug abuse related transmission of human T-lymphotropic virus type III/lymphadenopathy-associated virus. MMWR 35:152-155 (1986)

18. CDC., Safety of therapeutic immune globulin preparations with respect to transmission of human T-lymphotropic virus type III/lymphadenopathy-associated virus infection. MMWR 35: 231-233 (1986)

19. CDC., Hepatitis B vaccine: evidence confirming lack of AIDS transmission. MMWR 33:685-687 (1984)

20. Tedder, R.S., Uttley, A., Cheingsong-Popov, R. Safety of immunoglobulin preparation containing anti-HTLV-III. Lancet 1:815 (1985)

21. Lifson, A.R., Castro, K.G., McCray, E., et al., National surveillance of the acquired immunodeficiency syndrome in health care workers. JAMA (in press)

22. Anonymous. Needlestick transmission of HTLV-III from a patient infected in Africa. Lancet 1984; 2:1376-1377.

23. Stricof, R.L., Morse, D.L., HTLV-III/LAV seroconversion following a deep intramuscular needlestick injury. N Engl J Med 314:1115 (1986)

24. Oksenhendler, E., Harzic, M., Le-Roux, J.M., et al., HIV infection with seroconversion after a superficial needlestick injury to the finger. N Engl J Med 315:582 (1986)

25. Hirsch, M.S., Wormser, G.P., Schooley, R.T., et al., Risk of nosocomial infection with the human T-cell lymphotropic virus III (HTLV-III). N Engl J Med 312:1-4 (1985)

26. McCray, E., Cooperative Needlestick Surveillance Group. Occupational risk for the acquired immunodeficiency syndrome among health care workers. N Engl J Med 314:1127-1132 (1986)

27. Henderson, D.K., Saah, A.J., Azk, B.J., et al., Risk of nosocomial infection with human T-cell lymphotropic virus in a large cohort of intensively exposed health care workers. Ann Intern Med 104:644-647 (1986)

28. Gerberding, J.L., Bryant, C.E., Moss, A., et al., Risk of acquired immune deficiency syndrome (AIDS) virus transmission to health care workers (HCW): Results of a prospective cohort study. International Conference on Acquired Immunodeficiency Syndrome. Paris, France, (1986)

29. CDC., Acquired immune deficiency syndrome (AIDS): Precautions for clinical and laboratory staffs. MMWR 31:577-579 (1982)

30. CDC., Acquired immunodeficiency syndrome (AIDS): Precautions for health care workers and allied professionals. MMWR 32:450-451 (1983)

31. CDC., Summary: Recommendations for preventing transmission of infection with human T-lymphotropic virus type III/lymphadenopathy-associated virus in the workplace. MMWR 34:681-695 (1985)

32. CDC., Recommendations for preventing transmission of infection with human T-lymphotropic virus type III/lymphadenopathy-associated virus during invasive procedures. MMWR 35:221-223 (1985)

33. Friedland, G.H., Saltzman, B.R., Rogers, M.F., et al., Lack of transmission of HTLV-III/LAV to household contacts of patients with AIDS or AIDS related complex with oral candidiasis. N Engl J Med 314:344-349 (1986)

34. Thomas, P.T., Lubin, K., Enlow, R.W., et al., Comparison of HTLV-III serology, T cell levels, and the general health status of children whose mothers have AIDS with children of healthy inner city mothers in New York. International Conference on the Acquired Immunodeficiency Syndrome, Atlanta, Georgia, April (1985)

35. Fischl, M.A., Dickinson, G., Scott, C., et al., Evaluation of household contacts of adult AIDS patients. International Conference on the Acquired Immunodeficiency Syndrome, Atlanta, Georgia, April (1985)

36. Jason, J.M., McDougal, J.S., Dixon, G., et al., HTLV-III/LAV antibody and immune status of household contacts and sexual partners of persons with hemophilia. JAMA 255:212-215 (1986)

37. Kaplan, J.E., Oleske, J.M., Getchell, J.P., et al., Evidence against transmission of HTLV-III/LAV in families of children with AIDS. Ped Infect Dis 4:468-471 (1985)

38. Groopman, J., Salahuddin, S., Sarngadharan, M., et al., HTLV-III in saliva of people with AIDS related complex and healthy homosexual men at increased risk of AIDS. Science 226:447-449 (1984)

39. CDC., Recommendations for preventing possible transmission of human T-lymphotropic virus type III/lymphadenopathy-associated virus from tears. MMWR 34:533-534 (1985)

40. Ho, D.D., Byington, R.E., Schooley, R.T., et al., Infrequency of isolation of HTLV-III virus from saliva in AIDS. N Engl J Med 313:1606 (1985)

41. Drotman, D.P. Insect-borne transmission of AIDS? Questions and answers. JAMA 254:1085 (1985)

42. Drotman, D.P. Insect-borne transmission of AIDS? (Letters). JAMA 255:463-464 (1986)

43. Castro, K.G., Lieb, S., Narkunas, J., et al., The epidemiology of AIDS in Belle Glade, Florida. Epidemic Intelligence Service 35th Annual Conference, Atlanta, Georgia, April 14-18 (1986)

44. Lifson, A.R., Rogers, M.F., White, C., et al., Unrecognized modes of transmission of HIV?: AIDS in children reported without risk factors. Pediatric Infect Dis (in press)

7

Epidemiology of AIDS Outside the United States

R. A. Ancelle, J. B. Brunet

Five years after the first description of the acquired immunodeficiency syndrome (AIDS) (1)(2) in the United States of America (USA), cases have been reported in about 60 countries on five continents. Progressively, specific surveillance systems for AIDS have been established using, in accordance with the World Health Organization recommendations, the Centers for Disease Control (Atlanta, USA) case definition (3). However, at present, the epidemiology of AIDS worldwide is still difficult to assess due to large gaps in available information and because each country uses a different surveillance system to collect data. Available current data on AIDS outside of the United States is reviewed.

OVERALL SITUATION

By March 1986, detailed surveillance data were available from only a few countries, mainly in the Americas, Europe and Oceania. Fifty-seven countries have reported 23,919 cases to the World Health Organization (WHO), and another 23 countries have submitted reports but deny any cases. Eighty-two percent (82%) of the total reported cases were diagnosed in the USA and 10% were reported from 26 European countries. In Africa, only Kenya and South Africa have officially reported cases: 10 and 21 respectively. In Asia, China and Hong Kong reported one and three cases respectively in September 1985; Thailand had reported six cases by December 31, 1985; and Japan 14 cases by January 31, 1986 (4).

According to the Pan American Health Organization (5), there has been a steady increase in the number of cases recorded in Canada (0.3 per million population for the last six months of 1981, to 7.4 per million population for the same period of 1985), and Brazil (0.4 cases per million population for the last six months of 1982, to 1.6 per million population for the same period of 1985).

Most of the Caribbean Islands and the countries of South America have reported cases. In Haiti, cases were first recognized in 1979 (6); by June 1985, the prevalence rate per million population was 65, similar to the overall USA figure of 70 per million population.

The prevalence rate (per million) in Australia (the Oceania region) has increased from 0.06 in December 1982, to 9.0 in December 1985 (7).

In Europe (Table 1), the highest prevalence rates per million population were noted in Switzerland (15.4), Denmark (13.3) and France (10.4). Although the rate per million population is 14.0 in Belgium, this figure exaggerates the prevalence of truly endemic cases, since 70% of the cases reported in that country originated from Africa.

Cases are only just emerging from countries in the Eastern bloc. Lack of reporting may account for the absence of recorded AIDS cases in these countries, but it is also likely that limitations in foreign travel and disapproval of homosexuality have limited the emergence of the disease.

The considerable number of AIDS cases in patients originating from central Africa who were diagnosed in Belgium and France drew attention to the African continent (8)(9). Organized surveillance has only recently been set up and no data from these networks have been published to date. However, various studies show that the disease is epidemic in the Central African Republic, Kenya, Rwanda, Uganda, Zaire and Zambia (10)-(17), and AIDS has now become a major public health problem.

Prevalence rates are difficult to assess in Africa since studies were undertaken in limited areas over short periods. In 1983, the estimated prevalence rates were 150 to 200 cases per million population in Kinshasa, Zaire (17), and 800 cases per million population in Kigali, Rwanda (13).

These studies suggest that the virus is more widely distributed in certain populations of central Africa than it is in the United States or the European continent. In Africa, males and females are affected equally, and the risk groups are not those identified in Europe or the United States, but groups with multiple heterosexual contacts (12)(15). Better understanding of the epidemiology of AIDS in Africa will be gained when results of the surveillance systems become available.

For most countries the only available information is the number of cases. Therefore, the epidemiological features analysed in the following paragraphs will concern primarily Europe and are accurate as of December 31, 1985.

TABLE 1. Total Number of AIDS Cases Reported In 23 European Countries and Estimated Prevalence Rates Per Million Population

December 31, 1985

Country	Cases	Rate Per Million Population[a]
Austria	28	3.7
Belgium	139	14.0
Czechoslovakia	0	0
Denmark	68	13.3
Finland	10	2.0
France	573	10.4
Germany, Fed. Rep.	377	6.2
Greece	13	1.3
Hungary	0	0
Iceland	0	0
Ireland	8	2.2
Italy	140	2.4
Luxemburg	3	7.5
Netherlands	98	6.8
Norway	17	4.0
Poland	0	0
Portugal	18	1.7
Spain	83	2.2
Sweden	42	5.1
Switzerland	100	15.4
United Kingdom	287	5.1
U.S.S.R.	0	0
Yugoslavia	2	0.1
TOTAL	2006	

a Source of population figures: INED 1985

DISTRIBUTION OF CASES BY DISEASE CATEGORY AND DEATHS

In Europe, 1005 deaths were reported for 2006 cases (case-fatality rate: 50%). Two-thirds of cases (1327 cases) presented with one or more opportunistic infections; 20% (392 cases) with Kaposi's sarcoma alone; 12% (246 cases) with both opportunistic infections and Kaposi's sarcoma. Progressive multifocal leukoencephalopathy and various lymphomas were found in 41 cases. The overall fatality rates, irrespective of the duration of the disease, suggest that the prognosis is less severe for patients with Kaposi's sarcoma alone (fatality rate: 28%) than for other clinical forms (54% to 66%). This impression is confirmed by actuarial survival curves which show a survival rate of 80% at one year for patients with Kaposi's sarcoma alone (18).

DISTRIBUTION BY AGE AND SEX

In Europe, as in Australia, Brazil and Canada, males accounted for the majority of cases (91%). The M:F sex ratio was 10.5:1. Forty percent of cases occurred in the 30-39 year age group. Fifty-eight pediatric cases (children under 15 years) were reported in 11 European countries. Forty-one (71%) of these children had parents either with AIDS or belonging to a high risk group for AIDS; 16 were related to receipt of contaminated blood or blood products (eight hemophiliacs and eight blood transfusion recipients). No risk factors were identified in one case.

These data show that among pediatric cases in Europe, as in the USA, mother-to-child transmission predominates. The mechanisms of perinatal transmission of human immunodeficiency virus (HIV) still need to be studied, but it is believed that infection is possible during pregnancy, labor and delivery, or shortly after birth (19)-(23).

DISTRIBUTION BY RISK GROUP

The distribution of AIDS cases according to risk group, an indication of the possible means of disease acquisition, reveals marked regional differences.

Homosexuals/Bisexuals

AIDS was first described among homosexuals and bisexuals, and this group still remains the major target of the disease in Australia (89%: 141 cases out of 159), Brazil (74%: 499 out of 673), Canada (77%: 395 out of 511) and Europe (67%: 1342 out of 2006). The relative proportion of homosexual cases is similar in Europe and the USA (Figure 1).

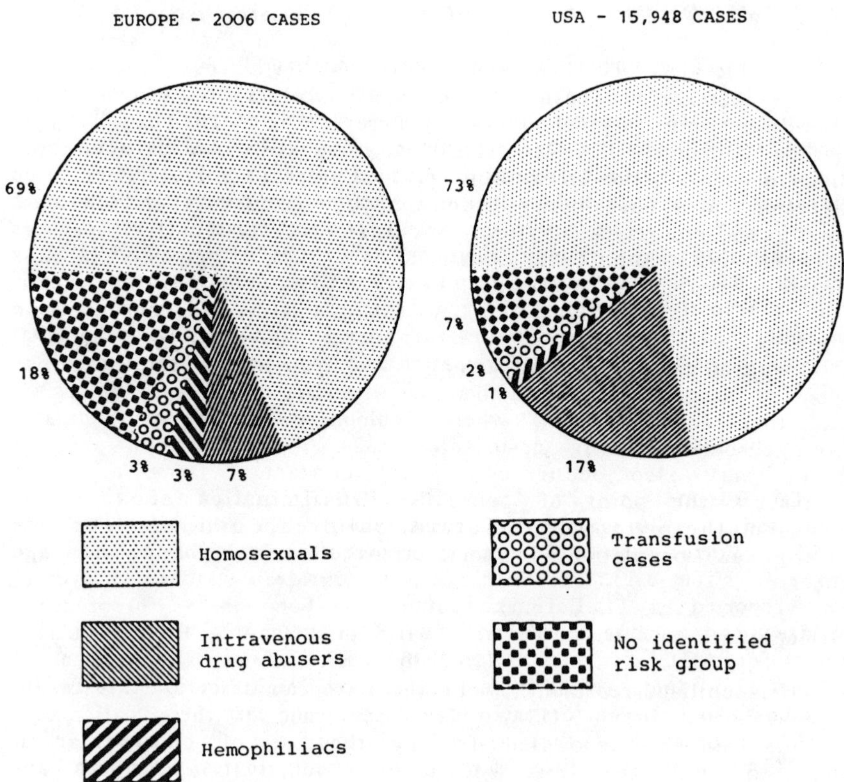

Figure 1. Distribution of cases reported in Europe and the USA by risk group - December 31, 1985.

Transfusion Recipients

Cases among transfusion recipients represent a low but significant proportion of cases: Brazil 1% (8 out of 673 cases), Canada 3% (16 out of 511) and Europe 3% (51 out of 2006). Although systematic screening of blood donors has been implemented in most countries, cases among transfusion recipients will still occur due to the long incubation period of the disease. The relative proportion for this group is also similar in Europe and the USA.

Intravenous Drug Abusers

In Canada, only one case out of the 511 has occurred in a heterosexual drug abuser. No cases have been reported in Australia. In Brazil, 2% of the 673 cases are related to intravenous drug abuse, and all of these patients were diagnosed in the two major cities, Rio de Janeiro and Sao Paulo.

In Europe, intravenous drug abusers represent 7% of the 2006 cases, and in the USA, 17% of the 15,948 cases reported by the same date. The relative proportion represented by this group has been stable in the USA since 1983 (24), whereas in Europe a marked increase has been observed since October 1984 when 2% of 559 cases were intravenous drug abusers (25). The gap between Europe and the USA is decreasing progressively with the rapid dissemination of the HIV virus among European drug abusers. High infection rates have been documented by serosurveys and in some European countries, by an increase in seropositivity rates between 1983 and 1985: Austria: 44% (26); France: 70% (27); Federal Republic of Germany: 4-6% (28); Italy: 6-76% (29); Spain: 11-48% (30); Switzerland: 16-32% (31); United Kingdom: 1.5-6.4% (31).

Transmission of HIV among drug abusers is facilitated by repeated needle-sharing and booting (drawing blood into a syringe and then re-injecting it) whereby blood rinses the contaminated syringe before being re-injected (32). Transmission in this group may also occur by sexual contact. Drug addiction represents the point of origin for dissemination of the virus from mothers to their future children, and also to the heterosexual population. In some areas this is becoming a major concern.

Hemophiliacs

Hemophiliacs represent 3% of the European cases and 1% of the cases reported in the USA. The occurrence of these patients in Europe can be accounted for by the use of clotting agents imported from the USA before viral inactivation methods and routine screening of blood for HIV antibodies were employed (33)(34). In Brazil, 4% of AIDS cases were diagnosed in this group.

Patients Not Belonging To Any Identified Risk Groups

In Canada, this group represents 13% of the total cases (69 cases out of 511), of which 74% originated from "endemic" areas.

In Europe, this group accounts for 18% of reported cases, and in the USA only 7%. This disparity can be explained since in Europe 70% of such patients, versus 3% in the USA, originated from countries where most AIDS cases occur outside of the identified risk groups (mainly central African countries and Haiti) (Figure 2) (35),(36). However, in Africa and Haiti, as in other countries, the principal identified modes of transmission are through sexual contact or through contaminated injections or blood transfusions (37).

DISTRIBUTION BY RISK GROUP AND COUNTRY OF DIAGNOSIS FOR 18 EUROPEAN COUNTRIES

Despite efforts to standardize surveillance systems, precise comparisons between countries in Europe are difficult. Furthermore, in countries where the disease is still rare, the current

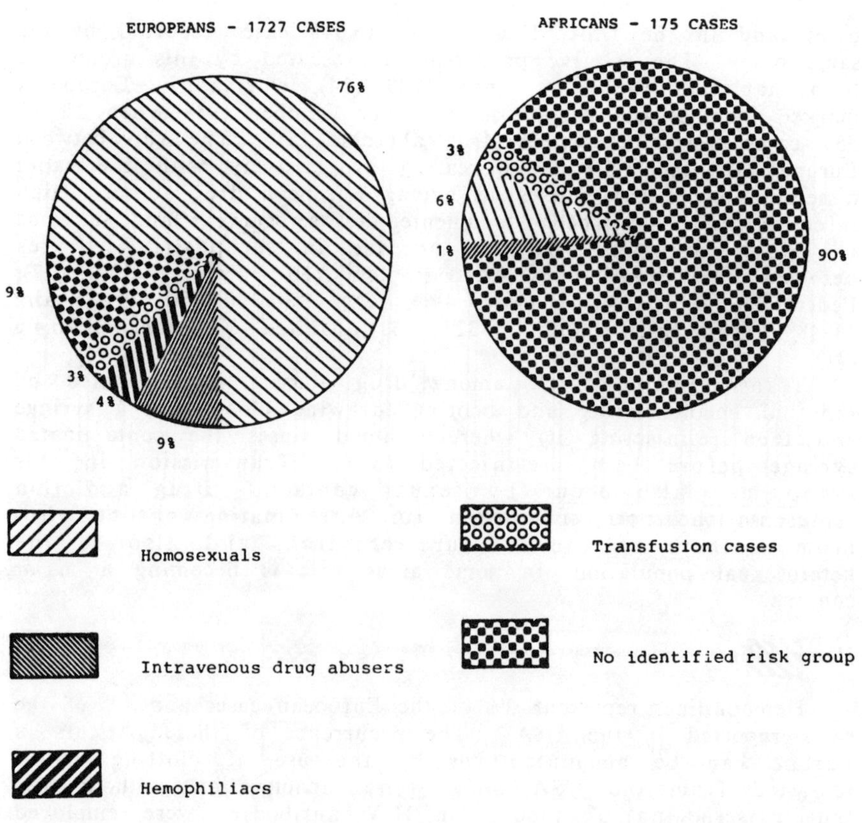

Figure 2. Comparison of risk groups of African and European cases diagnosed in Europe - December 31, 1985.

distribution may be modified significantly as the number of cases increases. Nevertheless, four distinct patterns are seen (Figure 3).

In most of the northern countries (Denmark, Finland, Netherlands, Norway, Sweden) male homosexuals account for over 80% of the total number of cases, and in some of these countries not all the risk groups are represented. On the other hand, in the countries with the greatest number of cases (Federal Republic of Germany, France, United Kingdom), homosexuals also account for the majority of cases, but all identified risk groups are found. In southern countries such as Italy and Spain, intravenous drug abusers account for a much larger fraction of cases, 43% of reported cases in each country. Finally, the proportion of patients from outside the identified risk groups is highest in Belgium and France, where many patients have originated in Africa, reflecting historical links between Africa and the two countries.

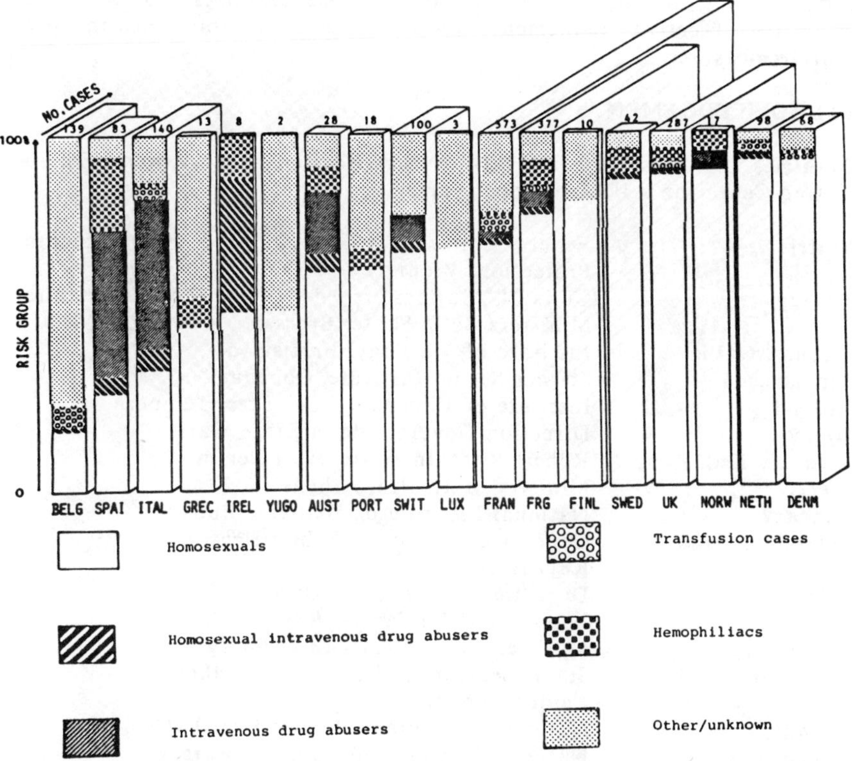

Figure 3. AIDS - Distribution of risk groups in European countries - December 31, 1985.

CONCLUSION

Given the restrictive nature of the case definition of AIDS, which identifies only those patients with the most severe clinical manifestations of the disease, the data provided here should be regarded as an indicator of the potential magnitude of the new public health problem created by the emergence and spread of HIV. Many countries are now facing an emerging epidemic. Surveillance data have evidenced significant regional epidemiologic differences in the importance of specific risk groups. Heterosexual populations are at grestest risk in central Africa and Haiti, while male homosexuals predominate in Australia, Brazil, Canada, Europe and the USA. Considerable variation in the distribution of risk groups are noted within countries in Europe. In northern European countries, most cases have been observed among homosexuals, whereas in the southern countries, such as Italy and Spain, cases have occurred mostly among intravenous drug abusers.

These observations underline the continued importance of accurate surveillance. Only through such data can an improved understanding of the spread of the disease be obtained which is vital to effective implementation of specific public health preventive measures.

ACKNOWLEDGEMENTS

Countries participating in the World Health Organization Collaborating Center on AIDS - Europe (Paris):

Austria	Federal Ministry of Health and Environmental Protection, Vienna
Belgium	Conseil Superieur de l'Hygiene Publique, Ministere de la Sante, Brussels
Czechoslovakia	Institute of Virology, Bratislava
Denmark	Statens Serum Institute, Copenhagen
Finland	Institute of Biomedical Sciences, Tampere
France	Direction Generale de la Sante, Paris
Germany Fed. Rep.	Robert Koch Institute, West Berlin
Greece	Ministry of Health, Athens
Hungary	National Institute of Hygiene, Budapest
Iceland	General Direction of Public Health, Reykjavik
Ireland	Department of Health, Dublin
Italy	Ministero della Sanita, Rome
Luxemburg	Ministere de la Sante, Luxemburg
Netherlands	Staatstoezicht op de Volksgezondheid, Leidfehendam
Norway	National Institute of Public Health, Oslo
Poland	National Institute of Hygiene, Warsaw
Portugal	Instituto Nacional de Saude, Lisbon
Spain	Ministerio de Sanidad y Consumo, Madrid
Sweden	National Bacteriological Laboratory, Stockholm
Switzerland	Office Federale de la Sante Publique, Berne
United Kingdom	Communicable Disease Surveillance Centre, London
USSR	Ministry of Public Health, Moscow
Yugoslavia	Federal Institute of Public Health, Belgrade

REFERENCES

1. CDC., Pneumocystis pneumonia - Los Angeles. MMWR 30: 250-252 (1981)

2. CDC., Kaposi's sarcoma and pneumocystis pneumonia among homosexual men - New York City and California. MMWR 30: 305-308 (1981)

3. CDC., Revision of the case definition of acquired immunodeficiency syndrome for national reporting. MMWR 34: 373-375 (1985)

4. WHO (Geneva) - May 1986 (unpublished data)

5. WHO. AIDS in the Americas - Update. Wkly Epidem Rec 61: 88 (1986)

6. Pape, J., Liautaud B., Thomas F., et al., Characteristics of the acquired immunodeficiency syndrome (AIDS) in Haiti. N Engl J Med 309: 945-950 (1983)

7. AIDS Coordination Unit, Department of Health, Sydney Australia. December 31, 1985 (unpublished)

8. Brunet, J. B., Bouvet, E., Leibowitch, J., et al., Acquired immunodeficiency syndrome in France. Lancet 1: 700-701 (1983)

9. Clumeck, N., Mascart-Lemoine, F., de Maubeuge, J., et al., Acquired immune deficiency syndrome in black Africans. Lancet 1: 642 (1983)

10. Brun-Vezinet, F., Rouzioux, C., Montagnier, L., et al., Prevalence of antibodies to lymphadenopathy-associated retrovirus in African patients with AIDS. Science 226: 453-456 (1984).

11. Lesbordes, J.L., McCormick, J.B., Beuzit, Y., et al., Aspects cliniques du SIDA en Republique Centrafricaine. Med Trop 45: 405-411 (1985)

12. Kreiss, J.K., Koech, D., Plummer, F.A., et al., AIDS virus infection in Nairobi prostitutes. N Engl J Med 314: 414-418 (1986)

13. Van de Perre, P., Rouvroy, D., Lepage, P., et al., Acquired immunodeficiency syndrome in Rwanda. Lancet 2: 62-65 (1984)

14. Van de Perre, P., Rouvroy, D., Lepage, P., et al., Female prostitutes: a risk group for infection with human T-cell lymphotropic virus type III. Lancet 2: 524-526 (1985)

15. Bayley, A.C., Dowing, R.G., Gheingson-Popov, R., et al., HTLV-III serology distinguishes atypical and endemic Kaposi's sarcoma in Africa. Lancet 1: 359-361 (1985)

16. Serwadda, D., Mugerwa, R., Sewankambo, N., et al., Slim disease: a new disease in Uganda and its association with HTLV-III infection. Lancet 2: 849-852 (1985)

17. Piot, P., Quinn, T., Taelman, H., et al., Acquired immunodeficiency syndrome in a heterosexual population in Zaire. Lancet 2: 65-69 (1984)

18. Brunet, J.B., Bouvet, E., Massari, V., Epidemiological aspects of acquired immunodeficiency syndrome in France. Ann NY Acad Sci 437: 334-339 (1984)

19. Lapointe, J., Michaud, J., Pekovic, D. et al., Transplacental transmission of HTLV-III virus. N Engl J Med 312: 1325-1326 (1985)

20. Cowan, M.J., Hellmann, D., Chudwin, D., et al., Maternal transmission of acquired immune deficiency syndrome. Pediatrics 73: 382-386 (1984)

21. Ziegler, J.B., Cooper, D.A., Johnson, R.O. et al., Postnatal transmission of AIDS-associated retrovirus from mother to infant. Lancet 1: 896-897 (1985)

22. Thiry, L., Sprecher-Goldberg, S., Jonckheer T., et al., Isolation of AIDS virus from cell-free breast milk of three healthy virus carriers. Lancet 2: 891-892 (1985)

23. Scott, G.B., Fischl, M.A., Klimas, N., et al., Mothers of infants with the acquired immunodeficiency syndrome: outcome of subsequent pregnancies. International Conference on AIDS, Atlanta, Georgia, 1985

24. CDC., Acquired Immunodeficiency syndrome - Update USA. MMWR 25: 12-23 (1986)

25. WHO., Acquired immunodeficiency syndrome - report on the situation in Europe by 15th October 1984. Wkly Epidem Rec 3: 16-19 (1985)

26. Fuchs, D., Blecha, H., Dienhardt, F., et al., High frequency of HTLV-III antibodies among heterosexual intravenous drug abusers in the Austrian Tyrol. Lancet 1: 1506 (1985)

27. Reynes, J., Quartanta, J.F., Pesce, A., et al., Prevalence elevee des anticorps anti-LAV/HTLV-III dans une population d'heroinomanes nicois. Presse Med 14: 2348-2349 (1985)

28. Gurtler, L.G., Wernicke, D., Eberle, J., Increase in prevalence of HTLV-III in haemophiliacs. Lancet 2: 1275 (1984)

29. Angarano, G., Pastore, G., Monno, L., et al., Rapid spread of HTLV-III infection among drug addicts in Italy. Lancet 2: 1302 (1985)

30. Rodrigo, J., Serra, M., Aguilar, E., et al., HTLV-III antibodies in drug addicts in Spain. Lancet 2: 156-157 (1985)

31. Mortimer, P., Vandervelde, E., Jesson, W., et al., HTLV-III antibody in Swiss and English intravenous drug abusers. Lancet 2: 449-450 (1985)

32. Des Jarlais, D., Friedman, S., Hopkins, W., Risk reduction for the acquired immunodeficiency syndrome among intravenous drug users. Ann Intern Med 103: 755-759 (1985)

33. Melbye, M., Froebel, K.S., Madhok, R., et al., HTLV-III seropositivity in European hemophiliacs exposed to factor VIII concentrate imported from the USA. Lancet 2: 1444-1446 (1984)

34. Rouzioux, C., Brun-Vezinet, F., Courouce, A.M., et al., Immunoglobulin G antibodies to lymphadenopathy - associated virus in differently treated French and Belgian hemophiliacs. Ann Intern Med 102: 476-479 (1985)

35. Biggar, R.J., Melbye, M., Kestens, L., et al., Seroepidemiology of HTLV-III antibodies in a remote population of eastern Zaire. Br Med J 290: 808-810 (1985)

36. Lamey, B., Melameka, N., Aspects Cliniques et epidemiologiques de la cryptococcose a Kinshasa. Med Trop 42: 507-511 (1982)

37. Mann, J., Francis, H., Kapita, B.M., Household transmission of HTLV-III in Zaire. International Conference on AIDS, Atlanta, April 1985

8
AIDS in Subsaharan Africa

Robert J. Biggar, Gerard Agius

The acquired immunodeficiency syndrome (AIDS) is now widely recognized to be an important public health problem in many parts of central and eastern Africa (1),(2). However, almost all areas outside of this AIDS epidemic zone have also already observed AIDS cases, suggesting that human immunodeficiency virus (HIV), the causative agent, has penetrated widely throughout the continent. If the epidemic continues unabated, this problem threatens to have grave repercussions both for the health care system and for the future development of nations in this region. It is therefore important to share the current status of knowledge about the AIDS problem in Africa, especially since many recent studies have added significantly to information on this topic. This chapter will focus only on HIV and not other related retroviruses that have recently been described as co-existing in this region. The impact of these other viruses on health is still under exploration, but so far, appears to be minor compared to that of HIV.

RECOGNITION OF THE PROBLEM

In 1980/81, physicians in Belgium and France observed a puzzling increase in the number of patients referred for medical problems from Zaire, Rwanda and other countries, who had unusual opportunistic infections such as cryptococcosis (3)-(5). When AIDS was reported in the United States in June 1981, the clinical similarities between the patients from Africa and those being described in the United States at that time (6)-(8) became apparent.

Although the African patients were found to have immunodeficiency problems of a type typically seen in AIDS patients (9), some researchers remained skeptical that the African disease had the same etiology, in part because the epidemiologic profile was different. Whereas almost all American and European cases were males, the African cases were appearing in women almost as frequently as men (3)-(5). Nevertheless, by 1983 the WHO Conference on AIDS in Europe recorded a remarkable surge of cases fitting the AIDS definition among Africans being evaluated in Europe (10). Investigators in Africa were able to confirm that a similar epidemic of diseases associated with immunosuppression was occurring in Kinshasa, Zaire (1983) (11) and Kigali, Rwanda (1984) (12). When HIV [then called human T-lymphotropic virus III (HTLV-III) or lymphadenopathy-associated virus (LAV)] was determined to be the causative agent of AIDS in early 1984, analysis of the African sera definitively showed that the causative agent for the parallel epidemics was the same virus (13), (14).

Lack of documentation has prohibited accurate assessment of when AIDS emerged in Africa as a clinical problem. From records of selected diseases in the Kinshasa area, both cryptococcosis and Kaposi's sarcoma began to increase in frequency in 1978/79 (11). However, other areas have not been studied. Furthermore, neither of these disorders provide a very sensitive indicator of AIDS, since AIDS has many other manifestations among Africans and, relative to elsewhere, there is a high background rate for both diseases in central Africa. Cases of AIDS-like illness among Europeans who had lived in Africa in 1976/77 have been reported (15),(16), although in one instance, evaluation of sera remaining from the subject showed no trace of antibody to HIV (personal communication, M. Melbye), casting doubt about the relationship of this case to AIDS. Thus, the earliest appearance of the AIDS epidemic that has been clinically documented in Africa is 1978/79, approximately the same time that AIDS appeared in the United States and Europe (17). However, the data from Africa in this regard must be regarded as very weak.

With the availability of tests for HIV antibody, it has now been possible to undertake retrospective studies of sera stored from earlier studies of the African population. Even here, data are not clearcut. Early studies based upon prototype tests for antibody to HIV had unexpected problems with reactivity and could not be confirmed later by more specific tests (1). Thus, some reports suggesting either a widespread or a high prevalence of antibody against HIV in sera from historic collections dating to the early 1970's were clearly in error (17a). With methodologic refinements, the specificity of the tests for HIV antibodies in African sera greatly improved.

Certainly, in all recent studies, HIV seropositivity in Africa prior to the mid 1970's was rare. The earliest sample considered unequivocally positive is a single sample from among several hundred Zairian persons bled in 1959 (18). In a study of mothers attending antenatal clinics in Kinshasa, Zaire, 0.25%

(2/805 sera) of the attendees were seropositive for HIV antibodies in 1970. By 1980, mothers at the same clinics had a 3.1% (15/489) prevalence, and by 1986, 5.7% (30/529) were seropositive (19). With a prevalence of 0.25% in 1970 (at least in this population), attempts to detect HIV infection further back in time will require huge studies. However, it may be useful to look in historic collections of sera from other areas of central Africa, since HIV infection may well have appeared elsewhere earlier than it appeared in Kinshasa.

The data to trace the spread of HIV infection within Africa are limited. Despite this, it is possible to document that the earliest place recording an epidemic increase in cases was Kinshasa, Zaire in 1978/79 (11). By 1982, a similar increase of aggressive Kaposi's sarcoma was noted in Lusaka, Zambia (20). When first sought in Rwanda in 1984, AIDS cases had already been seen (12), although in the opinion of the local doctors, they had not been common much earlier (personal data). The epidemic in Uganda stands out as an exception to most of the other areas, in that rural areas in the south of the country adjacent to Rwanda and Tanzania were affected as much as, or more than urban areas (Table 1) (21). The disrupted social order in the population of this area, which had been subjected to both protracted civil war and an invasion in the recent past, contributed to spread in this region. It was soon apparent that the area in Tanzania adjacent to Uganda also had a similar epidemic problem (22). Currently, at least one or more cases of AIDS have been found in most of the countries of Africa, but only in parts of the central and eastern areas of Africa is the incidence high.

Female prostitutes probably serve as a major contributor to the spread of HIV infection in subsaharan Africa. They are at high risk of becoming infected and travel widely. In Nairobi, Kenya, a relatively low prevalence area for HIV infection, almost all of the prostitutes first found to be seropositive were from Tanzania (23). The role of prostitutes in spreading HIV infection throughout the continent was further demonstrated by a report from Ghana, a country of West Africa with little AIDS. Of the first 72 seropositive persons, 63 (88%) were female, and 57 (90%) of these had been prostitutes that practiced their profession in other countries of Africa. In contrast, only one (1%) of 98 prostitutes who worked exclusively in Ghana was seropositive (24).

These studies raise questions about the origin of AIDS. African serum samples are the earliest samples known to be positive for HIV antibodies from anywhere in the world, which suggests that AIDS might have emerged in Africa. Additionally, Africa appears to harbor a number of other human retroviruses, raising the possibility that HIV is a mutant of one of these or a recombinant of several of them. Most of these viruses are still under investigation and their distribution and historical prevalence remain obscure.

Table 1. Prevalence of HIV Seropositivity in Selected Populations of Ugandan Adults (Blood Obtained 1985/86)

Group	Pos./tested	(%)
Health urban residents (Kampala)		
Bantu	110/716	(15.4%)
West Nile Nilotic people	7/43	(16.3%)
Hospital employees	41/410	(10.0%)
Healthy older persons not sexually active for five years	0/96	(0.0%)
AIDS patients in the rural Southeast	40/40	(100.0%)
Controls from rural Southeast	5/30	(17.0%)
Healthy rural residents West Nile district	1/77	(1.3%)
Traders from Tanzania	10/15	(66.7%)

Data derived from references 17a and 50.

SEROLOGIC CONSIDERATIONS

Researchers familiar with the pitfalls of working with sera from African patients have long been aware that it sometimes has a 'stickiness' rarely encountered in sera from American or European persons. The cause of this 'stickiness' is not well understood, but it has caused difficulties with many commonly used testing procedures, including the enzyme-linked immunosorbent assays and immunofluorescent tests, that served as the principal screening techniques for HIV antibodies. In the early tests for HIV antibody, these 'false positive' reactions from Africa were read as positive in part because confirmation tests with prototype Western blots yielded faintly reactive bands at appropriate sites. Initially, there was no experience to caution investigators that such reactions did not reflect true HIV antibody since they were not observed among Americans and Europeans and since it was plausible that Africans could be seropositive at low titer because of infection many years earlier. These hypotheses were soon shown to be in error by improvements in testing that distinguished between 'stickiness' and true positivity for HIV antibody.

With respect to African serology, it is noteworthy that malaria and no doubt other parasitic infections induce production of many of those factors which may contribute to 'stickiness', such as autoantibodies, immune complexes and high immunoglobulin levels (25). It is not a specific cross-reactivity with malaria which caused the problem. Results of studies based on these early prototype assays provided a misrepresentation of the distribution of HIV virus in the population, with especially high rates appearing in areas where parasitic diseases such as malaria were endemic in the population (25),(26).

Current commercially available tests now provide quite reliable evidence of the presence or absence of specific antibody against HIV. The major technical reservation is that new retroviruses continue to appear in Africa, and cross-reactivities to known and yet to be discovered viruses remain to be explored. The ability to establish definitive proof of antibody presence will not resolve a remaining problem, however, that of human error in testing, which is the largest cause of discrepancy between tests in our experience. Using modern test systems with good specificity, a large number of studies published in 1986 have provided an accurate description of HIV infection and hold the potential for blood screening and diagnostic services, if they can be widely applied in Africa. In some areas, lack of equipment and trained personnel capable of doing the somewhat complex procedures involved in these tests has contributed to limiting their current usefulness. However, the major drawback to practical implementation of these tests has been their cost, which is about $2 for each screening test in most assays and about ten times that for a confirmatory Western blot. In areas where the per capital health expenditure may be less than $10, that cost is prohibitive for practical use. Efforts currently in progress hold promise that an economical and effective field test may soon be available for use in Africa (27).

THE EPIDEMIOLOGY OF HIV AND AIDS

The observation that the sex ratio of African AIDS cases was nearly equal provided an early clue to the later finding that HIV in Africa was transmitted heterosexually in the great majority of cases. Much evidence now supports this contention. Studies in Zaire reported person-to-person chains of transmission in which males and females alternated (11). Early studies in Rwanda (28),(29) and later ones in Nairobi (23) concluded that prostitutes and men who frequented prostitutes were risk groups, and the prevalence among persons attending venereal disease clinics was markedly higher than that among the general public (Table 2) (23),(30). Among healthy subjects, such as blood donors, the prevalence was highest in the age-groups with greatest sexual activity, peaking in the early 30's for men and the late 20's for women (Figure 1) (2),(30). Among families, spouses but not other

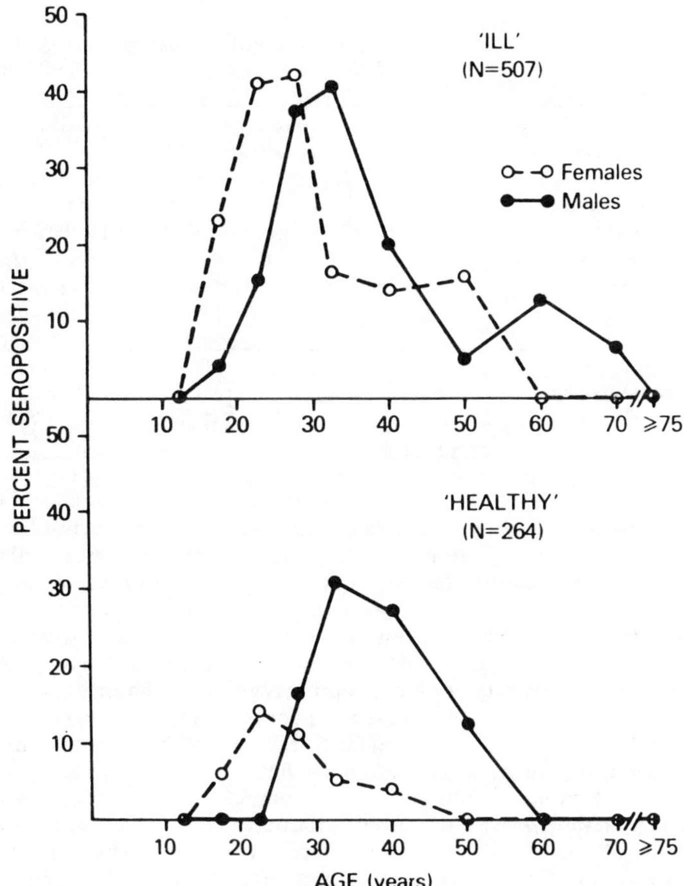

Figure 1. Seroprevalence of HIV antibody among healthy and 'ill' adults living in Lusaka, Zambia (blood obtained 1985).

Healthy- blood donors, antenatal clinic patients and hospital employees.

Ill- - - persons hospitalized for any reason or attending outpatient clinics (except antenatal clinics).

Table 2. Prevalence of HIV-Antibodies in Sexually Active Populations of Nairobi, Kenya.

Group	Year Studied 1980	1983/84	1985/86
Female prostitutes	5/116 (4%)	66/130 (51%)	126/215 (59%)
Men attending veneral disease clinics	2/118 (2%)	13/93 (14%)	19/107 (18%)
Pregnant women	0/111 (0%)	N.A.	15/735 (2%)

N.A. = Not available
Data from reference 23.

family members of seropositive subjects were much more likely to be positive than the general public (31). All of these observations support the importance of heterosexual transmission of HIV in Africa.

Venereal diseases have been a major problem in Africa (32), and HIV is no exception. Whether the actual presence of venereal disease or other aspects of personal hygiene enhance the possibility of infection between sexual partners (1) is unknown, but certainly HIV is transmitted effectively in the absence of any such condition. Groups with frequent heterosexual exposure are at greatest risk. Similar, although less compelling evidence of heterosexual transmission has now documented that heterosexual transmission of HIV occurs in all populations of the world. The risk of infection per exposure has not yet been determined. Given the high prevalence of HIV among sexually active persons of both sexes in Africa, it is unlikely to be very low. The almost equal prevalence of HIV among women and men in Africa could be construed to argue that infectivity is amost equally likely in both directions, but it is probable that men have a greater number of different sexual partners than women (and therefore greater exposure), and the equal sex ratio may be because male-to-female transmission is more efficient than female-to-male transmission.

While HIV infection may be a heterosexually transmitted venereal disease, other routes of infection are also possible, potentially escalating the number of cases as the prevalence in the population increases. In particular, blood donors in Africa, as elsewhere, are predominantly young adults, the group at highest risk of being seropositive. In areas where HIV infection is epidemic, as many as 5 to 20 percent of donors (usually male) are seropositive (30),(33),(34). From studies in the United States, blood from such donors is highly likely to transmit HIV infection (35),(36). Through this means, HIV infection has spread to groups otherwise at low risk of infection in Africa, particularly children and older adults (37),(38). In Africa, anemia from malaria or sickle cell disease has been a frequent indication for transfusion in childhood, and about one-third of seropositive children whose mothers are seronegative will have a history of transfusion in the relatively recent past (compared to only seven percent of seronegative children) (Table 3) (38a).

Table 3. Comparison of Potential Risk Factors for Adult AIDS Cases and Children Who Were Seropositive for HIV Antibody In Kinshasa, Zaire (1985/86)

Risk Factor	Adult AIDS Cases		Children HIV pos.	
	Male (141)*	Female (154)	2-14** (40)	0-2** (16)***
Foreign travel	19%	19%	--	--
AIDS-like case in household	4%	7%	--	--
AIDS-like illness in acquaintance	7%	11%	--	--
Previous venereal disease episode	35%	28%	--	--
Visit to healer/acupuncturist	14%	25%	0%	6%
Scarifications	21%	20%	25%	6%
Previous hospitalization	32%	41%	52%	50%
Operations	14%	11%	8%	60%
Medical injections (in past year)	78%	81%	95%	N.A.
Blood transfusions	4%	14%	60%	31%

* In parenthesis, the number of subjects studied.

** Age in years.

*** Data for seropositive infants with seronegative mothers only. However, 50% of seropositive infants had seropositive mothers.

NA = Not available.

Data derived from references 38, 38a, 60.

It is apparent that any group at risk of being transfused, such as peripartum women or trauma patients, are at increased risk of being exposed to HIV in proportion to the prevalence of the virus in the donor pool. However, in addition to the usual medically recognized indications for transfusion, in some areas of Africa, doctors have adopted the practice of giving small amounts of blood as 'tonic' for fatigue, depression, and other vague symptoms. Such practices, of questionable medical value, will contribute to the spread of HIV infection into other groups otherwise at low risk of being infected, such as older persons.

In the absence of a reliable, practical, and economical screening procedure to eliminate HIV-infected blood, the risks of transfusion must be weighed carefully against the need for blood. In addition, sources of donors for transfusion services need to be reviewed, because some groups may be especially likely to contribute HIV-infected blood, such as prisoners and perhaps military men. Without specific studies, it may be difficult to predict in advance which groups will be more likely to be seropositive.

Pregnancy will result in exposure of unborn children to HIV infection among seropositive mothers, and the high prevalence of HIV infection in young adult women [up to 10% of antenatal clinic attendees in some hospitals (30)] makes this a potentially serious public health problem in many urban areas. Studies to quantitate the risk of vertical transmission are underway. In women with AIDS or evidence of immunosuppression or who have previously had an infant who developed AIDS, the risk of AIDS in the infant may be as high as 50% (39),(40). It is also unclear when during pregancy or delivery infection takes place most commonly. Infection following delivery appears to be rare but can occur, as documented by an Australian case in which a mother seroconverted as a result of an infected transfusion given just after the delivery of her infant, but the infant nevertheless became infected, possibly through breast milk (41). HIV has been isolated from breast milk (42), although oral transmission of HIV infection is certainly very rare and probably only occurs under unusual conditions (43). Infants who become infected with HIV appear to have an accelerated progression to AIDS, the average time to AIDS being about 14 months compared to several years among adults (44). In Africa, there has been some suggestion that infants may also get HIV infection through contaminated needles, since the average number of injections given to seropositive infants of seronegative mothers was twice that given to seronegative infants of seronegative mothers (38a). However, in another study of seropositive children of seronegative mothers in Africa, no relationship was found with needle exposure (37).

Other practices have not yet emerged as major contributors to the magnitude of the HIV and AIDS problem in Africa, although there is reason for concern. In particular, shortages of needles and other medical equipment in many areas of Africa lead to reuse, often with minimal cleaning and no proper sterilization. This occurs both within the medical setting and through the practices of 'street healers' and persons doing tattooing for ritual or cosmetic reasons. In America, the actual risk from exposure to an infected needle is low, perhaps one transmission per thousand inadvertent punctures among health care workers (45). But the extent of exposure in Africa and the probability that such exposures result in a greater average contamination (because they are associated with pushing the inoculum through the unsterile needle) may cause this to be a more important problem among African patients exposed to contaminated needles. Efforts to promote good medical practices with respect to needle and equipment use and sterilization should be expanded, and staff need to be warned to be careful about accidental exposure themselves.

Among the possible causes of spread, the prospect of spread of HIV through insect vectors has raised considerable alarm. However, there is no evidence that insects transmit HIV infection, and certainly, if they ever do, this route of transmission is not a major contributor to the scope of the epidemic currently (1),(46). Evidence suggesting the possibility of insect-vectored transmission is that HIV has been demonstrated in the juices of bedbugs (but not mosquitos) freshly fed blood meals from an infected source (47). Evidence that this is not an important contributor relies on epidemiology. The pattern of HIV infection shows that the groups infected are those with venereal or blood exposure. Were insects to be an important source of HIV infection, the groups infected would include those with heavy exposure to them, such as children and the elderly in the same household, rural residents, and those with field occupations. These groups are relatively less infected than urban office workers of the upper and middle classes. However, such evidence does not eliminate the possibility that HIV infection could occasionally be transmitted through an insect vector.

Given the pattern of heterosexual transmission, it is now possible to construct a profile of the groups at highest risk of HIV infection in Africa, including prostitutes and those exposed to prostitutes or other very promiscuous persons. These are, in fact, the groups with the highest prevalence. In some areas of central African cities, the majority of prostitutes are seropositive (23),(28). Factors that affect access to or interest in promiscuous sexual activity will dominate the distribution of HIV. Thus, urban populations in which social mores are more relaxed (compared to village lifestyles) have a much higher prevalence of HIV infection. The affluent, educated and powerful persons are also more likely to be seropositive than the lower social classes (30). Military men and others who travel frequently should also be at greater risk, as is evident in the frequency of venereal diseases among these groups.

CLINICAL FEATURES OF AIDS IN AFRICA

African patients with HIV infection have developed virtually the entire spectrum of outcomes seen in Americans and Europeans with HIV infection (48). Following infection, seroconversion occurs probably within six to 12 weeks, sometimes associated with a flu-like illness (49). In the great majority, infection is probably a silent event or so non-specific and minimal in symptoms that it is not recognized. From careful prospective studies, particularly in Australia, some seroconverting persons are known to have a mild mononucleosis-like syndrome, including pharyngitis and fever (50). On blood examination, a small proportion of atypical lymphocytes may be found. Among Africans, seroconversion usually goes unnoticed. However, in one instance, a severe life-threatening encephalopathy occurred along with the more typical symptoms (51).

As among other populations, infection in Africans frequently provokes lymphadenopathy that is persistent and may cause concern for the patient or the doctor. Among healthy persons found to have mild lymphadenopathy in Zambia, HIV seropositivity was three-fold more frequent than among those without it (unpublished data). But the more severe cases will often be referred for biopsy to exclude hematologic malignancies, and among 14 patients referred to one tumor clinic for surgical evaluation of pronounced generalized lymphadenopathy 12 (86%) were seropositive (unpublished data). On biopsy, only non-specific hyperplasia is found in the HIV-associated cases (52). If further examined, such persons usually already have evidence of immunodeficiency, with low helper T-cell numbers being the predominant problem (unpublished data). In our studies, suppressor T-cell numbers tended to be somewhat higher in Africans than in Americans and Europeans, both in HIV-infected and non-infected persons.

With the immunodeficiency comes risk of lesser AIDS manifestations (Table 4) and of the frank opportunistic infections and Kaposi's sarcoma that constitute AIDS. The risk of developing AIDS among Africans who are HIV-infected has been little studied. Among a small group of subjects, only one percent of seropositive persons became AIDS cases in the first year of follow-up (53). However, we know that among seropositive American adults the risk of AIDS is nearly zero in the first two years after infection but probably closer to four to five percent per year thereafter (54). The actual types of infection that afflict HIV-infected Africans may be different, at least in distributional frequency, than occur among immunosuppressed patients in America and Europe because of the different range of potential pathogens that exist in Africa (48). Thus, cryptococcosis, tuberculosis due to *Mycobacterium tuberculosis*, and cryptosporidial diarrhea may be more common in Africans. *Pneumocystis carinii* pneumonia and cytomegalovirus infection appear to be somewhat less common, although this may be partly a function of difficulties in diagnosis. Some illnesses have not emerged as problems despite concerns that they might do so, including malaria and other parasitic diseases. This may be partly because HIV-infection is predominantly an urban problem so far, whereas malaria occurs predominantly in rural areas.

Among cancers, Kaposi's sarcoma is well known to be associated with HIV-induced immunodeficiency among Americans and Europeans. It is also a cancer that has long been endemic in parts of eastern and central Africa, particularly the Rift Valley areas

Table 4. Association Between HIV Seropositivity and Clinical Disorders Other Than Frank AIDS in Adult Patients in Lusaka, Zambia (1985)

Clinical Disorder	Pos./tested	(%)
Herpes zoster	4/5	(80%)
Oral thrush	6/12	(50%)
Diarrhea	23/88	(26%)
Tuberculosis	17/71	(24%)
Weight loss	45/230	(20%)
Fever	31/182	(17%)
Neurological problems	3/32	(9%)
Other problems	7/63	(11%)

Data derived from reference 30.

(1). This endemic form of African Kaposi's sarcoma is histologically similar to that of AIDS-associated Kaposi's sarcoma. However, the clinical course of the endemic form is generally different, being a slowly progressive, nodular disease of the distal extremities, whereas the HIV-associated form is a rapidly progressive, plaque-forming disease that affects the trunk/face and internal organs. The endemic form of Kaposi's in African is not HIV- (55) or immunodeficiency-related (56), but the typical AIDS-related form does occur among African AIDS patients and is associated with HIV infection (57) and immunodeficiency (58). Other malignancies such as B-cell lymphomas are recognized to be associated with immunosuppression due to HIV-infection in Americans (59). So far, these have not been noted to be a problem among Africans, although no systematic study has been undertaken.

For monitoring the epidemic, public health authorities in the United States and elsewhere have found it useful to compose a 'surveillance' definition of AIDS. The variation in the clinical spectrum of AIDS among Africans is less a problem than the lack of adequate facilities for definitive diagnosis of either HIV-induced immunodeficiency or of the subsequent illnesses to which these immunosuppressed persons are prey. We suggest the definition provided in Table 5, which is derived from, but not identical to that offered by Mann et al. (60). Even with such a definition, however, it is important for clinicians dealing with African patients to recognize that not all illnesses in seropositive subjects are related to AIDS or immunosuppression. In some areas, a large number of seropositive subjects will be relatively recently infected and not (as yet) immunosuppressed. Thus, many patients will have illnesses that respond normally to conventional and available therapies. Even in those with advanced immunodeficiencies associated with HIV infection, much can be done to promote recovery and ease pain and discomfort, despite an ominous prognosis.

Table 5. AIDS Definition Proposed for Use in Africa

For surveillance purposes, a case must have:

1. Absence of conditions that explain the patient's clinical or immunological status

2. At least one of three clinical criteria:

    a. A syndrome of profound weight loss (>10 percent of normal body weight) and either chronic diarrhea for at least two months or chronic/recurrent fever for at least one month and no other cause for these symptoms.

    b. An opportunistic infection included in the Centers for Disease Control definition of AIDS and/or disseminated Kaposi's sarcoma with internal invasion.

    c. Confirmed HIV-induced immunosuppression and life-threatening illnesses other than those recognized by the Centers for Disease Control

To be confirmed, a case must have:

1. HIV antibodies present;

2. Immunodeficiency measured by T-subset analysis indicating a depletion of T-helper cells.

Definition modified from reference 60.

FUTURE PROSPECTS

The epidemic in Africa threatens to be a public health disaster affecting not only the personal well being of the individuals but also the development of the region. According to some authorities, there may be several million persons already infected with the virus (2). We feel this number may overestimate the situation because HIV infection has been mainly studied in the high-prevalence urban areas, whereas the bulk of the population lives in the rural areas which have a substantially lower HIV-prevalence. Nevertheless, it is already a large and rapidly growing problem that will dominate the health concerns of countries in these areas for the rest of this century and well into the next, even in the most optimistic of projections.

There is an additional burden that goes beyond health care. The groups most at risk are those on whom these countries depend for the next generation of leaders, the urban educated elite. Assuming that infection in Africa has the same implications as infection in America and Europe, many of these will be lost just as they are coming to their peak productivity. The results could have a devastating impact on development.

Where HIV infection is already epidemic, epidemiology provides clues as to means for interdicting the spread of this infection. It must be recognized, however, that other venereal diseases have been difficult to combat in Africa, even when an effective cure is known and the duration of infectivity is relatively short. In HIV infection, no cure is known and infectivity may continue, at least intermittently, for life. Prevention is therefore paramount, and education to inform the general population of the routes of spread and measures to prevent exposure are essential. The problem of blood exposure is potentially solvable with widespread use of screening programs, but no method is yet known to prevent maternal-infant transmission, and AIDS is likely to be an increasingly important problem in pediatric clinics in the near future.

Where HIV infection has not yet been introduced or is only rarely present, the success of surveillance and education programs may be even greater. Populations where HIV will be first detected include venereal disease clinic attendees and groups with frequent heterosexual exposures such as prostitutes. Efforts to warn the local populace, particularly those who travel, of the transmission routes and means to protect themselves from infection, such as rigorous attention to condom use (61), should be even more effective in preventing introduction of infection than in reducing spread once HIV has been introduced. When seropositive persons are identified, all efforts should be made to educate them about the danger they may pose to their community through sexual activity or blood donations. In the event a prostitute is found, re-employment in a non-risk occupation will repay the effort many times over. Thus, countries that currently have minimal problems with AIDS cannot be complacent about their present good fortune.

The difficulties of managing HIV and AIDS in Africa must be handled by African authorities in ways which will vary according to local need and custom. However, outside help will be essential. Technically, there is a need for rapid, economical, and simple screening tests which are appropriate to use in the African context (27). The discovery of new, related human retroviruses such as LAV-2 and HTLV-IV will complicate this problem and force consideration of the yet unexplored ways in which these new agents will interact with HIV or cause illnesses by themselves. At this point, however, HIV is the major threat, and it is against this threat that technology must be mobilized. Both effective and affordable therapies and a practical vaccine will be essential for controlling HIV in Africa. Unfortunately, neither exists. In the meantime, interim measures such as behavior modification concentrating on reducing the number of partners and promoting the use of condoms or other anti-viral contraceptive measures will help, although obviously only sexual acts between uninfected persons can be considered truly safe. In addition, blood screening is a necessity for areas in which HIV is epidemic. Education to reinforce good medical practice in the use and re-use of equipment and to reduce the practice of 'street healers' will also be desirable.

Despite all of these, AIDS will continue to dominate the health and development of this area into the foreseeable future.

REFERENCES

1. Biggar, R.J., The AIDS problem in Africa. Lancet 1:79-83 (1986)

2. Quinn, T.C., Mann, J.M., Curran, J.W., et al., AIDS in Africa: an epidemiologic paradigm. Science 234:955-963 (1986)

3. Clumeck, N., Mascart-Lemone, F., de Maulbeuge, J., et al., Acquired immune deficiency syndrome in black Africans. Lancet 1:642 (1983)

4. Sonnet, J., De Bruyere, M., Syndrome de deficit acquis de l' immunite --acquired immunodeficiency syndrome (AIDS): etat de la question. Donnees personnelles de la pathologie observee chez des Zairois. Louvain Med 102:297-307 (1983)

5. Brunet, J.B., Bouvet, E., Chaperon, J., et al., Acquired immunodeficiency syndrome in France. Lancet 1:700-701 (1983)

6. Gottlieb, M.S., Schroff, R., Schanker, H.M., et al., *Pneumocystis carinii* pneumonia and mucosal candidiasis in previously healthy homosexual men: evidence of a new acquired cellular immunodeficiency. N Engl J Med 305:1425-1431 (1981)

7. Masur, H., Michelis, M.A., Greene, J.B., et al., An outbreak of community-acquired *Pneumocystis carinii* pneumonia: initial manifestation of cellular immune dysfunction. N Engl J Med 305:1431-1438 (1981)

8. Hymes, K.B., Cheung, T., Greene, J.B., et al., Kaposi's sarcoma in homosexual men: a report of eight cases. Lancet 2: 598-600 (1981)

9. Clumeck, N., Sonnet, J., Taelman, H., et al., Acquired immune deficiency syndrome in African patients. N Engl J Med 310:492-497 (1984)

10. Biggar, R.J., Bouvet, E., Ebbesen, P., et al., Epidemiology of AIDS in Europe. Eur J Cancer Clin Oncol 20:165-167 (1984)

11. Piot, P., Quinn, T.C., Taelman, H., et al., Acquired immunodeficiency syndrome in a heterosexual population in Zaire. Lancet 2:65-69 (1984)

12. Perre, P., Rouvroy, D., Lepage, P., et al., Acquired immunodeficiency syndrome in Rwanda. Lancet 2: 62-65 (1984)

13. Ellrodt, A., Barre-Sinoussi, F., Le Bras, Ph., et al., Isolation of human T-lymphotropic retrovirus (LAV) from Zairian married couple, one with AIDS, one with prodromes. Lancet 1:1383-1385 (1984)

14. Brun-Vezinet, F., Rouxioux, C., Montagnier, L., et al., Prevalence of antibodies to lymphadenopathy-associated retrovirus in African patients with AIDS. Science 226:453-456 (1985)

15. Bygbjerg, I.C., AIDS in a Danish surgeon (Zaire, 1976). Lancet 1:925 (1983)

16. Vandepitte, J., Verwilghen, R., Zachee, P., AIDS and cryptococcosis (Zaire, 1977). Lancet 1:925-926 (1983)

17. Melbye, M., Biggar, R.J., Ebbesen, P., Epidemiology--Europe and Africa. In: AIDS, A Guide to Clinicians. (Ebbesen, P., Biggar, R.J., Melbye, M., eds). Munksgaard/Saunders, Copenhagen, 29-41 (1985)

17a. Carswell, J.W., Sewankambo, N., Lloyd, G., et al., How long has the AIDS virus been in Uganda? Lancet 1:1217 (1986)

18. Nahmias, A.J., Weiss, J., Yao, X., et al., Evidence of human infection with an HTLV-III/LAV-like virus in central Africa, 1959. Lancet 1:1279-1280 (1986)

19. Desmyter, J., Goubau, P., Chamaret, S., et al., Anti-LAV/HTLV-III in Kinshasa mothers in 1970 and 1980. International Conference on Acquired Immunodeficiency Syndrome (AIDS), Paris, June (1986)

20. Bayley, A.C., Aggressive Kaposi's sarcoma in Zambia (1983) Lancet 1:1318-1320 (1984)

21. Serwadda, D., Mugerwa, R.D., Sewankambo, N.K., et al., Slim disease: a new disease in Uganda and its association with HTLV-III infection. Lancet 2:849-852 (1985)

22. Forthal, D.N., Mhalu, F.S., Dahoma, A., et al., AIDS in Tanzania. International Conference on Acquired Immunodeficiency Syndrome (AIDS), Paris, June (1986)

23. Kreiss, J.K., Koech, D., Plummer, F.A., et al., AIDS virus infection in Nairobi prostitutes: spread of the epidemic in East Africa. N Engl J Med 314:414-418 (1986)

24. Neequaye, A.R., Neequaye, J., Mingle, J.A., et al., Preponderance of females with AIDS in Ghana. Lancet 2:978 (1986)

25. Biggar, R.J., Gigase, P.L., Melbye, M., et al., ELISA HTLV retrovirus antibody reactivity associated with malaria and immune complexes in healthy Africans. Lancet 2:520-523 (1985)

26. Biggar, R.J., Possible nonspecific associations between malaria and HTLV-III/LAV. N Engl J Med 315:457-458 (1986)

27. Carlson, J.R., Martens, S.C., Yee, J.L., et al., A rapid, easy and economical screening assay for antibodies to the human immunodeficiency virus. Lancet 1:361-362 (1987)

28. Van de Perre, P., Clumeck, N., Carael, M., et al., Female prostitutes: A risk group for infection with human T-cell lymphotropic virus type III. Lancet 2:524-527 (1985)

29. Clumeck, N., Van de Perre, P., Carael, M., et al., Heterosexual promiscuity among African patients with AIDS. N Engl J Med 313:182 (1985)

30. Melbye, M., Njelesani, E.K., Bayley, A., et al., Evidence for heterosexual transmission and clinical manifestations of human immunodeficiency virus infection and related conditions in Lusaka, Zambia. Lancet 2:1113-1115 (1986)

31. Mann, J.M., Quinn, T.C., Francis, H., et al., Prevalence of HTLV-III/LAV in household contacts of patients with confirmed AIDS and controls in Kinshasa, Zaire. JAMA 256:721-724 (1986)

32. Rosenbert, M.J., Schult, K.F., Burton, N., Sexually transmitted diseases in sub-Saharan Africa. Lancet 2:152 (1986)

33. Van de Perre, P., Munyambuga, D., Zissis, G., et al., Antibody to HTLV-III in blood donors in Central Africa. Lancet 1:336-337 (1985)

34. Mann, J.M., Francis, H., Quinn, T.C., et al., Role of blood transfusions in transmission of HTLV-III infection in Zaire. Am J Epidem (In press)

35. Feorino, P.M., Jaffe, H.W., Palmer, E., et al., Transfusion-associated acquired immunodeficiency syndrome. Evidence for persistent infection in blood donors. N Engl J Med 312: 1293-1296 (1985)

36. Jaffe, H.W., Sarngadharan, M.G., DeVico, A.L., et al., Infection with HTLV-III/LAV and transfusion associated acquired immunodeficiency syndrome. JAMA 254:770-773 (1985)

37. Lepage, P., Van de Perre, P., Carael, M., et al., Are medical injections a risk factor for HIV infection in children? Lancet 2:1103-1104 (1986)

38. Mann, J.M., Francis, H., Davachi, F., et al., HTLV-III/LAV seroprevalence in pediatric inpatients 2-14 years old in Kinshasa, Zaire. Pediatrics 78:673-677 (1986)

38a. Mann, J.M., Francis, H., Davachi, F., et al., Risk factors of human immunodeficiency virus seropositivity among children 1-24 months old in Kinshasa, Zaire. Lancet 2:654-656 (1986)

39. Cowan, M.J., Hellman, D., Chudwin, D., et al., Maternal transmission of acquired immune deficiency syndrome. Pediatrics 73:382-386 (1984)

40. CDC., Recommendations for assisting in the prevention of perinatal transmission of human T-lymphotropic virus type III/Lymphadenopathy-associated virus and acquired immunodeficiency syndrome. MMWR 34:721-732 (1985)

41. Ziegler, J.B., Cooper, D.A., Johnson, R.O., et al., Postnatal transmission of AIDS-associated retrovirus from mother to infant. Lancet 1:896-898 (1985)

42. Thiry, L., Sprecher-Goldberger, S., Jonckheer, T., et al., Isolation of AIDS virus from cell-free breast milk of three healthy virus carriers. Lancet 2:891-892 (1985)

43. Biggar, R.J., The epidemiology of the human retroviruses and related clinical conditions. In AIDS: Modern Concepts and Therapeutic Challenges. (Broder, S., ed), Marcel Dekker, Inc., New York, p 91-121 (1986)

44. Scott, G.B., Fischl, M.A., Klimas, N., et al., Mothers of infants with the acquired immunodeficiency syndrome. Evidence for both symptomatic and asymptomatic carriers. JAMA 253:363-366 (1985)

45. Weiss, S.H., Biggar, R.J., The epidemiology of human retrovirus-associated illnesses. Mt. Sinai J Med 53:579-591 (1986)

46. Zuckerman, A.J., AIDS and insects. Br Med J 292:1094-1095 (1986)

47. Lyons, S.F., Jupp, P.G., Schoub, B.D., Survival of HIV in the common bedbug. Lancet 2:45 (1986)

48. Biggar, R.J., The clinical features of HIV infection in Africa. Br Med J 293:1453-1454 (1986)

49. Melbye, M., The natural history of human T lymphotropic virus-III infection: the cause of AIDS. Br Med J 292:5-12 (1986)

50. Cooper, D.A., Gold, J., Maclean, P., et al., Acute AIDS retrovirus infection: definition of a clinical illness associated with seroconversion. Lancet 1:537-540 (1985)

51. Biggar, R.J., Johnson, B.K., Musoke, S.S., et al., Severe illness associated with HIV seroconversion in an African. Br Med J 293:1210-1211 (1986)

52. Metroka, C.E., Cunningham-Rundles, S., Pollack, M.S., et al., Generalized lymphadenopathy in homosexual men. Ann Intern Med 99:585-591 1983.

53. Mann, J.M., Bila, K., Colebunders, R.L. et al., Natural history of human immunodeficiency virus infection in Zaire. Lancet 2:707-709 (1986)

54. Goedert, J.J., Biggar, R.J., Weiss, S.H., et al., Three-year incidence of AIDS in five cohorts of HTLV-III-infected risk group members. Science 231:992-995 (1986)

55. Biggar, R.J., Melbye, M., Kestens, L., et al., Kaposi's sarcoma in Zaire is not associated with HTLV-III infection. N Engl J Med 16:1051 (1984).

56. Bayley, A.C., Downing, R.G., Cheingsong-Popov, R., et al., HTLV-III serology distinguishes atypical and endemic Kaposi's sarcoma in Africa. Lancet 1:359-361 (1985)

57. Kesten, L., Melbye, M., Biggar, R.J., et al., Endemic African Kaposi's sarcoma is not associated with immunodeficiency. Int J Cancer 36:49-54 (1985)

58. Downing, R.G., Eglin, R.P., Bayley, A.C., African Kaposi's sarcoma and AIDS. Lancet 1:478-480 (1984)

59. Biggar, R.J., Horm, J., Lubin, J.H. et al., Cancer trends in a population at risk of AIDS. J Natl Cancer Inst 74:793-797 (1985)

60. Mann, J.M., Francis, H., Quinn, T.C., et al., Surveillance for AIDS in a Central African city: Kinshasa, Zaire. JAMA 255:3255-3259 (1986)

61. Mann, J., Quinn, T.C., Piot, P., et al., Condom use and HIV infection among prostitutes in Zaire. N Engl J Med 316:345 (1987)

Part II
Etiologic Agent

9
Retroviruses: Current Concepts of Structure and Function

John M. Coffin

Over the last two decades, retroviruses have proven to be remarkably rewarding organisms for study (1),(2). Quite apart from their role in important human diseases, these infectious agents have provided researchers with incisive tools for probing the molecular basis of carcinogenesis, and have revealed novel and important mechanisms of information transfer. The intellectual impetus of the discovery of reverse transcriptase in 1970, and the financial impetus of the war on cancer in the early 1970's, combined to convert retrovirology from an arcane corner of virology to a major growth industry.

Not surprisingly, much of the research emphasis has been on unique features of retroviruses relevant to cancer; eg. mechanisms of viral DNA and RNA synthesis as well as structure and function of viral and cellular oncogenes. Issues such as epidemiology, virion structure, immunology, pathogenesis of cytopathic viruses, among others, have not been completely ignored, but have received relatively little attention. The discovery that infection with a retrovirus, now called human immunodeficiency virus (HIV), is intimately associated with the causation of the acquired immunodeficiency syndrome (AIDS) is changing this emphasis dramatically, revitalizing interest in studies which consider retroviruses as infectious pathogens, rather than as transducing agents.

This chapter will attempt to provide background information concerning retrovirus-host cell interactions with an emphasis on virion and genome structure and molecular mechanisms of replication and pathogenesis.

DEFINITION

Retroviruses are most uniquely defined as those viruses with RNA genomes whose replication in via a DNA intermediate. In addition to this defining characteristic (the prefix retro refers to the use of a mechanism of information transfer [RNA to DNA] which is the reverse of the usual), retroviruses share many additional features, including the following:

1. The virion is always enveloped by a lipid bilayer derived from the host cell membrane and contains a surface glycoprotein spike as well as an internal, roughly spherical core. The core contains the genome as well as several enzymes - most prominently reverse transcriptase. Other virion enzymatic activities invariably include a ribonuclease H used for DNA synthesis, a DNA endonuclease needed for integration of viral DNA, and a protease used to generate the capsid proteins by cleavage of a precursor.

2. The retrovirus genome is unique in several respects. First, it is a 7-10kb molecule of RNA structurally resembling eukaryotic mRNA with a 5' capping group and 3' polyadenylate sequence. Second, it is present in the virion in two copies. Thus, retroviruses are the only known diploid viruses. Third, it always occurs in association with lower molecular weight RNA's, most notably a single molecule of tRNA which serves as a primer for DNA synthesis.

3. Finally, all major events in replication are unique to retroviruses. They include the following steps: synthesis of double-stranded linear viral DNA in the cytoplasm of the infected cell by a process that leads to the formation of long terminal repeats (LTR's); integration of viral DNA into cellular DNA to form the provirus, and transcription of the provirus, using cellular machinery, to form new RNA genomes and mRNA's. Signals provided within the LTR stimulate (and sometimes regulate) the activity of cellular RNA polymerase. This cycle permits a more intimate association of replication with cellular function than in any other group of viruses.

4. The retrovirus genome invariably contains three genes: the gag gene (for *g*roup-specific *a*nti*g*en) that encodes for the nucleocapsid proteins; the pol gene that encodes for the reverse transcriptase and other enzymatic proteins and the env gene which encodes for the envelope proteins.

NATURAL HISTORY

Retroviruses are widespread among vertebrates, and infectious virus has been isolated from fish, reptiles, birds, and mammals. Particles morphologically resembling virions have been detected in lower taxonomic classes as well; including insects and even tapeworms. Among mammals and birds virtually all species which have been examined sufficiently closely have yielded retroviruses. In a number of species such viruses are an important source of naturally-occurring disease (Table 1). Although retroviruses were initially identified with malignancies, it is apparent that they are associated with a wide variety of diseases, including ones that are degenerative or immunological in nature. The type of disease produced by a given virus may be influenced by the genetic makeup or age of the host. For example, some strains of avian leukosis (leukemia) virus strains induce B-lymphomas in most lines of chickens, but erythroleukemia in other lines of chickens (3),(4). Furthermore, only slightly different strains of avian leukosis virus induce osteopetrosis whereas others lead to viremia, but no disease at all (5). Thus, the pathogenic spectrum of a given retrovirus isolate is a particularly poor criterion for classification.

Table 1. Some Mammalian and Avian Retroviral Diseases

Species	Disease	Virus
Humans	T-cell leukemia/lymphoma Acquired immunodeficiency Syndrome (AIDS, AIDS related complex (ARC)	Human T-cell leukemia virus (HTLV) Human immunodeficiency virus (HIV)
Primates	Lymphoma	Gibbon ape leukemia virus (GALV)
Cattle	B-cell lymphoma	Bovine leukemia virus (BLV)
Sheep	Visna, Maedi	Visna
Goats	Arthritis, encephalitis	Caprine encephalitis virus (CaEV)
Horses	Anemia	Equine infectious anemia virus (EIAV)
Cats	T-cell lymphoma, immunodeficiency	Feline leukemia virus (FeLV)
Mice	T-cell lymphoma, paralysis, mammary carcinoma	Murine leukemia virus (MLV)
Chickens	B-cell lymphoma, erythroleukemia, osteopetrosis, wasting	Avian leukosis virus (ALV)

Compared to many other viruses, retroviruses are transmitted from one host to another inefficiently. This low transmission rate no doubt reflects the extreme lability of the virion. The half-life of Rous sarcoma virus in cell culture medium is on the order of a few hours, and all retroviruses are readily inactivated by mild detergent, gentle heating, drying, or moderately high or low pH. Thus, in many instances, transmission is by close physical contact involving exhange of blood or semen. In populations where a virus is endemic, the major mode of transmission is often vertical, by infection of the offspring with virus produced in the mother - via milk in mammals or virus released from the oviduct into the albumen of birds' eggs. A number of viruses have special adaptations for this sort of existence. Mammary tumor virus, for example, is expressed at high levels in lactating mammary glands but at much lower levels in other tissue.

Most retrovirus infections are characterized by latency periods measured in months to years. Such long latent periods are clearly what one would expect for a virus whose major modes of transmission are either vertical or via intimate contact, since a virus which killed its host before it could be transmitted would not survive very long in nature. Latency is also an inherent characteristic of retrovirus infection which inevitably involves integration of viral DNA into the host genome. Since retroviral infection can be completely eliminated only by destruction of all infected cells, such infections, once established, are likely to be permanent.

Retrovirus infection can even extend well beyond the life of a single infected host. Many species of vertebrates contain, as part of their genetic composition, inherited proviruses closely resembling those derived from infectious virus. These endogenous proviruses have been most intensively studied in chickens and mice, and have been found to be closely related to - and certainly derived from - exogenous viruses endemic to the same species. Nevertheless, they are very poorly expressed, generally due to secondary modification of the DNA (such as methylation). When expressed, many endogenous proviruses can give rise to a complete infectious virus, which, in general, is nonpathogenic. This nonpathogenicity presumably represents a specific adaptation, since an endogenous virus which even slightly diminished the reproductive potential of its host would be rapidly lost. Although endogenous viruses are stably associated with a given host genome (the loss rate for one such element has been estimated at $3x10^{-6}$per generation) (6), their numbers and locations differ from individual to individual indicating that they have been introduced relatively recently (post-speciation).

Retention of biological activity by endogenous proviruses indicates that they were derived by processes not greatly different from that of a normal virus life cycle; ie., by infection of germ line cells with virus (usually derived from another endogenous provirus). There are, in eukaryotic genomes, numerous elements with provirus-like structures for which no virus has yet been found. These are collectively called "retro-transposons" (7) implying that they move by reverse transcriptase but without leaving the cell. This mobility without virion release is almost certainly the case with elements such as Ty in yeast (8) and A-particles in mice. However, in some instances (such as the copia element of *Drosophila*) it is possible that there is an extracellular virus that has not yet been found.

TAXONOMY

For some time, the family retroviridae has been classified as shown in Table 2. This classification is based principally on pathogenic and morphological characteristics and can now be considered as being rather out of date. Recently, the nucleotide sequences of numerous retrovirus genomes have been determined including at least one representative of all listed taxa except spumavirinae. Analysis of this information reveals that within genera, the individual members are quite closely related in overall organization (refer to Figure 2, for example) and sequence. Groupings within higher taxa, however, do not reflect relationships revealed by nucleotide sequencing. For example, the avian and mammalian C-type viruses have similar virion morphology and pathogenic characteristics, and are thus usually grouped together. However, the nucleotide sequences of these viruses make it clear that the two groups are only very distantly related and that the avian viruses are more closely related to mouse mammary tumor virus, which has quite different biological properties. Similarly, HIV shares host range and other properties with human T-cell leukemia virus I (HTLV-I), but is quite different structurally and clearly belongs with the lentiviruses (visna and relatives) (9). A more accurate taxonomy would not use any classification higher than the current "genus" level and would include as separate genera all currently identified groups.

Table 2. Current Taxonomy of Retroviruses
Family: Retroviridae

Subfamily	Genus	Example
Oncovirinae	(Type C viruses)	Avian leukosis virus
		Murine leukemia virus
	(Type B viruses)	Mouse mammary tumor virus
	(Type D viruses)	Mason-Pfizer virus
		Simian AIDS virus
Lentivirinae	Lentivirus	Visna
	(unnamed)	Human immunodeficiency virus
Spumavirinae	Spumavirus	Simian foamy virus

VIRION STRUCTURE AND ASSEMBLY

Virions of retroviruses are similar but not identical in appearance. All contain a capsid within a roughly spherical envelope with more or less visible spikes (or peplomers) of glycoproteins. The capsids vary somewhat in structure and the original classification system into B, C, and D-type particles is based on details of capsid morphology. ("A" particles are strictly intracellular forms.) Lentiviruses and HIV have yet a different morphology. While the typical A, B, C and D particles contain roughly spherical capsids differing in the extent of condensation and in location within the envelope, HIV and the lentiviruses have a distinctive oblong-shaped capsid.

Virions of retroviruses have a fairly simple protein composition, usually containing only eight or nine proteins. Because of the fragility of the internal structures, details of capsid organization are not well known. Figure 1 depicts, in schematic fashion, what is currently known about virion structure. Virion structural genes and their products for selected retroviruses are listed in Table 3, and the distribution of sequences coding for the various retrovirus gene products is shown in Figure 2.

RETROVIRUS VIRION PROTEINS

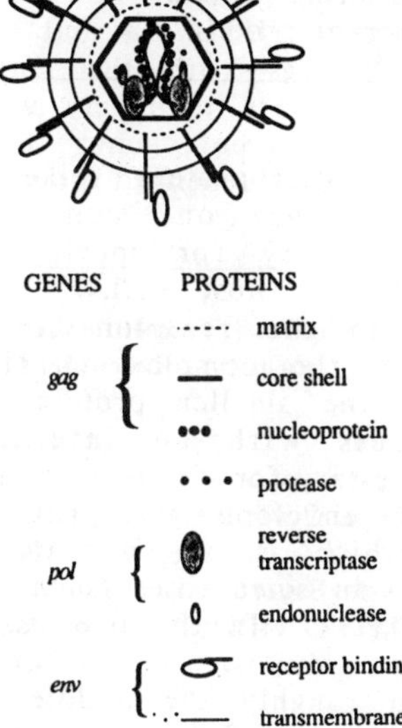

Figure 1. The retrovirus virion. This highly schematic sketch shows the approximate locations of the various virion components common to all retroviruses. Abbreviations: M = matrix protein; C = major core shell protein; N = nucleoprotein; P = protease; RT = reverse transcriptase; EN = endonuclease; RB = receptor binding protein; TM = transmembrane protein.

Table 3. Retrovirus Virion Proteins

Coding Regions			Gag		Pol		Env		
	Matrix		Core Shell	Nucleo-Protein	Protease	R.T.	EN	RB	TM
ALV(RSV)	p19	p10	p27	p12	p15	p58/92	p32	gp85	gp37
MLV	p15	p12	p30	p10	p14	p75	p45	gp70	p15(E)
HTLV	p19	x	p24	p15	*	*	*	gp60	p21
HIV	p17	x	p24	p15?	*	p55/61	*	gp120	gp41

* Cleavage sites have not been accurately determined.
x Not found in these viruses

ALV avian leukosis virus
RSV Rous sarcoma virus
MLV murine leukemia virus
HTLV-I human T-cell leukemia virus I
HIV human immunodeficiency virus
RT reverse transcriptase
EN endonuclease
RB receptor binding protein
TM transmembrane protein

The surface glycoprotein spike consists of two proteins (Figure 1.) The larger one contains the receptor binding activity and is necessary for specifying the initial interaction of the virus with the host cell. The smaller transmembrane protein is joined to the receptor binding protein by disulfide bonds and anchors the complex to the lipid envelope. The C-terminal end of the smaller protein spans the membrane and presumably interacts with an internal virus protein. This interaction is not necessary for virion formation.

The larger envelope glycoprotein contains the receptor-binding activity, which is of first importance in specifying the target animal and - in some cases (such as HIV) - the target cell to be infected (10),(11). In the one case that has been genetically defined (avian leukosis virus), receptor interaction specificity was found in roughly the middle third of the protein (12). The large glycoprotein also forms the major target for the immune response against virions and infected cells. Among different retroviruses it varies in apparent molecular weight from 60,000 to about 120,000, with the largest size found in AIDS viruses and lentiviruses. Much of this variation in size is due to different degrees of glycosylation: gp120's of HIV isolates are predicted to contain about two dozen carbohydrate side chains. Much of the remaining difference in molecular weight of the large envelope protein of the AIDS virus compared to other retroviruses may be accounted for by about 125 amino acids in "hypervariable" regions (13)-(17) (Figure 3). Both structural features may be relevant to the absence of a strong neutralizing immune response in HIV infected individuals (18),(19), since the hypervariable regions might allow rapid antigenic variation and the glycosylation sites might mask potentially antigenic regions (20).

The envelope glycoproteins are the products of the env gene, and their synthesis and processing are virtually identical among all retroviruses. The env gene products are translated from a spliced, subgenomic RNA and, like cellular glycoproteins, are synthesized on membrane-bound polyribosomes, followed by removal of an N-terminal signal peptide. Glycosylation and transport occur via the usual cellular pathways through the endoplasmic reticulum and Golgi apparatus where cleavage (by a cellular enzyme) into the two subunits occurs. A structure of about 24 uncharged amino acid residues in the smaller protein serves as a membrane anchor.

Coding Regions Of Retroviruses

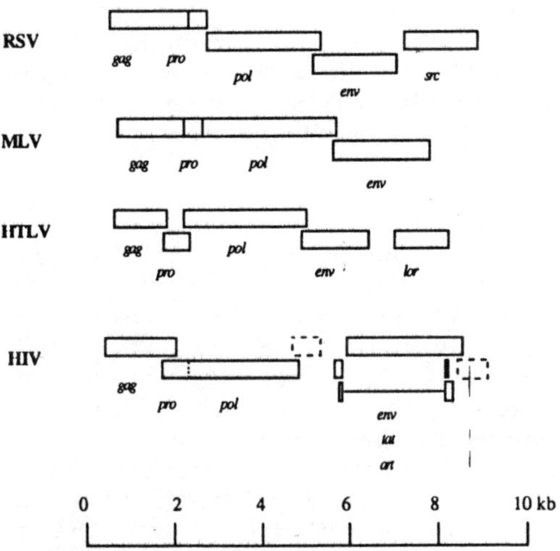

Figure 2. Retrovirus reading frames. Representatives of four different retrovirus groups are shown. The various identified open reading frames are indicated by boxes; where boxes overlap the same nucleotide sequence is translated from two or more different reading frames. Dividing lines denote termination codons or cleavage sites. Dotted boxes indicate reading frames encoding unnamed proteins of unknown function. Note the different relative positions of the gag, protease (pro) and pol domains among the four groups of viruses. Note also the multiple use of the env region of HIV.

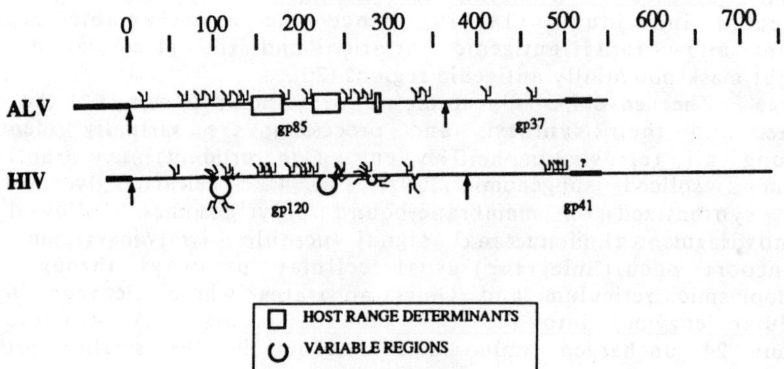

Figure 3. The organization of avian leukemia virus (ALV) and human immunodeficiency virus (HIV) env proteins. In both cases the larger fragment is the receptor binding protein; the smaller C-terminal protein the transmembrane region.

The internal proteins of the virion are all products of two genes, gag and pol (Table 3, Figure 1). The gag gene contributes the bulk of structural proteins which vary in number from three to five depending on the virus. The three invariant proteins for all retroviruses include (from N- to C-terminus): first, a probable "matrix" protein which lies adjacent to the membrane and probably interacts with it (sometimes via an added fatty acid group) to mediate budding; second, the largest gag product (p24 in HIV) which most likely forms the core shell visible in electron micrographs; and third a small, basic, protein which is found in close association with the genome RNA and which behaves as a nonspecific nucleic acid binding protein. Some, but not all, retroviruses have a fourth gag protein of unknown function located on the precursor between the matrix and capsid proteins.

The remaining virion proteins serve enzymatic, rather than structural roles. The first of these is a protease encoded C-terminal to the nucleic acid binding protein, but in various reading frames relative to gag and pol (Figure 2). Finally there are two or three polypetides derived from the pol gene which carry out synthetic and nucleolytic events early in replication (synthesis of viral DNA and some steps necessary for integration) (Table 4).

Table 4. Activities of the Pol Gene Products of Retroviruses

	Activity	Function
Large Fragment	DNA polymerase	Synthesis of viral DNA
	RNase H	Removal of template RNA
	"Nicking acitivty"	Generation of plus-strand primer
Small Fragment	Endonuclease ("integrase")	Required for integration

The processing of gag and pol proteins is fairly well understood and seems to be intimately connected with virion assembly and budding. In all retroviruses, the pol gene is expressed as a C-terminal extension of about 5-10% of the gag precursor molecules. Both gene products are cleaved via the virion protease, giving rise to the question of how the protease itself is generated. It now seems probable that the protease is active in the precursor form, but only slightly so, so that a critical mass of precursor has to assemble before cleavage begins. Once the initial cleavages take place, releasing active protease, the remaining cleavage would be relatively rapid. This scheme would agree with electron micrograph evidence which shows that there is a significant structural rearrangement (from an open to a condensed core) shortly after budding. By this model, assembly and budding would be of gag and gag-pol precursors, rather than cleavage products. This would ensure both an appropriate balance of the virus proteins in virions as well as the absence of active reverse transcription complexes within the infected cell (see below).

The assembly and release of virions by budding is an unusual process in at least two respects. First, with most retroviruses, assembly and budding occur simultaneously. Second, analysis of mutants shows that only a relatively small fraction of the virion proteins are required. Mutants lacking pol, env, and genome RNA still yield normal-appearing virions (except for the absence of surface projections). In fact, not even all of gag proteins are required since Rous sarcoma virus mutants lacking the C-terminal third (including the protease and about half the RNA-binding region) yield virus, albeit aberrant in appearance (21). Thus, capsid formation and budding are determined by only core and matrix proteins.

Until recently, the mechanisms by which pol was translated remained unclear. In all cases (except human T-cell leukemia virus 1 and 2, see below), nucleotide sequencing revealed that the gag and pol genes are directly adjoining and separated by a single termination codon, usually also with a change in reading frame. It was originally proposed that the bypassing of the terminator and shift of reading frame was a consequence of splicing of a small percent of the mRNAs to allow synthesis of a complete gag-pol precursor. Such a spliced RNA could not be detected, however, and it is now clear that novel (for eukaryotic cells) mechanisms of translation suppression account for the expression of pol in a fixed ratio to gag (22),(23). Apparently, under certain conditions which are not fully understood, ribosomes can either skip a terminator (in the case of murine leukemia virus, a glutamine residue is inserted in its place) or change reading frames. The frequency with which this aberration occurs determines the ratio of gag to gag-pol precursor synthesized. At the moment, this mechanism seems limited to retroviruses; no normal cell or other virus process in known to use it.

THE GENOME

As noted above, retrovirus genomes are synthesized and processed by the same mechanisms used for the synthesis of normal cell mRNA. Thus, the genomes physically resemble cell mRNAs: they have a sequence of about 200 adenosine residues at their 3' ends (poly A sequence), a capping group of the usual sort at their 5' end and are further modified by the presence of methylated adenosine residues (24). The overall organization of retrovirus genomes are similar to one another: the virion genes are always in the order gag-pol-env and differ only in mechanism of readthrough of pol and disposition of the protease reading frame (Figure 2). The function of additional reading frames is discussed below. In addition to the reading frames, all genomes contain a set of terminal regions essential for its function as a template for reverse transcription and for proper function (integration and transcription) of viral DNA (Figure 4). From 5' to 3' these include:

R: A directly repeated sequence (12-250 bases; 98 in HIV) found adjacent to the poly (A) at the 3' end. R serves a critical role during viral DNA synthesis to form a "bridge" for transfer of the growing chain from one end of the genome to the other.

U5: Unique sequence (80-200 bases) adjacent to R.

PB: The binding site for the tRNA primer which serves to initiate viral DNA synthesis soon after infection. The primer can be one of several different tRNA's (lysine tRNA in the case of HIV) and the primer binding site invariably consists of 18 bases perfectly complementary to the 3' end of the tRNA.

Leader region: The sequence betwen PB and the beginning of gag. It usually contains two well defined functions: a splice donor site for the generation of subgenomic mRNA's and a signal (sometimes called "psi") that specifies assembly into virions presumably by specifically interacting with a virus protein. The arrangment of these is usually (5') donor-packaging signal (3') so that spliced mRNA's lack the signal and thus are not packaged.

Except for the splice acceptor and some additional donor sites, there are no known processing signals within the coding regions of the retrovirus genome, although specific sequences can have effects on RNA splicing (see below).

Defined genome regions near the 3' end include:

PP: (For polypurine tract) a run of 10 or more guanine and adenosine residues which invariably mark the initiation site of plus-strand DNA synthesis, probably by providing a specific cleavage and primer site when present in a RNA-DNA hybrid.

U3: A unique region near the 3' end varying in length from about 200 to 1200 bases. Because it forms the upstream end of the LTR, U3 consists mostly of sequences relevant to initiation and regulation of transcription (see below).

R: Finally, the 3' end of the genome contains a second copy of the repeated sequence identical to that of the 3' end. Depending on the virus, either R or U3 contains a canonical signal (AAUAAA) for poly(A) addition.

In virions, the genome is invariably present in two copies joined to one another by base-pairing at multiple points, most strongly in a poorly defined region known as the dimer linkage structure near the 5' end. The function of this unusual arrangement is not known with certainty; it has the effect of causing a very high frequency of recombination (25); and an attractive idea is that the presence of two copies permits a high level of repair of damage to the relatively fragile single- stranded RNA.

REPLICATION

The replication of retroviruses can be divided into two phases: The first, including synthesis and integration of the provirus, is carried out principally by enzymes found in the virion; the second - including synthesis of progeny mRNA's and genomes - entirely by cellular systems (Figure 4). Given a virus that replicates in this fashion, the seemingly complex events of viral DNA synthesis can in fact be viewed as the simplest solution to two general problems: First, all DNA polymerases (including reverse transcriptase) require a pre-existing polymer to serve as primer for DNA synthesis. Second, cellular RNA polymerase II requires the presence of specific sequences upstream of the initiation site. Both of these problems dictate that the virus arrange a way to provide DNA sequences longer at the ends than the genome itself. The elegant solution achieved by the virus is to use the ability of the reverse transcription system to change templates (or "jump") to synthesize a DNA molecule con-

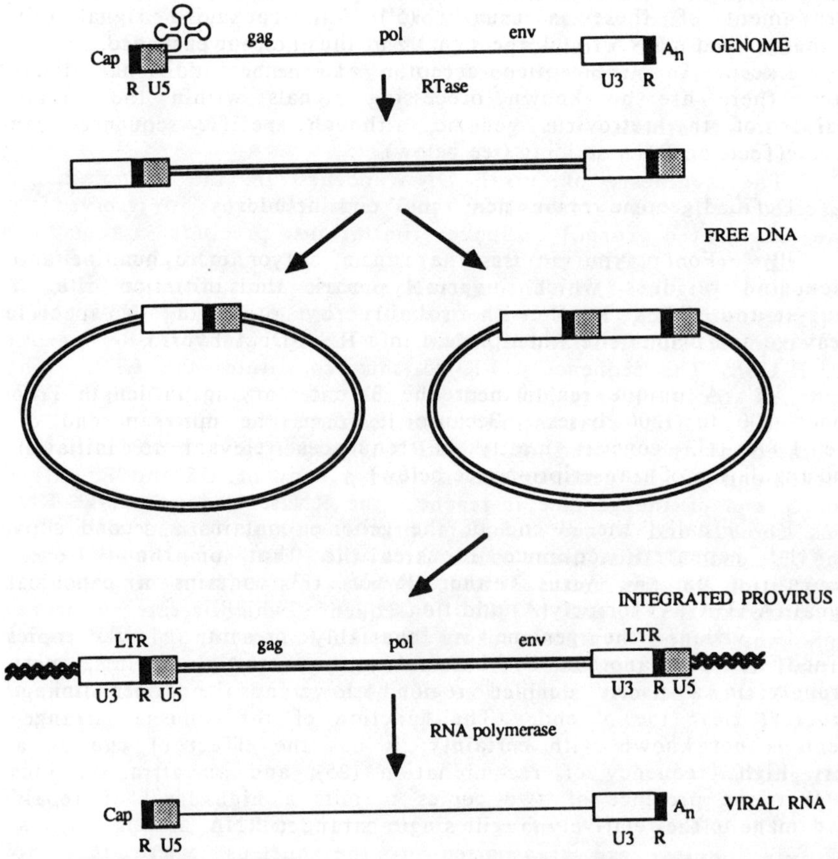

Figure 4. Schematic outline of the retrovirus replication cycle. Single lines indicate RNA; double lines viral DNA (with LTR sequences boxed); and wavy lines show cell DNA around the integration site. (Courtesy of S.A. Herman).

taining, as terminal repeats, sequences present only once near each end of the viral genome.

Initial Events

The entry of virus into cells is not very well understood. It clearly requires interaction of the env protein with a specific receptor, since the lack of the receptor (or its blockage) reduces infectivity by seven orders of magnitude or more. Penetration most likely occurs by receptor-mediated endocytosis, although this has not been demonstrated directly for any retrovirus. It is important to bear in mind that subsequent early events do not require the synthesis of any virus-coded proteins and that they take place within some sort of (poorly defined) structure derived from the viral capsid. Most of these events are catalyzed by the virion enzymes encoded by the pol gene.

Viral DNA Synthesis

The synthesis of viral DNA occurs in the cytoplasm of infected cells. [By convention, the term provirus is reserved for the integrated form.] Space limitations preclude a complete description of this process here, so only highlights will be presented (Figure 5). The overall process leads from a molecule of single-stranded RNA with the structure R-U5-genes-U3-R to a molecule of double-stranded DNA of the structure U3-R-U5-genes-U3-R-U5. The sequence U3-R-U5 thus constitutes the LTR. The ends of the LTR are defined by the sites of initiation of DNA synthesis. The first strand synthesized (the minus strand) is initiated at the 3' end of the tRNA primer and proceeds toward the 5' end of the genome, and is thus a copy of U5 and R. When the 5' end of the genome is reached, the RNase H removes the RNA just copied, and a new template primer pair is formed with R at the 3' end. This event constitutes the first jump, and permits completion of the minus strand. While this is happening, a nick is made at the 3' end of the PP sequence which creates a primer for plus strand synthesis using the U3-R portion of the minus strand DNA as template. A second jump to the end of the minus strand then permits completion of both strands and formation of the LTR's.

Integration

The linear DNA molecules (probably still in association with capsid proteins) are transported to the nucleus where they are circularized (Figure 6) either by direct joining of the ends or by homologous recombination between two LTR's. The next event is integration of the viral DNA into that of the host. The integration event is apparently a regular and indispensable part of the replication cycle and is another characteristic which distinguishes retroviruses from all other families. In contrast to DNA synthesis, integration has not yet been duplicated in vitro, and the mechanism is, therefore, much more poorly understood. Integration is a highly specific process, since the provirus is always joined in the same way to cellular DNA to provide a structure flanked by the LTR's. Invariably, there is a duplication of a short (4-6 base) sequence of cell DNA and a loss of two bases at the exposed end of each LTR. Figure 6 presents a hypothetical scheme which could lead to the structure found, involving staggered cuts in viral and cellular DNA which are subsequently repaired. Specificity for these cuts probably resides in the virus endonuclease, since this protein has been shown to be required for integration (26). The length of host cell DNA duplicated varies with the type of virus, and the enzyme can specifically

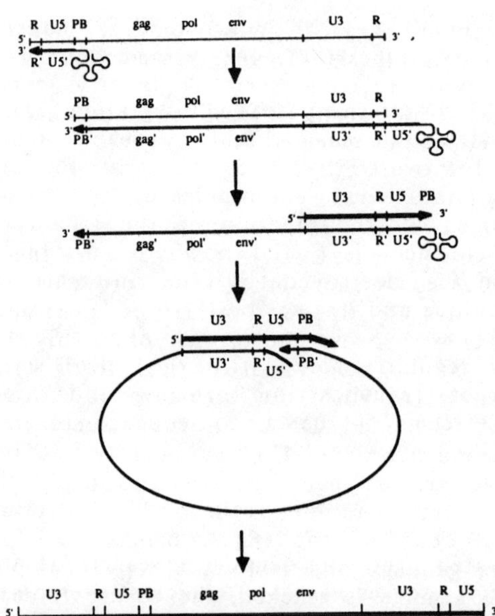

Figure 5. Viral DNA synthesis. Direction of synthesis is shown by arrows. Note the successive "jumps" of reverse transcripts; the first using the R sequence as a bridge, the second using a copy of the primer binding (PB) site. (Courtesy of S.A. Herman).

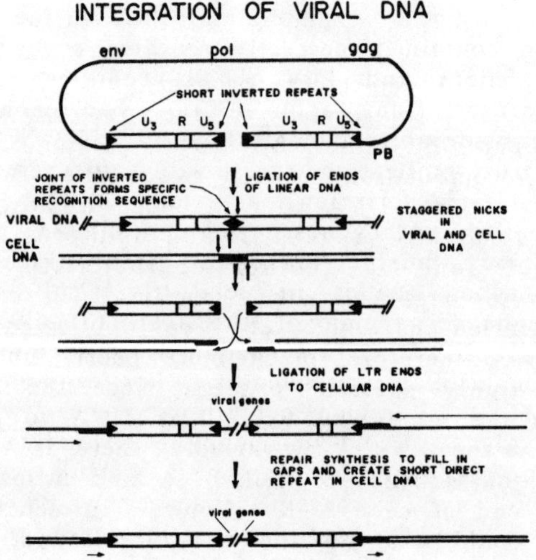

Figure 6. A possible scheme for integration of viral DNA. Note that this outline is based only on structural analysis. None of the enzymatic reactions suggested has been definitively characterized.

recognize the surrounding viral sequences (27). It must be emphasized that none of the other enzymes involved in this process has been identified.

The viral DNA intermediate to integration remained unknown until recently. It now seems highly probable that the relevant intermediate is the two-LTR circle and that the integration system (presumably the viral endonuclease) specifically recognizes the sequence formed by the junction of the LTR's (28),(29). This combination of sequences is found nowhere else in the viral DNA, and, furthermore, is destroyed by the integration process, rendering the event unique and irreversible.

Once integrated, the provirus is almost completely stable and is replicated regularly along with the cell DNA. There is no excision or direct transposition process and loss of provirus (when it occurs) seems to be a consequence of random deletion events.

Expression

Once integrated, the provirus behaves as though it were a cellular gene. It serves as an efficient template for mRNA synthesis by RNA polymerase II. For this purpose, much of the U3 region of the LTR consists of sequences which resemble cellular signals (Figure 7). Located 5' of the initiation site for RNA synthesis (or "cap" site) are standard consensus signals for eukaryotic transcription: a "TATA" box about 24 bases upstream, and a "CCAAT" box about 80 bases upstream. In addition, there are more or less well-defined enhancer elements which can stimulate synthesis from any promoter in relatively distance- and orientation-independent fashion. These are often present in multiple copies, as, for example. in the murine leukemia virus LTR which can contain a perfectly repeated sequence of about 70 base pairs in length and HIV which contains repeated binding sites for a transcription factor (30). The enhancer sequences can provide considerable biological specificity by affecting both the rate of virus replication (presumably by regulating the rate of initiation of transcription) as well as the cell specificity of replication and pathogenesis. For example, the differential ability of various murine leukemia virus strains to transform different cell types resides in relatively small sequence differences in the enhancer region of the LTR (31)-(33). In addition to specifying replication rate and tissue specificity, the LTR can also provide regulatory sequences. For example, the mammary tumor virus (MTV) U3 region contains sequences which respond to the action of glucocorticoid hormones, by binding the LTR's of human hormone-receptor complex and stimulating transcription. Similarly, HTLV-1 and 2 contain sequences which respond directly or indirectly to the "transactivating" influence of the lor protein (see below).

In addition to specifying the initiation of transcription and hence the 5' end of the viral transcript, the LTR also specifies the 3' end of the viral RNA. As with most eukaryotic RNA's, synthesis of viral RNA proceeds through the LTR into adjacent

FEATURES OF LTR's

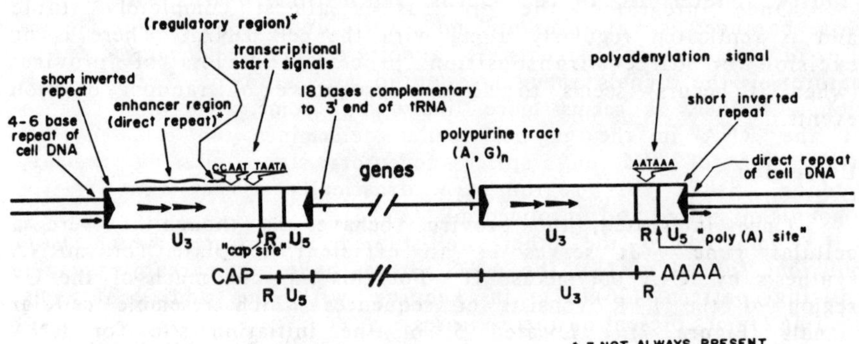

Figure 7. Structural features of LTR's. Note that although the LTR's are identical in sequence, the signals are only shown for the LTR in which they are important. Thus, initiation signals are shown only in the 5' LTR; 3' processing signals only in the 5' LTR.

cell DNA and the primary transcript is then rapidly cleaved and polyadenylated to generate the final 3' end. A consensus addition signal (AAUAAA) is invariably found within either U3 or R 16-20 bases upstream of the poly (A). Interestingly, a significant fraction of genomes can be derived from RNA polyadenylated at sites derived from adjoining host DNA (34).

As shown in Figure 7, the LTR thus contains a complex collection of signals used at various stages of virus replication. Despite the wide diversity of viruses and the virtually complete lack of sequence homology among different groups, all LTR's contain these signals and they can often be recognized this way.

Processing

The viral RNA transcripts that are made have three distinct fates. They can become new genomes; they can serve directly as mRNA for the gag and gag-pol precursors or they can be spliced to form env or other mRNA's. The spliced mRNA's invariably contain the 5' end of the genome (R-U5 and all or part of the leader) joined to one or more downstream regions, always including the original 3' end. The necessity of making such mRNA's raises an additional problem. Clearly there must be a balance among these uses; too much or too little splicing, for example, would be obviously deleterious to the virus replication. What determines this balance is, at present, not well understood. Inefficient use of the splicing signals is almost certainly not due to the nature of the signals themselves or to any kind of direct regulation. Rather, it seems more likely that some structural feature of the RNA in the gag-pol region determines the efficiency of utilization of the env splice acceptor, since altering the sequence within this region can drastically affect the relative amounts of spliced and unspliced mRNA (35).

Compared to the other well-studied retroviruses which have only one spliced mRNA, the AIDS viruses have a remarkably complex splicing pattern (36),(37), in keeping with the additional open reading frames present on these viruses.

Transactivation

Until recently, it seemed that expression of all the proviruses was accomplished entirely by factors and systems already existent in the cell prior to infection, for which the provirus and its transcript simply provided appropriate signals. Indeed, this property of the retrovirus infection cycle is crucial to the ability of some viruses to acquire oncogenes by exchanging host cell information for some or all of the coding sequence of the virus. This process would not be so readily feasible if these viruses required a viral gene product for expression. More recently it has been found that some of the "newer" retroviruses, including HTLV-I and II and HIV do not follow this formerly general rule. Rather, full expression of these viruses apparently requires the presence of one or more protein products of the virus genome itself. This phenomenon was first described with HTLV-I when it was found that reconstructed DNA's containing an HTLV-I LTR joined to a gene with a readily assayable product (chloramphenicol acetyl transferase) were expressed much more efficiently in HTLV-I infected than in uninfected cells (38). This effect was found to be due to the protein encoded by the lor (also called pX or tat-1) sequence (39)-(41). This nuclear protein causes the number of viral transcripts to be greatly increased, presumably by affecting the rate of initiation of transcription via interaction (possibly indirectly) with specific sequences in the U3 region of the LTR (42),(43).

When the same sort of experiment is done with HIV, a similar result is obtained: the expression of HIV-like DNA constructs is greatly stimulated by prior infection of the cell (44). This effect was initially also attributed to transcriptional activation. However, it now seems to be due to some post-transcriptional event, possibly the rate of translation (45). HIV, in fact, encodes two such activities. The first one described (tat or tat-III) has a target sequence within U5 and this presumably effects all viral mRNAs; the second (art) seems to be specific for gag and env expression (46). Both the tat and art proteins are encoded by use of different alternative reading frames in the same region of env (Figure 2) (47)-(50).

It is apparent that the tat gene is required for replication of HIV (51); however, the role of transactivation in the life of these retroviruses remains to be clarified. It is possible that the phenomena observed reveal only a portion of a more complex regluatory network in which (for example) the activity of the transactivating proteins themselves might be somehow regulated by interaction with a cell component. Indeed, both types of viruses seem to have quiescent phases in infected individuals in which viral expression is very difficult to detect. Alternatively, transactivation may allow higher levels of expression or a more rapid infection cycle than would be available with unmodified cell systems. It should be emphasized that transactivation has been studied almost solely using the artificial constructs and transfection methodology, which (although quite revealing) may only disclose a fraction of the overall picture. Experimentation using more complete infection cycles is needed to clarify the issue further.

PATHOGENESIS

The various retroviruses can induce a wide variety of different diseases in natural and experimental hosts. As noted in a prior section, the pathological consequences of infection include no disease, a variety of malignancies, various degenerative conditions and probably also conditions with an autoimmune basis. Due to intense effort in the past few years, there has been considerable progress in understanding the cellular, molecular, and sometimes even the biochemical bases of these diseases. The molecular basis of retrovirus oncogenesis is probably best understood, although rapid progress is being made toward an understanding of the degenerative conditions associated with AIDS and other cytopathic virus infections.

Malignancy

With the possible exception of the HTLV-bovine leukemia virus group (see below), all retroviral carcinogenesis is mediated by the action of oncogenes (or onc genes). Oncogenes can be defined as nucleotide sequences which are derived from normal cellular genes (c-onc genes or protooncogenes) and which have been altered in some way to confer on their products the ability to transform certain normal cells into tumor cells.

The activation event which converts a protooncogene into an oncogene can be one of three fundamentally different types. First, all or part of the nucleotide sequence can be inserted into the viral genome, usually in place of viral genes. This rare set of events gives rise to rapidly transforming viruses such as Rous sarcoma virus, Abelson murine leukemia virus, and simian sarcoma virus.

The second type of activation can occur following integration of a provirus into or near a protooncogenes. This type of event, although it probably occurs less than once per million infected cells can occur with high frequency in certain circumstances, as in chickens infected with avian leukosis virus or mice infected with murine leukemia virus or mouse mammary tumor virus. For example, integration within the c-myc gene is found in virtually all B-cell lymphomas induced by avian leukosis virus and in many T-lymphomas induced by murine leukemia virus. Similar or identical oncogenes can also apparently be activated by non-viral events. For example, chromosome breakage and rejoining may accomplish activation of c-myc in certain lymphoid tumors in mouse and man, and point mutations activate ras (another oncogene) in both spontaneous (or chemically-induced) tumors and with certain transforming viruses.

Experience with these retroviral diseases has demonstrated that normal cells contain at least 20-30 different genes which can be activated into oncogenes. It seems that many (perhaps all) protooncogenes may be involved in the normal regulation of the cell cycle - in particular in the response of the cell to growth factors, although a function has been assigned to only a few (all of which encode growth factors or their receptors). There are two important - not mutually exclusive - differences between activated oncogenes and their cellular ancestors. First, their control is altered so that they are under the influence of viral rather than the normal cellular transcriptional signals, leading to unregulated expression at higher levels in inappropriate cell types. Second, they have frequently suffered mutations - such as deletions or point mutations in regulatory domains.

In exception to the avian viruses, carcinogenesis by HTLV I and II and bovine leukemia virus seems not to involve the action of typical oncogenes; these viruses do not contain cell-derived sequences; and there seems to be no similarity of integration regions from one tumor to the next, as would be expected for insertional activation. Rather, it has been suggested that carcinogenesis might be due to transactivation of cellular protooncogenes mediated by the lor gene product. A recently suggested pair of targets for such transactivation is the T-cell growth factor, IL-2, as well as the cell receptor for it (C. Rosen, personal communication). It could be imagined that over-expression of these proteins could cause cells to be stimulated to divide in the complete absence of the usual IL-2 signal, but direct evidence for this mechanism remains scanty.

Cell Killing

Although retroviral infections need not lead to cell damage, the AIDS epidemic has forcefully brought home the importance of cytopathic infections in the biology of these viruses. At an organismal level, there are two distinct mechanisms for cell killing by retroviruses; direct cytopathogenic effects and immune responses against otherwise healthy cells expressing viral antigens. The latter interaction certainly occurs in some cases and may be of importance in "wasting" types of diseases associated with certain avian and feline leukemia virus infections. This issue has not yet been explored in great depth and is probably not important in AIDS.

Infection with a number of retroviruses - including HIV and even some oncoviruses - can lead to cell death in certain cell culture models. Two fundamentally different mechanisms have been proposed, both of which may be important in HIV infection. The first mechanism involves apparent "overreplication" of the virus. It has been repeatedly noted that cells infected with cytopathic retroviruses have excessive amounts of unintegrated DNA - hundreds of copies as compared to one or a few copies in non-cytopathic infection (52)-(55). Since retroviral DNA apparently does not contain signals for its own replication, the excess copies must probably arise by repeated cycles of transcription - reverse transcription either via complete infection cycles involving re-infection of a cell with virus produced by it or by a "short-circuit" cycle involving reverse transcription of newly synthesized RNA. Two features of the "usual" replication cycle serve to prevent the "short circuit" cycle from happening. First, cleavage of the gag and gag-pol precursor proteins into an active "mature" form does not take place until the virion is released (or about to be released) by the infected cell. Thus, an active reverse transcriptase-template complex seems never to be present within the cell. Second, expression of the env gene product at the cell surface confers a very high level of resistance to superinfection, preventing nascent viruses from reentering the same cell. Indeed, cytopathic variants of normally noncytopathic avian leukosis virus strains differ specifically in the particular receptor utilized for infection (12),(56), indicating that it may be more difficult to establish superinfection resistance with some retroviral receptors than others. In the case of HIV and most other cytopathic retroviruses, the mechanism of accumulation of viral DNA is not known.

Also not known is why excess viral DNA should be associated with cell killing. It may simply be that the excess of viral signals (such as binding sites for transcriptional or translational factors) renders these factors unavailable to the cells for their own purposes. Alternatively, the DNA itself may be toxic, or there may be a consequent high level of expression of some toxic viral gene products.

An alternative cytopathic mechanism is based on the observation that HIV-infected cultures contain numerous multicellular syncytia comprised of large numbers of cells fused together. Such cells can apparently form by interaction of the env protein on the surface of an infected cell with T4 protein on a neighboring cell, followed by membrane fusion analogous to that used for virus infection. This event has been observed directly on mixtures of T4 positive cells with cells expressing env protein (57),(58). It has been proposed that this mechanism would permit a relatively small number of infected cells to do considerable damage by incapacitating a much larger number of T4-positive uninfected cells.

EVOLUTION

Although HIV has clearly appeared as a human pathogen very recently, there is every reason to believe that retroviruses have been around for at least a substantial fraction of vertebrate evolution. Unlike most infectious agents, retroviruses have left "fossil" traces of prior association with their host in the form of endogenous proviruses in the germline. Although the endogenous proviruses which can be readily expressed as infectious virus seem to be relatively recently acquired (at least post speciation), recent experimentation has revealed additional, new classes of endogenous viruses in the DNA of several species, including humans. These are distantly related to the modern oncoviruses (such as murine leukemia virus) but are clearly of great antiquity since they have suffered many point mutations which would render their coding regions unusable, and even the LTR's (which should have been identical at the time of insertion) have diverged in sequence (59). Furthermore, the similarity of integration sites of some elements in humans and chimpanzees (60) implies their presence prior to divergence of the species (60). Thus, this association, at least of oncoviruses with primates would seem to be quite longstanding, and involve repeated waves of "endogenization" of proviruses. Unfortunately, other groups of retroviruses such as lentiviruses do not seem to have left such distant traces in the germ line.

Although clearly very ancient, retroviruses are also capable of very rapid variation and adaptation to new niches as evidenced by two recent examples. The first is the relatively frequent appearance of viruses containing oncogenes. These are presumably the consequence of a very rare series of events involving integration at specific sites and illegitimate recombination. Although the probability of any retrovirus infected cell giving rise to an oncogene containing virus could be substantially less than 10^{-10}, the consequences are readily visible and a very large number of animals can be easily screened by visiting a slaughterhouse or a veternarian, for example. Because the horizontal transmission of retroviruses is very poor, viruses as virulent as the transforming viruses almost certainly die with the animal in which they arose, unless they are given a good home by the curious virologist. Thus, the laboratory can be considered the niche to which these viruses have adapted.

The spread of HIV into the human population represents a

second example of recent retrovirus evolution. In this case the virus is most likely a variant of much older viruses, which probably existed in Africa in association with either a monkey or possibly an isolated human population (61)-(63). Its appearance internationally probably reflects changes in living conditions including increased international travel.

It should be clear from the above discussion that retroviruses have adapted to a wide variety of niches, and have done so despite their very low rate of transmission and the lability of the virion. The adaptability of these viruses is intimately related to special features of the replication cycle. Retrovirus replication involves a fairly high frequency of both point mutations and rearrangements, and an extraordinarily high frequency of recombination. The former presumably reflects infidelity of the replication systems (probably both RNA polymerase and reverse transcriptase) and gives rise to about one error per replication cycle (64). The recombination frequency seems to be a consequence of the diploid genome of retroviruses and the ability of the reverse transcriptase system to change templates during replication (25).

The result of this "genetic flexibility" is a significant amount of genetic variation within even a closely related population of viruses. Different HIV or avian leukosis isolates, for example, can differ by 5-10% from one another. The ability to generate this sort of variation may be important not only in allowing the viruses to adapt to new environments, but also to aid survival as in the apparently rapid sequence and possibly antigenic variation in HIV and some other viruses. It should be apparent that the rapid variability of these viruses must be borne in mind when developing strategies to deal with them.

CONCLUSIONS

The outbreak of AIDS has provided renewed impetus to obtaining a deeper knowledge of retrovirus biology. It should be apparent that although some areas are understood in considerable depth, such as the structure of the genome and mechanism of viral DNA synthesis, others remain quite obscure. As our understanding of the virology of AIDS has increased, many new and fascinating retrovirological problems have appeared, and many old problems (such as antigenic variation or mechanism of cell killing) which previously were relatively little studied, have moved into the forefront. Just as AIDS is quite different from all other infectious diseases, so is HIV quite different from all other retroviruses. Infection with this virus involves phenomena not seen before. Many questions remain unanswered. For example, what is the function of the two additional open reading frames, (both of which are expressed as protein)? What is the biochemical nature of the transactivation phenomenon? What is its biological role? What regulates the infection process? What is the reason for the poor neutralization in the face of an otherwise strong immune response? Does sequence variation in fact correspond to antigenic variation?

These questions and many others still confront the inquiring virologist, and the answers will be of both enormous practical and theoretical importance to understanding this devasting but fascinating disease.

REFERENCES

1. Weiss, R., Teich, N., Varmus, H.E., Coffin, J.M., (eds.) Molecular Biology of Tumor Viruses, Part III: RNA Tumor Viruses. Volume I. Cold Spring Harbor Press, Cold Spring Harbor, N.Y., (1982)

2. Weiss, R., Teich, N., Varmus, H.E., Coffin, J.M., Molecular Biology of Tumor Viruses. Part III: RNA Tumor Viruses. Second edition, Volume II. Cold Spring Harbor Press, Cold Spring Harbor, N.Y., (1985)

3. Robinson, H.L., Miles, B.D., Catalano, D.E., et al., Susceptibility to erbB-induced erythroblastosis is a dominant trait of 15_1 chickens. J Virol 55:617-622 (1985)

4. Nilsen, T.W., Maroney, P.A., Goodwin, R.G. et al., c-erbB activation in ALV-induced erythroblastosis: Novel RNA processing and promoter insertion result in expression of an amino-truncated EGF receptor. Cell 41:719-726 (1985)

5. Robinson, H.L., Blais, B.M., Tsichlis, P.N., et al., At least two regions of the viral genome determine the oncogenic potential of avian leukosis viruses. Proc. Natl. Acad. Sci. U.S.A. 79:1225-1229 (1982).

6. Copeland, N.G., Hutchinson, K.W., Jenkins N.A., Excision of the DBA ecotropic provirus in dilute coat-color revertants of mice occurs by homologous recombination involving the viral LTRs. Cell 33:379-387 (1982)

7. Baltimore, D., Retroviruses and retrotransposons: The role of reverse transcription in shaping the eukaryotic genome. Cell 40:481-482 (1985)

8. Boeke, J.D., Garninkel, D.J., Styles, C.A., et al., Ty elements transpose through an RNA intermediate. Cell 40:491-500 (1985)

9. Sonigo, P., Alizon, M., Staskus, K., et al., Nucleotide sequence of the visna lentivirus: Relationship to the AIDS virus. Cell 42:369-382 (1985)

10. Dalgleish, A.G., Beverley, P.R., Clapham, D.H., et al., The CD4 (T4) antigen is an essential component of the receptor for the AIDS virus. Nature 312:763-767 (1984)

11. Klatzmann, D., Barre-Sinoussi, F., Nugeyre, M.T., et al., Selective tropism of lymphadenopathy associated virus (LAV) for helper-inducer T lymphocytes. Science 225:59-63 (1984)

12. Dorner, A.J., Coffin, J.M., Determinants for receptor interaction and cell killing on the avian retrovirus glycoprotein gp85. Cell 45:365-374 (1986)

13. Alizon, M., Wain-Hobson, S., Montagnier, L., et al., Genetic varability of the AIDS virus: Nucleotide sequence analysis of two isolates from African patients. Cell 46:63-74 (1986)

14. Willey, R.L., Rutledge, R.A., Dias, S., et al., Identification of conserved and divergent domains within the envelope gene of the acquired immunodeficiency syndrome retrovirus. Proc Natl Acad Sci U.S.A. 83:5038-5042 (1986)

15. Starcich, B.R., Hahn, B.H., Shaw, G.M., et al., Identification and characterization of conserved and vairable regions in the envelope gene of HTLV-III/LAV, the retrovirus of AIDS. Cell 45:637-648 (1986)

16. Hahn, B.H., Shaw, G.M., Taylor, M.E., et al., Genetic variation in HTLV-III/LAV over time in patients with AIDS or at risk for AIDS. Science 232:1548-1553 (1986)

17. Hahn, B.H., Gonda, M.A., Shaw, G.M., et al., Genomic diversity of the acquired immune dificiency syndrome virus HTLV-III: Different viruses exhibit greatest divergence in their envelope genes. Proc Natl Acad Sci USA 82:4813-4817 (1985)

18. Robert-Guroff, M., Brown, M., Gallo, R.C., HTLV-III-neutralizing antibodies in patients with AIDS and AIDS-related complex. Nature 316:72-76 (1985)

19. Weiss, R.A., Clapham, P.R., Cheingsong-Popov, R., et al., Neutralization of human T-lymphotropic virus type III by sera of AIDS and AIDS-risk patients. Nature 316:69-72 (1985)

20. Coffin, J.M., Genetic variation in AIDS viruses. Cell 46:1-4 (1986)

21. Voynow, S.L., Coffin, J.M., Truncated gag-related proteins are produced by large deletion mutants of Rous sarcoma virus and form virus particles. J Virol 55:79-85 (1985)

22. Yoshinaka, Y., Katoh, I., Copeland, T.D., et al., Translational readthrough of an amber termination codon during synthesis of feline leukemia virus protease. J Virol 55:870-873 (1985)

23. Jacks, T., Varmus, H.E., Expression of the Rous sarcoma virus pol gene by ribosomal frameshifting. Science 230:1237-1242 (1985)

24. Kane, S.E., Beemon K., Precise localization of m^{6}A in Rous sarcoma virus RNA reveals clustering of methylation sites: Implications for RNA processing. Mol Cell Biol 5:2298-2306 (1985)

25. Coffin, J.M., Structure, replication and recombination of retrovirus genomes: some unifying hypotheses. J Gen Virol 42:1-26 (1979)

26. Donehower, L.A., Varmus, H.E., A mutant murine leukemia virus with a single missense codon in pol is defective in a function affecting integration. Proc Natl Acad Sci U.S.A. 81:6461-6465 (1984)

27. Duyk, G., Longiaru, M., Corinik, D., et al., Circles with two tandem long terminal repeats are specifically cleaved by pol gene-associated endonuclease from avian sarcoma and leukosis viruses: Nucleotide sequences required for site-specific cleavage. J Virol 56:589-599 (1985)

28. Panganiban, A.T., Temin, H.M., The terminal nucleotides of retrovirus DNA are required for integration but not virus production. Nature 306:155-161 (1983)

29. Panganiban, A.T., Temin, H.M., Circles with two tandem LTRs are precursors to integrated retrovirus DNAs. Cell 36:673-679 (1983)

30. Jones, K.A., Kadonaga, J.T., Luciw, P.A., et al., Activation of the AIDS retrovirus promoter by the cellular transcription factor, Spl. Science 232:755-759 (1986)

31. Chatis, P.A., Holland, C.A., Silver, J.E., et al., A 3' end fragment encompassing the transcriptional enhancers of nondefective Friend virus confers erythroleukemogenicity on Moloney leukemia virus. J Virol 52:248-254 (1984)

32. Rosen, C.A., Haseltine, W.A., Lenz, J., et al., Tissue selectivity of murine leukemia virus infection is determined by long terminal repeat sequences. J Virol 55:862-866 (1985)

33. Stocking, C., Kollek, R., Bergholz, U., et al., Point mutations in the U3 region of the longer terminal repeat of Moloney murine leukemia virus determine disease specificity of the myeloproliferative sarcoma virus. Virology 153:145-149 (1986)

34. Herman, S.A., Coffin, J.M., Differential transcription from the long terminal repeats of integrated avian leukosis virus DNA. J Virol (In press)

35. Miller, C.K., Temin, H.M., Insertion of several different DNAs in reticuloendotheliosis virus strain T suppresses transformation by reducing the amount of subgenomic DNA. J Virol 58:75-80 (1986)

36. Rabson, A.B., Daugherty, D.F., Venkatesan, S., et al., Transcription of novel open reading frames of AIDS retrovirus during infection of lymphocytes. Science 229:1388-1390 (1985)

37. Muesing, M.A., Smith, D.H., Cabradilla, C.O., Nucleic acid structure and expression of the human AIDS/lymphadenopathy retrovirus. Nature 313:450-458 (1985)

38. Sodroski, J.G., Rosen, C.A., Haseltine, W.A., Trans-acting transcriptional activation of the long terminal repeat of human T lymphotropic viruses in infected cells. Science 225:381-385 (1984)

39. Sodroski, J., Rosen, C., Goh, W.C., et al., A transcriptional activator protein encoded by the x-lor region of the human T-cell leukemia virus. Science 228:1430-1434 (1985)

40. Sodrowki, J.G., Goh, W.C., Rosen, C.A., et al., Trans-activation of the human T-cell leukemia virus long terminal repeat correlates with expression of the x-lor protein. J Virol 55:831-835 (1985)

41. Seiki, M., Hikioshi, A., Taniguchi, T., et al., Expression of the pX gene of HTLV-I: General splicing mechanism in the HTLV family. Science 228:1532-1534 (1985)

42. Rosen, C.A., Sodroski, J.G., Haseltine, W.A., Location of cis-acting regulatory sequences in the human T-cell leukemia virus type I long terminal repeat. Proc Natl Acad Sci U.S.A. 82:6502-6506 (1985)

43. Rosen, C.A., Sodroski, J.G., Kettman, R., et al., Activation of enhancer sequences in Type II human T-cell leukemia virus and bovine leukemia virus long terminal repeats to virus-associated trans-acting regulatory factors. J Virol 57:738-744 (1986)

44. Sodroski, J., Rosen, C., Wong-Staal, F., et al., Trans-acting transcriptional regulation of human T-cell leukemia virus type III long terminal repeat. Science 227:171-173 (1985)

45. Rosen, C.A., Sodroski, J.G., Goh, W.C., et al., Post-transcriptional regulation accounts for the trans-activation of the human T-lymphotropic virus type III. Nature 319:555-559 (1986)

46. Sodroski, J., Goh, W.C., Rosen, C., et al., A second post-transcriptional trans-activator gene required for HTLV-III replication. Nature 321:412-416 (1986)

47. Arya, S.K., Guo, C., Josephs, S.F., et al., Trans-activator gene of human T-lymphotropic virus type III (HTLV-III). Science 229:69-73 (1985)

48. Sodroski, J., Patarca, R., Rosen, C., et al., Location of the trans-activating region on the genome of human T-cell lymphotropic virus type III. Science 229:74-77 (1985)

49. Goh, W.C., Rosen, C., Sodroski, J. et al., Identification of a protein encoded by the trans activator gene tatIII of human T-cell lymphotropic retrovirus type III. J Virol 59:181-184 (1986)

50. Seigel, L.J., Ratner, L., Josephs, S.F., et al., Transactivation induced by human T-lymphotropic virus type III (HTLV-III) maps to a viral sequence encoding 58 amino acids and lacks tissue specificity. Virology 148:226-231 (1986)

51. Dayton, A.I., Sodroski, J.G., Rosen, C.A., et al., The trans-activator gene of the human T-cell lymphotropic virus type III is required for replication. Cell 44:941-947 (1986)

52. Keshet, E., Temin, H.M., Cell killing by spleen necrosis virus is correlated with a transient accumulation of spleen necrosis virus DNA. J Virol 31:376-388 (1979)

53. Mullins, J.I., Chen, C.S., Hoover, E.A., Disease-specific and tissue-specific production of unintegrated feline leukemia virus variant DNA in feline AIDS. Nature 319:333-336 (1986)

54. Shaw, G.M., Hahn, B.H., Arya, S.K., et al., Molecular characterization of human T-cell leukemia (lymphotropic) virus type III in the acquired immune deficiency syndrome. Science 226:165-1171 (1984)

55. Weller, S.K., Joy, A.E., Temin, H.M., Correlation between cell killing by members of some subgroups of avian leukosis virus and the transient accumulation of unintegrated linear viral DNA. J Virol 33:494-506 (1980)

56. Weller, S.K., Temin, H.M., Cell killing by avian leukosis viruses. J Virol 39:713-721 (1981)

57. Lifson, J.D., Reyes, G.R., McGrath, M.S., et al., AIDS retrovirus induced cytopathology: Giant cell formation and involvement of CD4 antigen. Science 232:1123-1127 (1986)

58. Sodroski, J., Goh, W.C., Rosen, C., et al., Role of the HTLV-III/LAV envelope in syncytium formation and cytopathicity. Nature 322:470-474 (1986)

59. Repaske, R., Steele, P.E., O'Neill, R.R., et al., Nucleotide sequence of a full-length human endogenous retroviral segment. J Virol 54:764-772 (1985)

60. Steele, P.E., Martin, M.A., Rabson, A.B., et al., Amplification and chromosomal dispersion of human endogenous retroviral sequences. J Virol 59:545-550 (1986)

61. Curran, J.W., Morgan, W.M., Hardy, A.M., et al., The epidemiology of AIDS: Current status and future prospects. Science 229:1352-1357 (1985)

62. Kanki, P.J., Barin, F., M'Boup, S., et al., New human T-lymphotropic retrovirus related to simian T-lymphotropic virus type III (STLV-IIIAGM). Science 232:238-243 (1986)

63. Kanki, P.J., Alroy, J., Essex, M., Isolation of T-lymphotropic retrovirus related to HTLV-III/LAV from wild-caught African green monkeys. Science 230:951-954 (1985)

64. Coffin, J.M., Tsichlis, P.N., Barker, C.S., et al., Variation in avian retrovirus genomes. Ann NY Acad Sci 354:410-425 (1980)

10

Feline Leukemia Virus: Current Status of the Feline Acquired Immune Deficiency Syndrome and Immunoprevention

Richard G. Olsen, Louis J. Lafrado, Mark G. Lewis, Lawrence E. Mathes, Keith Haffer, Richard Sharpee

Retrovirus-induced acquired immune deficiency has been recognized in numerous animal virus systems for more than a decade (1). These animal retroviruses, including feline leukemia virus (FeLV), murine leukemia virus (MuLV), and avian leukosis virus have as common outcomes of infection a loss of immune competence and induction of neoplasia. In depth investigations into retrovirus-mediated disease have, understandably, centered on the neoplastic aspects of infection. Immunosuppression, until recently, was viewed in terms of its contribution to tumor cell survival rather than as a disease entity in itself. The discovery of a retroviral etiology for the acquired immune deficiency syndrome (AIDS) in humans, however, has stimulated a re-examination of all retrovirus animal models for clues to understanding the pathogenesis, treatment and eventual prevention of this devastating human disease.

In this chapter we summarize what is known about the pathogenesis of immunosuppression in feline retrovirus infection in feline animal model systems. Because of the availability of numerous excellent reviews of the FeLV and FeLV diseases (1)-(5), this chapter will be restricted to those reports that focus on immunodeficiency related to FeLV and will introduce new data from our and other laboratories that may have important implications for retrovirus research in general, and for AIDS research in particular, especially for vaccine development.

IMMUNOLOGIC BASIS OF FELINE ACQUIRED IMMUNE DEFICIENCY SYNDROME (FAIDS)

Feline leukemia virus was first described by Jarrett et al. (6) in 1964. It was named in the tradition of other related oncornaviruses after the disease with which it was first identified. The name is unfortunate in that leukemia is perhaps the least frequent manifestation of virus infection (7). Far more prevalent are the non-neoplastic diseases caused by FeLV, including non-regenerative anemia, panleukopenia-like syndrome, thymic atrophy, hemolytic anemia and glomerulonephritis. FeLV-infected cats may display a complex clinical picture with one or more disease forms present.

Immunosuppression accompanies virtually all FeLV infections rendering the host susceptible to a myriad of opportunistic or pathogenic agents. An outcome of this "acquired immune deficiency" is the high rate of secondary viral, bacterial and parasitic infections associated with FeLV viremia in cats (8).

The association of opportunistic pathogens with FeLV infections was perhaps the first clue that FeLV viremic cats were immunodeficient (9)-(11). The actual description of the immunosuppressed state of viremic cats, however, emerged from allograft survival studies by Perryman et al. (12). The allograft rejection response in persistently infected kittens was delayed. This depressed cell mediated immune response correlated with severe thymic atrophy and paracortical lymphoid depletion.

Abrogation of immunity affects T- but not B-lymphocytes. With the onset of viremia, peripheral blood lymphocytes of cats do not respond normally to the T-lymphocyte mitogens and to the antigen keyhole limpet hemocyanin, whereas reactivity to staphylococcal protein A and to the B-cell mitogen lipopolysaccharide is comparable to uninfected cats (13)-(16). Similarly, concanavalin A receptor mobility on T-cells is depressed, while immunoglobulin receptor mobility on B-cells remains normal in viremic cats (17), (18). Dunlap et al. (17) found that cells could bind concanavalin A (Con A), but the normal capping response was inhibited. This suggested that the population of cells that was Con A responsive was either present and non-reactive or were not present. Grant et al. (19) established that an increased proportion of T cells was responsive to phytohemagglutinin in viremic cats. This observation again suggested that the lymphocyte population found in viremic cats was different from that in normal cats. This shift may be related to a selective loss or suppression of the Con A responsive T cells with a weaker suppression or increase in the phytohemagglutinin responsive population. Prior to these studies, Stiff and Olsen (20) had observed the loss of a short-lived suppressor cell function in viremic cats. This loss in suppressor function may explain the increase in responsive cells observed by Grant et al. (19).

Loss of cell function is not restricted to lymphocytes. Recent evidence from this laboratory has suggested a possible defect in the polymorphonuclear leukocyte (PMN) (21), a cell population responsible for host defense against bacterial and fungal diseases. This defect was demonstrated using a light release assay which measures the oxidative metabolic burst associated with stimulation of phagocytic cells by external factors. The activity is measured using a chemically enhanced luminescence or chemiluminescence (CL) (22). The chemiluminescence is the response of excited molecules returning to the ground state. Upon interaction with appropriate stimuli, neutrophils will undergo an oxidative metabolic burst with the subsequent generation of oxygen-derived radicals including superoxide anion, hypochlorite anion and hydroxyl radicals, all of which play a pivotal role in bacterial killing (22). Employing a luminogenic molecule, luminol, photons associated with the chemiluminescence response are quantifiable. The phagocytic chemiluminescence response has been proposed to be equivalent to the cells' cytocidal activity (23). Using this method, we have demonstrated a significant depression in the cytocidal activity of neutrophils from FeLV-infected cats compared to healthy controls (21). This depression of neutrophil function by FeLV may occur by two possible mechanisms: first, by direct infection of the granulocytic precursor cell by the virus, and/or second, by an association of the neutrophil with FeLV virions, viral proteins, or immune complexes. Alteration of neutrophil function has also been noted in retroviral diseases of human (AIDS) (24) and non-human (25) primates.

IMMUNOLOGIC STATUS OF FeLV CONVALESCENT CATS

The majority of cats exposed to FeLV resist infection and establish sound immunity to FeLV disease. However, cats with this status often have latent FeLV infection (26)-(29). Bone marrow cells may express FeLV-associated membrane antigen for a protracted period in the absence of detectable infectious virus in peripheral blood (30), and upon culturing in vitro, bone marrow cells often resume active virus production (26)-(29). Corticosteroid treatment of convalescent cats in vivo has in some cases activated latent infection in the bone marrow (27). The immunologic status of such cats is only now being thoroughly examined and much more research is necessary to define the long-term effects of latent FeLV infection.

As stated above, polymorphonuclear leukocytes from chronically infected cats show defective chemiluminescence and recent studies suggest that a defect in polymorphonuclear leukocyte function may continue to be present in a subpopulation of convalescent (non-viremic) FeLV-exposed cats. Lafrado and Olsen (31) have shown in time course experiments that cats recovering from a transient FeLV viremia exhibit a depression in in vitro polymorphonuclear leukocyte function during the viremic stage of infection that persists for at least one year post-infection. These data are important when considering the health status of cats with nonviremic (latent) FeLV infections. Our data suggest that there may exist a population of FeLV-exposed nonviremic cats which have successfully recovered from the initial insult but maintain a functional defect in the granulocytic cell lineage during the latent form of disease. This defect is plausible since the site of latent infection, according to the investigations of Rojko et al. (27), is predominantly the myelomonocytic precursors. Reduction in polymorphonuclear leukocyte phagocytic capacity may explain why a significant minority of FeLV-negative cats develop virus-negative (negative for expression of FeLV antigens) lymphosarcomas (32),(33). Twenty-nine percent of reported lymphosarcomas have been shown to be non-virus producers (33). Polymorphonuclear cell populations have been demonstrated to participate in tumor cell cytolysis by various investigators (34), (35). Hardy and his colleagues (33), as well as Neil and Onions (5), have suggested that nonproducer lymphosarcomas are a result of a "hit and run" effect of FeLV. Our data support this theory, but also suggest that the presence of nonproducer lymphosarcomas may be a consequence of decreased tumor surveillance by functionally incompetent neutrophils, and only indirectly related to FeLV infection.

PROPOSED MECHANISM OF FeLV-MEDIATED IMMUNOSUPPRESSION

A preponderance of data has accumulated to support at least three mechanisms of FeLV-mediated immunosuppression. Any one mechanism may function independently or in concert with others to render the infected animal severely immunosuppressed.

FeLV-Mediated Cytotoxicity

Thymic atrophy, lymphoid and myeloid depletion, hemolytic anemia, and/or non-regenerative anemia are common clinical findings in FeLV-viremic cats (7). Indeed, the clinical presentation of feline leukemia virus can be complex. FeLV-viremic cats may present with lymphoid cell depletion which may reverse to hyperplasia (36). Clinical manifestations are dependent in part upon the infecting subtype of FeLV, of which three (A,B,C) have been defined serologically.

Thymic atrophy is usually seen in FeLV-infected kittens and is often associated with a runting syndrome characterized by lymphoid depletion, retarded growth and opportunistic infection (7). Thymic atrophy may be a result, rather than a cause of immunosuppression, in that thymectomy does not leave kittens more susceptible to infection (37).

Lymphoid depletion is also a common clinical finding in FeLV-infected cats (4). Based on histological examination of lymphoid tissues, the T-cell dependent paracortical areas have the most pronounced lesions. Neutropenia and anemia are apparent outcomes of FeLV invasion of bone marrow where the virus grows well. FeLV infection can cause detectable cytolytic changes in myeloid, erythroid, and lymphoid progenitor cells. The outcome of infection is often depletion of cell populations which are essential for specific and non-specific host defenses.

Infected cats may have a form of disease in which aplastic anemia is characteristic (38). It has been proposed that aplastic anemia is a result of suppression of erythroid progenitors through a group C FeLV (FeLV-C) related cytolytic event in the bone marrow (39). Committed precursors of the granulocyte/macrophage cell lineage have also been shown to be depleted in cats infected with FeLV-C (36).

Cytolytic changes in FeLV infections may be due to an indirect effect on the rate of progenitor cell growth, through selected loss of a regulatory lymphocyte population. Alternatively, Hoover and colleagues (36) have shown that depletion of cortical follicular lymphocytes correlates with extinction of viral replication. These latter data suggest that pathogenesis is a result of a series of cytolytic events leading to depletion of the self-renewal capacity of lymphocytes.

Mullins et al. (40) have recently shown that the cytopathogenesis of FAIDS is closely associated with the presence of unintegrated FeLV viral DNA in bone marrow cells. This unintegrated viral DNA appears with the onset of FAIDS and has been shown to persist throughout the course of disease. These findings are significant in light of parallel observations in human AIDS (41). The occurrence of this variant of FeLV has been suggested to be a disease- and tissue-specific marker of FAIDS. Mullins attributes the mechanism of lymphocytotoxicity noted in feline AIDS to these unintegrated sequences in bone marrow cells.

In contrast, lymphomagenesis has recently been ascribed to FeLV proviral insertion within the c-myc region of feline DNA (42). Mullins et al. (43) have demonstrated viral transduction of the c-myc gene as etiologic in feline leukemias, a contrasting feature with the avian leukosis virus model in chickens in which transduction does not occur (44). The association of myc with FeLV results in myc activation which in turn results in the development of feline T-cell lymphomas.

FeLV-Associated Immunosuppressive Factors In Vitro

The observation that FeLV and FeLV p15E (an envelope protein) were immunosuppressive in vitro was made during research to develop a vaccine for this disease. Inactivated whole or disrupted FeLV, when used as an immunogen, proved to induce only a weak immune response in cats and was not protective against virulent virus challenge (45),(46). The combination of inactivated FeLV with FeLV-infected tumor cells promoted less of an immune response to antigens of FeLV than did tumor cells alone, and cats who received the combination were more susceptible to viral challenge with feline sarcoma virus than unvaccinated animals (47),(48). These studies suggested that FeLV, or a component of FeLV, was an active immunosuppressant.

These observations led us to examine FeLV for immunosuppressive factors and during these studies Hebebrand et al. (49) discovered that ultraviolet light-inactivated FeLV (UV-FeLV) was able to suppress cat lymphocytes. Additional studies using purified proteins from FeLV showed that a 15,000 dalton protein from the envelope of the virus was able to inhibit lectin and antigen-induced mitogenesis of both cat and human lymphocytes (50)-(52). These initial studies concentrated on such lymphocyte functions as lectin-induced mitogenesis (49),(52), antigen-induced mitogenesis (50), mixed lymphocyte reaction (53) and lectin receptor mobility (17),(54), all of which were found to be deficient in FeLV-infected cats and could be mimicked in vitro with UV-FeLV or FeLV-p15E. In vivo studies have also shown that both UV-FeLV and FeLV-p15E could suppress antibody development, presumably by an effect on T-helper lymphocytes (48),(52).

Since our first reports of in vitro suppression of lymphocyte function by FeLV and FeLV-p15E, a number of other retrovirus isolates have been tested similarly. To date, all retrovirus isolates tested show some degree of immunosuppression in an inactivated state (55)-(64). In general, most of these studies have concentrated on T-lymphocyte function. Limited investigations have been performed to test the effect of retroviruses on B-cell function. These studies have found that disrupted retroviruses have no direct effect on B-lymphocyte function tested either in vitro (18),(65) or in vivo (66). Cianciolo et al. (64) were the first to show that disrupted murine retroviruses could inhibit cells other than lymphocytes, demonstrating that disrupted Rauscher or Friend leukemia viruses (RLV) (FLV) could inhibit not only lymphocyte blastogenesis, but also macrophage chemotaxis, both in vitro and in vivo. These studies suggested that the observed in vitro retroviral suppression may not be cell-type specific. We have recently expanded our research to determine other cell types that may be affected by inactivated FeLV and FeLV-p15E. Wellman et al. (67) reported that FeLV and FeLV-p15E inhibited erythroid colony formation. These authors found that FeLV and FeLV-p15E were able to inhibit erythroid precursor cell proliferation selectively while having no effect on granulocyte macrophage progenitors. Lewis et al. (21) and Lafrado et al. (68) reported a loss in neutrophil chemiluminescence during FeLV infections and in normal neutrophils incubated with FeLV or FeLV-p15E. These findings may explain the observed increase in opportunistic bacterial infections observed in FeLV-infected cats. Basu et al. (69) have reported that FeLV and FeLV-p15E are able to inhibit human natural killer (NK) cell cytolysis, but not binding of NK cells to the target cells.

Cianciolo et al. (70),(71) showed that spontaneous and carcinogen-induced murine malignant cells synthesize a protein that is physiochemically and antigenically similar to retroviral p15E. Its immunosuppressive activity was identical to p15E in its ability to inhibit macrophage function. Since individuals with cancer have been shown to have abnormal immune responses, they examined human cancerous effusions for substances similar to p15E (72). They found that monocyte functions were blocked by a substance(s) present in the effusions and that this activity could be inhibited by monoclonal antibodies directed toward murine p15E. In addition, selected human malignant and mitogen-transformed cells were screened by indirect immunofluorescence with the anti-p15E monoclonal antibodies and both cell types were found to express a p15E related antigen (73). These studies suggest that a p15E-like protein may be present in many tumor cells, potentially disturbing the host's immune system. This also suggests that retroviruses may have, at some point in their evolution, acquired the gene for p15E production and incorporated it into their genome. Also, the expression of a p15E-like molecule by normal dividing cells suggests that it may be a control protein for normal cells (74).

The existence of an immunosuppressive transmembrane protein on all retroviral envelopes has led Cianciolo et al. (75) to determine if the protein molecules from different retroviral isolates contain conserved amino acid sequences. They found that the transmembrane component from a number of retroviruses including human T-cell leukemia virus I (HTLV-I), FeLV, bovine leukemia virus and murine leukemia virus all contain regions with significant homologies. They synthesized a 17 amino acid peptide that contains a conserved sequence and found that it could inhibit lymphocyte mitogenesis by an interleukin-2 (IL-2) dependent mechanism (75) and inhibit monocyte respiratory bursts (76). This peptide should be useful in providing a new means of investigating the mechanisms of retroviral induced immunosuppression.

The mechanism by which disrupted retroviruses or the envelope p15E protein cause suppression is not known, but previous studies have suggested that the cause may be a disruption of normal cellular signals at or near the cellular membrane surface. The loss of T-cell function associated with retroviral presence suggests a specific inhibition of a T-cell factor. Copelan et al. (77) found that IL-2 production and responses were inhibited by FeLV and FeLV-p15E, without associated changes in macrophage production of interleukin-I (IL-I), suggesting a specific action of FeLV on T-cell proliferation at the IL-2 level. Orosz et al. (78),(79) carried these studies further using a murine system. They showed that FeLV and FeLV-p15E not only blocked lymphocyte proliferation but, in addition, were associated with a reduction in the generation of cytotoxic T-cell activity. This loss was only observed if the virus or p15E was present during the time of initial allogeneic cell exposure. Once the cells were committed, the virus had no effect on their cytolytic action. They found that FeLV or FeLV-p15E could inhibit IL-2 stimulated growth of an IL-2 dependent cell line in a similar fashion to that observed by Copelan et al. (77). Although FeLV or FeLV-p15E must be present during the induction phase of the assay to have an immunosuppressive effect, they need be present for only six hours in the 48 hour assay. Further studies showed that FeLV had no effect on the IL-2 molecule or its binding, but was able to inhibit the IL-2 signal from entering the cell. Also, lymphocytes in the presence of FeLV could not be stimulated to produce IL-2, but lymphocytes previously committed to IL-2 production were not affected by the presence of this virus. In addition, gamma interferon production was inhibited by FeLV in vitro (79), and in vivo (80) in FeLV-infected cats. Basu et al. (69) have found that FeLV and FeLV-p15E are able to inhibit human natural killer (NK) cells and lymphokine activated killer (LAK) cell cytotoxicity, without having any effect on the binding of these cells to their target populations. Similar effects have been observed in the murine NK system (81) and in NK cells derived from human AIDS patients (82). These studies again suggest that p15E may exert its effect by interfering directly with the passage of an exogenous signal into a cell through the surface membrane, or possibly by indirectly inhibiting the surface membrane mobility, thereby inhibiting further cell functions.

The immunosuppression attributed to retroviral p15E mirrors the suppression associated with high prostaglandin E_2 (PGE_2) levels in cell culture. Lewis et al. (83) attempted to determine if FeLV or FeLV-p15E mediated its effect by stimulating an increase in prostaglandin production. Instead, they found that both prostaglandin inhibitors, such as aspirin and indomethacin, and PGE_2 itself could reverse the FeLV-associated suppression of Con A-stimulated mitogenesis and capping (18),(83). Further studies demonstrated that FeLV actually inhibited production of PGE_2 by purified monocytes in vitro (83). These observations suggest that prostaglandins are not directly associated with FeLV mediated immunosuppression.

Indeed, a common factor among the various drugs and chemicals found to reverse FeLV suppression of Con A stimulation of lymphocytes (i.e., colchicine (54), indomethacin or PGE_2) (17),(83) is that they all cause an increase in cAMP levels in cells (84)-(86). Using other drugs known to increase cAMP levels, Lewis et al. (87) were able to reverse the FeLV suppression of Con A-stimulated mitogenesis. These drugs include specific adenylate cyclase activators, forskolin, $GppNH_2$, cholera toxin, NaF and a cAMP analog, dibutryl cAMP. Drugs shown to inhibit phosphodiesterase, the enzyme used to degrade cAMP, were found to have no effect. These findings suggest that FeLV-p15E may have at least part of its effect by interfering with cAMP production, which is a central component of the second messenger system used for signal transfers across the cell surface membrane. If p15E is able to inhibit exogenous signal transfers by interference with cAMP production, many essential cellular processes would be disrupted.

Preliminary studies using the calcium ionophore A23187 indicate that p15E is able to inhibit Ca^{2+} ion from crossing into the cell. Lafrado et al. (68) have found that FeLV-p15E is able to inhibit activation of neutrophils by A23187. This activation occurs when the inophore allows Ca^{2+} ions to cross the cell membrane. This indicates that the inhibitory action of p15E on A23187 stimulation of neutrophils may be calcium associated. Calcium is a critical component for all known cellular signal transport mechanisms; without Ca^{2+}, a cell would appear to be unresponsive, analogous to the effect of p15E. As to why some cells are sensitive to p15E (e.g. T-lymphocyte) and others are not (e.g. B-lymphocyte), is still an open question.

FeLV-Associated Immunosuppressive Factors In Vivo

The immunosuppressive sequelae of FeLV viremia have been attributed, to some degree, to the presence of soluble serum factors that are either not of viral origin or not exclusively so. Variously identified as antibodies, free tumor antigen (in cats with tumors), or antigen-antibody complexes, these factors have been collectively referred to as "specific blocking factors" (SBF) (88). In humans, the presence of SBF in the serum has been reported to interfere with an effective immune response against tumor progression even in the presence of sensitized lymphocytes (89),(90). The exact composition of SBF remains unclear. Nelson et al. (91) have suggested that SBF are not antibodies but are immunosuppressive molecules produced by T-cells.

A considerable effort has been made to describe these factors and their effects in the feline leukemia model. Cockerell et al. (14) reported that serum from FeLV-infected cats suppressed Con A-induced blastogenesis of cat lymphocytes in vitro. Jones et al. (92) proposed that circulating immune complexes (CIC) were responsible for the immunosuppression noted in FeLV infections and demonstrated that removal of CIC through extracorporeal immunoadsorption resulted in clinical improvement in a significant number of treated cats. Removal of CIC from the serum of FeLV-viremic cats has also significantly improved humoral immune responses to FeLV (93),(94).

An alternative approach for determining the significance of soluble immunosuppressive factors was taken by Lewis et al. (21). These investigators exposed neutrophils from FeLV-free cats to latex beads previously opsonized with serum from either FeLV-viremic cats or healthy cats. They observed a significant suppression in latex bead-induced chemiluminescence when viremic serum was used as opsonin. Neutrophils from normal cats incubated with latex beads opsonized with FeLV-viremic serum responded in a range from 8% to 64% of the results obtained from the same cells incubated with beads opsonized with control serum. In titration experiments using viremic serum and normal serum, neutrophil chemiluminescence responses decreased with increasing concentration of viremic serum. While this experiment did not describe the nature of the serum factor present, a number of possibilities are suggested. A species of molecules similar to those suggested by Nelson et al. (91) may account for the suppression of chemiluminescence through blocking of neutrophil Fc receptors, thereby inhibiting neutrophil-IgG interaction. Alternatively, hypocomplementemia has been proposed to be responsible for the depression of neutrophil chemiluminescence responses (95) with loss of activation potential of neutrophil complement component receptors. The strongest candidates, however, are aberrant antigen-antibody complexes (CIC). Starkebaum et al. (96) demonstrated that CIC reduced the phagocytic capacity of human neutrophils. More recently, Verder et al. (97) have also described the effects of immune complexes on cytotoxic effector cell function in late-onset rubella syndrome. These authors demonstrated that removal of CIC improved both killer and natural killer cell functions with improvement in the condition of treated patients.

The role of CIC and/or SBF in feline leukemia disease remains an open question. Determination of the exact nature of these factors will be necessary to understand their role in the immunopathogenesis of FeLV infection.

IMMUNOTHERAPY AND IMMUNOPREVENTION

Ex Vivo Adsorption

As mentioned, immunosuppression in FeLV-infected cats may be accounted for, at least in part, by the presence of high levels of CIC or other SBF. CIC also have the potential to cause pathological lesions in other organ systems (98). Thus, efforts have been made to remove these CIC/SBF from the plasma.

Jones et al. (92) were the first to report the use of *Staphylococcus aureus* Cowan I in the removal of CIC through ex vivo immunoadsorption in FeLV infected cats. Protein A, found in the cell wall of the Cowan I strain *S. aureus* (99), possesses a number of biologically important activities. Prominent among these is the ability to bind with high affinity and avidity to the Fc region of immunecomplexed immunoglobulin G (IgG) from many animal species (100). This property of staphylococcal protein A has generated much interest in its use as a tool in immunotherapy. Jones et al. (92) perfused plasma of FeLV-viremic cats over a strain of this staphylococcus species, after the organism had been heat-killed and formalin-stabilized. This treatment was associated with clinical improvement in three of five FeLV-infected cats. The concentration of CIC in the serum of FeLV-infected cats was reduced with the concomitant removal of a presumptive immunoinhibiting factor (i.e., an antigen-antibody complex or another suppressor factor).

Subsequent to this preliminary observation, other evidence was reported supporting the efficacy of staphylococcal protein A as immunotherapy for FeLV-infected cats. Liu et al. (101),(102) demonstrated dramatic improvement in FeLV-infected cats when treated with this substance by ex vivo and in vivo immunoadsorption. Their studies indicated induction of cytotoxic antibody to FeLV protein gp70 by the ex vivo regimen. In addition, these authors reported remission of leukemia and loss of FeLV viremia in in vivo treatments with purified staphylococcal protein A. Induction of circulating gamma-IFN and complement-dependent cytotoxic antibodies was also noted. Relapse occurred, however, upon cessation of immunotherapy.

Snyder et al. (103) have suggested that perfusion of cat plasma over SPA stimulates increased titers of anti-FeLV antibody. Clearance of FeLV viremia was shown to correlate well with increased antibody titers to FeLV gp70. More recently, Harper et al. (104) have demonstrated that infusion of purified SPA results in an antitumor response in lymphosarcoma-bearing FeLV-infected cats. These results were supported by previous reports suggesting that staphylococcal protein A injections had an antitumor effect in canine mammary carcinoma (105). The tumor regression induced by staphylococcal protein A was transient with all tumors returning to pretreatment status, after discontinuing staphylococcal protein A treatment.

The precise mechanism of the immunomodulation induced by staphylococcal protein A is not known. However, a number of theories, in addition to CIC removal have been proposed. We postulate that the presence of CIC provides a negative feedback signal, thereby suppressing polyclonal activation of B-cells. Therefore, as a B-cell mitogen (106), staphylococcal protein A could activate the humoral immune response directly as well as through immunoadsorption and removal of CIC (negative feedback). Alternative hypotheses have suggested that the important factors are the reduction in viral antigen load, nonspecific immune stimulation, or removal of antibody regulating molecules such as anti-idiotype antibodies (103),(107).

Harper et al. (104) recently reported that direct intravenous infusion of staphylococcal protein A was associated with regression of lymphosarcoma in FeLV infected cats in the absence of a detectable antiviral immune reaction as indicated by lack of an increase in alpha and beta IFN levels. These data contrast with those of Liv et al. (102) (described above) who administered staphylococcal protein A into the peritoneal cavity. The reason for the discrepant findings is unknown, but recent data accumulated in this laboratory support some of the observations of Harper and colleagues (104). Intraperitoneal injection of staphylococcal protein A twice weekly for eight weeks failed to induce an antiviral immune response in the form of alpha- or beta-IFN. Harper et al. (104) reported an increase in absolute neutrophil count in the 24 hours following infusion of staphylococcal protein A with a return to pre-infusion levels after 24 hours. Our results (108) indicate that intraperitoneal injection of purified staphylococcal protein A results in granulocytosis in peripheral blood samples 48 hours after injection. Cats undergoing this therapy yielded neutrophils capable of producing a normal chemiluminescence response. The reason for this return to normal chemiluminescence response is not clear. If it is assumed that every stem cell is not FeLV-infected, then it is possible that staphylococcal protein A infusion results in recruitment of committed granulocyte progenitors which are uninfected with FeLV, resulting in an increase in virus-free neutrophils in the peripheral blood. Liu et al. (102) also reported improvement in bone marrow cytology during and after treatment with staphylococcal protein A. Improvement in in vitro lymphocyte activation has been observed when human lymphocytes were incubated with autologous serum treated with staphylococcal protein A (109).

While immunotherapy of FeLV-infected cats has shown promise, the efficacy of this modality as sole treatment of retroviral disease remains questionable. The lack of a clear understanding of the mechanism of FeLV-induced immunopathogenesis will delay development of a successful therapeutic regimen.

Vaccine for Feline Leukemia

The development of a protective immune response against FeLV provides life-long immunity to subsequent exposure to the virus. The protective immune response has been determined to consist of a humoral response towards both viral proteins and viral-related neoplastic disease (110). In addition, it is likely that a strong cell-mediated response against FeLV-infected cells is elicited, although none has been documented to date. The level of antibody directed towards the viral-associated antigens found on FeLV transformed cells correlates with protection against tumor development (11). In addition, high levels of virus-neutralizing antibody have been shown to protect cats against viral exposure (110), even when the antibody is colostral or received as passive immunotherapy (111)-(119). These findings indicate that a vaccine for FeLV needs to generate two types of humoral responses in the host; first, a strong antiviral response that will inhibit initial exposure, and second, a strong anti-tumor response to remove FeLV-infected cells.

Early vaccine preparations consisted of killed, or live attenuated FeLV. The preparations containing killed FeLV failed to induce protective levels of neutralizing antibodies or to protect from tumor development (45),(46),(117),(118). In fact, Schaller et al. (46) found that killed FeLV vaccinated cats were more susceptible to subsequent challenge with live FeLV than the non-vaccinated controls. These studies foreshadowed the findings that FeLV-p15E caused immunosuppression in vivo and in vitro. A live attenuated vaccine studied by Jarrett and co-workers (119) proved to be effective in inhibiting persistent infections in adult cats, but not in preventing the establishment of latent infections. In addition, the vaccine strain proved to be pathogenic to weaning kittens (118). Purified subunits of virus were even less effective at generating a protective response. Salerno et al. (120) showed that purified FeLV gp70 was ineffective at eliciting a protective immune response in cats, although guinea pigs responded well. However, recently Nunberg et al. (121) determined a 14 amino acid sequence in FeLV gp70 that specifically interacts with neutralizing antibody for all known FeLV subgroups.

In an attempt to generate a strong anti-tumor response, Jarrett et al. (119) inoculated four month-old kittens with the lymphoid tumor cell line FL-74, which is a producer of large quantities of Kawakami-Theilen-FeLV. These cats developed strong anti-tumor and anti-viral responses. However, this vaccine was pathogenic to neonatal kittens and the use of a live tumor cell as a vaccine proved to be unmarketable. In order to circumvent this problem, Olsen et al. (47),(48) and Heding et al. (122) used killed FL-74 cells as the immunogen. These preparations proved effective at eliciting good anti-tumor responses, but were unable to inhibit the development of persistent viremia upon challenge. The mixing of the killed FL-74 cells with inactivated FeLV proved to be even less effective, causing an increase in tumor development and death as compared to cats receiving the tumor cells alone (48).

The failure of inactivated virus or killed tumor cells to induce protective immunity led Olsen and his co-workers to concentrate on manipulating the FL-74 cells to induce release of FeLV-related antigens. Olsen et al. (123) had previously shown that the FeLV antigens cycled on the cell surface during the cell cycle. They theorized that the antigens were released into the medium and could be collected. Wolff et al. (124) determined that the tumor-related antigens could in fact be recovered from the culture fluids. Using these concentrated culture fluids, Lewis et al. (125) found that immunized cats developed good antibody responses towards FeLV tumor antigens and, in addition, good responses were observed to all of the viral structural proteins. Upon challenge, over 80% of the vaccinated animals were protected against persistent viremia and tumor development. The protection was afforded to cats of 12 weeks of age or older. Since this report, the process has been further refined by Norden Laboratories, Lincoln, NE, and is now available commercially, with continued field testing showing it to be safe and effective.

Recently, Mastro et al. (126) reported that cats immunized with this vaccine develop an antibody reacting with a 70 Kd protein present in the preparation which appears distinct, but related to, FeLV gp70. Although analysis of the vaccine preparation showed that it seemed to contain all of the proteins present in the mature virus, vaccinated cats generated a poor antibody response to purified proteins isolated directly from the virus. Upon in vivo challenge, however, vaccinated cats developed a rapid antibody response to purified viral protein. The investigators theorized that the viral protein present within the vaccine preparation may be different in conformation from that found in the mature virion. This argument is strengthened by the observation that the vaccine preparation is not immunosuppressive, even though p15E moieties are present and can be detected by monoclonal antibodies. Olsen et al. (127) speculated that the vaccine may contain env gene products that are either unprocessed, or in some way altered, allowing for the presence of p15E, without its immune-interfering effects.

For the vaccine to be effective in protecting cats from FeLV, it must be able to inhibit the establishment of a latent FeLV infection in bone marrow or other cells. Sharpee et al. (128) have studied the effects of vaccination on the establishment of latent infection. In their study, twelve vaccinated cats were challenged with Rickard-FeLV. These cats were protected from viremia and latent infections as tested by the method of Rojko et al. (20). In summary, these studies offer promising results and suggest that vaccination will be protective against any of the known disease syndromes associated with FeLV infection, including latency.

CONCLUSION

Feline leukemia and feline leukemia virus provide excellent opportunities for the evaluation of retroviral immunopathogenesis. This review has provided a basis for an understanding of current knowledge and future directions in the field. Most importantly research efforts in vaccine development for FeLV have provided both a precedent and a paradigm for development of vaccines in other retroviral diseases, such as human immunodeficiency virus (HIV) infection. Our data indicate that the development of vaccines for retroviral pathogens are indeed possible and practical.

ACKNOWLEDGMENTS

This research was supported in part by NCI grants CA-30338, CA-31547 and The American Cancer Society grant IN-16Y.

REFERENCES

1. Bendinelli, M., Matteucci, D., Friedman, H., Retrovirus-induced acquired immunodeficiency. Adv. Cancer Res 45:125-81 (1985)

2. Cerny, J., Essex, M., Mechanisms of immunosuppression by oncogenic RNA viruses. In: Naturally Occurring Biological Immunosuppressive Factors and Their Relationship to Disease (Neubauer, R., ed), CRC Press, Boca Raton, FL, p 233-256 (1979)

3. Olsen, R.G., Feline Leukemia. CRC Press, Boca Raton, FL (1981)

4. Rojko, J.L., Olsen, R.G., The immunobiology of the feline leukemia virus. Vet Immunol Immunopathol 6:107-165 (1984)

5. Neil, J.C., Onions, D.E., Feline leukemia viruses: Molecular biology and pathogenesis. Anticancer Res 5:49-64 (1985)

6. Jarrett, W.F.H., Crawford, E.M., Martin, W.B., et al., A virus-like particle associated with leukemia (lymphosarcoma). Nature (Lond) 202:567-569 (1964)

7. Hause, W.R., Olsen, R.G., Clinical aspects of feline leukemia disease. In: Feline Leukemia (Olsen, R.G., ed) CRC Press, Boca Raton, FL, p 89-114 (1981)

8. Cotter, S.M., Hardy, W.D., Jr., Essex, M., Association of feline leukemia virus with lymphosarcoma and other disorders in the cat. J Am Vet Med Assoc 166:449-454 (1985)

9. Hardy, W.D., Jr., Old, L.J., Hess, P.W., et al., Horizontal transmission of feline leukemia virus. Nature 244:266-269 (1973)

10. Jarrett, W., Jarrett, O., Mackey, L., et al., Horizontal transmission of leukemia virus and leukemia in the cat. J Natl Cancer Inst 51:833-841 (1973)

11. Essex, M., Sliski, A., Cotter, S.M., et al., Immunosurveillance of naturally occurring feline leukemia. Science 190: 790-792 (1975)

12. Perryman, L.E., Hoover, E.A., Yohn, D.S., Immunologic reactivity of the cat: Immunosuppression in experimental feline leukemia. J Natl Cancer Inst 49:1357-1365 (1972)

13. Cockerell, G.L., Hoover, E.A., Krakowka, S., Lymphocyte mitogen reactivity and enumeration of circulating B- and T-cells during feline leukemia virus infection in the cat. J Natl Cancer Inst 47:1995-1999 (1976)

14. Cockerell, G.L., Hoover, E.A., Inhibition of normal lymphocyte mitogenic reactivity by serum from feline leukemia virus-infected cats. Cancer Res 37:3985-3989 (1976)

15. Cockerell, G.L., Krakowka, S., Hoover, E.A., Characterization of feline T- and B-lymphocytes and identification of an experimentally induced T-cell neoplasm in the cat. J Natl Cancer Inst 57:907-913 (1976)

16. Rojko, J.L., Hoover, E.A., Finn, B.L., et al., Characterization and mitogenesis of feline lymphocyte populations. Int Arch Allergy Appl Immunol 68:226-232 (1982)

17. Dunlap, J.E., Nichols, W.S., Hebebrand, L.C., et al., Mobility of lymphocyte surface membrane concancavalin A receptors of normal and feline leukemia virus-infected viremic felines. Cancer Res 39:956-959 (1979)

18. Lewis, M.G., Fertel, R.H., Olsen, R.G., The reversal of feline retrovirus-induced suppression of lymphcoyte Con A receptor mobility by indomethacin and PGE_2. Leukemia Res 9:1105-1109 (1985)

19. Grant, C.K., Ernisse, B.J., Pontefract, R., Comparison of feline leukemia virus-infected and normal cat T-cell lines in interleukin 2-conditioned medium. Cancer Res 44:498-502 (1984)

20. Stiff, M.I., Olsen, R.,G., Loss of the short-lived suppressive function of peripheral leukocytes in feline retrovirus-infected cats. J Clin Lab Immunol 7:133-138 (1982)

21. Lewis, M.G., Duska, G.O., Stiff, M.I., et al., Polymorphonuclear leukocyte dysfunction associated with feline leukemia virus infection. J Gen Virol 67:2113-2118 (1986)

22. Allred, C.D., Margets, J., Hill, H.P., Lumino-induced neutrophil chemiluminescence. Biochim Biophys Acta 631:380-385 (1980)

23. Sassada, M., Johnston, R.B., Macrophage microbicidal activity. Correlation between phagocytosis-associated oxidative metabolism and the killing of candida by macrophages. J Exp Med 152:85-98 (1980)

24. Ras, G.J., Eftychis, H.A., Anderson, R., et al., Mononuclear and polymorphonuclear leukocyte dysfunction in male homosexuals with acquired immunodeficiency syndrome (AIDS). S Afr Med J 66:806-809 (1984)

25. Gardner, M.B., Personal communication. (1986)

26. Post, S.F., Warren, L., Reactivation of latent feline leukemia virus. Developments in cancer research, In: Feline Leukemia Virus (Hardy, W.D.J., Essex, M., McClelland, A.J., eds) Elseviers - Holland, New York, p 151-158 (1980)

27. Rojko, J.L., Hoover, E.A., Quackenbush, S.L., et al., Reactivation of latent feline leukemia virus infection. Nature 298:385-388 (1982)

28. Madewell, B.L., Jarrett, O., Recovery of feline leukemia virus from non-viremic cats. Vet Rec 112:399-442 (1983)

29. Pedersen, N.C., Meric, S.M., Ho., E., et al., The clinical significance of latent feline leukemia virus infection in cats. Feline Pract 14:32-48 (1984)

30. Rice, J.B., Olsen, R.G., Feline oncovirus-associated cell membrane antigen and feline leukemia virus group-specific antigen expression in bone marrow and serum. J Natl Cancer Inst 66:737-743 (1981)

31. Lafrado, L.J., Olsen, R.G., Demonstration of depressed polymorphonuclear leukocyte function in non-viremic FeLV infected cats. Cancer Invest 4:297-300 (1986)

32. Hardy, W.D., Jr., Zuckerman, E., McClelland, H.W., et al., The immunology and epidemiology of FeLV non-producer feline lymphosarcoma. In: Viruses and Naturally Occurring Cancers, 7th Gold Spring Harbor Conference on Cell Proliferation (Essex, M., Todaro, G.J., zur Hausen, H., eds), Cold Spring Harbor Press, Cold Spring Harbor, NY, p 677-698 (1980)

33. Hardy, W.D., Jr., McClelland, A.J., Zuckerman, E.E., et al., Development of virus non-producer lymphosarcomas in pet cats exposed to FeLV. Nature 288:90-92 (1980)

34. Lichtenstein, A., Spontaneous tumor cytolysis mediated by inflammatory neutrophils: Dependence upon divalent cations and reduced oxygen intermediates. Blood 67:657-665 (1986)

35. Lichtenstein, A., Kahle, J., Anti-tumor effect of inflammatory neutrophils: Characteristics of in vivo generation and in vitro tumor cell lysis. Int J Cancer 35:121-127 (1985)

36. Hoover, E.A., Mullins, J.I., Quackenbush, S.L., et al., Pathogenesis of feline retrovirus-induced cytopathic diseases: Acquired immune deficiency syndrome and aplastic anemia. In: Animal Models of Retrovirus Infection and Their Relationship to AIDS (Salzman, L.E., ed), Academic Press, Orlando, p 59-74 (1986)

37. Hoover, E.A., Krakowka, S., Cockerell, G.L., et al., Influence of thymectomy on the susceptibility of cats to feline leukemia virus and lymphosarcoma. Am J Vet Res 39:393-395 (1978)

38. Mackey, L., Jarrett, W., Jarrett, O., et al., Anemia associated with feline leukemia infections in cats. J Natl Cancer Inst 54:209-217 (1973)

39. Gasper, P.W., Hoover, E.A., Feline leukemia virus strain-specific abatement of erythroid burst-forming units (BFU-e). In: Leukemia Reviews International (Rich, M.E., ed), Marcell Decker, New York, Vol 1, p.71-72 (1983)

40. Mullins, J.I., Chen, C.S., Hoover, E.A., Disease-specific and tissue-specific production of unintegrated feline leukemia virus variant DNA in feline AIDS. Nature 319:333-336 (1986)

41. Shaw, G.M., Hahn, B.H., Arya, S.K., et al., Molecular characterization of human T-cell leukemia (lymphotropic) virus type III in the acquired immune deficiency syndrome. Science 226: 1165-1171 (1984)

42. Levy, L.S., Gardner, M.B., Casey, J.W., Isolation of a feline leukemia provirus containing the oncogene myc from a feline lymphosarcoma. Nature 308:853-856 (1984)

43. Mullins, J.I., Brody, D.S., Bimari, R.C., Jr., et al., Viral transduction of c-myc gene in naturally occurring feline leukemias. Nature 308:856-858 (1984)

44. Payne, G., Bishop, J.M., Varmus, H.E., Multiple arrangements of viral DNA and an activated host oncogene (c-myc) in bursal lymphomas. Nature 295:209-213 (1982)

45. Yohn, D.S., Olsen, R.G., Schaller, J.P., et al., Experimental oncornavirus vaccines in the cat. Cancer Res 36:646-651 (1976)

46. Schaller, J.P., Hoover, E.A., Olsen, R.G., Active and passive immunization of cats with inactivated feline oncornavirus. J Natl Cancer Inst 59:1441-1450 (1977)

47. Olsen, R.G., Hoover, E.A., Mathes, L.E., et al., Immunization against feline oncornavirus disease using a killed tumor cell vaccine. Cancer Res 36:3642-3646 (1976)

48. Olsen, R.G., Hoover, E.A., Schaller, J.P., et al., Abrogation of resistance to feline oncornavirus disease by immunization with killed feline leukemia virus. Cancer Res 37:2082-2085 (1977)

49. Hebebrand, L.C., Mathes, L.E., Olsen, R.G., Inhibition of concanavalin A stimulation of feline lymphocytes by inactivated feline leukemia virus. Cancer Res 37:4532-4533 (1977)

50. Hebebrand, L.C., Olsen, R.G., Mathes, L.E., et al., Inhibition of human lymphocyte mitogen and antigen response by a 15,000 dalton protein from feline leukemia virus. Cancer Res 39:443-447 (1979)

51. Mathes, L.E., Olsen, R.G., Hebebrand, L.C., et al., Abrogation of lymphocyte blastogenesis by a feline leukemia virus protein. Nature 274:687-688 (1978)

52. Mathes, L.E., Olsen, R.G., Hebebrand, L.C., et al., Immunosuppressive properties of a virion polypeptide, a 15,000 dalton protein from feline leukemia virus. Cancer Res 39:950-955 (1979)

53. Stiff, M.I., Olsen, R.G., Effect of retroviral protein on the one-way mixed lymphocyte reaction. J Gen Virol 64:957-959 (1983)

54. Nichols, W.S., Dunlap, J.E., Mathes, L.E., et al., Retrovirus immunosuppression in vitro: Evidence for possible cytoskeletal involvement in lymphocyte surface membrane-related abnormalities. Immunol Lett 1:67-71 (1979)

55. Fowler, A.K., Twardzik, D.R., Reed, C.D., et al., In vitro cellular immune suppression by C-type virion protein. Cancer Res 37:4529-4531 (1977)

56. Denner, J., Wunderlick, V., Bierwolf, O., Suppression of human lymphocyte mitogen response by disrupted primate retrovirus of type C and type D. Acta Biol Med Ger 39:19-26 (1980)

57. Hellman, A., Fowler, A.K., Twardzik, D.R., et al., Abolition of lymphocyte blastogenesis by oncornaviral components. In: Macrophages and Lymphocytes (Escobar, M.R., and Friedman, H., eds), Plenum, New York, Part B, p 99-109 (1980)

58. Denner, J., Wunderlick, V., Bierwolf, D., Suppression of human lymphocyte mitogen response by proteins of the type D retrovirus PMFV. Int J Cancer 37:311-316 (1986)

59. Israel, E., Yu, M., Wainberg, M.A., Non-specific effects of avian retrovirus co-incubated on lymphocyte function: abrogation of antigen-and mitogen-induced proliferative responsiveness. Immunology 38:41-50 (1979)

60. Langweiler, M., Cockerell, G.L., DeNoronha, F., Role of suppressor cells in feline leukemia virus-associated immunosuppression. Cancer Res 43:1957-1960 (1983)

61. Wainberg, M.A., Israel, E., Viral inhibition of lymphocyte mitogens. I. Evidence for the nonspecificity of the effect. J Immunol 124:64-70 (1980)

62. Wainberg, M.A., Spira, B., Boushira, M., et al., Inhibition by human T lymphotropic virus (HTLV-I) of T-lymphocyte mitogenesis: failure of exogenous T-cell growth factor to restore responsiveness to lectin. Immunology 54:1-7 (1985)

63. Weislow, O.S., Fisher, O.V., Twardzek, D.R., et al., Depression of mitogen-induced lymphocyte blastogenesis by baboon endogenous retrovirus-associated components. Proc Soc Exp. Biol 166:522-527 (1981)

64. Cianciolo, G.J., Mathews, T.J., Bolognesi, D.P., et al., Macrophage accumulation in mice is inhibited by low molecular weight products from murine leukemia virus. J Immunol 124: 2900-2905 (1980)

65. Mathes, L.E., Olsen, R.G., Immunobiology of feline leukemia virus disease. In: Feline Leukemia (Olsen, R.G., ed), CRC Press, Boca Raton, FL, p 77-88 (1981)

66. Trainin, Z., Wernicke, P., Urgar-Waror, H., et al., Suppression of the humoral antibody response on natural retrovirus infections. Science 220:858-859 (1983)

67. Wellman, M.L., Kociba, G.J., Lewis, M.G., et al., Inhibition of erythroid colony-forming cells by a Mr 15,000 protein of feline leukemia virus. Cancer Res 44:1527-1529 (1984)

68. Lafrado, L.J., Lewis, M.G., Mathes, L.E., et al., Suppression of in vitro neutrophil function by feline leukemia virus (FeLV) and purified FeLV-p15E. J Gen Virol (In press)

69. Basu, S., Lewis, M.G., Olsen, R.G., et al., Inhibition of human NK function by inactivated feline leukemia virus (submitted)

70. Cianciolo, G.J., Heberman, R.B., Snyderman, R., Depression of murine macrophage accumulation by low-molecular-weight factors derived from spontaneous mammary carcinomas. J Natl Cancer Inst 65:829-834 (1980)

71. Cianciolo, G.J., Lostrom, M.E., Tarr, M., et al., Murine malignant cells synthesize a 19,000 dalton protein that is physiochemically and antigenically related to the immunosuppressive retroviral protein, p15E. J Exp Med 158:885-900 (1983)

72. Cianciolo, G.J., Hunter, J., Silva, J., et al., Inhibitors of monocyte responses to chemotoxins are present in human cancerous effusions and react with monoclonal antibodies to the p15(E) structural proteins of retrovirus. J Clin Invest 68:831-844 (1981)

73. Cianciolo, G.J., Phipps, D., Snyderman, R., Human malignant and mitogen transformed cells contain retroviral p15E-related antigen. J Exp Med 159:964-969 (1984)

74. Cianciolo, G.J., Copeland, T.D., Oroszlan, S., et al., Inhibition of lymphocyte proliferation by a synthetic peptide homologous to retroviral envelope proteins. Science 230:453-455 (1985)

75. Snyderman, R., Cianciolo, G.J., Immunosuppressive activity of the retroviral envelope protein p15E and its possible relationship to neoplasia. Immunol Today 5:240-244 (1984)

76. Harrell, R.A., Cianciolo, G.J., Copeland, T.D., et al., Suppression of the respiratory burst of human monocytes by a synthetic peptide homologous to envelop proteins of human and animal retroviruses. J Immunol 136:3517-3520 (1986)

77. Copelan, E.A., Reinhart, J.J., Lewis, M., et al., The mechanism of retrovirus suppression of human T cell proliferation in vitro. J Immunol 131:2017-2020 (1983)

78. Orosz, C.G., Zinn, N.E., Olsen, R.G., et al., Retrovirus-mediated immunosuppression. I. FeLV-UV and specific FeLV proteins alter T-lymphocyte behavior by inducing hyporesponsiveness to lymphokines. J Immunol 134:3396-3403 (1985)

79. Orosz, C.G., Zinn, N.E., Olsen, R.G., et al., Retrovirus-mediated immunosuppression. II. FeLV-UV alters in vitro murine T-lymphocyte behavior by reversibly impairing lymphokine secretion. J Immunol 135:583-590 (1985)

80. Engelman, R.W., Fulton, R.W., Good, R.A., et al., Suppression of gamma interferon production by inactivated feline leukemia virus. Science 227:1368-1370 (1985)

81. Moody, D.J., Specter, S., Bendinelli, M., et al., Suppression of natural killer cell activity by Friend murine leukemia virus. J Natl Cancer Inst 72:1349-1356 (1984)

82. Bonavida, B., Katz, J., Gottlieb, M., Mechanism of defective NK cell activity in patients with acquired immunodeficiency syndrome (AIDS) and AIDS-related complex. I. Defective trigger on NK cells for NKCF production by target cells and partial restoration by IL-2. J Immunol 137:1157-1163 (1986)

83. Lewis, M.G., Fertel, R.H., Olsen, R.G., Reversal of feline retroviral suppression by indomethacin. Leuk Res 9:1451-1456 (1985)

84. Gemsa, G., Kramer, W., Brenner, M., et al., Induction of prostaglandin E release from macrophage by colchicine. J Immunol 124:376-380 (1980)

85. Kantor, H.S., Hampton, T.N., Indomethacin in submicromolar concentration inhibits cyclic AMP-dependent protein kinase. Nature 276:817-819 (1978)

86. Goodwin, J.S., Bromberg, S., Messner, R.P., Studies on the cyclic AMP response to prostaglandin in human lymphocytes. Cell Immunol 60:298-307 (1981)

87. Lewis, M.G., Fertel, R.H., Olsen, R.G., Reversal of retroviral induced suppression in vitro with substances that increase cyclic AMP levels. (in preparation)

88. Hellstrom, K.E., Hellstrom, I., Snyder, H.W., Jr., et al., Blocking (suppressor) factors, immune complexes, and extracorporeal immunoadsorption in tumor immunity. In: Contemporary Topics in Immunobiology (Salinas, F.A., Hanna, M.G., Jr., eds) Plenum Press, New York, Vol 15:213-238 (1985)

89. Baldwin, R.W., Price, M.R., Rabins, R.A., Significance of serum factors modifying cellular immune responses to growing tumors. Br J Cancer 28:37-47 (1973)

90. Bansal, S.C., Bansal, B.R., Thomas, H.L., et al., Ex vivo removal of serum IgG in a patient with colon carcinoma. Cancer 42:1-18 (1978)

91. Nelson, K., Hellstrom, I., Hellstrom, K.E., Tumor antigen-specific suppressor factors made by T cell hybridomas. In: T-cell hybridomas (Taussig, H.J., ed), CRC Press, Boca Raton, p 129-138 (1985)

92. Jones, F.R., Yoshida, L.H., Ladiges, W.C., et al., Treatment of feline leukemia and reversal of FeLV by ex vivo removal of IgG: A preliminary report. Cancer 46:675-84 (1980)

93. Engleman, R.W, Tyler, R.D., Trang, L.Q., et al., clinicopathologic responses in cats with feline leukemia virus-associated leukemia-lymphoma treated with staphylococcal protein A. Am J Pathol 118:367-378 (1985)

94. Snyder, H.W., Jr., Singhal, M.C., Ernst, N.R., et al., Extracorporeal perfusion of plasma over immobilized *Staphylococcus aureus* protein A as a treatment of retroviral infection and AIDS in man. In: Animal Models of Retrovirus Infection and Their Relationship to AIDS (Salzman, L.H., ed), Academic

Press, Orlando, p 403-419 (1986)

95. Kett, M.A., Wilton, E., Naama, J.K., et al., Circulating immune complexes associated with decreased complement-mediated inhibition of immune precipitation in sera from patients with bacterial endocarditis. Clin Exp Immunol 63:359-366 (1986)

96. Starkebaum, G., Jiminz, R.A.H., Arend, W.P., Effect of immune complexes on human neutrophil phagocytic function. J Immunol 128:141-147 (1982)

97. Verder, H., Dickmeiss, E., Haahr, S., et al., Late-onset rubella syndrome: coexistence of immune-complex disease and defective cytotoxic effector cell function. Clin Exp Immunol 63:367-375 (1986)

98. Phillips, T.M., Hobhan, T.V., Korac, S., et al., The pathophysiology of ciruculating immune complexes: Their role in host-tumor interactions and removal by immunoadsorption therapy. In: Contemporary Topics in Immunobiology (Salinas, F.A., Hanna, M.G., Jr., eds) Plenum Press, New York, Vol 15:111-137 (1985)

99. Kessler, S.W., Rapid isolation of antigens from cells with a staphylococcal protein A antibody absorbent: Parameters of the interaction of antigen-antibody complexes with protein A. J Immunol 115:1617-1629 (1975)

100. Forsgren, A., Sjoquist, J., Protein A from *Staphylococcus aureus*. 1. Pseudo-immune reaction with human gamma-globulin. J Immunol 97:822-827 (1966)

101. Liu, W.T., Engleman, R.W., Trang, L.Q., et al., Appearance of cytotoxic antibody to viral gp70 on feline lymphoma cells (FL-74) in cats during ex vivo immunoadsorption therapy: Quantitation, characterization, and association with remission of disease and disappearance of viremia. Proc Natl Acad Sci USA 81:3516-3520 (1984)

102. Liu, W.T., Good, R.A., Trang, L.Q., et al., Remission of leukemia and loss of feline leukemia virus in cats injected with staphylococcus protein A: Association with increased circulating interferon and complement-dependent cytotoxic antibody. Proc Natl Acad Sci (USA) 81:6471-6475 (1984)

103. Snyder, H.W., Jr., Singhal, M.C., Hardy, W.D., Jr., et al., Clearance of feline leukemia virus from persistently infected pet cats treated by extracorporeal immunoadsorption is correlated with an enhanced antibody response to FeLV gp70. J Immunol 132:1538-1543 (1984)

104. Harper, H.D., Sjoquist, J., Hardy, W.D., Jr., et al., Antitumor activity of protein A administered intravenously to pet cats with leukemia or lymphosarcoma. Cancer 55:1863-67 (1985)

105. Terman, D.S., Yamamoto, T., Mattioli, M., et al., Extensive necrosis of spontaneous canine mammary adenocarcinoma after extracorporeal perfusions over *Staphylococcus aureus* Cowan I. J Immunol 124:795-805 (1980)

106. Sakane, T., Greene, I., Protein A from *Staphylococcus aureus*: A mitogen for human T-lymphocytes and B-lymphocytes, but not L-lymphocytes. J Immunol 120:301-311 (1978)

107. Klausner, J.S., Miller, W.J., O'Brien, T.D., et al., Effects of plasma treatment with purified protein A and *Staphylococcus aureus* Cowan I on spontaneous animal neoplasms. Cancer Res 45:1263-1269 (1985)

108. Lafrado, L., Zack, P., Olsen, R., Effect of in vivo immunoadsorption therapy on the immunologic status of FeLV-infected cats. (Manuscript in preparation)

109. Spitzer, T.R., Lazarus, H.M., Effects of staphylococcal protein A-treated human leukemic serum on autologous leukemic blast growth and mitogenesis of lymphocytes. J Clin Immunol 4:455-460 (1984)

110. Hardy, Jr., W.D., Hess, P.W., MacEwen, E.G., et al., biology of feline leukemia virus in the natural environment. Cancer Res 36:582-588 (1976)

111. Hoover, E.A., Schaller, J.P., Mathes, L.E., et al., Passive immunity to feline leukemia: Evaluation of immunity from dams naturally infected and experimentally vaccinated. Infect Immun 15:49-54 (1977)

112. Jarrett, O., Russell, P.H., Stewart, M.F., Protection of kittens from feline leukemia virus infection by maternally-derived antibody. Vet Rec 101:304-305 (1977).

113. deNoronha, F., Schafer, W., Essex, M., et al., Influence of antisera to oncornavirus glycoprotein (gp71) and infection of cats with feline leukemia virus. Virology 85:617-621 (1978)

114. deNoronha, F., Grant, C.K., Leitz, H., et al., Ciruclating levels of feline leukemia and sarcoma viruses and fibrosarcoma regression in persistently viremic cats. Cancer Res 43:1663-1668 (1983)

115. deNoronha, F., Braggs, R., Schafer, W., et al., Prevention of oncornavirus-induced sarcomas in cats by treatment with antiviral antibodies. Nature 267:54-56 (1977)

116. Haley, P.J., Hoover, E.A., Quackenbush, S.L., et al., Influence of antibody infusion on pathogenesis of experimental feline leukemia virus infection. J Natl Cancer Inst 74:821-827 (1985)

117. Petersen, N.C., Theilen, G.H., Weimer, L.L., Safety and efficacy of living and killed feline leukemia virus vaccines. Am J Vet Res 40:1120-1126 (1979)

118. Salerno, R.A., Larson, V.M., Phelps, A.H., et al., Infection and immunization of cats with the Kawakami-Theilen strain of feline leukemia virus. Proc Soc Exp Biol Med 160:18-23 (1979)

119. Jarrett, W., Jarrett, O., Mackey, L., et al., Vaccination against feline leukemia virus using a cell membrane system. Int J Cancer 16:134-141 (1975)

120. Salerno, R.A., Lehman, E.D., Larson, V.M., et al., Feline leukemia virus glycoprotein vaccine: preparation and evaluation of immunizing potency in guinea pig and cat. J Natl Cancer Inst 61:1487-1497 (1978)

121. Nunberg, J.H., Rodgers, G., Gilbert, J.H., et al., Method to map antigenic determinant recognized by monoclonal antibodies: localization of a determinant of virus neutralization of the feline leukemia virus envelope protein gp70. Proc Natl Acad Sci (USA) 81:3675-3679 (1984)

122. Heding, L.D., Schaller, J.P., Blakeslee, J.R., Jr., et al., Inactivation of tumor cell-associated feline oncornavirus for preparation of an infectious virus-free tumor cell immunogen. Cancer Res 36:1647-1652 (1976)

123. Olsen, R.G., Milo, G.E., Schaller, J.P., et al., Influence of culture conditions on growth of FL-74 cells and feline oncornavirus-associated cell membrane antigen production. In Vitro 12:37-43 (1976)

124. Wolff, L.H., Mathes, L.E., Olsen, R.G., Recovery of soluble feline oncornavirus-associated cell membrane antigen from large volumes of tumor culture fluids. J Immunol Meth 26:151-156 (1979)

125. Lewis, M.G., Mathes, L.E., Olsen, R.G., Protection against feline leukemia by vaccination with a subunit vaccine. Infect Immun 34:888-894 (1981)

126. Mastro, J.M., Lewis, M.G., Mathes, L.E., Feline leukemia vaccine: Efficacy, content and probable mechanism. Vet Immunol Immunopathol 11:205-213 (1986)

127. Olsen, R.G., Lewis, M.G., Mastro, J., et al., Feline retrovirus vaccine. In: Leukemia: Recent Advances in Biology and Treatment (Gale, R.P., and Golde, D.W., eds) Alan R. Liss, Inc., New York, Vol 28:239-248 (1985)

128. Olsen, R.G., Lewis, M.G., Haffer, K., et al., Field experience with the feline leukemia vaccine. In: Animal Retroviruses (Essex, M., Restic, M., Kakoma, I., eds), Elsevier, Amsterdam (In press)

11
The Role of Human T-Lymphotropic Retroviruses in Leukemia and AIDS

Mangalasseril G. Sarngadharan, Phillip D. Markham

Human retrovirology has a relatively short history. However, the first evidence indicating the involvement of a retrovirus in the neoplastic disease of an animal was recorded around the beginning of this century. In 1908 Ellermann and Bang succeeded in transmitting the erythro-myeloblastic form of chicken leukemia by filtrates (1). Three years later Rous succeeded in transmitting the first solid tumor (chicken sarcoma) by a cell-free filtrate (2). The infectious agent, Rous sarcoma virus, is a retrovirus studied in great detail. The next major milestone in retrovirology was the discovery and isolation of the first mammalian retrovirus, the murine leukemia virus, from an inbred strain of mice (3). This was followed quickly by the isolation of other oncogenic retroviruses from inbred animals independently by Harvey, Kirsten and Moloney (4). The use of cell-free filtrates to transmit leukemogenic viruses into newborn or infant hosts was a fundamental approach developed by Gross and was later applied by Jarrett et al. to transmit and identify feline leukemia virus, the first leukemia virus that was identified as the cause of leukemia in an outbred mammal (5),(6). Retroviruses were subsequently identified in the etiology of naturally occurring leukemias and lymphomas of cows (7) and gibbons (8).

In all these animal systems a retrovirus was the cause of naturally occurring leukemias and lymphomas. As an analogy it was hypothesized that a retrovirus would sooner or later be identified as the etiological agent for many of the human leukemias and lymphomas. But it was not as easy to test the hypothesis as it was in the animal model systems. One major difference between most animal retroviral diseases and human leukemias was the clear absence of abundant viremia in humans. Therefore, even intensive examinations of cells and tissues from patients with a variety of malignancies did not reveal viral particles the way many diseased animal tissues did. Investigators who had gotten used to the familiar findings of the association of viremia with animal leukemias used the lack of such findings in the human leukemias to argue for the absence of retroviral involvement in human leukemias. However, there is at least one major exception to the rule of high level virus replication as a prerequisite for leukemogenesis. The infectious agent (bovine leukemia virus) could not be identified or isolated from blood of leukemic cows until the blood cells were put in culture after stimulation with phytohemagglutinin (PHA) (7).

The absence of established methods to cultivate human cells of different lineages interfered with serious attempts to isolate the infectious agent of human leukemias. Gallo and his associates at the National Cancer Institute approached the problem by looking for reverse transcriptase (RT) (9),(10) in cells and tissues of patients with leukemias and lymphomas. Fresh peripheral blood lymphocytes (PBL) of patients with leukemia were analyzed for RT. A preliminary finding of an RT-like activity in extracts of leukocytes from a patient with lymphoblastic leukemia (11) gave early encouragement to further careful study. A high molecular weight, Mg^{2+}-dependent RT from a patient with acute lymphoblastic leukemia (phenotype of the leukemic lymphocyte was unknown) was isolated and partially characterized (12). In retrospect, this may have been the first detection of a component of the human retrovirus subsequently isolated (13) from human adult T-cell leukemia (ATL), a disease uncommon in the United States.

Simultaneously with studies to improve the sensitivity of detection of RT and to distinguish it from cellular DNA polymerases, attempts were made in our laboratories to develop culture systems capable of growing human cells of various lineages. Culture conditioned media of PHA-treated human peripheral blood lymphocytes were found to have a specific factor that supported the growth of antigen (lectin)-stimulated T cells (14). This factor was termed T-cell growth factor, but is more commonly known as interleukin-2 (IL-2). For the first time, long-term cultures of normal or neoplastic T-cells became a reality, and the search for retrovirus involvement in human T-cell malignancies, feasible. A major difference was observed in the response to IL-2 between normal T cells and T cells of patients with certain leukemias involving mature T cells. Normal T cells developed the IL-2 receptor and responded to IL-2 only after activation with a lectin or an antigen (15), whereas certain leukemic T cells constitutively express IL-2 receptors on their surface (16) and respond to IL-2 without prior activation (17). Long-term cultures of human leukemic T cells yielded isolates of the first human retrovirus with a definite etiologic link to disease (13), (18). These viruses were termed human T cell leukemia (lymphotropic) viruses (HTLV) and the first member of the family (HTLV-

I) was identified as the cause of adult T-cell leukemia (ATL). Additional members of this retrovirus family have been subsequently identified and named HTLV-II, -III, etc. In the succeeding sections, we will describe the characteristics of these viruses, their disease association and epidemiology, and their relationship with other retroviruses.

HUMAN T-LYMPHOTROPIC VIRUS TYPE I (HTLV-I)

HTLV-I and Adult T-Cell Leukemia

The two initial isolates of HTLV-I were obtained from T-cell lines established from peripheral blood cells of two black patients originally diagnosed with aggressive variants of mycosis fungoides and Sezary cell leukemia respectively (13),(18). Later, it was appreciated that these patients really had ATL as described by Takatsuki and his colleagues in Japan (19)-(21), also called the "T-lymphosarcoma leukemia" among Caribbean black immigrants in London (22).

The new disease entity, called ATL, was first appreciated when careful subtyping of lymphomas and leukemias into T-cell and B-cell malignancies became possible. Takatsuki and colleagues noticed that the prevalence of T-cell malignancies in adults was relatively high in Japan (19)-(21) with clustering in the Southwestern parts of the country, notably in the Kyushu and Shikoku districts (23). This form of T-cell malignancy was generally aggressive; skin manifestations and hypercalcemia were frequent findings. Histopathologic studies suggested that this disease represented growth of mature T lymphocytes frequently with abnormal, convoluted nuclei similar to those seen in Sezary cell leukemia, a similar disease but with no apparent geographic clustering (24),(25). The nuclear convolutions of ATL usually have less depth to their indentation and have a more "lumpy" appearance than Sezary cells. Multinucleated giant cells represent a small percentage of the total tumor cell population in ATL patients. However, in many cases morphologic features are not definitive; for example, in some ATL cases nuclear convolutions are not apparent. In fact, the pathologic findings can be quite variable. For example, some cases may fit the diagnosis of diffuse histiocytic lymphoma, a mixed or large cell lymphoma of a T-cell type. Some features of the neoplastic T-cells, however, are more consistent, such as the expression of both the IL-2 receptors (26), and the helper/inducer T-cell antigen, known as OKT4 or leu3 (27),(28).

A similar T-cell malignancy which clustered among Caribbean black immigrants in London (22),(29) has been determined to be the same clinical entity as the Japanese ATL. Although uncommon, ATL is also found in the United States, where it has been referred to in the past as aggressive forms of mycosis fungoides and Sezary leukemia. In the United States, many of these cases have occurred among blacks either living in the Southwest or who originated from the Caribbean (30).

HTLV-I is a Horizontally Transmitted Human Retrovirus

After the initial isolation of HTLV-I in the United States (13), several additional isolates were obtained from ATL patients from around the world (18),(27),(31)-(35). Hybridization studies have indicated no homology between the genomes of HTLV-I and other known animal retroviruses. Moreover, HTLV-I cDNA (cDNA = DNA complementary to the viral RNA) failed to hybridize with normal human cellular DNA, indicating that HTLV-I is not an endogenous human retrovirus (36). The only cellular DNA that contained the proviral sequences were those obtained from primary cell cultures producing HTLV-I or those experimentally infected with the virus. These proviral sequences were also absent from cultured B-cells of the patient whose T-cells were the source of the original HTLV-I isolate (37). These results clearly demonstrated that this virus is not transmitted through the germ line and must be acquired by exogenous infection. In addition, they indicated the T-cell tropism of HTLV-I.

Genome Organization

More detailed molecular studies on HTLV-I became possible after successful cloning of the proviral DNA (38)-(40). The complete nucleotide sequence of the gene has been determined (40) and some unusual features of HTLV-I genome have been noted. In addition to the characteristic gag, pol, and env genes present in all replication competent retroviruses, the HTLV-I genome contains an extra sequence 3' to the env gene. This sequence was originally identified by Seiki et al. (40) as pX and was subsequently shown to code for a protein that trans-activates the viral LTR (long-terminal repeat), thereby regulating the transcription of the viral genome (41). The gene is, therefore, called a transactivator (tat) gene (Figure 1) (41).

Replication competent chronic leukemia viruses generally induce monoclonal tumors after a long latency period, thought to be caused by provirus integration proximal to certain cellular genes that, as a result, get cis-activated and provide the infected cell a growth advantage over uninfected cells (42). Thus, in spite of numerous and random integrations, possibly throughout the cellular genome, those near certain cellular genes lead to leukemic transformation and eventual clonal expansion of the infected cell. This mechanism for leukemogenesis has been demonstrated in retroviral induced B-cell lymphomas of chickens in which provirus integration next to the cellular myc gene activates a cellular gene and causes clonal proliferation of the infected cell (43),(44). The likelihood of integration at the proper site may be a function of the amount of virus available, accounting for the presence of significant viremia before development of leukemia in most animal systems.

In human ATL, virus integration is also monoclonal in individual patients. However, the site of integration is not constant for all patients (45),(46). Thus, there is a clear difference in the mechanism of leukemogenesis between HTLV-I and animal leukemia viruses. In HTLV-I infection, irrespective of the site of integration, the product of the tat gene transactivates the viral LTR for more abundant virus replication. It is hypothesized that the tat product interacts with a cellular gene conferring a selective growth advantage to the infected cell. A most probable cellular target might be the gene for IL-2 or its receptor. By DNA transfection experiments it has been shown that the product of the tat gene of HTLV-II (tat-II) activates the genes for both IL-2 and IL-2 receptor (47). Although IL-2 production is only observed in the initial period after activation, the expression of IL-2 receptor remains constitutive. In view of the brief nature of IL-2 gene expression, its involvement in leukemogenesis may be limited to the initiation of the leukemic transformation, and it may not be necessary for maintenance of the transformed state. Alternatively, activation of the IL-2 gene may be incidental, while the key event may be activation of the IL-2 receptor gene into continuous expression.

GENE ORGANIZATION OF HTLV-I

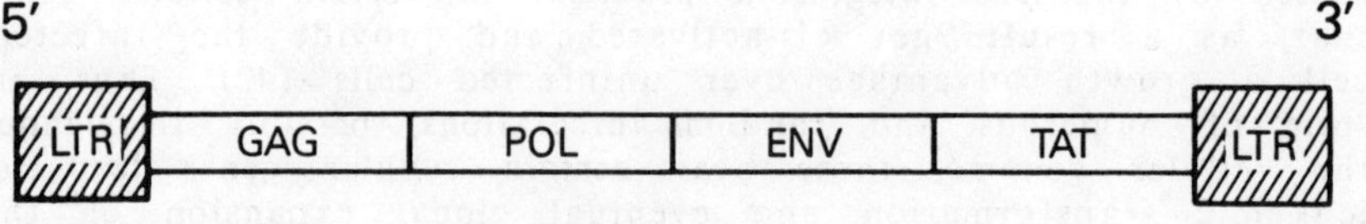

Figure 1. Genomic organization of HTLV-I.

It was reported that cells from ATL patients established in tissue culture, and some T cells transformed by HTLV-I in vitro, produce a factor named ATL-derived factor (ADF) (48) or IL-2-receptor augmenting factor (IAF) (49). ADF/IAF was capable of inducing IL-2 receptor (IL-2-R) expression on certain T cell lines (48) and on unstimulated normal peripheral blood lymphocytes (49). This activity was also produced by HTLV-II-infected cells (49). It is conceivable that the tat-activation of the IL-2-receptor gene may be indirect and may be mediated through the activation of ADF/IAF genes. This cascade of events could culminate in the expression of cell receptors essential for the response to IL-2 produced elsewhere in the body. As noted earlier, the constitutive expression of IL-2-receptors is a characteristic feature of all HTLV-I-positive ATL lymphocytes and helps to distinguish ATL from other malignancies involving mature T cells (16).

Isolation of HTLV-I from Primary Cultures of ATL-Patients

As mentioned previously, HTLV-I can be isolated from cultured T cells of ATL patients (14),(15). Neoplastic T-cells from ATL patients express the IL-2 receptor and therefore can be grown directly with IL-2 in suspension culture (17). Fresh peripheral blood cells were banded on Ficoll-Hypaque and grown in complete growth media supplemented with fetal calf serum and IL-2. These cell cultures were monitored at regular intervals for distinct morphological characteristics, for expression of virus (detected by the release of viral reverse transcriptase activity into supernatant fluids), and by electron microscopy. HTLV-I has the typical morphology of a type-C retrovirus and is released by budding from the cell membrane. The size of a mature particle is approximately 100 nm. The virus isolated from primary T cell cultures has been used to study its in vitro properties.

Comparative studies of various isolates were made on the basis of immunological cross-reactivities of the viral proteins, sequence homology by molecular hybridization, restriction endonuclease cleavage patterns of proviral DNA, and more recently by nucleotide sequence analyses. By these approaches, the majority of HTLV-I isolates were found, regardless of country of origin, to be identical (50).

Biological Properties of HTLV-I

The ability of HTLV-I to infect and transform fresh human T lymphocytes in vitro was suggested by Miyoshi et al. (31), and confirmed by subsequent studies (27),(51). The procedures used for these studies were similar to those used to initiate fresh leukemic T cells in cell culture. Leukocytes from normal sources, e.g., umbilical cord blood or adult bone marrow, were banded in Ficoll-Hypaque, and incubated with PHA to induce IL-2 receptors. These stimulated cells were then infected by cocultivation with HTLV-I-producing cells and grown in media supplemented with IL-2. Infected replicating cells became apparent within three to six weeks. In general, the transformed cells eventually no longer needed added IL-2, although the initial steps of transformation were facilitated by its inclusion in the growth medium. Adult peripheral blood leukocytes, in contrast to cord blood or bone marrow cells, were not susceptible to infection. Also, cell-free transmission was not as efficient as cocultivation for HTLV-I infection (P. Markham, unpublished results).

T lymphocytes infected in vitro with HTLV-I had several properties in common with primary T lymphocytes from HTLV-I-positive patients. For example, a percentage of cells from either source usually contained lobulated nuclei and some cells were polynucleated. HTLV-I-transformed cells expressed T-lymphocyte markers, including receptors for sheep erythrocytes (OKT11/leu5) and reacted with lymphocyte-specific monoclonal antibodies, e.g., (leu1, and often OKT3). Histochemically, these cells stained positive with an atypical globular-granular staining pattern for nonspecific esterase and acid phosphatase, and lacked granulocyte markers, e.g., myeloperoxidase, chloroacetate esterase, and Sudan Black staining. They also did not contain B-lymphocyte markers, e.g., surface immunoglobulin, Epstein-Barr virus nucleic acids or antigens. Like leukemic T lymphocytes from ATL patients, the HTLV-I- transformed cord blood T lymphocytes were usually OKT4/leu3a$^+$ (helper T-cell phenotype). Bone marrow T-lymphocytes transformed by HTLV-I in vitro, however, sometimes expressed surface markers usually found in other T-cell subsets. Thus, one encountered in these cultures cells expressing the helper/inducer phenotype (OKT4/leu3a$^+$), cytotoxic/suppressor phenotype (OKT8/leu2a$^+$) or those showing neither of these phenotypes (52). The surface phenotype of the primary T cells producing HTLV-I or the in vitro transformed T cells did not, however, strictly correlate with their expected functional characteristics. For instance, OKT4$^+$ HTLV-I producing T cells might not provide the expected helper/inducer function (53).

Even though it is clear that the prime cell target for HTLV-I is T lymphocytes of the helper/inducer subgroup (T4$^+$), other cell types have been infected with HTLV-I. For example, B lymphocytes established in culture from one patient with ATL were found to produce infectious virus (54). Also, HTLV-I was transmitted to the promyelocytic cell line HL-60 at a very low efficiency (55). Non-hematopoietic cells, e.g., fibroblasts, could also be infected by HTLV-I in vitro (56). T cells of the suppressor subgroup (T8$^+$) can, under certain conditions, be infected by HTLV-I. This appears possible if the virus is exposed to a population of immature cells, e.g., bone marrow leukocytes, or to cultures depleted of T4 cells (P. Markham, unpublished results). In a unique clinical situation, a patient was shown to have dual infection with HTLV-I and HTLV-III, and an HTLV-I transformed population of T8 cells was obtained, presumably as a consequence of a reduction in T4 cells by HTLV-III infection (57). From the point of view of developing animal model systems, cell lines from rabbits (58), hamsters (59), rats (60), and cats (61) were reported to be infected by HTLV-I. HTLV-I was also transmitted to rabbits in vivo by transfusion (62).

Effects of HTLV-I on Immune Function

Since a primary target of HTLV-I is the T-4 lymphocyte, a key immunoregulatory cell, any effect on the function of this population could have far reaching consequences on immune function aside from the development of ATL. It was noted that HTLV-I-transformed cells constitutively produced one or more of the following activities: macrophage migration enhancing factor, leukocyte migration inhibitory factor, migration enhancing factor, macrophage activating factor, differentiation inducing factor, colony stimulating factor, eosinophil growth and maturation activity, fibroblast activating factor; gamma interferon, and macrophage differentiating factor (63). In addition to these activities, preliminary tests suggested that biological activities related to IL-2, B cell growth factor, and platelet-derived growth factor could also be released in some instances. Clearly the constitutive production of some of these activities, if they occur in vivo, could greatly influence other elements of the immune system.

Like some other retroviruses (64) a number of reports suggested that infection by HTLV-I could adversely affect host immune functions, leading to an increased incidence of opportunistic infections and/or the development of malignancies other than ATL. Essex and his coworkers found that patients in an infectious diseases ward in an HTLV-I endemic region in Japan had almost three times the prevalence of antibodies to HTLV-I than the general population in that area (65). Likewise, an AIDS-like illness was detected in an HTLV-I positive patient from Japan more than a year prior to the development of ATL (66), and an increased incidence of herpetic infections was noted among seropositive patients in Panama (67). The loss of helper T-cell function due to HTLV-I infection was also suggested to play a role in the development of other types of malignancies. For example, an increased incidence of seropositivity to HTLV-I was noted among patients in the Caribbean with B-cell lymphoma (68) and possibly among patients with non-Hodgkins lymphoma and other hematopoietic cell cancers in Japan (69).

A direct effect on HTLV-I-infected cells was also seen. It was observed that regulatory T lymphocytes taken from ATL patients from Japan and from the Caribbean had reduced or no helper cell activity while several did retain some suppressor activity, i.e., affected B cell maturation in vitro (53). In addition, although most T-cell lines cloned from an HTLV-I infected ATL patient had specific cytotoxic activity against neoplastic T-cells expressing HTLV-I (providing the target tumor cells also expressed at least one HLA antigen (HLA-A1) in common with the effector cells) (70), one clone had lost its normal immune functions. When exposed to tumor cells expressing HTLV-I antigens, this clonal population ceased to proliferate and eventually died (71). This aberrant T-cell clone was found to have one copy of HTLV-I provirus per cell. Loss of normal immune regulation was also demonstrated by in vitro infection of helper T-cells and cytotoxic T-cells with HTLV-I and HTLV-II (72). Before infection, a cloned human helper T-cell line proliferated and provided "help" to B cells only in the presence of both a specific soluble antigen and histocompatible antigen-presenting cells. Following infection with either HTLV-I or HTLV-II, these cells responded with increased proliferation and indiscriminate stimulation of polyclonal immunoglobulin production by B cells regardless of the histocompatibility of the antigen presenting cell or the presence of the soluble antigen. Similarly, HTLV-I infection of the normal cytotoxic T-cell clone led to a diminution or loss of their cytotoxic function (72). These data suggest that HTLV-I-infection of T cells might induce immune deficiency and lead to polyclonal B-cell activation.

Other HTLV-I-Associated Diseases

Several lines of evidence have suggested that HTLV-I may be involved in the development of certain neurological disorders. In HTLV-I endemic regions of Japan, for example, a higher than expected percentage of patients with a myelopathy were found to be seropositive for HTLV-I (73),(74). Several of these patients had received blood transfusions from donors from HTLV-I endemic areas. This syndrome is now designated as HTLV-I-associated myelopathy. Similarly, HTLV-I infection has been associated in a high percentage of cases with a condition called tropical spastic paraparesis in patients from several countries in the Caribbean (75)-(77) and some areas of Africa (78).

Seroepidemiology of HTLV-I

In a preliminary survey of human sera, antibodies to HTLV-I were present in two patients with T-cell malignancies (originally diagnosed as cutaneous T-cell leukemia and later reclassified as ATL) and in the serum of the wife of one of the patients, but in none of 50 normal donors (79). A sero-survey from patients with a variety of T-cell malignancies in the United States indicated that HTLV-I was not associated with all T-cell neoplasms (80). However, an excellent correlation exists between ATL and the presence of serum antibodies to HTLV-I (65),(81),(82). Normal individuals and patients with B-cell leukemias and lymphomas lack antibodies to HTLV-I as do patients with T-cell malignancies that are not the typical HTLV-I type. In ATL-endemic geographic areas, the prevalence of antibody-positive asymptomatic carriers is significantly higher than in nonendemic areas. For instance, in Japan seroprevalence among normal subjects ranges from 0% in the Hokkaido district in the north to as high as 16% in the Nagasaki area and 15% in the Kagoshima area in the Kyushu district in the southwest (83). The prevalence of antibody-positivity paralleled remarkably well the clustering pattern of ATL (81)-(86). A second well-documented endemic area for HTLV-I-associated malignancies is in the Caribbean basin. In one study approximately 70% of patients with non-Hodgkin's lymphoid malignancies seen in Jamaica in one year had serum antibodies to HTLV-I (87). Similarly, antibodies to HTLV-I were found in nearly 100% of black

Caribbean immigrants in England with ATL (29),(88)-(90). In Jamaica, antibodies to HTLV-I are found in 2 - 10% of the normal population.

Antibody-positive adult T-cell malignancies with clinical features similar to those of typical ATL have been found sporadically in the United States and Israel (80), and a few cases have also been identified in Central and South America and in Africa. Antibody prevalence of 2 to 10% has been found among normal populations from Capetown (South Africa), Nigeria, Egypt, Tunisia and Ghana (91), suggesting that clusters of ATL cases may be anticipated in these regions.

Seroepidemiologic studies indicate that transmission of HTLV-I may require close or intimate contact, although, with a few exceptions, the means of transmission is still uncertain. Evidence for this assertion is the observation that after patients with ATL, antibody prevalence is highest in family members of ATL patients. In fact, in areas where ATL is not endemic family members are the only significant group of antibody-positive persons (92). Within families the data suggest that transmission occurs male to female and female to offspring (93). In numerous studies laboratory workers with contact with HTLV-I have been consistently negative for antibodies to HTLV-I. The single seropositive laboratory worker (90) known to date had antibodies to HTLV-I at least eight years before the virus was ever isolated in the laboratory. Antibodies to HTLV-I have been demonstrated in people receiving transfusions of HTLV-positive blood (94), and a high prevalence of antibodies has been found in hemophiliacs (95). The virus has also been isolated from intravenous drug users (Popovic and Gallo, unpublished data). Transmission might occur during sexual contact through lymphocytes in semen, by insect vectors, by blood transfusions, by contaminated needles during illicit drug use, by in vivo maternal-fetal exchange, and possibly through mother's milk.

Studies on HTLV-I seroprevalence among Japanese immigrants to Hawaii from Okinawa, an HTLV-I-endemic area, suggest that infection within the household occurs and that geographic area influences infection rate (96). A 20% seroprevalence for HTLV-I was observed in Okinawa immigrants and in their offspring born in Hawaii compared to 35% in similarly aged men who were lifetime residents of Okinawa. A control group of immigrants from Niigata, a nonendemic area of Japan, had extremely low seroprevalence rates, indicating that Hawaii itself is not an endemic area for HTLV-I. Factors that were significantly associated with seropositivity were years of residence in Japan before migration (migrants) and increasing age of offspring of the Okinawan migrants. Antibody titer was highest among Okinawa life time residents, intermediate among migrants and lowest among offspring of Okinawan migrants.

HUMAN T-LYMPHOTROPIC VIRUS TYPE II (HTLV-II)

A human T-lymphotropic retrovirus related to, but distinguishable from HTLV-I was originally isolated from a cell line established from a patient with a variant of hairy cell leukemia.

This was designated $HTLV\text{-}II_{MO}$ (97). It was subsequently detected in at least one other patient with a similar disease (98). The virus probably spreads through blood and blood products as it has been isolated from a patient with hemophilia A (99). Although there are some subtle morphological and biological differences, it has very important similarities to HTLV-I. It resembles HTLV-I in its genomic structure and organization, overall nucleotide sequence homology (about 40%), and in in vitro biological properties. Recent epidemiological evidence indicates that HTLV-II, like HTLV-I and HTLV-III (see below), is spreading in intravenous drug addict populations. However, many more epidemiologic studies need to be done with this virus as its disease associations are still unclear.

Like HTLV-I, HTLV-II transformed human and marmoset T cells when infected either by cocultivation with infected cells or by cell-free virus (100). The infected human cells were found to be T-lymphocytes of the T4 subtype. However, in vitro studies established that B-lymphoid cells were also susceptible to infection by HTLV-II.

Even though HTLV-II has been isolated only rarely, much is known concerning its genomic organization. Its genome has been cloned (101),(102) and sequenced (103),(104). Haseltine et al. (104) and others (105) compared the nucleotide sequence of the region between the env gene and the 3' LTR of HTLV-II with the corresponding sequence of HTLV-I. In addition to finding a high degree of homology between HTLV-I and -II in a 1000-nucleotide long region of this novel genetic element, they identified a long open reading frame capable of encoding polypeptides 357 amino acids long for HTLV-I and 337 amino acids long for HTLV-II, respectively (104). A protein of approximately 42kD was identified (106) in a cell line C81-66 (C63/CR) established from human cord blood T-cells by infection with HTLV-I (107). This cell line does not produce HTLV-I and only expresses a limited number of HTLV-I proteins (107). The p42 is not related to HTLV-I gag and env proteins (106) and is suggested to be a trans-acting factor that may be relevant in the transforming ability of HTLV-I. Similar findings were also reported by Slamon et al. for HTLV-II (108). A protein of 37-38kD is the corresponding product of the HTLV-II-trans-activator gene (106),(108). The genes coding for the trans-activator proteins are now called tat-I (HTLV-I) and tat-II (HTLV-II), respectively. Target sequences for the trans-activator proteins in the host cell genome are beginning to be identified and the mechanisms by which they might be involved in the process of cell transformation are under investigation. As outlined earlier, the tat-II product has been shown to stimulate the expression of both the IL-2 and IL-2 receptor genes (47).

HUMAN T-LYMPHOTROPIC VIRUS TYPE-III (HTLV-III)

It was apparent soon after recognition of AIDS as a distinct entity (109)-(111) that it was caused by an infectious agent transmitted by sexual intercourse or by blood or blood products (112),(113). Several factors also suggested that this agent could be a retrovirus with some properties similar to HTLV-I and HTLV-II. In addition to the mode of transmission, the agent responsible for AIDS was not removed by filtration. For instance, filtered blood products such as Factor VIII received by hemophiliacs, retained the infectious agent. The characteristic clinical feature of the disease is a defect in the cellular immune system. One of the earliest detected laboratory findings was a selective loss of the helper ($T4^+$) T-cell population resulting in an inversion of the helper/suppressor ($T4^+/T8^+$) ratio. Our prior experience with HTLV-I and HTLV-II, both of which have a preferred tropism for $T4^+$ lymphocytes, suggested to us that a retrovirus with a similar tropism was the most likely candidate to cause AIDS. In retrospect, these predictions proved correct, but there is one major difference in the biological outcome of the AIDS virus compared to either HTLV-I or II. HTLV-I and -II transform T-cells in vitro and make them immortal, whereas the AIDS agent is cytopathic to these same cells (see below).

Biological Properties of HTLV-III

Isolation of HTLV-III

Attempts to isolate the presumed virus from patients with AIDS and AIDS-related complex (ARC) and from other donors at risk for these diseases were initiated using procedures similar to those described earlier for the isolation of HTLV-I and -II (13), (18). Mitogen stimulated human mononuclear cells were grown in the presence of IL-2 and the cultures were monitored for viral reverse transcriptase activity in the supernatant fluids. Virus expression was also followed by transmission to fresh normal human adult peripheral blood, bone marrow, or umbilical cord blood T-lymphocytes (114)-(118), by electron microscopic observation of fixed, sectioned cells, and by immunological procedures initially using sera from seropositive donors and eventually with specific antisera to viral proteins. In early experiments, virus production was observed from time to time, but only transiently. A major advance in the study of AIDS occurred with the discovery that some established cell lines could be infected by HTLV-III (116).

Virus was usually detected in supernatant fluids within one to three weeks after establishing cultures of primary cells from AIDS or ARC patients or donors at risk for these diseases. Release of virus usually declined rapidly coinciding with loss of viable cells, especially those with the helper/inducer ($OKT4^+$/$Leu3a^+$) phenotype. Careful examination of cultured cells subsequently suggested that activation of viral synthesis required immune stimulation of infected cells (119). Stimulation in vitro could be provided by mitogen or added cells (allogeneic antigens).

HTLV-III has been isolated from hundreds of AIDS or ARC patients and from healthy individuals at risk for AIDS (117), (118) (Table 1). Isolation of virus as evidence of infection in the source material was always definitive. However, technical limitations inherent in the methodology limited the rate of

Table 1. Groups, Both Symptomatic and Asymptomatic From Which HTLV-III Has Been Isolated

Homosexual Men
IV Drug Abusers (male and female)
Hemophiliacs
Transfusion Recipients (male and female)
Prostitutes
Hetrosexually Active Men and Women
Spouses of HTLV-III-Infected Individuals
Children of "At Risk" Women
African and Haitian Immigrants to the U.S.
Health Care/Laboratory Workers with Exposure (very rare)
Seronegative "At Risk" Individuals (rare)

success. Certain manipulations of culture conditions were found to improve the outcome, e.g., cocultivation of patient cells with mitogen stimulated peripheral blood leukocytes from uninfected donors (our unpublished observation). Isolation of virus from cultured cells also was substantially facilitated by inclusion of hydrocortisone in the culture media. For example, in approximately 50% of samples from virus-positive AIDS or ARC patients, the amount of virus released was significantly increased when the culture was supplemented by 5ug/ml hydrocortisone. More importantly, in approximately 15% of AIDS specimens, the inclusion of hydrocortisone allowed the detection of virus that would otherwise have gone undetected (120).

Tissue Sources of HTLV-III

A summary of tissues and body fluids from which HTLV-III has been isolated is given in Table 2. The majority of HTLV-III isolations from leukocytes to date have been from peripheral blood leukocytes. However, in a small number of samples, infectious virus was also isolated from leukocytes obtained from bone marrow and lymph node tissues (117),(118). HTLV-III is probably involved in AIDS-related encephalopathy and other neurological disorders. In fact, proviral DNA has been detected in brain tissue (121) and virus has been isolated from brain, cerebrospinal fluid and other neurologic tissues (122)-(125). Consistent with the evidence for sexual transmission, HTLV-III was isolated from semen (126),(127), urine (our unpublished observation) and cervical secretions of some women at risk for AIDS (128 and our personal observation). HTLV-III was also isolated from saliva from healthy homosexual men who were at high risk for AIDS, and from ARC patients (129),(130). Virus has also been isolated from milk of infected mothers (131) and from cell-free plasma (132 and our personal observation). Cells other than T-lymphocytes were found to harbor infectious virus in vivo, e.g., circulating monocyte/macrophages, alveolar macrophages obtained by bronchoalveolar lavage (122),(133) and endothelial cells (134). An observation that emphasized the need for caution while working with tissues from infected individuals was the isolation of HTLV-III from tears (135), and from corneal endothelial and epithelial cells grown in tissue culture (136).

Table 2. Tissue Sources of HTLV-III Isolates

Peripheral Blood
Bone Marrow
Lymph Node
Thymus
Brain Phagocytic Cells
Circulating Monocyte/Macrophages
Alveolar Macrophages
Corneal Epithelial Cells
Corneal Endothelial Cells
Skin Langerhans Cells
Cell-Free Plasma
Saliva
Semen
Cerebrospinal Fluid
Tears
Urine
Cervical Fluids
Breast Milk

Target Cells, Virus Receptors, and Possible Reservoirs of Infectious Virus

It is well established that a primary target cell for HTLV-III is the T lymphocyte of the helper/inducer class defined by specific monoclonal antibodies (137),(138). On these and possibly other cells, e.g., monocyte-macrophages, the CD4 molecule (identified by the OKT4 series or other equivalent monoclonal antibodies) appears to serve as a primary receptor for the virus (137),(138) even though its expression on cells is apparently not always required (139). Transfection of the gene coding for the T4 molecule to T4-negative cells also permitted infection by HTLV-III to otherwise non-permissive cells (140). Molecular studies further demonstrated the direct binding of the 58kD CD4 molecule and a 110kD viral glycoprotein (presumably the envelope protein) (141).

As described previously, many cell types were observed to be infected by HTLV-III in vivo. A wide range of cell types are also susceptible to infection by HTLV-III in vitro. HTLV-I-transformed T4$^+$ lymphocytes were found to be especially susceptible to infection and in some instances particularly sensitive to cytopathic effect (142),(143). Other cell types include HTLV-I-transformed T8 positive lymphocytes (144), B-lymphotropic cells (145), lung, peripheral blood, or brain macrophages (122),(133), (146), endothelial cells (our personal observation), and some other hematopoietic cell lines, e.g., U937, HL60, and K562 (137), (147). Although some of these cell lines contain a low number of cells expressing the T4 antigen, the receptor(s) permitting infection remains to be determined. It was observed that cells from several (but not all) Epstein-Barr virus (EBV) genome-positive B-cell lines could be readily infected by HTLV-III regardless of the presence of detectable T4 surface markers (145). EBV genome-negative B-cells could not be infected. However, these cells were converted to an HTLV-III-receptive state by pre-infection with either transforming or non-transforming EBV. These observations support the possibility that either EBV-coded or -induced cellular proteins are involved in the formation of the receptor for HTLV-III in B lymphocytes.

Modes of Transmission of HTLV-III

The actual mechanisms of HTLV-III transmission (i.e., blood to blood, blood to mucous membrane, semen to mucous membrane) and their relative importance in the natural history of infection remain to be determined. It is well recognized that in the United States the prevalence of HTLV-III infection is highest among homosexual males, intravenous drug abusers, those receiving blood or blood products on a regular basis (e.g., hemophiliacs), and children of infected mothers (148). It is apparent that transmission of virus requires repeated intimate contact, or exchange of blood products and is not transmitted by casual contact, even within families (149)-(151). Of importance to the control of HTLV-III infection is the emerging realization that repeated heterosexual contact with infected people can also be a significant risk factor. Studies of sexual contacts of HTLV-III-infected patients in the U.S. military yielded compelling early evidence that HTLV-III and therefore resulting diseases could be heterosexually transmitted (152),(153). A larger study of the military population and their spouses further demonstrated heterosexual spread of HTLV-III (154), (Redfield, personal communication). The study found that the ratio of infected men to women was 2.5 to 1; much closer to that reported for some areas of Africa where heterosexual transmission is the significant mode of virus spread (155). It was also found that among married couples, if one partner proved to be infected by HTLV-III, his/her sexual partner had a 40-50% chance of becoming infected. This occurred regardless of whether the first to become infected was male or female. Other controlled studies of sexual partners have further emphasized that heterosexual contact with infected individuals may spread HTLV-III infection. Epidemiological studies of clusters of HTLV-III infected people in the U.S., including a highly publicized study in Belle Glade, Florida, and a similar study in Italy have been interpreted to mean that heterosexual transmission is a significant cause of infection (156)-(159).

Seroepidemiological Correlation Between HTLV-III Infection and AIDS

Retroviral infections are characterized by strong and prolonged humoral immune response in the host. As demonstrated earlier in the case of HTLV-I and HTLV-II infections (79),(81),(82),(97), screening for antibodies is a practical and efficient way of identifying viral infection. Therefore, one of the earliest studies that we undertook after the isolation and characterization of HTLV-III was to use the virus to detect serum antibodies in patients with AIDS and ARC and otherwise healthy individuals belonging to known risk groups for AIDS (160),(161). In addition to establishing the epidemiological evidence linking HTLV-III and AIDS, this served to develop a blood screening assay to detect individuals infected with HTLV-III.

Two procedures were used to identify serum antibodies. They were: (i) a simple enzyme-linked immunosorbent assay (ELISA) and (ii) a much more elaborate and more sensitive immunoblot (Western blot) assay. In the first assay, density banded HTLV-III was lysed with a nonionic detergent (NP-40 or Triton X-100) and 0.5 M NaCl, and the antigens in the lysate were allowed to adsorb onto the surface of wells in multi-well plastic plates. The plates were washed and properly treated to prevent nonspecific protein adsorption. When test sera containing antibodies to HTLV-III proteins were reacted with these plates, specific immune complexes involving human immunoglobulins were formed on the wells. These were then detected using enzyme-tagged immunoglobulins reactive against human immunoglobulins and capable of reacting with chromogenic substrates. The intensity of the color yield was measured using specially designed colorimeters and was correlated with the amount (titer) of anti-HTLV-III antibodies present in the human serum tested. Antibody-negative human sera did not react with the HTLV-III antigens on the plate and were removed during the washing and, therefore, did not "fix" the enzyme-tagged second antibody and no color was produced.

The ELISA test is highly sensitive and specific, but the quality of the antigen preparation is extremely important. Contaminating proteins in the virus lysate can result in false positive results, just as insufficient antigen levels can result in false negatives. An inherent drawback of the ELISA is that the color yield only represents an aggregate of all reactivities in the test serum and it does not attribute reactivities to individual antigens. Therefore, a contaminating nonviral antigen which might react with the test serum (e.g., some HLA proteins contaminating the antigen preparation) could cause a false positive test. On the other hand, in the Western blot test antigens are separated by sodium dodecyl sulfate-polyacrylamide gel electrophoresis (SDS-PAGE) and transferred to a nitrocellulose strip (162) before performing the immunological reaction. As a consequence, reactivities to individual antigens are clearly identified. A detailed understanding of the virion-derived structural and envelope antigens makes interpretation of the Western blot patterns easy. A truly positive ELISA sample always gives a positive reaction to one or more viral antigens in the Western blot. On the other hand, a false positive ELISA test will not be associated with a positive Western blot pattern. Such sera may show reactivity on Western blot that cannot be attributed to HTLV-III antigens. Western blot assays can thus be used as a good confirmatory test for ELISA-positive samples.

A very high level of antibody prevalence was observed in the initial ELISA tests for sera from AIDS and ARC patients. At the same time sera of normal subjects and those of patients with diseases unrelated to AIDS were clearly nonreactive (160). The specificity and sensitivity of the Western blot system was significantly higher than in the ELISA. In a blinded study of a panel of sera using a combination of ELISA and Western blot assays, the correlation between antibodies to HTLV-III and AIDS was 100%. At the same time, none of the controls was reactive (161).

Extensive serological studies have proven beyond doubt the association between HTLV-III infection and the development of AIDS. In addition, these studies clearly identified a spectrum of clinical states related to HTLV-III infection including an asymptomatic carrier state. Prospective studies of members of identified AIDS-risk groups reveal a natural history of HTLV-III infection that shows progression from the antibody-negative healthy carrier state to the antibody-positive healthy carrier state to subclinical immune perturbation to lymphadenopathy and AIDS (148). The contagious nature of the healthy carrier state has been clearly demonstrated by studies on transfusion related AIDS cases in which blood from such donors were identified as the sole source of HTLV-III infection in the recipients who otherwise had no known risk factors (163),(164). These serological studies also provided the data that led to implementation of blood screening by U.S. blood banks in the spring of 1985.

Western blot pattern varied from one HTLV-III-infected person to another and also varied with time for the same individual. Figure 2 shows some representative patterns observed. Lane 2 shows a serum with strong reactivities to the antigens p120, p66, p51, p41, p31, p24 and p17. The serum represented in lane 3 is missing strong reactivities to p24 and p17, but has all of the other reactivities seen in lane 2. Serum shown in lane 4 has only the reactivity to the protein p41. A clear understanding of the nature of these antigens (see below) is essential for a meaningful interpretation of Western blot results.

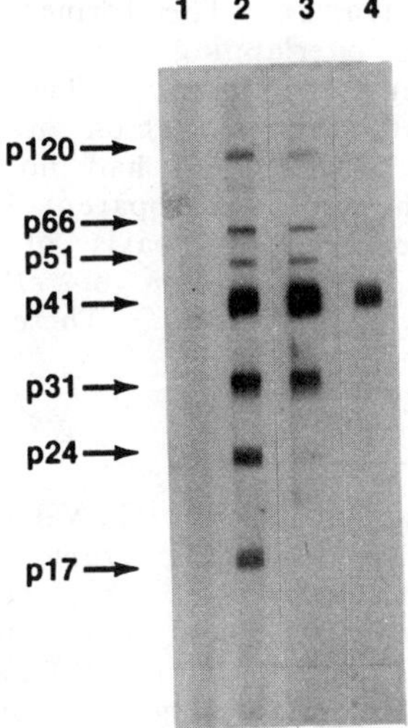

Figure 2. Detection of HTLV-III p41 by human sera in the immunoblot assay. Lysates of HTLV-III were fractionated by SDS-PAGE and blotted to nitrocellulose sheets. Strips were cut from these sheets containing a representative profile of viral antigens and were used in detecting antibodies in human sera to HTLV-III antigens (186). Lane 1, negative human control serum. Lane 2, serum of an ARC patient with multiple reactivities. Lanes 3 and 4, sera of AIDS patients containing antibodies to fewer viral antigens.

Molecular Properties of HTLV-III

Cloning of the HTLV-III Genome and Determination of its Nucleotide Sequence

Development of a continuous producer cell line for HTLV-III has helped to characterize in detail the molecular properties of the virus. Simultaneously with characterization of the protein components of the virus, investigators were actively exploring the genetic make-up of the virus. These studies led to the cloning of the viral genome (165). One clone (BH10) representing nearly the total length of the genome and two others (BH5 and BH8) that together represented the total sequences in BH10 were obtained by cloning the unintegrated DNA in acutely infected H9 cells (165). These clones were used to determine the complete nucleotide sequence of the HTLV-III proviral DNA (166). The HTLV-III sequence consists of 9,749 bases in which five large open reading frames were initially identified. By analogy with other retroviruses, three of these reading frames were identified as the gag, pol, and env genes. The other two largest open reading frames were called sor (for short open reading frame) and 3'orf (for 3' open reading frame). The former, contained between the pol and env genes and overlapping the pol gene by 86 bases, had no precedent in other retroviruses. The latter, 3' to the env gene and extending into the U3 region of the LTR, occupied the portion of the tat-I in HTLV-I but had no homology with it. Other reading frames which were not apparent from sequence data have since been identified on the basis of functional assays involving the transfection and expression of cDNA clones and of deletion mutants constructed in vitro. These are described in sections below.

Cloning of the Tat, Sor, and 3' Orf Genes

Nucleotide sequence analysis of the HTLV-III/LAV genome predicted at least two novel open reading frames (166)-(169) termed here sor and 3' orf. Existence of a third novel gene, termed tat, was inferred from the observation that expression of HTLV-III LTR-linked genes was enhanced in HTLV-III-infected cells relative to uninfected cells, suggesting the presence of a factor(s) in infected cells that acted in trans (170). The structure and location of these sequences in the HTLV-III genome were identified by obtaining functional cDNA clones and screening cDNA libraries with specific HTLV-III subgenomic probes. Several selected clones were characterized by restriction mapping, DNA sequencing, and functional and immunological testing. Three proviral DNA clones corresponding to the functional tat gene, 3'orf gene and sor gene were obtained (171),(172). The tat and 3'orf genes respectively code for 2.0 and 1.8 Kb messages and arise by double splicing - a feature novel for retroviruses but shared by the HTLV-bovine leukemia virus group of retroviruses. The sor gene transcripts may also involve double splicing. The functional tat gene consists of three exons with coding sequence in the second exon located between the pol and env genes. The tat gene encodes a polypeptide of 14kD apparent molecular weight. The in vitro synthesized 14kD protein is immunoreactive with antibodies in sera of individuals with AIDS and associated disorders, showing that the tat gene functions in vivo and is immunogenic. The results also show that no post-translational modifications are necessary for at least the immune reactivity of the tat proteins (172). The sor and 3'orf genes encode for polypeptides of 23kD and 27kD apparent molecular weights, respectively, which are also recognized by sera of some HTLV-III infected individuals. The above results clearly show that the tat, sor and 3'orf genes are expressed in vivo and their products are immunogenic (172). Using different approaches, similar results have been reported by others for the 3'orf protein (173),(174) and the sor protein (175),(176). The exact functions of the 3'orf and sor proteins in vivo remain to be determined. In addition to these, at least one other functional gene has been identified in the HTLV-III genome. This gene, described as art (anti-repressor of transcription) or trs (transregulator of splicing), encompasses the same nucleotide sequence as tat-III but is in a different reading frame (177),

(178). The function of this gene is described by one group (177) as an anti-repressor that acts to abrogate a negative control on the transcription of the viral gag and env proteins, while another group believes that the effect is a down regulation of splicing (178). Figure 3 shows a diagrammatic representation of the organization of the HTLV-III genome.

Characterization of HTLV-III Proteins

As noted earlier, antibody positive human sera recognized a large number of proteins in extracts of HTLV-III. Although these proteins were presumed to be of viral origin, we needed to establish their origin and to characterize their properties more directly. The task was made somewhat simpler through knowledge of the complete nucleotide sequence of the viral genome and thereby the predicted amino acid sequence of the products of the various viral genes. Multiple approachs to the study of these proteins were undertaken. Some proteins were purified from viral extracts by conventional chromatography procedures (179), while others were purified using specific monoclonal antibodies by immunoaffinity procedures. Amino acid sequences of these proteins were determined and these were compared with the deduced sequences of the different gene products. In addition, immunoprecipitation studies using specific monoclonal antibodies allowed the identification of the primary gene products and the pattern of their processing to proteins found in the mature virion. These findings are described in more detail below.

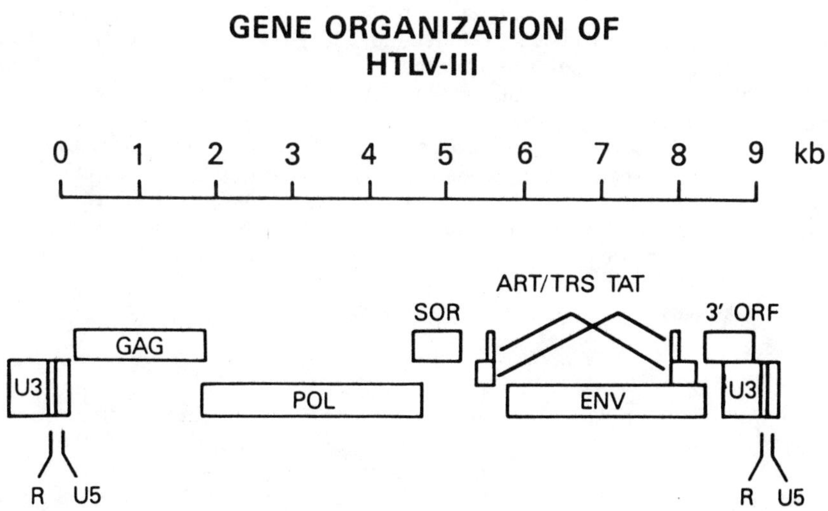

Figure 3. Genomic organization of HTLV-III.

Products of HTLV-III Gag Gene

An initiation site near the 5' end of the viral genomic RNA allows for translation of the gag gene resulting in synthesis of a precursor polyprotein, which upon post-translational cleavage gives rise to non-glycosylated structural proteins of 17, 24, and 15kD, respectively. As with HTLV-I and -II, the major immunogenic gag protein in HTLV-III is the 24kD protein p24, which constitutes the major protein fraction in the mature virion (179). N-terminal amino acid sequence of purified p24 showed this protein to represent the middle peptide derived from post-translational cleavage of the precursor polyprotein. N-terminal sequencing analysis of purified p17 instead showed the NH_2-terminal residue of p17 to be inaccessible to Edman degradation, suggestive of some kind of NH_2-terminal modification occurring post-transcriptionally (180).

To identify the gag precursor polyprotein in the cytoplasm of infected cells, we analyzed lysates of HTLV-III-producing cells by immunoprecipitation and SDS-PAGE. Log phase cultures of H9/ HTLV-III_B were labeled with [^{35}S]-cysteine overnight. The cells were lysed with detergents and the clarified extract was treated overnight with ascitic fluid from two independent anti-p24 hybridomas (181) and two independent anti-p17 hybridomas. The precipitates were collected and analyzed by SDS-PAGE. While the anti-p24 and p17 monoclonal antibodies precipitated the respective individual proteins, both also precipitated a common 53kD protein (180). Therefore, the same antigenic determinants recognized on the cleaved products are present on the p53 molecule. This result identifies the cellular p53 as the precursor of HTLV-III gag proteins. Similar immunoprecipitation studies of viral proteins metabolically labeled with [^{3}H]-myristic acid using anti-p17 and anti-p24 monoclonal antibodies precipitated a labeled pr53 gag. In addition, the anti-p17 antibody also precipitated a smaller amount of labeled p17. No incorporation of radioactivity was evident in the p24 precipitated by anti-p24 antibody. This analysis clearly demonstrates that p17 occupies the NH_2-terminal portion of HTLV-III gag precursor p53 and is N-myristylated. The myristyl moiety has been speculated to be a very important feature involved in the recognition by specific cellular membrane-bound molecules of retroviral proteins (182). This interaction would then be critical for assembly of viral proteins and packaging of mature virions.

Products of HTLV-III Pol Gene

Approximately 80 percent of all HTLV-III seropositive individuals have a serological reactivity to two peptides of 66 and 51kD when analyzed by Western blot. These two proteins were found to be antigenically unrelated to products of the gag or env gene. In one approach to determine their nature, we prepared a mouse hybridoma secreting a monoclonal antibody (M3364) directed against these antigens. The hybridoma was subjected to repeated cycles of subcloning in attempts to separate the two reactivities, but they could not be separated (183). This indicated that p66 and p51 share common determinants (Figure 4). We purified the antigen from an extract of HTLV-III by immunoaffinity chromatography using purified M3364 immunoglobulins coupled to activated CH-Sepharose. The bound proteins were eluted with 0.2 M glycine, pH 2.8 and analyzed by Western blot and Coomassie blue staining. P66 and p51 are the only proteins recognized in these fractions by an HTLV-III positive human serum and by Coomassie blue stain (Figure 5), showing that the purified proteins were homogeneous and immunoreactive. A portion of these fractions was subjected to amino acid sequencing by gas phase Edman degradation. The analysis generated single amino acid residues in 17 successive cycles. A comparison of the amino acid sequence observed with the sequence predicted from the known nucleotide sequence of HTLV-III, clone BH10 and BH5 showed a perfect match for a product of the pol gene segment between nucleotide 2130 and 2180 (183). These sequence data indicate that p66 and p51 have common amino-terminal amino acid sequences and that p51 must be derived from p66 by processive cleavage near the carboxy-terminus.

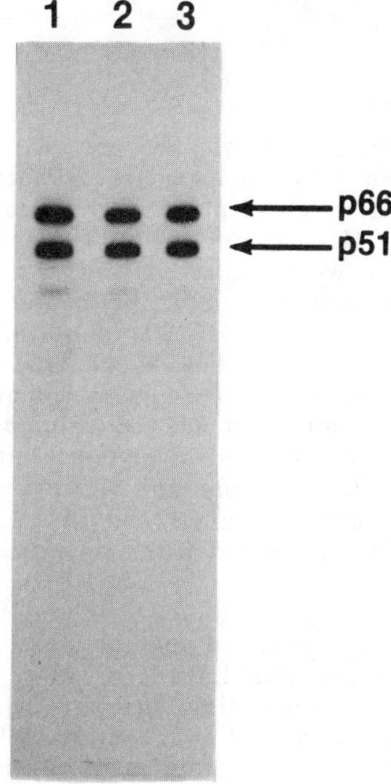

Figure 4. Detection of p66/p51 by mouse monoclonal antibody (M3364) in the immunoblot assay. Lanes 1, 2, and 3, supernatant fluids from three individual clones of the mouse hybridoma line M3364.

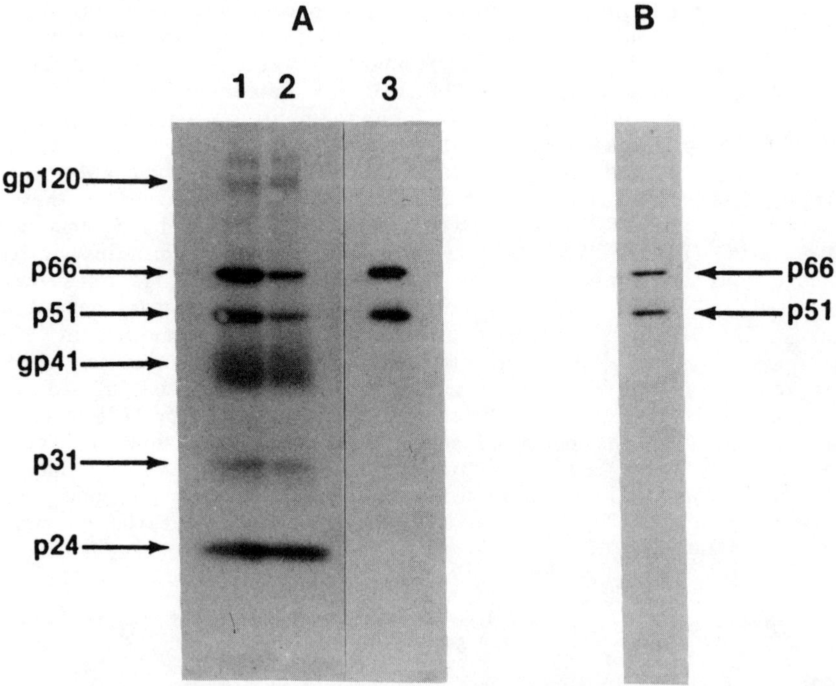

Figure 5. Purification of p66/p51 by immunoaffinity chromatography. Purified IgG from mouse monoclonal antibody M3364 was coupled to activated CH-Sepharose and prepared into a column. An extract of HTLV-III was applied to the IgG-Sepharose column. The unbound proteins were collected and the column was washed with the equilibration buffer. Proteins bound to the column were eluted with 0.2 M glycine, pH 2.8, containing 0.1 mM phenylmethylsulfonyl fluoride (PMSF) and 4 ml fractions were collected. (A) Western blot profiles on the unfractionated sample (lane 1), the fraction that did not bind to the column (lane 2), and a fraction eluted from the column with glycine buffer (lane 3). The antibody source was serum from an AIDS patient. (B) A sample identical to the one used in lane 2 of (A) was analyzed by acrylamide gel electrophoresis and stained with Coomassie blue.

Immunoaffinity purified p66/51 was assayed for RT activity. The enzyme reaction was linear for more than 60 minutes at 37°C (Figure 6), clearly indicating that at least one of the two proteins recognized by M3364 was active RT of HTLV-III. Whether both peptides are required to achieve full enzymatic activity or either peptide is independently active is not known at the moment. The fact that antibodies to HTLV-III RT are highly prevalent among virus-infected people presents a unique finding of a retroviral RT being so highly immunogenic in the course of natural infection.

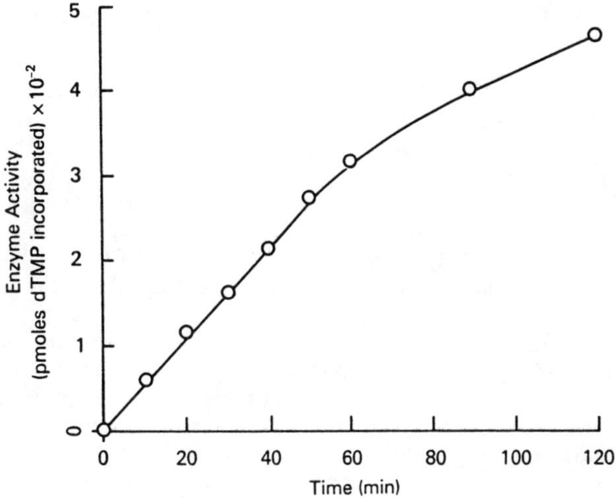

Figure 6. Kinetics of reverse transcriptase (RT) activity. Portions of fractions eluted from the immunoaffinity column (Figure 5) were neturalized and assayed for RT activity using oligo (dT) · poly (A) as the primer · template (183).

Nucleotide sequences 3' to the RT portion of the pol gene code for a 31kD endonuclease molecule (166),(184). This part of the pol gene was cloned into bacterial expression vectors for direct expression of the endonuclease and for expression as a fusion protein with human superoxide dismutase. The endonuclease and the fusion protein contained in the bacterial extracts were found to be immunoreactive when analyzed by a Western blot immunoassay using sera of AIDS patients (184). From initial results, the endonuclease appears to correlate well with RT in eliciting antibodies in the infected host.

Env Gene Products

HTLV-III env gene encodes information for two structural glycosylated proteins. These include gp120 as the amino terminal exterior component and gp41 as the carboxy-terminal transmembrane portion. They are initially synthesized in the form of a 160kD precursor polyprotein. Sera of HTLV-III infected individuals react with two glycoproteins, gp120 and gp41 present in viral preparations analyzed by Western blotting (Figure 7) (185). Moreover, gp41 is the antigen most consistently correlated with seropositivity to HTLV-III and the reactivity to it is the most persistent (160),(161). A hybridoma designated M25 secreted an antibody recognizing the same gp41 that was reactive with positive human sera (Figure 2) and was instrumental in characterizing this protein as indeed a viral component representing the transmembrane portion of the env gene (186). The precursor product relationship between gp160 and gp41 was established by immunoprecipitation followed by radiolabel sequencing of gp41. HTLV-III_B-producing H9 cells were labeled with either [^{3}H]-leucine or [^{3}H]-isoleucine overnight and the cell lysates immunoprecipitated with the M25 monoclonal antibody. The resulting immunoprecipitates were analyzed by SDS-PAGE (Figure 8) and the radioactive gp41 band was sliced out. The protein was then eluted and used for aminoterminal amino acid sequence analysis. Isoleucine was unambiguously assigned at position 4 of the first 24 cycles examined. Leucine occurred in cycles 7, 9, 12, 26, 33, and 34 out of 40 cycles analyzed (Figure 9). These sequences were compared with the nucleotide sequence of the env gene of HTLV-III. The amino acid sequence determined was a perfect match with the predicted sequence and it precisely located gp41 in the env gene of HTLV-III provirus clones BH10 and BH8. Furthermore, these sequencing data identify gp41 as the carboxy-terminal fragment generated by cleavage of gp160 between arg^{518} and ala^{519} (Figure 10).

Gp120 was purified in our laboratory from a lysate of HTLV-III by sequential chromatographic procedures using a Waters HPLC system (unpublished results). An aliquot of the purified gp120 appeared as a single protein band stained by a silver stain after SDS-PAGE (Figure 11A). The functional integrity of the purified protein was monitored by an absorption experiment. A human serum that gave a clear immunological reaction with gp120 on Western blots was preincubated with an aliquot of the purified gp120. The absorbed serum specifically lost reactivity to gp120, while retaining reactivities to other HTLV-III antigens (Figure 11B).

Radioimmunoprecipitation of metabolically labeled viral proteins in extracts of HTLV-III-producing cells with anti-HTLV-III positive patient sera bring down both the gp160 and gp120 along with other viral antigens (187). Allan et al. (188) separated these labeled gp160 and gp120 by electrophoresis and subjected each to automated Edman degradation. This yielded identical radiolabeled amino acid sequences for both gp160 and gp120 in the first 40 degradation cycles. A comparison of the experimentally observed positions of leucine, cysteine, and valine with the predicted amino acid sequence of HTLV-III gene products gave a perfect match for gp160 and gp120 to be products of the env gene of HTLV-III. The processing of gp160 thus involves a cleavage near the carboxy end of the molecule to generate the amino terminal gp120 and the carboxy terminal gp41.

Comments on Western Blot Confirmation of the HTLV-III-Antibody Test

A review of the Western blot reactions of a large number of antibody positive sera indicate that gp120 only reacts with a small percent of sera. This may lead to the erroneous conclusion that gp120 may not be as immunogenic as some other antigens that are more frequently identified by the immunoblot technique. When proteins of HTLV-III-producing cells are metabolically labeled with radioactive amino acids and reacted with antibody-positive human sera, the immunoprecipitates contain HTLV-III env and gag

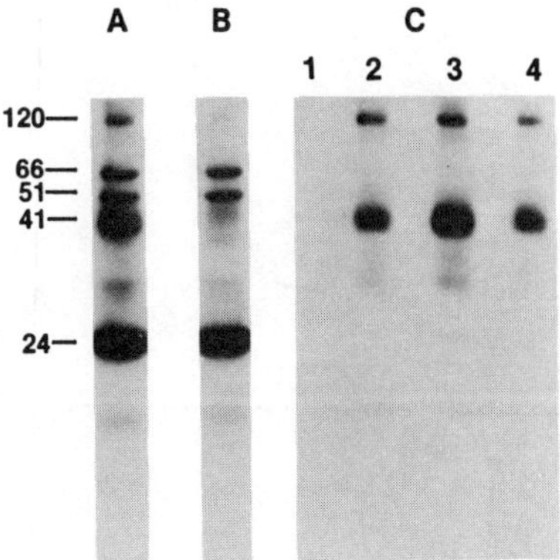

Figure 7. Sucrose density-banded HTLV-III was solubilized with Triton x-100 and NaCl and chromatographed on a column of lentil lectin-agarose. Bound glycoproteins were eluted with 0.5 M alpha-methylmannoside. Aliquots of the virus extract (A), the flowthrough fraction (B) and each of the first four alpha-methyl-mannoside-eluted fractions (C, Lanes 1-4) were analyzed by immunoblot assay with an HTLV-III antibody-positive human serum to identify the seroreactive antigens (185). Numbers on left are antigen sizes in thousands.

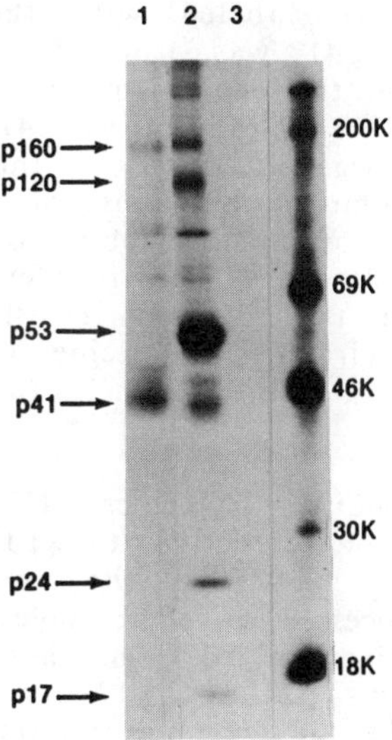

Figure 8. Immunoprecipitation of metabolically labeled HTLV-III proteins by AIDS sera and mouse monoclonal antibody to HTLV-III p41 (M25). Tissue culture cells were radioactively labeled by incubation for 18 hours with (^{3}H)-leucine. Lane 1, ascitic fluid from M25; Lane 2, serum from AIDS patient; Lane 3, negative human control serum.

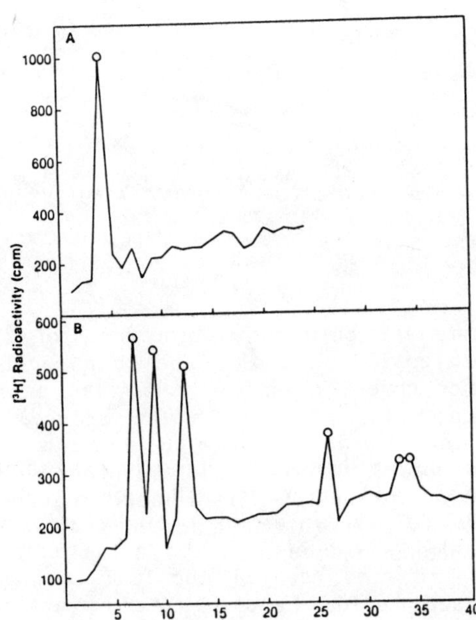

Figure 9. Amino terminal sequence analysis of p41 labeled with (A) [^{3}H]-isoleucine and (B) [^{3}H]-leucine. H9/HTLV-III$_B$ cells were labeled with the radioactive amino acids and the labeled p41 was isolated from cell extract by immunoprecipitation with the mouse monoclonal antibody M25 as described in Figure 8. The radioactive p41 band was identified by autoradiography and was sliced out of the gel and eluted with water containing 10 nmoles of apomyoglobin. The dialyzed proteins in the presence of apomyoglobin were subjected to semi-automated Edman degradation. The recovery of radioactivity in each cycle is given in the figure. Positive identifications are indicated by the open circles. Isoleucine was found in position 4 while leucine was found in positions 7, 9, 12, 26, 33 and 34.

proteins and their precursor molecules (187). Thus, even sera that show no Western blot reaction to gp120, precipitate gp120 from the cell extract. In fact, the env precursor molecule gp160, and the two processed envelope molecules gp120 and gp41, are all clearly identified in the immunoprecipitate (Figure 8). Similarly, the gag proteins p24 and p17 are accompanied by their common precursor p53 in the immunoprecipitate. This latter point is highly significant and often useful in some critical studies. Individuals seroconverting to HTLV-III often do not show a complete range of antibody reactivities. We have observed that they may show a reactivity to just p24 in the Western blot. There are instances in which a Western blot reactivity to a protein similar in size to viral p24 may be seen in sera of some

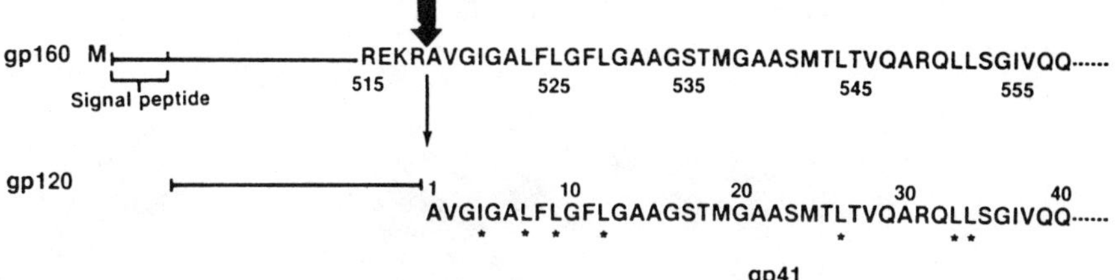

Figure 10. Diagram representing the processing of the primary env gene product into gp120 and gp41. The amino acids are represented by single letter codes. Numbers below the amino acid sequence of gp160 denote the positions in the deduced amino acid sequences for the primary gene product. Bold arrow indicates the identified cleavage site. Amino acid residues identified by asterisks are those determined by radiolabel sequence analysis (Figure 9). Numbers above the amino acids in gp41 denote the degradation cycle of the sequence procedure.

normal blood donors. Identification of the true antiviral reactivity can be made by analyzing the questionable serum by immunoprecipitation of the labeled extract of HTLV-III-producing cells. If the p24 reactivity is truly antiviral, the immunoprecipitate will show both the p24 and also its cellular precursor p53.

Genetic Variability of HTLV-III Genomes

A striking property of the HTLV-III genome is the extent of variability from one isolate to another. The molecular cloning of HTLV-III made it possible to analyze restriction enzyme maps of DNA from different HTLV-III isolates by Southern blotting. Extensive differences in the restriction enzyme sites were found between DNA from different isolates, in all parts of the viral genome (165),(189),(190). Genetic variability is of obvious importance in many aspects of the biology of HTLV-III relating to host immune surveillance. A detailed analysis of this problem was undertaken (190) using published information on the DNA sequence of several isolates of HTLV-III to establish the gene order and open reading frame distribution (166)-(168),(191),(192). The greatest differences were found to occur within the env gene and to some extent in the 3'orf. Outside the env and 3'orf genes, most differences were scattered point mutations, most of which were in the third base of codons and resulted either in no change in the amino acid sequence or in conservative amino acid substitutions. Other differences resulted from duplications in short stretches of DNA in the gag-pol overlap region. Differences in the 3'orf gene included frameshift deletions and premature termination signals.

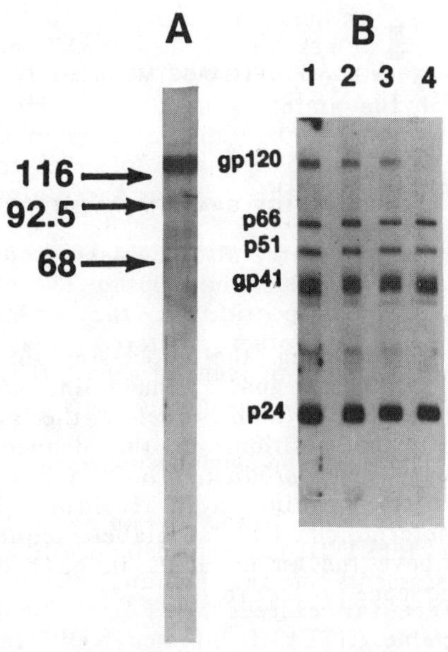

Figure 11. Purification and immunological identification of HTLV-III gp120. Gp120 was purified from an HTLV-III extract as described in the text. The purified sample was analyzed by SDS-PAGE and visualized by silver stain (A). The purified gp120 was used to absorb the Western blot reactivites of an HTLV-III-antibody positive human serum against HTLV-III antigens in a viral lysate (B). Lanes 1 and 3 are the reactivities with 5 and 1 *ul* aliquots of the unabsorbed serum. Lanes 2 and 4 are the patterns with 5 and 1 *ul* aliquots of the serum absorbed with gp120. Lane 4 shows a clear absorption specifically of the gp120 reactivity. The numbers in panel A represent molecular weights of standard proteins in thousands.

In addition to conservative point mutations, the differences within env genes included clustered and non-clustered non-conservative point mutations and small duplications and deletions. The former probably occur through reverse transcriptional errors while the latter likely reflect a copy choice mechanism whereby the reverse transcriptase switches templates during the course of transcription.

From the relatively low amount of diversity seen in non-env regions it is likely that changes in these regions would be deleterious for virus replication and are therefore selected against. It is evident that even within the env gene, high relative divergence is clustered within several regions and that regions of strong conservation are also present. Particularly notable is the conservation of all 18 cysteine residues in the large external membrane protein gp120 and of the three cysteine residues closest to the amino terminus of the transmembrane protein gp41. These cysteines could be very important to the three dimensional structure of the env proteins. The constant regions include most of the amino terminal 100 amino acids of the gp120, substantial regions of the middle portion of the gp120, 50-60 amino acids at the amino terminus of the gp41, and other scattered areas. Presumably these areas are also critical for virus replication and transmission.

Areas of hypervariability are also evident and include large areas from amino acids 150 to 200 and 300 to 380 of the env precursor polyprotein, the signal peptide at the amino terminus of the env precursor, and several other scattered areas. The degree of difference is great enough to suggest that these regions are not critical for viral replication and transmission.

Mechanisms of Cytopathic Effect and Immunosuppression

Considerable effort is being made to unravel the basic mechanisms responsible for HTLV-III-induced cell death and the generalized effect on all segments of the immune system. The overall immunosuppressive effect far exceeds what may be predicted from the number of detectable HTLV-III-infected cells in vivo. Both in vivo and in vitro observations suggest that events coincident or subsequent to expression of virus are responsible for most of the pathological developments. Many observations of a decrease in specific immune functions or immune markers even in the face of evidence of generalized, nonspecific immune activation have been made (193). Most notable is the quantitative loss of T4 helper T lymphocytes (194),(195). Although not necessarily confirmed when testing individual cell subtypes (196), reduced levels of lymphokines and gamma interferon were also reported (197). Defects in the function of selected cells included: reduced lymphoproliferative response to soluble antigens (196), defect in monocyte migration response to chemical stimuli (198), selective loss of HLA-restricted cytotoxic T lymphocyte (CTL) response (199), and reduced NK cell activity (200).

Use of pertinent immunological and hematological determinations, e.g., absolute number of helper T-lymphocytes, cellular immunity (delayed hypersensitivity), presence of antibody to HTLV-III proteins, etc., coupled with characteristic clinical symptoms including prolonged, atypical febrile illnesses (200a), chronic lymphadenopathy, thrush, or the presence of opportunistic infections, have led to the formulation of descriptive classification schemes of HTLV-III-related diseases (200b, 200c). These "staging" systems have proven useful in providing a uniform system for the clinical evaluation of patients and have facilitated an understanding of the natural history of HTLV-III infection.

With possible relevance to viral expression and development of disease, evidence for a state of immune activation was noted in AIDS and ARC patients. This included observations of increased HLA alloantigen induced CTL activity (199), elevated numbers of cells bearing activation markers (201), and increased levels of interferon alpha, and interferon induced oligoadenylate synthetase (202),(203). The significance of the specific observations in relation to the disease process and whether defects are a direct or indirect result of infection remain to be clarified. In vitro studies with HTLV-III-infected lymphocytes do suggest that immune stimulation may affect viral expression and cell death. It was reported that both primary T-lymphocytes from HTLV-III infected individuals and T-cells infected in vitro can be selected and grown in vitro without inducing the expression of virus. Immune (mitogen) stimulation, however, results in virus expression and concomitant cell death (119). Other observations suggest that the mode or type of immune stimulation may affect the time course of virus expression. For example, a comparison of the infectivity of HTLV-III in cultures of leukocytes stimulated with PHA or with HLA alloantigens (204) indicated that HLA-alloantigens were as effective as mitogens for establishing infection. However, HLA alloantigen stimulated, HTLV-III-infected cells tended to survive longer in cell culture and produced virus for a considerably longer period of time. This further suggested that HTLV-III does not necessarily exert a cytopathic effect under all conditions of infection. The cytopathic effect of this virus may be in part immune-mediated, with the polyclonal stimulation of T cells by mitogens leading to T cell-mediated destruction of infected cells. It is likely that unspecified co-actors could contribute to the cytopathic effect of HTLV-III-infection.

Mechanisms responsible for the cytopathic effect and generalized immune suppression are only beginning to be understood at the molecular level. Molecular manipulations of the viral genes have ruled out a direct involvement of several unique HTLV-III genes, e.g., sor, 3'orf, tat-III and art (205)-(208). For example, deletion of sor or 3'orf gene did not affect viral cytopathogenicity, and the presence of tat-III and art in the absence of env gene also did not result in cell death. At least some cell death has been attributed to the interaction of viral envelope glycoprotein on infected cells with the CD4 (T4 antigen) molecules on the same or on other cells, leading to cell fusion. Several lines of evidence demonstrate that this process requires both viral envelope and the T4 molecule. This fusion between HTLV-III env-positive cells and cells expressing T4 antigens was graphically illustrated using a two color immunofluorescence technique (209),(210). Cell fusion was blocked by antibody to T4 and by purified viral envelope gp120 (211). It was also suggested, at least in vitro, that conserved regions of the env gene product were involved, and that glycoproteins were needed for fusion as well as for infection of cells. At least some T4 cell death can, therefore, be attributed to HTLV-III env glycoprotein-mediated cell fusion and since infected cells can fuse with uninfected T4 positive cells, total cell death could be much more widespread than reflected only by the total number of infected cells. As suggested by others (194),(195), loss of these critical regulator T cells (helper/inducer) would certainly have far reaching consequences on cellular and humoral immunity.

Several other observations suggested that either viral coded proteins or a product of induced cellular genes might contribute to the loss of immune function in infected individuals. It was reported that some HTLV-III proteins may have an inhibiting effect on cell immune functions (64). Such effects have been demonstrated for other retroviral proteins (212). One candidate protein is the viral envelope, which was found to bind to the viral receptor on uninfected cells and to interfere with cell fusion and infection (211). Either soluble gp120, or intact virions could contribute to the systemic loss of immune functions by directly interfering with T4 cell functions, blocking cell surface sites needed for the recognition of cells or factors, or possibly by serving as a target for cytotoxic cellular interaction. A role for a virus-coded protein in pathogenesis was also suggested by the identification of an open reading frame whose 5'-end overlapped with the HTLV-III pol gene (unrelated to env) that shares some characteristics with a similar gene in visna virus, another cytopathic virus (175). Evidence was found that this gene is functional since it coded for a 23 kD protein which induced the production of antibody during natural infection (175).

The contribution of soluble factors to generalized immune dysfunction was further studied by testing products of infected cells. It was observed, for example, that peripheral blood mononuclear cells cultured from donors secrete factors capable of inhibiting mitogen-induced B cell maturation and immunoglobulin synthesis, and T cell proliferation (213 and our personal observation). A study of normal adult peripheral blood mononuclear cells infected by HTLV-III in vitro also demonstrated the liberation of factor(s) capable of inhibiting immunoglobulin synthesis and T cell activation. The production of both activities gradually declined more or less coinciding with overall cell death in the infected cultures (our personal observation). Whether these activities represent viral or cell gene products remain to be determined. However, if they are found to play a significant role in the pathogenesis of HTLV-III disease, their detection and control could be useful in the management of the disease.

Other HTLV-III-Associated Diseases

The involvement of HTLV-III in disorders of the central nervous system is well documented. Approximately 30% of patients with AIDS have neurological symptoms before death, and brain tissue obtained at autopsy from over 75% of AIDS patients shows neuropathological changes (214),(215). Virus has been observed and/or isolated from a variety of neurologic tissues including brain, CSF, and lumbar spinal cord (122)-(125). De novo synthesis of antibodies specific for HTLV-III was also found to occur behind the blood-brain barrier (216). The cells most commonly found to be infected in the neurologic tissue were lymphocytes and multinucleated giant cells (composed of monocytes/macrophages). Infection of endothelial cells lining brain capillaries was also indicated. Interestingly, inoculation of macaques with simian T lymphotropic virus type III (STLV-III), a virus similar to HTLV-III, frequently resulted in the development of encephalopathy (217). The mechanisms by which HTLV-III is involved in the development of neurological disorders are not known. In addition to the possibility of direct infection of nerve cells, the following indirect mechanisms may be considered: 1) production of factors by infected macrophages which affect normal cell function; 2) a hyperimmune response to viral antigens resulting in normal cell damage; and 3) basal ganglia calcification resulting from damage to infected endothelial cells. Regarding the possibility of soluble factors affecting neurological function, it was reported that neuroleukin, a lymphokine produced by lectin-stimulated T cells, exhibited both neuronal cell growth and lymphocyte modulation activity, and shares some sequence homology with a conserved portion of HTLV-III envelope (218). It is clear that strategies aimed at control of HTLV-III must include agents able to penetrate into the nervous system.

A number of neoplastic disorders are associated with HTLV-III infection and the development of AIDS (219). Kaposi's sarcoma (KS) was recognized as a manifestation of AIDS even in the earliest reported cases (220), and is in fact included as part of the clinical definition of AIDS, although AIDS-associated KS has been mostly limited to homosexual men (219). Among other malignancies reported, Burkitt-like lymphomas, non-Hodgkin's lymphomas, and other B-cell lymphomas appear to be the most prevalent (221)-(224).

The direct or indirect involvement of HTLV-III in malignancies remains to be determined. An indirect association mediated through resident EBV was suggested for some B cell neoplasms. For example, it has been noted that patients with AIDS, as well as some highly promiscuous healthy homosexual males have elevated levels of antibody to EBV and frequently develop fatal EBV-associated lesions (225)-(227). Furthermore, the presence of biologically active, transforming EBV was found in the plasma of AIDS patients, especially those with B cell-associated diseases. The presence of circulating infectious EBV correlated with a lack of EBV neutralizing antibody in the sera of these same patients (228). The increased EBV activity may be caused by the generalized immune suppression associated with HTLV-III infection or the formation of immune complexes which bind neutralizing antibody.

Control of the Spread of HTLV-III

Stability and Inactivation of HTLV-III in Laboratory and Clinical Environments

The stability of HTLV-III when exposed to several commonly encountered conditions was investigated (229)-(231). In the presence of human plasma, infectious HTLV-III can be recovered from dried material at room temperature, for surprisingly long periods of time, i.e., more than three days beginning with a titer of virus of 10^7 (the rate of inactivation being roughly 1 $\log_{10}TCID_{50}$ per 9 hr). This finding could have important implications for the transmission of virus by contaminated needles and syringes and in clinical situations involving contact with patient tissues or bodily products. Furthermore, in an aqueous environment infectious virus survived longer than 15 days at room temperature (23-27°C), and at 36-37°C the rate of inactivation was 1 log/83-116 min. (229). These findings are summarized in Table 3.

It was clear from these and other studies that infectious HTLV-III can be present following exposure to a number of environmental conditions encountered in a laboratory and/or clinical setting. Fortunately, HTLV-III behaves similarly to other enveloped retroviruses in its sensitivity to chemical disinfectants and detergents. Also summarized in Table 3 is the effect of several commonly used reagents, including sodium hypochlorite (bleach), ethanol, paraformaldehyde, quarternary ammonium chlorides, NP-40, and nonoxynol-9 (a non-ionic surfactant commonly used in spermicides) (232),(233). Anti-viral agents have also been tested on infected cells. For example, fixation with cold acetone (234) or with a combination of methanol and acetone (229) also abolished the ability to recover virus.

Prevention and Treatment of HTLV-III Disease

Intense multifaceted programs are in progress addressing the development of ways to prevent infection by HTLV-III, and to intervene in the pathological consequence of infection. Due to several characteristic peculiarities associated with HTLV-III specifically or to retroviruses in general, the process of developing a useful vaccine for preventing viral infection and spread is faced with many challenges. Unlike some infectious agents, use of whole or attenuated virus for immunization has only been considered with much trepidation for fear of the consequences from inadvertent use of incompletely inactivated virus, or possible regeneration of active virus by recombination with cellular genes or genes from other infecting agents. Furthermore, a direct immunosuppressive effect suggested for some viral proteins (212) may limit which proteins can be used and their manner of presentation. Since the envelope proteins would be expected to be primary targets for immune recognition, all or parts of the viral env-gene-coded proteins have received special attention.

A number of methods, each with its inherent advantages and disadvantages, are being used to test the immunogenicity of selected proteins, or combinations of proteins (235). These include: 1) the isolation and purification of selected viral proteins; 2) the chemical synthesis of selected proteins; 3) the introduction by genetic manipulation of selected viral genes into expression vectors for the synthesis of viral proteins; 4) use of certain viral genes as vectors for introducing HTLV-III env gene directly into host cells; and 5) production of anti-idiotypic antibody to serve as a primary immunogen.

Many of these studies include the testing of methods to optimize immunogenicity. For example, some success has been reported using immune-stimulating complexes (ISCOMS). These are

Table 3. Stability/Inactivation of HTLV-III

Treatment	Substrate	Infectious Titer/ Inactivation Rate	Reference
Heat			
37°C	media/human	1 log/83-116 min	(229),(230)
50°C	plasma or serum	1 log/24 min	(230)
56°C	plasma or serum	1 log/2-20 min	(229),(230)
60°C	plasma or serum	1 log/24 sec	(230)
pH.			
pH- 3	media	4 log/10 min	(231)
pH-13	media	5 log/10 min	(231)
Chemical			
H_2O_2 (0.3%)	media	6 log/10 min	(231)
Ethyl alcohol (50%)	media	5 log/10 min	(231)
Ethyl alcohol (70%)	50% plasma	10 log/min	(229)
Isopropyl alcohol (35%)	media	5 log/10 min	(231)
Paraformaldehyde (0.5%)	media	6 log/10 min	(231)
Quaternary ammonium chlorides (0.08%)	50% plasma	10 log/10 min	(229)
Sodium hypochlorite (bleach) (0.1%)	media	5 log/10 min	(229)
Sodium hypochlorite (bleach) (0.5%)	50% plasma	10 log/10 min	(229)
Iodine (wescodyne) (approximately 0.4% iodine)	media	5 log/10min	a
Nonidet P-40 (0.5%)	50% plasma	10 log/min	(229)
Tween-20 (2.5%)	media	0 log/10 min	(231)
Tri(n-butyl)phosphate/ sodium cholate	0.3%/0.2% anti-hemophiliac factor	1 log/5 min	(232)

[a] P. Sarin (personal communication).

small rosettes of protein and lipid which incorporate viral proteins in a way to, at least, partially mimic intact virions (236). Virus-neutralizing immune response has also been obtained in some animals inoculated with a recombinant vaccinia virus vector containing the env gene of HTLV-III (237),(238).

A number of species of animals have been tested for their ability to be infected by HTLV-III. The only non-human animal model giving promising results to date has been chimpanzees. These are susceptible to infection, develop viremia, and virus can be recovered from their blood cells. However, no pathological consequences have yet been reported. When inoculated with virus-infected tissues, partially purified virus or viral proteins, chimpanzees can also mount a substantial immune response (239)-(241). Of concern is the fact that chimpanzees are in limited supply and available animals must be used judiciously.

A number of anti-viral agents are also being tested for possible use for treatment. The chemotherapeutic approach has concentrated on special categories of pharmacological agents with demonstrated in vitro inhibiting effects on HTLV-III infection and/or replication. Potential agents must be relatively non-toxic to the host. Another consideration is the desirability of an agent having the potential of crossing the blood-brain barrier. Many of the drugs tested were known to inhibit viral RT (242),(243) an enzyme involved in the initial stage of retrovirus infection and replication. Several of these and other candidate drugs were tested for an effect on the replication of HTLV-III. For example, suramin (244),(245), ribavirin (246), 3'-azido-3'deoxythymidine (AZT) (247) and other nucleoside analogs (248), and rifamycin derivatives (249) were reported to block the infection of T-cells by HTLV-III in vitro. Alpha-interferon (250), phosphonoformate (251), and antimonotungstate (HPA-23) (252) were also reported to be effective. However, a polyanion such as HPA-23 should not be expected to be a specific inhibitor of RT and in fact should be a general inhibitor of many cellular enzymes. Other RT inhibitors that have been tested include a combination of the T cell stimulating compounds dithiocarb and inosine pranobex (253), and exogenous synthetic oligonucleotides complementary to viral RNA (254).

Preliminary clinical trials of suramin (255) and AZT (256)-(258) performed on AIDS or ARC patients yielded results encouraging to a chemotherapeutic approach to virus control. Of the compounds tested, the purine and pyrimidine nucleoside analogs appeared to be most promising in fulfilling viral inhibitory functions, being non-toxic, and effective in the central nervous system. Other primary agents e.g., dideoxycytidine and ribavirin, await rigorous in vivo testing. Treatment may require combined therapy with two or more agents for optimal effectiveness. It is generally believed that even with a safe and effective anti-viral agent, treatment will require an approach utilizing combined therapy. This may allow use of doses lower than will be effective individually, and therefore may prove beneficial while lowering risk of cumulative side effects. For example, in vitro studies with suramin and acyclovir (a nucleoside analogue commonly used to treat herpes viruses) suggested that combined use substantially reduced the concentration of each agent needed to inhibit viral infection (259).

RELATED PRIMATE RETROVIRUSES

Nonhuman Primate Retroviruses

A number of retroviruses related to HTLV-I or HTLV-III have been found in several species of non-human primates. For example, serum antibodies reactive with HTLV-I were found in wild-caught Japanese macaques (260)-(262). HTLV-I antibodies were also detected in other monkeys and apes, e.g., African green monkeys, rhesus monkeys, cynomolgus monkeys, and chimpanzees (263)-(268). Subsequent to serological studies, virus homologous to HTLV-I, called STLV-I, was isolated from several primate species (263), (269)-(271). A role for these primate viruses in the development of disease has not been clearly established. However, STLV-I was shown to transform lymphocytes in vitro and in a rare instance was isolated from an animal with a spontaneous lymphoid malignancy (272). This widespread prevalence in animals in Africa and other old World countries, and serological evidence that humans in some areas have also been exposed to these or closely related viruses (265),(273),(274) have led to speculation regarding the possible African origin of HTLV-I.

Several old World primates also were found to harbor a virus immunologically related to HTLV-III. This was named STLV-III. The virus isolated from apparently healthy African green monkeys is called $STLV\text{-}III_{AGM}$ (275). $STLV\text{-}III_{AGM}$ contains some proteins that are immunologically related to proteins of HTLV-III. Antibodies to a T lymphotropic retrovirus were seen from captive and wild-caught sooty mangabeys and a distinct virus was eventually isolated (276),(277). It is interesting that these isolates are not cytopathic in their natural hosts. A retrovirus probably identical to $STLV\text{-}III_{AGM}$ was isolated from rhesus macaque monkeys with lymphoma, splenomegaly, or opportunistic infections (278),(279). Also, macaques inoculated with $STLV\text{-}III_{AGM}$ developed an immune deficiency syndrome characterized by weight loss, a decrease in $T4^+$ peripheral blood lymphocytes, and opportunistic infections (217). A virus structurally related to STLV-III, although distinct except for some apparent homology in some core proteins, was isolated from one pig-tail macaque with poorly differentiated lymphoma (280). This virus was clearly distinguished from a type D retrovirus also found in macaques from primate centers, who suffer from an epidemic of immune deficiency associated with retroperitoneal fibromatosis (281).

OTHER HUMAN RETROVIRUSES

A retrovirus named HTLV-IV has been isolated from prostitutes in Senegal, West Africa (282). This virus cross-reacts with HTLV-III to some extent, but is more related to $STLV\text{-}III_{AGM}$

(282). A similar virus (SBL 6669) was recently isolated by Swedish scientists from the blood of an immunosuppressed West African patient (G. Biberfeld, personal communication). Another virus, referred to as LAV-2 (lymphadenopathy-associated virus-2) (283), was isolated from AIDS patients from Guinea-Bissau and Cape Verde. Sera from these patients cross-reacted with HTLV-III and more strongly with $STLV\text{-}III_{MAC}$. Unlike HTLV-IV, LAV-2 appears to be more cytopathic in vitro and to be associated with clinical AIDS in infected individuals.

CONCLUSIONS

The short history of human retrovirology has witnessed an explosive growth of unprecedented proportions. The field now attracts world-wide attention by thousands of scientists, public health officials, and those who formulate public policy. Shortly after the technology to grow human T-cells became available in 1976, the first key experiments to develop long-term cultures of human neoplastic T cells were conducted which, in turn, led to the isolation of the first human retrovirus. Unrelated to these developments, clinicians on a different continent were beginning to recognize a peculiar clustering of a certain aggressive form of T cell leukemia. It was quickly established that the first known human retrovirus was the causative agent. The experience gained with the study of this virus gave us insight into a possible cause of AIDS soon after it was recognized that the underlying feature of the syndrome was the loss of T-cell function. With the influx of scientists of diverse disciplines into the field, rapid progress is being made in understanding these viruses and the diseases they cause.

What has occurred so far has been an exhaustive exploitation of a critical, albeit very limited technology, i.e., the ability to grow human T cells in vitro. As similar technologies become available for growing and manipulating other types of human cells, we fully anticipate that similar breakthroughs in identifying etiologic agents for other diseases will follow. In essence, the field of human retrovirology is in its infancy.

REFERENCES

1. Ellermann, V., Bang, O., Experimentelle Leukaemie bei Huhnern. Centralbl f Bakt Abt I, (Orig.) 46:595-609 (1908)

2. Rous, P., Transmission of malignant new growth by means of a cell-free filtrate. JAMA 56:198 (1911)

3. Gross, L., "Spontaneous" leukemia developing in C3H mice following inoculation in infancy, with Ak leukemic extracts, or Ak-embryos. Proc Soc Exp Biol Med 78:27-32 (1951)

4. Weiss, R., Teich, N., Varmus, H.E. (eds.), RNA Tumor Viruses, Second Ed., Cold Spring Harbor Laboratory, Cold Spring Harbor, New York, (1982)

5. Jarrett, W.F.H., Martin, W.B., Crighton, G.W., et al., Leukemia in the cat. Transmission experiments with leukaemia (lymphosarcoma). Nature 202:566-567 (1964)

6. Jarrett, W.F.H., Crawford, E.M., Martin, W.B., et al., Leukemia in the cat: A virus-like particle associated with leukemia (lymphosarcoma). Nature 202:567-568 (1964)

7. Miller, J.M., Miller, L.D., Olson, C., et al., Virus-like particles in phytohemagglutinin-stimulated lymphocyte cultures with reference to bovine lympho-sarcoma. J Natl Cancer Inst 43:1297-1305 (1969)

8. Kawakami, T.G., Huff, S.D., Buckley, P.M., et al., C-type virus associated with gibbon lymphosarcoma. Nature New Biol 235:170-171 (1972)

9. Temin, H.M., Mizutani, S., RNA-dependent DNA polymerase in virions of Rous sarcoma virus. Nature 226:1211-1213 (1970)

10. Baltimore, D., Viral RNA-dependent DNA polymerase. Nature 226:1209-1211 (1970)

11. Gallo, R.C., Yang, S.S., Ting, R.C., RNA-dependent DNA polymerase of human acute leukemic cells. Nature 228:927-929 (1970)

12. Sarngadharan, M.G., Sarin, P.S., Reitz, M.S., et al., Reverse transcriptase activity of human acute leukaemic cells: Purification of the enzyme, response to AMV 70S RNA, and characterization of the DNA product. Nature New Biol 240:67-72 (1972)

13. Poiesz, B.J., Ruscetti, F.W., Gazdar, A.F., et al., Detection and isolation of type-C retrovirus from fresh and cultured lymphocytes of a patient with cutaneous T-cell lymphoma. Proc Natl Acad Sci USA 77:7415-7419 (1980)

14. Morgan, D.A., Ruscetti, F.W., Gallo, R.C., Selective in vitro growth of T-lymphocytes from normal human bone marrow. Science 192:1007-1008 (1976)

15. Ruscetti, F.W., Gallo, R.C., Human T-lymphocyte growth factor: Regulation of growth and function of T lymphocytes. Blood 57:379-394 (1981)

16. Waldmann, T.A., Greene, W.C., Sarin, P.S., et al., Functional and phenotypic comparison of human T-cell leukemia/lymphoma virus positive adult T cell leukemia with human T cell leukemia/lymphoma virus negative Sezary leukemia, and their distinction using anti-TAC. J Clin Invest 73:1711-1718 (1984)

17. Poiesz, B.J., Ruscetti, F.W., Mier, J.W., et al., T-cell lines established from human T-lymphocytic neoplasias by direct response to T-cell growth factor. Proc Natl Acad Sci USA 77:6815-6819 (1980)

18. Poiesz, B.J., Ruscetti, F.W., Reitz, M.S., et al., Isolation of a new type-C retrovirus (HTLV) in primary uncultured cells of a patient with Sezary T-cell leukemia. Nature 294:268-271 (1981)

19. Takatsuki, K., Uchiyama, J., Sagawa, K., et al., Adult T-cell leukemia in Japan, In: Topics in Hematology (Seno, S., Takaku, F., Irino, S., eds.), Excerpta Medica, Amsterdam, p 73-77 (1977)

20. Takatsuki, K., Uchiyama, T., Ueshima, Y., et al., Adult T-cell leukemia: further clinical observations and cytogeneic and functional studies of leukemic cells. Jpn J Clin Oncol 9:317-324 (1979)

21. Uchiyama, T., Yodoi, J., Sagawa, K., et al., Adult T-cell leukemia: clinical and hematologic features of 16 cases. Blood 50:481-492 (1977)

22. Catovsky, D., Greaves, M.F., Rose, M., et al., Adult T-cell lymphoma-leukemia in blacks from the West Indies. Lancet 1:639-642 (1982)

23. Tajima, K., Tominaga, S., Kuroishi, T., et al., Geographical features and epidemiological approach to endemic T-cell leukemia/lymphoma in Japan. Jpn J Clin Oncol 9(Suppl.):495-504 (1979)

24. Hanaoka, M., Clinical pathology of adult T-cell leukemia. Acta Haematol (Jpn.) 44:1420-1430 (1981)

25. Takatsuki, K., Uchiyama, T., Ueshima, Y., et al., Adult T-cell leukemia: proposal as a new disease and cytogenetic, phenotypic, and functional studies of leukemic cells. Gann 28:13-22 (1982)

26. Waldmann, T., Broder, S., Greene, W., et al., A comparison of the function and phenotype of Sezary T-cells with human T-cell leukemia/lymphoma virus (HTLV)-associated adult T-cell leukemia. Clin Res 31:5474-5480 (1983)

27. Popovic, M., Sarin, P.S., Robert-Guroff, M., et al., Isolation and transmission of human retrovirus (human T-cell leukemia virus). Science 219:856-859 (1983)

28. Yamada, Y., Phenotypic and functional analysis of leukemic cells from 16 patients with adult T-cell leukemia/lymphoma. Blood 61:192-199 (1983)

29. Blattner, W.A., Kalyanaraman, V.S., Robert-Guroff, M., et al., The human type-C retrovirus, HTLV, in blacks from the Caribbean region, and relationship to adult T-cell leukemia/lymphoma. Int J Cancer 30:257-264 (1982)

30. Blattner, W.A., Takatsuki, K., Gallo, R.C., Human T-cell leukemia/lymphoma virus and adult T-cell leukemia. JAMA 250:1074-1081 (1983)

31. Miyoshi, I., Kubonishi, I., Yoshimoto, S., et al., Type C virus particles in a cord T-cell line derived by co-cultivating normal human cord leukocytes and human leukemic T-cells. Nature 294:770-771 (1981)

32. Yoshida, M., Miyoshi, I., Hinuma, Y., Isolation and characterization of retrovirus from cell lines of human adult T-cell leukemia and its implication in the disease. Proc Natl Acad Sci USA 79:2031-2035 (1982)

33. Haynes, B.F., Miller, S.W., Palker, T.J., et al., Identification of human T-cell leukemia virus in a Japanese patient with adult cell leukemia and cutaneous lymphomatous vasculitis. Proc Natl Acad Sci USA 80:2054-2058 (1983)

34. Vyth-Drees, F.A., de Vries, J.E., Human T-cell leukemia virus in lymphocytes from a T-cell leukaemia patient originating from Surinam. Lancet 2:993 (1983)

35. Greaves, M.F., Verbi, W., Tilley, R., et al., Human T-cell leukemia virus (HTLV) in the United Kingdom. Int J Cancer 33:795-806 (1984)

36. Reitz, M.S., Poiesz, B.J., Ruscetti, F.W., et al., Characterization and distribution of nucleic acid sequences of a novel type-C retrovirus isolated from neoplastic human T lymphocytes. Proc Natl Acad Sci USA 78:1887-1891 (1981)

37. Gallo, R.C., Mann, D., Broder, S., et al., Human T-cell leukemia-lymphoma virus (HTLV) is in T- but not B-lymphocytes from a patient with cutaneous T-cell lymphoma. Proc Natl Acad Sci USA 79:4680-4683 (1982)

38. Manzari, V., Wong-Staal, F., Franchini, et al., Human T-cell leukemia-lymphoma virus (HTLV): cloning of an integrated defective provirus and flanking cellular sequences. Proc Natl Acad Sci USA 80:1574-1578 (1983)

39. Seiki, M., Hattori, S., Yoshida, M., Human adult T-cell leukemia virus: molecular cloning of the provirus DNA and the unique terminal structure. Proc Natl Acad Sci USA 79:6899-6902 (1982)

40. Seiki, M., Hattori, S., Hirayama, Y., et al., Human adult T-cell leukemia virus: complete nucleotide sequence of the provirus genome integrated in leukemia cell DNA. Proc Natl Acad Sci USA 80:3618-3622 (1983)

41. Sodroski, J.G., Rosen, C.A., Haseltine, W.A., Transacting transcriptional activation of the long terminal repeat of human T-lymphotropic viruses in infected cells. Science 325:381-385 (1984)

42. Wong-Staal, F., Gallo, R.C., The family of human T-lymphotropic leukemia viruses: HTLV-I as a cause of adult T cell leukemia and HTLV-III as the cause of acquired immunodeficiency syndrome. Blood 65:253-263 (1985)

43. Hayward, W.S., Neel, B.G., Astrin, S.M., Induction of lymphoid leukosis by avian leukosis virus: activation of a cellular onc gene by promoter insertion. Nature 290:475-480 (1981)

44. Neel, B.G., Hayward, W.S., Robinson, H.L., et al., Avian leukosis virus-induced tumors have common proviral integration sites and synthesize discrete new RNAs: oncogenesis by promoter insertion. Cell 23:323-334 (1981)

45. Hahn, B., Manzari, V., Columbini, S., et al., Common site of integration of HTLV in cells of three patients with mature T-cell leukemia-lymphoma. Nature 303:253 (1983)

46. Hahn, B., Manzari, V., Columbini, S., et al., Common site of integration of HTLV in cells of three patients with mature T-cell leukemia-lymphoma: A retraction. Nature 305:340 (1983)

47. Greene, W.C., Leonard, W.J., Wano, Y., et al., Trans-activator gene of HTLV-III induces IL-2 receptor and IL-2 cellular gene expression. Science 232:877-880 (1986)

48. Okada, M., Maeda, M., Tagaya, Y., et al., TCGF (IL-2)-receptor(s). II. Possible role at ATL-derived factor (ADF) on constitutive IL-2 receptor expression of HTLV-I(+) T cell lines. J Immunol 135:3995 (1985)

49. Nakamura, S., Taguchi, Y., Yodoi, J., et al., Interleukin-2-Receptor augmenting factor (IAF) expressed by HTLV-I and HTLV-II-infected and transformed cells but not by HTLV-III infected cells. (Submitted)

50. Wong-Staal, F., Gallo, R.C., Human T-lymphotropic retroviruses. Nature 317:395-403 (1985)

51. Markham, P.D., Salahuddin, S.Z., Kalyanaraman, V.S., et al., Infection and transformation of fresh human umbilical cord blood cells by multiple sources of human T-cell leukemia-lymphoma virus (HTLV). Int J Cancer 31:413-420 (1983)

52. Markham, P. D., Salahuddin, S.Z., Macchi, B., et al., Transformation of different phenotypic types of human bone marrow T-lymphocytes by HTLV-I. Int J Cancer 33:13-17 (1984)

53. Miedema, F., Terpstra, F.G., Smit, J.W., et al., Functional properties of neoplastic T cells in adult T cell lymphoma/leukemia patients from the Caribbean. Blood 63:477-481 (1984)

54. Longo, D. L., Gelmann, E. P., Cossman, J., et al., Isolation of HTLV-transformed B-lymphocyte clone from a patient with HTLV-associated adult T-cell leukaemia. Nature 310: 505-506 (1984)

55. Hiramatsu, K., Masuda, M., Yoshikura, H., Mode of transmission of human T-cell leukemia virus type I (HTLV-I) in a human promyelocytic leukemia HL60 cell. Int J Cancer 37:601-606 (1986)

56. Yoshikura, H., Nishida, J., Yoshida, M., et al., Isolation of HTLV derived from Japanese adult T-cell leukemia patients in human diploid fibroblast strain IMR90 and the biological characters of the infected cells. Int J Cancer 33:745-749 (1984)

57. Harper, M.E., Kaplan, M.H., Marselle, L.M., et al., Concomitant infection with HTLV-I and HTLV-III in a patient with T8 lymphoproliferative disease. N Engl J Med 315: 1073-1078 (1986)

58. Miyoshi, I., Yoshimoto, S., Kubonishi, I., et al., Infectious transmission of human T-cell leukemia virus to rabbits. Int J Cancer 35:81-85 (1985)

59. Akagi, I., Takata, H., Ohtsuki, Y., et al., Transformation of hamster spleen lymphocytes by human T-cell leukemia virus type I. Int J Cancer 37:775-779 (1986)

60. Tateno, M., Kondo, N., Itoh, T., et al., Rat lymphoid cell lines with human T cell leukemia virus production. I. Biological and serological characterization. J Exp Med 159: 1105-1116 (1984)

61. Hoshino, H., Tanaka, H., Shimotohno, K., et al., Immortalization of peripheral blood lymphocytes of cats by human T-cell leukemia virus. Int J Cancer 34:513-517 (1984)

62. Kotani, S., Yoshimoto, S., Yamato, K., et al., Serial transmission of human T-cell leukemia virus type I by blood transfusion in rabbits and its prevention by use of X-irradiated stored blood. Int J Cancer 37:843-847 (1986)

63. Salahuddin, S. Z., Markham, P. D., Lindner, S. G., et al., Lymphokine production by cultured human T-cells transformed by human T-cell leukemia-lymphoma virus. Science 223: 703-706 (1984)

64. Trainin, Z., Wernicke, D., Ungar-Waron, H., et al., Suppression of the humoral antibody response in natural retrovirus infections. Science 220:858 (1983)

65. Essex, M. E., McLane, M. F., Tachibana, N., et al., Seroepidemiology of human T-cell leukemia virus in relation to immunosuppression and the acquired immunodeficiency syndrome. In: Human T-cell Leukemia/ Lymphoma Virus, (Gallo, R.C., Essex, M., Gross, L., eds), Cold Spring Harbor Laboratory, Cold Spring Harbor, NY, p 355-362 (1984)

66. Kobayashi, M., Yoshimoto, S., Fujishita, M., et al., HTLV-positive T-cell lymphoma/leukaemia in an AIDS patient. Lancet 1:1361-1362 (1984)

67. Reeves, W., Saxinger, W.C., Clark, J., et al., Seroepidemiology of HTLV-I - Panama. J Infect Dis (In press)

68. Clark, J.W., Hahn, B.H., Mann, D.L., et al., Molecular and immunologic analysis of a chronic lymphocytic leukemia case with antibodies against human T-cell leukemia virus. Cancer 56:495-499 (1985)

69. Clark, J.W., Robert-Guroff, M., Ikehara, O., et al., Human T-cell leukemia-lymphoma virus type I and adult T-cell leukemia-lymphoma in Okinawa. Cancer Research 45:2849-2852 (1985)

70. Mitsuya, H., Guo, H-G., Megson, M., et al., Transformation and cytopathogenic effect in an immune human T-cell clone infected by HTLV-I. Science 223:1293-1296 (1984)

71. Mitsuya, H., Broder, S., Cytotoxic T-cells specific for human T-cell leukemia/lymphoma virus. In: Human T-cell Leukemia/Lymphoma Virus, (Gallo, R.C., Essex, M., Gross, L., eds), Cold Spring Harbor Laboratory, Cold Spring Harbor, NY p 229-235 (1984)

72. Popovic, M., Flomberg, N., Volkman, D.J., et al., Alteration of T-cell functions by infection with HTLV-I or HTLV-II. Science 226:459-462. (1984)

73. Osame, M., Usuku, K., Izumo, S., et al., HTLV-I associated myelopathy, a new clinical entity. Lancet 1:1031-1032 (1986)

74. Osame, M., Izumo, S., Igata, A., et al., Blood transfusion and HTLV-I associated myelopathy. Lancet 2:104-105 (1986)

75. Gessain, A., Barin, F., Vernant, J.C., et al., Antibodies to human T-lymphotropic virus type-I in patients with tropical spastic paraparesis. Lancet 2:407-410 (1985)

76. Rodgers-Johnson, P., Gajdusek, D. C., Morgan, O., et al., HTLV-I and HTLV-III antibodies and tropical spastic paraparesis. Lancet 2:1247-1248 (1985)

77. Bartholomew, C., Cleghoru, F., Charles, W., et al., HTLV-I and tropical spastic paraparesis. Lancet 2:99-100 (1986)

78. Gessain, A., Francis, H., Sonau, T., et al., HTLV-I and tropical spastic paraparesis in Africa. Lancet 2:698 (1986)

79. Kalyanaraman, V.S., Sarngadharan, M.G., Bunn, P.A., et al., Antibodies in human sera reactive against an internal structural protein of human T-cell lymphoma virus. Nature 294:271-273 (1981)

80. Gallo, R.C., Kalyanaraman, V.S., Sarngadharan, M.G., et al., Association of the human type-C retrovirus with a subset of adult T-cell cancers. Cancer Res 43:3892-3899 (1983)

81. Kalyanaraman, V.S., Sarngadharan, M.G., Nakao, Y., et al., Natural antibodies to the structural core protein (p24) of the human T-cell leukemia (lymphoma) retrovirus found in sera of leukemia patients in Japan. Proc Natl Acad Sci USA 79:1653-1657 (1982)

82. Robert-Guroff, M., Nakao, Y., Notake, K., et al., Natural antibodies to human retrovirus HTLV in a cluster of Japanese patients with adult T-cell leukemia. Science 215:975-978 (1982)

83. Robert-Guroff, M., Gallo, R.C., Establishment of an etiologic relationship between the human T-cell leukemia/lymphoma virus (HTLV) and adult T-cell leukemia. Blut 47:1-12 (1983)

84. Hinuma, Y., Komoda, H., Chosa, T., et al., Antibodies to adult T-cell leukemia-virus-associated antigen (ATLA) in sera from patients with ATL and controls in Japan: a nation-wide seroepidemiological study. Int J Cancer 29:631-635 (1982)

85. Hinuma, Y., Nagata, K., Misoka, M., et al., Adult T-cell leukemia: antigen in an ATL cell line and detection of antibodies to the antigen in human sera. Proc Natl Acad Sci USA 78:6476-6480 (1981)

86. Robert-Guroff, M., Schupbach, J., Blayney, D.W., et al., Sero-epidemiologic studies on HTLV-I. In: Human T-Cell Leukemia/Lymphoma Virus, (Gallo, R.C., Essex, M., Gross, L., eds) Cold Spring Harbor Press, Cold Spring Harbor, NY, p 285-295 (1984)

87. Blattner, W.A., Clark, J.W., Gibbs, W.N., et al., HTLV: epidemiology and relationship to human malignancy. In: Human T-Cell Leukemia/Lymphoma Virus, (Gallo, R.C., Essex, M., Gross, L., eds) Cold Spring Harbor Press, Cold Spring Harbor, NY, p 267-274 (1984)

88. Blattner, W.A., Blayney, D.W., Robert-Guroff, M., et al., Epidemiology of human T-cell leukemia/lymphoma virus. J Infect Dis 147:406-416 (1983)

89. Catovsky, D., Greaves, M.F., Rose, M., et al., Adult T-cell lymphoma-leukemia in blacks from the West Indies. Lancet 1:639-642 (1982)

90. Schupbach, J., Kalyanaraman, V.S., Sarngadharan, M.G., et al., Antibodies against three purified proteins of the human type-C retrovirus, human T-cell leukemia-lymphoma virus, in adult T-cell leukemia-lymphoma patients and healthy blacks from the Caribbean. Cancer Res 43:886-891 (1983)

91. Saxinger, W., Blattner, W.A., Lavine, P.H., et al., Human T-cell leukemia virus (HTLV-I) antibodies in Africa. Science 225:1473-1476 (1984)

92. Robert-Guroff, M., Kalyanaraman, V.S., Blattner, W.A., et al., Evidence for human T-cell lymphoma-leukemia virus infection of family members of human T-cell lymphoma-leukemia virus positive T-cell leukemia-lymphoma patients. J Exp Med 157:248-258 (1983)

93. Tajima, K., Tominaga, S., Suchi, T., et al., Epidemiological analysis on distribution of antibody to adult T-cell leukemia-virus-associated antigen (ATLA): possible horizontal transmission of adult T-cell leukemia virus. Gann 73:893-901 (1982)

94. Saxinger, W.C., Gallo, R.C., Possible risk to recipients of blood from donors carrying serum markers of human T cell leukemia virus. Lancet 1:1074 (1982)

95. Evatt, B.L., Stein, S.F., Francis, D.P., et al., Antibodies to human T cell leukaemia virus associated membrane antigens in haemophiliacs: evidence for infection before 1980. Lancet 2:698-700 (1983)

96. Blattner, W.A., Nomura, A., Clark, J.W., et al., Modes of transmission and evidence for viral latency from studies of human T-cell lymphotropic virus type 1 in Japanese migrant populations in Hawaii. Proc Natl Acad Sci USA 83:4895-4898 (1986)

97. Kalyanaraman, V.S., Sarngadharan, M.G., Robert-Guroff, M., et al., A new subtype of human T-cell leukemia virus (human T-leukemia virus-II) associated with a T-cell variant of hairy cell leukemia. Science 218:571-573 (1982)

98. Rosenblatt, J.D., Golde, D.W., Wachsman, W., et al., A second isolate of HTLV-II associated with atypical hairy cell leukemia. N Engl J Med 315:372-377 (1986)

99. Kalyanaraman, V.S., Narayanan, R., Feorino, P., et al., Isolation and characterization of a human T-cell leukemia virus type II from a hemophilia-A patient with pancytopenia. EMBO Journal 4:1455-1469 (1985)

100. Popovic, M., Kalyanaraman, V.S., Mann, D.L., et al., Infection and transformation of T cells by human T-cell leukemia/lymphoma virus of subgroups I and II (HTLV-I, HTLV-II). In Human T-cell Leukemia/ Lymphoma Virus, (Gallo, R. C., Essex, E., Gross, L., eds), Cold Spring Harbor Laboratory, NY, p 217-227 (1984)

101. Chen, I.S.Y., McLaughlin, J., Gasson, J.C., et al., Molecular characterization of genome of a novel human T-cell leukemia virus. Nature 305:502-505 (1983)

102. Gelmann, E.P., Franchini, G., Manzari, V., et al., Molecular cloning of a new unique human T-leukemia virus (HTLV-II_{MO}). Proc Natl Acad Sci USA 81:993-997 (1984)

103. Shimotohno, K., Takahashi, Y., Shimizu, N., et al., Complete nucleotide sequence of an infectious clone of human T-cell leukemia virus type II: An open reading frame for the protease gene. Proc Natl Acad Sci USA 82:3101-3105 (1985)

104. Haseltine, W.A., Sodroski, J., Patacra, R., et al., Structure of 3'-terminal region of Type-II human T-lymphotropic virus: evidence for new coding region. Science 225:419-421 (1984)

105. Wachsman, W., Shimotohno, K., Clark, S.C., et al., Expression of the 3' terminal region of human T-cell leukemia viruses. Science 226:177-179 (1984)

106. Lee, T.H., Coligan, J.E., Sodroski, J.A., et al., Antigens encoded by the 3'-terminal region of human T-cell leukemia virus: evidence for a functional gene. Science 226:57-61 (1984)

107. Salahuddin, S.Z., Markham, P.D., Wong-Staal, F., et al., Restricted expression of human T-cell leukemia-lymphoma virus (HTLV) in transformed human umbilical cord blood lymphocytes. Virology 129:51-64 (1983)

108. Slamon, D.J., Shimotohno, K., Kline, M., et al., Identification of the putative transforming protein of the human T-cell leukemia viruses HTLV-I and HTLV-II. Science 226: 61-65 (1984)

109. Gottlieb M.S., Schroff, R., Schanker H.M., et al., *Pneumocystis carinii* pneumonia and mucosal candidiasis in previously healthy homosexual men: evidence of a new acquired cellular immunodeficiency. N Engl J Med 305: 1425-1431 (1981)

110. Masur, H., Michelis, M.A., Greene, J.B., et al., An outbreak of community-acquired *Pneumocystis carinii* pneumonia: initial manifestation of cellular immune dysfunction. N Engl J Med 305:1431-1438 (1981)

111. Siegel, F.P., Lopez, C., Hammer G.S., et al., Severe acquired immunodeficiency in male homosexuals, manifested by chronic perianal ulcerative herpes simplex lesions. N Engl J Med 305:1439-1444 (1981)

112. Fauci, A.S., Macher, A.M., Longo, D.L., et al., Acquired immunodeficiency syndrome: epidemiologic clinical, immunologic and therapeutic considerations. Ann Intern Med 100: 92-106 (1984)

113. Francis, D.P., Curran, J.W., Essex, M., Epidemic acquired immune deficiency syndrome: Epidemiologic evidence for a transmissible agent. J Natl Cancer Inst 71:1-4 (1983)

114. Barre-Sinoussi, F., Chermann, J.-C., Rey, F., et al., Isolation of a T lymphotropic retrovirus from a patient at risk for acquired immune deficiency syndrome (AIDS). Science 220:868-871 (1983)

115. Gallo R.C., Salahuddin, S.Z., Popovic, M., et al., Frequent detection and isolation of cytopathic retroviruses (HTLV-III) from patients with AIDS and at risk for AIDS. Science 224:500-503 (1984)

116. Popovic, M., Sarngadharan, M.G., Reed, E., et al., Detection, isolation and continuous production of cytopathic human T lymphotropic retrovirus (HTLV-III) from patients with AIDS and pre-AIDS. Science 224:497-500 (1984)

117. Markham, P.D., Salahuddin, S.Z., Popovic, M., et al., Advances in the isolation of HTLV-III from patients with AIDS and AIDS-related complex and from donors at risk. Cancer Res 45:4588s-4591s (1985)

118. Salahuddin, S., Markham, P., Popovic, M., et al., Isolation of infectious human T-cell leukemia/lymphotropic virus type III (HTLV-III) from patients with acquired immunodeficiency syndrome (AIDS) or AIDS-related complex (ARC) and from healthy carriers: A study of risk groups and tissue sources. Proc Natl Acad Sci USA 82:5530-5534 (1985)

119. Zagury, D., Bernard, J., Leonard, R., et al., Long-term cultures of HTLV-III-infected T cells: A model of cytopathology of T-cell depletion in AIDS. Science 231:850-853 (1986)

120. Markham, P.D., Salahuddin, S.Z., Veren, K., et al., Hydrocortisone and some other hormones enhance the expression of HTLV-III. Int J Cancer 37:67-72 (1986)

121. Shaw, G.M., Harper, M.E., Hahn, B.H., et al., HTLV-III infection in brains of children and adults with AIDS encephalopathy. Science 227:177-181 (1985)

122. Gartner, S., Markovits, P., Markovitz, D.M., et al., The role of mononuclear phagocytes in HTLV-III/LAV infection. Science 233:215-219 (1986)

123. Levy, J.A., Shimabukuro, J., Hollander, H., et al., Isolation of AIDS-associated retrovirus (ARC) from cerebrospinal fluid and brain from patients with neurologic findings. Lancet 2:586-588 (1985)

124. Koenig, S., Gendelman, H.E., Orenstein, J.M., et al., Detection of AIDS virus in macrophages in brain tissue from AIDS patients with encephalopathy. Science 233:1089-1093 (1986)

125. Ho, D.D., Rota, T.R., Schooley, R.T., et al., Isolation of HTLV-III from cerebrospinal fluid and neural tissues of patients with neurologic syndromes related to the acquired immunodeficiency syndrome. N Engl J Med 313:1493-1497 (1985)

126. Zagury, D., Bernard, J., Leibowitch, J., et al., HTLV-III in cells cultivated from semen of two patients with AIDS. Science 226:449-51 (1984)

127. Ho, D.D., Schooley, R.T., Rota, T.R., et al., HTLV-III in the semen and blood of a healthy homosexual man. Science 226:451-453 (1984)

128. Vogt, M.W., Witt, D.J., Craven, D.E., et al., Isolation of HTLV-III/LAV from cervical secretion of women at risk for AIDS. Lancet 1:525-527 (1986)

129. Groopman, J.E., Salahuddin, S.Z., Sarngadharan, M.G., et al., HTLV-III in saliva of people with AIDS-related complex and healthy homosexual men at risk for AIDS. Science 226:447-449 (1984)

130. Lecatsas, G., Houff, S., Macher, A., et al., Retrovirus-like particles in salivary glands, prostate and testes of AIDS patients. Proc Soc Exp Biol Med 178:653-655 (1985)

131. Thiry, L., Sprecher-Goldberger, S., Jonckherr, T., et al., Isolation of AIDS virus from cell-free breast milk of three healthy virus carriers. Lancet 2:891-892 (1985)

132. Zagury, D., Fouchard, M., Vol, J.C., et al., Detection of infectious HTLV-III/LAV virus in cell-free plasma from AIDS patients. Lancet 2:505-506 (1985)

133. Salahuddin, S.Z., Rose, R.M., Groopman, J.E., et al., Human T lymphotropic virus type III infection of human alveolar macrophages. Blood 68:281-284 (1986)

134. Barnes, D.M. Brain endothelial cell infected by AIDS virus. Editorial. Science 233:418-419 (1986)

135. Fujikawa, L.S., Salahuddin, S.Z., Palestine, A.C., et al., Isolation of human T lymphotropic virus type III from the tears of a patient with the acquired immunodeficiency syndrome. Lancet 2:529-530 (1985)

136. Salahuddin, S.Z., Palestine, A.G., Heck, E., et al., Isolation of human T cell leukemia/lymphotropic virus type III from cornea. Am J Ophthalmol 101:149-152 (1986)

137. Dalgleish, A.G., Beverly, P.C.L., Clapham, P.R., et al., The CD4 (T4) antigen is an essential component of the receptor for the AIDS retrovirus. Nature 312:763-767 (1985)

138. Klatzmann, D., Champagne, E., Chamaret, S., et al., T-lymphocyte T4 molecule behaves as the receptor for human retrovirus LAV. Nature 312:767-769 (1985)

139. Hoxie, J.A., Flaherty, L.E., Haggarty, B.S., et al., Infection of T4 lymphocytes by HTLV-III does not require expression of the OKT4 epitope. J Immunol 136:361-363 (1986)

140. Madden, P.J., Dalgleish, A.G., McDougal, J.S., et al., The T4 gene encodes the AIDS virus receptor and is expressed in the immune system and the brain. Cell 47:333-348 (1986)

141. McDougal, J.S., Kennedy, M.S., Sligh, J.M., et al., Binding of HTLV-III/LAV to T4 cells by a complex of the 110K viral protein and the T4 molecule. Science 231:382-385 (1986)

142. Koyanagi, Y., Harada, S., Takahashi, M., et al., Selective cytotoxicity of AIDS virus infection towards HTLV-I-transformed cell lines. Int J Cancer 36:445-451 (1985)

143. Mitsuya, H., Guo, H.G., Cossman, J., et al., Functional properties of antigen-specific T-cells infected by human T-cell leukemia-lymphoma virus (HTLV-I). Science 225: 1484-1486 (1984)

144. DeRossi, A., Aldovini, A., Franchini, G., et al., Clonal selection of T lymphocytes infected by cell-free human T-cell leukemia/lymphoma virus type I: parameters of virus integration and expression. Virology 143:640-645 (1985)

145. Salahuddin, S.Z., Ablashi, D.V., Gonda, M.A., et al., HTLV-III (AIDS virus) infection of EBV genome-positive B-lymphoid cells with or without detectable T4 antigens. Int J Cancer (In press).

146. Nicholson, J.K.A., Cross, G.D., Callaway, C.S., et al., In vitro infection of human monocytes with human T lymphotropic virus type III/lymphadenopathy-associated virus (HTLV-III/LAV). J Immunol 137:323-329 (1986)

147. Levy, J.A., Shimabukuro, J., McHugh, T., et al., AIDS-associated retroviruses (ARV) can productively infect other cells besides human T helper cells. Virology 147:441-448 (1985)

148. Blattner, W.A., Biggar, R.J., Weiss, S.H., et al., Epidemiology of human T-lymphotropic virus type III and the risk of acquired immunodeficiency syndrome. Ann Intern Med 103:665-670 (1985)

149. Hirsch, M.S., Wormser, G.P., Schooley, R.T., et al., Risk of nosocomial infection with human T-cell lymphotropic virus III (HTLV-III). N Engl J Med 312:1-4 (1985)

150. Weiss, S.H., Saxinger, W.C., Rechtman, D., et al., HTLV-III infection among health care workers: Association with needle-stick injuries. JAMA 254:2089-2093 (1985)

151. Friedland, G.H., Saltzman, B.R., Rogers, M.F., et al., Lack of transmission of HTLV-III/LAV infection to household contacts of patients with AIDS or AIDS-related complex with oral candidiasis. N Engl J Med 314:344-349 (1986)

152. Redfield, R.R., Markham, P.D., Salahuddin, S.Z., et al., Frequent transmission of HTLV-III among spouses of patients with AIDS-related complex and AIDS. JAMA 253:1571-1573 (1985)

153. Redfield, R.R., Markham, P.D., Salahuddin, S.Z., et al., Heterosexually acquired HTLV-III/LAV disease (AIDS-related complex and AIDS). JAMA 254:2094-2096 (1985)

154. Barnes, D.M., Military statistics on AIDS in the US, Editorial. Science 233:283 (1986)

155. Quinn, T.C., Mann, J.M., Curran, J.L., et al., AIDS in Africa: An epidemiologic paradigm. Science 234:955-963 (1986)

156. Fischl, M.A., Dickinson, G.M., Scott, G.B., et al., Heterosexual and household transmission of the human T-lymphotropic virus type III. International Conference on Acquired Immunodeficiency Syndrome (AIDS). Paris, France (1986)

157. Des Jarlais, D.C., Chamberland, M.E., Yancovitz, S.R., et al., Heterosexual partners: A large risk group for AIDS. Lancet 2:1346-1347 (1984)

158. Norman, C., Sex and Needles, not insects and pigs, spread AIDS in Florida town. Editorial. Science 234:415-417 (1986)

159. Luzi, G., Ensoli, B., Turbessi, G., et al., Transmission of HTLV-III infection by heterosexual contact. Lancet 2: 1018 (1985)

160. Sarngadharan, M.G., Popovic, M., Bruch, L., et al., Antibodies reactive with human T-lymphotropic retroviruses (HTLV-III) in the serum of patients with AIDS. Science 224:506-508 (1984)

161. Safai, B., Sarngadharan, M.G., Groopman, J.E., et al., Seroepidemiological studies of HTLV-III in AIDS. Lancet 2:1438-1440 (1984)

162. Towbin, H., Staehelin, T., Gordon, J., Electrophoretic transfer of proteins from polyacrylamide gels to nitrocellulose sheets: Procedure and some applications. Proc Natl Acad Sci USA 76:4350-4353 (1979)

163. Groopman, J.E., Salahuddin, S.Z., Sarngadharan, M.G., et al., Virologic studies in a case of transfusion-associated AIDS. N Engl J Med 311:1419-1422 (1984)

164. Jaffe, H.W., Sarngadharan, M.G., DeVico, A.L., et al., Infection with HTLV-III/LAV and transfusion-associated acquired immunodeficiency syndrome. JAMA 253:770-773 (1985)

165. Hahn, B.H., Shaw, G.M., Arya, S.K., et al., Molecular cloning and characterization of the HTLV-III virus associated with AIDS. Nature 312:166-169 (1984)

166. Ratner, L., Haseltine, W., Patarca, R., et al., Complete nucleotide sequence of the AIDS virus, HTLV-III. Nature 313:277-284 (1985)

167. Sanchez-Pescador, R., Power, M.D., Barr, P.J., et al., Nucleotide sequence and expression of an AIDS-associated retrovirus (ARV-2). Science 227:484-492 (1985)

168. Wain-Hobson, S., Sonigo, P., Danos, O., et al., Nucleotide sequence of the AIDS virus, LAV. Cell 40:9-17 (1985)

169. Muesing, M.A., Smith, D.H., Cabradilla, C.D., et al., Nucleic acid structure and expression of the human AIDS/lymphadenopathy retrovirus. Nature 313:450-457 (1985)

170. Sodroski, J., Patarca, R., Rosen, C., et al., Location of the trans-activating region on the genome of human T-cell lymphotropic virus type III. Science 229:74-77 (1985)

171. Arya, S.K., Guo, C., Josephs, S.F., et al., Trans-activator gene of human T-lymphotropic virus type III (HTLV-III). Science 229:69-73 (1985)

172. Arya, K.S., Gallo, R.C., Three novel genes of human T-lymphotropic virus type III: Immune reactivity of their products with sera from acquired immune deficiency syndrome patients. Proc Natl Acad Sci USA 83:2209-2213 (1986)

173. Allan, J.S., Coligan, J.E., McLane, M.F., et al., A new HTLV-III/LAV encoded antigen detected by antibodies from AIDS patients. Science 230:810-813 (1985)

174. Franchini, G., Robert-Guroff, M., Wong-Staal, F., et al., Expression of the protein encoded by the 3' open reading frame of human T-cell lymphotropic virus type III in bacteria: Demonstration of its immunoreactivity with human sera. Proc Natl Acad Sci USA 83:5282-5285 (1986)

175. Lee, T.H., Coligan, J.G., Allan, J.S., et al., A new HTLV-III/LAV protein encoded by a gene found in cytopathic retroviruses. Science 231:1546-1549 (1986).

176. Kan, N.C., Franchini, G., Wong-Staal, F., et al., Identification of HTLV-III/LAV sor gene product and detection of antibodies in human sera. Science 231:1553-1555 (1986)

177. Sodroski, G., Goh, W.C., Rosen, C., et al., A second post-transcriptional trans-activator gene required for HTLV-III replication. Nature 321:412-417 (1986)

178. Feinberg, M.B., Jarrett, R.F., Aldovini, A., et al., HTLV-III expression and production involve complex regulation at the levels of splicing and translation of viral RNA. Cell 46:807-817 (1986)

179. Sarngadharan, M.G., Bruch, L., Popovic, M., et al., Immunological properties of the gag protein p24 of the acquired immunodeficiency syndrome retrovirus (human T-cell leukemia virus type-III). Proc Natl Acad Sci USA 82:3481-3484 (1985)

180. Veronese, F.D., Rahman, R., Copeland, T.D., et al., Characterization of the gag gene products of HTLV-III/LAV. (Submitted for publication)

181. Veronese, F.D., Sarngadharan, M.G., Rahman, R., et al., Monoclonal antibodies specific for p24, the major core protein of human T-cell leukemia virus type III. Proc Natl Acad Sci USA 82:5199-5202 (1985)

182. Schultz, A.M., Henderson, L.E., Oroszlan, S., et al., Amino terminal myristylation of the protein kinase $p60^{src}$, a retroviral transforming protein. Science 227:427-429 (1985)

183. Veronese, F.D., Copeland, T.D., DeVico, A.L., et al., Characterization of highly immunogenic p66/p51 as the reverse transcriptase of HTLV-III/LAV. Science 231:1289-1291 (1986)

184. Steimer, K.S., Higgins, K.W., Powers, M.A., et al., Recombinant polypeptide from the endonuclease region of the acquired immune deficiency syndrome retrovirus polymerase (pol) gene detects serum antibodies in most infected individuals. J Virol 58:9-16 (1986)

185. Sarngadharan, M.G., Veronese, F.D., Lee, S., et al., Immunological properties of HTLV-III antigens recognized by sera of patients with AIDS and AIDS-related complex and of asymptomatic carriers of HTLV-III infection. Cancer Res. 45:4574S-4577S (1985)

186. Veronese, F.D., DeVico, A.L., Copeland, T.D., et al., Characterization of gp41 as the transmembrane protein coded by the HTLV-III/LAV envelope gene. Science 229:1402-1405 (1985)

187. Kitchen, L.W., Barin, F., Sullivan, J.L., et al., Aetiology of AIDS-antibodies to human T-cell leukemia virus (type III) in haemophiliacs. Nature 312:367-369 (1984)

188. Allan, J.S., Colligan, J.E., Barin, F., et al., Major glycoprotein antigens that induce antibodies in AIDS patients are encoded by HTLV-III. Science 228:1091-1094 (1985)

189. Shaw, G.M., Hahn, B.H., Arya, S.K., et al., Molecular characterization of human T-cell leukemia (lymphotropic) virus type III in the acquired immune deficiency syndrome. Science 226:1165-1171 (1984)

190. Wong-Staal, F., Shaw, G.M., Hahn, B.H., et al., Genomic diversity of human T-lymphotropic virus type III (HTLV-III). Science 229:759-762 (1985)

191. Starcich, B.R., Hahn, B.H., Shaw, G.M., et al., Identification and characterization of conserved and variable regions in the envelope gene of HTLV-III/LAV, the retrovirus of AIDS. Cell 45:637-648 (1986)

192. Alizon, M., Sonigo, P., Barre-Sinoussi, F., et al., Molecular cloning of lymphadenopathy-associated virus. Nature 312:757-760 (1984)

193. Siegal, F.P., Immune function and dysfunction in AIDS. Semin Oncol 111:29-39 (1984)

194. Fauci, A.S., Macher, A.M., Longo, D.L., et al., Acquired immunodeficiency syndrome: Epidemiologic, clinical, immunological, and therapeutic considerations. Ann Intern Med 76:95-100 (1985)

195. Fahey, J.L., Prince, H., Weaver, M., et al., Quantitative changes in T helper or T suppressor/cytotoxic lymphocyte subsets that distinguish acquired immune deficiency syndrome from other immune subset disorders. Am J Med 76: 95-100 (1985)

196. Lane, H.C., Depper, J.M., Greene, W.S., et al., Quantitative analysis of immune functions in patients with the acquired immune deficiency syndrome. N Engl J Med 313: 79-84 (1985)

197. Murray, H.W., Rubin, B.G., Masur, H., et al., Impaired production of lymphokines and immune (gamma) interferon in the acquired immune deficiency syndrome. N Engl J Med 310: 883-889 (1984)

198. Smith, P.D., Ohara, K., Masur, H., et al., Monocyte function in the acquired immune deficiency syndrome. J Clin Invest 74:2121-2128 (1984)

199. Shearer, G.M., Salahuddin, S.Z., Markham, P.D., et al., Prospective study of cytotoxic T lymphocyte responses to influenza and antibodies to human T lymphotropic virus-III in homosexual men. J Clin Invest 76:1699-1703 (1985)

200. Rook, A.A., Masur, H., Frederick, W.R.J., et al., Interleukin-2 enhances natural killing activity and virion-specific cytotoxic lymphocyte activities of patients with the acquired immunodeficiency syndrome. Clin Res 31:351A (1983)

200a. Ho, D.D., Sarngadharan, M.G., Resnick, L., et al., Primary human T-lymphotropic virus type III infection. Ann Intern Med 103:880-883 (1985)

200b. Redfield, R.R., Wright, D.C., Tramont, E.C., The Walter Reed staging classification for HTLV-III infection. N Engl J Med 314:131-132 (1986)

200c. Haverkos, H.W., Gottlieb, M.S., Killen, J.Y., et al., Classification of HTLV-III/LAV-related diseases. J Infect Dis 152:1095 (1985)

201. Schroff, R.W., Gottlieb, M.S., Prince, H.E., et al., Immunological studies of homosexual men with immunodeficiency and Kaposi's sarcoma. Clin Immunol Immunopathol 27: 300-314 (1983)

202. DeStefano, E., Friedman, R.M., Friedman-Kien, A.E., et al., Acid-labile alpha interferon: A possible preclinical marker for the acquired immune deficiency syndrome in hemophiliacs. N Engl J Med 309:583-586 (1982)

203. Read, S.E., Williams, B.R.G., Coates, R.A., et al., Elevated levels of interferon-induced 2'-5' oligoadenylate synthetase in generalized persistant lymphadenopathy and the acquired immunodeficiency syndrome. J Infect Dis 152:466-472 (1985)

204. Shearer, G.M., Bernstein, D.C., Shaw, S., et al., Stimulation with alloantigens enhances retrovirus production by HTLV-III-infected peripheral blood leukocytes (submitted).

205. Fisher, A.G., Ratner, L., Mitsuya, H., et al., Infectious mutants of HTLV-III with changes in the 3' region and markedly reduced cytopathic effect. Science 233:655-659 (1986)

206. Sodroski, J., Goh, W.C., Rosen, C., et al., Replicative and cytopathic potential of HTLV-III/LAV with sor gene deletions. Science 231:1549-1553 (1986)

207. Dayton, A.I., Sodroski, J.G., Rosen, C.A., et al., The trans-activator gene of the human T cell lymphotropic virus type III is required for replication. Cell 44:941-947 (1986)

208. Sodroski, J., Goh, W.C., Rosen, C., et al., Role of HTLV-III/LAV envelope in syncytium formation and cytopathicity. Nature 322:470-474 (1986)

209. Lifsom, J.D., Reyes, G.R., McGrath, M.S., et al., AIDS retrovirus induced cytopathology: giant cell formation and involvement of CD4 antigen. Science 232:1123-1127 (1986)

210. Lifsom, J.D., Feinberg, M.B., Reyes, G.R., et al., Induction of CD4-dependent cell fusion by the HTLV-III/LAV envelope glycoprotein. Nature 323:725-728 (1986)

211. Matthews, T.J., Weinhold, K.J., Langlois, A., et al., Interaction between HTLV-III_B envelope gp120 and CD4: role of carbohydrate in binding and cell fusion. Science (In press)

212. Pahwa, S., Pahwa, R., Saxinger, C., et al., Influence of the human T-lymphotropic virus/lymphadenopathy-associated virus on functions of human lymphocytes: evidence for immunosuppressive effects and polyclonal B-cell activation by banded viral preparation. Proc Natl Acad Sci USA 82: 8198-8202 (1985).

213. Laurence, J., Mayer, L., Immunoregulatory lymphokines of T hybridomas from AIDS patients: Constitutive and inducible suppressor factors. Science 225:66-69 (1984).

214. Snider, W.D., Simpson, D.M., Nielsen, S., Neurological complications of acquired immune deficiency syndrome: analysis of 50 patients. Ann Neurol 14:403-418 (1983).

215. Levy, R.M., Bredesen, D.E., Rosenblum, M.L., Neurological manifestations of the acquired immunodeficiency syndrome (AIDS): experience at UCSF and review of the literature. J Neurosurg 62:475-495(1985)

216. Resnick, L., diMarzo-Veronese, F., Schupbach, J., et al., Intra-blood-brain-barrier synthesis of HTLV-III-specific IgG in patients with neurologic symptoms associated with AIDS or AIDS-related complex. N Engl J Med 313:1498-1504 (1985)

217. Letvin, N.L., Daniel, M.D., Sehgal, D.K., et al., Induction of AIDS-like disease in macaque monkeys with T-cell tropic retrovirus STLV-III. Science 230:71-73 (1985)

218. Gurney, M.E., Apatoff, B.R., Spear, G.T., et al., Neuroleukin: A lymphokine product of lectin-stimulated T cells. Science 234:597-581 (1986)

219. Biggar, R.J., Horn, J., Lubin, J.H., et al., Cancer trends in a population at risk of acquired immunodeficiency syndrome. J Natl Cancer Inst 74:793-797 (1985)

220. Hymes, K.B., Cheung, T., Greene, J.B., et al., Kaposi's sarcoma in homosexual men: A report of eight cases. Lancet 2:598-600 (1981)

221. Ziegler, J.L., Drew, W.L., Miner, R.C., et al., Outbreak of Burkitts-like lymphoma in homosexual men. Lancet 2: 631-633 (1982)

222. Levine, A.M., Meyer, P.R., Begardy, M.K., et al., Development of B-cell lymphoma in homosexual men. Ann Intern Med 100:7-12 (1984)

223. Snider, W.D., Simpson, D.M., Aronky, K.E., et al., Primary lymphoma of the nervous system associated with the acquired immunodeficiency syndrome. N Engl J Med 308:95 (1983)

224. Ziegler, J.L., Beckstead, J.A., Volberding, P.A., et al., Non-Hodgkin's lymphoma in 90 homosexual men. Relation to generalized lymphadenopathy and the acquired immunodeficiency syndrome. N Engl J Med 311:565-600 (1984)

225. Cheeseman, S.H., Sullivan, J.L., Brettler, D.B., et al., Analysis of cytomegalovirus and Epstein-Barr virus antibody responses in treated hemophiliacs: implications for the study of acquired immunodeficiency syndrome. JAMA 252:83-85 (1984)

226. Quinnan, G.V., Masur, H., Rook, A.H., et al., Herpesvirus infections in the acquired immune deficiency syndrome. JAMA 252:72-76 (1984)

227. Dummer, J.S., Bound, L.M., Singh, G., et al., Epstein-Barr virus induced lymphoma in cardiac transplant recipients. Am J Med 77:179-183 (1984)

228. Ablashi, D., Fladager, A., Markham, P.D., et al., Isolation of Epstein-Barr virus from the plasma of AIDS patients. (In press)

229. Resnick, L., Veren, K., Salahuddin, S.Z., et al., Stability and inactivation of HTLV-III/LAV under clinical and laboratory environments. JAMA 255:1887-1891 (1986)

230. McDougal, J.S., Martin, L.S., Cost, S.P., et al., Thermal inactivation of the acquired immunodeficiency syndrome virus, human T-lymphotropic virus-III/lymphadenopathy associated virus, with special reference to anti-hemophiliac factors. J Clin Invest 76:875-877 (1985)

231. Martin, L.S., McDougal, J.S., Loskoski, S.L., Disinfection and inactivation of the human T-lymphotropic virus type III/lymphadenopathy-associated virus. J Infect Dis 152:400-403 (1985)

232. Prince, A.M., Horowitz, B., Brotman, B., Sterilization of hepatitis and HTLV-III viruses by exposure to tri(N-butyl) phosphate and sodium cholate. Lancet 1:706-710 (1986)

233. Hicks, D.R., Martin, L.S., Getchell, J.P., et al., Inactivation of HTLV-III/LAV-infected cultures of normal human lymphocytes by nonoxynol-9 in vitro. Lancet 2:1422-1423 (1985)

234. Markham, P.D., Tondreau, S., Inactivation of HTLV-III_B by treatment of infected cells with acetone. (Submitted)

235. Gallo, R.C., Fischinger, P.J., Bolognesi, D.P., Vaccine strategies against human retroviruses associated with AIDS. In: Vaccine Intervention Against Virus Induced Tumors. (Goldman, J.M., Epstein, M.A., eds), MacMillan Company, London, p 81-91 (1986)

236. Morein, B., Sundquist, B., Hoglund, S., et al., ISCOM, a novel structure for antigenic presentation of membrane proteins from enveloped viruses. Nature 308:457-460 (1984)

237. Chakrabarti, S., Robert-Guroff, M., Wong-Staal, F., et al., Expression of the HTLV-III envelope gene by a recombinant vaccinia virus. Nature 320:535-537 (1986)

238. Hu, S-L., Kosowski, S.G., Dalrymple, J.M., Expression of AIDS virus envelope gene in recombinant vaccinia viruses. Nature 320:537-540 (1986)

239. Alter, H.J., Eichberg, J.W., Saxinger, W.C., et al., Transmission of HTLV-III infection from human plasma to chimpanzees: An animal model for AIDS. Science 226: 549-552 (1984)

240. Francis, D.P., Feorino, P.M., Broderson, J.R., et al., Infection of chimpanzees with lymphadenopathy-associated virus. Lancet 1:1276-1277 (1984)

241. Fultz, P.N., McClure, H.M., Swenson, R.B., et al., Persistent infection of chimpanzees with human T-lymphotropic virus type III/lymphadenopathy-associated virus: A potential model for acquired immunodeficiency syndrome. J Virol 58:116-124 (1986)

242. Chandra, P., Steel, L.K., Ebener, U., et al., Chemical inhibitors of oncoviral DNA polymerases: Biological implications and their mode of action. In: Inhibitors of DNA and RNA Polymerases. (Sarin, P.S., Gallo, R.C., eds) Oxford: Pergamon Press, p 47-89 (1980)

243. Hirsch, M.S., Kaplan, J.C., Prospects of therapy for infection with human T-lymphotropic virus type III. Ann Intern Med 103:750-755 (1985)

244. Mitsuya, H., Popovic, M., Yarchoan, R., et al., Suramin protection of T cells in vitro against infectivity and cytopathic effect of HTLV-III. Science 226:172-174 (1984)

245. Balzarini, J., Mitsuya, H., DeClercq, E., et al., Comparative inhibitory effects of suramin and other selected compounds on the infectivity and replication of human T-cell lymphotropic virus (HTLV-III)/lymphadenopathy-associated virus (LAV). Int J Cancer 37:451-457 (1986)

246. McCormick, J.B., Getchell, J.P., Mitchell, S.W., et al., Ribavirin suppresses replication of lymphadenopathy-associated virus in cultures of human adult T lymphocytes. Lancet 1:1367-1369 (1984)

247. Bolognesi, D., Barry, D.W., Broder, S., 3'-azido-3'-deoxythymidine (BWA509U). An antiviral agent that inhibits the infectivity and cytopathic effect of human T-lymphotropic virus type-III/lymphadenopathy-associated virus in vitro. Proc Natl Acad Sci USA 82:7096-7100 (1985)

248. Mitsuya, H., Broder, S., Inhibition of the in vitro infectivity and cytopathic effect of HTLV-III/LAV by 2',3'-dideoxynucleosides. Proc Natl Acad Sci USA 83:1911-1915 (1986)

249. Anand, R., Moore, J., Feorino, P., et al., Rifabutine inhibits HTLV-III. Lancet 1:97-98 (1986)

250. Ho, D.D., Hartshorn, K.L., Rota, T.R., et al., Recombinant human interferon alpha suppresses HTLV-III replication in vitro. Lancet 2:602-604 (1985)

251. Sandstrom, E.G., Kaplan, J.C., Byington, R.E., et al., Inhibition of human T-cell lymphotropic virus type III in vitro by phosphonoformate. Lancet 2:1480-1482 (1985)

252. Rozenbaum, W., Dormont, D., Spire, B., et al., Antimonotungstate (HPA 23) treatment of three patients with AIDS and one with prodrome. Lancet 1:450-451 (1985)

253. Pompidou, A., Zagury, D., Gallo, R.C., et al., In vitro inhibition of LAV/HTLV-III infected lymphocytes by dithiocarb and inosine pranobex. Lancet 2:1423 (1985)

254. Zamecnik, P.C., Goodchild, J., Taguchi, Y., et al., Inhibition of replication and expression of human T-cell lymphotropic virus type III in cultured cells by exogenous synthetic oligonucleotides complementary to viral RNA. Proc Natl Acad Sci USA 83:4143-4146 (1986)

255. Broder, S., Yarchoan, R., Collins, J.M., et al., Effects of suramin on HTLV-III/LAV infection presenting as Kaposi's sarcoma or AIDS-related complex: Clinical pharmacology and suppression of virus replication in vivo. Lancet 2:627-630 (1985)

256. Yarchoan, R., Klecker, R.W., Weinhold, K.J., et al., Administration of 3'-azido-3'-deoxythymidine, an inhibitor of HTLV-III/LAV replication, to patients with AIDS or AIDS related complex. Lancet 1:575-580 (1986)

257. Barnes, D., Editorial, Promising results halt trial of anti-AIDS drug. Science 234:15-16 (1986)

258. Wright, K., Editorial, First tentative signs of therapeutic promise. Nature 323:283 (1986)

259. Resnick, L., Markham, P.D., Veren, K., et al., Suppression of HTLV-III infectivity in vitro by a combination of acyclovir and suramin. J Infect Dis 154:1027-1039 (1986)

260. Miyoshi, I., Yoshimoto, S., Fujishita, M., et al., Natural adult T-cell leukemia virus infection in Japanese monkeys. Lancet 2:658 (1982)

261. Hayami, M., Ishikawa, K., Komuro, A., et al., ATLV antibody in cynomolgus monkeys in the wild. Lancet 2:620 (1983)

262. Ishida, T., Yamamoto, K., Kaneko, R., et al., Seroepidemiological study of antibodies to adult T-cell leukemia virus-associated antigen (ATLA) in free-ranging Japanese monkeys. Microbiol Immunol 27:297-301 (1983)

263. Miyoshi, I., Fujishita, M., Taguchi, H., et al., Natural infection in non-human primates with adult T-cell leukemia virus or a closely related agent. Int J Cancer 32:333-336 (1983)

264. Yamamoto, N., Hinuma, Y., Zur Hausen, H., et al., African green monkeys are infected with adult T-cell leukemia virus or a closely related agent. Lancet 1:290-291 (1983)

265. Hunsmann, G., Schneider, J., Schmitt, J., et al., Detection of serum antibodies to adult T-çell leukemia virus in non-human primates and in people from Africa. Int J Cancer 32:329-332 (1983)

266. Hayami, M., Komuro, A., Nozawa, K., et al., Prevalence of antibody to adult T-cell leukemia virus-associated antigen (ATLA) in Japanese monkeys and other non-human primates. Int J Cancer 33:179-183 (1984)

267. Guo, H-G., Wong-Staal, F., Gallo, R.C., Novel viral sequences related to human T-cell leukemia virus in T cells of a seropositive baboon. Science 223:1195-1197 (1984)

268. Dracopoli, N.C., Tarner, T.R., Else, J.G., et al., STLV-I antibodies in feral populations of east African vervet monkeys. Int J Cancer 38:373-378 (1984)

269. Komuro, A., Watanabe, T., Miyoshi, I., et al., Detection and characterization of simian retroviruses homologous to human T-cell leukemia virus type I. Virology 138:373-378 (1984)

270. Yamamoto, N., Kobayashi, N., Takauchi, K., et al., Characterization of African green monkey B-cell lines releasing an adult T-cell leukemia-virus-related agent. Int J Cancer 34:77-82 (1984)

271. Tsujimoto, H., Komuro, A., Ijima, K., et al., Isolation of simian retroviruses closely related to human T-cell leukemia virus by establishment of lymphoid cell lines from various non-human primates. Int J Cancer 35:377-384 (1985)

272. Homma, T., Kanki, P.J., King, N.W., Jr., et al., Lymphoma in macaques: association with virus of human T lymphotropic family. Science 225:716-718 (1984)

273. Saxinger, W.C., Blattner, W.A., Levine, P.H., et al., Human T-cell leukemia virus (HTLV-I) antibodies in Africa. Science 225:1473-1476 (1984)

274. Blattner, W.A., Saxinger, W.C., Gallo, R.C., HTLV-I, the prototype human retrovirus: epidemiologic features. Prog Clin Biol Res 182:223-245 (1985)

275. Kanki, P.J., Alroy, J., Essex, M., Isolation of T-lymphotropic retrovirus related to HTLV-III/LAV from wild caught African green monkeys. Science 230:951-954 (1985)

276. Fultz, P.N., McClure, H.M., Anderson, D.C., et al., Isolation of a T-lymphotropic retrovirus from naturally infected sooty mangabey monkeys. Proc Natl Acad Sci USA 83: 5286-5290 (1986)

277. Lowenstine, L.J., Pedersen, N.C., Higgins, J., et al., Seroepidemiologic survey of captive old-World primates for antibodies to human and simian retrovirus and isolation of a lentivirus from sooty mangabeys. Int J Cancer 38:563-574 (1986)

278. Kanki, P.J., McLane, M.F., King, N.W., et al., Serologic identification and characterization of a macaque T-lymphotropic retrovirus closely related to HTLV-III. Science 228:1199-1701 (1985)

279. Daniel, M.D., Letvin, N.L., King, N.W., et al., Isolation of T-cell tropic HTLV-III-like retrovirus from macaques. Science 228:1201-1204 (1985)

280. Benveniste, R.E., Arthur, L.O., Tsai, C-C., et al., Isolation of a lentivirus from a macaque with lymphoma: comparison with HTLV-III/LAV and other lentiviruses. J Virol 60:483-490 (1986)

281. Giddens, W.E., Tsai, C-C., Morton, W.R., et al., Retroperitoneal fibromatosis and acquired immunodeficiency syndrome in macaques. Am J Path 119:253-263 (1985)

282. Kanki, P.J., Barin, F., Boup, S., et al., New human T-lymphotropic retrovirus related to simian T-lymphotropic virus type-III (STLV-III_{AGM}). Science 232:238-243 (1986)

283. Clavel, F., Guetard, D., Brun-Vezinet, F., et al., Isolation of a new human retrovirus from West African patients with AIDS. Science 233:343-346 (1986)

12
Origins of HTLV-III (HIV)

P. J. Kanki, M. Essex

Over the last decade the field of retrovirology has expanded to include the first known human retroviruses. Presently, there are at least four distinct exogenous human retroviruses, at least two of which are unequivocably associated with significant human disease or cancer. A unique feature common to this group of human viruses is their affinity for growth in the T4 helper population of lymphocytes. Human T-lymphotropic virus type I (HTLV-I) has been found in certain geographically distinct regions of the world, particularly the southwest islands of Japan, the Caribbean basin and many regions of Africa (1),(2). In these areas, HTLV-I has been etiologically linked with a unique T-cell malignancy termed adult T-cell leukemia/lymphoma (ATLL) (1)-(4). HTLV-II was first described from a patient with a T cell variant of hairy cell leukemia - its definitive role in human disease is still not clear; it appears to be very closely related to HTLV-I (5).

There is now strong evidence for an etiologic relationship of HTLV-III/lymphadenopathy-associated virus (LAV) and AIDS (6)-(10). This member of the HTLV family is characterized by its cytopathic effect and T4 tropism in vitro; similarly, infection with the AIDS virus in people is hallmarked by the depletion of the T4 lymphocyte population and isolation of the virus from these cells (6). The tropism of HTLV-III/LAV for the T4 lymphocyte is not absolute and recent studies have shown its growth in cells of the monocyte/macrophage lineage. There are many features of the HTLV-III/LAV virus such as its unusual genetic structure and its apparent rapid mutation rate that are unique.

Previously there were no similar known viruses found naturally in animals.

In 1985, we described the identification and characterization in sub-human primates of such a related virus. This virus called simian T-lymphotropic virus type III (STLV-III) was isolated from macaque monkeys with an immunodeficiency syndrome similar to the human condition (11), (12). STLV-III infected Hut-78 cells (an established human mature T cell line) demonstrated a characteristic cytopathic effect with the formation of pleomorphic, multinucleated giant cells and Mg^{++} dependent reverse transcriptase activity in the supernatant of such cultures. STLV-III demonstrated an affinity for growth in T4 lymphocyte populations of either human or simian origin. Filtered cell-free supernatants from cells infected with STLV-III could efficiently infect fresh human T lymphocytes grown in the presence of T-cell growth factor. Typical type C retroviral particles were observed budding from and aggregated around infected cells. Mature, extracellular viral particles had a cylindrical-shaped nucleoid, similar to that of HTLV-III/LAV.

The similarities and cross-reactivity of STLV-III viral proteins to the major proteins of HTLV-III/LAV indicated the close relationship of these viruses, not shared by any other known retrovirus including the ungulate lentiviruses. We serologically identified and characterized the proteins of STLV-III by radioimmunoprecipitation and sodium dodecyl sulfate polyacrylamide gel electrophoresis (RIP/SDS-PAGE) techniques (11)-(14). Virus specific proteins of approximately 160 kilodaltons (kd), 120kd, 64kd, 55kd, 53kd, 32kd, 31kd, 24kd, and 15kd were identified, all similar in size to the major gag, env, pol and 3'orf encoded proteins of HTLV-III/LAV (11), (13), (14). The same viral antigens were similarly recognized by select STLV-III positive simian and HTLV-III/LAV positive human reference serum samples. Monoclonal antibodies directed to the major core protein of HTLV-III/LAV, p24, also cross-reacted with a similar protein species in STLV-III, and although the electrophoretic mobility of this protein was somewhat slower, it was conventionally designated the p24 of STLV-III. Select monkey sera with antibodies to STLV-III were also capable of immunoprecipitating the major gag encoded proteins of HTLV-III/LAV, p55 and p24. These sera showed minimal cross-reactivity with the gp120 and gp160 of HTLV-III/LAV, thus demonstrating the apparent type specific immunoreactivity of the env-encoded glycoproteins, consistent with observations in other retrovirus systems.

The similarities of the STLV-III virus to HTLV-III/LAV indicated that these viruses might have evolved from a common progenitor virus. The STLV-III virus was first isolated from captive ill macaques, these primates being indigenous to areas of Asia. Evidence for significant HTLV-III/LAV infection in humans in these parts of the world was rare. In contrast, there were numerous reports of AIDS-like diseases and HTLV-III/LAV infection in areas of Central Africa, and many of the retrospective studies suggested that cases of AIDS were seen as early as 1970 (15)-

(18). We therefore considered the possibility that HTLV-III/LAV infection in humans might have emerged in Africa, potentially resulting from a chance transmission of simian virus to man. There are numerous species of African Old World primates and we investigated the possibility that these species might harbor an STLV-III virus. The recognition that there existed in nature a simian counterpart to HTLV-I, termed STLV-I, also lent credence to this hypothesis.

In 1985 we described the high prevalence of antibodies to STLV-III in healthy wild-caught African green monkeys (*Cercopithecus sp.*) but not in other African primates such as the chimpanzee (*P. troglodytes*), baboon (*Papio sp.*), Patas monkey (*Erthrocebus patas*), or colobus monkey (*Colobus polykomos*) (14). We were successful in isolating infectious virus from seven of eight antibody positive African green monkeys (13). The viral protein characteristics of the STLV-III of African green monkeys ($STLV\text{-}III_{AGM}$) were similar to those already described for $STLV\text{-}III_{mac}$. Present data on over a thousand serum samples from African green monkeys and related species indicate that 30-70% of these animals possess antibodies to STLV-III proteins. In all cases these seropositive monkeys have been apparently healthy without evidence of immunosuppression. This was in apparent contrast with our studies on captive macaques, where serologic data compiled from three different primate centers indicate that STLV-III was not a highly prevalent virus in populations of Asian macaque monkeys. In addition, all seropositive macaques to date have had some clinical or pathological evidence of disease. Of hundreds of samples tested from apparently healthy macaques both wild-caught and captive, we found no serologic evidence of exposure to STLV-III (19). Future studies will determine if STLV-III represents a virus that naturally infects macaque species or if it is possible that it has been artificially introduced to these species in captive situations, potentially from STLV-III infected African primates. From a biological standpoint the STLV-III's of macaque and African green monkey represent two important model systems for the study of AIDS. Virus isolation, serology, and inoculation studies of STLV-III in the macaque host indicate that this related virus is closely associated with an immunodeficiency syndrome that has similar features to human AIDS. In contrast, the African green monkey system is most interesting because of the apparent lack of disease in this primate host. Detailed comparative studies in the pathogenesis of $STLV\text{-}III_{AGM}$ infection may indicate whether this represents a unique virus or virus-host adaptation, such that these monkeys can mount an effective immune response that protects against disease development.

The close relationship between STLV-III and HTLV-III/LAV suggested that human retroviruses might exist that would be more closely related to STLV-III than to the prototype AIDS virus, HTLV-III/LAV. It was well-recognized that African green monkeys were widespread throughout most of sub-Saharan Africa. Several serologic studies indicated that the serologic profiles of U.S.

HTLV-III positive individuals were characteristic of HTLV-III viral antigen, with a more variable and limited reactivity to the cross-reactive epitopes of STLV-III. Conversely, African green monkey sera recognized the STLV-III viral proteins quite specifically with only limited cross-reactivity to HTLV-III antigens. Using this type of differential serologic analysis we studied numerous serum samples from people in different parts of Africa.

In some regions of Africa, HTLV-III/LAV, like other sexually transmitted agents, appears to infect both males and females at elevated rates. Antibody prevalence seems to be higher in certain groups such as female prostitutes and their contacts (15)-(18). Serum samples were obtained from healthy prostitutes at routine medical examinations in Dakar, Senegal. At the time of sampling none of the individuals showed any signs of AIDS or a related disease. The serologic studies of the healthy Senegalese prostitutes and controls revealed an unusual antibody profile to HTLV-III/LAV antigen that had not been described previously (20),(21). By both Western blot analysis and RIP/SDS-PAGE these sera showed reactivity to gag related antigens of HTLV-III/LAV with minimal or no reactivity to the env-encoded antigens. Most notably, all such samples showed reactivity with all of the major antigens of STLV-III. Their selective and weak reactivity with HTLV-III/LAV antigens suggested cross-reactive antibodies directed to the conserved epitopes of both viruses. We postulated that a virus infecting apparently healthy people in Senegal would be very closely related to STLV-III$_{AGM}$, with more epitopes shared with the simian virus than with the representative U.S. strain of HTLV-III/LAV. Our present knowledge of the biology and epidemiology of this family of viruses indicates that the existence of such variant strains may not be unique to Senegal. In fact, our data suggest that earlier reports of antibody reactivity directed only to the p24 gag protein of HTLV-III/LAV in various human populations could reflect exposure to such variant strains.

A new human T-lymphotropic virus, termed HTLV-IV, isolated from these people has shown retroviral type particles, in vitro growth characteristics, and major viral proteins similar to those of the STLV-III/HTLV-III/LAV group of retroviruses (21). The serologic data suggest that this virus shares more common epitopes with STLV-III$_{AGM}$ than with the prototype HTLV-III/LAV that infects people in the U.S. and Europe. A retrospective serologic study suggests that HTLV-IV was present in Dakar, Senegal in the mid-70's (21). Thus, evidence to date indicates that HTLV-IV may have been present in at least a small proportion of people in West Africa for over a decade in the absence of AIDS or a related disorder. To our knowledge, AIDS has only rarely been observed in Dakar, Senegal in the last year. All of the individuals in the present study with evidence of exposure to HTLV-IV were subjected to a physical examination and were apparently healthy at the time of sampling. This is in sharp contrast to the seroepidemiologic data from other parts of the world, where evidence of exposure to HTLV-III/LAV is closely linked with the development of AIDS and related clinical syndromes.

AIDS is caused by a human T-lymphotropic virus, HTLV-III/LAV, which has many characteristics that appear unique to this class of retroviruses. This devastating disease can only be effectively prevented or cured with a better understanding of the pathobiology of this complex virus. Many retroviruses found in outbred mammal systems provide valuable model systems for the study of AIDS. The STLV-III viruses appear to be closely related to HTLV-III/LAV with common epitopes in all the major antigens of this virus. The further identification and characterization of these cross-reactive epitopes may be directly applicable to vaccine development. The availability of a primate species infected with a related virus that either resists disease development (African green monkey) or succumbs to an AIDS-like syndrome (rhesus macaque) provides two models that should enhance our understanding of the pathobiology of these viruses.

Similarly, HTLV-IV may represent a virus with altered or different pathogenic potential in people. Further studies on HTLV-IV infected people and the seroepidemiology of this virus will be necessary before we can fully understand the biologic behavior of this new human T-lymphotropic virus. The determination of the critical portions of the virus that are responsible for these apparent differences in pathogenicity will be most important. It is quite likely that many new members of the human T-lymphotropic virus family will be found in the future, perhaps with a wide range of pathogenicity. As we learn more about the evolution of this general family of viruses we will better understand how the unique pathogenicity of the HTLV-III/LAV virus has evolved and how it can better be prevented through vaccine and therapeutic efforts.

REFERENCES

1. Poiesz, B., Ruscetti, F.W., Gazdar, A.F., et al., Detection and isolation of type-C retrovirus particles from fresh and cultured T-cell lymphoma. Proc Natl Acad Sci 77:7415-7419 (1980)

2. Miyoshi, I., Kubonishi, I., Yoshimoto, S., et al., Type C virus particles in a cord T-cell line derived by co-cultivating normal human cord leukocytes and human leukemia T-cells. Nature 296:770-771 (1981)

3. Yoshida, M., Miyoshi, I., Hinuma, Y., Isolation and characterization of retrovirus from cell lines of human adult T-cell leukemia and its implications in the disease. Proc Natl Acad Sci 79:2031-2035 (1982)

4. Essex, M., McLane, M.F., Tachibana, N., et al., Seroepidemiology of human T-cell leukemia virus in relation to immunosuppression and the acquired immunodeficiency syndrome. In: Human T-cell Leukemia Viruses (Gallo, R.C., Essex, M., Gross, L., eds), Cold Spring Harbor Press, Cold Spring Harbor, New York, p 355-361 (1984)

5. Kalyanaraman, V.S., Sarngadharan, M.G., Robert-Guroff, M., et al., A new subtype of human T-cell leukemia virus (HTLV-III) associated with a T-cell variant of hairy cell leukemia. Science 218:571-573 (1982)

6. Popovic, M., Sarngadharan, M., Read, E., et al., Detection, isolation, and continuous production of cytopathic retroviruses (HTLV-III) from patients with AIDS and pre-AIDS. Science 224:497-500 (1984)

7. Gallo, R., Salahuddin, S., Popovic, M., et al., Frequent detection and isolation of cytopathic retroviruses (HTLV-III) from patients with AIDS and at risk for AIDS. Science 224: 500-503 (1984)

8. Schupbach, J., Popovic, M., Gilden, R.V., et al., Serological analysis of a subgroup of human T-lymphotropic retroviruses (HTLV-III) associated with AIDS. Science 224:503-506 (1984)

9. Sarngadharan, M., Popovic, M., Bruch, L., et al., Antibodies reactive with human T-lymphotropic retroviruses (HTLV-III) in the serum of patients with AIDS. Science 224:506-508 (1984)

10. Barre-Sinoussi, F., Chermann, J.C., Rey, F., et al., Isolation of a T-lymphotropic retrovirus from a patient at risk for acquired immune deficiency syndrome (AIDS). Science 220:868-871 (1983)

11. Kanki, P.J., McLane, M.F., King, N.W., et al., Serologic identification and characterization of a macaque T-lymphotropic retrovirus closely related to human T-lymphotropic retroviruses (HTLV) type III. Science 228:1199-1201 (1985)

12. Daniel, M.D., Letvin, N.L., King, N.W., et al., Isolation of a T-cell tropic HTLV-III-like retrovirus from macaques. Science 228:1201-1204 (1985)

13. Kanki, P.J., Alroy, J., Essex, M., Isolation of T-lymphotropic retrovirus related to HTLV-III/LAV from wild-caught African green monkeys. Science 230:951-954 (1985)

14. Kanki, P.J., Kurth, R., Becker, W., et al., Antibodies to simian T-lymphotropic retrovirus type III in African green monkeys and recognition of STLV-III viral proteins by AIDS and related sera. Lancet 1:1330-1332 (1985)

15. Piot, P., Taelman, H., Minlangu, K.B., et al., Acquired immunodeficiency syndrome in a heterosexual population in Zaire. Lancet 2:65-69 (1984)

16. VandePerre, P., Lepage, P., Kestelyn, P., et al., Acquired immunodeficiency syndrome in Rwanda. Lancet 2:62-65 (1984)

17. Clumeck, N., Robert-Guroff, M., VandePerre, P., et al., Seroepidemiologic studies of HTLV-III antibody prevalence among selected groups of heterosexual Africans. JAMA 254:2599-2602 (1985)

18. VandePerre, P., Clumek, N., Carall, M., et al., Female prostitutes: a risk group for infection with human T-cell lymphotropic type III. Lancet 2:524-526 (1985)

19. Chou, M-J., Kanki, P.J., Essex, M., (Unpublished data)

20. Barin, F., M'Boup, S., Denis, F., et al., Serological evidence for virus related to simian T-lymphotropic retrovirus III in residents of West Africa. Lancet 2:1387-1389 (1985)

21. Kanki, P.J., Barin, F., M'Boup, S., et al., New human T-lymphotropic retrovirus (HTLV-IV) related to simian T-lymphotropic virus type III_{AGM} (STLV-III_{AGM}). Science 232:238-243 (1986)

13
Experimental Models of HIV Infection

Patricia N. Fultz, W. John W. Morrow

Acquired immunodeficiency syndrome (AIDS) usually develops several years after infection with a virus variously called lymphadenopathy-associated virus (LAV) (1), human T-lymphotropic virus type III (HTLV-III) (2),(3), or AIDS-associated retrovirus (ARV) (4). More recently, the name human immunodeficiency virus (HIV) has been proposed for this virus. The immunodeficiency caused by HIV apparently results from cytopathic effects of the virus on its primary target cells, T-helper lymphocytes, which are identified by monoclonal antibodies to T4 and Leu3 antigens (5)-(7). HIV also replicates in macrophages (8), as do two other retroviruses, visna (9) and equine infectious anemia virus (10). All three of these viruses are classified as lentiviruses and exhibit limited nucleic acid homology (11),(12) and antigenic cross-reactivity (13).

Historically, animal models have been valuable in elucidating the pathogenesis of viral infections, in determining mechanisms of resistance and susceptibility to viruses, and in testing vaccines and drugs for prophylactic and therapeutic efficacy. Several animal models have been developed for studying the pathogenesis of retroviruses. One of these is infection of cats with feline leukemia virus (FeLV), which can result in immunodeficiency and subsequent opportunistic infections (14), similar to those seen in AIDS patients. In addition, FeLV is T-cell tropic, but unlike HIV, FeLV also replicates in B-cells, polymorphonuclear leukocytes, platelets, and other cell types, including epithelial cells (15). While HIV, FeLV, and some other retroviruses share properties such as cell tropism and cytopathogenicity, an apparent major difference between HIV and many retroviruses is the extensive genomic heterogeneity that has been observed among isolates of HIV (16),(17). Because much of the observed heterogeneity is in the env region that encodes the major viral surface protein, the development of a vaccine that can protect against the myriad strains of HIV may be difficult. Therefore, a model system in which an animal can be readily infected with HIV is extremely important for eventual testing of prototype vaccines. This chapter summarizes progress in the development of animal models for studying the pathogenesis of HIV and for testing vaccines and drugs that might either prevent infection or alter its course.

PRIMATE MODELS

Over the past two to three years, various nonhuman primate species have been tested for susceptibility to infection by HIV. Animals of various species were inoculated with peripheral blood mononuclear cells (PBMC), tissue homogenates, or plasma from AIDS patients or with the virus itself (after HIV was identified as the etiologic agent of AIDS). Infection was considered to have occurred if seroconversion was documented and virus was recovered from PBMC. Among the primates tested, infection was consistently achieved only with the chimpanzee (*Pan troglodytes*) (18)-(21).

Infection in Chimpanzees

In general, infection of chimpanzees with tissue from AIDS patients or with various strains of HIV results in seroconversion within approximately six weeks while virus can be recovered from lymphocytes within one to two weeks of inoculation. Both IgM and IgG antibody responses to HIV occur (18),(21). The majority of the chimpanzees received intravenous (iv.) injections, although some were inoculated by intracerebral (ic.), intramuscular (im.), intraperitoneal (ip.), or subcutaneous (sc.) routes, as well as intravenously (20). One chimpanzee became infected after exposure of its vaginal mucosa to virus, but another chimpanzee apparently never became infected following two exposures of its oral mucosa to virus (22). Outcomes of infection, i.e., times of seroconversion and initial virus isolation, have been similar in all cases, irrespective of the route of infection (Table 1).

Differences in the amount of time necessary for seroconversion and initial virus isolation have been observed, however, with different isolates of HIV. Inoculation of five chimpanzees with ARV resulted in latent periods of four to nine months before seroconversion occurred and virus could be isolated from lymphocytes. As already stated, seroconversion and virus isolation after inoculation of strains of HTLV-III, LAV, or immunodeficiency-associated virus (IDAV-2) or even some human tissue homogenates, occurred within days or weeks. The long latent period associated with ARV has been documented by independent invest-

Table 1. Seroconversion and Virus Isolation in Chimpanzees Inoculated with HIV or Tissues from AIDS Patients

		Number of Chimpanzees			
			Virus	Sero-	
Inoculum	Route[a]	Inoculated	Positive	converted	Reference
Human AIDS Tissue					
brain	ic, iv	4	2	3	20
plasma	iv	5	0	4	18,20
AIDS Virus					
HTLV-III	iv	7	7	7	20
LAV	iv	15	10	15	20,21
	mucosa[b]	2	1	1	22
IDAV-2	iv	2	0	2	20
ARV	iv	5	5	5	-[c]
Total[d]		40	25(63)	37(93)	

a Some of the chimpanzees received virus by intraperitoneal, intramuscular or subcutaneous injection, in addition to intravenously.
b Either oral or vaginal mucosa was exposed to LAV.
c Unpublished data of Fultz et al., and Levy and Morrow et al.
d Values in parentheses are percentages of the total number infected.

Abbreviations: ic = intracerebral; iv = intravenous; HTLV-III = human T-cell lymphotropic virus type III; LAV = lymphadenopathy-associated virus; IDAV = immunodeficiency-associated virus; ARV = AIDS associated retrovirus.

igators. The ARV inoculum was either cell-free virus or autologous lymphocytes infected in vitro and was injected iv., as were other HIV isolates. These results suggest that different isolates of HIV may have different pathogenic or replicative properties in vivo.

Two uninfected chimpanzees were housed for more than one year with cage mates infected with LAV and from which virus was recovered routinely. One animal showed no evidence of acquiring infection during 16 months of cage exposure. The second animal had a transient LAV-specific IgM response (by enzyme immunoassay and immunofluorescence assay [IFA]) three months after his cage mate was infected; however, this uninfected chimpanzee has not seroconverted to IgG and virus has not been isolated from PBMC during 20 months of exposure (21). These data would support the belief that HIV is not spread by casual contact.

Symptoms of Disease in Chimpanzees

Although no chimpanzee infected with HIV has developed overt disease, chimpanzees did develop several symptoms known to be associated with acute or asymptomatic infection in humans. These included physical, hematologic and immunologic abnormalities, which were always transient and resolved spontaneously. Reduction in rate of weight gain was significant among juvenile chimpanzees infected with LAV and generally occurred during a six month period following initial infection (21). Failure to gain weight persisted for varying periods of time, and one chimpanzee gained no weight for 16 months after inoculation of LAV. In contrast, one juvenile infected with ARV showed no change in rate of weight gain as of 12 months after inoculation (Fultz, unpublished data).

We observed several hematologic and immunologic abnormalities in seven juvenile chimpanzees infected with LAV (Table 2). The most prevalent abnormalities were neutropenia (defined as less than 1200 neutrophils/mm^3 and less than 20% of total white blood cells) and an increased number of T8 cells. The latter was considered significant if the increase occurred during the first six months after infection and persisted for at least two consecutive months. We and Gajdusek et al. (20) have also documented lymphocytosis in some infected animals. In general, however, lymphocyte counts and numbers of T4 and T8 cells (and thus T4:T8 ratios) fluctuated throughout the course of infection (21),(23). Natural killer (NK) cell activity generally was high in ARV-infected chimpanzees, with dramatic increases in NK killing immediately following injection of the virus.

The only obvious clinical symptom in infected chimpanzees has been lymphadenopathy. In our experience with juvenile chimpanzees, we observed only variable, transient enlargement of inguinal

Table 2. Symptoms Associated with HIV Infection in Humans in LAV-infected Chimpanzees (N=7)

Symptom	Number of Animals with Symptom
increase in T8 cells	5
weight loss/failure to thrive	4
neutropenia	4
lymphadenopathy	3
thrombocytopenia	1
hypergammaglobulinemia	1
rash (truncal)	1
diarrhea	0

Data are from references 19 and 21, and unpublished results of Fultz et al.

and axillary lymph nodes, which is often seen in uninfected chimpanzees. However, for one chimpanzee given human plasma, Alter et al. (18) reported enlargement of cervical and inquinal lymph nodes, the latter to a maximum of 6 cm x 3 cm, that persisted for 32 weeks. A lymph node biopsy specimen from this animal showed severe lymphoid hyperplasia with enlarged germinal centers. During the period of maximum lymphadenopathy, mitogenic responses to phytohemagglutinin (PHA) and pokeweed mitogen (PWM) were diminished, and T4:T8 ratios varied from a low of 0.43 to a high of 1.22. Although total number of lymphocytes in this animal were comparable to preinfection counts, the percentage of total T cells, identified by OKT3 monoclonal antibodies, was often depressed compared with the percentage in uninfected controls.

Of the 40 chimpanzees reported to have been infected with various isolates of HIV, all are clinically well up to three years after infection.

Immune Status of Infected Chimpanzees

Immune responses in chimpanzees infected with HIV showed no T- or B-cell impairment, and only occasional decreased responses to mitogenic stimulation have been noted (see above). During 18 months of infection, the responses of two chimpanzees infected with LAV to concanavalin A, PWM, PHA or *Staphylococcus aureus* remained stable and within normal limits (Fultz, unpublished data). Also, IgG virus-specific antibody titers in infected animals generally reached maximum levels within six months of infection and remained at high levels for more than two years.

Virologic Status of Infected Chimpanzees

Once infection with HIV was established in chimpanzees, the virus persisted despite high titers of antiviral antibodies. Most of the virus appeared to be cell-associated throughout infection, since virus was isolated infrequently from serum or plasma samples (21). This observation differs from what has been found in human infection where infectious virus has been cultured from 50% of serum and plasma samples (24),(25). In addition, we have failed to detect virus in saliva obtained on throat swabs of LAV-infected chimpanzees (21, unpublished data).

In our experience with LAV infection of chimpanzees, virus can be recovered routinely from PBMC by cocultivation with human PHA-stimulated white blood cells (21). By monitoring the supernatants of cocults for reverse transcriptase (RT) activity (26), we could recover virus at monthly intervals from animals infected for two years. However, during the period from one month to 12 months after infection, we found that the number of infected PBMC decreased from approximately 10^4 infected cells per 10^7 PBMC to 1 to 10 infected cells per 10^7 PBMC (Figure 1). Whether the number of infected cells will change during different disease states, i.e., if a chimpanzee develops AIDS or AIDS-related complex, remains to be seen.

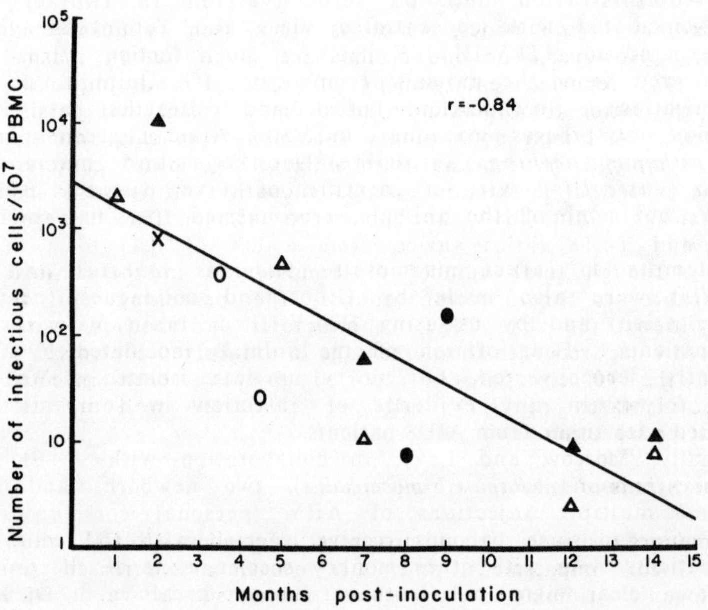

Figure 1. Time-dependent decrease in the number of virus-infected peripheral blood lymphocytes in chimpanzees after inoculation of LAV. Different symbols represent data obtained from different individual chimpanzees. (Reprinted with permission from Reference 21).

OLD AND NEW WORLD MONKEYS

Gajdusek et al. (20) inoculated the following Old and New World monkey species with isolates of HTLV-III and LAV: rhesus macaques (*Macaca mulatta*), stump-tailed macaques (*M. arctoides*), cynomolgus macaques (*M. fascicularis*), bonnet macaques (*M. radiata*), capuchin monkeys (*Cebus albifrons*) squirrel monkeys (*Saimiri sciureus*), and patas monkeys (*Erythrocebus patas*). None of the animals seroconverted and HTLV-III was isolated only sporadically from peripheral blood lymphocytes of three rhesus macaques (that did not seroconvert).

Results of experiments to infect rhesus macaques have been variable. We injected nine rhesus monkeys with various combinations of plasma and lymphocytes from AIDS patients and four rhesus with cell-free LAV (unpublished data). None of the animals seroconverted and virus was not recovered from lymphocytes, although the monkeys were given 10 times more LAV than routinely used to infect chimpanzees. In addition, we have never demonstrated in vitro replication of LAV or ARV in lymphocytes from rhesus macaques. In collaboration with M. Gardner and colleagues, Morrow and Levy gave two newborn and two adult macaques multiple injections of ARV, as well as PBMC and a spleen extract from an AIDS patient. There was no evidence of infection by seroconversion or by recovery of virus. Researchers at the Food and Drug Administration detected seroconversion in two of three rhesus inoculated with concentrated virus and autologous lymphocytes exposed to HTLV-III in vitro, but no infectious virus could be recovered from the animals' lymphocytes (G. Quinnan, personal communication). In addition, Purcell and colleagues have inoculated not only rhesus macaques, but also African green monkeys (*Cercopithecus aethiops*), squirrel monkeys and marmosets (*Mystax fusicollis*) with a mixture of five distinct isolates of HIV, but none of the animals seroconverted (personal communication).

Attempts to infect marmosets (*Saquinas labratus* and *M. fusicollis*) were also made by Gibbs and colleagues (personal communication) and by us using HTLV-III or brain material from AIDS patients. Four of ten of the animals inoculated by Gibbs apparently seroconverted, but no virus was isolated. We were unable to obtain any evidence of infection in four marmosets inoculated with tissue from AIDS patients.

Finally, Morrow and Levy, in collaboration with J. Eichberg, gave six baboons (*Papio cynocephalus*), two newborns and four juveniles, multiple injections of ARV (personal communication). Four years ago some baboons received peripheral blood cells from AIDS patients. As with other monkey species, none of the animals has shown clear signs of seroconversion or presence of virus by RT activity in lymphocytes cocultivated with human PBMC. All the baboons are clinically healthy.

In summary, some investigators have been able to demonstrate transient infections in rhesus macaques, but less than 50% of inoculated rhesus macaques have seroconverted and recovery of virus was achieved from even fewer animals. Therefore, it is generally agreed that rhesus macaques and other species of monkeys are not suitable models for pathogenesis studies with HIV or for testing vaccines or therapeutic drugs.

SMALL-ANIMAL MODELS

Several investigators have attempted to reproduce an AIDS-like disease in a variety of small laboratory animals. A small-animal model would greatly facilitate certain areas of research and would allow for more thorough experimentation, permiting analysis of the responses of a group of animals rather than the response of a single animal, which often is the case when using chimpanzees. One of the most comprehensive studies with small animals was done over the past 3-1/2 years by one of us (W.J.W.M.) with Jay Levy; that work is summarized below.

Mice

Newborn mice of the BALB/c, ICR, WS, C3H or C57Bl strains were injected either with human mononuclear cells from AIDS patients or with ARV. In some cases whole blood, platelets, bone marrow, plasma, ultracentrifuged plasma pellets and spleen cell suspensions were used to infect mice by ip., sc., or ic. routes. Comparisons were made with control groups of animals that were similarly injected with cells from healthy, non-homosexual volunteers or fluids from uninfected tissue cultures.

An unexplained mortality rate of approximately 18% (compared with that for control groups) was observed in a 12 month period (Table 3). The deaths that occurred appeared to be due to varying causes, including tumors and opportunistic infections. Runting and diarrhea were observed many times. Nevertheless, the circumstances leading to these diseases have not been determined. ARV could not be detected convincingly in lymphocyte or blood cultures from any of the animals, and seroconversion was equivocal, as tested by IFA, and could not be confirmed by immunoblot. In one attempt to adapt a variant of the virus to mice, ARV was passaged at two-week intervals through seven generations of newborn BALB/c mice. RT activity in spleen cultures was measured throughout the course of the experiment; however, at no time was RT activity noted. We conclude that ARV is not readily adaptable to infection of murine lymphocytes.

Rats, Guinea Pigs, Hamsters and Rabbits

Fisher 344 rats, Hartley guinea pigs, Golden Syrian hamsters, and New Zealand White rabbits were inoculated using the same protocols used for mice. Essentially no unexplained mortalities or secondary diseases were seen in any of these groups of animals (Table 4). Hamsters and guinea pigs did not seroconvert, as tested by IFA (27). Two litters of rabbits (12 animals) were inoculated with ARV. After six months some serum samples were weakly positive by IFA, although Western blot analysis could not positively confirm this finding.

Table 3. Deaths Occurring in Mice Inoculated with AIDS Retrovirus Between Infancy and 12 Months of Age

	Group	Deaths	% Mortality[a]
Experimental			
	BALB/c	47/251	18.7
	C3H	5/30	16.7
	ICR or WS	7/41	17.1
	Total	59/322	18.3
Control			
	BALB/c	3/58	5.2
	C3H	0/18	0.0
	ICR or WS	2/15	13.3
	Total	5/91	5.5

a $0.01 < p < 0.025$ (chi-square test) inoculated animals compared to uninoculated controls.

CONCLUSIONS

Testing of various small animal and nonhuman primate species indicates that the chimpanzee is the only reliable model of infection with HIV. Since there appear to be differences in the pathogenesis of various isolates of the virus, the challenge inoculum in any vaccine trial should probably be a strain, such as LAV, that has been shown to establish infection repeatedly. Although HIV infection has not resulted in progressive disease in any chimpanzee, certain symptoms associated with infection in humans have been observed. In addition, the incubation time before onset of AIDS can be more than five years in persons infected with HIV and may be just as long in chimpanzees. Using the chimpanzee model system, studies are in progress to determine if cofactors, such as other viruses, multiple exposures to HIV or continued antigenic stimulation, play a role in development of disease. However, because of the expense of maintenance and the limited availability of chimpanzees, models of infection and disease using other retroviruses and other species of animals probably will be needed to understand fully the pathogenesis of HIV.

The closest relatives of the human AIDS virus appear to be the recently described simian T-lymphotropic viruses (STLV-III or SIV) isolated from several species of Old World monkeys (28)-(30). These viruses are morphologically, biologically and anti-

Table 4. Species of Rodents Tested for Experimental Infection with ARV*

Animal	Group	% Mortality[a]
Rats	Test	0/30
	Control	0/21
Guinea pigs	Test	0/14
	Control	0/4
Hamsters[b]	Test	0/16
	Control	0/8

* ARV = AIDS-associated retrovirus

a Number of animals monitored during the period between 35 days and 12 months of age.

b A particularly high attrition rate (approximately 30%) occurred in the hamsters in the middle and later stages of infancy (between 10-35 days old), and poor development was noted in some animals. This problem occurred in both test and control groups. The deaths probably were due to bad mothering, but the ic. route of injection used in these animals may also have contributed to the morbidity and mortality.

genically related to HIV, and some of these isolates already have been shown to cause disease and an immunodeficiency syndrome in experimentally infected rhesus macaques (31). The STLV-III-macaque model will make it possible to do studies (such as testing of therapeutic drugs) that are not possible using chimpanzees. Much effort currently is being directed towards developing STLV-III model systems as alternative ways to learn more about the pathogenesis of AIDS and related viruses.

ACKNOWLEDGMENTS

We wish to express our appreciation to J. Levy, R. Purcell, J. Eichberg, G. Quinnan and C. Gibbs for personal communications of unpublished data; J. Levy for encouragement; M. Gardner and N. Lerce for participation in some rhesus experiments; and to P. Baker for secretarial assistance.

REFERENCES

1. Barre-Sinoussi, F., Chermann, J.C., Rey, F., et al., Isolation of a T-lymphotropic retrovirus from a patient at risk for acquired immune deficiency syndrome (AIDS). Science 220:868-871 (1983)

2. Popovic, M., Sarngadharan, M.G., Read, E., et al., Detection, isolation, and continuous production of cytopathic retroviruses (HTLV-III) from patients with AIDS and pre-AIDS. Science 224:497-500 (1984)

3. Gallo, R.C, Salahuddin, S.Z., Popovic, M., et al., Frequent detection and isolation of cytopathic retroviruses (HTLV-III) from patients with AIDS and at risk for AIDS. Science 224: 500-503 (1984)

4. Levy, J.A., Hoffman, A.D., Kramer, S.M., et al., Isolation of lymphocytopathic retroviruses from San Francisco patients with AIDS. Science 225:840-842 (1984)

5. Dalgleish, A.G., Beverley, P.C.L., Clapham, P.R., et al., The CD4 (T4) antigen is an essential component of the receptor for the AIDS retrovirus. Nature 312:763-767 (1984)

6. Klatzmann, D., Barre-Sinoussi, F., Nugeyre, M.T., et al., Selective tropism of lymphadenopathy-associated virus (LAV) for helper-inducer T lymphocytes. Science 225:59-63 (1984)

7. McDougal, J.S., Kennedy, M.S., Sligh, J.M., et al., Binding of HTLV-III/LAV to $T4^+$ T cells by a complex of the 110K viral protein and the T4 molecule. Science 231:382-385 (1986)

8. Levy, J.A., Shimabukuro, J., McHugh, T., et al., AIDS-associated retroviruses (ARV) can productively infect other cells besides human T helper cells. Virology 147: 441-448 (1985)

9. Narayan, O., Wolinsky, J.S., Clements, J.E., et al., Slow virus replication: the role of macrophages in the persistence and expression of visna viruses of sheep and goats. J Gen Virol 59:345-356 (1982)

10. Crawford, T.B., Cheevers, W.P., Klevjer-Anderson, P., et al., in: Persistent Viruses: ICN-UCLA Symposium in Molecular and Cellular Biology (Stevens, J.G., Todaro, G.J., Fox, C.F., eds) Vol XI, Academic Press, New York, p 727-749 (1978)

11. Gonda, M.A. Wong-Staal, F., Gallo, R.C., et al., Sequence homology and morphologic similarity of HTLV-III and visna virus, a pathogenic lentivirus. Science 227:173-177 (1985)

12. Stephens, R.M., Casey, J.W., Rice, N.R., Equine infectious anemia virus gag and pol genes: relatedness to visna and AIDS-virus. Science 231:589-594 (1986)

13. Montagnier, L., Chermann, J.C., Barre-Sinoussi, F., et al., A new human T-lymphotropic retrovirus: Characterization and possible role in lymphadenopathy and acquired immune deficiency syndromes. In: Human T-cell Leukemia/Lymphoma Virus (Gallo, R.C., Essex, M.E., Gross, L., eds) Cold Spring Harbor Laboratory, Cold Spring Harbor, p 363-379 (1984)

14. Hardy, W.D., Immunopathology induced by the feline leukemia virus. Springer Semin Immunopathol 5:75-106 (1982)

15. Rojko, J.L., Hoover, E.A., Mathes, L.E., et al., Pathogenesis of experimental feline leukemia virus infection. J Natl Cancer Inst 63:759-768 (1979)

16. Wong-Staal, F., Shaw, G.M., Hahn, B.H., et al., Genomic diversity of human T-lymphotropic virus type III (HTLV-III). Science 229:759-762 (1985)

17. Benn, S., Rutledge, R., Folks, T., et al., Genomic heterogeneity of AIDS retroviral isolates from North America and Zaire. Science 230:949-951 (1985)

18. Alter, H.J., Eichberg, J.W., Masur, H., et al., Transmission of HTLV-III infection from human plasma to chimpanzees: an animal model for AIDS. Science 226:549-552 (1984)

19. Francis, D.P., Feorino, P.M., Broderson, J.R., et al., Infection of chimpanzees with lymphadenopathy associated virus. Lancet 2:1276-1277 (1984)

20. Gajdusek, D.C., Gibbs, C.J., Jr., Rodgers-Johnson, P., et al., Infection of chimpanzees by human T-lymphotropic retroviruses in brain and other tissues from AIDS patients. Lancet 1:55-56 (1985)

21. Fultz, P.N., McClure, H.M., Swenson, R.B., et al., Persistent infection of chimpanzees with HTLV-III/LAV: a potential model for acquired immunodeficiency syndrome. J Virol 58:116-124 (1986)

22. Fultz, P.N., McClure, H.M., Daughtarty, H., et al., Vaginal transmission of human immunodeficiency virus (HIV) to a chimpanzee. J Infect Dis 154:896-900 (1986)

23. Eichberg, J.W., Alter, H.J., Dreesman, G.R., Longitudinal study of HTLV-III-infected chimpanzees by lymphocyte subpopulation analysis. J Med Primatol 14:317-326 (1985)

24. Ho, D.D., Byington, R.E., Schooley, R.T., et al., Infrequency of isolation of HTLV-III virus from saliva in AIDS. N Engl J Med 313:1606 (1985)

25. Levy, J.A., Kaminsky, L.S., Morrow, W.J.W., et al., Infection by the retrovirus associated with the acquired immunodeficiency syndrome: clinical, biological and molecular features. Ann Intern Med 103:694-699 (1985)

26. Hoffman, A.D., Banapour, B., Levy, J.A., Characterization of the AIDS-associated retrovirus reverse transcriptase and optimal conditions for its detection in virions. Virology 147:326-335 (1985)

27. Kaminsky, L.S., McHugh, T., Stites, D., et al., High prevalence of antibodies to AIDS-associated retroviruses (ARV) in acquired immune deficiency syndrome and related conditions and not in other disease states. Proc Natl Acad Sci 82:5535-5539 (1985)

28. Daniel, M.D., Letvin, N.L., King, N.W., et al., Isolation of T-cell tropic HTLV-III-like retrovirus from macaques. Science 228:1201-1204 (1985)

29. Kanki, P.J., Alroy, J., Essex, M., Isolation of T-lymphotropic retrovirus related to HTLV-III/LAV from wild-caught African green monkeys. Science 230:951-954 (1985)

30. Fultz, P.N., McClure, H.M., Anderson, D.C., et al., Isolation of a T-lymphotropic retrovirus from naturally infected sooty mangabey monkeys (*Cercocebus atys*). Proc Natl Acad Sci USA 83:5286-5290 (1986)

31. Letvin, N.L., Daniel, M.D., Sehgal, P.K., et al., Induction of AIDS-like disease in macaque monkeys with T-cell tropic retrovirus STLV-III. Science 230:71-73 (1985)

14
Laboratory Detection of Human Immunodeficiency Viruses

Stanley H. Weiss

The characterization in 1984 of a new human retrovirus, the third member of the human T-lymphotropic virus family (HTLV-III), is the foundation for understanding the acquired immunodeficiency syndrome (AIDS) epidemic (1)-(3). The evidence is overwhelming that HTLV-III infection is necessary for a person to develop AIDS. The spectrum and natural history of HTLV-III infection remain the subject of vigorous research efforts.

A nomenclature committee has suggested use of the term human immunodeficiency virus (HIV) for this generic class of viruses. Material developed from specific isolates (e.g., HTLV-IIIB, LAV-1 [lymphadenopathy-associated virus], ARV-2 [AIDS associated retrovirus]) and any tests based upon these reagents are to continue to include the prior nomenclature to indicate the viral strain. Since the vast majority of reagents in world-wide use as well as the comparative analyses to date are from the H9 clone of the HTLV-IIIB virus, the term HTLV-III remains appropriate for most laboratory assays. For simplicity, HIV will be used in this chapter despite its limitations (4). The existent research and commercial assays now available to detect evidence of HIV exposure are briefly reviewed.

An approach to the rational use and interpretation of these new tests is provided.

APPROACHES TO THE DETECTION OF INFECTIOUS AGENTS

A laboratory measure which directly detects the presence of an infectious agent is highly desirable. For some agents, such as hepatitis B virus (HBV), large quantities of viral antigen are produced during active infection and tests which effectively measure viral antigen are available. But for many other viral agents antigen may not be directly detectable even during active infection (5).

The presence or absence of antibodies may be used to indicate whether or not a host response to the agent has occurred. The presence of antibodies should not be interpreted as indicating resolution of infcction; many viruses are characterized by persistence. In the case of retroviruses such as HTLV-I and HIV, antibodies can indicate previous infection leading to the integration (and survival) of the viral genome within the host cell's DNA. Thus, the presence of antibodies can be a highly significant marker both of latent and of active infection.

ANTIBODY DETECTION

The enzyme linked immunoabsorbent assay (ELISA, or EIA) had been previously successfully employed for detecting HTLV-I antibodies (6). This framework was important in developing serologic assays for HIV (7),(8), leading to the development of a prototype HIV ELISA which was reproducible, sensitive and specific (9). The research breakthrough enabling production of purified HTLV-III in large quantities was integral to the development of these assays (2).

Several commercial companies have been licensed by the Food and Drug Administration (FDA) for marketing HTLV-III and LAV-1 antibody ELISA kits to screen donated blood products in the U.S. These kits are also utilized at "alternative test sites". Such sites exist specifically to provide persons who consider themselves at increased risk for HIV infection to be tested voluntarily, and the U.S. Public Health Service has recommended HIV testing for some persons at increased risk (10). Although the intended purposes in the blood bank and clinical/diagnostic settings are similar, the practical applications are quite different. In the former situation, one wishes to screen out any blood that is potentially infected with HIV; one wishes to minimize false negatives in order to assure a continuing safe supply of blood products. In the latter clinical instance, the primary purpose is to correctly counsel persons concerning whether or not they have been infected. However, both medical and non-medical considerations regarding HIV testing have led to a perceived impact far greater than most other laboratory tests. HIV testing is perceived as an invasive procedure in our society. Fears concerning the medical implications of reactive test results and concerning potential social risk in the event of a break in confidentiality have foundation (3). False positive results similarly raise special concern. A written informed consent procedure in advance of testing has been recommended to address these issues (3).

Since most health care professionals who order HIV tests currently will have only limited familiarity with the tests, it is highly desirable for the laboratory report to both provide the clinician with considerable guidance concerning the limitations of the test results, and indicate the desirablity of further consultation with the laboratory (or blood bank) director, infectious disease specialist, or other expert. Such an expert should be able to assist the clinician in employing standard principles of decision theory to apply the battery of licensed and unlicensed (research) tests appropriately and efficiently to a given situation. Confidentiality concerns may severely limit the information provided to the testing laboratory by the referring professional. The types of tests and considerations regarding them are discussed below.

Comparison of Screening Assays

The ELISA is currently the only licensed HIV antibody detection procedure in the U.S. The first generation of commercially refined antibody kits have sensitivities and specificities (see Table 1 for definitions and reference (9) for formulae) of approximately 98% (11),(12). However, valid data comparing various antibody ELISA kits is extremely limited and is complicated by the absence of a generally accepted "gold" (or even "silver") standard (see Table 1). Licensure required correct identification of sera in a test panel, but that panel was limited in extent and was designed as but one of several essential minimum requirements. Different manufacturers have used different panels of sera in their field evaluations. Therefore, apparent observed differences may merely reflect differences in patient selection and not true differences among the tests.

Lacking an established reference laboratory standard, a prototype HIV assay was assessed on the basis of clinical-epidemiologic considerations, which included a panel of sera drawn from healthy blood donors prior to the AIDS epidemic who were considered "true negatives" (9). In contrast, the subsequent FDA assessment of vendor products has relied upon current blood donors (13)-(15). Thus, the operative assumption "all blood donors are true negatives" is known to be false. Unfortunately, this leads to the paradoxical situation that perfect specificity (no false positives) is attained only for a test which detects absolutely no positives among current blood donors! Comparison of tests by "the numbers" alone, for either of these reasons, could lead to highly misleading conclusions and undesirable results.

In the absence of gold standards, the true sensitivity and specificity for the detection of HIV antibodies remain imprecise. Furthermore, these assays primarily detect IgG, not IgM (or IgA) antibodies. Several independent reports suggest that HIV antigenemia and/or IgM antibodies sometimes precede the expression of IgG antibodies, reflecting an eminently plausible biologic scenario. Thus, even if an IgG assay were perfectly sensitive, some persons truly infected could not be detected by such a test. The frequency, duration, and importance of this (IgG) seronegative window remain the subject of investigation.

Table 1. Epidemiologic Assessment of Tests: Definitions

Sensitivity* -	The probability that a test result will be positive if infection is present.
Specificity* -	The probability that a test result will be negative if infection is not present.
"Gold" (Reference) Standard -	A definitive means of categorization, widely accepted by experts in the field, for absolutely defining the presence or absence of a condition (such as HIV infection).
"Silver" (Criterion) Standard -	The best currently available (or the accepted) standard, which is expected to be superceded as technology advances; used as an interim reference standard when a "gold" standard either does not exist or is otherwise unavailable.

* Laboratory personnel frequently use these terms differently, with the terms applied to detection and strength of a "test signal" (e.g., titer) rather than the epidemiologic, statistical definitions above.

Predictive Value

One should note that sensitivity and specificity as defined by the epidemiologist for laboratory tests (Table 1) reflect aspects of the test configuration as defined by the manufacturer, and remain constant for all approved uses. Much more important to the user, in practice, are the positive and negative predictive values. These will vary depending upon the (estimated) "true" positivity proportion in the population being tested (a "gold standard" would be employed to determine this proportion) or, when dealing with an individual patient, upon the "prior probability of infection/seropositivity" or the "prior probability of disease" (PPD) (15).

Table 2. Evaluation of Potential Sources of Error with HIV ELISA Screening Tests

I. Procedural Error

A) Physical mixing up of specimens during testing (retesting correctly labelled sera would reveal a discrepancy).
B) Subsequent incorrect linkage of test results (testing of a newly acquired specimen from the same subject would reveal a discrepancy).

II. Technical Error During Testing

A) Erroneous dilution (or omission) of sera or reagents
B) Splashing during test sera or reagent addition, or pipet contamination
C) Washing errors
D) Incorrect absorbance measurement (e.g., wrong wavelength; bubbles on wet plate or scratches on plate; equipment or electronic malfunction)

III. Test Kit Error

A) Variability in kit reactivity (related to vendor quality control)
B) Instability or deterioration of reagents

IV. False Positive Results

These may occur in association with certain clinical conditions. In such circumstances, specific confirmatory tests are especially important.

A) Recognized Problems

1)* HLA-antibodies: (related to technical aspects of the viral purification process of only some manufacturers' test kits [e.g.,? multiparous women]).
2) Repetitive freeze/thaws (e.g., some stored sera)

* For some screening tests, these conditions may not pose problems (see text).

Table 2. Evaluation of Potential Sources of Error with HIV ELISA Screening Tests (Continued)

3) Other retroviruses:
Probably significant - STLV-III, HTLV-IV, and LAV-2
? Significant - HTLV-I; HTLV-II
?? Other retroviruses

4)* Heating of sera

5) Persons with autoantibodies (e.g., ? antinuclear antibodies as in systemic lupus erythematosus, or antimitochondrial antibodies)

B) Speculated as problems

1) ? Alcoholic hepatitis
2) ? African sera ("sticky sera")
3) ? Hypergammaglobulinemia

V. False Negative Results

A) HIV-specific antibodies may decline as a function of severity of HIV related immune dysfunction.
B) Viremic patients who have not (yet?) developed (IgG) antibodies - probably including those persons most recently exposed/infected.
C) Hypogammaglobulinemia (including congenital conditions) as a variant of (B) above.
D) ? States of antigen excess.
E) ? Heating of sera.

VI. Dichotomous Interpretation of Results:

The test is actually a continuous measurement: the chance of misclassification varies with the relative test reactivity strength of the sample.

A) Non-reactive
B) Weakly reactive
C) Strongly reactive

* For some screening tests, these conditions may not pose problems (see text).

STLV = Simian T-lymphotropic virus; HTLV = Human T-cell lymphotropic/leukemia virus; HIV = Human immunodeficiency virus

Test Performance

Receiver operator characteristic ("ROC") curve analysis is a useful method for comparing the performance of assays when congruent definitions of sample groups have been provided, and to assess claims of vendor improvement. Such analysis, for example, reveals that a purportedly improved prototype ELISA (16) probably in fact had poorer performance than a predecessor (9).

Procedural errors can be one of the most frequent causes of test error (Table 2). When samples are solely identified by code, and in the absence of full automation, the risk of procedural errors may be further magnified. In such settings, strict guidelines will generally need to be implemented. With the institution of HIV testing in blood banks and clinical laboratories, the most frequent cause of erroneous results have been technical and procedural errors (Table 2). Thus, improvements in theoretic test performance characteristics alone may not significantly improve performance in practice due to "user failure".

False ELISA Reactivity

The currently available first generation ELISA kits use purified disrupted whole virus. Purification to remove (human or bacterial) cellular contaminants is an essential step in the manufacturing process. High-titer HLA-antibody sera can be used to assess preparation purity for tests based upon virus produced in human cell lines, such as H9/HTLV-IIIB. (For viral components produced through recombinant methods in bacteria such as *Escherichia coli* (17), analogous measures which detect residual bacterial contaminants are necessary.) Evaluation of the prototype HIV ELISA suggested the potential for false positive reactions on the basis of HLA class II reactivity; there was very little such reactivity with the prototype assay itself, reflecting high antigen purity (9),(18). Problems associated with false HLA reactivity were noted subsequent to licensure for (at least) two commercial assays (19),(20). Methods to reduce such reactivity have been developed (21) and the next generation of HIV whole virus ELISAs are expected to be more specific.

Repetitive freezing and thawing of sera increases the probability of false positive reactions (decreased specificity, usually primarily due to weak reactives), and may potentially also decrease the sensitivity. The recommendations of manufacturers to use their kits on fresh sera are appropriate. If sera is heated in an attempt to inactivate virus, both assay sensitivity and specificity are impaired for several of the commercial screening assays. Thus, whenever inferior quality sera is tested, whether for research or clinical purposes, special care must be taken in interpreting and in reporting the ELISA results.

An analysis of specific clinical conditions that have given difficulties for certain tests in practice and knowledge concerning the design of these tests (and thus the theoretical problems) can help guide the discriminating laboratory manager in judiciously selecting a commercial kit (Table 2).

Control Assays

HIV antibody detection involves the use of preparations containing the HIV virus. An analogous assay may be run without HIV antigen, providing a comparison (control) assay for the evaluation of reactivity. Absence of reactivity on the control assay implies that the primary assay reactivity was related to HIV itself, providing an increased level of confidence that the primary assay reactivity reflects true positivity. This technique has been effectively utiltized in research studies for ELISA (e.g., the proprietary H9 control plate), immunofluorescence, and western blot methods, and serves routinely as a parallel control in radioimmunoprecipation.

While reactivity on the control assay indicates the presence of some reactivity to non-viral constituents (e.g., related to HLA antibodies or antinuclear antibodies), it can not rule out the posssibility of concomitant true reactivity. Thus, false positivity can not be presumed and alternative HIV assays may need to be employed to discriminate between true and false positivity. The clinical history may also be helpful in this evaluation. Similarly, tests which directly detect conditions associated with false reactivity (e.g., HLA antibodies) should not be relied upon to rule out true positivity (18),(20).

Reactivity Strength

The whole virus ELISA detects reactivity to any of a variety of viral components. AIDS patients with opportunistic infections have been shown to be significantly less reactive by ELISA than AIDS patients with Kaposi's sarcoma (9). This probably reflects the observation that during the course of HIV infection, humoral immunity may become impaired and lower levels of specific antibody produced. Persons with HIV-associated lymphadenopathy tend to be very strongly reactive by ELISA, as well as by immunofluorescence (22).

The relative titers of viral component-specific antibodies probably vary over time in individuals. This can be anticipated to lead to systematic differences in ELISA reactivity and detection rates among varying populations or patient groups, but the critical tests to differentiate these antibodies quantitatively remain under research development. Furthermore, in some persons HIV antigen may be produced in sufficient quantity to form immune complexes with HIV antibodies and reduce antibody reactivity strength.

Special Problems

Studies undertaken in Africa suggested non-specific, weak HIV ELISA reactivity which was more common among persons with high antibody titers against species of malaria (23). The specificity issues noted above certainly apply to Africa as well. Additionally, the apparent non-specific association may have been partially related to an insufficient accounting for the interval changes in the research assay (24). Other investigators have also found African sera to be unusally reactive in ELISAs (25), suggesting that the higher immunoglobulin levels in this population may, in effect, systematically shift the standardization curve for African sera as compared to U.S. and European sera. With African sera a competitive ELISA which is marketed commercially has out-performed other screening methodologies in recent research studies (26).

Other related retroviruses, human and/or non-human, may well account for low level reactivities in Africa as well. The finding of very low titer antibodies to HTLV-IIIB in stored sera from Uganda is consistent with such a possibility (27). Infrequently, high titer HTLV-I antibodies can lead to falsely reactive HIV screening results (9). With the continuing discovery of additional retroviruses such as HTLV-IV, HTLV-V, STLV-IV (simian T-lymphotropic virus), and LAV-2, ongoing research is likely to clarify gradually these cross-reactivity issues.

Schema for the Interpretation of HIV ELISA Results

The (estimated) probability of infection prior to testing (the "pre-test" probability) is essential for the appropriate interpretation of a test result whatever the purpose - clinical, counseling or research. This estimate dramatically impacts upon the attained predictive value after testing (or "post-test" probability).

When the prior probability is high (as for risk group members from hyper-endemic regions), the positive predictive value of a strongly reactive ELISA is very high. A weakly or moderately reactive result, although still likely to be truly positive, mandates further testing. Thus, the actual ELISA value and not simply a reactive/non-reactive result should always be obtained from the testing laboratory. In contrast, a non-reactive result has only a moderate negative predictive value, so that it is important to rule out technical or procedural error (Table 2), recheck the clinical history, and possibly employ alternative and/or more sensitive assays before accepting a surprising negative result as final.

For a well non-risk group member, such as a blood donor, the negative predictive value of a non-reactive ELISA result is extremely high. In the event of a reactive result, procedural or technical error should be ruled out. Thus, standard blood bank policy for a reactive result is to repeat the test in duplicate. A repetitively strongly reactive result is likely to be a true positive, but additional confirmatory tests are often necessary to attain an acceptable positive predictive value. (Care must be taken, however, since assays are not generally strictly independent, so that pure Bayesian analysis will lead to overestimation of predictive values).

A moderate or weakly reactive result suggests the need for clinical re-assessment, and thus further discussion with the subject. Is there a possibility that the result reflects an early seroconversion, so that repeat testing in several weeks might clarify an equivocal result? Does the subject have a condition associated with false positive reactions? In the latter instance, a negative direct confirmatory test (e.g., Western blot) is strong evidence for true negativity. In the event that even the repeat clinical history indicates no accepted risk factor (so that the pre-test probability remains very low), then even an initial positive confirmatory test implies only a low positive predictive value, so that further evaluation remains appropriate (e.g., by reference research laboratories).

Immunofluorescence

Antibodies against viruses are commonly detected in clinical laboratories by indirect immunofluorescence assays (IFA). For HIV, IFA is currently available only as a research tool. Acetone-fixed HIV-infected and uninfected (control) cells are typically applied to slides or isolated wells, incubated with test sera, and counter-stained (e.g. with fluorescein-conjugated anti-human IgG). A dilution series of a given serum is usually run to assess strength (titer) of reactivity. The reactions are viewed microscopically as a fluorescent stain (black and white reproduction of a typical positive result, Figure 1).

The fluorescent staining pattern, when read by a skilled observer, is quite informative. Anti-nuclear antibody and anti-mitochondrial antibody reactivity patterns may be causes of non-HIV reactivity. However, the titration-endpoints of the reactions on the infected and uninfected cells can be compared. This information is then synthesized as a positive or negative result. Reactions against both infected and uninfected cells suggest non-specific reactivity, but it is unclear whether or not such an IFA pattern might occur concomitantly with true (but weak) HIV-specific antibody, such as might prevail in high-risk-group members with high anti-HLA titers (18).

Spectrum of HIV Antibodies

Several confirmation assays enable the visualization of specific antibody reactivities. With the sequencing of the nucleic acid structure of several isolates of HIV, the functional structure of this RNA virus is being unveiled rapidly. Analysis of the genome indicates the presence of several "open reading frames" (Figure 2), which have been related to essential viral components: 1) gag - the viral core, 2) pol - the enzyme reverse transcriptase (which is essential in creating a DNA copy of the viral RNA), 3) env - the envelope of the virus, including the glycoprotein (gp) membrane, 4) tat - a trans-acting protein related to the control of viral replication. Serologic work based on cloned monoclonal reagents (28)-(30) along with concordance to predictions based on the viral genome has provided an evolving picture of the relationship of various component viral proteins to HIV (Table 3). These components vary in inherent immunogenicity and their relationship to disease state remains incompletely understood. The 14 kilodalton tat-III gene product is not com-

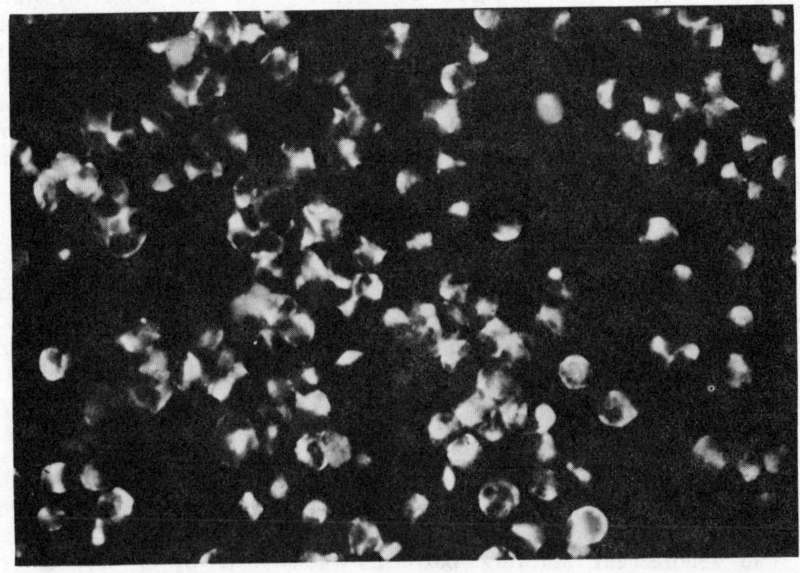

Figure 1. Indirect immunofluorescence assay (IFA). A typical positive HIV IFA result. Immunofluorescence appears white. (Courtesy of Drs. Francis K. Mundon and Daniel H. Zimmerman, Electro-Nucleonics, Inc., Columbia, MD.)

monly detected by standard techniques.

Western Blot

While the disrupted whole virus ELISA detects HIV antibodies, the precise spectrum remains undetermined. The Western blot (WB), also known as immunoblot, procedure has become a mainstay in confirmation since it readily permits visualization of the component antibody reactivities (7),(8).

Preparation of the WB begins with purification of HIV from culture materials, followed by dissociation of the concentrated HIV with detergent. These steps involve the selective loss of some viral components such as gp120. The material is then resolved by polyacrylamide gel electrophoresis, so that the components are separated by their molecular weights, and electrophoretically transferred to a support medium such as nitrocellulose paper. Individual strips are reacted with test or control sera, and developed to reveal bands where the serum antibodies have bound to the resolved viral proteins. The development process involves either photographic plates to reveal radioactivity (e.g., a strip radioimmunoassay) (31) or chemical incubation (e.g., biotin-avidin technique). The latter approach has gained

Table 3. Some Common HIV-Related Immunogenic Proteins

Protein (p) or Glycoprotein (gp) Name (Based on Size*)	Sometimes Referred To In Earlier Literature As	Relationship to HIV Genome
gp 160	--	env
gp 120	gp 110	env
p 66	p 61, p 64	pol
pr 53 gag	p 55	gag
p 51	p 53	pol
gp 41	(gp 41-45)	env
p 24	p 25	gag
p 17	p 15**, p18	gag

* In kilodaltons
** A p15 antigen also exists but is poorly immunogenic

commercial favor due to the shorter processing time and the elimination of radioactive materials. Although prototype and standard WB techniques do not reveal the larger envelope components gp120 and gp160, recent refinements enable detection at some laboratories (Figure 3).

Radioimmunoprecipitation

The radioimmunoprecipitation (RIP) technique requires HIV to be grown in cell culture in the presence of a radioactive label, purified, and disrupted (32)-(34). Standard techniques lead to poor labelling of gp41, but lentil-lectin enhancement or alternative radiolabels may be utilized if gp41 detection by RIP is desired (Figure 4). The material is reacted with the test serum, isolated by precipitation, fully washed, resolved electrophoretically, and developed to analyze the radioactivity pattern. The entire process takes several days to over a week, and requires considerable technical skill. Since RIP reliably detects gp120 and gp160 antibodies, it is the reference standard for these large envelope antibodies (Figure 4). RIP analysis routinely includes a comparison against control material from a radiolabelled cell culture that was grown without HIV, to differentiate cellular from viral reactivity.

Utilization and Interpretation of WB and RIP

The great confirmatory powers of WB and RIP lie in their ready demonstration of the specific HIV-related antibodies and in

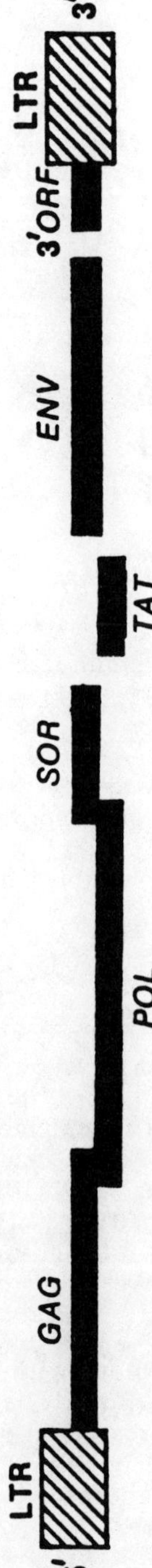

Figure 2. Organization of HIV genome.

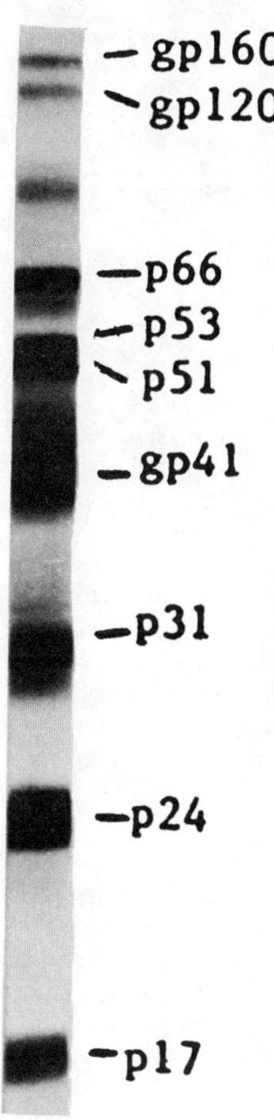

Figure 3. Western blot. Western blot with enhancement of gp120 and gp160 reactivity. Fine detail is typically better appreciated in original WB than in reproduction (e.g., p51 and pr53gag are clearly separated in the original). (Courtesy of Dr. Steve Alexander, Biotech Research Laboratories, Inc., Rockville, MD)

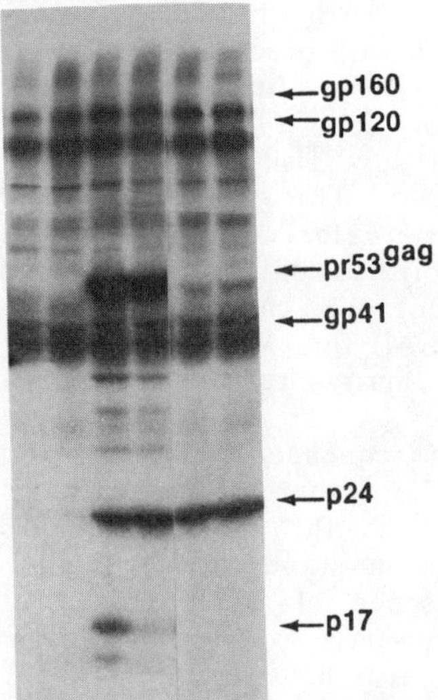

Figure 4. Radioimmunoprecipitation. Typical positive sera from six subjects by radioimmunoprecipitation on HIV-infected cells, demonstrating routine gp41 detection with enhanced methods. Lanes 1 and 2, env reactivity without gag. Lanes 3 and 4, env and gag with strongly reactive gag-precursor reactivity. Lanes 5 and 6, env and gag with weak gag-precursor reactivity. (Courtesy of Dr. Fulvia di Marzo Veronese, Bionetics Research, Rockville, MD)

the pattern itself. When classic patterns (Figures 3 and 4) are present, positivity is a virtual certainty. When several related antibodies are detected, the pattern again may be presumed to have high predictive value. Thus, the newer WB's which enhance gp120 and gp160 detection are helpful in classifying some potentially ambiguous sera (Weiss SH, Alexander S, et al. unpublished data). A broad gp41 WB band is generally acceptable as adequate confirmation but additional testing of very low risk group sera may be necessary. In contrast, a solitary sharp (thin) WB band at p40 is likely to indicate reactivity unrelated to HIV. An experienced virologist and laboratory can be crucial in making this critical but subjective distinction. As in other areas of medicine, adequate training in subtle differences is essential. Significant variation in WB sensitivity and interpretation still exist (35),(36). Apparent WB reactivity may not be confirmed by reference WB laboratories, so that aberrant findings should be pursued (37).

In the absence of gp41 on classic WB, there is widespread agreement that the combination of p24 and pr53gag provide reliable confirmation. However, the interpretation of standard WB's with isolated p24 reactivity is controversial (38). Some laboratories have noted this as the sole reactivity, and in some instances subsequent testing has proven consistent with early HIV infection (39,40). Such data have been used to argue that p24 core antibody frequently precedes envelope antibodies.

Some persons with solitary p24 bands may be found among historic blood donor sera (9) and instances of prolonged persistent p24 reactivity in low risk subjects have been noted (Wormser GP, unpublished data). This persistent reactivity pattern can be associated with a relatively sharp (i.e., atypical) p24 region (Weiss SH, unpublished data). Whereas the CDC has accepted p24 alone as sufficient WB confirmation of sera which are repeatedly reactive by ELISA, the Walter Reed Army Institute of Research laboratory and many retrovirologists treat such reactions as equivocal.

The observed sequence of development of HIV antibodies is dependent upon the inherent technical sensitivities of the assays employed as well as the biology of infection. Thus, the absence of gp41 antibody on standard WB should not be interpreted as ruling out the presence of other env antibodies. Some sera which have appeared to have antibodies solely to the p24 core antigen can be shown to also have env reactivity with RIP and other newer assays (Figure 4; and Weiss SH, unpublished data).

The interpretation of other WB and RIP patterns in terms of specificity and sensitivity for HIV infection remain uncertain (41)-(43). Persons without evidence of HIV antibodies or with unusual WB reactivity patterns have sometimes been found to be HIV-infected by culture (41),(43).

NEUTRALIZING ANTIBODIES

HIV antibodies are detectable which have neutralizing properties in vitro, e.g. inhibition of syncytial formation (44)-(46). Although at least some AIDS patients also have such antibodies, the protective role, if any, of the antibodies detected by these methods remains to be determined. These assays currently remain a purely research tool, but have found particular application in the HIV vaccine developmental efforts. Antibodies to purified thymosin alpha-1 have shown some preliminary evidence of neutralizing capability in vitro as well (47).

HIV DETECTION: IN SITU HYBRIDIZATION, ANTIGEN ASSAYS, CULTURE

The technique of in situ hybridization offers a direct approach for localization of HIV nucleic acid sequences in cellular preparations (48)-(50). The limited proportion of infected cells in vivo, the low viral sequence copy number per cell, and the need to examine slide preparations by hand with light microscopy have served to limit its application outside highly sophisticated research laboratories.

Parenteral needle-stick injuries among health care and laboratory workers exposed to HIV have led to HIV transmission only infrequently (4),(51),(52). This suggests that the usual infectious titer of HIV in peripheral blood is much lower than for hepatitis B virus, and that an HIV antigen assay needs to be extraordinarily sensitive to be useful. In vitro hybridization experiments have also indicated that HIV infected cells are rare in blood, brain and lung (48)-(50), so that detection of HIV antigen in tissue homogenates will likely also require sensitive assays. Massive viremia, if it occurs at all, appears to be unusual. Sensitive in vitro HIV antigen detection systems are under development (35),(53)-(56). However, rigorous assessment of such assays in terms of specificity and reproducibility remain necessary. Demonstration that such an assay specifically measures viral antigen will be a challenging task in so far as there are no independent laboratory criteria. Thus, claims regarding research or clinical utility will require very close scrutiny for each proposed application. For example, specificity of a given assay is likely to prove greater in an acellular sterile body fluid such as cerebrospinal fluid than in stool or saliva. Preliminary results suggest that circulating HIV antigen may precede detectable HIV antibodies and that antigen may thereafter become non-detectable, only to reappear in some persons with severe clinical immunosuppression (56),(57).

HIV virus isolation by cell culture involves the use of carefully selected permissive cell lines such as some malignant T-cell lines or co-cultivation with normal lymphocytes which have been stimulated with mitogens and maintained with T-cell growth factor (and sometimes alpha-interferon) (1),(2),(58). These culture techniques enhance viral titer. Recently, some HIV isolates with a propensity for growth in monocyte/macrophage lines have been described, and may reflect differences in cellular biology among HIV isolates (59)-(61). The presence of retroviruses is detected by testing the culture at periodic intervals for specific Mg^{++}-dependent reverse transcriptase activity in the medium and/or viral antigen detection (as described above). These findings are then further confirmed by detection of viral antigens within the cultured cells, as by electron microscropy and/or with monoclonal reagents. Cultures may reveal either active or latent HIV infective states. These methods require advanced technology within the context of adequate provisions for biosafety and are not feasible beyond the research setting. The cost is great, and the laboratory equipment and skilled research technicians are extremely limited. The limited sensitivity and difficulty of HIV cultures does not allow wide-spread use for the determination of HIV carrier states.

SUMMARY

The armamentarium of HIV detection systems has grown rapidly over the last two years. Future developments are likely to include assays based on panels of monoclonal antibodies (with the expectant promise of further improved sensitivity and specificity) and ever more rapid test turn-around time (e.g., screening formats such as dot-blots or latex agglutination which can yield screening results in seconds (62), analogous to home pregnancy kits). HIV testing alternatives will continue to move from the research bench to the clinical laboratory. The judicious choice of these tools will depend upon an increased understanding of the dynamics of HIV infection, critical head-to-head comparison testing, and cost-benefit decision analyses.

REFERENCES

1. Gallo, R.C., Salahuddin, S.Z., Popovic, M., et al., Frequent detection and isolation of cytopathic retroviruses (HTLV-III) from patients with AIDS and at risk for AIDS. Science 224:500-503 (1984)

2. Popovic, M., Sarngadharan, M.G., Read, E., et al., Detection, isolation, and continuous production of cytopathic retrovirus (HTLV-III) from patients with AIDS and pre-AIDS. Science 224:497-500 (1984)

3. Landesman, S.H., Ginzburg, H.M., Weiss, S.H., The AIDS epidemic. N Engl J Med 312:521-525 (1985)

4. Weiss, S.H., Biggar, R.J., The epidemiology of human retrovirus-associated illnesses. Mount Sinai J Med 53:579-591 (1986)

5. Dodd, R.Y., Donor screening and epidemiology. Prog Clin Biol Res 182:389-405 (1985)

6. Saxinger, W.C., Gallo, R.C., Application of the indirect enzyme-linked immunosorbent assay microtest to the detection and surveillance of human T-cell leukemia-lymphoma virus. Lab Invest 49:371-377 (1983)

7. Sarngadharan, M.G., Popovic, M., Bruch, L., et al., Antibodies reactive with human T-lymphotropic retroviruses (HTLV-III) in the serum of patients with AIDS. Science 224:506-508 (1984)

8. Schupbach, J., Popovic, M., Gilden, R.V., et al., Serologic analysis of a subgroup of human T-lymphotropic retroviruses (HTLV-III) associated with AIDS. Science 224:503-505 (1984)

9. Weiss, S.H., Goedert, J.J., Sarngadharan, M.G., et al., Screening test for HTLV-III (AIDS-agent) antibodies: Specificity, sensitivity, and applications. JAMA 253:221-225 (1985)

10. CDC., Additional recommendations to reduce sexual and drug abuse-related transmission of human T-lymphotropic virus type III/lymphadenopathy-associated virus. MMWR 35:152-155 (1986)

11. Marwick, C., Use of AIDS antibody test may provide more answers. JAMA 253:1694-1699 (1985)

12. Sivak, S.L., Wormser, G.P., Predictive value of a screening test for antibodies to HTLV-III. Am J Clin Pathol 85:700-703 (1986)

13. Petricciani, J.C., Seto, B., et al., An analysis of serum samples positive for HTLV-III antibodies. N Engl J Med 313: 47-48 (1985)

14. CDC., Results of human T-lymphotropic virus type III test kits reported from blood collection centers - United States, April 22 - May 19, 1985. MMWR 34:375-376 (1985)

15. Weiss, S.H., Goedert, J.J., Screening for HTLV-III antibodies: the relation between prevalence and positive predictive value. JAMA 253:3397 (1985)

16. Carlson, J.R., Bryant, M.L., Hinrichs, S.H., et al., AIDS serology testing in low- and high-risk groups. JAMA 253: 3405-3408 (1985)

17. Chang, T.W., Kato, I., McKinney, S., et al., Detection of antibodies to human T-cell lymphotropic virus-III (HTLV-III) with an immunoassay employing a recombinant *Escherichia coli*-derived viral antigenic peptide. Biotechnology 3: 905-909 (1985)

18. Weiss, S.H., Mann, D.L., Murray, C., et al., HLA-DR antibodies and HTLV-III antibody ELISA testing. Lancet 2:157 (1985)

19. Kuhnl, P., Seidl, S., Holzberger, G., HLA DR4 antibodies cause positive HTLV-III antibody ELISA results. Lancet 1: 1222-1223 (1985)

20. Hunter, J.B., Menitove, J.E., HLA antibodies detected by ELISA HTLV-III antibody kits. Lancet 2:387 (1985)

21. Arthur, L.O., Bess, J.W., Barrett, C.F., et al., Removal of HLA DR antigens from HTLV-III preparations using immunoaffinity chromatography. J Cell Biochem suppl 10A:226 (abstract) (1986)

22. Kaminsky, L.S., McHugh, T., Stites, D., et al., High prevalence of antibodies to AIDS-associated retrovirus in AIDS and related conditons but not in other disease states. Proc Natl Acad Sci (USA) 82:5535-5539 (1985)

23. Biggar, R.J., Gigase, P.L., Melbye, M., et al., ELISA HTLV retrovirus antibody reactivity associated with malaria and immune complexes in healthy Africans. Lancet 2:520-523 (1985)

24. Blaser, M.J., Cohn, D.L., Cody, H., et al., Counterimmunoelectrophoresis for detection of human serum antibody to HTLV-III. J Immunologic Methods 91:181-186 (1986)

25. Gazzolo, L., Robert-Guroff, M., Jennings, A., et al., Type-I and type-III HTLV antibodies in hospitalized and out-patient Zairians. Int J Cancer 36:373-378 (1985)

26. Melbye, M., Njelesani, E.K., Bayley, A., et al., Evidence for heterosexual and clinical manifestations of human immunodeficiency virus infection and related conditions in Lusaka, Zambia. Lancet 2:1113-1115 (1986)

27. Saxinger, W.C., Levine, P., Dean, A.G., et al., Evidence for exposure to HTLV-III in Uganda prior to 1973. Science 227: 1036-1038 (1985)

28. di Marzo Veronese, F., Copeland, T.D., DeVico, A.L., et al., Characterization of highly immunogenic p66/p51 as the reverse transcriptase of HTLV-III/LAV. Science 231:1289-1291 (1986)

29. Wright, C.M., Felber, B.K., Paskalis, H., et al., Expression and characterization of the trans-activator of HTLV-III/LAV virus. Science 234:988-992 (1986)

30. di Marzo Veronese, F., Sarngadharan, M.G., Rahman, R., et al., Monoclonal antibodies specific for p24, the major core portein of human T-cell leukemia virus type III. Proc Natl Acad Sci USA 82:5199-5202 (1985).

31. Towbin, H., Staehelin, T., Gordon, J., Electrophoretic transfer of proteins from polyacrilamide gels to nitrocellulose sheets: procedures and some applications. Proc Natl Acad Sci USA 76:4350-4354 (1979)

32. Robey, W.G., Safai, B., Oroszlan, S., et al., Characterization of envelope and core structural gene products of HTLV-III with sera from AIDS patients. Science 228:593-595 (1985)

33. Barin, F., McLane, M.F., Allan, J.S., et al., Virus envelope protein of HTLV-III represents the major target antigen for antibodies in AIDS patients. Science 228:1094-1096 (1985)

34. Allan, J.S., Coligan, J.E., Barin, F., et al., Major glycoprotein antigens that induce antibodies in AIDS patients are encoded by HTLV-III. Science 228:1091-1093 (1985)

35. Saxinger, W.C., Rose, A., Oral presentation. FDA/NIH/CDC workshop: Experience with HTLV-III antibody testing - Update on: screening, laboratory and epidemiologic correlations. Bethesda, MD, July 31, 1985.

36. Saxinger, W.C., Rose, A.H., Tarone, R.E., et al., Variability in Western blot performance among laboratories with major HTLV-III/LAV test experience. (submitted)

37. Saag, M.S., Britz, J., Asymptomatic blood donor with a false positive HTLV-III Western blot. N Engl J Med 314:118 (1986)

38. Carlson, J.R., Hinrichs, S.H., Levy, N.B., et al., Evaluation of commercial AIDS screening test kits. Lancet 1:1388 (1986)

39. Saah, A.J., Sensitivity of the ELISA for HIV antibodies during early stages of infection. Presented at the NIH Consensus Development Conference on the impact of routine HTLV-III antibody testing of blood and plasma donors on public health. Bethesda Md, July 7-9, 1986.

40. Biggar, R.J., Johnson, B.K., Musoke, S.S., et al., Severe illness associated with appearance of antibody to human immunodeficiency virus in an African. Br Med J 293:1210-1211 (1986)

41. Petricciani, J.C., Seto, B., Wells, M., et al., An analysis of serum samples positive for HTLV-III antibodies. N Engl J Med 313:47-48 (1985)

42. Esteban, J.I., Shih, J.W.K., Tai, C.C., et al., Importance of Western blot analysis in predicting infectivity of anti-HTLV-III/LAV positive blood. Lancet 2:1083-1086 (1985)

43. Ward, J.W., Grindon, A.J., Feorino, P.M., et al., Laboratory and epidemiologic evaluation of an enzyme immunoassay for antibodies to HTLV-III. JAMA 256:357-361 (1986)

44. Robert-Guroff, M., Brown, M., Gallo, R.C., HTLV-III-neutralizing antibodies in patients with AIDS and AIDS-related-complex. Nature 316:72-74 (1985)

45. Weiss, R.A., Clapham, P.R., Cheingsong-Popov, R., et al., Neutralization of human T-lymphotropic virus type III by sera of AIDS and AIDS-risk patients. Nature 316:69-72 (1985)

46. Faulkner-Valle, G.P., de Rossi, A., Gassa, O.D., et al., LAV/HTLV-III neutralizing antibodies in the sera of patients with AIDS, lymphadenopathy syndrome and asymptomatic seropositve individuals. Tumori 72:219-224 (1986)

47. Sarin, P.S., Sun, D.K., Thornton, A.H., et al., Neutralization of HTLV-III/LAV replication by antiserum to thymosin alpha-1. Science 232:1135-1137 (1986)

48. Harper, M.E., Marselle, L.M., Gallo, R.C., et al., Detection of HTLV-III-infected lymphocytes in lymph nodes and peripheral blood from AIDS patients by in situ hybridization. Proc Natl Acad Sci USA 83:772-776 (1986)

49. Chayt, K.J., Harper, M.E., Marselle, L.M., et al., Detection of HTLV-III RNA in lungs of patients with AIDS and pulmonary involvement. JAMA 256:2356-2359 (1986)

50. Stoler, M.H., Eskin, T.A., Benn, S., et al., Human T-cell lymphotropic virus type III infection of the central nervous system: a preliminary in situ analysis. JAMA 256:1260-1264 (1986)

51. Weiss, S.H., Saxinger, W.C., Rechtman, D., et al., HTLV-III infection among health care workers: Association with needle-stick injuries. JAMA 254:2089-2093 (1985)

52. Moss, A., Osmond, D., Bacchetti, P., et al., Risk of seroconversion for acquired immunodeficiency syndrome (AIDS) in San Francisco health workers. J Occupational Med 28:821-824 (1986)

53. Paul, D.A., Falk, L.A., Detection of HTLV-III antigens in serum. J Cell Biochem suppl 10A:224 (abstract) (1986)

54. Falk, L., Paul, D., Knigge, M., Detection of HTLV-III antigens in lysates of peripheral blood/lymph node mononuclear cells. J Cell Biochem suppl 10A:200 (abstract) (1986)

55. Hedenskog, M., Ward, B., Dewhurst, S., et al., Testing for AIDS retrovirus (HTLV-III/LAV) antibodies and antigens by indirect immunofluorescence. J Cell Biochem suppl 10A:201 (abstract) (1986)

56. Goudsmit, J., de Wolf, F., Paul, D.A., et al., Expression of human immunodeficiency virus antigen (HIV-Ag) in serum and cerebrospinal fluid during acute and chronic infection. Lancet 2:177-180 (1986)

57. Allain, J.P., Laurian, Y., Paul, D.A., et al., Serologic markers in early stages of human immunodeficiency virus infection in hemophiliacs. Lancet 2:1233-1236 (1986)

58. Salahuddin, S.Z., Markham, P.D., Popovic, M., et al., Isolation of infectious human T-cell leukemia/lymphotropic virus type III (HTLV-III) from patients with acquired immunodeficiency syndrome (AIDS) or AIDS-related complex (ARC) and from healthy carriers: A study of risk groups and tissue sources. Proc Natl Acad Sci USA 82:5530-5534 (1985)

59. Gartner, S., Markovits, P., Markovitz, D.M., et al., The role of mononuclear phagocytes in HTLV-III/LAV infection. Science 233:215-219 (1986)

60. Gartner, S., Markovits, P., Markovitz, D.M., et al., Virus isolation from and identification of HTLV-III/LAV-producing cells in brain tissue from a patient with AIDS. JAMA 256: 2365-2371 (1986)

61. Streicher, H.Z., Joynt, R.J., HTLV-III/LAV and the monocyte/ macrophage. JAMA 256:2390-2391 (1986)

62. Carlson, J.R., Mertens, S.C., Yee, J.L., et al., Preliminary communication: Rapid, easy and economical screening test for antibodies to the human immunodeficiency virus. Lancet 1: 361-362 (1987)

15
Predictive Values of Antibody Tests for HIV

Steven L. Sivak

Serologic tests have been developed to detect antibodies to human immunodeficiency virus (HIV) and have been in general use since mid-1985 (1). These tests have been used to study the epidemiology of infection, to determine the prevalence of HIV infection in various groups, and to screen donated blood in an attempt to prevent transfusion-related acquired immunodeficiency syndrome (AIDS) (2). It is assumed that the presence of antibodies to the virus represents active infection. Donated blood found to be positive for antibodies to the virus is discarded and donors of these units notified of their positive antibody status (2). It is hoped that with screening, the incidence of AIDS related to blood transfusion will approach zero. The success of such screening programs will depend greatly upon the accuracy of the testing procedure.

Serology for HIV antibodies is also being utilized as a diagnostic tool in evaluation of individual patients. Since the presence of antibodies may have significant implications for those tested, possibly leading to major modifications in sexual behavior, lifestyle, interpersonal relationships and requirements for medical attention (3), accurate interpretation of test results is necessary.

The accuracy of a test depends in part on the test characteristics (4),(5). These are defined as the sensitivity and specificity of the test. The sensitivity is simply the proportion (or percent) of individuals with disease who have a positive test or: the number of positive tests divided by the number of individuals with disease tested. This is also known as the true positive rate.

The specificity of a test is the proportion of individuals without disease who have a negative test or: the number of negative tests divided by the number of individuals without disease tested. This is also known as the true negative rate (4),(5).

The sensitivity and specificity of a test are, therefore, determined by subjecting two groups of individuals to a test: one group that is known to have the disease and one group that does not.

The sensitivity and specificity do not determine the likelihood that a positive test represents a true positive result or that a negative test represents a true negative result. These values are defined by the predictive value of a positive test and the predictive value of a negative test, respectively. The predictive value of a positive test is: the number of true positive results/total number of positive results. According to a corollary of Bayes' Theorem of conditional probability, this is equal to:

$$\frac{(P \times \text{Sensitivity})}{(P \times \text{Sensitivity}) + [(1-P) \times (1-\text{Specificity})]}$$

where P = the prevalence of disease (or the likelihood of the disease being present before the test is performed) in the group (or individual) tested. P is also known as the pretest probability of disease.

Similarly, the predictive value of a negative test is: the number of true negative results/total number of negative results which is equal to:

$$\frac{(1-P) \times \text{Specificity}}{[(1-P) \times \text{Specificity}] + [P \times (1-\text{Sensitivity})]}$$

It is apparent from these equations that the prevalence or likelihood of infection with HIV before a test is performed will be an important factor in the predictive value of test results. (A complete discussion of Bayes' Theorem is beyond the scope of this chapter. The interested reader is referred to references 4 and 5 in the bibliography).

Antibodies to HIV are most often detected by two techniques, an enzyme linked immunosorbent assay (ELISA), and by Western blot analysis (6). Although the latter detects antibodies to specific viral antigens and is thought to be more sensitive and more specific, it is labor intensive and less readily available (7). The ELISA detects antibodies to disrupted whole virus. In the United States as of April 1985, ELISA tests were commercially available from three companies and were the most widely used tests for screening (1). The performance characteristics of three test kits are listed in Table 1. Sensitivity varies from 93.4% to 99.6% and specificity from 99.2% to 99.8%.

Apparent differences in the performance of the individual kits may not be real since determination of test characteristics was done using different groups of sera. It is known that antibodies to HIV may decrease over time. If more sera from

TABLE 1. Test Characteristics for ELISA Kits Produced by Three Manufacturers to Detect Antibodies to HIV (Ref. 1).

Manufacturer*	Sensitivity	Specificity
Electro-Nucleonics	99.6%	99.2%
Abbott	93.4%	99.8%
Litton	98.9%	99.6%

* Abbott Laboratories, North Chicago, Illinois; Electro-Nucleonics, Inc., Fairfield, New Jersey; Litton Industries, Sunnyvale, California.

patients who were late in the course of AIDS are included in the test sample of only one of the tests, the sensitivity of that test may appear to be lower than its true value. Also, if sera from asymptomatic volunteers infected with HIV are inadvertently included in a group thought to be free of infection, then that test's specificity will be falsely lowered (1).

Prevalence data on HIV infection for various groups at risk for infection are available from studies which utilized the Western blot technique for antibody detection and are shown in Table 2 (8),(9). If one assumes that the Western blot test is 100% sensitive and 100% specific, then these studies may be considered to indicate the true prevalence of infection. The data listed for intravenous drug abusers were obtained from patients in Switzerland (8) but is consistent with the range of prevalence rates from studies done in the United States (6). Information concerning homosexual and bisexual men from both Switzerland and San Francisco was also included since there is a wide range for prevalence rates of infection with HIV in this group. It has been estimated that the prevalence of HIV infection in the general United States population at no known risk is less than .05%. This figure is based on preliminary data from screening blood donors and from published calculations (6),(10).

Using this information along with the principles of Bayes' Theorem, one can calculate the predictive values of test results obtained with each of the three ELISA tests for individuals belonging to different risk groups or the general population at low risk for infection with HIV (Table 3). In general terms, as the pretest probability of infection with HIV increases, the predictive value of a test improves and the predictive value of a negative test falls. If the pretest probability of infection (prevalence of infection) with HIV falls, then the predictive value of a positive test declines and the predictive value of a negative test rises.

TABLE 2. Prevalence Rates for Infection with HIV Based Upon Data Utilizing the Western Blot Technique For Antibody Detection.

Group	Prevalence (Reference)
HOMOSEXUAL OR BISEXUAL MEN	
San Francisco	65% (11)
Switzerland	10% (8)
HEMOPHILIACS	62% (9)
INTRAVENOUS DRUG ABUSERS	36% (8)
NO KNOWN RISK	0.05% (6),(10)

Each of the available tests for detection of antibodies to HIV displays a high degree of sensitivity and specificity and hence the predictive value of a positive test is high when there is at least a moderate chance of infection before the test is performed. Even with only a 10% pretest probability of infection, a positive test is more than 90% accurate with all of the available tests. As the pretest probability approaches 40%, the predictive value of a positive test exceeds 99%.

It is important to note, however, that if an ELISA test is used for an individual from a population that has a low prevalence of infection, such as a blood donor or other individual at no known risk for infection with HIV, the predictive value of a positive test is rather poor. Here, a positive test will be truly positive only between 5% and 19% of the time. It would be ill advised, therefore, to conclude that a positive ELISA test result meant infection with HIV without confirmation with a more specific technique such as the Western blot analysis.

The prevalence of infection with HIV varies according to risk group, year of testing and geographic location. The range of values listed in Table 2 is broad enough (from 0.05% to 65%) to be useful to estimate predictive values for specific populations not shown, if the prevalence of infection is known.

Such theoretical determinations of predictive values have been confirmed by early data from blood donor screening programs. In one study, only 5% of positive sera were confirmed as true positives by the Western blot technique and in another study, this figure was 23% (6),(12). On the other hand, ELISA positive sera from high risk individuals have been confirmed positive more than 85% of the time (6).

The predictive value of a negative result is excellent when the pretest probability of a test is low. When the pretest probability of infection with HIV is less than 35%, the accuracy of a negative test is greater than 98% for all tests. If, however, an individual tested is a member of a group with a high

TABLE 3. Predictive Value of Screening Tests for HIV Antibody*

Risk Group	Manufacturer	Predictive Value Test Positive	Predictive Value Test Negative
Homosexual or Bisexual Men			
San Francisco	E-N**	99.57%	99.26%
	Abbott	99.88%	89.06%
	Litton	99.78%	97.99%
Switzerland	E-N	93.26%	99.96%
	Abbott	98.10%	99.27%
	Litton	96.49%	99.88%
Hemophiliacs	E-N	99.51%	99.35%
	Abbott	99.87%	90.26%
	Litton	99.75%	98.23%
Intravenous Drug Abusers	E-N	98.59%	99.77%
	Abbott	99.62%	96.41%
	Litton	99.29%	99.38%
No Known Risk	E-N	5.86%	99.999%
	Abbott	18.94%	99.997%
	Litton	11.01%	99.999%

* Predictive value of a positive test is the likelihood that a positive test is a true positive result. Similarly, the predictive value of a negative test is the probability that the test is truly negative.

** E-N = Electro-Nucleonics

likelihood of infection with HIV, say >60%, there may be as great as a 10% chance that a negative test is falsely negative. It has been reported that members of high risk groups for HIV infection have volunteered to donate blood in order to obtain an antibody screen at no cost (13). This use of blood banks is to be strongly discouraged since, because of the reasons mentioned, it may lead to a paradoxical increase in the number of transfused units of contaminated blood despite routine screening for HIV antibody.

In summary, it is the predictive value of a test that determines its accuracy and clinical value. The predictive value is not only dependent upon the test characteristics but also on the likelihood of infection before the test is performed. Although the three commercially available ELISA test kits for HIV antibody evaluated possess a high degree of sensitivity and specificity, the predictive value of a positive test is poor when used in an individual with an exceedingly low pretest probability of infection, such as a member of the general United States population at no known risk for infection with HIV. Since a diagnosis of HIV infection has very serious implications, confirmation of a positive ELISA with the Western blot technique (or other suitable confirmatory test) is mandatory in individuals at low risk. If the test is positive in an individual who is a member of a high risk group for infection with HIV, then further testing is not essential. Because the predictive value of a negative test in high risk individuals is suboptimal, further testing may be necessary if there is a strong clinical suspicion of HIV infection. Members of high risk groups must continue to refrain from donating blood.

REFERENCES

1. Petricciani, J.C. Licensed tests for antibody to human T-lymphotropic virus type III: Sensitivity and specificity. Ann Intern Med 103:726-729 (1985)

2. CDC., Provisional Public Health Service inter-agency recommendations for screening donated blood and plasma for antibody to the virus causing acquired immunodeficiency syndrome. MMWR 34:1-5 (1985)

3. CDC., Prevention of acquired immune deficiency syndrome (AIDS); Report of inter-agency recommendations. MMWR 32: 101-103 (1983)

4. Fink, D.J., Galen, R.S., Probabilistic approaches to clinical decision support, In: Computer Aids to Clinical Decisions. (Williams BT, ed), CRC Press; Boca Raton, FL, p 1-43 (1982)

5. Weinstein, M.C., Fineberg, H.V., ed. Clinical Decision Analysis, W. B. Saunders Company, Philadelphia, Pa, p 75-131 (1980)

6. CDC., Recommendations for assisting in the prevention of perinatal transmission of human T-lymphotropic virus type III/lymphadenopathy associated virus and acquired immunodeficiency syndrome. MMWR 34:721-732 (1985)

7. Weiss, S.H., Goedert, J.J., Sarngadharan, M.G., et al., Screening test for HTLV-III (AIDS agent) antibodies. JAMA 253: 221-225 (1985)

8. Schupbach, J., Haller, O., Markus, V., et al. Antibodies to HTLV-III in Swiss patients with AIDS and pre-AIDS and in groups at risk for AIDS. N Engl J Med 312:265-70 (1985)

9. Goedert, J.J., Sarngadharan, M.G., Eyster, M.E., et al., Antibodies reactive with human T-cell leukemia viruses in the serum of hemophiliacs receiving factor VIII concentrate. Blood 65:492-495 (1985)

10. Sivak, S.L., Wormser, G.P. How common is HTLV-III infection in the United States? N Engl J Med 313: 1352-1353 (1985)

11. CDC., Antibodies to a retrovirus etiologically associated with AIDS in populations with increased incidences of the syndrome. MMWR 33:377-379 (1984)

12. Schoor, J.B., Berkowitz, A., Cumming, P.D., et al., Prevalence of HTLV-III antibody in American blood donors. N Engl J Med 313: 384-385 (1985)

13. Perkins, J.T., Janda, W.M., Does antibody screening of donors increase the risk of transfusion-associated AIDS? N Engl J Med 313:115-116 (1985)

Part III
Immunology of HIV Infection

16
The Immune Deficiency of AIDS

Frederick P. Siegal

The acquired immune deficiency syndrome, AIDS, is a newly recognized disorder of the immune system remarkable for its severity and permanence. A variety of relatively rare "primary" immune deficiency disorders were known, as reflected in a classification of the World Health Organization (1), before the recognition of AIDS. Most of these disorders are thought to be hereditary, though some, like AIDS, probably reflect environmental influences, including viral infections of several types.

AIDS is remarkable among immunodeficiency diseases, both because of its clearly infectious nature and its onset only after its adult victims have had an opportunity to incorporate a large variety of commensal or latent microorganisms into their microbial entourage. It is these organisms, by and large, that create clinically important illness. Precedent for the clinical pattern of illness associated with the acquired cellular immunodeficiency seen in AIDS patients lies in individuals immunosuppressed for organ transplantation and in the occasional patient who has the syndrome of thymoma with immunodeficiency. There are striking parallels among these disorders in the "opportunistic" clinical complications of the immune system failure.

The panoply of opportunistic infections and cellular proliferative processes (neoplasms?) in AIDS initially directed the attention of clinical immunologists towards cell-mediated immunity, since this is the component of the immune system that deals chiefly with the obligate and facultative intracellular pathogens predominating in AIDS. More recently, defective antibody production has been appreciated to exist in such patients, despite the absence of a clinically-recognizable antibody deficiency syndrome in most adults. Children with AIDS often present with infections more usually seen in antibody deficiency states, for reasons to be discussed later.

The purpose of this review is to outline the immunologic abnormalities seen in AIDS and to place them in perspective. The defects of cellular and humoral immunity that characterize AIDS have been quite well defined over the past six years of study, and can be seen now as a continuum of decline of several host defense mechanisms.

PATHOGENESIS

Immune functions apparently fail as a direct consequence of infection with human immunodeficiency virus (HIV) in a gradual process that culminates in increasingly evident susceptibility to opportunistic infection. Depletion of lymphoid cells that express the T-4 (CD-4) molecule on their surface is the most obvious manifestation. The mechanisms whereby this process proceeds clearly involve direct cytotoxic infection of certain cells within the immune system. Virus appears to be activated to proliferate and kill latently infected T cells during immune stimulation of these cells. Thus, functional depletion of T cell clones critical to the host defense may occur before full T cell depletion. However, the quantity of cells productively infected has been considered by some to be too low at any one time (on the order of 1/10,000 cells) to account for the profound depletion observed (2). Other mechanisms have, therefore, been postulated to account for the severe deficits that occur. Surface expression of HIV by cells in the process of productive infection may entrap uninfected circulating cells having receptors for virus (CD-4, T-4), leading to in vivo syncytium formation and trapping or killing of the adhering cells (3). Secondary effects such as the liberation of virus-specified or infection-induced immunosuppressive and myelosuppressive factors may also be contributing factors. Some of these may be analogous to the viral gene products of other retroviruses, such as p15(E) of feline leukemia virus, which are known to be immunosuppressive in vitro and in vivo (4). It is of considerable interest that certain of the immune dysfunctions observed in vitro may be reproduced by incubation of uninfected lymphoid cells with purified HIV that has been disrupted, suggesting that not all the effects of the virus require the direct cytopathic actions of living virus (5). Autoimmune mechanisms have been postulated, and antilymphocyte antibodies have been widely demonstrated, particularly in homosexual men (6),(7), but the evidence that they play an important role in lymphoid cell depletion is unconvincing, and they may be more a marker of homosexuality than of HIV infection (8).

HIV exerts profound effects on the complex systems of host defense at almost all levels of function. Although perhaps its principal target is the lymphocyte population expressing the CD-4 molecule (9)-(11), other cells, some of which express this marker and others which apparently do not, are also involved. These include monocyte-macrophages (12), dendritic lymphoid cells involved in self-recognition and antigen presentation (13) and cells within the central nervous system (14)-(16). HIV infection also leads to profound effects on cells that have not yet been shown to be directly infected with the virus, including certain thymus-independent, non-T, large, granular lymphocytes that are crucial to containment of infections with intracellular pathogens (17), (18), and hematopoietic progenitor cells (CFU-GM) (19). The histology of the thymus is profoundly affected during this infection, possibly rendering effective spontaneous reconstitution of thymus-dependent immunity a doubtful prospect (20).

Current evidence suggests that a significant proportion of subjects who have been infected with HIV will have a gradually progressive fall in immune functions over time. Limited experience with cohort studies indicates that duration of infection is a major, though not necessarily the only, determinant of progression of immune deficiency (21). Estimates of outcome based on these studies suggest that at least 50% of subjects seropositive for HIV will become clinically affected at some level.

DETERMINANTS OF CLINICAL ILLNESS IN HIV INFECTION

Expression of illness in retroviral infection can be correlated closely with the degree of measurable immune deficiency. Linear declines in many markers of host defense and hematopoiesis are observed that follow simple clinical staging systems on which many clinicians can agree (Figure 1) (18). The development of severe, systemic opportunistic infections (OI) (22) is a consequence of progression of the immune deficits to critically low and reasonably reproducible levels (18),(23). Before this occurs, clinical manifestations (sometimes referred to as "lesser AIDS") may develop, which may be attributable to either identifiable, usually commensal microorganisms (e.g., minor oral candidiasis) or reactivation of latent viruses (e.g. *Herpes simplex* virus, varicella-zoster virus) in a self-limited clinical event. Other clinical findings (e.g. chronic diarrhea, night sweats, weight loss and wasting) may be unexplained, but are probably related to other commensals of the "normal flora" which become relatively invasive in the presence of a failing host defense system.

Some disease manifestations (e.g., pulmonary tuberculosis) occur in normals as well as in patients with severe cellular immune deficiency; as such, they are not considered to be definitive evidence for AIDS under the surveillance definition promulgated originally by the Centers for Disease Control (CDC). But they may, nevertheless, represent early expression of clinically important cellular immunodeficiency, as in the tuberculin-positive subject who develops reactivation tuberculosis when treated for autoimmune disease with corticosteroids (24).

Disease in the central nervous system (CNS) can be caused by opportunistic organisms (e.g. *Toxoplasma gondii*, cryptococcus, papovaviruses) or by HIV itself (14),(15). Some patients develop encephalopathic changes (cerebral atrophy on computed to-

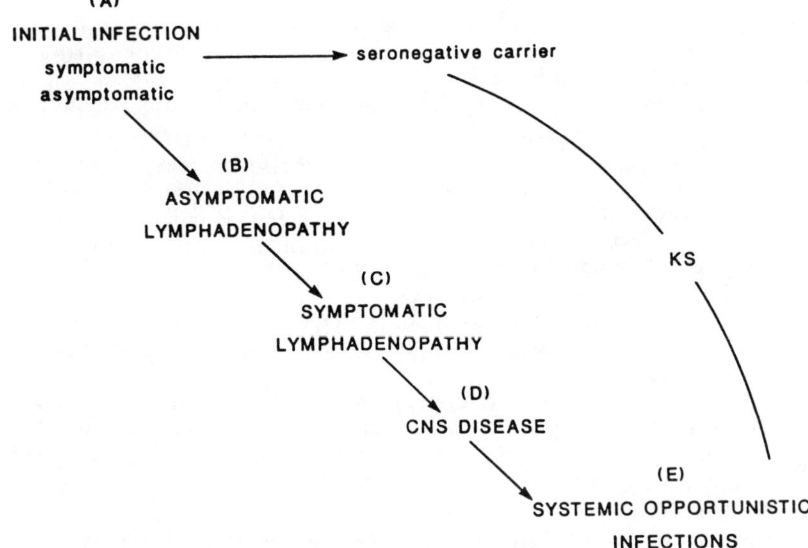

Figure 1. Clinical spectrum of AIDS retrovirus infection.

mography, abnormal neurologic findings, dementia) or myelopathy in the absence of definable opportunistic diseases. In some of these, HIV has been demonstrated in brain or in spinal cord. Most of these subjects have severe cellular immune deficits, suggesting that clinically important manifestations of the neurotropism of the AIDS retrovirus might be the result of opportunism. However, some individuals having relatively spared immune systems have developed CNS disease attributed to HIV involvement of the brain, suggesting that infection of nervous tissues is, like involvement of the immune system, only a matter of duration of infection with the agent (25).

The neoplastic processes complicating HIV infection should be considered to be opportunistic diseases, most likely reflecting, as do the infections, the resident microflora and past history of the individual patient. Virtually all have been described as complications of other immune deficiency states, including congenital and acquired primary immune deficiencies (e.g., Wiskott-Aldrich syndrome, Bruton's agammaglobulinemia, common variable immunodeficiency, thymoma with immunodeficiency). These same complications have been observed among subjects medically immunosuppressed for organ transplantation (26),(27). Many are thought to reflect inductive processes mediated with viruses other than HIV, most notably human papilloma viruses and herpes viruses.

Kaposi's sarcoma (KS) holds a relatively unique place in the spectrum of AIDS. Although it is a case-defining disorder, it may, unlike other opportunistic diseases, develop in subjects with minimal, or even no measurable immunodeficiency. Almost all of those who develop this complication of AIDS are homosexual men. It also has been seen in some homosexual men who lack antibodies to HIV (unpublished personal observation). Worsening prognosis of the disease is, however, closely associated with increasing degrees of immune deficit (28). These observations suggest that a cofactor epidemiologically associated with homosexuality is involved, which interacts with immunodeficiency in the pathogenesis of KS. Some evidence for genetic cofactors also exists (see below). Since the genetic predisposition is associated with the major histocompatibility complex, it possibly reflects selective immunologic incapacity to resist the cofactor, i.e., a "lacunar" immunodeficiency. For example, KS among the elderly has long been recognized to be most frequent among Jewish and Italian men. KS that arose in younger persons in the contact of renal transplantation also occurred almost exclusively in these ethnic groups (26).

Lymphoproliferative disorders including Hodgkin's disease, non-Hodgkin's lymphomas and certain other neoplastic complications of HIV infection generally occur among individuals exhibiting significant, and sometimes profound immune deficits. In addition to herpes viruses and papilloma viruses, coinfection with the transforming human T lymphoma-leukemia ("lymphotropic") viruses I and II (HTLV-I, HTLV-II) may participate in the pathogenesis of some types of neoplasia (29).

CHARACTERISTICS OF NORMAL CELLULAR IMMUNITY

Most clinicians still think of cell-mediated immunity against intracellular organisms as fully described by the interaction of microbial antigens with T cells, which recruit and activate monocyte-macrophages through lymphokines, leading to formation of round-cell infiltrates and granulomas and eventuating in effective killing of intracellular pathogens. While this pathway plays an essential effector role, the functions of dendritic lymphoid cells, macrophages and probably B cells (all Ia-bearing cells) in antigen presentation to the T cell, interactions among clonally expanded helper, suppressor and cytotoxic T cells and B lymphocytes, and their soluble products (interferon-gamma, interleukins 1 and 2, antibodies, helper, and suppressor factors, and other soluble mediators -- the lymphokines) constitute the adaptive part of the cellular host defense. These mechanisms are considered "adaptive" because B and T lymphoid cells recognize antigen via highly specific receptor molecules, and clonally expand to adapt to the challenge of specific antigen. (It is worth recalling that antibodies, generally involved in "humoral" host defenses such as opsonization, are involved in host defense against certain viruses not only through neutralization, but also probably through antibody-dependent cellular cytotoxicity, when they recognize virus-coded cell surface neoantigens characteristic of infected host cells.)

Also contributing to resistance to intracellular pathogens is the class of large, granular lymphocytes (LGL), previously included among "null" or "third population" lymphoid cells. Such cells have not been totally classified, but they do not express certain lineage markers of T and B cells and probably lack the highly specific receptor molecules associated with adaptive immune responses. Instead, these cell populations are normally present and active from the first months of postnatal life and provide a basis for host defense even in the immunologically virgin organism. They function in the absence of prior exposure to antigen and clonal expansion. As such, they are considered to be components of a "natural" as opposed to adaptive immune system. LGL are known to include cell populations engaged in the production of interferon-alpha, in antibody-dependent cellular cytotoxicity and in some forms of natural cytotoxicity (natural killer or NK cells). Current data also suggest that LGL-derived lymphokines, among them alpha-interferon, participate in the activation of macrophages, in the maturation of cytotoxic T lymphocytes and in the augmentation of NK cell activity. As such, they can activate the final common effector mechanisms of cellular immunity in ways similar to antigen-activated T cells.

DEFECTS OF IMMUNITY IN AIDS

Immune Responses in AIDS Patients

In vivo abnormalities in AIDS have been observed in most functions studied. Skin test anergy to common recall antigens that usually reveal delayed-type hypersensitivity (DTH) is generally present in fulminant AIDS. Progressively weakening DTH is observed during development of the syndrome (18),(30)-(32). It is worth recalling that anergy is a quantitative term, since more concentrated antigen may elicit a response not evident with more dilute reagents (e.g. 5 vs 250 TU tuberculin). The presence of anergy suggests that some part of the arc from antigen recognition through recruitment of inflammatory cells is defective. Some preservation of skin reactivity has been observed even with microbial antigens derived from agents causing active infection (e.g. candida skin tests positive in the face of oral and esophageal thrush). The interpretation of this finding is not clear, but might suggest either that only crucial clonal deletion (not loss of all antigen-reactive clones) is important in facilitating opportunistic infections, or that cellular activities involved in delayed-type hypersensitivity are not central to the host defense defects involved in AIDS (30). Systematic study of recall DTH responsiveness during the course of HIV infection demonstrates that gradual declines occur with increasing degrees of clinical illness; however, skin anergy does not appear to predict the development of systemic opportunistic infections, as do certain other measures of cell mediated immunity (18).

Primary immunization to elicit DTH commonly employs skin-sensitizing haptens such as 2,4-dinitrochlorobenzene (DNCB) or 2,4-dinitrofluorobenzene (DNFB). These reagents bind to skin proteins, or perhaps directly to antigen-presenting, Ia-bearing cells (Langerhans cells, monocyte/macrophages, B cells) in the skin, leading to clonal selection and expansion of antigen-reactive T cells. The development of a contact dermatitis upon challenge one month later suggests intact cellular immunity. No published data on DNCB sensitization are available (33), but it is this author's impression from limited studies that patients with AIDS and possibly some within its incubation period cannot be sensitized. A paucity of Langerhans cells in skin biopsies has been reported, as well as an inability of these cells to express Ia antigens (34). This latter function may be dependent on lymphokines such as interferons. Moreover, these antigen-presenting cells may be themselves infected by HIV, as the dendritic lymphoid cells of lymph nodes appear to be (13).

Perhaps as a reflection of the above, patients with AIDS frequently fail to produce granulomas effectively. Disorganized inflammatory responses, often characterized by overwhelming numbers of microorganisms, are seen in infected tissues on biopsy or at post-mortem examination. The knowledge that granuloma formation is often deranged should encourage the pathologist to carry out specialized stains for microorganisms that would otherwise not seem indicated.

Studies of stratified patient groups as well as serial follow-up indicate that gradual declines in white cell count, neutrophil count and lymphocyte count occur during HIV infection (18). Leukopenia becomes increasingly prominent during progression through the spectrum of HIV infection, and may provide a useful clue that serious clinical problems are to be expected. At least late in the disease, leukopenia is undoubtedly multifactorial, involving poor marrow reserves and release of granulocytes (19),(35), myelosuppression related to drugs (for example, trimethoprim-sulfamethoxazole), and peripheral destruction of neutrophils and other formed elements either via immune adherence through cell-bound immune complexes or through true antineutrophil antibodies.

Lymphopenia develops largely as a consequence of the selective depletion of the CD-4 positive helper-inducer T cell subset, normally the predominant lymphoid cell type. Decreases in CD-8^+ (suppressor-cytotoxic) cells and B cells (which remain in the same proportions relative to T cells in blood) also occur (18),(23),(32). Evidence that numerical declines in CD-4+ cells are important in the pathogenesis of opportunistic infections comes from studies showing that when the number of these circulating cells is reduced below 250-300/mm^3, serious opportunistic infections begin to develop (18),(23). Most likely, the recirculating pool reflects the total body availability in tissues of these important antigen-recognizing T cells, which play a keystone role in the generation of many other immune responses (9).

Diffuse elevations of all three major immunoglobulin classes, though chiefly of IgG and IgA, are usually present in the disease, and frequently in patients who eventually progress to full-blown AIDS (36)-(40). Serum IgD is also raised and is considered a useful marker of this disorder (40). Oligoclonal Ig bands have been described in serum as well as in cerebrospinal fluid (41),(42). Hypergammaglobulinemia reflects in part direct polyclonal activation of B cells by structural glycoproteins of HIV (5). Of considerable interest is a significant sequence homology between env gp120 of HIV and the newly described neuronal growth factor and polyclonal B cell activator, neuroleukin (43). Similarities between the retroviral and normal cellular products may explain some of the effects HIV has on both brain and the B cell immune response in AIDS; HIV may bind to the same receptors as does neuroleukin. Epstein-Barr virus (EBV), long known to be capable of driving B cells to differentiate into plasmacytoid cells also probably contributes to the hypergammaglobulinemia. The lack of an effective T cell suppression of EBV and EBV-infected B cells has been demonstrated in AIDS, most likely related to ineffective suppressor-inducer T cells or inadequate generation of cytotoxic T cells (44). This defect would also be expected to predispose to B cell activation by EBV, and possibly to the involvement of EBV in the pathogenesis of lymphomas.

In contrast to the sometimes massive hypergammaglobulinemia, specific antibody titers to some infecting pathogens appear to be lower than expected. Active toxoplasmosis, for example, has been seen in AIDS patients lacking serum antibodies, and IgM antibodies fail to appear in the face of infection with toxoplasma and cytomegaloviruses (CMV) (45),(46). The lack of IgM antibody has been taken to suggest a deficit of antibody production, but may only reflect the recrudescent, rather than primary, nature of the infections cited.

Perhaps more impressive is the failure of AIDS patients (and of those in the prodromal phases in some studies) to produce primary antibody responses to immunogens not previously encountered. Immunization with keyhole limpet hemocyanin (KLH), pneumococcal vaccine and bacteriophage phi-X 174 have resulted in only minimal antibody responses in overt AIDS (47)-(50), reflecting the requirement for helper T cells in the process of clonal selection, expansion and maturation that leads to the production of high-affinity antibodies. In the particular case of phi-X 174, a thymus-dependent immunogen, the antibody responses in both children and adults with HIV infection are blunted, and the shift from IgM to IgG antibody also fails (49),(50). Even the relatively thymus-independent antigens in pneumococcal vaccine are poorly immunogenic in patients with HIV-induced immunodeficiency, suggesting that defective B cell responses (independent of the helper T cell deficits) may play a role in the humoral immunodeficiency (50).

IgG subclass deficiencies have been described in children with AIDS, although without a consistent pattern; adults with AIDS do not appear to have recognizable subclass deficits (51).

SPECIAL FEATURES OF CHILDREN WITH CONGENITAL AIDS AND ARC

The child with congenital HIV infection presents initially with bacteremias and recurrent episodes of sometimes unexplained pneumonitis, failure-to-thrive, dermatitis and other findings common to children with severe, combined immunodeficiency (SCID) (52)-(54). In adults with AIDS, bacteremias and pneumonias suggestive of an antibody deficiency syndrome are much less frequent, occurring perhaps in 5-10% of cases (55). Most adults with AIDS, and children (e.g., hemophiliacs) who acquire the AIDS retrovirus well after birth have difficulty primarily with intracellular pathogens, reflecting the relative importance of deficits in cellular immune mechanisms (18),(22).

Perhaps the reason for this is the demonstrable inability of children and adults to mount a primary immune response (see above). Anamnestic responses do not occur in those failing to mount primary responses, presumably because of the lack of memory B cells. Consequent to this failure of antibody production, any newly colonizing microorganism, including those defended against chiefly by opsonizing or neutralizing antibodies, would be expected to cause disease. The clinical syndrome in children thus includes antibody deficiency manifestations and can to some extent be ameliorated by provision of passive humoral immunity through the use of intravenous immune (gamma) globulin (56). There is, however, no evidence that immune globulin therapy, even in children, has a long-term beneficial effect.

In contrast, the adult or older child who develops AIDS later in life has already made many primary and secondary immune responses, through deliberate immunization or natural colonization, by the time the defects of helper T cells supervene; he has relatively normal cohorts of memory B cells for common pathogens. Secondary responses yielding high-affinity antibodies in this setting are apparently far less impaired, despite demonstrable abnormalities of B cell function. Nevertheless, since activation of effector cells of cellular immunity depends upon the active collaboration of the by then defective antigen-recognizing T cells and the LGL involved in cell mediated immunity, the principal opportunistic organisms are intracellular pathogens.

EFFECTS OF LYMPHOCYTE INFUSION OR MARROW TRANSPLANT

Most attempts to reconstitute AIDS patients by syngeneic or allogeneic bone marrow transplantation (57)-(60) or peripheral blood lymphocytes (58),(61) have failed. The failure of such interventions was historically important, supporting the infectious agent hypothesis of AIDS by suggesting that the putative agent was infecting donor cells. Initially, immunosuppressive conditioning was avoided because of the severe immunocompromise and neutropenia already present in the patients, though it was carried out in one attempt (60). The lack of conditioning may have played a role in failure of engraftment or reconstitution, but most patients were severely ill, and at least three had circulating cytotoxins (57) that may also have been important. It is striking that in none of these cases was significant graft-vs-host disease (GvHD) observed. The reasons for this are not known, nor is it clear why so few examples of GvH reactions (none has been really well documented) have been reported, despite the fact that many AIDS patients have been multiply transfused without developing this complication. The severity of the recipients' immune deficiency would seem an ideal setting for both ease of engraftment and the genesis of GvHD. HIV may selectively destroy those donor cells responding to recipient antigens that would otherwise mediate GvH reactions. Alternatively, the host cellular components (identified as NK cells active against *Herpes simplex* viruses (62)) implicated in inducing GvH reactions may be damaged or absent in AIDS patients (38). It would nevertheless seem judicious, when possible, to utilize irradiated blood components in the management of patients with this cellular immunodeficiency. The fact that even identical twin transplants failed to engraft successfully is perhaps the best argument that the presence of HIV itself in the recipient contributed to graft failure, either by infecting stem cells or by destroying lymphoid and other cells during their differentiation and activation.

Two in vivo attempts at reconstitution have led to conversion of DTH responses in the recipient that were concordant with those responses present in the marrow or lymphocyte donor. That lymphocyte or stem cell infusion sufficient to reconstitute DTH had no evident clinical effects supports the earlier observations that DTH appears to be poorly correlated with host defense in AIDS. Still more recently, three subjects treated with the antiviral drug, suramin, have been transplanted at times when HIV appeared to be suppressed. One of these patients, who had KS without OI, appears to have benefited, while the other two did not (63).

IMMUNOGENETICS AND AIDS

The association of KS with HLA-DR5 was first noted by Friedman-Kien and his colleagues (39) and has been confirmed by several laboratories studying ethnically-matched controls (64). The mechanism of this relationship is not defined. This disorder has been concentrated, among Caucasians, in Italians and Ashkenazi Jews, both in the classical form in the elderly male and, interestingly, also in those who developed KS in the context of immunosuppression for organ transplantation. There is still some question as to the restriction of the DR5 association in gay men to these ethnic groups. Of considerable interest is the finding that KS was most closely associated with DR5 in the early days of the AIDS epidemic. In successive cohorts, the DR5 frequency fell until it was actually below that of the control population, suggesting that those most susceptible on immunogenetic grounds were among its first victims (65); later sufferers possibly lack the genetic susceptibility factor. The immunogenetics of AIDS is outside the scope of this review, but it remains a major in vivo phenomenon that requires further study.

THYMIC FUNCTION IN AIDS

Thymic hormone levels are altered in AIDS patients in a seemingly paradoxical way. Thymulin (facteur thymique serique) is depressed in the sera of the majority of patients (66), while circulating thymosin alpha-1 is generally elevated (67). Intriguingly, the thymosin alpha-1 polypeptide has been shown to include an amino acid sequence homology with HIV gag p17 (68). Antibodies to thymosin alpha-1 neutralize HIV, inhibiting its infectivity for H-9 cells. The presence of circulating gag gene products may now explain the apparent elevation of thymosin by enzyme immunoassay, through cross reactivity between the two molecular species. Could this virus-encoded material affect the traffic or maturation of lymphoid cells destined to enter the thymus?

The morphology of the thymus has been altered significantly (20); there is considerable evidence for damage to thymic epithelium, as well as loss of Hassal's corpuscles (69),(70). Thymic involution (as in stress or in adenosine-deaminase deficiency) does not usually involve the loss of these bodies, which, in contrast, fail even to appear in most cases of severe, combined immunodeficiency (SCID) in infancy. Thymic morphology can be defined better through biopsy than at autopsy, since the multitude of changes that occur consequent to stress obscure the morphologic alterations associated with the disease itself. In AIDS, immunoglobulin and complement components have been shown to bind directly to thymus epithelium in vivo, suggesting an autoimmune attack on the gland (70). HIV may be found, like HTLV-I, to mimic the surface of thymic epithelial cells. HTLV-I p19 is found normally on the membrane of thymic epithelial cells (70),(71). This apeing of thymic epithelium by HTLV-I may provide a mechanism by which that human retrovirus interacts with and infects T cells.

These peculiarities of the thymus, though clearly not central to the immune defect of AIDS, could play a role in the pathogenesis of immune depletion in the syndrome. Haynes et al. have pointed out (71) that antithymic antibodies with certain specificities, by reacting also with cells at other sites of T cell traffic within the body, might lead to a more broadbased and significant defect of cellular immunity than would anatomic thymectomy alone. Adult thymectomy, by itself, does not exert a promptly depressive effect on cellular immunity.

HIV has not yet been shown directly to infect thymic cells (70). However, by analogy with similar cells elsewhere, one might expect the Ia+ dendritic cells in the cortex and the CD-4-bearing maturing T cells within the gland to be susceptible to infection. Whether thymic epithelium itself is involved is not yet known (70),(72). Because of the profound disturbances in the thymus during HIV infection, thymus transplantation could be a prerequisite to successful immune reconstitution, when bone marrow transplantation is attempted in AIDS patients under cover of antiviral agents. Thymic transplantation alone has been unsuccessful in AIDS (73),(74).

FUNCTIONS OF LARGE GRANULAR LYMPHOCYTES

Large granular lymphoid cells (LGL) are a nonadherent, functionally heterogeneous population that are distinguishable from T and B cells morphologically, by surface markers, and by density. Most express Ia antigens and Fc receptors for IgG, but lack definitive markers of T cells, though they may share some features (such as Leu-2/T-8) with T lymphocytes. In general, the effector functions associated with "natural" immunity reside in LGL. These cells lack the highly specific T and B cell antigen receptors, evidently recognizing foreign or tumor-specific cell surface structures through yet-to-be-defined binding sites. Natural killer (NK), killer (K cells functioning in antibody-dependent cellular cytotoxicity), lymphokine-activated killer (LAK) cells (75)-(77) and interferon-alpha (IFN-alpha) producing (18) cells are found in this subset of mononuclear cells, which, in sum, account for around 10% of normal lymphoid cells. Each of these cell types is defined by a function measurable in vitro. In addition, circulating dendritic lymphoid cells, rich in surface Ia molecules, and important as accessory cells for antigen presentation to and activation of T cells, are included among the LGL. Each of these more-or-less distinct cell types evidently accounts for a very small proportion of blood lymphoid cells and little is known of their localization to normal (78), lymphomatous (78) or HIV-infected (79) lymphoid tissue.

Equally obscure is the importance to the whole organism of any of the functionally-defined cell types found among the LGL. NK cells are thought to be involved in resistance to tumors. Evidence for this comes particularly from the susceptibility to certain neoplasms of inbred mouse strains lacking these cells. In addition, children with the Chediak-Higashi syndrome appear deficient in such cells and have a propensity to the development of neoplasms. LAK cells, generated in vitro from among the LGL of patients with certain carcinomas, are capable of producing tumor remissions in vivo in both experimental animals and in humans (75)-(77). Both NK cells and K cells may play a role in the containment of virus-infected cells, the effective killing of which inhibits the proliferation and spread of viruses (80),(81). Evidence that NK cells are important in real life comes from the observation that very young children, who are deficient in NK activity, are especially susceptible to *Herpes simplex* virus until the NK activity reaches normal levels at around two weeks of age (82).

LGL, whose exact hematopoietic lineages are not yet defined, represent an important component of the natural, as opposed to the "adaptive" cellular immune system (see above). These cell functions are present in the very young, immunologically virgin animal or human, even in the absence of memory T cells, and appear thereby to represent an early line of defense against invading microorganisms. Speculatively, they may represent a very ancient host defense system that predates the evolution of thymus-dependent immunity.

In AIDS, functional and phenotypic assays for NK, K (ADCC) and interferon-alpha producing cell types have been carried out in many laboratories (18),(81),(83)-(90). Other functional assays have not yet been done, so that little is known about dendritic lymphoid cells, or of the potential for LAK cell activation, which could be useful for the control of KS.

NK cells are defined by their ability to kill certain target cells in vitro. The most commonly employed target cell type is a myeloid leukemia line, K-562. Another, less widely known, is the *Herpes simplex*-infected fibroblast (38),(62),(80). NK activity against these two prototype targets is not restricted, as is T cell-mediated cytotoxicity, by self class I histocompatibility antigens (HLA-A, -B and -C). The cells carrying out the killing of the two target cell types are distinguishable. NK cell function declines by stage of disease in some studies, and is significantly lower in patients with overt AIDS than it is among individuals having lesser degrees of clinical illness (18),(38),(84),(86). However, in our hands, the means for both assays remain within the normal range, on a per-cell basis. Nevertheless, the number of lytic units per milliliter of blood is often significantly depressed because of reduced numbers of lymphoid cells (38). Thus, depression of NK activity at the level of the whole organism may be a determinant of certain complications of AIDS.

Such constructs are supported by many of the studies cited above, in which markers of NK cells have been employed rather than functional assays. The monoclonal antibody, Leu-7 (HNK-1), recognizes NK cells and cells involved in ADCC. Leu-11a monoclonal antibodies recognize an epitope on Fc receptors shared by granulocytes and NK cells. Most NK activity is accounted for by cells bearing the Leu-11 recognition site (81),(84), some of which are Leu-7 positive and others, negative. Normally, around 43% of Leu-7$^+$ cells share the T cell phenotype, Leu-4$^+$ (81). In late-stage HIV infections, the absolute numbers of NK cells are reduced and those present have been shown to have an immature phenotype (Leu-7$^+$, Leu-4$^+$, T-8$^+$) that correlates with depressed per-cell function against K562 (81).

Antibody-dependent cellular cytotoxicity is one mechanism by which mononuclear cells can destroy abnormal cells within the body. Virus-infected cells often express viral gene products or virus-induced cell surface alterations that the adaptive immune system recognizes, resulting in the production of IgG antibodies. Many hematopoietic cells, including neutrophils, monocytes and LGL, have receptors for the Fc portion of IgG (FcR) that permit their binding to any IgG antibody-coated cell. If the FcR-bearing cell has cytotoxic capacity, it can function in antibody-dependent cellular cytotoxicity (ADCC). ADCC has not been proven to be a crucial host defense system in vivo, but it is thought to play a role in the containment of some common infections which result in a modification of the cell surface (e.g., adenovirus), and tumors that invoke an antibody response. It might be an important potential effector mechanism in the containment of retroviral infection including HIV. ADCC is also thought important in homograft rejection, e.g. in renal transplantation. Perhaps because of the ubiquity and variety of cells involved in ADCC, this mechanism appears to be relatively conserved in patients with AIDS (83). Obviously, its utility depends on the presence of specific antibody of the IgG isotype, which is sometimes lacking in patients, especially children, who have advanced helper T cell deficiency.

IFN-alpha generation by a subset of LGL in response to exposure to *Herpes simplex* virus or *Herpes simplex*-infected cells appears to be a marker for a cell subset important in host defense against intracellular pathogens (see above) (17),(18).

This function resides in an LGL subset that lacks surface markers of NK (Leu-11a, Leu-7, HNK-1) but expresses Ia (18),(91). Removal of T cells in vitro increases the per-cell output of IFN-alpha, which suggests that the function of these cells, unlike that of so many immune cells, is independent of T cell help. In AIDS patients with OI, IFN-alpha generation by LGL in response to *Herpes simplex* antigens is severely depressed (17), and the development of OI is predicted by the loss of function of this cell type (18). The important role of this thymus-independent component of cellular immunity in the containment of OI is of special interest to the immunologist. Until analysis of patients with AIDS, cell mediated immunity was generally considered to be totally controlled by T cells, indeed widely spoken of as "T-cell immunity". In certain AIDS patients, the LGL producing IFN-alpha are capable of protecting against OI even when T cell function is severely depressed (18). In general, both the IFN-alpha generating cell and the T cell must be severely dysfunctional before OI develop. From this finding, one can infer that this cell type activates effector cells of cell mediated immunity in a way analogous to that of T cells, through the release of lymphokines. It has been suggested that this alternative mode of activating effector cells in the host defense against intracellular microorganisms reflects a redundant system, old in evolutionary terms, much as the complement system is now known to have a "classical" and an older "alternative" pathway, each capable of activating its final common effector arm.

It is worth drawing a distinction between the production of IFN-alpha in vitro in response to a specialized (*Herpes simplex* virus) stimulus, which is an index of LGL function, and the observation that serum acid-labile alpha IFN is often elevated in patients in the spectrum of HIV infection (92). Although both involve IFN-alphas, these findings appear to be mutually independent; elevated acid-labile IFN-alpha activity in serum does not predict the ability of LGL to produce IFN-alpha in vitro. Most likely, different cellular functions are involved; quite clearly, the species of IFN-alpha differ in the two systems (93).

FUNCTIONS OF MYELOID CELLS

The myeloid hematopoietic lineage is affected numerically over the course of HIV infection, as noted above Deficits of marrow release and mobilization of neutrophils in response to stress is blunted (35), although in the presence of severe pyogenic infections, significant leukocytosis and a "shift to the left" can occur. Suppression of the generation of polymorphonuclear leukocytes by soluble factors has been described, and an 84 kd glycoprotein defined that may be a natural regulator of hematopoiesis (19),(94). This is probably not a retroviral gene product, but is found in greatly increased amounts in supernatants of cultured bone marrow from patients with AIDS and AIDS related complex (ARC). Since patients with AIDS do not generally suffer from systemic candidal or bacteremic pseudomonas infections, even when quite neutropenic, defects of neutrophil chemotaxis, phagocytosis and intracellular killing (other than those consequent to antibody deficiency) are probably not of major importance in the pathogenesis of the syndrome. Studies of intrinsic neutrophil function have, perhaps appropriately, been very limited and generally have yielded normal results (72).

Little or nothing is known about the activities of eosinophils and basophils during HIV infection. Presumably, their function remains intact, judging from the occasional exacerbation of atopy in patients with AIDS, as well as the frequent presence of eosinophilia during drug reactions and other events conventionally associated with allergy. It is of interest that experimentally the generation of eosinophilia in animal models has been quite thymus-dependent, so it is somewhat surprising to find sometimes striking degrees of eosinophilia among severely immunocompromised AIDS patients.

Thrombocytopenia, a common finding in HIV infection (95), is covered elsewhere in this volume. Functionally, the platelets that remain must be fully competent, judging from the lack of clinically important bleeding seen in patients with these syndromes even when platelet counts are less than 20,000/mm^3.

MONOCYTE-MACROPHAGE FUNCTION IN AIDS

Unlike other hematopoietic cells, the monocyte appears to withstand HIV rather well. However, despite the finding that numbers of monocytes are stable over the span of HIV infection, there is evidence that HIV finds an important haven in these cells, which some believe (96) are the cell type to be infected earliest. Moreover, HIV strains isolated from monocyte-macrophages appear to be particularly adapted to these cells and to infect CD-4 positive lymphocytes less well than other monocytes. The infected monocyte may carry HIV infection to the central nervous system (96).

A proportion of blood monocytes normally expresses surface CD-4 determinants, probably accounting for the vulnerability of this cell type to infection by HIV. Interestingly, in patients with HIV infection, the normal numbers of circulating monocytes lack this marker. It is possible that the monocytes internalize their CD-4 molecules after interaction with HIV or its envelope glycoprotein, yet are not destroyed by the interaction, unlike the T-4 lymphocyte. Otherwise, to explain the numerical preservation of monocytes, one needs to assume that the marrow's ability to produce monocytes is far better than its capacity to produce helper T cells and neutrophils under the influence of HIV, with less mature monocytes failing to express this receptor molecule for HIV. Ia expression on monocytes is also depressed (97).

Monocytes in AIDS patients are largely functional, despite their surface marker alterations. Their ability to respond to some lymphokines is apparently unabated, judging from their capacity to kill intracellular pathogens when provided, ex vivo, with appropriate signals from crude lymphokine-containing supernatants or from the macrophage activator, IFN-gamma (98). Such data support the concept that the recognition limb of the immune system, rather than the effector limb, is most important in the pathogenesis of the severe intracellular infections that characterize AIDS. In contrast to macrophage activation, however, macrophage chemotaxis has been reported to be defective (99),(100), suggesting that dissociations among responses to different lymphokine signals may occur in the same effector cell. In a survey of several monocyte functions including phagocytosis, hexose-monophosphate shunt activation, ADCC and killing of WEHI cells, response to chemotactic stimuli was uniquely disturbed (100). Monocyte killing of melanoma cell lines in vitro in the presence of IFN-gamma and lipopolysaccharide, or lipopolysaccharide alone, is also intact among AIDS patients with KS (101). Phagocytosis and intracellular killing of fungi by blood monocytes from AIDS patients is intact (102). Alveolar macrophages from bronchoalveolar lavage specimens of AIDS patients also can be activated to increase peroxide production and kill phagocytosed toxoplasma by lymphokine containing supernatants and exogenous IFN-gamma (103).

HOST DEFENSE AGAINST HIV

HIV cleverly infects or inactivates the very components of the immune system likely to resist its ravages. In its ability to bind to certain structures of the CD-4 molecule, it mimics the activity of Ia molecules, which are also thought to interact with CD-4 and enhance normal interactions between antigen-presenting cells of the immune system and helper T cells. There is now some evidence that sequence homologies exist between Ia and p120, a component of the major envelope glycoprotein of HIV (104). If this is true, the virus might elude the immune system by mimicking "self". However, it seems clear that the immune system is not fooled by this, as abundant antibody to HIV-encoded gene products, including env, is made during the course of infection. The presence of IgG antibody indicates that helper T cells are quite capable, at least early in infection, of recognizing these antigens and clonally expanding to meet the challenge. Specific helper T cells are essential for the production of high-affinity IgG antibodies to any protein antigen.

A central question is whether immune resistance to HIV exists and whether it accounts for the differences in course of disease observed among its victims. So far, conflicting data are available concerning the effects of neutralizing antibodies (NA) on HIV. In some studies, relatively low titers of virus-neutralizing antibodies are found in most people with HIV infection, but their presence is not related to resistance, nor do people with higher antibody levels do better clinically (104)-(106). However, in at least one series, long survival in children with congenital HIV infection is related to the presence of NA (107). This could reflect either the importance of neutralization or the presence of earlier infection among those fetuses who were unable to make antibodies, as they were immunologically sicker. Late-stage adults with AIDS sometimes seem to lose previously high levels of antibody to certain retroviral antigens.

It is not known whether the presence of preformed passive antibody would prevent infection by HIV or modify its course, as is the case with measles, polio or hepatitis B. The utility of hyperimmune AIDS immune globulin may ultimately be testable, as such a preparation will soon become available. Were it to prove effective, one would have to conclude that free virus, rather than latently infected lymphocytes, was the principal infectious unit, an hypothesis that seems untenable at present.

Since HIV is an obligate intracellular pathogen whose products are expressed on the membrane of the infected cell, cellular immunity would seem most likely to contain it. Unfortunately, demonstrating cell mediated immunity against HIV appears to be difficult, possibly chiefly for technical reasons. One group has shown ADCC against infected but not uninfected H-9 target cells using sera that contain antibodies to HIV (83). Not surprisingly, cells of both normal and HIV-infected subjects sustain this type of function in vitro. As with antibodies, no survival advantage has as yet been associated with this in vitro function.

Lymphocyte proliferation in response to crude and relatively purified HIV is demonstrable in cells from a minority of infected donors, but in most, only when interleukin-2 is added to expand the responsive memory cells. In contrast, cytomegalovirus responses by the same subjects' cells are brisk and obvious (108). Attempts to demonstrate the presence of cytotoxic T lymphocytes in infected persons have been mostly unsuccessful. If one assumes the antigens to be adequate, one is confronted with the intriguing possibility that HIV selectively destroys the specific T memory cells that might abrogate an HIV infection, because of preferential, irreversible binding of such cells to HIV-infected cells through two receptors (the antigen receptor of the T cell and the T-4 molecule). This could lead to selective clonal deletion, leading to an early loss of T memory cells directed against HIV. This loss might not occur so soon as to prevent a primary and secondary antibody response that could then be sustained without additional T cell help through preferential polyclonal B cell activation by HIV. Perhaps a better possibility is that cell mediated immunity to HIV does exist early in infection, but does not play an effective role in viral containment by the immune system. Virus latency and pathogenetic mechanisms that permit escape from immune surveillance (as with visna virus (109)), may be important.

Indirect evidence that this may be so comes from studies of the development of AIDS dementia, which does not behave as if HIV were an OI. The immune functions we expect to contain intracellular pathogens are sometimes still reasonably well sustained at the point at which severe CNS disease is already clinically evident (25).

OVERVIEW

HIV infection leads to profound alterations within the immune system at many levels. Most of the clinical syndromes now associated with this virus are known to be opportunistic, because of their previous occurrence in patients with primary and secondary immune deficiencies before the advent of AIDS. Lymphomas, KS, lymphocytic interstitial pneumonitis and, of course, all of the more obviously infectious processes observed in people with AIDS have been described previously as consequential to naturally occurring or iatrogenic disorders of the host defense system. Unfortunately, an adequate understanding of most of these immune disorders has been retarded by their variability and relative rarity, which have made any statistical, and in general, prospective analysis extremely difficult. In contrast, the immune defects of AIDS are not only highly stereotyped, but develop in a more-or-less predictable pattern following HIV infection. As a result, statistically interpretable data bases have permitted analysis of this highly complex disorder to the point that, after only seven years of study, AIDS is as well understood as perhaps any of the primary immune defects that have been described in the last three decades.

Because it is one of the most intensively studied microbial agents of humans, we now recognize that HIV has evolved several molecular structures through which it interacts with and probably damages the immune system. One site, functionally at least, mimics Ia (class II) antigens of the major histocompatibility complex which bind to the CD-4 molecule. Another may imitate a lymphokine product of T cells that normally activates B cells and stimulates the growth of neural tissue. Yet another resembles the thymic hormone, thymosin alpha-1, sufficiently that anti-hormone antibodies can neutralize virus infectivity. Possibly a fourth structure cross reacts with a thymic epithelial component. No doubt more interactions will become identified as analysis at the molecular level continues. Already, HIV may be considered paradigmatic of the evolution of the host-parasite relationship.

An understanding of the nature of the immune defects of AIDS and its precursor clinical states not only permits better comprehension of the entire syndrome, but has shed considerable light on host defense mechanisms in humans. An improved understanding of the complex interactions of lymphoid cells in the generation of what is called cellular immunity has already been elucidated through study of this otherwise devastating disease. If this knowledge can be translated into the means of immune reconstitution, presumably via combinations of antiviral agents and biological response modifiers or hematopoietic cell transplantation, still more will be learned. In turn, knowledge gained in this area should have important repercussions in efforts being made against other immune, hematologic and neoplastic diseases.

ACKNOWLEDGMENT

Supported in part by grants from the U.S. Public Health Service, DHHS, CA-40527, and from the New York State AIDS Institute. The author is grateful to Marta Siegal, JD, Kanti R. Rai, MD, Rabia Mir, MD and Carlos Lopez, PhD for continued forbearance and helpful comments.

REFERENCES

1. WHO Scientific Group on Immunodeficiency. Primary Immunodeficiency Diseases. Meeting Report. Clin Immunol Immunopath 28:450-475 (1983)

2. Shaw, G.M., Hahn, B.H., Arya, S.K., et al., Molecular characterization of human T-cell leukemia (lymphotropic) virus type III in AIDS. Science 226:1165 (1984)

3. Lifson, J.D., Reyes, G.R., McGrath, M.S., et al., AIDS retrovirus induced cytopathology: Giant cell information and involvement of CD4 antigen. Science 232:1123-1127 (1986)

4. Mathes, L.E., Olsen, R.G., Hebebrand, L.C., et al., Abrogation of lymphocyte blastogenesis by a feline leukaemia virus protein. Nature 274:687-689 (1978)

5. Pahwa, S., Pahwa, R., Saxinger, C., et al., Influence of the human T-lymphotropic virus/lymphadenopathy-associated virus on functions of human lymphocytes: Evidence for immunosuppressive effects and polyclonal B-cell activation by banded viral preparations. Proc Nat Acad Sci (USA) 82:8198-8202 (1985)

6. Tomar, R.H., John, P.A., Hennig, A.K., et al., Cellular targets of antilymphocyte antibodies in AIDS and LAS. Clin Immunol Immunopath 37:37-47 (1986)

7. Dorsett, B., Cronin, W., Chuma, V., et al., Anti-lymphocyte antibodies in patients with the acquired immune deficiency syndrome. Amer J Med 78:621-626 (1985)

8. Warren, R.Q., Johnson, E.A., Donnelly, R.P., et al., Analysis of anti-peripheral blood mononuclear cell antibodies in sera from AIDS, ARC and healthy homosexuals, Abstract, Clinical Immunology Society, Baltimore, Maryland, October 11 (1986)

9. Fauci, A.S., Immunologic abnormalities in the acquired immunodeficiency syndrome (AIDS). Clin Res 32:491-499 (1984)

10. Dalgleish, A.G., Beverley, P.C.L., Clapham, P.R., et al., The CD4 (T4) antigen is an essential component of the receptor for the AIDS retrovirus. Nature 312:763-767 (1984)

11. Quinnan, G.V., Siegel, J.P., Epstein, J.S., et al., Mechanisms of T-cell functional deficiency in the acquired immunodeficiency syndrome. Ann Intern Med 103:710-714 (1984)

12. Gyorkey, F., Melnick, J.L., Sinkovics, J.G., et al., Retrovirus resembling HTLV in macrophages of patients with AIDS. Lancet 1:106 (1985)

13. Armstrong,, J.A., Horne, R., Follicular dendritic cells and virus-like particles in AIDS-related lymphadenopathy. Lancet 2:370-372 (1984)

14. Shaw, G.M., Harper, M.E., Hahn, B.H., et al., HTLV-III infection in brains of children and adults with AIDS encephalopathy. Science 227:177-182 (1985)

15. Levy, J.A., Shimabukuro, J., Hollander, H., Isolation of AIDS-associated retroviruses from cerebrospinal fluid and brain of patients with neurological symptoms. Lancet 2:586-588 (1985)

16. Ho, D., Sarngadharan, M.G., Resnick, L., et al., Primary human T-lymphotropic virus type III infection. Ann Intern Med 103:880-883 (1985)

17. Lopez, C., Fitzgerald, P.A., Siegal, F.P., Severe acquired immune deficiency syndrome in male homosexuals: Diminished capacity to make interferon-alpha in vitro associated with severe opportunistic infections. J Infect Dis 148:962-966 (1983)

18. Siegal, F.P., Lopez, C., Fitzgerald, P.A., et al., Opportunistic infections in acquired immune deficiency syndrome result from synergistic defects of both the natural and adaptive components of cellular immunity. J Clin Invest 78:115-123 (1986)

19. Leiderman, I.Z., Greenberg, M.L., Adelsberg, B.R., et al., A novel hematopoietic inhibitory protein from cultured AIDS bone marrow. UCLA Symposium on Molecular and Cellular Biology 9:111 (1986)

20. Davis, A.E., The histopathological changes in the thymus gland in the acquired immune deficiency syndrome. Ann NY Acad Sci 437:493-502 (1984)

21. Darrow, W.W., Presentation, NIAID Meeting on Cofactors in AIDS, Bethesda, MD, (1986)

22. Armstrong, D., Gold, J.W.M., Dryjanski, J., et al., Treatment of infections in patients with the acquired immunodeficiency syndrome. Ann Intern Med 103:738-743 (1985)

23. Taylor, J., Afrasiabi, R., Fahey, J.L., et al., Prognostically significant classification of immune changes in AIDS with Kaposi's sarcoma. Blood 67:666-671 (1986)

24. Pitchenik, A.E., Cole, C., Russell, B.W., et al., Tuberculosis, atypical mycobacteriosis, and the acquired immunodeficiency syndrome among Haitian and non-Haitian patients in South Florida. Ann Intern Med 101:641-645 (1984)

25. Siegal, F.P., Lopez, C., Fitzgerald, P.A., et al., Involvement of central nervous system during infection with HTLV-III/LAV may be consequent to immunodeficiency. International Congress on Immunology, Toronto, Canada, (1986)

26. Penn, I., Kaposi's sarcoma in organ transplant recipients: Report of 20 cases. Transplantation 27:8-11 (1979)

27. Harwood, A.R., Osoba, D., Hofstader, S.L., et al., Kaposi's sarcoma in recipients of renal transplants. Amer J Med 67: 759-765 (1979)

28. Safai, B., Johnson, K.G., Myskowski, P.L., et al., The natural history of Kaposi's sarcoma in the acquired immunodeficiency syndrome. Ann Intern Med 103:744-750 (1985)

29. Harper, M.E., Kaplan, M.H., Marselle, L.M., et al., Concomitant infection with HTLV-1 and HTLV-III in a patient with T8 lymphoproliferative disease. N Engl J Med 315:1073-1078 (1986)

30. Siegal, F.P., Normal delayed-type skin reactions in early stages of acquired cellular immunodeficiency. N Engl J Med 307:184 (1982)

31. Cohen, R.L., Oliver, D., Pollard-Sigwanz, C., Leukopenia and anergy as predictor of AIDS. JAMA 255:1289 (1986)

32. Hersh, E.M., Mansell, P.W., Reuben, J.M., et al., Immunological characterizations of patients with acquired immune deficiency syndrome, acquired immune deficiency syndrome-related symptom complex, and a related life-style. Cancer Res 44:5894-5901 (1984)

33. McLeod, W.A., Jeffries, E., Boyko, W., Screening for acquired immune deficiency syndrome with dinitrochlorobenzene. Can Med Assoc J 130:100-101 (1984)

34. Belsito, D.V., Sanchez, M.R., Baer, R.L., et al., Reduced Langerhans' cell Ia antigen and ATPase activity in patients with the acquired immunodeficiency syndrome. N Engl J Med 310:1279-1282 (1984)

35. Greenberg, M.L., Siegal, F.P., Neutrophil production, release and distribution in patients with the acquired immune deficiency syndrome (AIDS). Cell and Tissue Kinet 16:611-612 (1983)

36. Gottlieb, M.S., Schroff, R., Schanker, H.M., et al., *Pneumocystis carinii* pneumonia and mucosal candidiasis in previously healthy homosexual men. N Engl J Med 305:1425-1431 (1981)

37. Masur, H., Michelis, M.A., Greene, J.B., et al., An outbreak of community-acquired *Pneumocystis carinii* pneumonia. N Engl J Med 305:1431-1438 (1981)

38. Siegal, F.P., Lopez, C., Hammer, G.S., et al., Severe acquired immunodeficiency in male homosexuals, manifested by chronic perianal ulcerative *Herpes simplex* lesions. N Engl J Med 305:1439-1444 (1981)

39. Friedman-Kien, A.E., Laubenstein, L.J., Rubenstein, P., et al., Disseminated Kaposi's sarcoma in homosexual men. Ann Intern Med 96:693-700 (1982)

40. Chess, Q., Daniels, J., North, E., et al., Serum immunoglobulin elevations in AIDS: IgG, IgA, IgM, IgD. Diag Immunol 2:148-153 (1984)

41. Piechowiak, H., Hehlmann, R., Abb, J., et al., Changing biclonal gammopathy due to different lymphocyte clones in acquired immunodeficiency syndrome with Kaposi's sarcoma. Klin Wochenschr 63:1083-1086 (1985)

42. Papadopoulos, N.M., Lane, H.C., Costello, R., et al., Oligoclonal immunoglobulins in patients with the acquired immunodeficiency syndrome. Clin Immunol Immunopath 35:43-46 (1984)

43. Gurney, M.E., Apatoff, B.R., Spear, G.T., et al., Neuroleukin: A lymphokine product of lectin-stimulated T cells. Science 234:574-581 (1986)

44. Birx, D.L., Redfield, R.R., Tosato, G., Defective regulation of Epstein-Barr virus infections in patients with acquired immunodeficiency syndrome (AIDS) or AIDS-related disorders. N Engl J Med 314:874-879 (1986)

45. Luft, B.J., Conley, F., Remington, J.S., et al., Outbreak of central-nervous system toxoplasmosis in Western Europe and North America. Lancet 1:781-784 (1983)

46. Dylewski, J., Chou, S., Merigan, T.C., Absence of detectable IgM antibody during cytomegalovirus disease in patients with AIDS. N Engl J Med 309:493 (1983)

47. Lane, H.C., Masur, H., Edgar, L.C., et al., Abnormalities of B-cell activation and immunoregulation in patients with the acquired immunodeficiency syndrome. N Engl J Med 309:453-458 (1983)

48. Pahwa, S.G., Quilop, M.T., Lange, M. et al., Defective B-lymphocyte function in homosexual men in relation to the acquired immunodeficiency syndrome. Ann Intern Med 101:757-763 (1984)

49. Junker, A.K., Ochs, H.D., Collier, A.C., et al., Abnormal immune responses in homosexual men with chronic generalized lymphadenopathy. Pediatr Res 18:258A (1984)

50. Bernstein, L.J., Ochs, M.D., Wedgwood, R.J., et al., Defective humoral immunity in pediatric acquired immune deficiency syndrome. J Pediat 107:352-357 (1985)

51. Church, J.A., Lewis, J., Spotkov, J.M., IgG subclass deficiencies in children with suspected AIDS. Lancet 1:279 (1984)

52. Shannon, K.M., Ammann, A.J., Acquired immune deficiency syndrome in childhood. J Pediatr 106:332-342 (1985)

53. Oleske, J., Minnefor, A., Cooper, R., Jr. et al., Immune deficiency syndrome in children. JAMA 249:2345-2349 (1983)

54. Rubenstein, A., Sicklick, M., Gupta, A., et al., Acquired immunodeficiency with reversed T_4/T_8 ratios in infants born to promiscuous and drug-addicted mothers. JAMA 249: 2350-2356 (1983)

55. Polsky, B., Gold, J.W.M., Whimbey, E., et al., Bacterial pneumonia in patients with the acquired immunodeficiency syndrome. Ann Intern Med 104:38-41 (1986)

56. Minnefor, A., Oleske, J., Zabala, M., et al., International Conference on Acquired Immunodeficiency Syndrome (AIDS), Atlanta, GA (1984)

57. Hassett, J.M., Zaroulis, C.G., Greenberg, M.L., et al., Bone marrow transplantation in AIDS. N Engl J Med 309:665 (1983)

58. Lane, H.C., Masur, H., Longo, D.L., et al., Partial immune reconstitution in a patient with the acquired immunodeficiency syndrome. N Engl J Med 311:1099-1103 (1984)

59. Mitsuyasu, R.T., Volberding P., Groopman, J., et al., Syngeneic bone marrow transplantation for patients with AIDS and Kaposi's sarcoma. Blood 62:226A (1983)

60. Mitsuyasu, R.T., Volberding, P., Groopman, J., et al., Bone marrow transplantation from identical twins in the treatment of AIDS and Kaposi's sarcoma. J Cell Biochem 26:Suppl 8A:22 (1984)

61. Davis, K.C., Hayward, A., Ozturk, G., et al., Lymphocyte transfusion in a case of acquired immunodeficiency syndrome. Lancet 1:599-600 (1983)

62. Lopez, C., Sorrel, M., Kirkpatrick D., et al., Association between pre-transplant natural killer cells and graft-vs-host disease after stem-cell transplantation. Lancet 2: 1103-1106 (1983)

63. Fauci, A.S., Presentation at International Congress of Immunology, Toronto, Canada, July 5-10 (1986)

64. Pollack, M.S., Gold, J., Metroka, C.E., et al., HLA-A,B,C and DR antigen frequencies in acquired immunodeficiency syndrome (AIDS) patients with opportunistic infections. Hum Immunol 11:99-103 (1984)

65. Rubinstein, P., Rothman, W.M., Friedman-Kein, A., Immunologic and immunogenetic findings in patients with epidemic Kaposi's sarcoma. Antibiot Chemother 32:87-98 (1984)

66. Dardenne, M., Bach J-F., Safai, B., Low serum thymic hormone levels in patients with AIDS. N Engl J Med 309:48-49 (1983)

67. Hersh, E.M., Reuben, J.M., Rios, A., et al., Elevated serum thymosin alpha I levels associated with evidence of immune dysregulation in male homosexuals with a history of infectious diseases or Kaposi's sarcoma. N Engl J Med 308:45-46 (1983)

68. Sarin, P.D., Sun, D.K., Thornton, A.H., et al., Neutralization of HTLV-III/LAV replication by antiserum to thymosin alpha 1. Science 232:1135 (1986)

69. Elie, R., Laroche, A.C., Arnoux, E., Thymic dysplasia in AIDS. N Engl J Med 308:841-842 (1983)

70. Savino, W., Dardenne, M., Marche, C., et al., Thymic epithelium in AIDS. Amer J Path 122:302-307 (1986)

71. Haynes, B.F., Robert-Guroff, M., Metzgar, R.S., et al., Monoclonal antibody against human T-cell leukemia virus p19 defines a human thymic epithelial antigen acquired during ontogeny. J Exp Med 157:907-920 (1983)

72. S. Fikrig, personal communication. (1986)

73. Dwyer, J.M., McNamara, J.G., Sigal, L.H., et al., Immunological abnormalities in patients with the acquired immune deficiency syndrome (AIDS) - a review. Clin Immunol Rev 3: 25-129 (1984)

74. Ciobanu, N., Paietta, E., Karten, M., et al., Thymus fragment transplantation in the acquired immunodeficiency syndrome. Ann Intern Med 103:479 (1985)

75. Lotze, M.T., Gromm, E.A., Mazumder, A., et al., Lysis of fresh and cultured autologous tumor by human lymphocytes cultured in T-cell growth factor. Cancer Res 41:4420-4425 (1981)

76. Grimm, E.A., Mazumder, A., Zhang, H.Z., et al., Lymphokine-activated killer cell phenomenon. Lysis of natural killer-resistant fresh solid tumor cells by interleukin 2-activated autologous human peripheral blood lymphocytes. J Exp Med 155:1823-1841 (1982)

77. Itoh, K., Tilden, A.B., Balch, C.M., Lysis of human solid tumor cells by lymphokine-activated natural killer cells. J Immunol 136:3910-3915 (1986)

78. Miller, M.L., Tubbs, R.R., Fishleder, A.J., et al., Immunoregulatory Leu-7$^+$ and T8$^+$ lymphocytes in B-cell follicular lymphomas. Hum Path 15:810-817 (1984)

79. Wood, G.S., Burns, B.F., Dorfman, R.F., et al., The immunohistology of non-T cells in the acquired immunodeficiency syndrome. Amer J Path 120:371-379 (1985)

80. Ching, C., Lopez, C., Natural killing of *Herpes simplex* virus type I-infected target cells: normal human responses and influence of anti-viral antibody. Infect Immun 26:49-56 (1979)

81. Landay, A., Poon, M-C., Abo, T., et al., Immunologic studies in asymptomatic hemophilia patients: Relationship to AIDS. J Clin Invest 71:1500-1504 (1983)

82. Siegal, F.P., Functional ontogeny of human lymphoid cells as a factor in maternal-fetal tolerance. Amer J Reprod Immunol 1:65-68 (1981)

83. Traylor, D., Kennedy, M., Andersen P., et al., "Natural" cell-mediated cytotoxicity among a group of HTLV-III seropositive hemophiliacs. Presentation at meeting of Clinical Immunology Society, October 11 (1986)

84. Creemers, P.C., Stark, D.F., Boyko, W.J., Evaluation of natural killer cell activity in patients with persistent generalized lymphadenopathy and acquired immunodeficiency syndrome. Clin Immunol Immunopath 36:141-150 (1985)

85. Gerstoft, J., Dickmeiss, E., Mathiesen, L., Cytotoxic capabilities of lymphocytes from patients with the acquired immunodeficiency syndrome. Scand J Immunol 22:463-470 (1985)

86. Baron, G.C., Klimas, N.G., Fischl, M.A., et al., Decreased natural cell-mediated cytotoxicity per effector cell in acquired immunodeficiency syndrome. Diagn Immunol 3:197-204 (1986)

87. Poli, G., Introna, M., Zamboni, F., et al., Natural killer cells in intravenous drug abusers with lymphadenopathy syndrome. Clin Exp Immunol 62:128-135 (1985)

88. Cunningham-Rundles, S., Metroka, C.E., Safai, B., et al., Cytotoxic effector mechanisms in AIDS. Adv Exp Med Biol 187:97-110 (1985)

89. Rook, A.H., Hooks, J.J., Quinnan, G.V., et al., Interleukin 2 enhances the natural killer cell activity of acquired immunodeficiency syndrome patients through a gamma-interferon-independent mechanism. J Immunol 134:1503-1507 (1985)

90. Hersh, E.M., Gutterman, J.U., Spector, S., et al., Impaired in vitro interferon, blastogenic, and natural killer cell responses to viral stimulation in acquired immune deficiency syndrome. Cancer Res 45:406-410 (1985)

91. Fitzgerald, P.A., Mendelsohn, M., Lopez, C., (Submitted for publication)

92. Destefano, E., Friedman, R.M., Friedman-Kien, A.E., et al., Acid-labile human leukocyte interferon in homosexual men with Kaposi's sarcoma and lymphadenopathy. J Infect Dis 146: 451-455 (1982)

93. Lopez, C., Fitzgerald, P.A., Siegal, F.P., et al., Unpublished data.

94. Leiderman, I.Z., Greenberg, M.L., Adelsberg, B.R., et al., An inhibitor of granulopoiesis in acquired immunodeficiency syndrome. (Submitted for publication).

95. Yu, J-R., Lennett, E.T., Karpatkin, S., Anti-$F(ab^1)_2$ antibodies in thrombocytopenic patients at risk for acquired immunodeficiency syndrome. J Clin Invest 77:1756-1761 (1986)

96. Ho, D.D., Rota, T.R., Hirsch, M.S., Infection of monocyte/ marcrophages by human T lymphotropic virus III. J Clin Invest 77:1712-1715 (1986)

97. Heagy, W., Kelley, V.E., Strom T.B., at al., Decreased expression of human class II antigens on monocytes from patients with AIDS. J Clin Invest 74:2089-2096 (1984)

98. Murray, H.W., Hillman, J.K., Rubin, B.Y., et al., Patients at risk for AIDS-related opportunistic infections. N Engl J Med 313:1504-1510 (1985)

99. Smith, P.D., Ohura, K., Masur, H., et al., Monocyte function in the acquired immune deficiency syndrome: Defective chemotaxis. J Clin Invest 74:2121-2128 (1984)

100. Poli, G., Bottazzi, B., Acero, R., et al., Monocyte function in intravenous drug abusers with lymphadenopathy syndrome and in patients with acquired immunodeficiency syndrome: Selective impairment of chemotaxis. Clin Exp Immunol 62:136-142 (1985)

101. Kleinerman, E.S., Ceccorulli, L.M., Zwelling, L.A., et al., Activation of monocyte-mediated tumoricidal activity in patients with acquired immunodeficiency syndrome. J Clin Oncol 3:1005-1012 (1985)

102. Washburn, R.G., Tuazon, C.U., Bennett, J.E., Phagocytic and fungicidal activity of monocytes from patients with acquired immunodeficiency syndrome. J Infect Dis 151:565-566 (1985)

103. Murray, H.W., Bellene, R.A., Libby, D.M., et al., Activation of tissue macrophages from AIDS patients. In vitro responses of AIDS alveolar macrophages to lymphokines and interferon-gamma. J Immunol 135:2374 (1985)

104. Weiss, R.A., Clapham, P.R., Cheingsong-Popov, R., et al., Neutralization of human T-lymphotropic virus type III by sera of AIDS and AIDS-related patients. Nature 316:69-72 (1985)

105. Robert-Guroff, M., Brown, M., Gallo, R.C., HTLV-III-neutralizing antibodies in patients with AIDS and AIDS-related complex. Nature 316:72-74 (1985)

106. Rasheed, S., Norman, G.L., Gill, P.S., et al., Virus-neutralizing activity, serologic heterogeneity, and retrovirus isolation from homosexual men in the Los Angeles area. Virol 150:1-9 (1986)

107. Oleske, J., Robert-Guroff, M., Personal Communication (1986)

108. Piazza, P., Rappocciolo, G., Guerrini, M., et al., Cell-mediated immune response to HIV antigen in homosexual men. Presentation at Clinical Immunology Society Meeting (1986)

109. Ruscetti, F.W., Mikovits, J.A., Kalyanaraman, V.S., et al., Analysis of effector mechanisms against HTLV-I- and HTLV-III/LAV-infected lymphoid cells. J Immunol 136:3619- 3624 (1986)

17
T-Cell Immunity in AIDS

Susanna Cunningham-Rundles, Rudolph Bedford, Craig E. Metroka

When the present pandemic of the acquired immune deficiency syndrome (AIDS) was first described in 1981, leukopenia and lymphopenia were reported as prominent laboratory findings in patients with opportunistic infections (OI) (1)-(4). In contrast, low normal to normal numbers of circulating leukocytes and lymphocytes were often seen in patients with AIDS who had Kaposi's sarcoma (KS) at initial presentation (5),(6). Persistent generalized lymphadenopathy syndrome (LAS) in homosexual men was also found to be rarely accompanied by decreased leukocyte or lymphocyte counts (7). However, in both KS and LAS patients leukocytes, neutrophils and lymphocytes have been observed to decrease continuously over time. Safai et al. (8) in a longitudinal study found that higher initial leukocyte and lymphocyte counts were directly correlated with survival at two years ($p<0.05$). In their study, 55% of patients with a normal number of lymphocytes at presentation were alive at two years, in contrast to only 30% of patients with low lymphocyte counts. Whether this difference in outcome is a function merely of differences in duration of infection with human immunodeficiency virus (HIV) or whether there are additional factors affecting the rate and depth of immunosuppression is unclear (7),(9)-(11). Clearly there is great clinical variability in the course of disease in different groups of patients. Patients with OI, for example, in general have a much more rapid downhill course.

Since the isolation and characterization of HIV (12)-(14), the unique significance of the T helper/inducer lymphocyte subset has become clearer as HIV has a tropism for this cellular subset. Although reduced absolute counts as well as relative proportions of helper inducer T lymphocytes have been seen invariably in patients with OI, this is not the case with patients with KS, some of whom despite being HIV antibody positive have had normal values for three years in the context of stable clinical disease. Why the counts are relatively preserved in certain patients is unclear at this time but of great potential importance. The relationship between helper/inducer lymphocytes in peripheral blood, the functional capacity of the immune system, and clinical course is of fundamental interest. Study of these issues, however, may be influenced by the choice of immunologic function to be investigated, the method of study adopted and the specific patient population recruited. Methods in which defined cellular subsets are concentrated to a fixed number can be useful in determining intrinsic functional activity, whereas study of mononuclear cells without further separation may give information on cellular interactions that may more accurately mimic in vivo interactions.

PATHOLOGIC CHANGES OF LYMPHOID ORGANS IN AIDS

Pathological descriptions of thymic tissue from AIDS patients have featured severe glandular involution with thymocyte depletion, absence of a defined cortex or medulla, and loss of Hassall's corpuscles. Davis (15) has described this process as an organ specific immune complex attack on Hassall's corpuscles, thymic epithelial cells and thymic lymphocytes. Thus, both the thymic lymphocytes (originating in bone marrow and fetal liver), as well as the epithelial cells responsible for production of thymosin alpha-1, thymosin beta 3, thymosin beta 4, thymopoietin and thymulin, are attacked by either HIV or by other disease related processes.

Although gradual atrophy of the thymus gland occurs as part of the normal aging process, even in the very elderly, thymic epithelium remains plump and both Hassall's corpuscles and architecture do not change. In AIDS patients, in addition to the unusual depletion of thymic structures, there is a distinctly abnormal cellular infiltrate in which the predominant cell type is the lymphocyte in children and the plasma cell in adults. The infiltrating plasma cells produce polyclonal IgG which binds to Hassall's corpuscles and to epithelial cells. The changes are reminiscent of severe combined immunodeficiency disease (Nezelof syndrome) and the graft-versus-host-reaction. The finding of elevated thymosin alpha-1 in LAS and AIDS (16) may imply that an increased production of thymic factors occurs initially as a compensation for tissue depletion. Treatment of patients with thymic factors, specifically thymosin fraction 5 (TF5), has been found to enhance T cell responses but not to affect the helper-inducer to cytotoxic-suppressor, $T4^{+}/T8^{+}$, ratio (17). Somewhat less significant effects have been seen using thymosin alpha 1 and thymopoietin or thymulin. However, significant increases in both total T lymphocytes and T cell subpopulations have been reported by Trainin et al. (18) using thymic humoral factor (THF) in patients with AIDS related complex (ARC). These data suggest that thymic factors may be potentially useful in extending the period of latency and by inference, that the abnormal regulation of thymic factors during the autoimmune-like destruction of the thymus may profoundly accelerate the development of immunodeficiency.

The lymph node is also a site of profound changes in AIDS. We originally observed that lymphocytes from lymph nodes of patients with LAS were often able to respond to activators in vitro when peripheral blood lymphocytes were not (19). Lymph node histology was characterized by explosive follicular hyperplasia involving both cortex and medulla with attenuation of the mantle zone. Although initially the follicles were apparently composed of normal reactive constituents, additional biopsies in some patients suggested that with time, an increase in large cells (both cleaved and noncleaved) and immunoblasts, was seen. Eventually, follicular regression with hyalinization of the germinal centers was observed. Untimately, some patients developed Burkitt's lymphoma, immunoblastic sarcoma, or Kaposi's sarcoma.

The bone marrow may also show abnormalities in AIDS. Many of our patients with LAS presented with anemia and when bone marrow aspiration was performed, hyperplastic bone marrow was the most common finding. In what appeared to be more advanced cases, severe bone marrow hypoplasia or marked left shift in the myeloid series was observed. Finally, evidence of lymphoblastic infiltration was seen in some cases. Often this evolved into B cell lymphomas, a characteristic development in about 10% of LAS patients (7),(20),(21).

Clinically, patients with AIDS appear to have both T and B cell immune deficits, although the T cell defect is usually more prominent. Some of the characteristic infections in AIDS, including those caused by *Mycobacterium avium-intracellulare, Mycobacterium tuberculosis, Nocardia asteroides* and *Salmonella species* are well known opportunistists in T cell deficiency states. Infections associated with B cell dysfunction such as those caused by *Streptococcus pneumoniae* and *Hemophilus influenzae*, are also very common in AIDS patients and may be accompanied by a poor antibody response (22).

LYMPHOCYTE SUBSET IMBALANCE

Recognition of lymphocyte subset imbalance in AIDS provided an early marker of the syndrome in advance of identification of the etiologic retrovirus. Reduced $T4^+$ cells (helper/inducer T lymphocytes) and increased $T8^+$ cells (suppressor/cytotoxic T cells) were observed initially among homosexual patients and also among homosexual persons at risk for AIDS (22).

Serial examination of persons seropositive for HIV has shown that in some individual cases $T4^+/T8^+$ ratios may alter from the inverted state to normal (23),(24). However, this event appears to be only temporary in individuals followed to date and may reflect bone marrow stimulation that cannot be sustained indefinitely. Studies of lymphocyte subset balance in lymph nodes of patients with AIDS has shown that the same decreased ratio may be observed there (25) and that T suppressor/cytotoxic cells may be present in large numbers in mantles and follicular centers, areas normally occupied predominately by B cells.

Although lymphopenia is not common among infants with AIDS, Scott et al. (26) found marked inversion of T cell subsets with disease progression. Two of 14 infants, however, showed normal T lymphocyte subsets initially despite the presence of active *Pneumocystis carinii* pneumonia.

Several groups have also observed a reduced $T4^+/T8^+$ ratio due principally to increased $T8^+$ cells in adult patients with LAS or ARC, with a progressive reduction in $T4^+$ lymphocytes over time (6),(21),(26),(27). This trend has been seen in patients with blood transfusion acquired HIV disease. We recently studied 29 patients with thalassemia major where we observed that only two patients had lymphocyte subset percentages outside of the normal range. However, four patients had an inverted $T4^+/T8^+$ lymphocyte subset ratio and all of these patients had antibody to HIV. Three patients with a normal $T4^+/T8^+$ ratio (one had low $T3^+$%) also had HIV antibodies. Interestingly, all three had poor T lymphocyte proliferative response to phytohemaglutinin (PHA) (28). In general, blood transfusion associated AIDS has been accompanied by the same changes in lymphocyte subsets seen in other AIDS patients.

There is a suggestion that a relative reduction rather than an absolute reduction of $T4^+$ cells is a critical event. This seems to be the case particularly in infants where rapid expansion of the hematopoietic system is possible and replacement through differention from precursor cells can occur. However, little data on early changes have been available to date in other HIV infected patients except in repeatedly transfused persons with thalassemia or hemophilia. Since other immunoregulatory processes may be occurring in addition to retrovirus infection in these settings, more studies are needed to expand our knowledge of the early disease process.

The Helper/Inducer T-Lymphocyte

The $T4^+$ lymphocyte subset is effectively exhausted during the course of HIV disease. For example, among 26 patients with AIDS (either OI, or KS with concurrent OI) recently studied in this laboratory, the mean percentage of $T4^+$ cells was 6.25% in contrast to 42.9% for normal controls. The range for normals was 22% to 65% in contrast to 0 to 18.7% among patients. During sequential bleeds the $T4^+$ population tended to disappear entirely. As shown in Figure 1, relatively more $T4^+$ cells were seen among patients with KS alone (mean = 17.7%) and among patients with LAS (mean = 20.7%), compared to patients with OI (mean = 6.25%). In fact, in patients with KS the range of percentages of T4 positive lymphocytes was similar to LAS patients. Lymphocyte functional responses, however, could not be directly related to percentage of $T4^+$ or $T8^+$ lymphocytes as illustrated in Table 1 for response to PHA in patients with LAS. Similarly, when absolute numbers of lymphocyte subsets were examined in relationship to functional response in vitro, no correlation was seen among patients with AIDS for response to PHA or interleukin-2 (IL-2) (Table 2). Lane et al. (29) have shown that purified populations ($T4^+$ and $T8^+$) of cells from some AIDS patients proliferate normally in the presence of mitogen although unfractionated cells do not. However, these purified populations responded poorly to soluble antigen. These data suggested that unfractionated cells from AIDS patients were subject to some sort of suppressor effect and that there was an intrinsic deficiency of response to soluble antigen as well. In agreement with the concept of a suppressor factor, we observed that monocyte depleted peripheral blood mononuclear cells from AIDS or LAS patients, which were incubated to allow a period of recovery before stimulation, could, in fact, be induced to greatly improved if not to normal levels of lymphocyte activation to PHA in vitro (30), (31).

Table 1. Lack of Correlation Between Percentage of Lymphocyte Subsets ($T4^+$,$T8^+$) and Response to PHA In Vitro in LAS Patients

Case	$T4^+$	$T8^+$	Proliferative Response[a]
1	29.7	30.0	8,608
2	15.9	55.0	3,827
3	21.9	43.9	18,432
4	20.1	49.2	10,297

[a]cpm x 10^{-3}
PHA = Phytohemagglutinin
LAS = Lymphadenopathy syndrome

Since proliferative responses in vitro occur in connection with a cascade of events associated with the initial activation step, several groups have studied the possible role of soluble T-cell mediators on development of the proliferative response. A potentially important factor is IL-2 but unfortunately there is lack of agreement concerning production of this mediator by lymphocytes from AIDS patients in vitro since both low (32),(33) and normal (34) IL-2 production has been observed using slightly different methodology. Augmentation of proliferative response by exogenous IL-2 in AIDS has also been seen by some workers (32) but not by others (34). Since both production and utilization of

IL-2 occur in activated cultures, the disparities in these studies may reflect kinetic effects that need to be investigated more thoroughly in order to assess the whole metabolism of IL-2. A study by Prince et al. (34) has shown decreased IL-2 receptor expression in AIDS patients which was directly correlated with the $T4^+/T8^+$ ratio. Low T cell responses to soluble antigens and alloantigens were transiently restored in some patients with ARC and AIDS by treatment with recombinant IL-2 in vivo (35).

Table 2. Comparison of Relative and Absolute (Abs) Lymphocyte Subsets and Proliferative Response in Vitro

Case	Abs Lym per mm^3	% T4+	Abs T4+ per mm^3	% T8+	Abs T8+ per mm^3	Proliferative Response PHA	IL-2
1	300	3.3	10	49	146	11,680	395
2	810	0.1	0·8	82	664	3,171	816
3	830	10.8	90	60	498	1,107	325
4	910	1.1	10	25	228	8,578	1,917
5	1,090	6.0	65	53	578	13,364	2,369
6	1,090	10.5	114	78	850	11,419	ND
7	1,200	7.0	84	76	912	18,316	1,823
8	1,600	11.1	178	76	1,216	4,228	60
9	1,900	7.8	148	67	1,273	14,371	6,859

PHA = Phytohemagglutinin
IL-2 = Interleukin-2
ND = Not done
Lym = Lymphocyte

Since a key role of sensitized T cells in host defense is to secrete interferons which in turn stimulate the antimicrobial activity of monocytes and NK cells against intracellular pathogens, much consideration has been given to the possible role of aberrant interferon production in AIDS. Murray et al. (36) reported reduced interferon gamma production and Lopez et al. reported reduced interferon alpha production (37) in in vitro studies. In contrast, Eyster et al. reported elevated interferon alpha in serum of AIDS patients in an unusual acid labile form (38). Although these data may appear contradictory at first, they are not, since peripheral blood lymphocytes (largely T lymphocytes), the source of interferon in vitro, need not be the origin of interferon in serum in vivo (which could come from lymphoid organs). Furthermore, it is entirely possible that an early increased production of interferon in vivo might be associ-

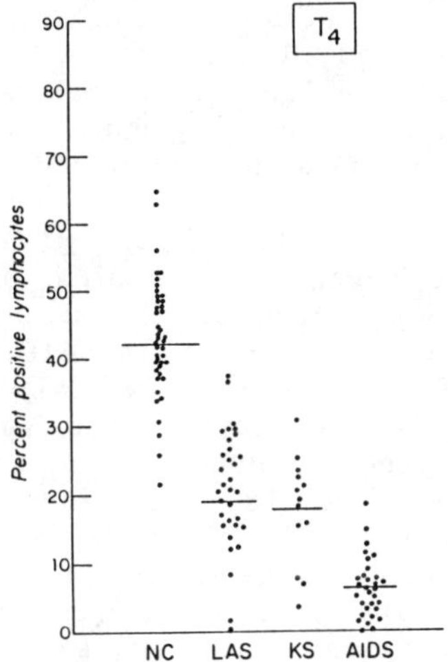

Figure 1. Percentages of T4$^+$ lymphocytes in peripheral blood of patients with LAS, KS, or AIDS (OI or KS with OI) compared to normal controls. Data obtained by flow cytometry of whole blood (Ortho Spectrum III)

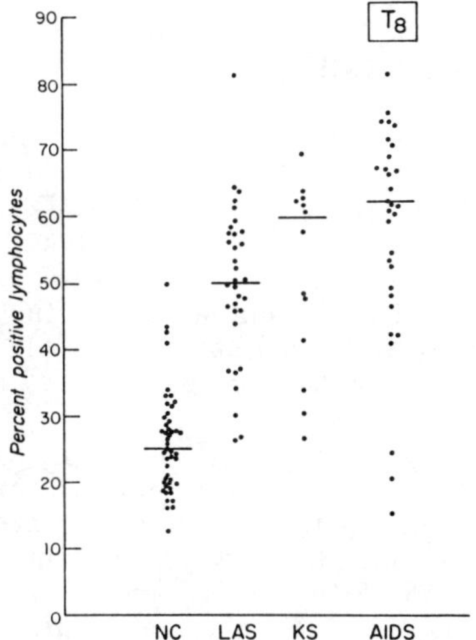

Figure 2. Percentages of T8$^+$ lymphocytes in peripheral blood of patients with LAS, KS, or AIDS (OI or KS with OI) compared to normal controls. Data obtained by flow cytometry of whole blood (Ortho Spectrum III).

ated with subsequent refractoriness of the same cellular population challenged in vitro. Lack of interferon production in vitro or the presence of high serum levels has been associated with disease progression in AIDS. We have observed that the serum interferon level was directly associated with clinical outcome in AIDS patients with KS (31). Since recent work in this laboratory (39) indicates that activated B cells in AIDS patients produce large quantities of acid labile interferon, it is likely that both impaired T cell production of gamma interferon and hyperactive B cell production of alpha interferon could occur simultaneously.

T-B cell interaction is affected by HIV infection of the $T4^+$ cells so that the T cell help required for immunoglobulin production is reduced (40). However, the major consequence of T cell alteration on B cell activation in AIDS may be closely related to absence of T suppressor activity directed against Epstein-Barr virus (EBV) infected B cells since it is believed that a subset of $T4^+$ cells (inducer) is a necessary additional component to the activity of $T8^+$ cells in preventing expansion of EBV infected B cells (41).

Several lines of evidence link decline of T cell immunity and evolution of AIDS but the critical changes that occur are not actually known. Virtually all cases of LAS which evolve into AIDS do so in rather abrupt steps. However, as described above, poor functional response, reduced $T4^+/T8^+$ ratio, elevated serum interferon, and impared interferon production in vitro have prognostic significance. Furthermore, therapies which arrest disease affect T cell populations or T cell function at least transiently suggesting a close association between depressed immune function and disease development.

The Suppressor/Cytotoxic T-Cell

Loss (or relative loss) of the $T4^+$ subset in AIDS, ARC and LAS has been widely recognized as a dominant feature. However, in early disease, inversion of the $T4^+/T8^+$ ratio can precede loss of the normal percentage of $T4^+$ lymphocytes. Clearly, this implies an imbalance effected through a disproportionately increased number of $T8^+$ lymphocytes. In fact, analysis of $T8^+$ expression in groups of patients with AIDS, ARC and LAS reveals that the $T8^+$ lymphocyte percentage may exceed levels seen in the normal population.

Data shown in Figure 2 for 45 healthy controls, 34 patients with LAS, 13 patients with AIDS-KS, and 26 patients with either KS and OI or OI alone, indicate the differences between groups. The mean percentage of $T8^+$ cells in controls was 25%, in contrast to 50% for LAS, 58% for KS and 62% for AIDS patients with OI. These data indicate that a relative increase in the cytotoxic/ suppressor cell population is common in HIV infection.

Both $T4^+$ and $T8^+$ lymphocytes normally proliferate in response to PHA which may account for the general lack of usefulness of response to PHA in predicting clinical course. A chief issue is the functional identity of the $T8^+$ cell, which is proportionately expanded in AIDS. Is this a suppressor cell or a cytotoxic cell? What function does it carry out? Does this reflect amplification of a single population or more than one? Is the $T8^+$ population the same in all groups of AIDS associated disease?

Suppressor T lymphocytes are known to be activated during the normal immunologic response process as well as to account for pathologically reduced immune responses. Current evidence suggests that there are at least several types of suppressor T lymphocytes, both specific and nonspecific. Normal suppressor T lymphocytes can be demonstrated in vitro by stimulating unseparated lymphocytes with concanavalin A and adding the stimulated cells back to autologous unstimulated cells which are then in turn activated with PHA. Compared to cell preparations incubated with PHA without activated suppressor T cells (actually carried out by adding sham activated cells), response is sharply reduced. Since AIDS patients respond poorly to T lymphocyte mitogens, one might assume that T suppressor cells could not be activated by this means in vitro. Interestingly, this does not appear to be so as at least certain T suppressor cells are functionally active in AIDS (Table 3). Since patients with LAS characteristically have had multiple exposures to common infective agents, e.g., cytomegalovirus, it seems possible that down regulation of immune response in vivo could be mediated in part by an amplified normal population of T suppressor cells.

Table 3. Relative Induction of Suppressor Cells in AIDS-KS, LAS and Controls

Case[a]		Intrinsic[b]	Autologous Suppressor Cells	Percent Inhibition
1	KS	7,882	4,428	44.0
2	LAS	7,956	3,730	53.0
3	LAS	14,120	5,700	59.6
4	KS	9,780	4,231	57.0
5	Control	19,972	11,378	43.0
6	Control	20,542	14,480	30.0
7	Control	19,870	9,924	50.1

a Mononuclear cells from peripheral blood were used in all cases except case #3 where lymph node tissue was the source of the cells.

b Intrinsic response to phytohemagglutinin carried out with autologous sham induced suppressor cells added back to responding population.

KS = Kaposi's sarcoma; LAS = Lymphadenopathy syndrome

Attempts to diminish the negative effects of such a suppressor population were undertaken using low dose X-irradiation (cesium source), which is known to inactivate suppressor cells in animal models. Control responses to PHA were reduced proportionately to the dose of irradiation, whereas in 12 cases of AIDS, seven showed a marked increase after low dose X-irradiation, and four showed lesser improvement in response (Table 4).

Table 4. Effect of Irradiation on Suppressor Cell Activity in AIDS

	0[a]	178[a]	89[a]	45[a]	Percent Change at 45 Rads
Control	26,032	18,681	21,170	24,863	5% Decrease
AIDS-KS	17,956	15,708	18,009	20,917	16% Increase
AIDS-KS	8,337	5,231	7,986	9,984	20% Increase
AIDS-KS	14,210	14,011	14,432	17,301	22% Increase
AIDS	10,986	10,031	12,001	13,419	22% Increase
AIDS-KS	13,468	13,334	14,698	15,449	15% Increase
Cancer[b]	8,311	5,613			

[a] Total rads
[b] A non-AIDS patient with cancer did not show an enhanced response.

As mentioned previously T-B cell cooperativity is altered in AIDS. Recently Birx et al. (42) demonstrated that AIDS patients' T cells in vitro increased immunoglobulin production induced by EBV and that this increase correlated with high numbers of EBV infected B-cells in the peripheral circulation of the AIDS patients. Loss of T cell suppression of outgrowth of B cells infected with EBV was noted. These effects appeared to be mediated through loss of $T4^+$ cells and alteration of $T8^+$ cells such that control of B cell activation was progressively lost. This phenomenon is particularly notable in patients with LAS and probably accounts for the elevated incidence of B cell lymphomas. The $T8^+$ population normally contains cytotoxic cells capable of mediating target specific lysis, the cytotoxic T lymphocyte (CTL). We have observed paradoxically that lymphocytes from AIDS patients are capable of increased lysis of spontaneously derived AIDS cell lines that contain multiple copies of the EBV genome (39). However, these CTL are clearly insufficient to reduce circulating EBV activated B cells. Quinnan et al. (43) have analyzed the interaction of CTL in control of viremia and progressive cytomegalovirus (CMV) disease in AIDS. The results of these important studies suggest that CMV specific CTL were virtually absent in AIDS and that failure to induce this cell in vitro was associated with both intrinsically deficient interleukin-2 production by T4^{+} cells and inhibition of IL-2 production by a serum blocking factor. These data also support the hypothesis that the T8^{+} lymphocyte in AIDS does not function normally.

Many studies on AIDS patients have been based on examination of clinical populations in whom disease processes had been ongoing for indeterminate periods of time prior to presentation. Nicholson (44) demonstrated that homosexual men without HIV infection had a rather marked lymphocytosis (35% increase above heterosexual controls), observed in both T4^{+} and T8^{+} subpopulations, possibly as a result of multiple antigenic exposure. Double labelling of T lymphocyte subsets showed that the homosexual men had increased T4^{+} cells bearing Ia^{+} antigen (Leu 8^{+}). This population of cells consists of feedback suppressor inducer cells which also provide some help in in vitro antibody responses. This same population was decreased in LAS patients. In AIDS patients both Ia^{+} and Ia^{-} subsets of T4^{+} cells were reduced. These data suggest a progressive loss of T4^{+} subsets in AIDS patients underline the need for understanding baseline immune parameters preceding HIV infection in the evaluation of the natural history of this retroviral infection. Further studies can be expected to focus on differences in the potential evolution of HIV disease in specific settings so that a rational basis for therapeutic intervention can be developed.

CONCLUSIONS

During the past seven years of study on T cell immunity in AIDS, there has been a gradual transition in focus from concepts of lymphocyte depletion associated with lack of immune response, toward analyses of intrinsic alteration in cellular function both at the subpopulation level and at the level of cell-cell interaction. The effect of HIV infection on regulation of immune response has become a central issue.

The T-lymphocyte subset ratio has continued to provide a useful indication of HIV disease. In some settings, e.g. blood transfusion associated HIV infection, inversion of the T4^{+}/T8^{+} ratio may precede reduction of the absolute T4^{+} cell number by some months. Imbalance of lymphocyte subsets has usually been associated with reduced immune function in vitro. Increase of T8^{+} lymphocytes accompanies loss of T4^{+} cells. This relative increase accounts for subset imbalance in cases were the percentage of T4^{+} cells is still within normal limits and is a striking feature of the syndrome. Identification of the functions mediated by the T8^{+} population and their role in disease evolution is an important research topic. These studies may ultimately clarify the basis of B cell deregulation in AIDS.

The role of the thymus and alteration in thymic hormone production in HIV infection is an important issue, since thymic epithelium and architecture, as well as thymic lymphocytes, are affected in the disease process. Although thymic factor replacement has not been successfully carried out, preliminary studies indicate that this ultimately may be possible.

Future studies on T-cell immunity in AIDS will focus on the mechanism of the effects of HIV infection on T-cell function. Better characterization of differences in altered immunoregulation in clinical subgroups is needed as well.

REFERENCES

1. Siegal, F.P., Lopez, C., Hammer, G.S., et al., Severe acquired immunodeficiency in male homosexuals manifested by chronic perianal ulcerative *Herpes simplex* lesions. N Engl J Med 305:1439-1444 (1981)

2. Gottlieb, M.S., Schroff, R., Schanker, H.M., et al., *Pneumocystis carinii* pneumonia and mucosal candidiasis in previously healthy homosexual men: Evidence of a new acquired cellular immunodeficiency. N Engl J Med 305:1425-1431 (1981)

3. Masur, H., Michelis, M.A., Green, J.B., et al., A community acquired outbreak of *Pneumocystis carinii* pneumonia: initial manifestation of cellular immune dysfunction. N Engl J Med 305:1431-1438 (1981)

4. Wormser, G.P., Krupp, L.B., Hanrahan, J.P., et al., Acquired immunodeficiency in male prisoners: New insights into an emerging syndrome. Ann Intern Med 98:297-303 (1983)

5. Urmacher, C., Myskowski, P., Ochoa, M., et al., Outbreak of Kaposi's sarcoma with cytomegalovirus infection in young homosexual men. Am J Med 72:569-575 (1982)

6. Friedman-Kien, A.E., Laubenstein, L.J., Rubinstein, P., et al., Disseminated Kaposi's sarcoma in homosexual men. Ann Intern Med 96:693-700 (1982)

7. Metroka, C.E., Cunningham-Rundles, S., Pollack, M.S., et al., Generalized lymphadenopathy in homosexual men. Ann Intern Med 99:585-592 (1982)

8. Safai, B., Johnson, K.G., Myskowski, P., et al., Natural history of Kaposi's sarcoma in the acquired immunodeficiency syndrome. Ann Intern Med 103:744-750 (1985)

9. Guinan, M.E., Thomas, P.A., Pinsky, P.F., et al., Heterosexual and homosexual patients with the acquired immunodeficiency syndrome. Ann Intern Med 100:213-218 (1984)

10. Abrams, D.I., Lewis, B.J., Volberding, P.I., Lymphadenopathy: Endpoint or prodrome? Update of a 24-month prospective study. Ann NY Acad Sci 437:207-215 (1984)

11. Francis, D.P., Jaffe, H.W., Fultz, P.N., et al., The natural history of infection with the lymphadenopathy associated virus/human T-lymphotropic virus type III. Ann Intern Med 103:719-722 (1985)

12. Gallo, R.C., Sarin, P.S., Gelmann, E.P., et al., Isolation of human T-cell leukemia virus in acquired immune deficiency syndrome (AIDS). Science 220:865-867 (1983)

13. Safai, B., Grossman, J.E., Popovic, M., et al., Seroepidemiological studies of human T-lymphotropic retrovirus type III in acquired immunodeficiency syndrome. Lancet 1:1438-1440 (1984)

14. Gallo, R.C., Salahuddin, S.Z., Popovic, M., et al., Frequent detection and isolation of cytopathic retroviruses (HTLV-III) from patients with AIDS and at risk for AIDS. Science 224: 500-503 (1984)

15. Davis, A.E., The histopathological changes in the thymus gland in the acquired immune deficiency syndrome. Ann NY Acad Sci 437:493-502 (1984)

16. Hersh, E.M., Rubin, J.M., Rios, A., et al., Elevated serum thymosin alpha 1 levels associated with evidence of immune dysregulation in male homosexuals with a history of infectious disease or Kaposi's sarcoma. N Engl J Med 308:45-46 (1983)

17. Naylor, P.H., Schulof, R.S., Sztein, M.B., et al., Ann NY Acad Sci 437:88-99 (1984)

18. Trainin, N., Burstein, Y., Buchner, V., et al., Viruses, Immunity and Immunodeficiency (Szentivanyi, A., Friedman, H., eds), Plenum Press, New York (In press)

19. Cunningham-Rundles, S., Safai, B., Metroka, C., et al., Lymphocyte effector function in vitro in the acquired immune deficiency syndrome. In: AIDS: The Epidemic of Kaposi's Sarcoma and Opportunistic Infections (Friedman-Kien, A.E., Laubenstein, L.J., eds), Masson, USA, p 153-159 (1984)

20. Ziegler, J.L., Beckslead, J.A., Volberding, P.A., et al., Non-Hodgkin's lymphoma in 90 homosexual men. Relation to generalized lymphadenopathy and the acquired immunodeficiency syndrome. N Engl J Med 311:565-570 (1984)

21. Levine, A.M., Meyer, P.B., Begandy, M.K., et al., Development of B cell lymphomas in homosexual men. Ann Intern Med 100:7-13 (1984)

22. Kornfeld, H., Vande Stouve, R.A., Lange, M., et al., T-lymphocyte subpopulation in homosexual men. N Engl J Med 307:729-734 (1982)

23. Laurence, J., Ban-vezinet, F., Schutzer, S.E., et al., Lymphadenopathy associated viral antibody in AIDS. N Engl J Med 311:1269-1273 (1984)

24. Gerstoft, J., Dickmeiss, E., Bentsen, K., The prognosis of asymptomatic homosexual men with decreased T helper to T suppressor ratio. Scand J Immunol 19:275-283 (1984)

25. Modlin, R.L., Meyer, P.R., Ammanu, A.J., et al., Altered distribution of B and T lymphocytes in lymph nodes from homosexual men with Kaposi's sarcoma. Lancet 2:769-771 (1983)

26. Scott, G.B., Buck, B.E., Leterman, J.G., et al., Acquired immunodeficiency syndrome in infants. N Engl J Med 310:76-81 (1984)

27. Detels, R., Schwartz, K., Visscher, B.B., et al., Relationship between sexual practices and T-cell subsets in homosexually active men. Lancet 609 (1983)

28. Cunningham-Rundles, S., Giardina, P., Hilgartner, M.W., Immunological analysis of patients with thalassemia major at risk for AIDS. (Manuscript in preparation)

29. Lane, H.C., Depper, J.M., Greene, W.C., Qualitative analysis of immune function in patients with the acquired immunodeficiency syndrome. N Engl J Med 313:79-84 (1985)

30. Cunningham-Rundles, S., Safai, B., Metroka, C.E., et al., Modulation of immune response. In: The Acquired Immunodeficiency Disease Syndrome, A.R. Liss, NY. Prog in Leuk Biol J, p 175-184 (1986)

31. Vadhan-Raj, S., Wong, G., Grecco, C., et al., Immunological variables as predictors of prognosis in patients with Kaposi's sarcoma and the acquired immunodeficiency syndrome. Cancer Res 46:417-425 (1986)

32. Ciobanu, N., Welte, K., Kruger, G., et al., Defective T cell response to PHA and mitogenic monoclonal antibodies in male homosexuals with acquired immunodeficiency syndrome and its in vitro correction by interleukin-2. J Clin Immunol 3:332-340(1983)

33. Kirkpatrick, C.H., Davis, K.C., Horsburgh, C.R., et al., Interleukin-2 production by persons with the generalized lymphadenopathy syndrome or the acquired immune deficiency syndrome. J Clin Immunol 5:31-37 (1985)

34. Prince, H.E., Kermani-Arab, A., Fahey, J.L., Depressed interleukin-2 receptor expression in acquired immune deficiency and lymphadenopathy syndromes. J Immunol 133:1313-1317 (1984)

35. Ernst, M., Korn, P., Flad, H.D., et al., Effects of systemic in vivo interleukin-2 (IL-2) reconstitution in patients with acquired immune deficiency syndrome (AIDS) and AIDS related complex (ARC) in phenotypes and functions of peripheral blood mononuclear cells. J Clin Immunol 6:170-181 (1986)

36. Murray, H.W., Rubin, B.Y., Masur, H., et al., Impaired production of lymphokines and immune (gamma) interferon production in the acquired immunodeficiency syndrome. N Engl J Med 310:883-889 (1984)

37. Lopez, C., Fitzgerald, P.A., Siegal, F.P., Severe acquired immune deficiency syndrome in male homosexuals: Diminished capacity to make interferon alpha in vitro associated with severe opportunistic infections. J Infect Dis 148:962-966 (1983)

38. Eyster, M.E., Goedert, J.J., Poon, M-C., et al., Acid-labile alpha interferon: A possible preclinical marker for the acquired immunodeficiency syndrome in hemophilia. N Engl J Med 309:583-586 (1983)

39. Cunningham-Rundles, S., Metroka, C.E., Safai, B., et al., Cytotoxic effector mechanisms in AIDS. In: AIDS-Associated syndromes (Gupta, S., ed), Plenum, NY, p 97-110 (1985)

40. Beniviste, E., Schroff, R., Stevens, R.H., et al., Immunoregulatory T cells in men with a new acquired immunodeficiency syndrome. J Clin Immunol 3:359-367 (1983)

41. Konttinen, Y.T., Bleustein, H.G., Zuaifler, N.J., Regulation of the growth of Epstein-Barr virus B cells. I. Growth regression by E rosetting cells from VLA-positive donors is a combined effect of autologous mixed lymphocyte culture reaction and activation of $T8^+$ memory cells. J Immunol 134:2287- 2293 (1985)

42. Birx, D.L., Redfield, R.R., Tosato, G., Defective regulation of Epstein-Barr virus infection in patients with acquired immunodeficiency syndrome (AIDS) or AIDS-related disorders. N Engl J Med 314:874-879 (1986)

43. Quinnan, C.T., Siegel, J.P., Epstein, J.S., et al., Mechanisms of T-cell functional deficiency in the acquired immunodeficiency syndrome. Ann Intern Med 103:710-714 (1985)

44. Nicholson, J.K.A., McDougal, J.S., Spira, T.J., Alterations of functional subsets of T helper and T suppressor cell populations in acquired immunodeficiency syndrome (AIDS) and chronic unexplained lymphadenopathy. J Clin Immunol 5:269-274 (1985)

18
B-Cell Abnormalities in AIDS: Role of HIV and Epstein-Barr Virus

David J. Volsky, Patrick K. Lai

The acquired immunodeficiency syndrome (AIDS) is characterized by severe abnormalities at virtually every level of the immune system, including defects in T lymphocyte function, altered B cell and monocyte activity, and various abnormalities of humoral immunity (1)-(3). Development and progression of these defects result in increased susceptibility to opportunistic infections and malignancies which are the leading cause of death in AIDS. Recently reported studies suggest that many of the immune abnormalities observed in AIDS-related conditions (ARC) may be directly caused by infection with human immunodeficiency virus (HIV), the primary etiologic agent of the syndrome (4)-(8). Foremost among these is the decrease in the number and function of circulating T4-positive helper/inducer T lymphocytes, which is believed to be due to cytolysis resulting from HIV infection and massive virus replication in these cells (9)-(11). Another target for HIV infection are cells of the monocyte/macrophage series, which have also been found to express the T4 receptor and support replication of the virus (12)-(14).

While the interaction between HIV and $T4^+$ T lymphocytes and macrophages, and the immunologic dysfunctions related to these two cell types, have been the focus of extensive research, the nature and cause of B cell abnormalities in AIDS are much less well understood. Yet, these abnormalities are as ubiquitous and severe as the T cell or macrophage defects, including, for example, polyclonal B cell activation and elevated immunoglobulin levels, increased spontaneous B cell proliferation and differentiation, decreased de novo antigen responses, and increased frequency of B cell lymphomas (Table 1).

Some of the B cell abnormalities in AIDS are consistent with the effects of reactivation of latent Epstein-Barr virus (EBV), as observed during chronic infectious mononucleosis and during immunosuppressive states following organ transplantation (15), (16). However, several recent reports emphasize the important role HIV may play directly in these changes. In this chapter, we review the B cell abnormalities in AIDS-related conditions, discuss the role of EBV and HIV, and advance a hypothesis that a direct interaction between HIV and EBV within human B lymphocytes may contribute to the initiation and intensification of B cell defects in AIDS. Several other reviews deal with various aspects of B cell abnormalities and their role in the pathogenesis of AIDS (2),(3),(17)-(19).

Table 1. Pathological Features Associated With Abnormal Function, Regulation or Control of B Lymphocytes in AIDS

Feature	Reference
Elevated serum immunoglobulin levels	20-26, 31, 77, 81
Increased spontaneous immunoglobulin secretion by individual B cells (polyclonal B cell activation)	22, 32, 34, 79
Increased level of circulating immune complexes	21, 78, 84
Decreased de novo antigen response	22, 32-34
Increased spontaneous proliferation and differentation	30, 34, 79
Increased titer of anti-EBV antibodies	29-31
Increased proportion of EBV-positive cells in peripheral blood	19, 29, 30, 43-47
High incidence of non-Hodgkin's lymphoma	48-54, 80, 82, 83

EBV = Epstein-Barr virus

EVIDENCE FOR B CELL DISREGULATION IN AIDS AND AIDS-RELATED CONDITIONS

AIDS-related B cell abnormalities can be divided into two interrelated broad categories (Table 1): A) defects in B cell function and B) B-lymphoproliferative disorders and malignancies resulting from defective control of spontaneous B cell proliferation.

Defects in B Cell Function

The most obvious abnormality of B cell function in AIDS is a polyclonal B cell hyperactivation. Hypergammaglobulinemia has been established as one of the earliest findings in AIDS (20)-(22). Elevated levels of IgG and IgA are usually present with generally normal levels of IgM (20)-(22). The presence of elevated immunoglobulin levels and a normal to elevated proportion of B lymphocytes was initially incorrectly considered to be indicative of intact B-cell mediated immunity in AIDS. This notion was further supported by the occurrence of normal to elevated levels of antibodies to specific viral agents, such as HIV (23)-(26) or EBV (27)-(31). However, more detailed studies demonstrated that B cells from AIDS patients, although present in normal numbers and capable of spontaneous immunoglobulin production, are defective in their ability to respond in vitro to T cell-independent B cell mitogens such as *Staphylococcus aureus* Cowan I (32). B cell response to challenge with new antigens in vivo, such as pneumococcal polysaccharide or keyhole limpet hemocyanin, has also been found to be severely impaired (33), (34). Thus, the elevated levels of IgG and IgA in AIDS seem to be the result of chronic polyclonal B cell activation, leaving a smaller proportion of undifferentiated cells to respond to new activation signals. This lack of response may explain why antibody tests have not regularly been helpful in diagnosing certain opportunistic infections, such as toxoplasmosis (35), coccidioidomycosis (36), or invasive cytomegalovirus (CMV) infections (37). Interestingly, antibody responses to HIV and EBV are basically preserved (23)-(31), indicating that infection with these two agents precedes development of the defective B cell responses. These observations also suggest that therapeutic strategies based on increasing the humoral immune response against HIV in AIDS or ARC patients may not be successful.

B-Lymphoproliferation and B-Cell Malignancies

B-cell maturation proceeds in a step-wise manner involving at least three successive stages: activation of resting B cells, proliferation, and differentiation into immunoglobulin-secreting plasma cells (38). Under normal circumstances, most B lymphocytes remain in the resting non-induced state (38). The hyperactivation of B lymphocytes in individuals at risk for AIDS and in AIDS patients implies a dramatic shift in the equilibrium of the B cell maturation pathway toward increased proliferation and terminal differentiation. In this respect, the B-cell dysfunction in AIDS resembles the B-lymphoproliferative disorders which occur in systemic lupus erythematosus, chronic infectious mononucleosis (15), or certain inherited immune deficiency syndromes (39).

Three different lines of evidence suggest that AIDS-related conditions are associated with B-lymphoproliferation.

1. Many individuals infected with HIV (and therefore considered at risk for AIDS) develop persistent generalized lymphadenopathy (PGL) within several months after infection (40)-(42). Typical sites for peripheral lymphadenopathy include the axillary and inguinal areas, as well as the preauricular, postauricular, and epitrochlear node groups. In addition, many patients have splenomegaly, increased retroperitoneal lymphadenopathy or thickening of the rectal mucosa consistent with a chronic proctitis (40)-(42). Histologic examination of lymph nodes reveals profound abnormalities in the germinal centers as reflected by follicular hyperplasia and germinal center hypertrophy, both usually confined to the B-cell zones of the lymphoid tissues (42). In addition to lymph nodes, another site for extensive B-lymphoproliferation may be the intestinal mucosa. As described recently by Kotler et al. (28), histologic evidence of lymphoproliferation consisting of increased numbers of follicular center-like cells, was found in the intestinal mucosa of 17 patients with AIDS or ARC and in two additional homosexual men with antibodies to HIV.

2. Besides generalized B cell hyperplasia as observed in lymph nodes and rectal mucosa, HIV-seropositive individuals and AIDS patients have evidence for a lymphoproliferative disease associated specifically with EBV (19),(29),(30),(43)-(47). EBV-driven lymphoproliferations are particularly frequent in infants and children with AIDS (43). The increase in the proportion of EBV^+ cells can be detected either directly by hybridization with EBV DNA probes (43), or inferred from assays measuring the number of spontaneously outgrowing EBV-transformed cells from blood (29),(30),(44),(45). In patients with ARC and AIDS, estimates of the mean frequency of circulating EBV-infected B cells range from 6 to 21 per 10^6 B cells, as compared to 1-2 per 10^6 B cells in normal healthy individuals (44),(45). The presence of large numbers of circulating EBV-infected cells is also reflected by the high frequency of isolation of EBV-positive lymphoblastoid cell lines during culture of peripheral blood lymphocytes from HIV-positive individuals (19),(46). It should be noted, however, that the frequency of spontaneously outgrowing EBV-positive cells is about three orders of magnitude smaller than the number of cells reported to produce immunoglobulin spontaneously in AIDS patients (6-21 per 10^6 vs. 10^3 - 10^4 per 10^6 circulating B lymphocytes, respectively) (44),(45),(47), indicating that EBV-infected cells may not account for the entire population of activated B cells in these patients.

3. In addition to benign B cell hyperplasia, a sizable proportion of AIDS patients develop malignant lymphomas, the second most common malignancy in AIDS patients (48)-(54). In most cases, the malignancies are defined as high-grade non-Hodgkin's B-

cell lymphomas (NHLs) which are disseminated in unusual extranodal sites such as the central nervous system or rectum, and show many features resembling the malignancies seen in organ transplant and inherited immunodeficiency patients. The phenotype is B cell without exception. Furthermore, a large proportion of B cell malignancies observed in AIDS patients have the characteristics of Burkitt's lymphoma, including the characteristic chromosomal translocations involving the c-myc oncogene (48),(52),(54). Of 39 cases of non-Hodgkin's lymphomas in homosexual men summarized by Erenberg (54), 14 (36%) were of Burkitt's lymphoma-like type. Interestingly, all of AIDS-related Burkitt's lymphoma cases reported so far have been associated with the presence of EBV genome in the tumor cells (51),(54), similar to the close association between EBV and Burkitt's lymphoma in endemic areas of Africa (55). In contrast, non-AIDS associated Burkitt's lymphoma cases outside of the high incidence areas are usually EBV genome-negative (55). The etiology of non-Burkitt's B-cell lymphomas is unclear. Systematic studies for the presence of EBV and other viral agents in these malignancies need to be performed. As of June 1985, the Centers for Disease Control added high-grade B-cell lymphoma outside of the central nervous system to the surveillance criteria for AIDS (56). Primary brain lymphoma had already been part of the original surveillance criteria.

POSSIBLE MECHANISMS FOR B-CELL ABNORMALITIES IN AIDS

The data summarized in the previous section suggest that B cell dysfunction in AIDS involves all three stages of B cell development and may as well include defects in the regulatory feedback T-cell suppressor mechanism. Clearly, the central B cell defect appears to be the chronic hyperactivation of B lymphocytes and the resulting hypergammaglobulinemia, lymphoproliferative disease and malignancies. Such hyperactivation could occur as a secondary response to exposure to various opportunistic pathogens. However, the absence of functional helper T lymphocytes in the presence of an excess of functional suppressor T cells, makes this possibility unlikely. Furthermore, AIDS patients have been shown to have a diminished ability to develop specific humoral immunity to new antigens, again suggesting a chronic primary defect in the stimulation process of B lymphocytes. An alternative and perhaps more consistent scenario would involve a primary B cell defect resulting from infection with, or exposure to, an agent that could act as a polyclonal B cell activator in the absence of functional helper T lymphocytes and with abundant activated T suppressor cells. The following sections will evaluate whether two viral agents closely associated with AIDS-related conditions, HIV and EBV, may play a pivotal role, alone or together, in the induction and maintenance of B cell defects in AIDS.

INVOLVEMENT OF EPSTEIN-BARR VIRUS

EBV, a ubiquitous human herpesvirus discovered in 1964, is

the cause of infectious mononucleosis (IM) and a major factor in Burkitt's lymphoma and nasopharyngeal carcinoma (55),(57). The virus is unique among herpesviruses in its tropism for B-lymphocytes and its capacity to transform cells into permanently growing cell lines. Approximately 80 to 90 percent of adults have been infected with EBV (58). Because of its cell-transforming and oncogenic potential, EBV should be considered a dangerous pathogen. However, under usual circumstances multiple humoral and cellular immune mechanisms have evolved to cope efficiently with this organism. These include: humoral immunity to EBV capsid, nuclear and membrane antigens; EBV-specific, HLA-restricted memory T-cells activated by a lymphocyte-detected membrane antigen (LYDMA); antibody-dependent cellular cytotoxicity (ADCC); and non-HLA-restricted natural killing (NK) (59). In the absence of immune surveillance, as seen in such clinical situations as children with inherited immune deficiencies (39), immune-suppressed organ transplant recipients (16), and AIDS patients, EBV-infected lymphocytes proliferate rapidly, often causing fatal polyclonal or monoclonal lesions.

Recent experiments suggest that HLA-restricted T cell recognition of EBV-infected cells is the prime mechanism for control of EBV induced transformation and proliferation of B cells (60). Helper T-lymphocytes play a major role in this control mechanism (60). Infection and lysis of helper/inducer T-lymphocytes by HIV (9)-(11) is likely to damage the fine homeostatic balance between EBV and its host, allowing the rapid proliferation of EBV-carrying B cells seen in AIDS-associated disorders (29)-(31),(44),(45). Since it is well-known that EBV is a polyclonal T cell-independent B cell activator (59), the increased proportion of EBV-infected cells could account, at least in part, for the hyperimmunoglobulinemia observed in AIDS patients.

Further evidence for defective regulation of EBV infection in AIDS-related disorders stems from studies on the pattern of EBV-specific antibody responses in HIV-positive individuals. Several recent studies in patients with ARC and AIDS describe an increased prevalence of serum IgG and IgA antibodies to EBV capsid antigens, increased levels of IgG (but not IgA) antibodies to EBV early antigen, and high levels of antibodies to EBV nuclear antigen, EBNA (27),(29),(30),(45),(61). Compared with healthy controls, AIDS patients are more likely to have EBV present in cultures of oropharyngeal secretions (29). Many of the findings in AIDS-related conditions such as elevated levels of circulating EBV-infected cells and absence or low EBV-specific cytotoxicity, are very similar to those seen in patients with acute infectious mononucleosis (15). However, the low levels of IgM antibodies to VCA and the high titers of anti-EBNA antibodies are more indicative of EBV reactivation rather than primary infection. Interestingly, defective regulation of EBV infection may not be limited to patients with ARC or AIDS, whose T cell dependent immunity is severely impaired. In a recent study by Renaldo et al., increased levels of serum IgG antibodies to EA and VCA EBV antigens were also observed in asymptomatic homosexual men (31). These results suggest that infection with EBV is an important cofactor in conditions leading to the development of AIDS, and that HIV infection itself may reactivate latent EBV, thereby resulting in increased titers of antibodies to this herpesvirus.

The major consequence of EBV reactivation in HIV-positive individuals is the appearance of abnormally large numbers of EBV-infected B cells in the circulation. This EBV-driven B lymphoproliferation may be in part responsible for at least three other B cell abnormalities observed in AIDS: polyclonal B cell activation resulting in hypergammaglobulinemia, B cell hyperplasia of lymph nodes and rectal mucosa, and B-cell malignancies. Since EBV-immortalized B cells may undergo an indefinite number of cell divisions [in the absence of cell-mediated anti-EBV immunity (59),(60)], the probability of the occurrence of chromosomal aberrations leading to permanent activation of c-myc or other oncogenes would be increased. Chromosomal translocations involving the c-myc locus are considered necessary for the development of Burkitt's lymphoma in endemic (African) and non-endemic areas (62),(63). The pathogenesis of Burkitt's-like lymphoma in AIDS may therefore involve initial polyclonal expansion of the B cell population due to reactivation of EBV in the setting of decreased cellular immunity against EBV-infected cells, with subsequent emergence of a transformed monoclonal population characterized by a translocated c-myc oncogene. Another important consequence of the presence of an increased number of immortalized B lymphocytes in the circulation is the potential reservoir they provide for chronic HIV infection (see below).

INVOLVEMENT OF HUMAN IMMUNODEFICIENCY VIRUS

HIV is considered to be the primary etiologic agent of immunodeficiency in AIDS (7),(8). The immunopathogenic effects of HIV are thought to be due to the cytopathic interaction of the virus with the helper/inducer T lymphocyte subset expressing the T4 (CD4) viral receptor (7),(11). Given the central role of helper T lymphocytes in the function of the cellular immune system, impairment of these cells by HIV infection may have deleterious suppressive effects on the function of other components of the immune system that require T4 cell "help", such as suppressor/cytotoxic T lymphocytes or monocytes.

The expected effect of the helper T lymphocyte dysfunction on B lymphocytes would be decreased stimulation, proliferation and immunoglobulin secretion. The observed hyperactivation of B lymphocytes in the absence of T lymphocyte help (20)-(22) has been attributed in part to polyclonal B cell activation by EBV and thought to occur independently of HIV infection. However, recent studies have shown that human B lymphocytes can also be infected by HIV (19),(46),(64), and that exposure of B cells to HIV may actually have an immunostimulatory effect on these cells (65)-(67), as opposed to the immunosuppressive effect of the virus on T lymphocytes. This phenomenon was first indicated by studies of Pahwa et al. who evaluated the effects of disrupted HIV preparations on normal lymphoid cells (65). Peripheral blood lymphocytes were exposed to a disrupted HIV preparation obtained by detergent solubilization and homogenization of sucrose gradient-banded HIV. Relatively dilute concentrations of this preparation were found to stimulate immunoglobulin secretion by peripheral blood lymphocytes and at the same time block B cell differentiation in response to other known polyclonal B cell activators, such as pokeweed mitogen and EBV (65). In a subsequent study by the same investigators (64), this stimulatory effect of HIV was found to require the presence of T cells, suggesting that one of the mechanisms contributing to the B cell hyperactivation in AIDS could be via an HIV-induced T-dependent B cell activation, perhaps mediated by disrupted viral particles or by viral glycoproteins present in the circulation. The T cell dependence of B cell activation by HIV has also been demonstrated in a study by Yarchoan and colleagues in which they found that peripheral blood lymphocytes, but not purified B cells, produced immunoglobulin when exposed to HIV in vitro (45).

In contrast to the above-described studies, Schnittman and colleagues found no T cell requirement for HIV-induced activation of human B lymphocytes (67). Using three separate virus isolates, these investigators demonstrated that exposure of purified B cell preparations to infectious HIV induced marked proliferation, differentiation and immunoglobulin secretion, comparable to that seen with other T cell independent polyclonal B cell activators (67). The reasons for this discrepancy are unclear, but they could be due to HIV strain differences. T cell-independent B lymphocyte activation would likely require induction of resting B cells by virus binding and/or infection. HIV isolates are known to differ in their host cell range (68). The specific human T-lymphotropic virus III (HTLV-III) isolate from H9 cells used in the studies of Pahwa et al. and Yarchoan et al. (45),(65),(66) might be incapable of interacting with resting B cells.

Regardless of the precise mechanism of B cell activation by HIV, the above described studies clearly demonstrate that HIV, like EBV, is able to induce polyclonal B cell activation, thereby potentially contributing to the hypergammaglobulinemia and increased level of immune complexes that are characteristic of AIDS-related conditions.

The finding that exposure to infectious HIV causes B cell proliferation (67) should be noted with particular interest, especially in light of the known cytopathic/cytocidal effect of the virus on human T lymphocytes (10),(11). Although the B-lymphoproliferative effect of HIV could merely be the result of virus binding rather than infection [the effect can be achieved with non-infectious virus preparations (65)(66)], the nature of the interaction between HIV and B lymphocytes should be investigated in detail. While approximately one-third of B cell lymphomas observed in AIDS are of the Burkitt's lymphoma type and are associated with the EBV genome (53),(54), the etiology of the other B cell malignancies in AIDS is unknown. HIV-induced chronic activation of EBV-negative B cells could potentially lead to B cell lymphoma by increasing the probability of chromosomal aberrations in vigorously proliferating cells, as postulated for "receptor-mediated leukemogenesis" (69),(70) and African Burkitt's lymphoma (62),(63).

COINFECTION OF B LYMPHOCYTES WITH EBV AND HIV: POSSIBLE ROLE IN THE PATHOGENESIS OF AIDS

Not all of the B cell abnormalities observed in AIDS-related conditions can readily be explained by the effects of EBV or HIV infection alone. For example, an increase in the number of EBV-positive B lymphocytes also occurs in HIV-positive asymptomatic individuals whose immune system contains practically intact levels of the accessory and cytotoxic T cells required for controlling EBV-positive B cell proliferation. One explanation for this observation is based on a model of coinfection of B lymphocytes by EBV and HIV. That HIV can superinfect EBV-positive B cells in vitro was first demonstrated by Montagnier and colleagues in 1984 (64), prompting the suggestion that EBV positive B-lymphocytes may serve as a reservoir for HIV persistence and dissemination in vivo (64). This finding has been supported by data from our laboratory showing that B lymphoblastoid cell lines coinfected with EBV and HIV can regularly be isolated from peripheral blood of HIV-positive individuals (19),(46). Based on these results, we have proposed a hypothetic mechanism for the maintenance of chronic infection by HIV that provides an explanation for the long-term persistence of HIV with continuing dissemination of the virus into helper T lymphocytes, and the gradual increase in EBV-driven B cell lymphoproliferation, immunoglobulin secretion, and lymphoma. The hypothesis, schematically summarized in Figure 1, contains the following elements:

1. Primary infection of helper T4 lymphocytes with HIV results in virus replication in these cells and cytolysis (I A-C).
2. B lymphocytes containing latent EBV genome (II A) undergo a constant cycle of EBV-driven proliferation (II B, D), and elimination by host cellular immune defenses (II A, C, E). Helper T lymphocytes interact in recognizing lymphocyte-detected membrane antigen (LYDMA) on the surface of EBV-infected cells and in providing help for cytotoxic T-lymphocytes against the virus infected cells (II B, D). During this interaction, EBV-infected B-lymphocytes become infected with HIV released by helper T-lymphocytes (II B). Most of the EBV-positive, HIV-positive B cells are probably eliminated by the immune system (II C), but a minority of cells survive and begin to proliferate (II D).
3. Newly regenerated helper T-lymphocytes approach the proliferating EBV-positive, HIV-positive B-lymphocytes and become infected with HIV present in the B-cells (II D - III D). HIV-infected helper T cells are lysed (III E), while EBV-positive, HIV-positive B cells continue to circulate (II E). As the immune system weakens with each cycle (I-III, A-E) more proliferating B cells (i.e., lymphadenopathy) and fewer helper T lymphocytes (i.e., reduced $T4^+/T8^+$ ratio) will be found in the circulation.

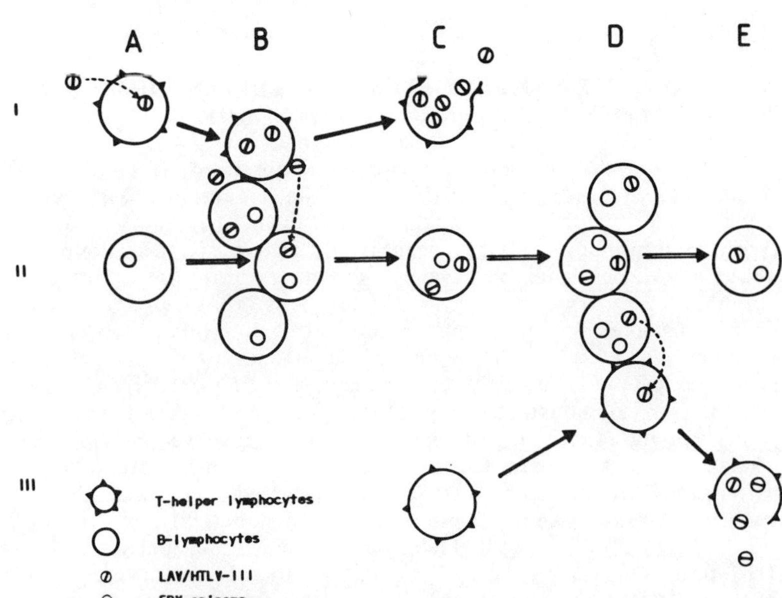

Figure 1. Scheme showing hypothetical interaction between EBV-infected B-lymphocytes and helper/inducer T lymphocytes in the process of maintaining chronic HIV infection. For details see text. LAV/HTLV-III = lymphadenopathy-associated virus/human T-lymphotropic virus III.

The hypothesis described above does not exclude the occurrence of a similar cycle of immune interactions resulting from coinfection of the same host cell with both HIV and an infectious agent other than EBV. Most AIDS patients have concomitant infection with cytomegalovirus (3),(53),(61), and a recent study by Laure and colleagues demonstrated evidence for the presence of hepatitis B virus DNA sequences in fresh and cultured lymphocytes from patients with AIDS (71).

Possible superinfection of EBV-positive B lymphocytes with HIV may also explain the dramatic increase in the level of antibodies to EBV early and late antigens in HIV seropositive individuals and AIDS patients. Results of recent experiments in our laboratory suggest that infection of EBV-positive B cells by HIV may directly affect the EBV life cycle. As shown in Table 2, the B-lymphoblastoid cell lines (LCL-EB), as well as the EBV-positive cell line P3HR-1 of Burkitt's lymphoma origin, showed a significant increase in the proportion of early antigen positive and viral capsid antigen positive cells three to four days after exposure to HIV. These results suggest that HIV may activate latent cellular EBV infection resulting in stimulation of the immune system to produce antibodies to EBV proteins.

Table 2. EBV Antigen Expression and Proliferation of EBV-Containing Cell Lines Infected by HIV

Cell Lines	Treatment	Prolifer-ation CPM*	Percent Cells Positive for EBV Antigen			
			EA-R	EA-D	VCA	MA
$LCL\text{-}EB_1$	----	13797	<1	<1	<1	n.d.
	TPA	7531	5	4	3	1
	HIV	14308	4	4	2	1
$LCL\text{-}EB_2$	----	16676	<1	<1	<1	n.d.
	TPA	14118	10	4	5	1
	HIV	13401	7	5	3	1
P3HR-1	----	n.t.	3	2	<1	n.t.
	TPA	n.t.	15	10	10	n.t.
	HIV	n.t.	10	12	6	n.t.

The EBV-transformed B lymphoblastoid (LCL-EB) cells were infected by HIV at 37°C for one hour. Mock-infected LCL-EB served as negative controls. The cells were cultured in RPMI-1640 medium supplemented with antibiotics and 10% fetal calf serum. Cells grown in medium containing 20 ng/ml tumor promoting agent (TPA) served as positive controls. At different time points, cells were assessed for the rate of proliferation and the expression of EBV antigens. Also studied was the EBV-positive cell line P3HR-1 of Burkitt's lymphoma origin.

n.d. = not detected; n.t. = not tested; EA-R = early antigens of restricted form; EA-D = early antigens of diffuse form; VCA = viral capsid antigens; MA = membrane antigen of EBV.

* Proliferation of LCL-EB was assessed after a 6 hr. pulse with ^{3}H-thymidine 24 hours after infection with HIV. CPM = mean counts per min.

The possibility of molecular interaction between HIV and EBV in the same host cell would not be without precedent. Two recent reports have described activation of HIV long terminal repeat (LTR) sequences by DNA viruses, including *Herpes simplex* virus-I and varicella-zoster virus (72),(73). Both intact *Herpes simplex* virus-I (72) and recombinant plasmids containing DNA fragments from various DNA-core viruses (73) were able to increase expression of a chloramphenicol acteyl-transferase (CAT) gene directed by HIV LTR (72),(73). The observed transient stimulation of chloramphenicol acetyl-transferase synthesis by heterologous viral DNA's has been attributed to viral regulatory proteins acting in trans to activate the HIV promoter (72),(73). It is not clear from these experiments, however, whether HIV itself would trans-activate other viruses. HIV has been shown to encode two potent trans-acting factors, TAT^{HIV} and art/trs, that increase HIV gene expression (74)-(76); these conceivably might transactivate expression of other viral DNA's. Certainly more experiments are required to evaluate these possibilities. Whatever the mechanism, molecular interactions between HIV and viral cofactors in AIDS could determine the duration and outcome of the asymptomatic HIV infection that precedes development of the full-blown syndrome.

SUMMARY

B cell defects play an important role in the pathogenesis of AIDS. Hyperactivation of B lymphocytes results in spontaneous proliferation and immunoglobulin secretion on one hand, and defective normal responses to new activation signals on the other. B cell hyperplasia contribute to the lymphadenopathy syndrome and intestinal lymphoproliferative disease, and not rarely evolve into B cell malignancies, often of the EBV-related Burkitt's lymphoma type. Many of the B cell abnormalities in AIDS are caused by primary and reactivated EBV infection. HIV may contribute directly to polyclonal B cell activation and B lymphoproliferative disease. Molecular interaction between HIV and EBV in B cells could aggravate the effects of each virus separately.

ACKNOWLEDGMENTS

The authors' experiments described in this chapter were supported by grants CA 37465 and CA 43464 from the National Institutes of Health and by a grant from the American Foundation for AIDS Research (AmFAR). The authors are grateful to J. Sonnabend, F. Sinangil and M. Stevenson for fruitful discussions, and to T. Chaudry for typing the manuscript.

REFERENCES

1. Fauci, A.S., Macher, A.M., Longo, D.L., et al., Acquired immunodeficiency syndrome: epidemiologic, clinical, immunologic and therapeutic considerations. Ann Intern Med 100:92-106 (1983)

2. Bowen, D.L., Lane, H.C., Fauci, A.S., Immunologic abnormalities in the acquired immunodeficiency syndrome. In: Acquired Immunodeficiency Syndrome (Klein, E., ed), Karger, Basel, p 207-223 (1986)

3. Pinching, A.J., The immunology of AIDS and HIV infection. Clinics Immun Aller 6:645-660 (1986)

4. Barre-Sinoussi, F., Chermann, J.C., Rey, F., et al., Isolation of a T-lymphotropic retrovirus from a patient at risk for acquired immune deficiency syndrome (AIDS). Science 220: 868-870 (1983)

5. Gallo, R.C., Salhuddin, S.Z., Popovic, M., et al., Frequent detection and isolation of cytopathic retroviruses (HTLV-III) from patients with AIDS and at risk for AIDS. Science 224: 500-503 (1984)

6. Levy, J.A., Hoffman, A.D., Kramer, S.M., et al., Isolation of lymphocytopathic retroviruses from San Francisco patients with AIDS. Science 225: 840-842 (1984)

7. Wong-Staal, F., Gallo, R.C., The family of human T-lymphotropic leukemia viruses: HTLV-I as the cause of adult T cell leukemia and HTLV-III as the cause of acquired immunodeficiency syndrome. Blood 65:253-263 (1985)

8. Montagnier, L., Lymphadenopathy-associated virus: From molecular biology to pathogenicity. Ann Intern Med 103:689-693 (1985)

9. Gottlieb, M.S., Schroff, R., Schanker, H.M., et al., *Pneumocystis carinii* pneumonia and mucosal candidiasis in previously healthy homosexual men: Evidence of a new acquired cellular immunodeficiency. N Engl J Med 305:1426-1431 (1981)

10. Klatzmann, D., Barre-Sinoussi, F., Nugeyre, M.T., et al., Selective tropism of lymphadenopathy-associated virus (LAV) for helper-inducer T lymphocytes. Science 225:59-63 (1984)

11. Lifson, J.D., Reys, G.R., McGrath, M.S., et al., AIDS retrovirus induced cytopathology: Giant cell formation and involvement of CD4 antigen. Science 232:1123-1127 (1986)

12. Rieber, P., Reithmuller, G., Loss of circulating T4+ monocytes in patients infected with HTLV-III. Lancet 1:270 (1986)

13. Gartner, S., Markovitz, P., Markovitz, D.M., et al., The role of mononuclear phagocytes in HTLV-III/LAV infection. Science 233:215-219 (1986)

14. Ho, D.D., Rota, T.R., Hirsch, M.S., Infection of monocyte/macrophages by human T lymphotropic virus type III. J Clin Invest 77:1712-1715 (1986)

15. Straus, S.E., Tosato, G., Armstrong, G., et al., Persisting illness and fatigue in patients with evidence of Epstein-Barr virus infection. Ann Intern Med 102:7-13 (1985)

16. Hanto, D.W., Firzzera, G., Gajl-Peczalska, J.K., et al., Epstein-Barr virus, immunodeficiency, and B cell lymphoproliferation. Transplantation 39:461-472 (1985)

17. Zolla-Pazner, S., B cells in the pathogenesis of AIDS. Immuno Today 5:289-291 (1984)

18. Purtilo, D.T., Lipscomb, H., Krueger, G., et al., Role of Epstein-Barr virus in acquired immune deficiency syndrome. In: AIDS-Associated Syndrome. (Gupta, S., ed), Plenum Press, New York, p 53-66 (1984)

19. Volsky, D.J., Sonnabend, J., Casareale, D., Hypothesis: How Epstein-Barr virus (EBV) may contribute to the induction of acquired immune deficiency syndrome (AIDS) by LAV/HTLV-III. In: Leukemia: Recent Advances in Biology and Treatment, Alan R. Liss, Inc., New York, p 187-200 (1985)

20. Carr, R., Veitch, S.D., Edmond, E., et al., Abnormalities of circulating lymphocyte subsets in haemophiliacs in an AIDS-free population. Lancet 1:1431-1434 (1984)

21. Nicholson, J.K.A., McDougal, J.S., Jaffe, H.W., et al., Exposure to human T-lymphotropic virus type III/lymphadenopathy-associated virus and immunologic abnormalities in asymptomatic homosexual men. Ann Intern Med 103:37-42 (1985)

22. Sieber, G., Tecihmann, H., Ludwig, W.D., et al., B-cell function in AIDS. Blut 51:143-144 (1985)

23. Sirianni, M.C., Rossi, P., Scarpath, B., et al., Immunological and virological investigation in patients with lymphadenopathy syndrome and in a population at risk for AIDS, with particular focus on the detection of antibodies to HTLV-III. J Clin Immunol 5:361-370 (1985)

24. Hehlmann, R., Kreeb, G., Erfle, V., et al., IgG-antibodies to HTLV-III with AIDS, LAS and persons at risk of AIDS in West Germany. Blut 50:13-18 (1985)

25. Kaminsky, L.S., McHugh, T., Stites, D., et al., High prevalence of antibodies to acquired immune deficiency syndrome (AIDS)-associated retrovirus (ARV) in AIDS and related conditions but not in other disease states. Proc Natl Acad Sci USA 82:5535-5539 (1985)

26. Hedenskog, M., Dewhurst, S., Ludvigsen, C., et al., Testing for antibodies to AIDS-associated retrovirus (HTLV-III/LAV) by indirect fixed cell immunofluorescence: Specificity, sensitivity and applications. J Med Virol 19:325-334 (1986)

27. Lipscomb, H., Tatsumi, E., Harada, S., et al., Epstein-Barr virus and chronic lymphadenopathy in male homosexuals with acquired immunodeficiency syndrome (AIDS). AIDS Res 1:59-82 (1983)

28. Kotler, D.P., Sinangil, F., Scholes, J.V., et al., Epstein-Barr virus-associated lymphoproliferation in rectal mucosa of patients with the acquired immunodeficiency syndrome. Gastroenterology (In press)

29. Sumaya, C.V., Boswell, R.N., Ench, Y., et al., Enhanced serological and virological findings of Epstein-Barr virus in patients with AIDS and AIDS-related complex. J Infect Dis 154: 864-870 (1986)

30. Ragona, G., Sirianni, M.C., Soddu, S., et al., Evidence for disregulation in the control of Epstein-Barr virus latency in patients with AIDS-related complex. Clin Exp Immunol 66:17-24 (1986)

31. Rinaldo, C.R., Kingsley, L.A., Lyter, D.W., et al., Association of HTLV-III with Epstein-Barr virus infection and abnormalities of T lymphocytes in homosexual men. J Infect Dis 154:556-561 (1986)

32. Pahwa, S.G., Quilop, M.T.J., Lange, M., et al., Defective B-lymphocyte function of homosexual men in relation to the acquired immunodeficiency syndrome. Ann Intern Med 101:757-763 (1984)

33. Ammann, A.J., Schiffman, G., Abrams, D., et al., B-cell immunodeficiency in acquired immune deficiency syndrome. JAMA 251:1447-1449 (1984)

34. Tsang, P.H., Zanjani, M.D., Warner, N., et al., Restoration of impaired B- and T-lymphocyte subsets and functions in vitro by isoprinosine in prodromal homosexuals and AIDS patients. J Clin Lab Immunol 20:159-165 (1986)

35. Luft, D.J., Conley, R., Remington, J.S., Outbreak of central nervous system toxoplasmosis in Western Europe and North America. Lancet 1:781-783 (1983)

36. Roberts, C.J., Coccidioidomycosis in acquired immune deficiency syndrome. Depressed humoral as well as cellular immunity. Am J Med 76:734-736 (1984)

37. Dylewski, J., Chan, S., Merigan, T.C., Absence of detectable IgM antibody during cytomegalovirus disease in patients with AIDS. N Engl J Med 309:493 (1983)

38. Hamaoka, T., Ono, S., Regulation of B-cell differentiation: Interactions of factors and corresponding receptors. Ann Rev Immunol 4:167-204 (1986)

39. Purtilo, D.T., Immune deficiency predisposing to Epstein-Barr virus-induced lymphoproliferative diseases: The X-linked lymphoproliferative syndrome as a model. In: Advances in Cancer Res, Academic Press, New York, NY, Vol 34:279-311 (1981)

40. Metroka, C.E., Cunningham-Rundles, S., Pollack, M.S., et al., Generalized lymphadenopathy in homosexual men. Ann Intern Med 99:585-591 (1983)

41. Abrams, D.I., Lewis, B.J., Beckstead, J.H., et al., Persistent diffuse lymphadenopathy in homosexual men: endpoint or prodrome? Ann Intern Med 100:801-808 (1984)

42. Abrams, D.I., AIDS-related conditions. Clinics Immun Aller 6:581-599 (1986)

43. Andiman, W.A., Eastman, R., Martin, K., et al., Opportunistic lymphoproliferations associated with Epstein-Barr viral DNA in infants and children with AIDS. Lancet 2:1390-1393 (1985)

44. Birx, D.L., Redfield, R.R., Tosato, G., Defective regulation of Epstein-Barr virus infection in patients with acquired immunodeficiency syndrome (AIDS) or AIDS-related disorders. N Engl J Med 314:874-879 (1986)

45. Yarchoan, R., Redfield, R.R., Broder, S., Mechanisms of B cell activation in patients with acquired immunodeficiency syndrome and related disorders. J Clin Invest 78:439-447 (1986)

46. Casareale, D., Sinangil, F., Hedenskog, M., et al., Establishment of retrovirus-, Epstein-Barr virus-positive B-lymphoblastoid cell lines derived from individuals at risk for acquired immune deficiency syndrome (AIDS). AIDS Res 1:253-270 (1984)

47. Lane, H.C., Masur, H., Edgar, L.C., et al., Abnormalities of B-cell activation and immunoregulation in patients with the acquired immunodeficiency syndrome. N Engl J Med 309:453-458 (1983)

48. Doll, D.C., List, A.F., Burkitt's lymphoma in a homosexual. Lancet 1:1026-1027 (1982)

49. Chaganti, R.S.K., Jhanvar, S.C., Koziner, B., et al., Specific translocations characterize Burkitt's like lymphoma of homosexual men with the acquired immunodeficiency syndrome. Blood 61:1269-1272 (1983)

50. Ziegler, J.L., Miner, R.C., Rosenbaum, E., et al., Outbreak of Burkitt's like lymphoma in homosexual men. Lancet 2:631-633 (1982)

51. Levine, A.M., Meyer, P.R., Begandy, M.K., et al., Development of B cell lymphoma in homosexual men. Clinical and immunologic findings. Ann Intern Med 100:7-13 (1984)

52. Groopman, J.E., Sullivan, J.L., Mulder, C., et al., Pathogenesis of B cell lymphoma in a patient with AIDS. Blood 67: 612-615 (1986)

53. Levine, A.M., Gill, P.S., Rasheed, S., AIDS-related malignant B cell lymphomas, In: AIDS--Modern Concepts and Therapeutic Challenges. (Broder, S., ed), Marcel Dekker, Inc., New York & Basel., p 233-243 (1986)

54. Ernberg, I., The role of Epstein-Barr virus in lymphomas of homosexual males. In: Acquired Immunodeficiency Syndrome. (Klein, E., ed), Karger, Basel, p 301-318 (1986)

55. de-The, G., Role of Epstein-Barr virus in human diseases: Infectious mononucleosis, Burkitt's lymphoma, and nasopharyngeal carcinoma. In: Viral Oncology. (Klein, G., ed), Raven Press, New York, p 769-798 (1980)

56. CDC., Revision of the case definition of acquired immunodeficiency syndrome for national reporting - United States. MMWR 34:21-23 (1985)

57. Adams, A., Molecular biology of the Epstein-Barr virus. In: Viral Oncology. (Klein, G., ed), Raven Press, New York, p 683-713 (1980)

58. Henle, W., Henle, G.E., Horwitz, C.A., Epstein-Barr virus specific diagnostic tests in infectious mononucleosis. Hum Pathol 5:551-559 (1974)

59. Pearson, G., Epstein-Barr Virus: Immunology, In: Viral Oncology. (Klein, G., ed), Raven Press, New York, p 739-768 (1980)

60. Rickinson, A.B., Moss, D.J., Wallace, L.E., et al., Long-term T-cell-mediated immunity to Epstein-Barr virus. Cancer Res 41:4216-4221 (1981)

61. Purtilo, D.T., Linder, J., Volsky, D.J., Acquired immune deficiency syndrome (AIDS). Clinics Lab Med 6:3-26 (1986)

62. Klein, G., The role of gene dosage and genetic transpositions in carcinogenesis. Nature 294:313-318 (1981)

63. Battey, J., Moulding, C., Taub, R., et al., The human c-myc oncogene: Structural consequences of translocation into the IgH locus in Burkitt's lymphoma. Cell 34:779-787 (1983)

64. Montagnier, L., Gruest, J., Chamaret, S., et al., Adaption of lymphadenopathy-associated virus (LAV) to replication in EBV-transformed B-lymphoblastoid cell lines. Science 225:63-65 (1984)

65. Pahwa, S., Pahwa, R., Saxinger, C., et al., Influence of the human T-lymphotropic virus/lymphadenopathy-associated virus on functions of human lymphocytes: Evidence for immunosuppressive effects and polyclonal B-cell activation by banded viral preparations. Proc Natl Acad Sci, USA 82:8198-8202 (1985)

66. Pahwa, S., Pahwa, R., Good, R.A., et al., Stimulatory and inhibitory influences of human immunodeficiency virus on normal B lymphocytes. Proc Natl Acad Sci, USA 83:9124-9128 (1986)

67. Schnittman, S.M., Lane, H.C., Higgins, S.E., et al., Direct polyclonal activation of human B lymphocytes by the acquired immune deficiency syndrome virus. Science 233:1084-1086 (1986)

68. Volsky, D.J., Sakai, K., Stevenson, M., et al., Retroviral etiology of the acquired immune deficiency syndrome (AIDS). AIDS Res 2:(Supp. 1)S35-S48 (1986)

69. Weissman, I.C., McGrath, M.S., Retrovirus lymphomagenesis: relationship of normal immune receptors to malignant cell proliferation. Curr Top Microbiol Immunol 98:103-113 (1982)

70. Ihle, J.N., Lee, J.C., Possible immunological mechanisms in C-type viral leukemogenesis in mice. Curr Top Microbiol Immunol 98:58-103 (1982)

71. Laure, F., Zagury, D., Saimot, A.G., et al., Hepatitis B virus DNA sequences in lymphoid cells from patients with AIDS and AIDS-related complex. Science 229:561-563 (1985)

72. Mosca, J.D., Bednarik, D.P., Raj, N.B.K., et al., Nature 325: 67-70 (1987)

73. Gendelman, H.E., Phelps, W., Feigenbaum, L., et al., Trans-activation of the human immunodeficiency virus long terminal repeat sequence by DNA viruses. Proc Natl Acad Sci, USA 83: 9759-9763 (1986)

74. Sodroski, J., Rosen, C., Wong-Staal, F., et al., Trans-acting transcriptional regulation of human T-cell leukemia virus type III long terminal repeat. Science 227:171-173 (1985)

75. Feinberg, M.B., Jarrett, R.F., Aldovini, A., et al., HTLV-III expression and production involve complex regulation at the levels of splicing and translation of viral RNA. Cell 46: 807-817 (1986)

76. Sodroski, J., Goh, W.C., Rosen, C., et al., A second post-transcriptional trans-activator gene required for HTLV-III replication. Nature 321:421-417 (1986)

77. Francioli, P., Clement, F., Vaudois, C.H., B_2-micro-globulin and immunodeficiency in a homosexual man. N Engl J Med 307: 1402-1403 (1982)

78. Euler, H.H., Kern, P., Loffler, H., et al., Precipitable immune complexes in healthy homosexual men, acquired immune deficiency syndrome and related lymphadenopathy syndrome. Clin Exp Immunol 59:267-275 (1985)

79. Lane, H.C., Fauci, A.S., Immunologic aspects of the acquired immunodeficiency syndrome. In: Advances in Host Defense Mechanisms. Acquired Immunodeficiency Syndrome (AIDS). Raven Press, New York, Vol 5, p 131-148 (1985)

80. Katz, B.Z., Andiman, W.A., Eastmon, R., et al., Infection with two genotypes of Epstein-Barr virus in an infant with AIDS and lymphoma of the central nervous system. J Infect Dis 153:601-604 (1986)

81. Schroff, R.W., Gottlieb, M.S., Prince, H.E., et al., Immunological studies of homosexual men with immunodeficiency and Kaposi's sarcoma. Clin Immunol Immunopathol 27:300-314 (1983)

82. Peterson, J.M., Tubbs, R.R., Savage, R.A., et al., Small non-cleaved B cell Burkitt's like lymphoma with chromosome t (8; 14) translocation and Epstein-Barr virus nuclear-associated antigen in a homosexual man with acquired immune deficiency syndrome. Am J Med 78:141-148 (1985)

83. Ioachim, H.L., Cooper, M.C., Lymphomas of AIDS. Lancet 1:96 (1986)

84. Lightfoot, M., Folks, T., Redfield, R., et al., Circulating IgA immune complexes in AIDS. Immunol Invest 14:341-345 (1985)

19
Cellular Cytotoxicity in AIDS

Susanna Cunningham-Rundles

The hallmark of the acquired immunodeficiency syndrome (AIDS) is the loss of cellular immune function (1)-(4). This single characteristic provided the original clue that led to the realization that destruction of the immune system was central to the development and evolution of the various opportunistic infections and tumors that constitute the clinical presentation of AIDS (5).

Impaired cellular immune function was also noted in homosexual patients with generalized lymphadenopathy who lived in endemic regions and shared lifestyle factors with AIDS patients (6),(7). Until the discovery and isolation of the retrovirus associated with AIDS, human T cell lymphotropic virus III/lymphadenopathy-associated virus (HTLV-III/LAV), now known as human immunodeficiency virus (HIV), the relationship between generalized lymphadenopathy, which in appropriate context became known as the lymphadenopathy syndrome (LAS) and true AIDS, was not clear. We and others (8)-(10) postulated a direct connection but had to defer conclusions until patients progressed to AIDS.

The discovery of HIV provided a marker for defining patients with LAS. Over time, now effectively seven years, more than 25% of our patients with LAS have developed AIDS and many more have shown signs of progression within the syndrome, e.g., development of constitutional symptoms. Although studies on the behavior of the retrovirus suggest a very long latency (9)-(12), a very major question is whether or not the condition of HIV infection must, of necessity, lead to the development of AIDS. Since the only apparent requirement for HIV replication is activation of the host cell, it seems unlikely that this could fail to occur except rarely, especially in patients who have the degree of exposure to common infectious agents that characterize patients with LAS.

The appearance of opportunistic infections (13)-(19) and worsening clinical course may be preceded by the development of constitutional systems weeks or months before. In our experience one marker of this process is the presence of serum interferon alpha (IFN-alpha), predominantly, if not exclusively, of the acid labile type (20). The period of time from observation of elevated serum IFN-alpha in patients with LAS to the onset of frank AIDS was three to 18 months. Since patients with AIDS related Kaposi's sarcoma (KS) and patients with AIDS associated opportunistic infections may also have elevated serum IFN-alpha levels similar to that occurring in LAS, a link between IFN-alpha and the onset of AIDS was postulated.

The central question that emerges from these observations is: What determines the critical boundary between LAS and AIDS? The basis for the latency of HIV, if it were clarified, might provide a ground for rational therapy. The studies presented here explore the relationship of cell mediated cytotoxicity to the immunological abnormalities found in AIDS.

LYMPHOCYTE SUBSET ALTERATION AND FUNCTIONAL IMMUNE RESPONSE

Infection and replication of HIV within the helper/inducer T lymphocyte, the $T4^+$ subset, seems to occur in most, although not all, patients significantly exposed to HIV, and is probably absolutely essential for the development of antibodies to the retrovirus. In a recent study of 12 patients with thalassemia evaluated for potential HIV infection, three were found to have an inverted $T4^+/T8^+$ ratio and all three, but none of the other nine, had antibodies to HIV. In these cases, the $T4^+$ percentage was in the low normal range (Table 1). The percentage of cytotoxic/suppressor T lymphocytes ($T8^+$) was not actually elevated with respect to the normal range but was greater than that of the $T4^+$ cells so that an inverted ratio was obtained. In full blown AIDS, the absolute numbers of total lymphocytes and lymphocyte subsets are reduced, but the relative proportions of the $T4^+$ and $T8^+$ positive T lymphocyte subsets tend to balance out roughly so that the percentage of $T3^+$ cells (total T-cells) observed does not show significant alteration from normal. These data are shown in Figure 1 for patients with AIDS and healthy controls. The decline of the $T4^+$ population in AIDS is reflected in diminished lymphocyte proliferative response. Increase in the relative proportion of the $T8^+$ population could potentially result in enhanced suppressor cell activity, increased natural killer (NK) activity, or in proliferation of cells unable to mediate normal function as a consequence of altered immunoregulation. However, AIDS patients and patients with LAS have normal (not enhanced or reduced) expansion of Con A induced suppressor cells in vitro (21), suggesting that this suppressor cell popula-

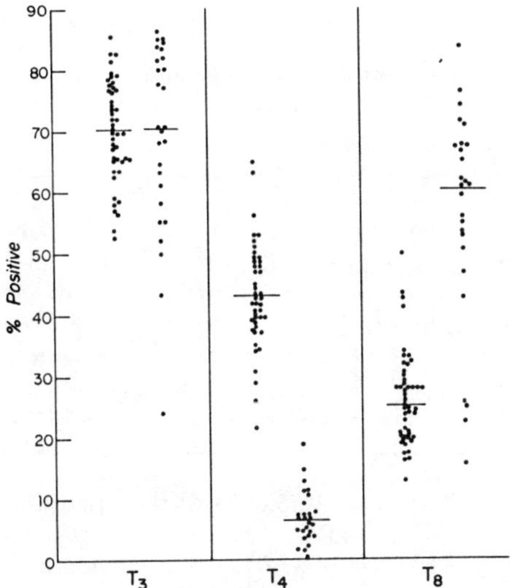

Figure 1. Relative proportions of T lymphocytes in controls (left hand column of each panel) and AIDS patients (right hand column of each panel). Data were obtained by flow cytometry with monoclonal antibodies. Horizontal lines indicate median.

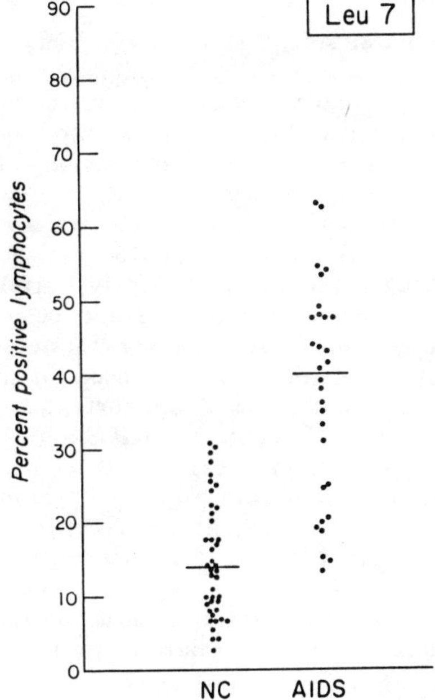

Figure 2. Increase of Leu 7^+ lymphocyte subpopulation in AIDS. Data show controls (NC) and AIDS patients. The percentage of Leu 7^+ cells was determined by flow cytometry. Horizontal lines indicate median.

Table 1. T Lymphocyte Subsets and Natural Killer Function in Transfusion Associated HIV Disease

Case	Percent Positive*			Ratio	Endogenous NK**
	$T3^+$	$T4^+$	$T8^+$	$T4^+/T8^+$	E:T 100:1
1	56.5	22.1	27.8	0.79	3.9
2	70.8	24.1	32.2	0.75	4.9
3	64.8	22.7	33.8	0.67	4.1

* Normal ranges: $T3^+$ (n=45) 53.0% - 85.0%, median = 70.0%
$T4^+$ (n=45) 21.5% - 65.0%, median = 42.0%
$T8^+$ (n=45) 13.0% - 50.5%, median = 25.0%

** Endogenous NK: Percent specific release following four hour assay against K562, normal range (n=90) 15.3% - 78.0%, median = 32.5%.

tion is not disproportionately activated. In addition, Birx et al. (22) have shown that in AIDS T cell suppression of Epstein-Barr virus (EBV) is virtually absent in vitro. Since essentially all homosexual patients with AIDS have antibodies to EBV, this is a highly relevant observation. Thus, expansion of the T suppressor cell population per se in AIDS seems unlikely.

The case for cytotoxic effector cell expansion would seem more likely since even in very ill AIDS patients for whom the clinical impression suggests an imminently fatal outcome, endogenous NK activity against the K562 target cell may be detected in vitro. We have used the Leu 7 marker to determine whether or not the NK population might be increased disproportionately in AIDS. The data shown in Figure 2 support the possibility of enhanced expression of Leu 7^+ cells in AIDS. The data show an increased percentage of cells bearing the Leu 7^+ phenotype. This increase was independent of absolute lymphocyte count and was not correlated with it. In healthy controls the percentage of Leu 7^+ cells ranged from 5% to 32% with a median of 16% of total lymphocytes. In contrast, 16 of 27 AIDS patients had a percentage of Leu 7^+ cells greater than 35%. This surface marker analysis suggests that the relative proportion of NK cells is increased in AIDS.

NATURAL KILLER ACTIVITY IN AIDS

NK activity is known to be an endogenous property of unstimulated lymphocytes, which is expressed as lysis of appropriate target cells bearing a broad range of foreign cell surface antigens of bacterial, viral or tumor origin. The potential role of this system in host defense in AIDS is of interest. In the system used for our investigations, lymphocytes are isolated and concentrated to measure intrinsic functional activity. The signaling system which regulates NK activity is known to involve interferon which is also made and secreted by the large granular NK cell. NK activity is thus self-regulating (although other cell types and other mediators may offset or counterbalance this effect). Since IFN-alpha is present in serum in LAS prior to the onset of AIDS, and can also be demonstrated in frank AIDS, it seemed possible that this substance might drive NK amplification and expansion. We had previously observed that acid labile IFN-alpha would augment NK activity of lymphocytes of healthy persons in vitro (23). Furthermore, Biron et al. reported that IFN's-alpha, beta, and gamma induce blastogenesis of NK cells in vivo in a mouse model (24). In addition to analyzing baseline endogenous NK activity, experiments attempting to amplify NK in vitro using recombinant interferon-alpha (IFN-r-alpha) were also carried out. The results of these experiments are summarized in Figure 3. NK cells from the AIDS patient population showed marked variation in individual cytotoxicity. Median cytotoxicity of the AIDS patient group was 16% with a range of 5.6% to 51.8%, and 11 patients (44%) had activity below 15%. In contrast, normal control killing always exceeded 15% and the median cytotoxicity was 32.5%, with a range of 15.3% to 78.0%. Addition of IFN-r-alpha to patient lymphocytes in vitro produced little effect, whereas among controls, the median was increased to 48% with a range of 24% to 81.2%. These observations are consistent with the hypothesis that the NK system in AIDS is in an "exhausted" or refractory state possibly as a result of prior activation early in the course of HIV disease.

Study of patients with LAS and less severely ill AIDS patients with KS has shown that refractory response to IFN-r-alpha in vitro is not a characteristic only of individuals with poor endogenous activity but can be marked in patients with normal endogenous function as well. Representative data are shown in Table 2.

The data suggest a different level of regulational defect than that reflected in direct assay against the target. It is possible that the development of refractory response to IFN-alpha in vitro reflects the end stage of a process that occurred in vivo and which may have been mediated by physiological IFN.

MODULATION OF CYTOTOXICITY IN AIDS

As discussed above, response to NK inducers in vitro may be absent in the presence of normal endogenous activity. In a trial of IFN-r-alpha in vivo in AIDS patients with KS, we observed that the patients who showed enhanced NK activity in vivo post therapy had also been able to show an enhanced response in vitro prether-

Table 2. Relative Augmentation of NK Activity In Vitro by IFN-r-alpha in LAS and AIDS-KS

Case	Endogenous NK*			IFN-r-alpha Augmented NK**		
	100:1	50:1	25:1	100:1	50:1	25:1
1-LAS	10.1	4.8	4.7	8.4	7.5	5.7
2-LAS	67.9	54.9	43.5	69.5	65.1	53.1
3-LAS	8.5	2.7	3.0	11.7	6.2	6.5
4-LAS	7.1	2.5	2.0	20.6	9.9	9.2
5-LAS	23.3	13.0	7.7	30.3	23.9	14.3
6-KS	19.8	9.5	5.8	33.1	27.9	16.2

* Against K562 at effector:target ratios as shown.
** As above with 800 I.U. IFN-r-alpha.

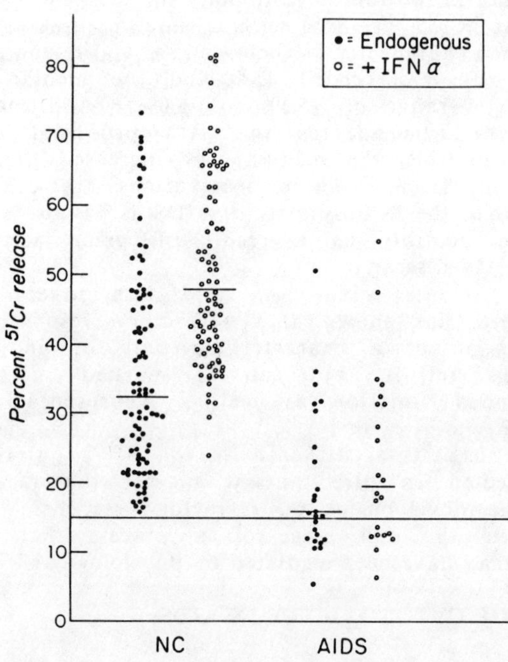

Figure 3. Natural killer activity against the K562 tumor target in AIDS. Data are given as percent ^{51}Cr release (cytotoxicity) following four hour Cr release assay in the presence and absence of 800 I.U. IFN-r-alpha in vitro. Short horizontal lines indicate median.

apy, but that the converse was untrue. Some patients who had NK augmentation in vitro did not respond in vivo (25). Retrospective analysis of immune response to IFN-r-alpha treatment, showed that patients who had a better response to lymphocyte activators in vitro and did not have detectable serum levels of IFN-alpha, clinically responded to therapy more frequently, and survived longer than did patients with poorer response in vitro and with detectable levels of serum IFN-alpha. Furthermore, the group with better immune function in vitro was much less likely to develop opportunistic infections. These data suggest that residual immune response and regulatory state of the NK/interferon system might be a critical factor in the evolution of AIDS as well as have prognostic implications in fully established disease (26), (27).

Restoration of immune function in vitro in AIDS was undertaken using a chemical immunomodulator, CL246,738, 3,6-bis (2-piperidinoethoxy) acridine trihydrochloride (American Cyanamid, Lederle Laboratories Division), in an effort to assess its potential use in vivo. Previous studies (28) had suggested a potential for this drug in enhancing immune function of lymphocytes in vitro. Initial studies were undertaken using preculture of mononuclear cells from patients with HIV infection with different concentrations of CL246 for 18 hours, followed by washing and assay against the K562 target. Data from a representative experiment are shown in Figure 4. As shown, augmentation with CL246 was achieved with concentrations less than 0.1 ug/ml. Following these and other studies, a Phase I trial with AIDS patients was undertaken. Although no definable clinical benefits were obtained, there was a marked effect on the NK system in more than 50% of the patients. One such example, for a patient who received 3 mg/kg in a single dose, is shown in Figure 5. Initially, endogenous NK activity was at the borderline of normal and showed marked augmentation by day 14. By day 28 post administration, decline in activity to baseline was seen. In the patient group as a whole, increased activity was seen 21 to 28 days following therapy. Increase in Leu 7^+ cells was also observed in most patients but this finding could not be correlated with enhanced NK activity. Interferon-alpha was detected in serum following CL246, suggesting that CL246 is an interferon inducer as previously suggested in animal model studies. Overall response of NK activity to IFN in vitro did not change in the patient group after CL246 therapy, probably because all patients had advanced disease.

CONCLUSION

The expression of cytotoxicity as indicated by NK function in AIDS suggests that down regulation and the development of a refractory state may occur relatively early in HIV infection. Expansion of cytotoxic function may be possible experimentally in vivo as well as in vitro using signals that can work beneficially with preexisting signals. These studies and others (29)-(31) support the concept that biological response modulation may be

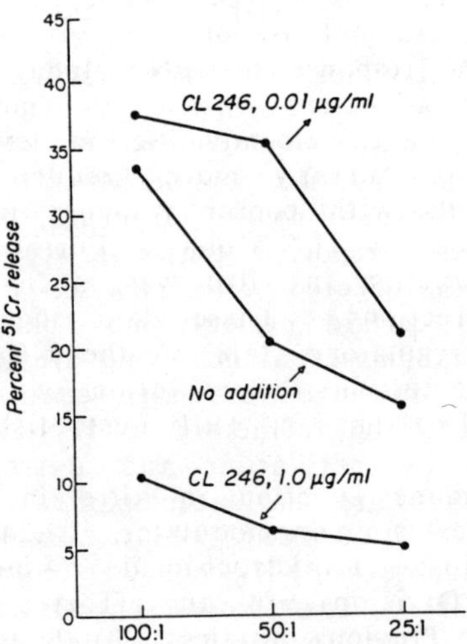

Figure 4. Effect of CL246 in vitro on NK activity. Data are given as percent ^{51}Cr release (vertical axis) at three effector: target ratios (horizontal axis). Experiments with CL246 reflect preculture followed by washing prior to assay.

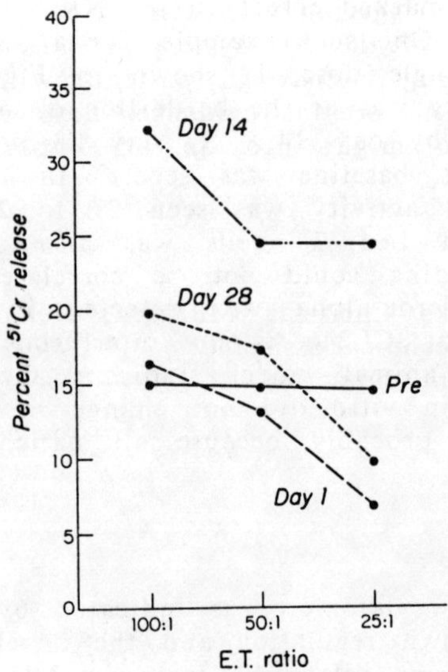

Figure 5. Endogenous NK activity in vitro following CL246 in vivo in an AIDS patient. Data are shown as percent cytotoxicity against K562 at three effector-target (ET) ratios.

possible in AIDS through the deliberate triggering of cells that are both intrinsically more resistant to the virus and can mediate host defense activities, perhaps acting directly against virus infected cells to reduce viral burden.

AIDS provides a unique opportunity to assess the potential role of the NK system and its possible interaction with specific cytotoxic T cells in responding to internal challenge (32),(33). Ruscetti et al. (32) have reported that NK cells are capable of in vitro lysis of HIV-infected cells. If so, the NK activation which is conserved in certain patients may be prognostically significant. Asymptomatic homosexual men who are HIV antibody positive are often observed to have very high endogenous NK activity, and at the same time, to be refractory to IFN-alpha augmentation in vitro, suggesting NK activation and dysregulation in early disease. These changes are not accompanied by loss of cells bearing markers for Leu 7 or Leu 11 (34). Evidence for defective release of cytolytic factors by NK cells has come from the work of Bonavida et al. (35). This work suggests that intrinsic alteration of NK cells is an important feature of AIDS. Several investigators (31),(33),(34) have reported NK activation in vitro in AIDS with interleukin-2 (IL-2). These reports suggest that regulatory defects rather than deficient cell numbers are associated with cytotoxic effector deficiency in AIDS. Interferon-alpha treatment of AIDS patients has been accompanied by increased NK activity. Similarly, in vivo IL-2 therapy has resulted in augmented NK activity (36),(37). The relationship of this augmentation to gamma IFN production remains unclear although in vitro studies (31) suggest that activation could occur through an interferon independent triggering mechanism.

The ultimate role of the NK system in AIDS development or in its potential to prolong latency in patients with HIV disease is unknown. In light of present evidence, however, it seems likely that the NK system might provide an important resource for modulation and therapy.

ACKNOWLEDGMENT

The author thanks Christina Millburn, Helen Link, and Kim Sokolski for excellent technical assistance.

These studies were supported by New York State AR163 and GMHC, New York.

REFERENCES

1. Gottlieb, M.S., Schroff, R., Schanker, H.M., et al., *Pneumocystis carinii* pneumonia and mucosal candidiasis in previously healthy homosexual men: Evidence of a new acquired cellular immunodeficiency. N Engl J Med 305:1425-1431 (1981)

2. Masur, H., Michelis, M.A., Greene, J.B., et al., A community acquired outbreak of *Pneumocystis carinii* pneumonia: initial manifestation of cellular immune dysfunction. N Engl J Med 305:1431-1438 (1981)

3. Siegal, F.P., Lopez, C., Hammer, G.S., et al., Severe acquired immunodeficiency in male homosexuals manifested by chronic perianal ulcerative *Herpes simplex* lesions. N Engl J Med 305:1439-1444 (1981)

4. Masur, H., Michelis, M.A., Wormser, G.P., et al., Previously healthy women with opportunistic infection as the initial manifestation of a community acquired cellular immunodeficiency. Ann Intern Med 97:533-539 (1982)

5. Gallo, R.C., Sarin, P.S., Gelmann, E.P., et al., Isolation of human T-cell leukemia virus in acquired immune deficiency syndrome (AIDS). Science 220:865-867 (1983)

6. Stahl, R.E., Friedman-Kien, A., Dubin, R., et al., Immunologic abnormalities in homosexual men. Relationship to Kaposi's sarcoma. Am J Med 73:171-178 (1982)

7. CDC., Diffuse, undifferentiated non-Hodgkin's lymphoma among homosexual men. MMWR 31:277-279 (1982)

8. Ziegler, J.L., Drew, W.L., Miner, R.C., Outbreak of Burkitt's like lymphoma in homosexual men. Lancet 2:261-263 (1982)

9. Metroka, C.E., Cunningham-Rundles, S., Pollack, M.S., et al., Generalized lymphadenopathy in homosexual men. Ann Intern Med 99:585-591 (1982)

10. Guarda, L.A., Butler, J.J., Mansell, P., et al., Lymphadenopathy in homosexual men. Morbid anatomy with clinical and immunologic correlations. Am J Clin Pathol 79(5):559-568 (1983)

11. Pinching, A.J., McManus, T.J., Jeffries, D.J., et al., Studies of cellular immunity in male homosexuals in London. Lancet 2:126-130 (1983)

12. Abrams, D.I., Lewis, B.J., Volberding, P.I., Lymphadenopathy: Endpoint or prodrome? Update of a 24-month prospective study. Ann NY Acad Sci 137:207-215 (1984)

13. Roberts, C.J., Coccidioidomycosis in acquired immune deficiency syndrome. Depressed humoral as well as cellular immunity. Am J Med 76(4):734-736 (1984)

14. Vieira, J., Frank, E., Spira, R.J., et al., Acquired immune deficiency in Haitians: opportunistic infections in previously healthy Haitians. N Engl J Med 308:125-129 (1983)

15. Elliott, J.H., Hoppes, S.L., Platt, M.S., The acquired immunodeficiency syndrome and *Mycobacterium avium-intracellulare* bacteremia, in a patient with hemophilia. Ann Intern Med 98:290-293 (1983)

16. Greene, J.B., Sidhu, G.S., Lewin, S., et al., *Mycobacterium avium-intracellulare*: a cause of disseminated life-threatening infection in homosexuals and drug abusers. Ann Intern Med 97(4):539-546 (1982)

17. Jaffe, H.W., Choi, K., Thomas, P.A., et al., National case-control study of Kaposi's sarcoma and *Pneumocystis carinii* pneumonia in homosexual men: Part 1. Epidemiologic results. Ann Intern Med 99:145-151 (1983)

18. Small, C.B., Klein, R.S., Friedland, G.H., et al., Community-acquired opportunistic infections and defective cellular immunity in heterosexual drug abusers and homosexual men. Am J Med 74:433-441 (1983)

19. Poon, M.C., Landay, A., Prasthofer, E.F., et al., Acquired immunodeficiency syndrome with *Pneumocystis carinii* pneumonia and *Mycobacterium avium-intracellulare* infection in a previously healthy patient with classic hemophilia. Clinical, immunologic, and virologic findings. Ann Intern Med 98: 287-290 (1983)

20. Metroka, C.E., Sonnabend, J.A., Cunningham-Rundles, S., et al., Acid labile interferon-alpha in homosexual men: A preclinical marker for opportunistic infection. (Manuscript submitted)

21. Cunningham-Rundles, S., Safai, B., Metroka, C., et al., Lymphocyte effector function in vitro in the acquired immune deficiency syndrome. In: AIDS: The Epidemic of Kaposi's Sarcoma and Opportunistic Infections. (Friedman-Kien, A.E., Laubenstein, L.J., eds), Masson, New York, p 153-159 (1984)

22. Birx, D.L., Redfield, R.R., Tosato, G., Defective regulation of Epstein-Barr virus infection in patients with acquired immunodeficiency syndrome (AIDS) or AIDS-related disorders. N Engl J Med 314:874-879 (1986)

23. Cunningham-Rundles, S., Analysis of mechanisms of immune suppression in the acquired immune deficiency syndrome. In: The Acquired Immune Deficiency Syndrome and Infections of Homosexual Men. (Ma, P., Armstrong, D., eds), Yorke Medical Books, NY (In press)

24. Biron, C.A., Sonnenfeld, G., Welsh, R.M., Interferon induces natural killer cell blastogenesis in vivo. J Leuk Biol 35: 31-37 (1984)

25. Krown, S.W., Real, F.Y., Cunningham-Rundles, S., et al., Preliminary observations on the effect of recombinant leukocyte alpha interferon in homosexual men with Kaposi's sarcoma. N Engl J Med 308:1071-1076 (1983)

26. Vodhan-Raj, S., Wong, G., Grecco, C., et al., Immunological variables as predictors of prognosis in patients with Kaposi's sarcoma and the acquired immunodeficiency syndrome. Cancer Res 46:417-425 (1986)

27. Krown, S.E., Real, F.Y., Vadhan-Raj, S., et al., Kaposi's sarcoma and the acquired immune deficiency syndrome. Cancer 57:1662-1665 (1986)

28. Cunningham-Rundles, S., Metroka, C., Schneider, J., et al., Immune deregulation in the lymphadenopathy syndrome. Serono Symposium, Recent Advances in Primary and Acquired Immunodeficiency Disease (Aviti, F., ed.), Raven Press, NY. p 257-267 (1985)

29. Prince, H.E., Kermani-Arab, A., Fahey, J.L., Depressed interleukin-2 receptor expression in acquired immune deficiency and lymphadenopathy syndromes. J Immunol 133:1313-1317 (1984)

30. Cunningham-Rundles, S., Metroka, C.E., Safai, B., et al., Cytotoxic effector mechanisms in AIDS. In: AIDS-Associated Syndromes. (Gupta, S., ed), Plenum, New York, p 97-110 (1985)

31. Rook, A.H., Hooks, J.J., Quinnan, G.V., et al., Interleukin 2 enhances the natural killer cell activity of acquired immunodeficiency syndrome patients through a gamma interferon independent mechanism. J Immunol 134:1504-1507 (1985)

32. Ruscetti, F.W., Mikovits, J.A., Kalyanaraman, V.S., et al., Analysis of effector mechanisms against HTLV-I and HTLV-III/LAV infected lymphoid cells. J Immunol 136:3619-3624 (1986)

33. Creemers, P.C., Stark, D.F., Boyko, W.J., Evaluation of natural killer cell activity in patients with persistent generalized lymphadenopathy and acquired immunodeficiency syndrome. Clin Immunol Immunpathol 36:141-150 (1985)

34. Wright, S.C., Role of natural killer cytotoxic factors in the mechanism of target cell killing by natural killer cells. J Clin Immunol 6:1-8 (1986)

35. Reddy, M., Pinyavat, N., Grieco, M.H., Interleukin-2 augmentation of natural killer cell activity in homosexual men with acquired immune deficiency syndrome. Infect Immun 44:339-343 (1984)

36. Lotze, M.T., Frana, L.W., Sharrow, S.O., et al., In vivo administration of purified human interleukin-1. I. Half-life and immunologic effects of the jurkat cell line derived interleukin-2. J Immunol 134:157-166 (1985)

37. Ernst, M., Korn, P., Flad, H.D., et al., Effects of systemic in vivo interleukin-2 (IL-2) reconstitution in patients with acquired immune deficiency syndrome (AIDS) and AIDS related complex (ARC) in phenotypes and functions of peripheral blood mononuclear cells. J Clin Immunol 6:170-181 (1986)

20
Serological Factors in the Pathogenesis of AIDS

Linda E. Miller, Anne K. Hennig, Patricia A. John, Bruce E. Kloster, Russell H. Tomar

The frequency of exposure to human immunodeficiency virus (HIV) has been high in groups known to be at increased risk for developing the acquired immune deficiency syndrome (AIDS) (1). Furthermore, it has been estimated that 1-2% of individuals in the United States who are currently infected with this virus will progress within one year to develop AIDS (1).

To date, no prognostic marker is available to identify those individuals infected with HIV who will ultimately develop AIDS (2),(3). Those clinical observations or laboratory measurements with some predictive value (for example, follicular involution in lymph nodes, oral candidiasis, herpes zoster, hypocholesterolemia, lymphopenia, or reversal of the T4/T8 ratio) do not have satisfactory reliability and/or do not detect changes early enough to be useful as prognostic markers (2)-(7). A reliable prognostic sign would be valuable in determining when a therapeutic protocol should be initiated and who should receive it, since all current treatment regimens are experimental and pose variable and often unknown risks to subjects.

To this end, we have been studying various factors present in the sera of AIDS patients and some individuals at risk for developing AIDS. These serological factors appear to precede the development of AIDS and may possibly contribute to the pathogenesis of this disease. In this chapter, the following topics will be discussed: (a) anti-lymphocyte antibodies (ALA), (b) serum inhibitory factors, and (c) paraproteins.

ANTI-LYMPHOCYTE ANTIBODIES (ALA)

In 1981, we found that sera from our first three AIDS patients contained antibodies which were cytotoxic to lymphocytes (8). These antibodies were demonstrated with a modified microcytotoxicity assay using normal human peripheral blood lymphocytes as targets (8). Subsequently, in a blinded study, coded serum samples from 10 AIDS patients, five presumably healthy heterosexual females, five presumably healthy heterosexual males, and five presumably healthy homosexual males submitted by the Centers for Disease Control were evaluated. Of the 10 AIDS samples, nine were positive or suspicious for the presence of anti-lymphocyte antibodies, while none of the heterosexual controls was positive (8). Three of the homosexual male "controls" had positive or suspicious results. Two of these individuals were available for follow-up. One was later found to have an inverted T4/T8 ratio, and decreased in vitro lymphocyte proliferation to four of five antigens tested. The other individual had a normal T4/T8 ratio, but developed generalized lymphadenopathy and had decreased in vitro lymphocyte proliferation to four of four antigens tested.

An indirect immunofluorescence assay was developed later and proved to be more sensitive in detection of ALA (9). Briefly, normal human peripheral blood lymphocytes are incubated with a 1:4 dilution of patient serum, washed, incubated with a fluorescein-conjugated $F(ab^1)_2$ goat-anti-human-immunoglobulin, and washed again. Fluorescence was measured by flow cytometry. As shown in Figure 1, ALA are present in most AIDS patients and in some lymphadenopathy syndrome (LAS) patients when tested by this method. Additional experiments using lymphocyte targets from a number of different donors in both the immunofluorescence and the microcytotoxicity assays for ALA have indicated that these antibodies are not directed against HLA antigens or sex-linked determinants (8) (9).

Since the T4(+) subset of T lymphocytes is preferentially decreased in AIDS patients, we examined whether the ALA were specifically directed against this lymphocyte subset (9). Patients' sera were incubated with normal human peripheral blood lymphocytes, and screened for ALA using a double label immunofluorescence assay. The assay employed a phycoerythrin-conjugated anti-Leu3a antibody to detect T4(+) lymphocytes, and a fluorescein-conjugated goat $F(ab^1)_2$ anti-human immunoglobulin to detect cell-bound ALA. As shown in Table 1, two of the AIDS/LAS patients tested possessed antibodies directed selectively against Leu3a(+) cells, while sera from six of the patients contained reactivity against both Leu3a(+) and Leu3a(-) cells.

In order to elucidate further the cell specificity of the ALA, a number of well-characterized continuous cell lines were used as targets in the single label immunofluorescence assay described above (9). The targets used were the T cell lines: MOLT-4, GM3639, and Hut 78; the B cell line, GM 3638; the human T-cell lymphotropic virus I (HTLV-I)-infected T cell line, Hut

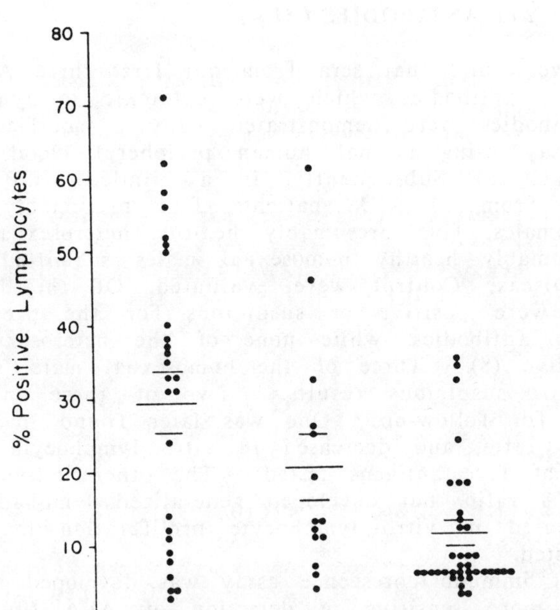

Figure 1. Mononuclear cells obtained from laboratory personnel were separated on a Ficoll-Hypaque gradient and reacted with sera from AIDS or LAS patients or controls. After appropriate incubation and washes, the cells were then reacted with fluorescein-labeled goat anti-human immunoglobulin. Each point represents the percentage of fluorescent-positive cells incubated with serum from a different individual. (Reprinted with permission from ref. 9)

102B2; and the Epstein-Barr virus (EBV)-transformed B cell line WEB-B. Antibody titers from individual AIDS and LAS patients against these cell lines are shown in Table 2.

Nine of 16 AIDS patients and five of the 10 LAS patients tested gave positive results with the Hut 102B2 cell line, most likely due to cross-reactivity with HIV antigens (10)-(12). Sera from seven of the 16 AIDS patients (44%) and six of the 10 LAS patients (60%) demonstrated reactivity against one or more non-HTLV-infected cell lines. The cellular specificity of the ALA appeared to be broad, since different patterns of reactivity were demonstrated by individual sera, some of which reacted against both T and B cell lines, some against T cells only, and some against B cells only.

Our results are in agreement with those of Williams et al. (13) and Pruzanski et al. (14), who demonstrated the presence of ALA in AIDS patients with reactivity against both T and B lymphocytes. In contrast, other laboratories have found that AIDS

Table 1. Double Labeling of Cells with Phycoerythrin-Conjugated anti-Leu 3a and Fluorescein-Conjugated Goat Anti-Human Immunoglobulin (Ig)

Percentage of cells in each patient sample.

Sera	Leu 3a+		Leu 3a-		ALA detected[a]
Controls	Ig-	Ig+	Ig-	Ig+	
1	26	2	49	21	-
2	25	2	50	21	-
3	24	2.5	49	22	-
4	23	2.5	51	21	-
5	26	2	49	20	-
Mean±SD	24.8±1.3	2.2±0.3	49.6±0.9	21±0.78	-
AIDS					
6	25	3.3*	49.5	20	Leu 3a+ only
7	26	8*	43*	22	Leu 3a+ only
8	21	4*	49	24*	Leu 3a+ & Leu 3a-
9	24	5*	42*	27*	Leu 3a+ & Leu 3a-
10	21	12*	33*	34*	Leu 3a+ & Leu 3a-
LAS					
11	21	13*	33*	32*	Leu 3a+ & Leu 3a-
12	18*	13*	37*	31*	Leu 3a+ & Leu 3a-
13	22	7*	45*	24*	Leu 3a+ & Leu 3a-
14	23	2	52	20	None detected

a Cell populations with surface-bound anti-lymphocyte antibodies (ALA) were determined to be those groups of Ig+ cells whose percentages were significantly greater than the mean of the values from the corresponding control group.

* ≥ 3 S.D. from mean of controls

(Reprinted with permission from ref. 9)

patients have antibodies which react with T cells only (15)-(17). Clearly, further studies need to be performed in order to obtain a more complete understanding of specificity of these antibodies.

The significance of ALA is unknown. Antibodies to lymphocytes have been noted in many disease states. ALA's have been observed transiently during viral infections, with a concurrent decrease in T cell numbers, which then return to normal during patient recovery (18). ALA with specificity directed against T cell subsets have been detected in sera of patients with juvenile rheumatoid arthritis (19), and ALA capable of reacting with both T and

Table 2. Antibody Titers of AIDS and LAS Patients Against Cell Lines[a]

			HTLV-I+	T Cell Lines			B Cell Lines	
No.	DX	Risk	Hut 102	Hut 78	MOLT-4	GM3639	GM3638	WEB-B
1	AIDS	Transfusion	40 [b]	10	10	< 10	< 10	10
2	AIDS	Homosexual	≥ 80 [b]	40	10	< 10	10	20
3	AIDS	Homosexual	≥ 80 [b]	20	10	20 [b]	10	20
4	AIDS	Homosexual	20	40	10	10	20	10
5	AIDS	Homosexual	< 10	20	< 10	10	< 10	< 10
6	AIDS	Homosexual	20	10	10	40 [b]	≥ 80 [b]	20
7	AIDS	Homosexual	20	20	20	< 10	40 [b]	10
8	AIDS	Homosexual	10	< 10	< 10	< 10	10	10
9	AIDS	Homosexual	20	< 10	20	< 10	10	10
10	AIDS	IV Drug	≥ 80 [b]	20	< 10	20 [b]	10	20
11	AIDS	IV Drug	40 [b]	< 10	≥ 80 [b]	< 10	10	20
12	AIDS	IV Drug	20	< 10	< 10	10	10	20
13	AIDS	IV Drug	≥ 80 [b]	20	≥ 80 [b]	≥ 80 [b]	20	≥ 80 [b]
14	AIDS	IV Drug	≥ 80 [b]	40	20	10	10	< 10
15	AIDS	IV Drug	≥ 80 [b]	< 10	20	< 10	10	20
16	AIDS	IV Drug	≥ 80 [b]	≥ 80 [b]	< 10	< 10	20	20
17	LAS	Homosexual	10	10	< 10	< 10	< 10	10
18	LAS	Homosexual	20	10	< 10	< 10	20	20
19	LAS	Homosexual	10	≥ 80 [b]	10	< 10	20	10
20	LAS	Homosexual	10	10	20	20 [b]	≥ 80 [b]	20
21	LAS	Homosexual	10	10	< 10	< 10	10	20
22	LAS	Homosexual	≥ 80 [b]	40	< 10	20 [b]	20	20
23	LAS	IV Drug	≥ 80 [b]	40	20	≥ 80 [b]	≥ 80 [b]	≥ 80 [b]
24	LAS	IV Drug	40 [b]	10	< 10	< 10	10	20
25	LAS	IV Drug	≥ 80 [b]	20	20	< 10	≥ 80 [b]	40 [b]
26	LAS	Hemophiliac	≥ 80 [b]	10	40 [b]	< 10	40 [b]	≥ 80 [b]
Range of Controls (n=21)			(<10-20)	(<10-40)	(<10-20)	(<10-10)	(<10-20)	(<10-20)

a Expressed as reciprocal of last serum dilution showing positive fluorescence.

HUT 102B2 = T4+, Leu 1+, Ia+, Tac+, T11±, T3-, T8-, T6-, B1-, SIg-;
HUT 78 = T3+, T4+, B1±, T8-, T6-, T11-, Tac-;
MOLT 4 = T8+, T6+, T4±, T11±, T3-, B1-, Ia-, Tac-;
GM 3639 = Leu 1+, T3-, T4-, T8-, T6-, B1-, Ia-, Tac-;
GM 3638 = B1+, SIg+, Ia+, T3-;
WEB-B = B1+, SIg+, Ia±, T3-, Tac-.

b Beyond range of controls for target cell line.

(Reprinted with permission from ref. 9)

B cells have been found in sera of patients with systemic lupus erythematosus (20),(21). Both of these diseases are characterized by defects in immune regulation, and it is possible that ALA may contribute to these abnormalities by reacting with specific lymphocyte subsets. On the other hand, it has been speculated that ALA may be produced as a result of a breakdown in immunoregulatory mechanisms (22).

These speculations might also be applied to the ALA observed in AIDS. If, as our findings suggest, there are multiple antibodies produced against a variety of antigens, this would suggest the existence of a generalized immunoregulatory defect, which would likely be a secondary phenomenon associated with primary HIV infection. The hypergammaglobulinemia seen in AIDS, as well as the B cell unresponsiveness to specific antigens (23), may be manifestations of such an alteration in immunoregulation. B cell function in this disease might be affected directly, as suggested by the work of others on T-cell independent B-cell activation (24)-(27) or indirectly, through control of B cell activation by T cells (28) . If the ALA in AIDS prove to be specifically directed against immunoregulatory lymphocyte subsets, this would suggest the possibility of involvement of ALA in the pathogenesis of this disease.

SERUM INHIBITORY FACTORS

Sera or plasma from AIDS patients have been reported to contain inhibitory activity against mitogen- or alloantigen-induced lymphocyte proliferation (29)-(33). Our laboratory has shown that sera from AIDS patients inhibit in vitro proliferation of normal peripheral blood lymphocytes in response to the mitogen, phytohemagglutinin (PHA) (29),(30). This inhibitory effect was evident when sera were added as late as 18 hours after culture initiation, and could be diluted, but not overcome, by mixing AIDS and control sera. Consistent results were obtained when sera were tested with lymphocytes from a number of different donors, indicating that inhibition was not dependent on a donor-related property of normal lymphocytes. The amount of inhibition demonstrated was found to depend on the serum/cell ratio and the amount of mitogen used in culture. Figure 2 illustrates this inhibitory effect of AIDS sera.

Our laboratory has also observed inhibition with sera from approximately 40% of LAS patients and 30% of hemophiliac patients, two of whom later developed AIDS. Thus, while serum inhibitory factors may be secondary to AIDS, these findings suggest that serum inhibition may precede or even participate in the development of the fully expressed disease. It is possible that serum inhibitory factors may contribute to the decreased responsiveness of lymphoid cells to a variety of immunologic stimuli, as well as to the lymphopenia seen in AIDS patients. The latter concept is supported by results from experiments designed to remove serum inhibitory activity by plasmapheresis (29),(34). As seen in Figure 3, plasmapheresis on one AIDS patient decreased serum inhibitory activity. Two weeks following pheresis, serum

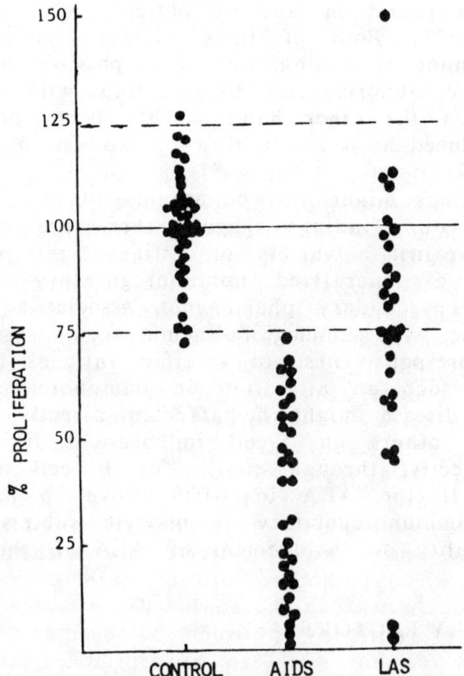

Figure 2. Effect of serum from AIDS or LAS patients on the proliferation of normal peripheral blood mononuclear cells stimulated with PHA. Cultures of 4 x 10^5 cells were incubated with 12.5% serum from normal controls or patients with AIDS or LAS, and stimulated with 25 ug/ml PHA. The mean of the net cpm of cultures with control sera represents 100% normal proliferation. The range of the control values is equal to 100% ± 2 SD of the mean. Each point represents the percentage of proliferation of cultures containing serum from one control, AIDS patient, or LAS patient.

inhibitory activity returned to the pre-pheresis level. Concomitant with the decrease in serum inhibitory activity was an increase in circulating T4 lymphocytes, which fell to pre-pheresis levels as the serum inhibition increased. These observations suggested that the pheresis procedure had removed a factor which played an etiologic role in the T4 lymphopenia (29),(34).

While the identity of the serum factor(s) responsible for the inhibitory activity is not known, several possibilities may be proposed. Laurence et al. have described a suppressor factor produced during a 48-hour culture of peripheral blood mononuclear cells from AIDS patients in the absence of mitogens (35). This factor inhibited T cell proliferation in response to pokeweed mitogen. These findings were extended by Laurence and Mayer (36), who used T cells from an AIDS patient to produce hybridomas which secreted factors suppressing pokeweed mitogen-driven immunoglobulin production. The suppression observed was not directly related to HIV virion production by the hybridoma lines (36). It is possible that the factor(s) we have found bear some similarities to those studied by Laurence and his colleagues.

Alternatively, the phenomenon of serum inhibition seen in AIDS patients may involve viral antigens. Inhibitory effects have been reported for an envelope protein from the feline leukemia virus (FeLV), which causes disorders with similarities to AIDS in cats (37)-(39). Studies have shown that serum from FeLV-infected cats contains a viral protein, p15E, which inhibits lymphocyte function (37)-(39). Preparations derived from a number of other retroviruses have been shown to inhibit mitogen-induced proliferation of human or murine lymphocytes (39)-(43). Recently, Pahwa et al. (44) have reported that purified preparations from supernatants of HIV-infected cell cultures inhibit polyclonal B cell activation and T cell proliferation in response to PHA. It is possible that these viral components may be circulating in the sera of AIDS patients, and contribute to the inhibitory activity.

Another mechanism which may be responsible for serum suppression in AIDS may involve interference with a cell surface receptor involved in lymphocyte proliferation. Such interference might be due to ALA, which could be directed against the receptor. Binding of antibody to such a receptor could prevent interaction of the receptor with an appropriate ligand, and thus block proliferative responses. This mechanism may involve interference with the action of interleukin-2 (IL-2). As indicated earlier, AIDS sera added to cultures of normal cells several hours after mitogen stimulation still inhibit proliferation (29), indicating suppression of a secondary proliferative mechanism. Since proliferation of IL-2-dependent continous T-cell lines is inhibited by AIDS sera (30),(32),(45), interference with the action of IL-2 is implicated. This interference may occur at the level of IL-2 synthesis. Inhibition of mitogen-induced lymphocyte proliferation by retroviral preparations has been associated with decreased IL-2 production (41),(42). In addition, several investigators have found that IL-2 synthesis is diminished in AIDS patients (46)-(50). Farmer et al. (33) and Siegal et al. (51) suggested that AIDS plasma/sera inhibited the production and/or release of IL-2 by control cells. However, we have observed that addition of exogenous IL-2 to either mitogen-stimulated peripheral blood mononuclear cells or IL-2 dependent continuous T-cell lines did not overcome suppression (30), suggesting that the inhibitory activity may be at the level of binding of IL-2 to its receptors, or subsequent cellular events.

Decreased proliferation might be due to a reduction in cell surface membrane IL-2 receptors. It has been reported that peripheral blood mononuclear cells from AIDS patients express reduced levels of IL-2 receptors (46),(49),(52)-(54) and that these levels correlate with decreased lymphocyte proliferation in mitogen-stimulated cultures (52)-(54) and in autologous mixed lymphocyte reactions (49). In addition, binding of IL-2 to available cell surface IL-2 receptors may be inhibited. Soluble

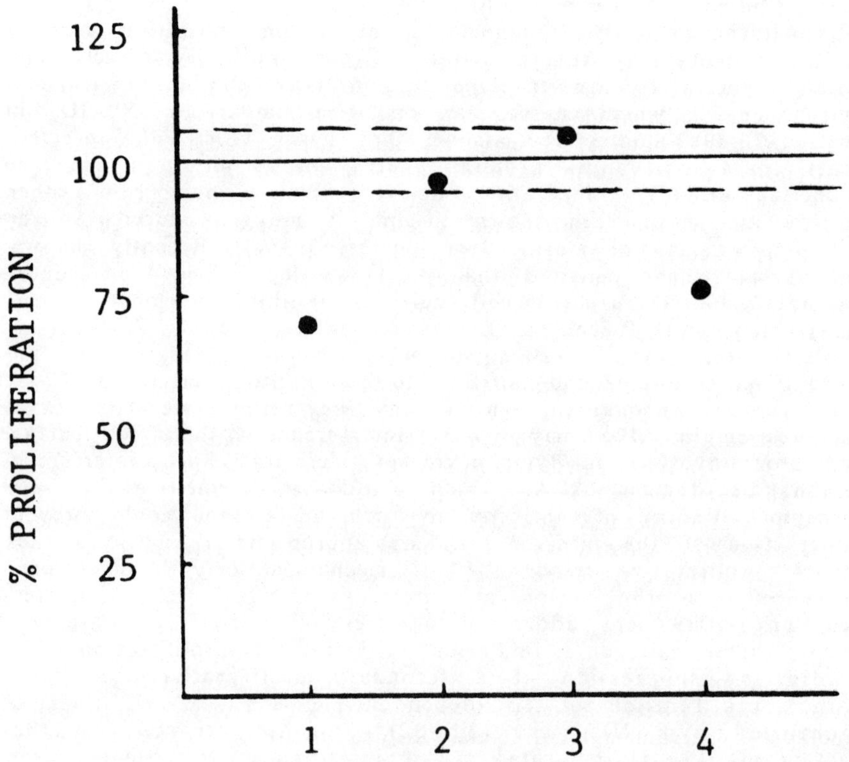

Figure 3. Effect of plasmapheresis on serum inhibition. Serum samples were obtained from one AIDS patient before the pheresis procedure (1), the following morning (2), one week (3), and two weeks (4) after pheresis. These sera and three control sera were tested on parallel cultures of 2 x 10^5 peripheral blood mononuclear cells from a healthy donor stimulated with PHA. The percent proliferation of cultures in each serum sample was calculated by comparison with cultures in control sera as described in ref. 29. Here, the range of proliferation of cultures in control sera (mean ± 2SD) is indicated by the dotted lines, and each point represents proliferation of cultures in the respective patient's serum sample. Although the pre-pheresis serum decreased proliferation of cultures when compared to control sera, samples obtained the morning following pheresis and one week later allowed control-level proliferation of cultures of this concentration of cells. However, by two weeks after pheresis, serum inhibition had returned to prepheresis levels.

IL-2 receptors, circulating in the serum of AIDS patients, may be involved in this inhibitory mechanism.

Dr. David Nelson and his colleagues at the National Institutes of Health found that surface IL-2 receptors from HTLV-I-infected cells (Hut 102B2) were shed into the culture supernate (55),(56). After developing an ELISA assay for soluble interleukin-2 receptors (sIL2R), these investigators determined that patients with various lymphoid malignancies had elevated sIL2R levels when compared to controls (57). Using this same assay, we have found that AIDS patients and other subjects who have antibodies to HIV also have elevated levels of sIL2R (unpublished findings).

Although the significance of these observations is unknown, we hypothesize that the elevated sIL2R may be involved in down-regulating immune responses in patients infected with HIV. Expression of surface IL-2 receptors has been shown to occur as a result of lymphocyte activation (58). It has been suggested that soluble interleukin-2 receptors, released from activated lymphocytes, might regulate immune responses by competing with cell-bound IL-2 receptors for the growth factor IL-2 (56). Thus, the elevated sIL2R levels seen in AIDS patients and others infected with HIV might inhibit proliferation of lymphocytes in vitro through this mechanism, as well as contribute to the decreased immune responsiveness found in these patients. We are currently exploring the possibility of whether sIL2R participate in the serum inhibition manifested by AIDS patients.

PARAPROTEINS

A number of abnormalities in the humoral arm of the immune system have been associated with AIDS. These abnormalities include hypergammaglobulinemia, failure to respond to primary in vivo immunizations, and defects in in vitro B cell activation (23),(24),(59). Consequently, we explored the possibility that sera from AIDS patients might also contain paraproteins, as another manifestation of B cell dysfunction.

Using serum immunoelectrophoresis, we found that over one-half of our AIDS and LAS patients had a monoclonal protein, which was IgG-kappa in the majority of cases (60). Our results, obtained from 15 AIDS and nine LAS patients, are shown in Table 3.

The significance of paraproteins in AIDS is not known. Paraproteinemia has been observed in patients with other primary immunodeficiency diseases (61)-(63). The frequent occurrence of B cell lymphomas in AIDS and LAS patients (64)-(66) and the reported cases of plasmacytosis (67) and plasmacytoma (68) in AIDS may be related to these findings. Whether these B cell abnormalities are primary manifestations of AIDS or secondary to the T cell defects or infections associated with AIDS is not clear. In a recent case report of an AIDS patient with a B cell lymphoma, Groopman et al. presented data which suggested that the pathogenesis of this lymphoma was linked to infection with Epstein-Barr virus, which in turn, was facilitated by infection

Table 3. Immunoelectrophoresis Results in AIDS and LAS

Results of Immunoelectrophoresis	Number of Patients AIDS(15)[a]	LAS(9)	Total(24)
No Abnormality	4	1	5
Indeterminate	3	2	5
IgG-Kappa M[b] Proteins	8	4	12
IgG M[b] Protein	0	2	2
All M[b] Proteins	8	6	14

a Total number of patients in each group in parentheses.
b Monoclonal

(Reprinted with permission from ref. 60)

with HIV (66). Clearly, more work needs to be done to elucidate the significance of paraproteins in AIDS.

SUMMARY

Our laboratory has been investigating the following serological factors and their possible roles in AIDS: (a) ALA; (b) serum inhibitory factors; and (c) paraproteins. Our studies to date indicate that the ALA associated with AIDS appear not to be specifically directed against one lymphocyte subset, but rather against multiple cellular antigens. As such, ALA may be present as a manifestation of the breakdown of immunoregulatory mechanisms characteristic of AIDS. In turn, ALA may contribute to the pathogenesis of AIDS by inhibiting the function of various cells of the immune system. We have observed that AIDS serum inhibits proliferation of normal lymphocytes in response to PHA. While the identity of the inhibitory factor(s) in AIDS serum is unknown, it is possible that this suppressive activity may be attributed to ALA, viral antigens from HIV, or sIL2R. Finally, we have observed paraproteins in AIDS sera, primarily of the IgG-kappa type. These monoclonal immunoglobulins may be produced as one of the manifestations of B cell dysfunction in AIDS.

While the roles of these serological factors in AIDS are unknown, it is possible that some or all of the factors may be involved in the pathogenesis of this disease, since they are present in a significant percentage of individuals at risk for developing AIDS, such as LAS patients and hemophiliacs who have been infected with HIV. These factors may prove to be useful in monitoring patients to help determine which individuals exposed to HIV will ultimately develop the full disease.

REFERENCES

1. Curran, J.W., Morgan, W.M., Hardy, A.M., et al., The epidemiology of AIDS: current status and future prospects. Science 229:1352-1357 (1985)

2. Cavaille-Coll, M., Messiah, A., Klatzmann, D., et al., Critical analysis of T cell subset and function evaluation in patients with persistent generalized lymphadenopathy in groups at risk for AIDS. Clin Exp Immunol 57:511-519 (1984)

3. Francis, D.P., Jaffe, H.W., Fultz, P.N., et al., The natural history of infection with the lymphadenopathy-associated virus/human T-lymphotropic virus type III. Ann Intern Med 103:719-722 (1985)

4. Fernandez, R., Mouradin, J., Metroka, C., et al., The prognostic value of histopathology in persistent generalized lymphadenopathy in homosexual men. N Engl J Med 309:185-186 (1983)

5. Klein, R.S., Harris, C.A., Small, C.B., et al., Oral candidiasis in high-risk patients as the initial manifestation of the acquired immunodeficiency syndrome. N Engl J Med 311:354-358 (1984)

6. Gottlieb, M.S., Wolfe, P.R., Fahey, J.L., et al., The syndrome of persistent generalized lymphadenopathy: experience with 101 patients, In: AIDS-Associated Syndromes (Gupta, S., ed.), Adv Exp Med Biol 187:85-91 (1985)

7. Abrams, D.I., Mess, T., Volberding, P.A., Lymphadenopathy: end-point or prodrome? Update of a 36-month prospective study, in: AIDS-Associated Syndromes (Gupta, S., ed.), Adv Exp Med Biol 187:73-84 (1985)

8. Kloster, B.E., Tomar, R.H., Spira, T.J., Lymphocytotoxic antibodies in the acquired immune deficiency syndrome (AIDS). Clin Immunol Immunopathol 30:330-335 (1984)

9. Tomar, R.H., John, P.A., Hennig, A.K., et al., Cellular targets of antilymphocyte antibodies in AIDS and LAS. Clin Immunol Immunopathol 37:37-47 (1985)

10. Kloster, B.E., Tomar, R.H., Stockman, J.A., et al., Antibodies to human T-cell lymphotropic virus-I membrane antigens and inverted T4/T8 ratios in hemophiliacs. Amer J Clin Path 83:450-456 (1985)

11. Essex, M., McLane, M.F., Lee, T.H., et al., Antibodies to cell membrane antigens associated with human T-cell leukemia virus in patients with AIDS. Science 220:859-862 (1983)

12. Schupbach, J., Popovic, M., Gilden, R.V., et al., Serological analysis of a subgroup of human T-lymphotropic retroviruses (HTLV-III) associated with AIDS. Science 224:503-505 (1984)

13. Williams, R.C., Masur, H., Spira, T.J., Lymphocyte-reactive antibodies in acquired immune deficiency syndrome. Clin Immunol 4:118-123 (1984)

14. Pruzanski, W., Jacobs, H., Laing, L.R., Lymphocytotoxic antibodies against peripheral blood B and T lymphocytes in homosexuals with AIDS and ARC. AIDS Research 1:211-220 (1984)

15. Kiprov, D.D., Busch, D.F., Simpson, D.M., et al., In: Acquired Immune Deficiency Syndrome (Gottlieb, M., Groopman, J., eds), Alan R. Liss, Inc., New York, p 299-308, (1984)

16. Pollack, M.S., Callaway, C., LeBlanc, D., et al., In: Non-HLA Antigens in Health, Aging, and Malignancy (Cohen, E., Singal, D.P., eds), Alan R. Liss, Inc., New York, p 209-213 (1983)

17. Dorsett, B., Cronin, W., Chuma, V., et al., Anti-lymphocyte antibodies in patients with acquired immune deficiency syndrome. Amer J Med 78:621-626 (1985)

18. DeHoratius, R.J., Lymphocytotoxic antibodies. Prog Immunol 4:151-174 (1980)

19. Morimoto, C., Reinherz, E.L., Borel, Y., et al., Autoantibody to an immunoregulatory inducer population in patients with juvenile rheumatoid arthritis. J Clin Invest 67:753-761 (1981)

20. Morimoto, C., Reinherz, E.L., Distaso, J.A., et al., Relationship between SLE T cell subsets, anti-T cell antibodies, and cell function. J Clin Invest 73:689-700 (1984)

21. Williams, R.C., Bankhurst, A.D., Montano, J.D., IgG antilymphocyte antibodies in SLE detected by ^{125}I protein A. Arth Rheum 19:1261-1270 (1976)

22. Kammer, G.M., Impaired T cell capping and receptor regeneration in active SLE. J Clin Invest 72:1686-1697 (1983)

23. Seligmann, M., Chess, L., Fahey, J.L., et al., AIDS--an immunologic reevaluation. N Engl J Med 311:1286-1291 (1984)

24. Lane, H.C., Masur, H., Edgar, L.C., et al., Abnormalities of B cell activation and immunoregulation in patients with the acquired immunodeficiency syndrome. N Engl J Med 309:453-458 (1983)

24. Lane, H.C., Masur, H., Edgar, L.C., et al., Abnormalities of B cell activation and immunoregulation in patients with the acquired immunodeficiency syndrome. N Engl J Med 309:453-458 (1983)

25. Kirchner, H., Tosato, G., Blaese, R.M., et al., Polyclonal immunoglobin secretion by human B cells exposed to EBV in vitro. J Immunol 122:1310-1313 (1979)

26. Miller, G., The oncogenicity of Epstein-Barr virus. J Infect Dis 130:187-203 (1974)

27. Aucouterier, P., Couderc, L.J., Gouet, D., et al., Serum immunoglobulin G subclass dysbalances in the lymphadenopathy syndrome and acquired immune deficiency syndrome. Clin Exp Immunol 63:234-240 (1986)

28. Gupta, A., Novick, B.E., Rubenstein, A., Restoration of suppressor T-cell functions in children with AIDS following intravenous gamma globulin treatment. Amer J Dis Child 140:143-146 (1986)

29. Hennig, A.K., Tomar, R.H., Inhibition of in vitro lymphocyte proliferation by serum from acquired immune deficiency syndrome patients depends on the ratio of cells to serum in culture. Clin Immunol Immunopathol 33:258-267 (1984)

30. Hennig, A.K., Tomar, R.H., Serum from AIDS patients inhibits mitogen-stimulated lymphocyte proliferation: characterization of the inhibition. Fed Proc 44:7643a (1985)

31. Cunningham-Rundles, S., Michelis, M.A., Masur, H., Serum suppression of lymphocyte activation in vitro in acquired immunodeficiency disease. J Clin Immunol 3:156-165 (1983)

32. Donnelly, R.P., Tsang, K.Y., Galbraith, G.M.P., et al., Inhibition of interleukin-2 induced T cell proliferation by sera from patients with the acquired immune deficiency syndrome. J Clin Immunol 6:92-101 (1986)

33. Farmer, J.L., Gottlieb, A.A., Nishihara, T., Inhibition of interleukin 2 production and expression of the interleukin 2 receptor by plasma from acquired immune deficiency syndrome patients. Clin Immunol Immunopathol 38:235-243 (1986)

34. Tomar, R.H., Kloster, B.E., Lamberson, H.V., Plasmapheresis increases T4 lymphocytes in a patient with AIDS. Amer J Clin Path 81:518-521 (1984)

35. Laurence, J., Gottlieb, A.B., Kunkel, H.G., Soluble suppressor factors in patients with acquired immune deficiency syndrome and its prodrome. J Clin Invest 72:2072-2081 (1983)

36. Laurence, J., Mayer, L., Immunoregulatory lymphokines of T hybridomas from AIDS patients: constitutive and inducible suppressor factors. Science 225:66-69 (1984)

37. Copelan, E.P., Rinehart, J.J., Lewis, M., et al., The mechanism of retrovirus suppression of human T cell proliferation in vitro. J Immunol 131:2017-2020 (1983)

38. Orosz, C.G., Zinn, N.E., Olsen, R.G., et al., FeLV-UV and specific FeLV proteins alter T lymphocyte behavior by inducing hyporesponsiveness to lymphokines. J Immunol 134:3396-3403 (1985)

39. Snyderman, R., Cianciolo, G.J., Immunosuppressive activity of the retroviral envelope protein p15E and its possible relationship to neoplasia. Immunol Today 5:240-244 (1984)

40. Denner, J., Wunderlich, V., Bierwolf, D., Suppression of human lymphocyte mitogen response by proteins of the type-D retrovirus PMFV. Int J Cancer 37:311-316 (1986)

41. Wainberg, M.A., Vydelingum, S., Boushira, M., et al., Reversible interference with TCGF activity by virus particles. Clin Exp Immunol 57:663-670 (1984)

42. Wainberg, M.A., Vydelingum, S., Margolese, R.G., Viral inhibition of lymphocyte mitogenesis: interference with the synthesis of functionally active T cell growth factor (TCGF) activity and reversal of inhibition by the addition of same. J Immunol 130:2372-2378 (1983)

43. Fowler, A.K., Twardzik, D.R., Reed, C.D., et al., Inhibition of lymphocyte transformation by disrupted murine oncornavirus. Cancer Res 37:4529-4531 (1977)

44. Pahwa, S., Pahwa, R., Saxinger, C., et al., Influence of the human T-lymphotropic virus/lymphadenopathy-associated virus on functions of human lymphocytes: evidence for immunosuppressive effects and polyclonal B-cell activation by banded viral preparations. Proc Natl Acad Sci 82:8198-8202 (1985)

45. Donnelly, R.P., Tsang, K.Y., Fudenberg, H.H., et al., Inhibition of interleukin 2-induced T cell proliferation by serum from patients with the acquired immune deficiency syndrome (AIDS). Fed Proc 44:6601a (1985)

46. Tsang, K.Y., Fudenberg, H.H., Galbraith, G.M.P., et al., Partial restoration of impaired interleukin-2 production and Tac antigen expression in AIDS patients by isoprinosine treatment in vitro. J Clin Invest 75:1538-1544 (1985)

47. Murray, H.W., Rubin, B.Y., Masur, H., et al., Impaired production of lymphokines and immune (gamma) interferon in the acquired immunodeficiency syndrome. N Engl J Med 310:884-889 (1984)

48. Lifson, J.D., Benike, C.J., Mark, D.F., et al., Human recombinant interleukin-2 partly reconstitutes deficiency in vitro immune responses of lymphocytes from patients with AIDS. Lancet 1:698-702 (1984)

49. Ebert, E.C., Stoll, D.B., Cassens, B.J., et al., Diminished interleukin 2 production and receptor generation characterize the acquired immunodeficiency syndrome. Clin Immunol Immunopathol 37:283-297 (1985)

50. Reuben, J.M., Hersh, E.M., Murray, J.L., et al., IL-2 production and response in vitro by the leukocytes of patients with acquired immune deficiency syndrome. Lymphokine Res 4:103-116 (1985)

51. Siegal, J.P., Djeu, J.Y., Stocks, N.I., et al., Sera from patients with the acquired immune deficiency syndrome inhibit production of interleukin-2 by normal lymphocytes. J Clin Invest 75:1957-1964 (1985)

52. Prince, H.E., Kermani-Arab, V., Fahey, J.L., Depressed interleukin-2 receptor expression in acquired immune deficiency and lymphadenopathy syndromes. J Immunol 133:1313-1317 (1984)

53. Ciobanu, N., Welte, K., Kruger, G., et al., Defective T cell response to PHA and mitogenic monoclonal antibodies in male homosexuals with acquired immunodeficiency syndrome and its in vitro correction by interleukin 2. J Clin Immunol 3:332-340 (1983)

54. Munn, C.G., Reuben, J.M., Hersh, E.M., et al., T cell surface antigen expression on lymphocytes of patients with AIDS during in vitro mitogen stimulation. Cancer Immunol Immunother 18:141-148 (1984)

55. Rubin, L.A., Kurman, C.C., Fritz, M.E., et al., Soluble interleukin-2 receptors are released by human lymphoid cells in vitro. Clin Res 33:388a (1985)

56. Rubin, L.A., Kurman, C.C., Fritz, M.E., et al., Soluble interleukin 2 receptors are released from activated human lymphoid cells in vitro. J Immunol 135:3172-3177 (1985)

57. Rubin, L.A., Kurman, C.C., Fritz, M.E., et al., Serum levels of soluble interleukin-2 receptors are elevated in patients with certain lymphoreticular malignancies. Clin Res 33:457a (1985)

58. Cantrell, D.A., Smith, K.A., The interleukin-2 T cell system: a new growth model. Science 224:1312-1316 (1984)

59. CDC., Update: Acquired immunodeficiency syndrome - United States. MMWR 34:245-248 (1985)

60. Heriot, K., Hallquist, A.E., Tomar, R.H., Paraproteinemia in patients with acquired immunodeficiency syndrome (AIDS) or lymphadenopathy syndrome (LAS). Clin Chem 31:1224-1226 (1985)

61. Geha, R.S., Schneeberger, E., Galien, J., et al., Synthesis of a M component by circulating B lymphocytes in severe combined immunodeficiency. N Engl J Med 290:726-728 (1984)

62. Dictor, M., Fasth, A., Olling, S., Abnormal B cell proliferation associated with combined immunodeficiency, cytomegalovirus, and cultured thymus grafts. Am J Clin Pathol 82:487-490 (1984)

63. Bushell, A.C., Whicher, J.T., Yuille, T., The progressive appearance of multiple urinary Bence Jones proteins and serum paraproteins in a child with immune deficiency. Clin Exp Immunol 38:64-69 (1979)

64. Snider, W.D., Simpson, D.M., Aronyk, K.E., et al., Primary lymphoma of the nervous system associated with the acquired immune deficiency syndrome (letter). N Engl J Med 308:45 (1983)

65. Ziegler, J., Beckstead, J.A., Volberding, P.A., et al., Non-Hodgkin's lymphoma in 90 homosexual men. N Engl J Med 311: 565-570 (1984)

66. Groopman, J.E., Sullivan, J.L., Mulder, C., et al., Pathogenesis of B cell lymphoma in a patient with AIDS. Blood 67: 612-615 (1986)

67. Franco, C.M., Hendrix, L.E., Lokey, J.L., Bone marrow abnormalities in the acquired immune deficiency syndrome (letter). Ann Intern Med 101:275-276 (1984)

68. Israel, A.M., Koziner, B., Straus, D.J., Plasmacytoma and the acquired immune deficiency syndrome. Ann Intern Med 99:635-636 (1983)

Part IV
Clinical Manifestations

21
HIV Infection and Persistent Generalized Lymphadenopathy

Usha Mathur-Wagh, Donna Mildvan

As early as 1979 and 1980, with the emergence of the epidemic of acquired immunodeficiency syndrome (AIDS), investigators in New York and California began observing a new entity of persistent generalized lymphadenopathy (PGL) in otherwise healthy homosexual men (1). Similarities between many of the epidemiologic and clinical features of this entity and those of AIDS were evident (2),(3). Both occurred in young, sexually active homosexual men residing in New York and California. Sexually transmitted diseases, such as gonorrhea, syphilis, amebiasis and hepatitis were common, and the use of recreational drugs widely prevalent in both groups. Among the first AIDS cases reported to the Centers for Disease Control (CDC), 69% of Kaposi's sarcoma and 48% of *Pneumocystis carinii* pneumonia (PCP) patients had lymphadenopathy before or at the time of diagnosis (4). Furthermore, a retrospective analysis of lymph node biopsies from selected New York City hospitals showed that cases of unexplained lymph node hyperplasia had increased 75% over the period between 1977 and 1981, with the largest increase occurring between 1980 and 1981 in males aged 16 to 44 years (5). Clinically, PGL patients displayed findings which were strikingly similar to, though less severe than, those encountered in AIDS (6)-(8).

To characterize further the relationship between PGL and AIDS, longitudinal studies in homosexual men were initiated. When several patients belonging to the earliest such study were found to progress to AIDS while under observation, it became apparent that PGL in fact represented a prodrome of AIDS in these patients (9). This observation was the first of many which extended the spectrum of illness associated with the new epidemic beyond that of the original descriptions of AIDS. Indeed, a diverse array of clinical manifestations, including asymptomatic immunodeficiency, autoimmune thrombocytopenia, the syndrome of "wasting" or "constitutional disease", as well as neurological syndromes, have been found to occur (10)-(14). It is also noteworthy that the etiologic retrovirus of AIDS, now designated human immunodeficiency virus (HIV), was first isolated from the lymph node of a patient with PGL (15), and subsequently, from patients with the entire spectrum of findings (16)-(20).

Although first described in homosexual men, the syndrome of PGL has also been documented in persons belonging to other risk groups for AIDS such as intravenous drug abusers, sexual partners of patients infected with HIV, and hemophiliacs (21)-(23). However, most of the current data regarding the epidemiologic, clinical and laboratory aspects of PGL are derived from longitudinal studies in homosexual or bisexual men, which represent the basis for the present review (24)-(34).

DEFINITION

PGL is defined as palpable lymphadenopathy of 1 cm or greater size involving two or more extrainguinal sites and persisting for more than three months in the absence of a concurrent illness or condition other than HIV infection to explain the findings. Recently, PGL has been categorized as group III of the CDC classification system for HIV infections (35). Based on current information it seems that PGL may be complicated by AIDS in 12 to 34% of patients followed longitudinally for four to five years (24)-(34). Whether in the remaining patients PGL represents a milder and/or stable form of infection with HIV, remains to be determined.

The syndrome of PGL must be differentiated from that of "wasting", which has been designated "constitutional disease", Group IV-a, in the new CDC classification system (35). Patients with overriding constitutional disease, unlike those with uncomplicated PGL, have prominent systemic signs and symptoms: weight loss of greater than 10% of baseline, chronic unexplained fever or diarrhea of greater than one month's duration. PGL patients may progress to constitutional disease, usually with concomitant involution of lymphadenopathy. In contrast to PGL, the syndrome of constitutional disease appears to represent a true prodrome of AIDS, since the majority (≥75%) of patients progress to AIDS in one to 20 months (mean four months) after this diagnosis (12).

CLINICAL FEATURES

Lymphadenopathy may either be discovered by the patient or noted during a routine physical examination in an asymptomatic individual. Alternatively, symptoms such as fatigue, malaise, low grade fever (≤100.5°F) and occasional night sweats, may accompany the lymphadenopathy in 35% to 75% of patients (24)-(34). These symptoms are usually mild and intermittent in nature and are generally not associated with significant morbidity. In addition, some studies report a history of viral-like illness associated with sore throat, fever and myalgias, in 25 to 33% of patients within two months of onset of lymphadenopathy (26),(28). A number of dermatologic findings such as facial seborrhea, bullous impetigo, tinea versicolor, and cutaneous fungal infections have also been described in up to 50% of patients with PGL (26),(28),(34). Lymph nodes are characteristically firm, non-tender and freely mobile, ranging from 1 to 5 cm in size and involving multiple sites such as the cervical, supraclavicular, posterior auticular, submandibular, axillary, epitrochlear and inguinal regions. Fluctuations in lymph node size may occur for no apparent reason. However, a consistent increase in a single lymph node to three or four times the original size may predate the onset of Kaposi's sarcoma or lymphoma, whereas a significant reduction in all nodal groups, occasionally with virtual disappearance of palpable adenopathy, may suggest an impending opportunistic infection (24). While a decrease in lymph node size over time seems also to occur in clinically stable PGL patients, a change in lymph node size, especially in the presence of new or worsening systemic symptoms, should prompt the initiation of a thorough evaluation, including lymph node biopsy, to exclude malignancy or early opportunistic infection.

Although palpable splenomegaly has been noted in fewer than one-third of all patients with PGL (24),(26),(34), this finding may be demonstrated in up to 75% of patients in whom abdominal CAT scans are performed (28).

LABORATORY FINDINGS

Laboratory abnormalities reported in patients with PGL are very similar although less severe than those described in patients with AIDS (6)-(8). The most common hematologic abnormalities reported include leukopenia (white blood cell count <4800/mm^3) in 10 to 41% (24),(28),(30),(34) and lymphopenia (lymphocyte count <1500/mm^3) in 38 to 62% of patients (24),(30),(34) presenting with PGL. Anemia and thrombocytopenia when present are mild and noted in fewer than 20% of patients (24),(26),(30). Bone marrow biopsies performed in a relatively small proportion of patients have revealed hypercellular marrows with an increase in the number of mature lymphocytes, plasma cells and eosinophils (26).

In approximately 10% of patients with PGL, a low serum cholesterol (28) and mild abnormalities of serum transaminases in the absence of hepatitis B surface antigen have been documented (26),(28). Antibodies to hepatitis B surface and/or core antigens are described in a large proportion (60 to 83%) of patients (24),(28),(30). In addition, a majority of patients with PGL have serologic evidence of past infection with a number of herpes viruses: antibodies to the virus capsid antigen (VCA) of Epstein-Barr virus (EBV) were documented in virtually 100% (24),(30),(34) and complement fixing antibodies to cytomégalovirus (CMV) and *Herpes simplex* virus (HSV) were reported in 93 to 100% (24),(26),(28),(30),(32),(34), and 90 to 94% of patients (24),(26) respectively.

Although PGL is presently defined by the typical constellation of clinical findings in association with a positive diagnostic test for HIV infection, the proportion of patients testing positive for HIV antibody among early PGL cohorts accrued before serologic testing became available, has varied from 75% (36) to 96% (30),(34), as a function of the sensitivity and type of assay.

A variety of immunologic abnormalities involving both T and B lymphocytes have been documented in patients with PGL. The most characteristic 'T' cell abnormality is a striking reduction in the proportion of T4+ cells and an increase in the number of T8+ cells leading to a reversal of the T4/T8 ratio in the majority of patients (24). The mean T4/T8 ratios vary from 0.42 to 1.09 (24),(28),(30),(34) and the mean absolute number of T4+ cells from 293 to 419/mm^3 (24),(34) in different studies. In addition, impaired in vitro 'T' lymphocytic responses to activation by mitogens and antigens, such as phytohemagglutinin (PHA), pokeweed mitogen (PMW), candida and *Escherichia coli* antigens, and a reduction in the natural killer (NK) cell activity have been observed in up to 50% of patients (26),(30). Polyclonal increases in serum gamma globulins, with varying degrees of elevations in immunoglobulins G, M, and A, as a manifestation of 'B' cell activation, have also been described in 31 to 75% of patients (24),(26),(28),(30).

Typically, lymph node histology reveals follicular hyperplasia involving the cortex, paracortex and the medullary regions (24). The follicles may vary in size and shape and show an increased number of normal mitoses. Capillary proliferation with prominence of endothelial cells is observed in a majority of cases (24),(26),(30). Routine bacteriologic, viral, fungal and mycobacterial cultures are all negative. Occasionally, in some patients with PGL, lymph node histology is characterized by follicular involution with small, hypocellular and sometimes hyalinized follicles (37). However, this histologic picture is more characteristic of the findings in patients with constitutional disease or frank AIDS, and thus represents a more advanced stage of illness than that associated with the follicular hyperplasia of uncomplicated PGL. HIV may be recovered from body fluids and lymph nodes of patients with PGL, and HIV particles have been identified in follicular dendritic cells (38).

Analysis of histocompatibility allodeterminants performed in three different investigations revealed the presence of HLA-DR5 antigen in a large proportion (35 to 53%) of patients with PGL (28),(30),(39). An increased frequency of the HLA-DR5 allotype has also been described in patients with Kaposi's sarcoma (40).

CLINICAL OUTCOME

A summary of the outcomes of PGL patients followed in various longitudinal studies is described in Table I. Three longitudinal studies of PGL from New York City, initiated in February, July, and November of 1981, have demonstrated comparable progression rates to AIDS of 33% 23% and 34% respectively (25),(27),(31). However, a San Francisco study of PGL initiated in November 1981, has shown the much lower progression rate of only 12% (29). Two additional studies from Atlanta and Los Angeles initiated in January 1982, have also reported similar rates of progression to AIDS of 16% and 18% respectively (33),(34). Multiple factors such as the duration of infection with HIV, period of follow-up of PGL patients, and study inclusion criteria might all be responsible for the differences in these AIDS progression rates. Moreover, differences in the extent and frequency of possible co-factor exposure, such as nitrite inhalant use by homosexual men with PGL, could also account for variations in the progression rates to AIDS as well as for specific disease manifestations (25),(41).

As shown in Table 1, different studies have identified a number of historical, clinical and laboratory features documented at presentation to be predictive of ultimate AIDS outcome. The most common entry parameters associated with an ultimately poor prognosis and described by more than one investigator include the presence of constitutional symptoms, leukopenia, lymphopenia, and a reduction in the absolute number of T4+ cells.

SUMMARY

The syndrome of PGL is one manifestation of infection with HIV and has been well characterized among homosexual and bisexual men. Approximately one-third of all patients with PGL may progress to AIDS when followed for up to five years. The differentiation of PGL from another AIDS-related entity "constitutional disease" is important since the latter represents a true prodrome of AIDS in the majority of patients. In addition to lymphadenopathy, the presence of other clinical and laboratory abnormalities, including constitutional symptoms, leukopenia, lymphopenia, and a reduction in the number of T4+ cells, appears to identify a subgroup of PGL patients who are at particularly high risk for the development of AIDS. Patients with these additional findings represent an important subpopulation for study of the possible beneficial effects of antiviral and immune enhancing agents directed against the underlying HIV infection.

Table 1. Studies of AIDS Risk Group Patients with Persistent Generalized Lymphadenopathy

Investigators Location (Ref. No.)	Study Period	No. of PGL Patients	No. (%) Progressing to AIDS*	Entry Parameters Predictive of a Poor Outcome
Mathur-Wagh et al. New York (24),(25)	Feb. 1981- June 1986	42	14 (33%)	heavy nitrite use, night sweats, constitutional symptoms, splenomegaly, anergy, leukopenia, decreased T4 cells.
Gold et al. New York (30),(31)	July 1981- Dec. 1985	91	21 (23%)	decreased lymphocytic proliferative responses, anemia, thrombocytopenia, lymphopenia, increased IgA.
Metroka et al. New York (26),(27)	Nov. 1981- June 1986	90	31 (34%)	constitutional symptoms, oral candidiasis, leukopenia, lymphopenia increased interferon alpha, anemia.
Abrams et al. San Francisco (28),(29)	Nov. 1981- June 1986	200	24 (12%)	antecedent thrush, history of herpes zoster, leukopenia, thrombocytopenia, elevated ESR
Fishbein et al. Altanta (32),(33)	Jan. 1982- Jan. 1986	78	14 (18%)	constitutional symptoms, decreased T4 cells.
Gottlieb et al. Los Angeles (34)	Jan. 1982- June 1986	101	30 (30%)	chronic diarrhea, oral candidiasis, leukopenia, lymphopenia, decreased T4 cells.

* During study period.

REFERENCES

1. Mildvan, D., Mathur, U., Enlow, R.W., et al., Persistent generalized lymphadenopathy among homosexual males. MMWR 31:249-251 (1982)

2. Gottlieb, M.S., Schanker, H.M., Fan, P.T., et al., Pneumocystis pneumonia - Los Angeles. MMWR 30:250-252 (1981)

3. Friedman-Kien, A., Laubenstein, L., Marmor, M., et al., Kaposi's sarcoma and pneumocystis pneumonia in homosexual men - New York City and California. MMWR 30:305-308 (1981)

4. CDC., Acquired immunodeficiency syndrome activity. Unpublished surveillance data.

5. Miller, B., Stansfield, S.K., Sack, M.M., et al., The syndrome of unexplained generalized lymphadenopathy in young men in New York City: Is it related to the acquired immune deficiency syndrome? JAMA 251:242-246 (1984)

6. Mildvan, D., Mathur, U., Enlow, R.W., et al., Opportunistic infections and immune deficiency in homosexual men. Ann Intern Med 96:700-704 (1982)

7. Gottlieb, M.S., Schroff, R., Schanker, H.M. et al., *Pneumocystis carinii* pneumonia and mucosal candidiasis in previously healthy homosexual men: evidence of a new acquired cellular immunodeficiency. N Engl J Med 305:1425-1431 (1981)

8. Siegal, F.P., Lopez, C., Hammer, G.S., et al., Severe acquired immunodeficiency in male homosexuals, manifested by chronic perianal ulcerative *Herpes simplex* lesions. N Engl J Med 305:1439-1444 (1981)

9. Mathur, U., Enlow, R.W., Spigland, I., et al., Generalized lymphadenopathy: A prodome of Kaposi's sarcoma in male homosexuals? Interscience Conference on Antimicrobial Agents and Chemotherapy, Miami Beach, Florida (1982)

10. Kornfield, M., Stouwe, R.A., Lange, M., et al., T lymphocyte subpopulations in homosexual men. N Engl J Med 307:729-731 (1982)

11. Morris, L., Distenfeld, A., Amorosi, E., et al., Autoimmune thrombocytopenic purpura in homosexual men. Ann Intern Med 96:714-717 (1982)

12. Mathur-Wagh, U., Mildvan, D., Prodromal syndromes in AIDS. Ann NY Acad Sciences 437:184-191 (1984)

13. Mildvan, D., Acquired immune deficiency syndrome (AIDS) or an opportunistic infection? Toward a clinical definition of AIDS. (Ma, P., Armstrong, D., eds) The Acquired Immune Deficiency Syndrome and Infections in Homosexual Men. Yorke Medical Books, New York, p 240-252 (1983)

14. Snider, W.D., Simpson, D.M., Nielson, S., et al., Neurological complications of acquired immune deficiency syndrome: Analysis of 50 patients. Ann Neurol 14:403-418 (1983)

15. Barre-Sinoussi, F., Chermann, J.C., Rey, F., et al., Isolation of a T-lymphotropic retrovirus from a patient at risk of acquired immune deficiency syndrome (AIDS). Science 220: 869-871 (1983)

16. Chermann, J.C., Barre-Sinoussi, F., Montagnier, L., Characterization and possible role in AIDS of a new T-lymphotropic retrovirus. In: Acquired Immune Deficiency Syndrome. UCLA Symposium on Molecular and Cellular Biology. Alan R. Liss, New York, p 31-46 (1984)

17. Gallo, R.C., Salahuddin, S.Z., Popovic, M., et al., Frequent detection and isolation of cytopathic retroviruses (HTLV-III) from patients with AIDS and pre-AIDS. Science 224:500-503 (1984)

18. Popovic, M., Sarngadharan, M.G., Read, E., et al., Detection, isolation, and continuous production of cytopathic retroviruses (HTLV-III) from patients with AIDS and pre-AIDS. Science 224:497-500 (1984)

19. Sarngadharan, M.G., Popovic, M., Bruch, I., et al., Antibodies reactive with human T-lymphotropic retroviruses (HTLV-III) in the serum of patients with AIDS. Science 224: 506-508 (1984)

20. Levy, J.A., Hoffman, A.D., Kramer, S.M., et al., Isolation of lymphocytopathic retroviruses from San Francisco patients with AIDS. Science 225:840-842 (1984)

21. Wormser, G.P., Krupp, L.B., Hanrahan, J.P., et al., Acquired immune deficiency in male prisoners. New insights into an emerging syndrome. Ann Intern Med 98:297-303 (1983)

22. Evatt, B.L., Ramsey, R.B., Lawrence, D.N., et al., The acquired immune deficiency syndrome in patients with hemophilia. Ann Intern Med 100:499-504 (1984)

23. Harris, C., Butkus-Small, C., Klein, R., et al., Immunodeficiency in female sexual partners of men with the acquired immune deficiency syndrome. N Engl J Med 308:1181-1184 (1983)

24. Mathur-Wagh, U., Enlow, R.W., Spigland, I., et al., Longitudinal study of persistent generalized lymphadenopathy in homosexual men: relation to acquired immunodeficiency syndrome. Lancet 1:1033-1038 (1984)

25. Mathur-Wagh, U., Mildvari, D., Van Camp., J., et al., Persistent generalized lymphadenopathy in homosexual men: a comparison of two cohorts. International Conference on Acquired Immunodeficiency Syndrome (AIDS), Paris, France (1986)

26. Metroka, C.E., Cunningham-Rundles, S., Pollack, M.S., et al., Generalized lymphadenopathy in homosexual men. Ann Intern Med 99:585-591 (1983)

27. Metroka, C.E., Cunningham-Rundles, S., Krim, M., et al., A four year prospective study of clinical and immunological parameters of patients with generalized lymphadenopathy. International Conference on Acquired Immunodeficiency Syndrome (AIDS), Paris, France (1986)

28. Abrams, D.I., Lewis, B.J., Beckstead, J.H., et al., Persistent diffuse lymphadenopathy in homosexual men: Endpoint or prodrome? Ann Intern Med 100:801-808 (1984)

29. Senechek, D.R., Abrams, D.I., Status of lymphadenopathy syndrome: a retrospective chart review of 303 patients. International Conference on Acquired Immunodeficiency Syndrome (AIDS), Paris, France (1986)

30. Gold, J.W.M., Weikel, C.S., Godbold, J., et al., Unexplained persistent lymphadenopathy in homosexual men. A longitudinal study. JAMA 254:930-935 (1985)

31. Gold, J.W.M., Armstrong, D., Continuing high risk for AIDS in a cohort of homosexual men with persistent unexplained lymphadenopathy. International Conference on Acquired Immunodeficiency Syndrome (AIDS), Paris, France (1986)

32. Fishbein, D.B., Kaplan, J.E., Spira, T.J., et al., Unexplained lymphadenopathy in homosexual men. A longitudinal study. JAMA 254:930-935 (1985)

33. Kaplan, J.E., Spira, T.J., Fishbein, D.B., et al., Lymphadenopathy syndrome in homosexual men. International Conference on Acquired Immunodeficiency Syndrome (AIDS), Paris, France (1986)

34. Gottlieb, M.S., Wolfe, P.R., Fahey, J.L., et al., The syndrome of persistent generalized lymphadenopathy: Experience with 101 patients. Adv Exp Med Biol 187:85-91 (1985)

35. CDC., Classification system for human T-lymphotropic virus type III/lymphadenopathy-associated virus infections. MMWR 35:334-339 (1986)

36. Mathur-Wagh, U., Mildvan, D., Yancovitz, S.R., et al., Persistent generalized lymphadenopathy in homosexual men: A 4 year follow-up and results of LAV serology measured by IgG ELISA. International Conference on Acquired Immunodeficiency Syndrome (AIDS), Atlanta, Georgia (1985)

37. Fernandez, R., Mouradian, J., Metroka, C., et al., The prognostic value of histopathology in persistent generalized lymphadenopathy in homosexual men. N Engl J Med 309:185-186 (1983)

38. Tenner-Racz, K., Racz, P., Dietrich, M., et al., Altered follicular dendritic cells and virus-like particles in AIDS and AIDS-related lymphadenopathy. Lancet 1:105-106 (1985)

39. Enlow, R.W., Nune, Roldan, A., LoGalbo, P., et al. Increased frequency of HLA-DR5 in lymphadenopathy stage of AIDS. Lancet 2:51-52 (1983)

40. Friedman-Kien, A.E., Laubenstein, L.J., Rubenstein, P., et al., Disseminated Kaposi's sarcoma in homosexual men. Ann Intern Med 96:693-700 (1982)

41. Mathur-Wagh, U., Mildvan, D., Senie, R., Follow-up at 4 1/2 years on homosexual men with generalized lymphadenopahty. N Engl J Med 313:1542-1543 (1985)

22
Pulmonary Manifestations of AIDS

Stuart M. Garay

Almost simultaneously, in late 1980 and early 1981, clinicians and epidemiologists in New York City, Los Angeles and San Francisco recognized an unusual pattern of opportunistic diseases occurring in predominantly young homosexual men. The initial reports of 26 previously healthy young homosexual men diagnosed with Kaposi's sarcoma and 15 diagnosed with *Pneumocystis carinii* pneumonia (PCP) were published by the Centers for Disease control (CDC) in its *Morbidity and Mortality Weekly Report* during June and July 1981 (1),(2). Since that time there has been an extraordinary escalation in the number of reported cases. As of the end of 1986 more than 29,000 patients had been diagnosed to have the acquired immunodeficiency syndrome (AIDS) in the United States. AIDS represents the severe end of the clinical spectrum of infection with the retrovirus, human immunodeficiency virus (HIV). This review will focus on the pulmonary manifestations associated with AIDS, an important topic since the lung is a critical target organ in over one-half of all AIDS cases.

ROLE OF THE IMMUNOLOGIC DEFECT

Many of the pulmonary infections seen in patients with AIDS represent endogenous reactivation of previously dormant organisms, which are unmasked by the defect in cellular immunity (3). For example, there is evidence that PCP is acquired as an asymptomatic infection by large numbers of well persons but only develops into a clinical pneumonia with the onset of immunosuppression. Similarly, the observation that Haitians, as well as intravenous drug abusers from endemic areas for tuberculosis, often present with *Mycobacterium tuberculosis* as the initial manifestation of their immune defect, favors the concept of endogenous reactivation. A histologic correlate to the presence of underlying impaired cellular immunity is the absence of granuloma formation in tissues involved with infection by organisms that usually elicit a granulomatous response in persons with normal im- munity. Such impaired granuloma formation may be found in AIDS patients with *M. tuberculosis.*

Deficient cellular immunity may also be important for the development of Kaposi's sarcoma, as has been suggested by the occurrence of this tumor in non-AIDS patients who have been immunosuppressed for renal transplantation or other causes. In addition, the humoral immune impairment found in AIDS predisposes to certain bacterial pneumonias, such as those caused by *Streptococcus pneumoniae* or *Hemophilus influenzae.*

Analysis of alveolar lavage cells in AIDS patients with PCP has revealed an increased cellular content, with the number of neutrophils and lymphocytes both in excess of the normal range found in healthy controls (4)-(6). The predominant cell type is the lymphocyte, but the usual OKT4/OKT8 ratio is reduced, due to an increase in total OKT8 cells (4),(5). Of interest, the total OKT4 cell count is often normal, despite a significant decrease in numbers of OKT4 cells in the peripheral blood. An increased number of IgG-secreting cells and higher IgG levels than in healthy controls, are also found in lavage fluid of AIDS patients (5). However, no characteristic cell profile is diagnostic of a specific pulmonary complication in AIDS. Nor is there any direct relationship between the type or quantity of cells present to respiratory symptoms, roentgenographic abnormalities or survival from pulmonary disease (6). The exact role of these immunologic and cellular alterations in the pathogenesis of pulmonary disease in AIDS remains to be elucidated.

DIAGNOSTIC APPROACH

In the non-AIDS immunocompromised patient, infection is responsible for three-quarters of the pulmonary complications. In the pre-AIDS era the diagnostic yield from fiberoptic bronchoscopy (utilizing transbronchial biopsy and brush biopsy) in the evaluation of such patients with an abnormal chest radiograph was approximately 50 percent compared to 70 percent from open lung biopsy (7),(8). Even at autopsy an exact etiologic diagnosis could not be made in 15 to 20 percent of cases, the final diagnosis being "non-specific pneumonitis."

With this background, the National Heart, Lung, and Blood Institute (NHLBI) convened a workshop in October 1983 to assess diagnosis and treatment of pulmonary complications in AIDS patients (9). The six participating medical centers (New York University Medical Center, University of California at San Francisco, University of California at Los Angeles, Memorial-Sloan

Kettering Hospital, Mount Sinai Medical Center - New York, and Harlem Hospital) had cared for a total of 1,067 patients with AIDS between November 1980 and July 1983 (representing one-half of the total AIDS patients in the United States at that time). From this group, 441 patients (41 percent) were found to have pulmonary disorders (Table 1). *Pneumocystis carinii* pneumonia either alone or coexisting with one or more infections was the most common pulmonary complication. This was seen in over three-quarters of patients. Approximately one-fifth of all patients had pulmonary opportunistic infections other than PCP. A small percentage of patients had pulmonary involvement with Kaposi's sarcoma. Fiberoptic bronchoscopy proved to be an effective means for diagnosing infections. Overall, 91 percent of pulmonary opportunistic infections were diagnosed by fiberoptic bronchoscopy: PCP (95 percent); *M. avium-intracellulare* (78 percent); cytomegalovirus (85 percent); legionella (95 percent); and fungal pneumonias (82 percent). The yield from the various diagnostic procedures done during bronchoscopy was assessed with respect to the diagnosis of PCP: transbronchial biopsy had the highest yield (93 percent), while brush biopsy had the lowest (39 percent). Bronchoalveolar lavage had a yield of 79 percent. Subsequent studies have confirmed the diagnostic utility of alveolar lavage for PCP with detection rates approaching that of transbronchial biopsy (10)-(15). Significantly greater quantities of fluid are used for the lavage technique as compared with the usual bronchial washings. The bronchoscope is wedged in a middle or lower lobe subsegmental bronchus and 100 to 150 ml of sterile, nonbacteriostatic, room temperature saline is instilled in 20-30 ml boluses. Suctioning after each bolus recovers 50 to 75 percent of the total instillate. Most patients tolerate the procedure with only transient worsening of gas exchange and chest radiograph. The yield from combined bronchoscopic techniques approaches 95 percent.

Because the organism load (especially for PCP) in AIDS patients is usually very high, less "invasive" diagnostic approaches have been sought. The utility of sputum examination for pneumocystis organisms was originally studied by Toth et al. in the pre-AIDS era (16) and found to be low. In contrast, investigators in San Francisco and Miami have recently reported a positive sputum yield of 78% and 55%, respectively in AIDS patients with PCP (17),(18). Others, however, have reported a much lower yield (19). The differences may be due to variation in induction methods (types of nebulizers used), or in techniques for processing specimens; the expertise of the individuals reviewing the slides may also be an important variable since organisms are sparse in sputum. Utilization of a fiberoptic suction catheter, as well as various other types of suction catheters in intubated patients, may also provide a less invasive means for diagnosis; but their routine use as a primary diagnostic approach is still being evaluated (20). Newer techniques such as monoclonal antibody staining of lavage fluid or sputum may add to the sensitivity of these diagnostic approaches (20a).

Table 1. Types and Frequency of Pulmonary Disorders in 441 Patients with AIDS

Pulmonary Disorder	No. of Patients	%
Pneumocystis carinii pneumonia	373	85
Without coexisting infection	255	58
With coexisting infection *	118	27
Cytomegalovirus	50	11
Mycobacterium avium-intracellulare	37	8
Mycobacterium tuberculosis	15	3
Legionella	9	2
Cryptococcus	8	2
Other	3	0.7
Other pulmonary infections	68	15
M. avium-intracellulare	37	8
Cytomegalovirus	18	4
Cytomegalovirus/M. avium-intracellulare	5	0.9
Cytomegalovirus/cryptococcus	1	0.2
Pyogenic bacteria	11	2
Legionella	10	2
Fungi	6	1
M. tuberculosis	4	0.9
Herpes simplex	2	0.5
Toxoplasmosis	1	0.2
Kaposi's sarcoma *	36	8

* All patients with Kaposi's sarcoma had an associated pulmonary infection noted above.

(Modified from Reference 9)

Bronchoscopy gives non-diagnostic findings in less than 10% of AIDS patients (and/or those at risk for AIDS) who have proven pulmonary disorders. Therefore, open lung biopsy should be reserved for those patients with progressive pulmonary disease, for whom both alveolar lavage and transbronchial biopsy are unrevealing. Open lung biopsy should also be considered for patients with coagulopathies or who require mechanical ventilation, if alveolar lavage can not be done or is non-diagnostic. Our experience with 30 patients during the past five years at New York University Medical Center suggests that when open lung biopsies are performed in this setting, one-third yield PCP, one-quarter are non-diagnostic revealing marked interstitial and alveolar abnormalities, one quarter demonstrate pulmonary Kaposi's sarcoma, and the remainder yield either miscellaneous infections, including those caused by cytomegalovirus and mycobacteria, or the rare entity of lymphocytic interstitial pneumonia (LIP) (Table 2) (21). Recently, it has been suggested that some cases of non-specific interstitial pneumonitis are directly caused by HIV infection (21a). At the present time clinicians are divided on the question of whether open lung biopsies should be performed in this patient population in light of the limited yield of treatable conditions and the overall poor prognosis.

Based upon the preceding data concerning diagnosis, an algorithm for the assessment of pulmonary manifestations of AIDS is suggested (Figure 1) (21b).

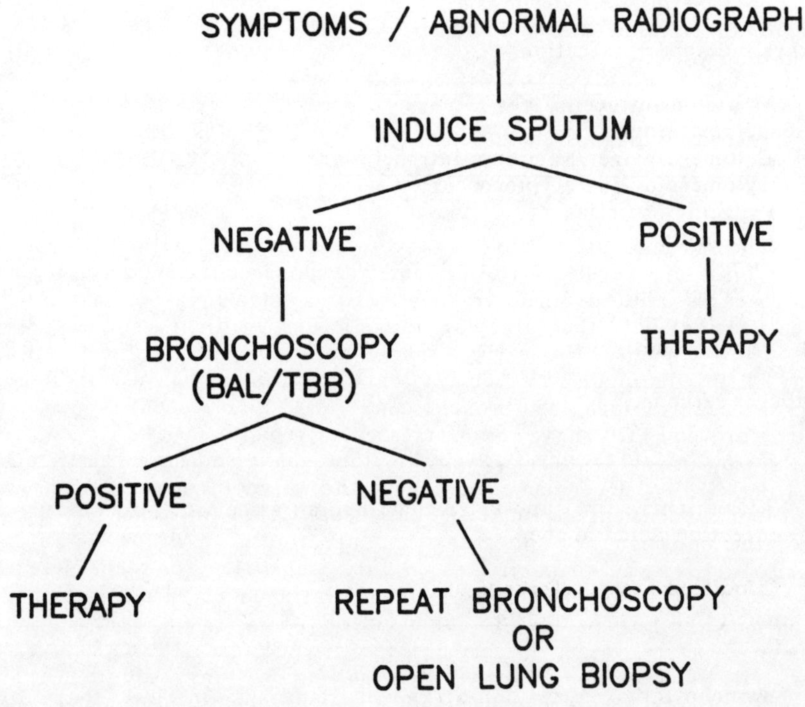

Figure 1. Algorithm for a diagnostic approach for suspected *Pneumocystis carinii* pneumonia and other pulmonary disorders in patients with AIDS. BAL = Bronchoscopic alveolar lavage; TBB = Transbronchial lung biopsy.

Table 2. Open Lung Biopsy Findings in 30 AIDS Patients at New York University Medical Center

Diagnosis by Open Lung Biopsy	Non-Diagnostic Lavage*	Non-Diagnostic Lavage & Trans-bronchial Biopsy*
Pneumocystis	3	3
Pneumocystis & Kaposi's sarcoma	1	
Pneumocystis & cytomegalovirus		1
Pneumocystis & M. avium-intracellulare	1	
Kaposi's sarcoma		7
Lymphoma		1
M. tuberculosis	1	
Cytomegalovirus	1	
Hemophilus influenzae pneumonia		1
Non-specific interstitial fibrosis	2	3
Lymphocytic interstitial pneumonitis		3
Non-diagnostic		2

* Preceding diagnostic studies.

The patient at risk for AIDS who presents with non-specific symptoms of fever, malaise, and dyspnea but a normal chest radiograph should initially undergo a non-invasive assessment. Measurement of the alveolar-arterial 0_2 gradient, single breath diffusing capacity for carbon monoxide, and gallium lung scanning may help distinguish which patients require an invasive diagnostic procedure such as bronchoscopy (9),(22)-(24). Most patients with proven PCP have an increased alveolar-arterial oxygen gradient (mean = 47 torr), even if they have normal chest radiographs (9). Exercise increases the alveolar-arterial oxygen gradient in patients with PCP but usually not in other AIDS associated pulmonary opportunistic infections. Although an abnormal diffusing capacity is highly sensitive for the diagnosis of PCP, it is non-specific. Thus, intravenous drug abusers, a high risk group for the development of AIDS, often have low diffusing capacity values in the absence of PCP or AIDS. Data from the NHLBI Workshop revealed that gallium-67 lung scanning had a sensitivity of 98 percent for PCP; however, the specificity was only 47 percent. Several subsequent studies have demonstrated the utility of gallium lung scanning, especially when the chest radiograph is normal (25)-(29) (Figures 2a and 2b). Diffuse uptake suggests PCP, whereas focal uptake suggests mycobacterial or bacterial infection (26). A graded scoring system improves the specificity of gallium-67 scanning for PCP to 90 percent (22).

Images are graded for intensity of pulmonary uptake: grade 1, normal (intensity less than or equal to adjacent soft tissues); grade 2, minimally abnormal (intensity greater than adjacent soft tissue but less than hepatic uptake); grade 3, abnormal (intensity equivalent to hepatic uptake); and grade 4, significantly abnormal (intensity greater than hepatic uptake). Patients with uptake equal to grades 1 or 2 do not usually have PCP, while grades 3 or 4 are highly suggestive for this pneumonia.

OPPORTUNISTIC INFECTIONS

Pneumocystis Carinii Pneumonia

Clinical Presentation

Pneumonia due to *Pneumocystis carinii* is the most common life-threatening infection in patients with AIDS. It occurs at least once in over 60 percent of patients and approximately one-quarter of initial episodes are fatal (30). The median survival time for AIDS patients with PCP is 35 weeks, compared to 125 weeks in patients with Kaposi's sarcoma (30a). A high degree of suspicion for PCP is necessary, since patients were often previously healthy and the illness often develops insidiously. Fever, cough, and dyspnea are non-specific complaints that may occur for many weeks to a few months before the patient seeks medical attention. In a comparative study, the median duration of symptoms in AIDS patients with PCP was 28 days versus five days in non-AIDS immunosuppressed patients (31). Occasional findings include chills, chest tightness and scanty sputum production. Analysis of the first 180 patients with PCP admitted to New York University Medical Center revealed that a subacute presentation occurred in about one-third of patients (Table 3). Physical findings were usually unremarkable except for tachypnea and a mean temperature elevation of 39°C. Laboratory studies were usually unrevealing except for lymphopenia and abnormalities in gas exchange. The mean initial arterial pO_2 was 73 torr with a mean alveolar-arterial oxygen gradient of 44 torr (Table 4). Though hypoxemia is usually present, it is often milder than in non-AIDS patients. An unexpected laboratory finding in our patients was an increase in serum lactic dehydrogenase, which may be secondary to alveolar damage (32). The chest radiograph typically shows diffuse, bilateral, reticular or reticulonodular infiltrates, although infiltrates may be confined to upper or lower lobes and may be unilateral on presentation (Figures 3-6) (Table 4) (33),(34). Between five and ten percent of patients present with normal chest radiographs. Rarely, spontaneous pneumothorax has been observed as an initial presentation. This appears to be due to the occasional finding of cystic parenchymal changes complicating an otherwise unremarkable episode of PCP (Figure 7). While enlarged hilar or mediastinal lymph nodes have been described in many patients, these findings are probably due to associated infections or tumors such as tuberculosis or Kaposi's sarcoma. Similarly, apical infiltrates and cavitation

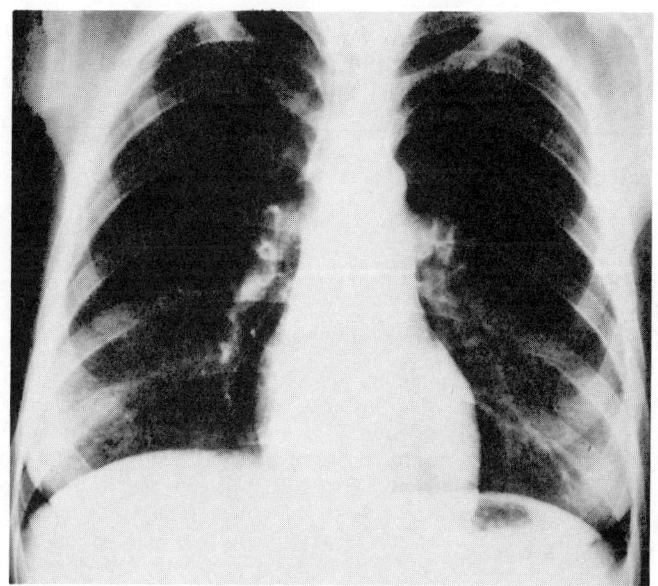

Figure 2a. *Pneumocystis carinii* pneumonia in a patient with a normal chest radiograph.

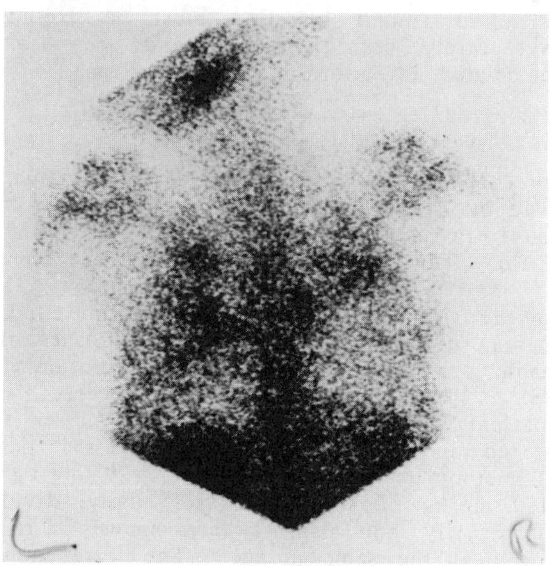

Figure 2b. *Pneumocystis carinii* pneumonia. Gallium scan of the thorax obtained at the same time as the radiograph shown above. Considerable uptake is present throughout the lungs bilaterally. Lavage documented *Pneumocystis carinii* organisms.

Table 3. Pneumocystis Carinii Pneumonia Symptoms: Experience with 180 Patients of New York University Medical Center

Fever (greater than 38°C	175 (97%)
Cough	155 (86%)
less than 2 weeks	98
2 - 4 weeks	26
4 - 8 weeks	20
greater than 8 weeks	11
Dyspnea	137 (76%)
less than 2 weeks	85
2 - 4 weeks	29
4 - 8 weeks	18
greater than 8 weeks	5

have been described (35),(35a). However, other etiologies such as tuberculosis and fungal infection must be excluded. Pleural effusions have rarely been described, and are also more likely due to other associated infections or Kaposi's sarcoma.

Treatment

In the pre-AIDS era, trimethoprim-sulfamethoxazole had emerged as the drug of choice for PCP. As of the end of 1986, it is still the usual initial therapy, but over one-half of patients treated with this drug cannot complete an entire course of treatment due to toxicity and/or failure to improve (36). Toxicity due to trimethoprim-sulfamethoxazole has included leukopenia, thrombocytopenia, diffuse erythematous skin rashes including the Stevens-Johnson syndrome, hepatotoxicity, azotemia, and drug fever (36)-(38). These complications have occurred in 18 to 65 percent of patients, in sharp contrast to the lesser frequency of toxicity reported in non-AIDS immunosuppressed patients. The dosage for trimethoprim-sulfamethoxazole is 20 mg/kg of trimethoprim and 100 mg/kg of sulfamethoxazole daily, divided into four doses. It is usually administered intravenously but can be administered orally at the same dosage. The intravenous route may be preferred because therapeutic failure has been attributed to poor absorption of the oral preparation resulting in inadequate blood levels. Folinic acid should not be given routinely to patients receiving trimethoprim-sulfamethoxazole, as there is no evidence that the vitamin prevents or reverses the cytopenias observed in AIDS patients. There is a small theoretical risk that folinic acid could impair the efficacy of the antibiotic, although this has been challenged recently. The cytopenias which occur with trimethoprim-sulfamethoxazole in AIDS patients appear to have an immunologic rather than a metabolic basis. Although both trimethoprim-sulfamethoxazole and pentamidine may cause leukopenia, the mechanism is probably different with the two agents; experience has shown that it is safe to switch patients to pentamidine while leukopenic from trimethoprim-sulfamethoxazole.

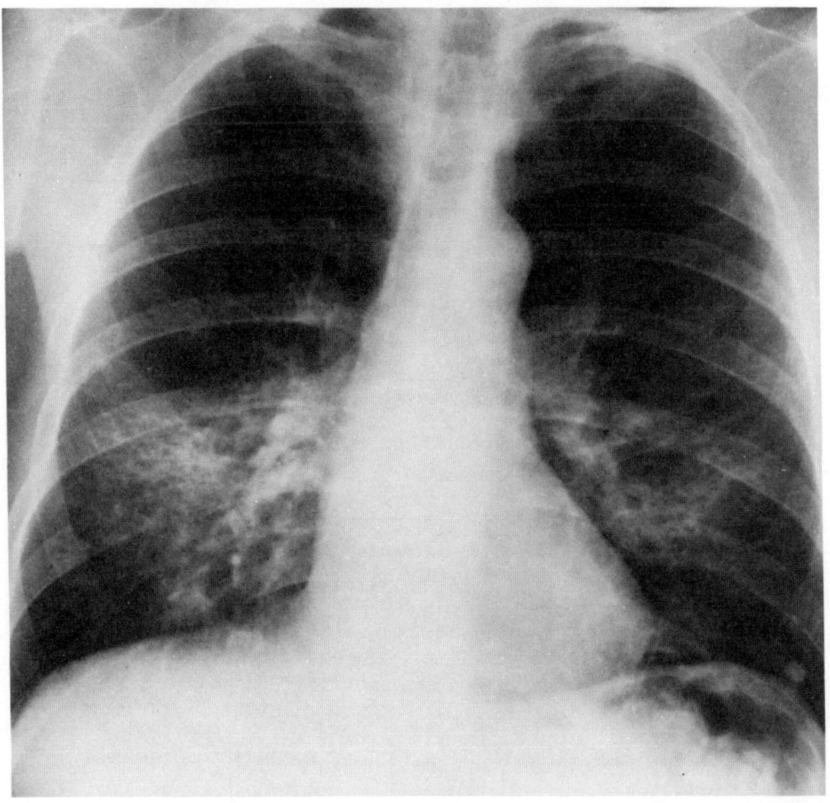

Figure 3. *Pneumocystis carinii* pneumonia. Posterior-anterior radiograph shows typical appearance of bilateral, perihilar and bibasilar reticular infiltrates, without evidence of adenopathy or effusions.

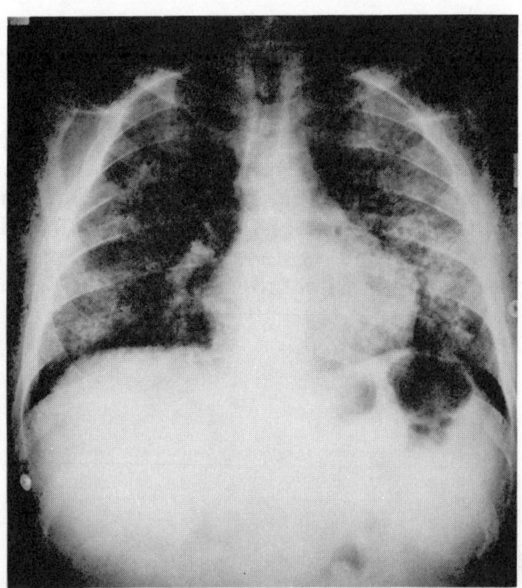

Figure 4a. *Pneumocystis carinii* pneumonia. Posterior-anterior chest radiograph demonstrates diffusely symmetrical reticular infiltrates with early focal coalescence.

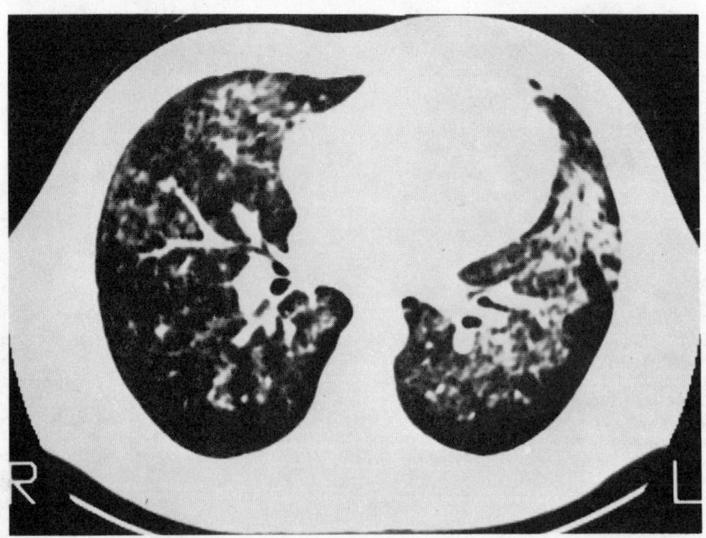

Figure 4b. *Pneumocystis carinii* pneumonia. Same patient as in Figure 4a. 1.5 cm thick CT section through the mid-lung fields documents predominately reticular appearing parenchymal disease with marked sparing of the lung periphery, especially posteriorly. Despite this interstitial reticular appearance, pathologically, the primary abnormality is intraalveolar.

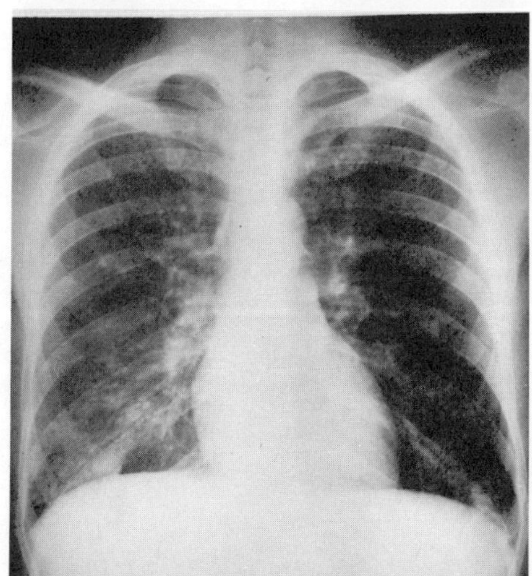

Figure 5a. *Pneumocystis carinii* pneumonia. Posterior-anterior chest radiograph. There is asymmetric pulmonary consolidation, especially prominent in the right lower lobe. Transbronchial biopsy documented *Pneumocystis carinii* pneumonia.

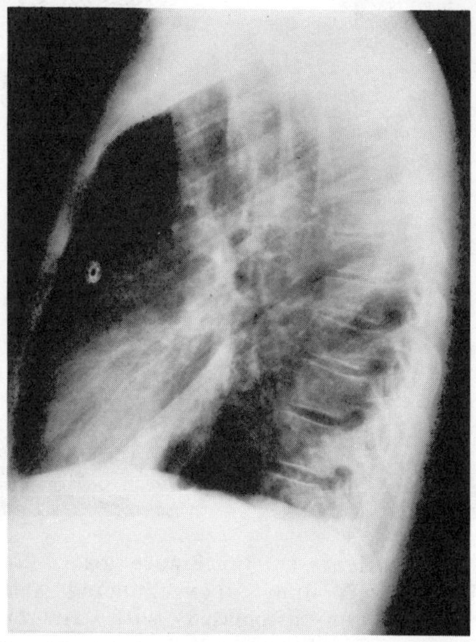

Figure 5b. *Pneumocystis carinii* pneumonia. Lateral chest radiograph of same patient as in Figure 5a.

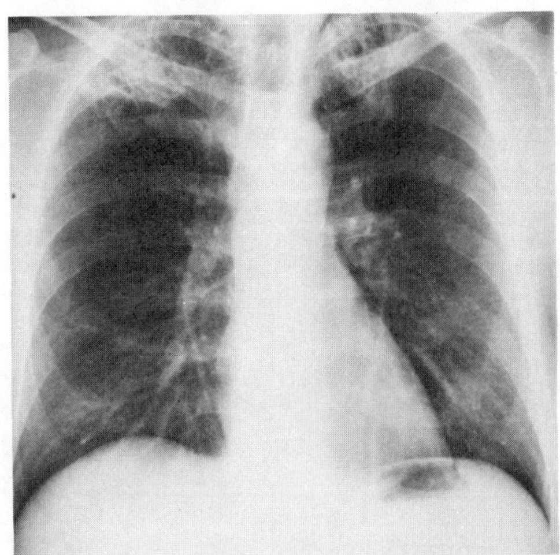

Figure 6a. *Pneumocystis carinii* pneumonia. Posterior-anterior radiograph shows atypical pattern of bilateral lung disease restricted to the apices, initially suggestive of mycobacterial infection.

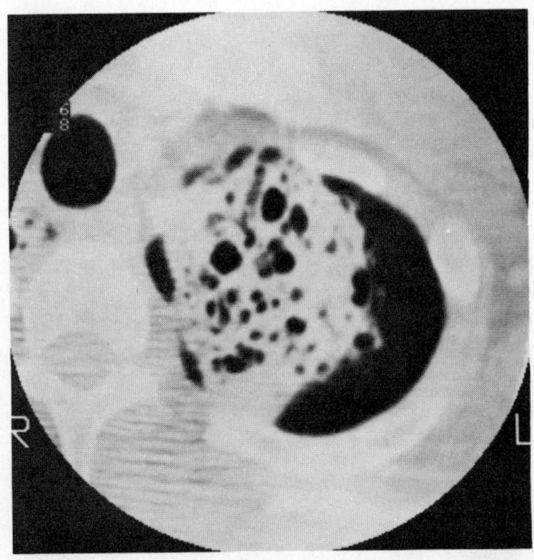

Figure 6b. Same patient as in Figure 6a. Enlargement of a section through the left lung apex showing sharply demarcated parenchymal consolidation associated with air bronchograms and discrete cavities. Transbronchial biopsy proven *Pneumocystis carinii* pneumonia - all cultures for mycobacteria were negative.

Table 4. Results of Physical Examination, Chest Radiograph and Selected Laboratory Tests in 180 AIDS Patients with Pneumocystis carinii Pneumonia at New York University Medical Center

	Mean (± SD)	Range
Physical Findings		
Temperature (^{o}C)	39 (± 1)	37.5-40
Respiratory (rate/min)	23 (± 5)	15-45
Laboratory Findings		
Arterial PO_2 (torr)	73 (± 7)	37-107
Alveolar-arterial O_2 gradient (torr)	44 (± 8)	0-76
Total leukocyte count (/mm^3)	5500 (± 1230)	1600-18,700
Absolute lymphocyte count (/mm^3)	591 (± 410)	0-3726
Lactic dehydrogenase (IU/L)	465 (± 67)	115-1650
Roentgenographic Findings	**Number**	
Bilateral interstitial	77	
Mixed interstitial/alveolar	45	
Peri-hilar interstitial	26	
Unilateral alveolar/interstitial	24	
Normal	8	

Most patients who do not tolerate trimethoprim-sulfamethoxazole because of toxicity can complete a two to three week course of pentamidine. However, approximately one-half of patients who fail to improve with trimethoprim-sulfamethoxazole, also fail to improve with pentamidine. Toxicity due to pentamidine includes azotemia, hepatotoxicity, hypoglycemia, orthostatic hypotension, drug fever, and occasional leukopenia. With the change in administration from intramuscular to intravenous use, sterile abscesses are no longer seen. Pentamidine isethionate is administered once daily at a dose of 4 mg/kg per day. Therapy with either trimethoprim-sulfamethoxazole or pentamidine should be administered for at least four days before considering a change of treatment; change should be considered only if there is clinical deterioration, since the rate of response is slow in AIDS patients. Simultaneous treatment with both drugs does not improve survival and toxicities are often additive. Three additional drugs, diaminodiphenylsulfone (dapsone), an anti-leprosy drug, difluoromethylornithine (DFMO), a drug used to treat trypanosomiasis, and trimetrexate, a methotrexate analog, are currently being investigated for their efficacy in PCP, especially for refractory cases (39)-(41),(41a). Whether or not these agents are associated with fewer side effects is an important question.

The rate of response to therapy has been analyzed in AIDS patients and is slower than in non-AIDS patients (30)-(32),(42). Typically, patients defervesce on the fifth to eighth day of treatment; arterial oxygen tension improves by at least 10 torr between days seven and 13; and chest radiographs show significant clearing of infiltrates by days 10 to 13. Treatment with either trimethoprim-sulfamethoxazole or pentamidine should be continued for at least 14 to 21 days. The optimal duration for therapy is uncertain, since it is not clear what constitutes a cure of PCP in these patients (43),(44). The relapse rate for PCP in AIDS patients has ranged from 20 to 30 percent. Repeat bronchoscopic analysis has revealed persistent cyst organisms even after three weeks of treatment. It is not known whether persistence of these cyst forms represents an increased risk for relapse.

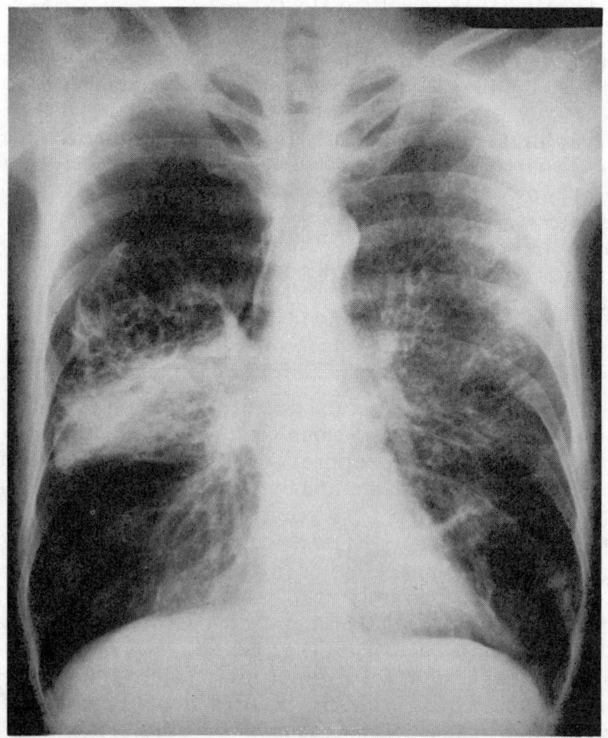

Figure 7. *Pneumocystis carinii* pneumonia. Spontaneous pneumothorax in a patient with extensive cystic changes in both upper lung fields, more prominent on the left. While non-specific, these cystic changes may be seen in patients with *Pneumocystis carinii* pneumonia and pose an increased risk of pneumothorax following transbronchial biopsy.

Arterial oxygen tension, alveolar-arterial oxygen gradient, and serum lactate dehydrogenase levels before therapy are useful prognostic indicators for survival in AIDS patients with PCP (31),(32). When survivors were compared with non-survivors, the former had a mean arterial oxygen tension of 72 versus 56 torr for the latter, a mean alveolar-arterial oxygen gradient of 42 versus 55 torr, and a mean serum LDH level of 394 versus 717 (IU/L) (Figure 8). Higher serum albumin levels and absolute lymphocyte counts were also seen in survivors. In contrast, there was no difference between those who lived and those who died with respect to mean duration of symptoms, physical findings and initial total leukocyte count.

Low dosage trimethoprim-sulfamethoxazole has been effective in preventing overt PCP in non-AIDS immunosuppressed patients. Unfortunately, a significant percentage of AIDS patients do not tolerate this drug. Pyrimethamine-sulfadoxine (fansidar) has recently been proposed as an effective prophylactic agent with fewer side effects (45),(46). Madoff et al. reported no cases of recurrent PCP in 28 patients treated with one tablet weekly for a mean of 28 weeks (45). Results of trimethoprim-sulfamethoxazole prophylaxis are anecdotal. Confirmation of the efficacy of pyrimethamine-sulfadoxine, as well as trimethoprim-sulfamethoxazole, in AIDS patients awaits the results of randomized trials, currently in progress. More recently prophylaxis utilizing nebulized or intramuscular pentamidine has been proposed and is under investigation (46a).

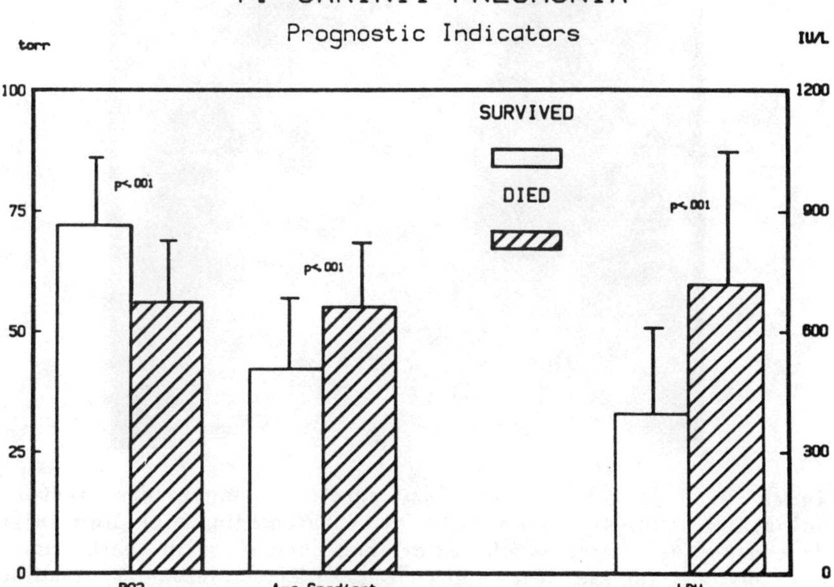

Figure 8. Prognostic indicators for survival from initial episodes of *Pneumocystis carinii* pneumonia in AIDS patients.

Mycobacterial Infections

Mycobacterium tuberculosis infection occurs in about 10 percent of AIDS patients. This infection appears to be more common in intravenous drug abusers and Haitian patients, as opposed to homosexual or bisexual men. In most patients tuberculosis is diagnosed several months prior to, or concomitant with, the diagnosis of AIDS (47),(48). Although the clinical presentation is variable, there is a consistent lack of apical and/or cavitary disease on chest radiograph, despite a high yield for *M. tuberculosis* from sputum cultures (Figure 9) (49). Histologic examination of the lung usually does not reveal acid-fast organisms, despite positive cultures from this site. Granulomata may or may not be present. *M. tuberculosis* can be isolated from at least one extrapulmonary site in about 50 percent of patients. Most patients respond to conventional therapy, i.e., isoniazid and rifampin, if treated early and for a prolonged period.

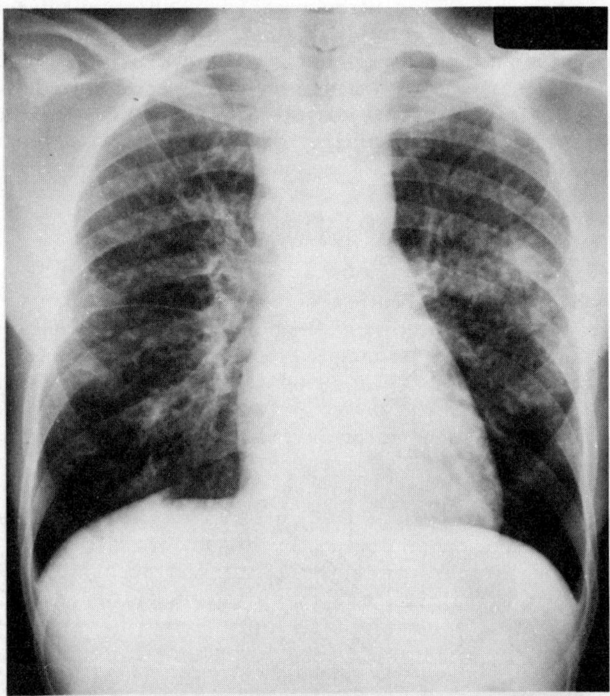

Figure 9. *Mycobacterium tuberculosis.* Posterior-anterior radiograph shows evidence of diffuse mediastinal and hilar adenopathy associated with ill-defined densities in both lungs, most obvious in the left upper lobe. These radiologic findings are most suggestive of primary infection despite epidemiologic evidence suggesting reactivation as the primary mechanism of infection.

Mycobacterium avium-intracellulare infection in AIDS patients is quite different from that in non-immunocompromised patients (50)-(52). In normal hosts the infection is primarily a pulmonary process characterized by slowly progressive local lesions which appear radiologically as cavities or patchy nodular infiltrates. Most patients are between 50 and 60 years of age, have a high prevalence of chronic obstructive pulmonary disease, and have mild or non-specific symptoms, shortness of breath or cough. In contrast, in AIDS patients this infection is usually widely disseminated. Whether or not the initial portal of entry is the lung, is unknown, but the most important clinical involvement is often non-pulmonary. Biopsies of lymph nodes or bone marrow are often more revealing than those from lung. Blood, bone marrow, stool, and urine cultures are also of value. Alveolar lavage cultures frequently grow *M. avium-intracellulare* in the absence of any histological evidence of infection in the lung. When pathologic findings are present, they are usually in the form of poorly formed granulomata without caseating necrosis. The radiographic findings may be normal or may demonstrate mediastinal adenopathy, miliary patterns, pulmonary nodules, and patchy alveolar and interstitial infiltrates. No therapeutic regimen has shown clinical or microbiological efficacy (53). The investigational agents ansamycin, and cloflazimine have excellent in vitro activity and are often administered with at least two other anti-tuberculous drugs. Unfortunately, persistently positive blood cultures for *M. avium-intracellulare* are seen despite this therapy (54).

Cytomegalovirus

Cytomegalovirus infection is the most frequent opportunistic infection found in autopsied AIDS patients. Pre-mortem, approximately one-quarter of bronchoscopic lavage specimens contain cytomegalovirus as demonstrated by culture or cytological methods, often in association with *P. carinii* (9). Cytomegalovirus pneumonia is a much rarer event than is culture positivity of respiratory secretions. Evidence for pulmonic infection should be based on histologic findings with demonstration of typical inclusion bodies, rather than culture results alone, since tissue specimens may be contaminated by blood or saliva. Radiographically, cytomegalovirus pneumonia is characterized by bilateral interstitial infiltrates, indistinguishable from those of PCP. When extensive cytomegalovirus pneumonia is present, it is usually a terminal complication and histologic evidence of dissemination to other organs is present. There is no effective treatment for this pneumonitis. Hydroxymethylpropoxymethylguanine (DHPG), a nucleoside analog related to acyclovir, has been shown to be a highly effective inhibitor of cytomegalovirus replication in vitro and has proved effective in cytomegalovirus retinitis. Our limited experience treating cytomegalovirus pneumonitis has been mildly encouraging (54a).

Fungi

Fungal pneumonias are unusual, often occurring in less than five percent of AIDS patients in association with disseminated infection (9),(55). *Cryptococcus neoformans* is the most common cause. In non-compromised hosts, peripheral nodules are usually seen. In AIDS patients, pulmonary cryptococcosis may present as a localized pneumonia, resulting in a lobar infiltrate radiographically; with dissemination (usually meningitis) an interstitial or miliary pattern may be observed. *C. neoformans* has been recovered from alveolar lavage fluid culture; histopathologic evidence of infection is variable but has been observed on transbronchial biopsy as well as open lung biopsy specimens. Disseminated *Histoplasma capsulatum* infection in AIDS patients occurs most frequently in those patients who live or originate from endemic areas (56)-(58),(58a), though we have seen patients who deny travel to such areas. When abnormal, chest radiographs reveal interstitial infiltrates or even miliary nodules. Histologic sections of lung demonstrate mild interstitial inflammation of the alveolar septae with focal nodules of chronic inflammatory cells containing histiocytes. Staining with Gomori's methenamine silver reveals small (3 to 5 *u*m), black, round structures that may be misinterpreted as *P carinii* cysts. Culture of lavage fluid or lung tissue, however, yields *H. capsulatum*. Rarely, *Nocardia asteroides* (which is not a true fungus), *Coccidioides immitis*, *Candida species* and *Aspergillus species* are responsible for pulmonary infections in AIDS patients. Nocardia infection usually presents as a unilateral lobar or segmental cavitating infiltrate, which may occur in association with mycobacterial disease (58b). Diagnosis is made by culture of sputum or lavage fluid or by histopathologic examination of a biopsy specimen. Like histoplasmosis, disseminated coccidiodomycosis usually occurs in AIDS patients living in endemic areas (59),(60). Following inhalation of airborne arthrospores pulmonary infection ensues with hematogenous dissemination to extrapulmonary sites. Single or multiple thin walled cavities may be seen radiographically. Biopsy specimens demonstrate poorly formed granulomata with thick-walled, 30 to 60 micron spherules containing numerous endospores, which are identified by periodic acid-Schiff stain. Cultures of alveolar lavage fluid grow *C. immitis*. Surprisingly, invasive candidiasis and aspergillosis are rare in AIDS patients, which accounts for their infrequent pulmonary involvement. On occasion, *Candida sp.* may invade bronchial walls and pulmonary parenchyma without significant inflammatory reaction. There is one report of aspergillus infection of the bronchial tree causing a transmural necrotizing bronchitis associated with a hyphal pseudomembrane and peribronchial and vascular invasion (61).

Bacteria

Primary bacterial pneumonias are quite unusual in AIDS patients. In the NHLBI Workshop only 11 (2%) of 441 patients had a primary bacterial pneumonia (9). However, since 1983 it has been increasingly recognized that certain bacterial pneumonias occur with greater frequency in AIDS patients compared to the general population (62),(63). Responsible organisms include *Streptococcus pneumoniae* and *Hemophilus influenzae.* Bacterial pneumonias are often associated with bacteremia. During a brief nine month period in 1983, legionella pneumonia was reported with increased frequency in AIDS patients in New York City. Since that time legionella pneumonia has rarely been seen. It should be remembered that AIDS patients, like normal hosts, may encounter infectious agents which occur sporadically in a given environment; such may have been the case with legionella.

Miscellaneous Infections

Rarely, pulmonary infections in AIDS patients have been caused by other infectious agents such as: *Toxoplasma gondii*, cryptosporidium, adenovirus, *Herpes simplex*, and varicella-zoster (64). Cryptosporidium is a unicellular protozoan belonging to the Coccidia family. While gastrointestinal involvement resulting in severe diarrhea is more often seen, at least three well documented cases of pulmonary disease have been described (65)(66). There is no effective treatment. When *Pneumocystis carinii*, mycobacteria, cytomegalovirus and fungal infections have been excluded as diagnostic possibilities, these unusual infections should be considered. Alternatively, Kaposi's sarcoma may be responsible for respiratory complaints and radiographic findings.

PLEURAL INVOLVEMENT IN AIDS PATIENTS

Clinically apparent pleural involvement is unusual. If present, the most likely cause is Kaposi's sarcoma. Rarely, pleural effusions may occur due to *C. neoformans, Aspergillus species, M. tuberculosis* or *Legionella species.* Spontaneous pneumothorax is a rare presentation for PCP (66a),(66b).

LYMPHOPROLIFERATIVE DISEASE

AIDS-Related Lymphoma

In most series, a significant percentage of AIDS-related lymphomas are primarily extranodal in distribution. Pathologically, involvement is most frequently noted in the central nervous system, gastrointestinal tract, liver, spleen or bone marrow. Thoracic involvement is relatively rare and often difficult to document (67). Mediastinal and hilar lymphadenopathy may be absent (Figures 10a and 10b). In a series of 70 autopsied AIDS patients reported by Marchevsky et al., only two (3%) patients were docu-

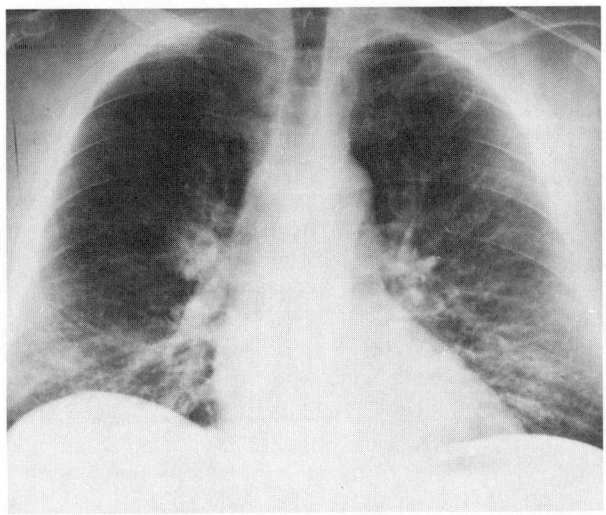

Figure 10a. Non-Hodgkin's lymphoma. Posterior-anterior radiograph. A well-defined mass is seen near the right hilum.

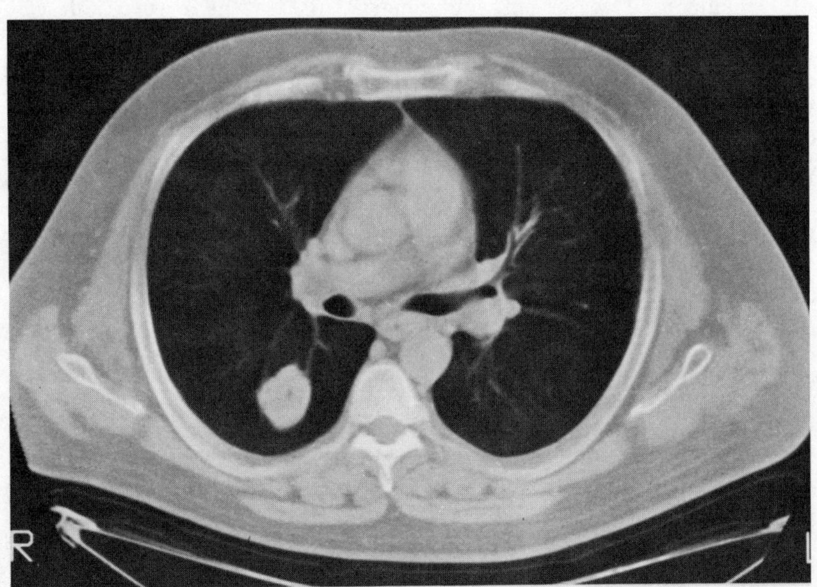

Figure 10b. CT section through the mid-lung field of same patient as in Figure 10a. A well defined soft tissue mass is demonstrated in the superior segment of the right lower lobe. No other abnormalities are present. Open lung biopsy documented lymphoma.

mented to have pulmonary lymphoma; in both cases chest roentgenogram showed bilateral interstitial changes, which in one case was associated with a left pleural effusion (68).

Lymphocytic Interstitial Pneumonitis

First described in 1966 by Carrington and Liebow, lymphocytic interstitial pneumonia (LIP) is a pathologic term used to describe an intense interstitial infiltration of the lung by lymphocytes, plasma cells, and immunoblasts. Classic LIP has often been associated with Sjogren's syndrome and rarely with systemic lupus erythematous. It has also been described in conjunction with a number of other disorders considered to be of immune origin: myasthenia gravis, pernicious anemia, chronic active hepatitis, and the auto-erythrocyte sensitization syndrome. Lymphocytic interstitial pneumonia has now been reported in patients with AIDS, particularly in children (69)-(73),(73a). In adults, it is extremely rare (three [0.7%] of 440 patients with pulmonary manifestations of AIDS seen at the New York University Medical Center from 1980-1985) (73). Its clinical and radiographic presentation is indistinguishable from that of pulmonary opportunistic infections (Figure 11). Transbronchial lung biopsy is usually non-diagnostic; the diagnosis is made by open lung biopsy. There is diffuse infiltration of the alveolar septa and peribronchiolar areas by lymphocytes, plasma cells with Russell bodies, plasmacytoid lymphocytes and immunoblasts. Vascular involvement occurs without necrosis or angiodestruction. Nodular aggregates of lymphoid cells with germinal centers are seen. There is some evidence to suggest that a viral etiology may be responsible for this entity in both AIDS and non-AIDS patients. Preliminary evidence suggests either the Epstein-Barr virus or HIV is the inciting agent in AIDS patients (21a). While some patients have responded without specific therapy, others have improved with immunosuppressive therapy (cyclophosphamide and/or prednisone).

RESPIRATORY FAILURE

A high percentage of AIDS patients develop respiratory failure at some time during the course of their illness. The NHLBI Workshop evaluated the outcome of endotracheal intubation and mechanical ventilation (9). Most patients had advanced PCP with severe and refractory hypoxemia; the mortality rate was 86 percent. Several recent studies have confirmed this high mortality rate in intubated AIDS patients (74)-(77),(77a). The most common etiology is PCP. The poor prognosis of patients with AIDS who require mechanical ventilation has raised difficult ethical and economic questions regarding the appropriateness of intensive care intervention (78). The inherent uncertainty regarding the outcome of any individual patient precludes any uniform recommendation.

Patients with AIDS and PCP manifest a clinical syndrome of hypoxemic respiratory failure indistinguishable from other forms of acute respiratory distress syndrome (ARDS) (Figure 12). Path-

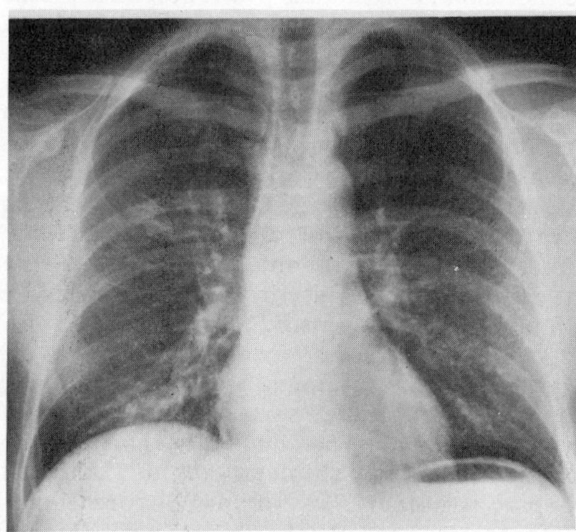

Figure 11. Lymphocytic interstitial pneumonitis (LIP). Posterior-anterior radiograph, very subtle, increased linear, parenchymal markings are present bilaterally; a nodular density is also present in the right upper lobe. These findings, including the presence of a nodular density, are non-specific. Open-lung biopsy documented LIP.

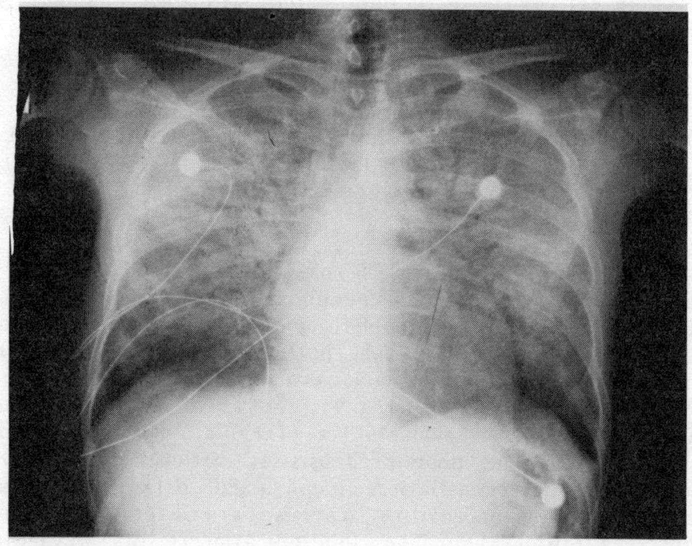

Figure 12. *Pneumocystis carinii* pneumonia/ARDS. Posterior-anterior radiograph shows diffuse air-space disease in a patient with respiratory failure, indistinguishable from other forms of the acute respiratory distress syndrome.

ologically, the spectrum of lung injury and response is also similar to ARDS. Physiologically, these patients require high inspired oxygen concentrations. They develop significant anatomic shunting (usually greater than 25 percent) as well as ventilation-perfusion mismatches, and a significantly diminished static thoracic compliance (usually less than 20cm H_2O). As with other forms of ARDS, the use of positive end-expiratory pressure (PEEP) has been advocated to maintain adequate oxygen saturation and avoid toxic inspired oxygen levels. Hemodynamic difficulties and barotrauma are frequently experienced in such AIDS patients (77). Pre-terminally, patients often develop progressive hypercapnia with increased dead space to tidal volume ratios (77).

Patients with AIDS who require intubation and mechanical ventilation pose special problems because of potential environmental contamination with blood and other body fluids. As a result, they are a cause of severe anxiety to many of the health professionals caring for them in intensive care units. Appropriate educational programs regarding modes of transmission of the disease and institution of appropriate preventive measures will allay most of these fears. In the intensive care unit these patients should be assigned private rooms. Personnel caring for these patients should wear gowns, gloves, masks and protective eyewear when in contact with respiratory tract secretions. Physicians performing fiberoptic bronchoscopy should exercise the same precautions, and the bronchoscope should be disinfected with high level disinfectants such as acid gluteraldehyde (or gas sterilized) after each use. Expired air from mechanical ventilators may disseminate airborne pathogens, and the ventilator exhaust should be vented to the outside whenever possible. Alternatively, a filter should be placed in the expired gasline. Contaminated surfaces can be disinfected with appropriate disinfectant solutions (e.g., hypochlorite).

PULMONARY KAPOSI'S SARCOMA

Clinical Presentation

Prior to the onset of AIDS, pulmonary Kaposi's sarcoma was a rare entity. According to the NHLBI Workshop, pulmonary Kaposi's sarcoma was an unusual pre-mortem finding, despite the frequency of cutaneous and lymph nodal Kaposi's sarcoma (9). In contrast, autopsy studies have shown that Kaposi's sarcoma is often present in the lungs (69),(79). The discrepancy is most likely due to the difficulty in pre-mortem diagnosis. Pulmonary involvement occurs in approximately 20 percent of AIDS patients with Kaposi's sarcoma (80). In one-half of these patients the diagnosis of AIDS was made less than five months earlier. Most patients have previous and/or concurrent pulmonary opportunistic infections and are usually bisexual or homosexual men.

The clinical presentation of pulmonary Kaposi's sarcoma may be indistinguishable from that of pulmonary opportunistic infecttions with respect to symptoms, physical findings, chest radiographs and gas exchange abnormalities (80),(81). Most patients present with fever, non-productive cough and dyspnea. Occasionally patients present with hoarseness and hemoptysis. The physical examination usually reveals cutaneous lesions of Kaposi's sarcoma, while the chest examination is unremarkable. Although most patients are hypoxemic, gas exchange abnormalities may be due to previous or concurrent opportunistic pneumonias.

In the pre-AIDS era, radiographic descriptions of pulmonary Kaposi's sarcoma noted hilar and mediastinal adenopathy, nodular infiltrates and pleural effusions. Reports involving AIDS patients have shown these radiographic presentations and have suggested that a non-specific, diffuse interstitial pattern, indistinguishable from *Pneumocystis carinii* pneumonia, may occur as well (Figures 13, 14a and 14b). The most common findings are either bilateral fluffy nodular infiltrates or mixed interstitial and alveolar infiltrates. Occasionally, a unilateral interstitial or alveolar process or an entirely normal chest radiograph is present. Pleural effusions are found in approximately 30 percent of patients and may be unilateral or bilateral. They are usually exudative and serosanguinous; cytological examination is non-diagnostic. Pleural biopsy is also unrevealing, since the lesions occur sporadically on the visceral and parietal pleura. Mediastinal nodal involvement may be due to Kaposi's sarcoma, but may also be caused by concurrent mycobacterial infection or non-Hodgkin's lymphoma.

As previously noted, it is difficult to arrive at a pre-mortem diagnosis of pulmonary Kaposi's sarcoma. In contrast to the experience with opportunistic infections in AIDS patients, fiberoptic bronchoscopy has a low diagnostic yield (25 percent). When present, endobronchial tumors appear as multiple red or violaceous lesions which are slightly raised and vascular. Visual appearance provides a tentative diagnosis. These lesions are often quite dangerous to biopsy with risk of profuse hemorrhage (82). The difficulties encountered in diagnosis utilizing transbronchial biopsy may be due to the fact that the sarcomatous lesions are focal, less cellular than most tumors and are scattered throughout the pulmonary interstitium. For the same reasons, open lung biopsy may fail to provide the diagnosis. Thus, unsuspected lesions are often found at postmortem examination (83).

Clinical Course

Once the diagnosis of pulmonary Kaposi's sarcoma is established, the mean duration of survival varies from five to eight months. Most patients with pulmonary Kaposi's have already received chemotherapy for previously diagnosed cutaneous or visceral involvement. While chemotherapy may be responsible for prolonged survival in some patients during their non-pulmonary phase, it is less successful for pulmonary involvement. Despite the progressive nature of pulmonary Kaposi's sarcoma, chemotherapy may provide some short-lived (two to four months) palliation. Combination chemotherapy has included adriamycin, vinblastine, bleomycin, vincristine, VP-16 as well as interferon. Death is not always due to pulmonary involvement with Kaposi's sarcoma; patients often succumb to concurrent or subsequent pulmonary opportunistic infection.

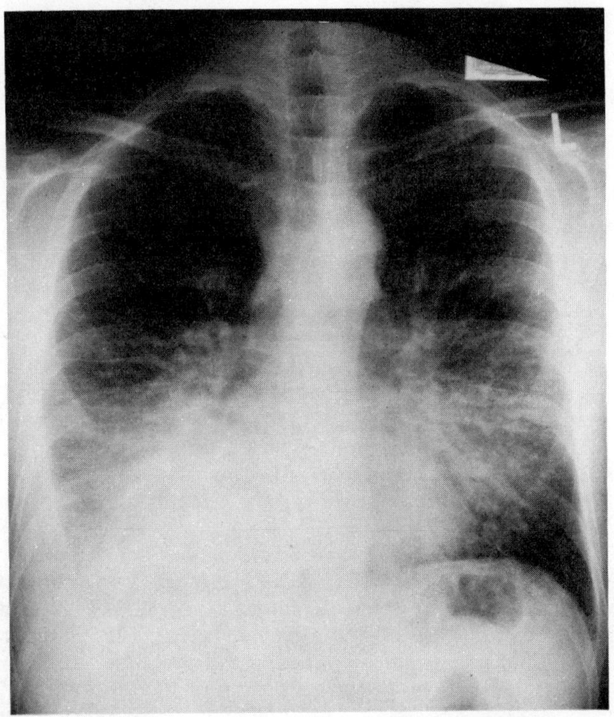

Figure 13. Kaposi's sarcoma. Posterior-anterior radiograph shows diffuse parenchymal infiltrates associated with a moderate sized right pleural effusion. There is a suggestion of subtle mediastinal widening. Open-lung biopsy documented Kaposi's sarcoma.

CONCLUSION

During the first five and one-half years of the AIDS epidemic, certain patterns have emerged with respect to the pulmonary manifestations of AIDS. Many unanswered questions still remain. The predominance of *Pneumocystis carinii* pneumonia has become apparent; the reason for this has not. Why some patients fail to respond to trimethoprim-sulfamethoxazole or pentamidine and why these drugs (especially trimethoprim-sulfamethoxazole) are associated with unusually frequent adverse reactions, remain perplexing daily clinical problems. Furthermore, the role and form of prophylactic therapy to prevent pneumocystis infection still need

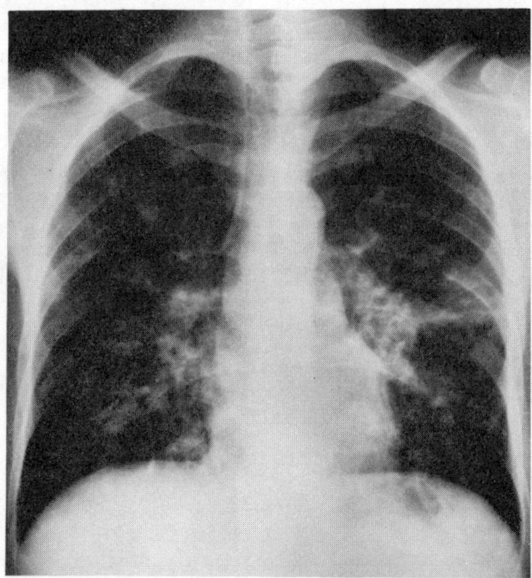

Figure 14a. Kaposi's sarcoma. Posterior-anterior radiograph. Ill-defined bilateral nodular densities are seen.

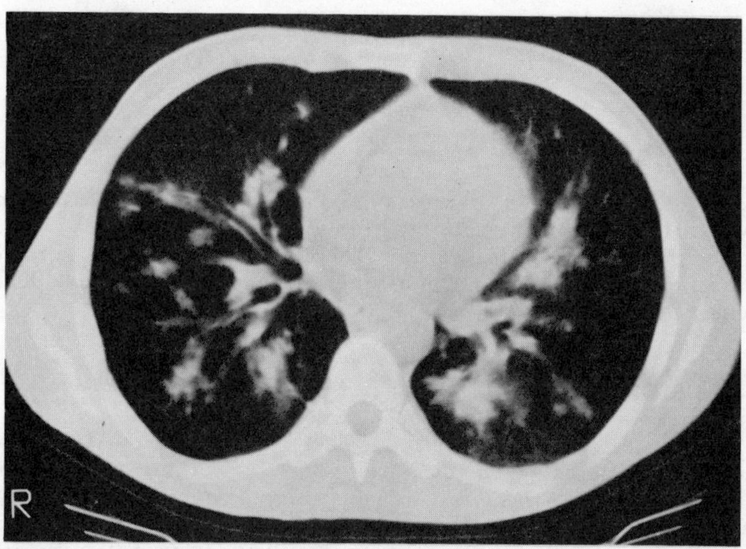

Figure 14b. Same patient as in Figure 14a. CT section documents the presence of poorly marginated parenchymal opacities scattered throughout the lungs, non-specific in appearance. Open-lung biopsy showed Kaposi's sarcoma.

to be addressed. The presence potentially of other infectious organisms, such as *M. tuberculosis*, *M. avium-intracellulare*, cytomegalovirus, fungi and pyogenic bacteria, make empiric antibiotic therapy unsatisfying and possibly dangerous. Improved methods to diagnose and treat pulmonary Kaposi's sarcoma await further research. While noninvasive means to diagnosis must be stressed, invasive approaches must not be forsaken. Because this epidemic is still evolving, caution must be taken not to preclude diagnostic modalities that may recognize changing patterns of opportunistic infections as well as discover new pathologic entities; the recent awareness of LIP and HIV-associated interstitial disease are examples of this. Finally, the devastating prognosis for AIDS patients with respiratory failure must be dealt with on an individual and realistic basis by patient, family and physician.

REFERENCES

1. CDC., Pneumocystis pneumonia - Los Angeles. MMWR 30:250-252 (1981)

2. CDC., Kaposi's sarcoma and Pneumocystis pneumonia among homosexual men - New York and California. MMWR 30:305-308 (1981)

3. Blaser, M.J., Cohn, D.L., Opportunistic infections in patients with AIDS: Clues to the epidemiology of AIDS and the relative virulence of pathogens. Ref Infect Dis 8:21-30 (1986)

4. Wallace, J.M., Barbers, R.G., Oishi, J.S., et al., Cellular and T-lymphocyte subpopulation profiles in bronchoalveolar lavage fluid from patients with acquired immunodeficiency syndrome and pneumonitis. Am Rev Respir Dis 130:786-790 (1984)

5. Young, K.R., Jr., Rankin, J.A., Naegel, G.P., et al., Bronchoalveolar lavage cells and proteins in patients with the acquired immunodeficiency syndrome. Ann Intern Med 103:522-533 (1985)

6. White, D.A., Gellene, R.A., Gupta, S., et al., Pulmonary cell populations in the immunosuppressed patient. Bronchoalveolar lavage findings during episodes of pneumonitis. Chest 88: 352-359 (1985)

7. Matthay, R.A., Moritz, E.D., Invasive procedures for diagnosing pulmonary infection. A critical review. Chest Clinics 2:3-17 (1981)

8. Singer, C., Armstrong, D., Rose, P.P., et al., Diffuse pulmonary infiltrates in immunosuppressed patients: prospective study of 80 cases. Am J Med 66:110-120 (1979)

9. Murray, J.F., Felton, C.P., Garay, S.M., et al., Pulmonary complications of the acquired immunodeficiency syndrome. N Engl J Med 310:1682-1688 (1984)

10. Broaddus, C., Dake, M.D., Stulbarg, M.S., et al., Bronchoalveolar lavage and transbronchial biopsy for the diagnosis of pulmonary infections in the acquired immunodeficiency syndrome. Ann Intern Med 102:747-752 (1985)

11. Stover, D.E., White, D.A., Romano, P.A., et al., Diagnosis of pulmonary disease in acquired immunodeficiency syndrome (AIDS): role of bronchoscopy and bronchoalveolar lavage. Am Rev Respir Dis 130:659-662 (1984)

12. Blumenfeld, W., Wagar, E., Hadley, W.K., Use of the transbronchial biopsy for diagnosis of opportunistic pulmonary infections in acquired immunodeficiency syndrome (AIDS). Am J Clin Pathol 81:1-5 (1984)

13. Golden, J.A., Hollander, H., Stulbarg, M.S., et al., Bronchoalveolar lavage as the exclusive diagnostic modality for *Pneumocystis carinii* pneumonia in patients with the acquired immunodeficiency syndrome. Chest 90:18-22 (1986)

16. Ognibene, F.P., Shelhamer, J., Gill, V., et al., The diagnosis of *Pneumocystis carinii* pneumonia in patients with the acquired immunodeficiency syndrome. Am Rev Respir Dis 129:929-932 (1984)

15. Hartman, B., Koss, M., Hui, A., et al., *Pneumocystis carinii* pneumonia in the acquired immunodeficiency syndrome (AIDS). Chest 87:603-607 (1985)

16. Toth, G., Balogh, E., Belay, M., Tracheal smear in pentamidine treated plasma-cell pneumonia. Acta Paed Acad Scient Hung 7:339-372 (1966)

17. Bigby, T., Margolskee, D., Curtis, J., et al., The usefulness of induced sputum in the diagnosis of *Pneumocystis carinii* pneumonia in patients with acquired immunodeficiency syndrome. Am Rev Respir Dis 133:515-518 (1986)

18. Pitchenik, A.E, Ganjei, P., Torres, A., et al., Sputum examination for the diagnosis of *Pneumocystis carinii* pneumonia in the acquired immunodeficiency syndrome. Am Rev Respir Dis 133:226-229 (1986)

19. Brown, S.M., Sithole, L., Aranda, C., Induced sputum in the diagnosis of *Pneumocystis carinii* pneumonia. Am Rev Respir Dis 133:A180 (1986)

20. Caughey, G., Wong, H., Gamsu, G., et al., Non-bronchoscopic bronchoalveolar lavage for the diagnosis of *Pneumocystis carinii* pneumonia in the acquired immunodeficiency syndrome. Chest 88:659-662 (1985)

20a. Kovacs, J.A., Gill, V., Swan, J., et al., Prospective evaluation of a monoclonal antibody in diagnosis of *Pneumocystis carinii* pneumonia. Lancet 2:1-2 (1986)

21. Fitzgerald, W., Bevelaqua, F., Garay, S., et al., Open lung biopsy in the acquired immunodeficiency syndrome. Chest (In press)

21a. Chayt, K.J., Harper, M.E., Marselle, L.M., et al., Detection of HTLV-III RNA in lungs of patients with AIDS and pulmonary involvement. JAMA 256:2356-2359 (1986).

21b. Murray, J.F., Garay, S.M., Hopewell, P.C., et al., Pulmonary complications of the acquired immune deficiency syndrome: An update. Report of the Second National Heart, Lung and Blood Institute Workshop. Am Rev Respir Dis 135:504-509 (1987)

22. Coleman, D.L., Hattner, R.S., Luce, J.M., et al., Correlation between gallium lung scans and fiberoptic bronchoscopy in patients with suspected *Pneumocystis carinii* pneumonia and the acquired immunodeficiency syndrome. Am Rev Respir Dis 130:1166-1169 (1984)

23. Hopewell, P.C., Luce, J.M., Pulmonary involvement in the acquired immunodeficiency syndrome. Chest 87:104-112 (1985)

24. Stover, D.E., White, D.A., Romano, P.A., et al., Spectrum of pulmonary diseases associated with the acquired immune deficiency syndrome. Am J Med 78:429-437 (1985)

25. Tuazon, C.V., Delaney, M.D., Simon, G.L., et al., Utility of gallium scintigraphy and bronchial washings in the diagnosis and treatment of *Pneumocystis carinii* pneumonia in patients with the acquired immune deficiency syndrome. Am Rev Respir Dis 132:1087-1092 (1985)

26. Kramer, E.L., Sanger, J.J., Garay, S.M., et al., Chest gallium scans in patients with acquired immunodeficiency syndrome. J Nucl Med (In press)

27. Barron, T.F., Birnbaum, B.A., Shane, L.B., et al., *Pneumocystis carinii* pneumonia studied by Gallium-67 scanning. Radiology 154:791-794 (1984)

28. Levin, M., McLeod, R., Young, Q., et al., *Pneumocystis* pneumonia: importance of gallium scan for early diagnosis and description of a new immunoperoxidase technique to demonstrate *Pneumocystis carinii*. Am Rev Respir Dis 128: 182-185 (1983)

29. Moses, S.G., Baker, S.R., Seldin, M.F., Diffuse pulmonary gallium accumulation with a normal chest radiogram in a homosexual man with *Pneumocystis carinii* pneumonia. A case report. Clin Nucl Med 8:608-609 (1983)

30. Haverkos, H.W., Assessment of therapy for *Pneumocystis carinii* pneumonia. PCP Therapy Project Group. Am J Med 76:501-505 (1984)

30a. Rivin, B.E., Monroe, J.M., Thomas, P.A., AIDS outcome: a first follow-up. N Engl J Med 311:857 (1984)

31. Kovacs, J.A., Hiemenz, J.W., Macher, A.M., et al., *Pneumocystis carinii* pneumonia: a comparison between patients with the acquired immunodeficiency syndrome and patients with other immunodeficiencies. Ann Intern Med 100:663-671 (1984)

32. Garay, S.M., Belenko, M., Schwiep, F., et al., Initial episode of *Pneumocystis carinii* pneumonia. International Conference on the Acquired Immunodeficiency Syndrome, Atlanta, Georgia (1985)

33. McCauley, D.I., Naidich, D.P., Leitman, B.S., et al., Radiographic patterns of opportunistic lung infections and Kaposi's sarcoma in homosexual men. Am J Roentg 139:647-651 (1982).

34. Naidich, D.P., Garay, S.M., Leitman, B.S., et al., Radiographic manifestation of pulmonary disease in the acquired immunodeficiency syndrome. Sem Roentg 22:14-30 (1987)

35. Milligan, S.A., Stulbarg, M.S., Gamsu, G., et al., *Pneumocystis carinii* pneumonia radiographically simulating tuberculosis. Am Rev Respir Dis 132:1124-1126 (1985)

35a. Barrio, J.L., Suarez, M., Rodriquez, J.R., et al., *Pneumocystis carinii* pneumonia presenting as cavitating and noncavitating solitary pulmonary nodules in patients with the acquired immunodeficiency syndrome. Am Rev Respir Dis 134: 1094-1096 (1986)

36. Wharton, M., Coleman, D.L., Wofsy, C.B., et al., Trimethoprim-sulfamethoxazole or pentamidine for *Pneumocystis carinii* pneumonia in the acquired immunodeficiency syndrome. Ann Intern Med 105:36-44 (1986)

37. Gordin, F.M., Simon, G.L., Wofsy, C.B., et al., Adverse reactions to trimethoprim-sulfamethoxazole in patients with the acquired immunodeficiency syndrome. Ann Intern Med 100: 495-499 (1984)

38. Small, C.B., Harris, C.A., Friedland, G.H., et al., The treatment of *Pneumocystis carinii* pneumonia in the acquired immunodeficiency syndrome. Arch Intern Med 145:837-840 (1985)

39. Leoung, G.S., Mills, J., Hopewell, P.C., et al., Dapsone-trimethoprim for *Pneumocystis carinii* pneumonia in the acquired immunodeficiency syndrome. Ann Intern Med 105:45-48 (1986)

40. Golden, J.A., Sjoerdsma, A., Sant, D.V., *Pneumocystis carinii* pneumonia treated with alpha-difluoromethylornithine. West J Med 141:613-616 (1984)

41. Dietrich, D.T., Chachoua, A., Greene, J., et al., Eflornithine treatment of resistant *Pneumocystis carinii* pneumonia in AIDS patients. International Conference on the Acquired Immunodeficiency Syndrome, Paris, France (1986)

41a. Kovacs, J.A., Allegra, J.A., Chabner, B.A., et al., Potent anti-pneumocystis and anti-toxoplasma activity of the new lipid soluble anti-folate trimetrexate. International Conference on the Acquired Immunodeficiency Syndrome (AIDS), Paris, France (1986)

42. Engelberg, L.A., Lerner, C.W., Tapper, M.L., Clinical features of *Pneumocystis carinii* pneumonia in the acquired immunodeficiency syndrome. Am Rev Respir Dis 130:698-694 (1984)

43. Shelhamer, J.H., Ognibene, F.P., Macher, A.M., et al., Persistence of *Pneumocystis carinii* in lung tissue of acquired immunodeficiency syndrome patients treated for pneumocystis pneumonia. Am Rev Respir Dis 130:1161-1165 (1984)

44. DeLorenzo, L.J., Maguire, G.P., Wormser, G.P., et al., Persistence of *Pneumocystis carinii* pneumonia in the acquired immunodeficiency syndrome. Evaluation of therapy by follow-up transbronchial biopsy. Chest 88:79-82 (1985)

45. Madoff, L.C., Sgavuzzo, D., Roberts, R.B., Fansidar secondary prophylaxis of *Pneumocystis carinii* pneumonia in AIDS patients. Clin Res 34:524A (1986)

46. Gottlieb, M.S., Knight, S., Mitsuyasu, R., et al., Prophylaxis of *Pneumocystis carinii* infection in AIDS with pyrimethamine-sulfadoxine. Lancet 2:398-399 (1984)

46a. Bernard, E.M., Donnelly, H.J., Huang, A., et al., Successful prevention and treatment of experimental *Pneumocystis carinii* pneumonia with aerosol pentamidine. International Conference on the Acquired Immunodeficiency Syndrome (AIDS), Paris, France (1986)

47. Louie, E., Rice, L.B., Holzman, R.S., Tuberculosis in non-Haitian patients with acquired immunodeficiency syndrome. Chest 90:542-545 (1986)

48. Pitchenik, A.E., Cole, C., Russell, B.W., et al., Tuberculosis, atypical mycobacteriosis and the acquired immunodeficiency syndrome among Haitian and non-Haitian patients in South Florida. Ann Intern Med 101:641-648 (1984)

49. Pitchenik, A.E., Robinson, H.A., The radiographic appearance of tuberculosis in patients with the acquired immunodeficiency syndrome (AIDS). Am Rev Respir Dis 131:393-396 (1985)

50. Zakowski, P., Fligiel, S., Berlin, O.G.W., et al., Disseminated *Mycobacterium avium-intracellulare* infection. JAMA 249:2980-2982 (1982)

51. Greene, J.B., Sidhu, G.S., Lewin, S., et al., *Mycobacterium avium-intracellulare*: A cause of disseminated life-threatening infection in homosexuals and drugs abusers. Ann Intern Med 97:539-544 (1982)

52. Marinelli, D.L., Albelda, S.M., Williams, T.M., et al., Nontuberculous mycobacterial infection in AIDS: Clinical, pathologic and radiographic features. Radiology 160:77-82 (1986)

53. Hawkins, C., Kiehn, T.E., Whimbey, E., et al., Treatment of *M. avium-intracellulare* infection in AIDS. International Conference on the Acquired Immune Deficiency Syndrome (AIDS), Atlanta, Georgia (1985)

54. Macher, A.M., Kovacs, J.A., Gill, V., et al., Bacteremia due to *Mycobacterium avium-intracellulare* in the acquired immunodeficiency syndrome. Ann Intern Med 99:782-785 (1983)

54a. Chachoua, A., Dieterich, D.T., Wernz, J., et al., CMV infections in patients with AIDS treated with 9-1,3 dihydroxy-2 propoxymethyl guanine. International Conference on the Acquired Immunodeficiency Syndrome (AIDS), Paris, France (1986)

55. Zuger, A., Louie, E., Holzman, R.S., et al., Cryptococcal disease in patients with the acquired immunodeficiency syndrome. Ann Intern Med 104:234-240 (1986)

56. Wheat, L.J., Salma, T.G., Zeckel, M.L., Histoplasmosis in the acquired immunodeficiency syndrome. Am J Med 78:203-210 (1985)

57. Small, C.B., Hewlett, D., Duncanson, F.P., et al., The acquired immunodeficiency syndrome and disseminated histoplasmosis in a non-endemic area. International Conference on the Acquired Immunodeficiency Syndrome (AIDS), Atlanta, U.S.A., (1985)

58. Taylor, M., Baddour, L., Alexander, J., Disseminated histoplasmosis associated with the acquired immunodeficiency syndrome. Am J Med 77:579-580 (1984)

58a. Johnson, P.C., Sarosi, G.A., Septimus, E.J., et al., Progressive disseminated histoplasmosis in patients with the acquired immune deficiency syndrome: A report of 12 cases and a literature review. Sem Respir Inf 1:1-8 (1986)

58b. Rodriquez, J.L., Barrio, J.L., Pitchenik, A.E., Pulmonary nocardiosis in the acquired immunodeficiency syndrome. Chest 90:912-914 (1986)

59. Roberts, C., Coccidiodomycosis in acquired immunodeficiency syndrome. Am J Med 76:743-746 (1984)

60. Kovacs, A., Forthal, D.N., Kovacs, J.A., et al., Disseminated coccidiodomycosis in a patient with acquired immune deficiency syndrome. West J Med 140:447-449 (1984)

61. Pervez, N.K., Kleinerman, J., Kattan, M., et al., Pseudomembranous necrotizing bronchial aspergillosis. Am Rev Respir Dis 131:961-963 (1985)

62. Simberkoff, M.S., Sadr, W.E., Rahal, Jr., J.J., *Streptococcus pneumoniae* infections and bacteremia in patients with acquired immunodeficiency syndrome, with report of a pneumococcal vaccine failure. Am Rev Respir Dis 130:1174-1176 (1984)

63. Polsky, B., Gold, J.W.M., Whimby, E., et al., Bacterial pneumonia in patients with the acquired immunodeficiency syndrome. Ann Intern Med 104:38-41 (1986)

64. Brodie, H.R., Drew, W.L., Hopewell, P.C., et al., Adenovirus pneumonia in homosexual males. Ann Rev Respir Dis 129:188A (1984)

65. Ma, P., Villanueva, T.G., Kaufman, D., et al., Respiratory cryptosporidiosis in the acquired immunodeficiency syndrome. JAMA 252:1298-1301 (1984)

66. Brady, E.M., Margolis, M.L., Korzeniowski, O.M., Pulmonary cryptosporidiosis in acquired immunodeficiency syndrome. JAMA 252:89-90 (1984)

66a. Goodman, P.C., Daley, G., Minagi, H., Spontaneous pneumothorax in AIDS patients with *Pneumocystis carinii* pneumonia. Am J Roentgen 147:29-31 (1986)

66b. Sherman, M., Levin, D., Briedbart, D., *Pneumocystis carinii* pneumonia with spontaneous pneumothorax. Chest 90:609-610 (1986)

67. Stern, R.G., Gamsu, G., Golden, J.A., et al., Intrathoracic adenopathy: Differential feature of AIDS and diffuse lymphadenopathy syndrome. Am J Roentg 142:689-692 (1984)

68. Marchevsky, A., Rosen, M.J., Chrystal, G., et al., Pulmonary complications of the acquired immunodeficiency syndrome. Hum Path 16:659-670 (1985)

69. Grieco, M.H., Chinoy-Acharya, P., Lymphocytic interstitial pneumonia associated with the acquired immunodeficiency syndrome. Am Rev Respir Dis 131:952-955 (1985)

70. Solal-Celigny, P., Coudere, L.J., Herman, D., et al., Lymphoid interstitial pneumonitis in acquired immunodeficiency syndrome-related complex. Am Rev Respir Dis 131:956-960 (1985)

71. Andiman, W.A., Martin, K., Rubinstein, A., et al., Opportunistic lymphoproliferations associated with Epstein-Barr viral DNA in infants and children with AIDS. Lancet 2:1390-1393 (1985)

72. Saldana, M.J., Mones, J., Buck, B.E., Lymphoid interstitial pneumonia in Haitian residents of Florida. Chest 84:347 abstract (1983)

73. Laubenstein, L.J., Kamelhar, D.L., Garay, S.M., et al., Lymphoid interstitial pneumonia in adult AIDS: Treatment with cytoxan and prednisone. International Conference on the Acquired Immune Deficiency Syndrome (AIDS), Paris, France (1986)

73a. Morris, J.C., Rosen, M.J., Marchevsky, A., et al., Lymphocytic interstitial pneumonia in patients with the acquired immune deficiency syndrome. Chest 91:63-67 (1987)

74. Luce, J.M., Hopewell, P.C., The acquired immunodeficiency syndrome: a San Francisco perspective. Intens Care Med 11:172-173 (1985)

75. Rosen, M.J., Cucco, R.A., Teirstein, A.S., Outcome of intensive care in patients with the acquired immunodeficiency syndrome. J Intens Care Med 1:55-60 (1986)

76. Maxfield, R.A., Sorkin, I.B., Fazzini, E.P., et al., Respiratory failure in patients with acquired immunodeficiency syndrome and *Pneumocystis carinii* pneumonia. Crit Care Med 14:443-449 (1986)

77. Garay, S.M., Respiratory failure in AIDS. Am Rev Respir Dis 133:A344 (1986)

77a. Wachter, R.M., Luce, J.M., Turner, J., et al., Intensive care of patients with the acquired immunodeficiency syndrome: outcome and changing patterns of utilization. Am Rev Respir Dis 134:891-896 (1986)

78. Stover, D.E., Intensive care for AIDS victims: A new dilemma. J Intens Care 1:4 (1986)

79. Niedt, G.w., Schinella, R.A., Acquired immunodeficiency syndrome: a clinicopathologic study of 56 autopsies. Arch Pathol Lab Med 109:727-734 (1985)

80. Garay, S.M., Belenko, M., Fazzini, E., et al., Pulmonary manifestations of Kaposi's sarcoma. Chest 91:39-43 (1987)

81. Ognibene, F.P., Steis, R.G., Macher, A.M., et al., Kaposi's sarcoma causing pulmonary infiltrates and respiratory failure in the acquired immunodeficiency syndrome. Ann Intern Med 102:471-475 (1985)

82. Pitchenik, A.E., Fischl, M.A., Saldana, M.J., Kaposi's sarcoma of the tracheobronchial tree. Chest 87:122-124 (1985)

83. Meduri, G.V., Stover, D.E., Lee, M., et al., Pulmonary Kaposi's sarcoma in the acquired immune deficiency syndrome. Clinical, radiographic and pathologic manifestations. Am J Med 81:11-18 (1986)

23
Pneumocystis carinii Infection in AIDS

Anthony F. Suffredini, Henry Masur

Pneumocystis carinii has achieved grim prominence as the most important pulmonary pathogen associated with the acquired immunodeficiency syndrome (AIDS). Over 65% of patients with AIDS will ultimately develop pneumocystis pneumonia and each episode carries a 10 to 50% mortality rate (1),(2). It is anticipated that in 1986 over 10,000 cases of pneumocystis pneumonia will occur in AIDS patients, and that in 1991, 75,000 to 100,000 cases will occur (1),(3). Thus, it is appropriate to devote considerable attention to the prevention, diagnosis, and therapy of this protozoan process in an effort to decrease the morbidity and mortality which pneumocystis infection causes in this population.

Despite intense interest in attempting to unravel the biology and pathophysiology of pneumocystis, the clinician remains confronted with several puzzling features of the illness. The organism cannot be reliably cultured (4)-(7). Serologic testing for diagnostic purposes is imprecise and insensitive (8),(9). In AIDS patients the signs and symptoms of the illness are frequently subtle and indistinct and often dissociated from the lung's histopathologic appearance (10),(11). There is no reliable mechanism to determine drug sensitivities. Standard therapies are frequently associated with significant toxicities limiting their usefulness (12),(13). Recurrent episodes of pneumonia are uniquely common in AIDS patients and simultaneous occurrence with other pulmonary processes, such as pulmonary Kaposi's sarcoma or cytomegalovirus pneumonitis, complicates management of the illness (2),(14),(15). Faced with these uncertainties, the clinician must have an appreciation of the unique characteristics and behavior of *P. carinii* and its resultant pulmonary disease in patients with AIDS.

HISTORY

Several excellent reviews are available detailing the historical aspects of *P. carinii* as a pulmonary pathogen (16)-(20). *Pneumocystis carinii* was first described by Chagas (1909) and later Carini (1910), though both considered the cysts to be stages in the life cycle of the trypanosome. Subsequently the Delanoes (1912) correctly identified the cysts as a new protozoan species in the lungs of Parisian sewer rats (18). The relationship of pneumocystis to human disease was not established until later, when in 1942, Van der Meer and Berg in Europe noted the association of pneumocystis and interstital plasma cell pneumonitis (21). During the post World War II era in Europe, epidemics of plasma cell pneumonitis occurred in nurseries and orphanages and carried a 50% mortality with supportive treatment (16),(17). With improvement in living conditions and general nutrition, this devastating illness decreased in incidence though mortality per episode remained high. The first U.S. case was not described until 1956 (22). During the following decade, pathologists learned how to recognize the organism and 107 cases were reported in the United States (23). From 1967 to 1970, 184 cases were reported to the Centers for Disease Control occurring in immunocompromised children and adults with underlying malignancies, congenital immunodeficiency disorders, or organ transplants (24). No effective therapy was available until the introduction of pentamidine in Europe in 1958. This therapy dramatically decreased the mortality rate for infants with plasma cell pneumonitis from 50 to 3% (25).

After pentamidine became available in the US in 1967, the recovery rate for pneumocystis pneumonia rose to 42% in the first 163 pentamidine treated cases (24). The next major therapeutic advance occurred in the 1970's when Hughes showed that trimethoprim-sulfamethoxazole (TMP-SMX) was efficacious in treating pneumocystis pneumonia and was associated with a 75 to 80% response rate (26),(27). There were few other major diagnostic or therapeutic advances until the 1980's. The AIDS epidemic in the early 1980's was a catalyst for increasing interest in this infection, as it had become a disease marker for AIDS. The incidence of pneumocystis pneumonia has increased dramatically, reflecting a growing population of patients at risk for this and certain other opportunistic infections.

BIOLOGY

Pneumocystis can be found in numerous mammalian species and is almost always limited to the lung (18),(19). Ultrastructurally, three forms exist, trophozoites, cysts, and sporozoites. The trophozoites are pleomorphic in appearance and are 1 to 4*u*m in diameter. They stain well with the Giemsa staining technique in pulmonary secretions or lung imprints but not in conventional formalin fixed (5 to 10*u*) paraffin sections of lung. Their internal structures include a nucleus, endoplasmic reticulum, mitochondria, and tubular extensions of the cytoplasm called filopodia (18),(28)-(30). Cysts are 4 to 6*u*m in diameter with a thick wall that stains with methenamine silver or toluidine blue, although the internal structures do not. Up to eight sporozoites are found within the cysts and are thought to mature upon release and develop into trophozoites (31). The sporozoites are not seen with methenamine silver or toluidine blue stains but can be visualized by phase contrast microscopy and electron microscopy (30),(31). They can be seen in pulmonary secretions or lung imprints if Giemsa stain is used, although the cyst wall does not stain well.

The exact taxonomic position of pneumocystis remains uncertain as it has characteristics of both a protozoan and a fungus (18),(20). It is unicellular and appears to lead an exclusively extracellular existence. Several investigators have described short term propagation of rat pneumocystis in cell cultures, yet to date, no long term propagation of human or rat pneumocystis in vitro has been achieved (4)-(7). The inability to serially cultivate the organism in vitro remains a major obstacle for improving our understanding of the organism, its immunology, and growth requirements.

Animal models are the mainstay of investigations of pneumocystis and host interaction. Rats are most commonly used but other animal species including mice, rabbits, and guinea pigs have been utilized as models of infection (32),(33). Rats treated with corticosteroids develop progressive pulmonary disease over a six to eight week period. The addition of a low protein diet enhances the immunosuppressive effects of steroids. Infection is felt to represent reactivation of a latent focus due to the immunodepressant effects of the steroids and low protein diet. Rats kept in a germ free environment from birth do not develop pneumocystis pneumonitis when placed on the above regimen. Germ free rats, however, will develop a primary infection with pneumocystis by exposure to unfiltered air or exposure to other rats with pneumocystis pneumonia (34).

IMMUNOLOGY

Animal Models

The immune surveillence system that regulates the development of *P. carinii* infection after initial exposure to the organism is composed of at least three elements: antibodies against pneumocystis, T-lymphocytes, and macrophages.

Antibodies to pneumocystis are initially absent in young rats or mice but appear as the rodents grow older, presumably reflecting respiratory droplet exposure and subclinical infections (35). The usual serum antibody response in animals is primarily immunoglobulin G and its production is dependent on the presence of specific T-lymphocytes (36). When steroid therapy is withdrawn in the corticosteroid-induced rat model, high antibody levels will develop in serum and bronchoalveolar lavage fluid. *P. carinii* cysts in bronchoalveolar lavage fluid from rats are found to be coated with IgG, IgA, and IgM (35). The antibodies that appear systemically and locally function as opsonins enabling the tissue macrophages to ingest and destroy the trophozoites (37).

T-lymphocytes have an active role in the control of pneumocystis infection. Murine antibody production against pneumocystis requires the presence of an intact thymus (36). Human T-cell lymphocytes in vitro undergo proliferation in the presence of *P. carinii* cysts and trophozoites. This response is dependent on the presence of monocytes (38). T-lymphocytes may also serve to activate macrophages which serve as the primary effector cells in the control of the pneumocystis infection.

Further evidence of the importance of T lymphocytes in the control of pneumocystis infection is demonstrated in the rat experimental model using cyclosporin as the sole immunosuppressant. This fungal metabolite causes inhibition of selective subsets of T-lymphocytes and yet provokes an overt pneumocystis pneumonitis (39). Changes in lymphocyte subpopulations have been found to occur during development and recovery from experimental pneumocystosis. Corticosteroid treated rats show peripheral blood lymphopenia with reversal of T-helper to T-suppressor lymphocyte ratios. Upon withdrawal of corticosteroids the lymphocyte subpopulations return to normal and the pneumocystis infection is cleared from the rat lungs (40).

The role of other immune effector mechanisms in the host's response to pneumocystis is unclear. Neutrophils and eosinophils are not characteristically seen in the histopathologic response to pneumocystis pneumonitis and are thus not felt to play a major role in the control of this infection (41).

Human Immunology

The relative importance of cell mediated and humoral immunity in the control of pneumocystis infection in humans is difficult to assess because both elements of the immune system are usually suppressed by the underlying immunosuppressive therapy or disease. In vitro data on the role of different effector cells in human disease is sparse (37),(38). Congenital immunodeficiencies, however, provide some insight into the role of cell mediated and humoral immune deficiencies in the pathogenesis of pneumocystis pneumonia (16). Bruton's agammaglobulinemia, congenital hypogammaglobulinemia, or pure B-cell defects have all been associated with pneumocystis pneumonia. Patients with combined T-cell and B-cell deficiencies seem to have a greater predisposition to pneumocystis than those with pure B-cell dysfunction alone (24). The few cases of pneumocystis pneumonia in patients with chronic granulomatous disease are probably more related to disordered mononuclear cell function than neutrophil dysfunction (42).

Conflicting results exist regarding the human serologic response to pneumocystis. This is in part due to the uncertain specificity of the antigen substrates used in the tests currently available. Early investigations showed that antibodies to pneumocystis were found in 30-40% of immunosuppressed patients with pneumocystis pneumonia, 5-10% of close contacts, and very few of the general population (43). Later studies using an indirect immunofluorescent antibody assay noted a high prevelance of antibody to pneumocystis in the general population (44),(45). These results are difficult to reconcile. Since there is no unequivocal reference standard for the presence of latent pneumocystis infections, it cannot currently be determined how many healthy individuals have subclinical pneumocystis infection or what percent of patients with pneumocystis pneumonia have reactivated a latent focus as opposed to acquiring primary disease. Recent developments using a monoclonal antibody to pneumocystis antigens may alleviate the difficulty of directly isolating a pure antigen and provide more specific data regarding the serologic response of humans to pneumocystis infection (46).

Several investigators have noted a lymphocyte predominance in the bronchoalveolar lavage of AIDS patients, most of whom had pneumocystis pneumonia (47)-(50). A smaller proportion of patients with pneumocystis pneumonia have had a neutrophil predominance in the lavage fluid even though no evidence of concurrent bacterial infection was found (47)-(50). The T-lymphocyte abnormalities present in peripheral blood (reduced helper T-lymphocytes and increased suppressor T-lymphotyctes) also appeared in the lungs of patients with pneumocystis pneumonitis (48),(49). Both blood and lavage samples have shown an increased number of IgG and IgA releasing cells and higher levels of IgG and IgA compared to normal controls (49). No cell profile however was characteristic of any particular pneumonia and no differences were found in AIDS patients without symptoms or radiographic findings compared to those with these abnormalities present (48),(50).

PATHOGENESIS OF PNEUMOCYSTIS PNEUMONIA

Alveolar Cell-Pneumocystis Interaction in Rodents.

The interaction of pneumocystis with the lung has been closely studied in the rat. Ultrastructural studies demonstrate that pneumocystis trophozoites develop an intimate association with the type I alveolar epithelial cells of the lung (28). Fusion or specialized filopodial attachment of the host and trophozoite cell membranes does not appear to occur (51). Recent studies have shown that the cell membranes of the trophozoite appear to interdigitate with the plasma membrane of the alveolar cell (52).

Several investigators (28),(29),(52),(53) have demonstrated that pneumocystis trophozoites are able to injure selectively the alveolar epithelial cells in the absence of any host inflammatory response. Selective attachment of the trophozoite to the type I pneumocyte can be demonstrated in rats after eight days of treatment with corticosteroids. During the following four weeks, focal necrosis of the type I pneumocyte occurs, preceded by the appearance of a subepithelial bleb and denuding of the alveolar capillary membrane. Increased premeability in the alveolar capillary membrane in the area of the degenerating type I pneumocyte can be shown using horseradish peroxidase as an ultrastructural marker of increased protein content in bronchoalveolar lavage fluid (53),(54). Upon tapering the steroids, a characteristic host inflammatory response occurs showing increased prominence of the alveolar macrophages and progressive lymphocyte infiltration and fibrosis (41). Increased lung surfactant catabolism occurs and may lead to a lowering of lung compliance, which may contribute to the development of respiratory failure (54),(55).

Alveolar Cell-Pneumocystis Interaction in Humans

The interaction of the pneumocystis organism with human lungs is not as precisely defined as in the above animal models. The hallmark histopathologic feature of pneumocystis pneumonia is diffuse alveolar damage which is a nonspecific response of the lung to multiple different injurious agents (56). Histologically, it is characterized by an exudative and proliferative response of the lung. A spectrum of pulmonary damage has been described in association with pneumocystis organisms varying from little or no host response to that of severe alveolar damage characterized by disruption of the alveolar capillary membrane, edema, hemmorrhage, proteinaceous exudates, hyaline membranes, fibrosis, type II alveolar cell proliferation and interstitial infiltration with lymphocytes and macrophages (56)-(58). Each of these extremes of inflammatory response can be associated with either sparse or copious organisms (11),(57). Though most pathologic descriptions of pneumocystis pneumonia emphasize the presence of a frothy or foamy honeycombed exudate within the alveolar space, it is present in only 50% of cases (56),(57), (59).

Electron microscopic studies of human pneumocystis have confirmed the intimate association of the trophozoite with the type I alveolar cell (31). Studies in AIDS patients with pneumocystis pneumonia have demonstrated that the albumin and total protein content of the bronchoalveolar fluid is significantly elevated suggesting an increased permeability of the alveolar capillary membrane (49). The finding of intravascular protein leakage across the alveolar capillary membrane is consistent with prior observations made in animals suggesting that the alveolar epithelial membrane is selectively damaged by pneumocystis (29),(53), (54).

Post-mortem studies in AIDS patients frequently show the presence of more than one pulmonary pathologic process. In patients with pneumocystis pneumonia, diffuse alveolar damage with fibrosis is frequently seen, although the contribution by other injurious agents such as oxygen toxicity, drug effect, or viral infection is unknown (15),(60).

CLINICAL MANIFESTATIONS

Prior to 1981, reports of pneumocystis infection in humans were found primarily in patients with immunologic deficiencies due to predisposing conditions such as premature birth, protein malnutrition, congenital immunodeficiency syndromes, collagen vascular disease, neoplasms, and organ transplantation (24). The annual attack rate in patients with neoplasms or renal transplants during 1967-1970 was estimated to be 0.01% and 1.1%, respectively (24).

The highest incidence of pneumocystis infection (22 to 42%) was seen in children who underwent intensive multiple agent chemotherapy, particularly those with acute lymphocytic leukemia (61). Clusters of cases were occasionally seen on oncology wards and renal transplant units (62),(63). Recurrent disease was unusual and the occurrence of concomitant infection, except for a variable incidence of cytomegalovirus infection, was low (64), (65).

Pneumocystis pneumonia is the most common opportunistic infection recognized in AIDS patients. Among all AIDS patients, 63% presented with pneumocystis pneumonia as their initial manifestation of AIDS (1),(2). The National Heart, Lung, and Blood Institute (NHLBI) Workshop report on pulmonary complications of AIDS described the pulmonary disease findings in 1067 patients from six participating institutions (2). Four hundred and forty one (41%) had serious pulmonary disorders with pneumocystis pneumonia occurring in 373 (84%). Simultaneous pulmonary infection by other agents such as cytomegalovirus, *Mycobacterium avium-intracellulare*, *Mycobacterium tuberculosis*, Legionella, or *Cryptococcus neoformans* occurred in 32% of these patients.

Pneumocystis pneumonia is a much more insidious disease in AIDS patients. When compared to patients with other immunosuppressive diseases, AIDS patients presenting with pneumocystis pneumonia had a longer duration of symptoms, lower respiratory rate, and higher room air arterial oxygen tension (10). The exact incidence and duration of asymptomatic or subclinical disease is unknown in AIDS patients. In San Francisco, an area with a high incidence of clinical AIDS, 189 consecutive autopsies of men and woman aged 20 to 50 years dying from other causes were evaluated for the presence of subclinical pneumocystis infection and none was found, although 18% of the subjects tested were positive for human immunodeficiency virus (HIV) antibody (66). A 5 to 16% incidence of unsuspected or undiagnosed pneumocystis pneumonia has been found on post-mortem examinations of patients dying with AIDS (15),(60).

An appreciation of the subtle nature of pneumocystis infection in AIDS patients is important, as the patients who are more likely to survive are those with less respiratory distress at the time of presentation as measured by respiratory rate, arterial oxygen content, and alveolar-arterial oxygen gradient (10),(67), (68). Because pneumocystis infection represents a major treatable disease entity in AIDS patients, a decrease in morbidity and mortality can probably be achieved by early diagnosis and therapy before progression to severe respiratory failure.

DIAGNOSIS

Diagnostic approaches to the AIDS patient with pulmonary

symptoms are based on noninvasive screening tests used to heighten clinical suspicions of an active pulmonary process and specific procedures that provide pulmonary secretions or tissue to confirm a diagnosis.

It is important to establish a specific diagnosis of pneumocystis pneumonia rather than to treat empirically (2). Anti-pneumocystis drugs are associated with adverse reactions in over 60% of patients (12),(13). There are several difficult issues involved in establishing a diagnosis of pneumocystis pneumonia. First, among patients with equivocal symptoms, what economical screening tests are useful to decide who should have a specific diagnostic procedure? In 125 AIDS patients with pneumocystis pneumonia evaluated with chest radiographs, pulmonary function tests and gallium scans, all patients except one, had at least one abnormal noninvasive test (69). Second, if a diagnostic procedure is needed, which should be done?

Chest Radiograph

In patients with AIDS the presence of a clearly abnormal chest radiograph is an indication to proceed to a procedure that can provide a specific histologic diagnosis. Further screening tests will usually serve only to delay a definitive diagnosis. The usual radiographic pattern of pneumocystis in immunocompromised patients is bilateral perihilar or diffuse interstitial infiltrates, although this finding is nonspecific (70). Documented pneumocystis pneumonia has also been recognized in association with an asymmetric distribution, lobar consolidation, pseudonodular infiltrates, cavities, or cystic appearing infiltrates, and occasionally, a normal appearing radiograph (16),(70),(71). All of these patterns can be seen in AIDS patients with pneumocystis pneumonia. The most common radiographic features are diffuse interstital infiltrates (60-75%) or interstitial - alveolar infiltrates (30%) with varying degrees of severity (14),(72)-(74). Atypical radiographic presentations including lobar consolidation have been noted in up to 10% of AIDS patients with pneumocystis pneumonia (72),(74).

Nuclear Medicine Procedures

Gallium-67 citrate scans represent a sensitive, expensive, though nonspecific screening test for active pulmonary disease in AIDS patients. This technique can be used to evaluate the patient presenting with pulmonary symptoms and a normal or minimally abnormal chest radiograph. The scan is conventionally performed 48 to 72 hours after injection of the radiolabeled isotope. Twenty-four hour scans are often equally useful. The sensitivity for pneumocystis pneumonia approaches 90 to 98%, although its specificity ranges from 40 to 47% (2),(69),(75). Pneumocystis pneumonia has been reported with normal or minimally abnormal scans, but typically the lung fields show diffuse symmetric pulmonary uptake that is at least equal to bone marrow uptake. Repeat scans do not appear to correlate well with the presence of pneumocystis after initiation of therapy because of persistent uptake of the radioisotope (76),(77).

Alternative nuclear medicine scanning techniques to assess the presence of active pulmonary disease are being developed. Ventilation scans performed with small sized radiolabeled aerosolized solutes may offer some advantage over gallium scanning as a rapid screening test to determine which patients should be considered for bronchoscopy. Aerosolized diethylenetriamine pentacetate (DTPA) labeled with technetium 99 has been noted in preliminary studies to be a sensitive though nonspecific marker of active pulmonary disease in selected AIDS patients with pneumocystis pneumonia (78),(79).

Serologic Testing

Serologic testing to detect antibody or circulating antigens have no clinical value in diagnosing pneumocystis pneumonia in any clinical setting (8),(9). As currently applied the above tests lack sensitivity, specificity, and have poor predictive value. Further work needs to be done to characterize the pneumocystis antigen and antibody to make these tests clinically relevant.

Pulmonary Function Testing

Arterial blood gases, lung spirometry, and diffusing capacity of carbon monoxide provide relatively sensitive though nonspecific tests of pulmonary impairment. In 159 patients with pneumocystis pneumonia only 8% had a normal alveolar-arterial partial pressure of oxygen gradient (less than 15 mmHg) (2). Exercise induced widening of the gradient may increase the sensitivity of this test but presumably not its specificity (14).

Pulmonary function tests in patients with pneumocystis pneumonia typically show a decrease in lung volumes (vital capacity and total lung capacity), an increase in flow rates (forced expired volume in one second to forced vital capacity ratio), and a decreased diffusing capacity. Although statistically significant differences occur in these measurements between AIDS patients with and without pneumocystis pneumonia, there is substantial overlap between both groups (14),(80). A decrease in diffusing capacity with a normal chest radiograph has been noted to occur with pneumocystis pneumonia, yet it may also occur with other conditions, such as intravenous drug abuse (74),(80).

Tissue Stains

The definitive diagnosis of pneumocystis pneumonia is dependent on demonstration of *P. carinii* cysts or trophozoites in samples of lung secretions or lung parenchyma. Methods used to document the presence of pneumocystis include light microscopic techniques using conventional stains, and microscopy using immunologic stains, phase contrast microscopy, and electron microscopy (30),(31),(46),(56),(81). The choice of technique depends on the

Table 1. Demonstration of Forms of Pneumocystis Carinii in Pulmonary Specimens Using Brightfield Microscopy and Various Staining Techniques

Pulmonary Specimen and Staining Technique	Ability to Stain Pneumocystis		
	Cyst Wall	Sporozoite	Trophozoite
Bronchoalveolar lavage			
Hematoxylin and Eosin	-	-	-
Methenamine Silver	+	-	-
Toluidine Blue O	+	-	-
Gram Weigert	+	-	-
Cresyl Echt Violet	+	-	-
Giemsa	-	+	+
Lung Imprint			
Hematoxylin and Eosin	-	-	-
Methenamine Silver	+	-	-
Toluidine Blue O	+	-	-
Gram Weigert	+	-	-
Cresyl Echt Violet	+	-	-
Giemsa	-	+	+
Lung Histology-Paraffin Sections (5-10 microns)			
Hematoxylin and Eosin	-	-	-
Methenamine Silver	+	-	-
Toluidine Blue O	+	-	-
Gram Weigert	+	-	-
Cresyl Echt Violet	+	-	-
Giemsa	-	-	-
Lung Histology-Plastic Sections (1 micron)			
Hematoxylin and Eosin	-	-	-
Methenamine Silver	+	-	-
Toluidine Blue O (after sulfation)	+	-	-
Toluidine Blue O (no sulfation)	-	+	+
Giemsa	-	+	+

equipment and expertise available, as well as the amount of time, cost, sensitivity and specificity of the individual procedures.

Light microscopy is used by most laboratories. Two types of toluidine blue 0 stain are used to stain the cyst forms of pneumocystis and can be used on histologic sections and samples of tissue imprints or secretions. The modified toluidine blue 0 stain uses the sulfation reagent employed in the cresyl echt violet stain of *P. carinii* and has the advantage of being rapid, using simple reagents, and is associated with less background artifact than the standard toluidine blue 0 stain (81). Methenamine silver outlines cysts on histologic samples or on tissue imprints or secretions. Both of these staining techniques stain fungi which can be confused with *P. carinii* cysts by inexperienced observers. Pneumocystis cysts are distinguished from fungal forms by the absence of budding, their intraalveolar location, and more oval shape (81). A control slide with pneumocystis cysts is necessary to avoid false negatives for both the toluidine blue 0 and methenamine silver stains.

The Gram Weigert method also stains cyst forms on histologic sections, tissue imprints, or secretions. Retained crystal violet by cell nuclei may make interpretation difficult. Stains for trophozoites and sporozoites used on tissue imprints or pulmonary secretions include the Giemsa, modified methylene blue, and Gram stain. With these stains, the trophozoites or sporozoites are difficult to see and background staining artifact may complicate their interpretation (81),(82).

The Papanicolaou stain has been used on bronchial washings and lavage fluid. Pneumocystis cysts appear as an amphophilic amorphous granular mass (83). A modification of the Papanicolaou smear views the material under ultraviolet light. The cysts emit bright fluorescence permitting localization and identification. This procedure may complement the use of other conventional stains (84).

The recent development of an immunofluorescent monoclonal antibody provides a rapid, simple, and specific technique for detection of *P. carinii* cysts in clinical specimens (46). Monoclonal antibodies generated by human *P. carinii* cysts react only with a specific epitope of the pneumocystis antigen. The antibody does not react with host cells or other organisms such as yeast. Because of its specificity, this technique has major implications for the future study of pneumocystis.

Sputum Examination

Based on previous experience in immunosuppressed patients other than AIDS patients with pneumocystis pneumonia, examination of expectorated sputum or transtracheal aspirates had a low yield (6 to 13%) for detection of *P. carinii* (24),(85). Several investigators have been able to induce sputum in AIDS patients. By staining smears with Giemsa stains they have been able to detect *P. carinii* in 55 to 73% of proven cases (86),(87). The procedure varies slightly among different investigators. Patients breath hypertonic saline (3 or 5%) administered by an ultrasonic nebulizer for 10-20 minutes. Recovered sputum is then either cytocentrifuged and stained with methenamine silver or smeared directly onto a slide and stained with a modified Giemsa stain. The negative predictive value of the test is approximately 50%. Cryptococcus has also been occasionally noted in sputum. In some patients, subsequent bronchoscopies diagnosed other pulmonary processes not detected by sputum examination, including Kaposi's sarcoma, *Cryptococcus neoformans*, and cytomegalovirus. A variation of the above method has been described in a case report using ultraviolet light examination of Papanicolaou stained sputum in an AIDS patient (88).

Sputum examination represents a simple first step in evaluating an AIDS patient who, because of an abnormal screening test, is at risk for pneumocystis. If sputum induction is unsuccessful or negative, then further diagnostic evaluation with bronchoscopy is indicated. Because sputum induction may miss other treatable pathogens, the patient whose diagnosis rests solely on the findings of sputum examination must be followed closely to assess the clinical response to therapy. Further, the clinician must consider whether this limited clinical information will be adequate for his particular patient. If documentation of pulmonary Kaposi's sarcoma, cytomegalovirus infection or another pulmonary infectious agent is important for therapeutic or prognostic information, than it may not be time or cost efficient to attempt sputum induction when bronchoscopy is needed anyway.

Fiberoptic Bronchoscopy

Fiberoptic bronchoscopy has been demonstrated to be the most successful single diagnostic tool used to evaluate the AIDS patient with pulmonary disease and has been especially useful in diagnosing pneumocystis pneumonia. The National Heart, Lung and Blood Institute workshop on pulmonary complications of AIDS reported that 95% of the 373 episodes of pneumocystis pneumonia were diagnosed by fiberoptic bronchoscopy. This retrospective evaluation noted that when four diagnostic studies were done with specimens obtained from fiberoptic bronchoscopy (tough imprints, fixed tissue, brushings and lavage), no case of pneumocystis pneumonia was missed (2). Other retrospective evaluations have noted an overall sensitivity of 85% using one or more of the following procedures: transbronchial biopsy, washings, touch imprints, and brushings (89).

When evaluated prospectively bronchoalveolar lavage has been noted to have an 87 to 89% sensitivity for diagnosis of pneumocystis pneumonia (90)-(92). Lavage combined with transbronchial biopsies increased the sensitivity rate to 94-100% (91),(92). The negative predictive value of bronchoscopy for pneumocystis pneumonia when both bronchoalveolar lavage and transbronchial biopsy are performed and no pneumocystis is found, is greater than 90% (92). In patients with adequate lavage and transbronchial biopsy specimens, this degree of reliability of a negative result strongly suggests an alternative diagnosis.

Complications associated with bronchoalveolar lavage and transbronchial biopsy include hemoptysis, pneumothorax, fever with chills, or transient new pulmonary infiltrates. The occurrence of pneumothorax can be minimized by the skillful bronchoscopist and by performance of biopsies under fluoroscopic guidance. Contraindications to transbronchial biopsy include a significant bleeding diathesis (platelet count less than 50,000/mm^3 or prothrombin time greater than three seconds above control values), severe hypoxemia (inability to maintain an arterial partial pressure of oxygen greater than 100 torr on an inspired oxygen concentration of 100%) or positive end expiratory pressures greater than five cm H_2O while on mechanical ventilation. In some of these patients bronchoalveolar lavage alone can be a useful diagnostic procedure.

Nonbronchoscopic Lung Lavage

Variations in the technique of fiberoptic bronchoalveolar lavage have been described using: 1) a control (movable) tipped catheter placed into the lung segments fluoroscopically (93); 2) lung lavage by catheters passed blindly in intubated patients into lung segments (94); or 3) endobronchial lavage using conventional endotracheal suctioning techniques (95),(96). These techniques hold some promise as potentially quick and cost effective diagnostic methods. However, their sensitivity, specificity, and safety need to be assessed in larger studies. When bronchoscopy is unavailable, they may be a valuable means of evaluating a patient who is deteriorating rapidly.

Transthoracic Needle Aspiration

Percutaneous needle aspiration of the lung has been reported as a diagnostic method in patients with AIDS, but its use as a routine diagnostic procedure is hampered by the high rate of associated pneumothoraces (97). In a series of 13 patients for whom adequate specimens were obtained, 11 were found to have pneumocystis. Other pathogens identified included cytomegalovirus, *Mycobacterium avium-intracellulare* and bacteria. Unfortunately, despite the advantage of being less costly and time consuming than fiberoptic bronchoscopy, pneumothorax occurred in 44% of the cases and 19% required chest tube thoracostomy. As currently performed percutaneous needle aspiration of the lung can not be recommended as a routine procedure in AIDS patients with pulmonary disease.

Open Lung Biopsy

It is unusual for properly performed bronchoalveolar lavage and transbronchial biopsies to fail to detect infection with pneumocystis. Open lung biopsy may be a useful diagnostic procedure in patients whose respiratory status is deteriorating and in whom fiberoptic bronchoscopy is contraindicated or nondiagnostic. Alternatively, when a second diagnosis is being considered that has therapeutic or prognostic significance for the patient, such as pulmonary Kaposi's sarcoma, an open lung biopsy may provide necessary clinical information. The procedure, however, has a moderate degree of morbidity and mortality (as high as 10% in critically ill patients) associated with it. Therefore, open lung biopsy should be reserved for those clinical situations where the patient will clearly benefit from a definitive diagnosis that cannot be attained with other diagnostic procedures (2), (98).

Summary of Diagnostic Approaches

The individual usefulness of any diagnostic test relates in part to the skill of the operators performing the procedure, the methods available for processing the lung material, and the technical capabilities of the pathologist and microbiologist evaluating the tissue or fluid samples. Further considerations influencing the clinicians choice of a diagnostic test should include: 1) the degree of invasiveness and morbidity associated with the procedure; 2) the ability to perform the procedure as an outpatient; 3) the clinical implications of the data gleaned from the study; 4) the time lost processing material from a potentially inconclusive test; 5) the hospital resources available to perform the procedure (operating room time, fluoroscopy); 6) the expense involved; and 7) the condition of the patient undergoing the procedure (bleeding diathesis, hypoxemia, depression).

The clinician caring for a patient with AIDS and abnormal pulmonary findings must make diagnostic decisions that are influenced by the specific circumstances regarding the availability of various diagnostic procedures in the health care facility. In clinically stable patients with either an abnormal chest radiograph, or an equivocal or normal chest radiograph but abnormal pulmonary signs or symptoms and an abnormal screening test, sputum induction may be attempted as a screening procedure. If this is negative or sputum cannot be induced, than fiberoptic bronchoscopy should be performed.

If the results of transbronchial biopsies and bronchoalveolar lavage are negative and the patient is clinically stable, than it is reasonable to observe the patient prior to embarking on repeat or further diagnostic workup. We have found that up to 32% of the AIDS patients evaluated with fiberoptic bronchoscopy have had no evidence of a treatable infectious pulmonary process and histopathologically show only changes of nonspecific interstitial pneumonitis (99). The etiology of this entity in AIDS patients is uncertain but in other groups of immunocompromised patients with diffuse pulmonary infiltrates it is presumed to be related to drug toxicity (especially chemotherapeutic agents), effects of radiation therapy, viral infection, oxygen toxicity, or to the underlying disease itself (100),(101). The patient with rapidly progressive respiratory failure, or one who develops significant clinical deterioration, may require further diagnostic evaluation with either a repeat fiberoptic bronchoscopy or an open lung biopsy.

THERAPY

Trimethoprim-Sulfamethoxazole

The usual initial therapy of pneumocystis pneumonia is

trimethoprim-sulfamethoxazole (TMP-SMX). Its efficacy has been well documented in children and adults with underlying malignancies or organ transplants (102),(103). Seventy to eighty percent of these patients will respond clinically and radiologically to intravenous TMP-SMX (20mg TMP/100mg SMX/kg/d, given in four equal doses) within four days (103),(104). In children TMP-SMX has been shown to be as effective as pentamidine isethionate with fewer adverse effects (27). Fourteen percent of non-AIDS patients treated for pneumocystis pneumonia experienced side effects and these were primarily rashes and gastrointestinal side effects, with rare episodes of hematologic or hepatic abnormalities (102).

Early in the AIDS epidemic it became apparent that differences existed in the presentation and the clinical response to anti-pneumocystis therapy of AIDS patients with pneumocystis pneumonia compared to non-AIDS patients. AIDS patients were noted to experience a longer time from the onset of illness to diagnosis (median 25 days versus five to six days) and required a longer duration of therapy (19 days versus 11 to 14 days) than non-AIDS patients with tumors or organ transplants. The relapse rate was noted to be higher in AIDS patients after their original episode of pneumonia (10),(105). Several investigators noted that the immediate outcome of pneumocystis pneumonia in AIDS was not worse than in non-AIDS patients with the understanding that this patient group required a longer duration of therapy and experienced frequent relapses (10),(105)-(107).

Serum drug levels should be monitored in critically ill patients because they may not absorb orally administered drugs well. Other factors such as abnormal renal function or unusual volumes of drug distribution may make therapeutic levels unpredictable even with intravenous administration. Peak levels of 5 to 10ug/ml of TMP and 100 to 150ug/ml of SMX, drawn 90 minutes after administration of the drug have been documented in successfully treated non-AIDS patients (108).

Sixty to 75% of AIDS patients treated with TMP-SMX will develop adverse reactions to the drug usually during the second week (10),(12),(13),(105)-(107),(109),(110). These adverse side-effects include rash, fever, leukopenia, thrombocytopenia, and transaminase elevations. Therapy will need to be changed to an alternate medication in 30 to 60% of the patients experiencing adverse reactions.

The reason for the increased incidence of adverse side-effects to TMP-SMX in AIDS patients is unknown but the adverse effects rapidly resolve upon discontinuation of the drug. Folinic acid (5 to 10mg/d) appears to be ineffective when given prophylactically or therapeutically to AIDS patients with cytopenias who are being treated with TMP-SMX (10),(110),(111). Hematologic abnormalities of patients due to folate deficiency, however, respond readily to folinic acid. Daily administration of folinic acid in immunosuppressed rats with pneumocystis pneumonia did not, however, interfere with the therapeutic action of TMP-SMX (112).

Pentamidine Isethionate

Prior to 1974, pentamidine isethionate (4 mg/kg/day) was the only therapy available for the treatment of pneumocystis pneumonia. Its principal mechanism of action may be inhibition of DNA synthesis and a minor mechanism may be through an effect on folate synthesis (113). In an early series of patients reported to the Centers for Disease Control from 1967-70, 42% of patients with pneumocystis pneumonia responded to pentamidine though adverse reactions occurred in 47% of the patients (24). The most common adverse reactions were renal insufficiency (23%) and local reactions from intramuscular administration including pain at the injection site and sterile abscesses (18%). Less common side effects included abnormal liver function tests, hypoglycemia, hypocalcemia, hematologic abnormalities, skin rashes, and rarely insulin dependent diabetes mellitus.

Studies evaluating the treatment of non-AIDS patients with pneumocystis pneumonia with either TMP-SMX or pentamidine, found that clinical response rates were similar though more adverse reactions occurred with intramuscular pentamidine (27),(102),(103),(114). More recently, studies in AIDS patients have been unable to demonstrate any significant difference in the clinical response of patients with first episode pneumocystis pneumonia randomized to receive TMP-SMX or pentamidine. Adverse effects occurred with equal frequency in both groups of patients (13),(115).

Pentamidine was only rarely given intravenously in the past because of reports of an association of this route of administration, with seizures, hypotension, and death (113). With the increased need for pentamidine in AIDS patients and the desire to minimize patient discomfort, its intravenous use was reevaluated. It has been shown to be well tolerated without significant hypotension when given as a slow infusion in 150 ml of 5% dextrose in water over one hour (116),(117).

Retrospective analysis has shown that several days may elapse between initiation of therapy and achievement of measureable levels of pentamidine in the lung (118). Aerosolization of pentamidine may provide a more rapid method of drug administration with less systemic side effects. Studies performed using a rat model of pneumocystis pneumonia have shown that aerosolized pentamidine has an anti-pneumocystis effect with low extrapulmonary uptake of the drug (119). This technique may prove to be less toxic than parenteral use of the drug but its clinical efficacy in humans remains to be demonstrated.

Alpha Difluoromethylornithine

There are few well-studied alternate therapies for pneumocystis infection. AIDS patients with pneumocystis pneumonia who were unable to tolerate TMP-SMX or pentamidine, have shown clinical improvement in several clinical trials with alpha difluoromethylornithine (DFMO), an irreversible inhibitor of ornithine decarboxylase (120)-(124). Patients were given two weeks of intravenous DFMO (400mg/kg/d) followed by oral therapy (300mg/kg/d) for two to six weeks. A clinical response rate of 72% overall was found in 53 AIDS patients who received the drug on a compassionate basis for more than 14 days (124). Patients requiring mechanical ventilation had a lower clinical response rate (0 to 40%) (121),(122). Side effects included cytopenias, anemia, gastrointestinal disturbances, hepatitis, and hearing loss.

Dapsone

Dapsone has been shown to be a useful alternate therapy in a murine model of pneumocystis pneumonia particularly when given in combination with trimethoprim (125). When given alone to AIDS patients with pneumocystis pneumonia, dapsone was found to be less effective than standard therapy (126). However, when given in conjunction with trimethoprim, dapsone was as effective as standard therapy (127). Its potential role as a prophylactic agent remains to be determined. Hypersensitivity reactions, hemolysis and methemoglobinemia are the major side-effects.

A diformyl derivative of dapsone, 4'4'sulfonylbisformanilide, has been used in conjunction with trimethoprim in a rat model of pneumocystis pneumonia and was noted to be as effective as TMP-SMX for therapy and prophylaxis (128). It potentially has less toxicity and fewer side-effects than dapsone.

Trimetrexate

Trimetrexate is a lipid soluble antifolate which may offer an alternative therapy with distinct advantages over conventional therapy. It has been found to be a more potent inhibitor of murine pneumocystis dihydrofolate reductase than trimethoprim or pyrimethamine. Because of its lipid soluble properties trimetrexate can enter both mammalian and protozoan cells in contrast to methotrexate which is transported into mammalian cells but not protozoan cells. Trimetrexate must be given with leucovorin to prevent hematologic toxicity. Eight of 10 AIDS patients with pneumocystis pneumonia treated with trimetrexate alone, or in combination with sulfamethoxazole, showed favorable clinical responses (129).

Carbutamide

Other classes of drugs showing potential as therapeutic agents are the sulfonylureas. Carbutamide, a sulfonylurea structurally related to tolbutamide, has been shown in a rat model to be as effective as TMP-SMX in treating and preventing pneumocystis pneumonia (130).

Treatment Recommendations

TMP-SMX is the usual initial therapy for pneumocystis pneumonia and if no response is found after four to five days, alternate therapy with pentamidine should be initiated (2). Animal experiments and retrospective studies in AIDS patients do not support an additive effect of pentamidine and TMP-SMX in combination over each drug alone (105),(131).

Therapeutic endpoints in the treatment of pneumocystis pneumonia in AIDS patients are less clear than in other immunocompromised patients. Non-AIDS patients treated with TMP-SMX show clinical (fall in temperature, improved arterial oxygenation) and radiographic signs of improvement within four days after the initiation of therapy (103). Pneumocystis cysts are rarely seen on repeat biopsies performed after several days of therapy (104).

Patients with AIDS appear to require a more prolonged course of therapy in order to clear the pneumocystis infection (10), (11),(105),(107),(132). Repeat fiberoptic bronchoscopy will show persistent pneumocystis cysts in 40-60% of AIDS patients after two to three weeks of therapy (2),(11),(13),(132). One study has shown that patients showing clinical improvement with histopathologic persistence of the organism after three weeks of therapy, did not relapse during a three month follow-up period (13). After receiving therapy, patients with persistent pneumocystis infection cannot be distinguished from those who have cleared the infection, on the basis of clinical signs, radiographic appearance, or gallium scans (11),(76),(77),(132). Histopathologic resolution of the alveolar inflammation correlates poorly with any clinical parameter (11). Repeat bronchoscopic evaluation to document persistent infection may be of research interest but does not appear to have practical importance except in special clinical circumstances when patients deteriorate or when there is suspicion of a complicating disease process (133). Most clinicians base their decision to continue anti-pneumocystis therapy on the clinical and radiographic signs of improvement (2),(133). Two to three weeks of therapy is given as the minimum duration of therapy.

PROPHYLAXIS

The patient with persistently impaired immunity remains at risk for recurrent pneumocystis upon discontinuing therapy (133). Prophylaxis with low doses oral TMP-SMX (5mg TMP - 25mg SMX/kg/day) given in two equally divided does has been found to be effective in a controlled trial of children at risk for pneumocystis (134). Because of the high incidence of side-effects noted in AIDS patients unrelated to dosage or serum levels, alternate therapies have been sought as effective prophylaxis (12).

Preliminary trials are being conducted using pentamidine (4mg/kg) every four weeks as anti-pneumocystis prophylaxis. If the initial data are confirmed in larger studies, pentamidine may have a role as a prophylatic agent in selected patients, although cumulative toxicities may represent a potential complication of its use (135),(136).

Pyrimethamine plus sulfadoxine (fansidar) has been used in limited studies as an alternate means of prophylaxis in AIDS patients. One tablet was administered weekly. Nine of 12 patients tolerated therapy for three to 12 months and none had a recurrence of pneumocystis pneumonia (137). In a controlled trial, 28 patients were followed for a mean of 27 weeks and none developed recurrent pneumocystis infection whereas 5/17 controls not receiving prophylaxis developed pneumocystis pneumonia (138). Though its long half-life (130 hours) facilitates administration on a weekly basis, the occurrence of adverse reactions to the drug can be severe and prolonged in patients who receive this therapy (139).

PROGNOSIS

The prognosis of AIDS patients with pneumocystis pneumonia needs to be evaluated in terms of the acute illness as well as for the overall prognosis for the immune deficiency syndrome. Early therapeutic intervention prior to severe respiratory failure has been associated with a better prognosis. Clinical or laboratory features at presentation with favorable prognostic importance include a lower respiratory rate, higher room-air arterial oxygen tension, lower alveolar arterial oxygen gradient, higher lymphocyte counts, higher albumin levels, and a normal chest radiograph (10),(67),(68).

Patients with acute respiratory failure who need endotracheal intubation and mechanical ventilation have a poor prognosis (14),(140),(141). Only 14% of patients with severe respiratory failure survived to leave the hospital in the National Heart, Lung and Blood Institute (NHLBI) Workshop report (2). The intensive-care unit course of these patients can be complicated by hypotension, barotrauma, and the occurrence of other infections (142),(143). Amelioration of respiratory failure due to pneumocystis pneumonia using corticosteroids has been described in several reports. It remains unclear at this time which patients will clearly benefit from this therapy (144)-(146).

Survival analysis of 1391 AIDS patients in New York City, from 1981-1984, noted that cumulative survival varied in accordance with the manifestations of AIDS. The median cumulative survival of patients with Kaposi's sarcoma alone was 125 weeks, with both Kaposi's sarcoma and pneumocystis pneumonia 61 weeks, and pneumocystis pneumonia alone 35 weeks (147). These sobering statistics must be considered when evaluating the appropriateness of intensive-care unit facilities for the patient with AIDS.

The ethical dilemmas of caring for patients in this situation have recently been outlined (148),(149). In general, physicians must rely on their own personal experience and that of expert consultants to decide on the appropriateness of aggressive medical interventions. As there are uncertainties with the disease process, intensive-care unit interventions may be indicated, if such heroic measures are consistent with a well informed patient's wishes. It is important to define clearly the clinically achievable goals of medical therapy and communicate them to the patient so that informed choices regarding medical therapy can be made (149). When it is apparent that medical therapy offers little benefit to the patient, supportive care to control pain, dyspnea or other discomforts becomes the therapeutic goal. Patients should be given a clear description of their overall prognosis and made aware of supportive facilities in the hospital and community. Providing adequate information to the patient may allow them to make a realistic assessment of their illness and avoid unnecessary use of intensive care units for terminally ill patients (141),(150).

Pneumocystis pneumonia remains a major therapeutic challenge in AIDS patients. Areas of research that may have a significant impact on this infection include: 1) studies on propagation of the organism in vitro; 2) investigation of the biologic properties of human pneumocystis dihydrofolate reductase; 3) studies on the diagnostic use of monoclonal antibodies against human pneumocystis and their application in seroepidemiologic studies of populations at risk; and 4) trials of newer therapeutic agents, possibly in combination with approaches to immune reconstitution.

REFERENCES

1. CDC., Update: Acquired immunodeficiency syndrome (AIDS) - United States. MMWR 35:17-21 (1986)

2. Murray, J.F., Felton, C.P., Garay, S.M., et al., Pulmonary complications of the acquired immune deficiency syndrome: report of a National Heart, Lung, and Blood Institute Workship. N Engl J Med 310:1682-1688 (1984)

3. Public Health Service. Coolfont report: a PHS plan for prevention and control of AIDS and the AIDS virus. Public Health Rep 101:341-348 (1986)

4. Cushion, M.T., Walzer, P.D., Cultivation of *Pneumocystis carinii* in lung-derived cell lines. J Infect Dis 149:644 (1984)

5. Latorre, C.R., Sulzer, A.J., Norman, L.G., Serial propagation of *Pneumocystis carinii* in cell line culture. Appl Environ Microbiol 33:1204-1206 (1977)

6. Pifer, L.L., Woods, D., Hughes, W.T., Propagation of *Pneumocystis carinii* in vero cell culture. Infect Immun 20:66-68 (1978)

7. Smith, J.W., Eichholtz, R., Miller, J., et al., Culture method for determining in vitro susceptibility of rat *Pneumocystis carinii* to pentamidine isethionate and trimethoprim-sulfamethoxazole. Annual Meeting of the American Society for Microbiology, New Orleans, Louisiana (1983)

8. Hughes, W.T., Serodiagnosis of *Pneumocystis carinii*. Chest 87:700 (1985)

9. Maddison, S.E., Walls, K.W., Haverkos, H.W., et al., Evaluation of serologic tests for *Pneumocystis carinii* antibody and antigenemia in patients with the acquired immune deficiency syndrome. Diag Microbiol Infect Dis 2:69-73 (1984)

10. Kovacs, J.A., Hiemenz, J.W., Macher, A.M., et al., *Pneumocystis carinii* pneumonia: a comparison between patients with the acquired immunodeficiency syndrome and patients with other immunodeficiences. Ann Intern Med 100:663-671 (1984)

11. Shelhamer, J.H., Ognibene, F.P., Macher, A.M., et al., Persistence of *Pneumocystis carinii* in lung tissue of acquired immunodeficiency syndrome patients treated for pneumocystis pneumonia. Am Rev Respir Dis 130:1611-1615 (1984)

12. Gordin, F.M., Simon, G.L., Wofsy, C.B., et al., Adverse reactions to trimethoprim-sulfamethoxazole in patients with the acquired immunodeficiency syndrome. Ann Intern Med 100:495-499 (1984)

13. Wharton, J.M., Coleman, D.L., Wofsy, C.B., et al., Trimethoprim-sulfamethoxazole or pentamidine for *Pneumocystis carinii* pneumonia in the acquired immunodeficiency syndrome: a prospective randomized trial. Ann Intern Med 105:37-44 (1986)

14. Stover, D.E., White, D.A., Romano, P.A., et al., Spectrum of pulmonary diseases associated with the acquired immune deficiency syndrome. Am J Med 78:429-437 (1985)

15. Welch, K., Finkbeiner, W., Alpers, C.E., et al., Autopsy findings in the acquired immune deficiency syndrome. JAMA 252:1152-1159 (1984)

16. Burke, B.A., Good, R.A., *Pneumocystis carinii* infection. Medicine (Baltimore) 52:23-51 (1973)

17. Gajdusek, D.C., *Pneumocystis carinii* as the cause of human disease: historical perspective and magnitude of the problem. In: Symposium on Pneumocystis carinii Infection NCI Monograph 43 (Robbins, J.B., DeVita, V.T., Dutz, W., eds) National Cancer Institute, Washington, DC, p 1-10 (1973)

18. Hughes, W.T., Pneumocystis pneumonia: a plague of the immunosuppressed. J Hopkins Med J 143:184-192 (1978)

19. Young, L.S., ed, *Pneumocystis carinii* Pneumonia: Pathogenesis, Diagnosis, Treatment. Marcel Dekker, New York (1984)

20. Walzer, P.D., *Pneumocystis carinii* infection. South J Med 70:1330-1337 (1977)

21. Van der Meer, G., Brug, S.L., Infection par pneumocystis chez l'homme et chez les animaux. Ann Soc Belg Med 22:301-307 (1942)

22. Dauzier, G., Willis, T., Barnett, R.N., *Pneumocystis carinii* in an infant. Am J Clin Pathol 26:787-793 (1956)

23. LeClair, R.A., Descriptive epidemiology of interstitial pneumocystic pneumonia: an analysis of 107 cases from the United States, 1955-1967. Am Rev Respir Dis 99:542-547 (1969)

24. Walzer, P.D., Perl, D.P., Krogstad, D.J., et al., *Pneumocystis carinii* pneumonia in the United States: epidemiologic, diagnostic, and clinical features. Ann Intern Med 80: 83-93 (1974)

25. Ivady, G., Paldy, L., Koltay, M., et al., *Pneumocystis carinii* pneumonia. Lancet 1:616-617 (1967)

26. Hughes, W.T., Feldman, S., Sanyal, S.K., Treatment of *Pneumocystis carinii* pneumonitis with trimethoprim-sulfamethoxazole. Can Med Assoc J 112:Suppl: 47S-50S (1975)

27. Hughes, W.T., Feldman, S., Chaudhary, S.C., et al., Comparison of pentamidine isethionate with trimethoprim-sulfamethoxazole in the treatment of *Pneumocystis carinii* pneumonia. J Pediatr 92:285-292 (1978)

28. Lanken, P.N., Minda, M., Pietra., G.G., et al, Alveolar response to experimental *Pneumocystis carinii* pneumonia in the rat. Am J Pathol 99:561-588 (1980)

29. Yoneda, K., Walzer, P.D., Interaction of *Pneumocystis carinii* with host lungs: an ultrastructural study. Infect Immun 29:692-703 (1980)

30. Ruffolo, J.J., Cushion, M.T., Walzer, P.D., Techniques for examining *Pneumocystis carinii* in fresh specimens. J Clin Micro 23:17-21 (1986)

31. Haselton, P.S., Curry, A., Ranklin, E.M., *Pneumocystis carinii* pneumonia: a light microscopical and ultrastructural study. J Clin Path 34:1138-1146 (1981)

32. Walzer, P.D., Young, L.S., Clinical relevance of animal models of *Pneumocystis carinii* pneumonia. Diag Microbiol Infect Dis 2:1-6 (1984).

33. Walzer, P.D., Schnelle, V., Armstrong, D., et al., Nude mouse: a new experimental model for *Pneumocystis carinii* infection. Science 197:177-179 (1977)

34. Hughes, W.T., Natural mode of acquisition for de novo infection with *Pneumocystis carinii.* J Infect Dis 145:842-848 (1982)

35. Walzer, P.D., Rutledge, M.E., Humoral immunity in experimental *Pneumocystis carinii* infection. J Lab Clin Med 97: 820-833 (1981)

36. Walzer, P.D., Rutledge, M.E., Serum antibody responses to *Pneumocystis carinii* among different strains of normal and athymic mice. Infect Immun 35:620-626 (1982)

37. Masur, H., Jones, T.C., The interaction in vitro of *Pneumocystis carinii* with macrophages and L-cells. J Exp Med 147:157-170 (1978)

38. Herrod, H.G., Valenski, W.R., Woods, D.R., et al., The in vitro response of human lymphocytes to *Pneumocystis carinii* antigen. J Immunol 126:59-61 (1981)

39. Hughes, W.T., Smith, B., Provocation of infection due to *Pneumocystis carinii* by cyclosporin A. J Infect Dis 145:767 (1982)

40. Walzer, P.D. LaBine, M., Redington, T.J., et al., Changes in lymphocyte subpopulations during development of and recovery from experimental *Pneumocystis carinii* pneumonia. Clin Res 31:378A (1983)

41. Walzer, P.D., Powell, R.D., Yoneda, K., et al., Growth characteristics and pathogenesis of experimental *Pneumocystis carinii* pneumonia. Infect. Immun 27:928-937 (1980)

42. Pedersen, F.K., Johansen, S., Rosenkvist, J., et al., Refractory *Pneumocystis carinii* infection in chronic granulomatous disease: successful treatment with granulocytes. Pediatrics 64:935-938 (1979)

43. Norman, L., Kagan, I.G., Some observations on the serology of *Pneumocystis carinii* infections in the United States. Infect Immun 8:317-321 (1973)

44. Meuwissen, J.H.E.Th., Tauber, I., Leeuwenberg, A.D.E.M., et al., Parasitologic and serologic observations of infection with *Pneumocystis carinii* in humans. J Infect Dis 136: 43-49 (1977)

45. Pifer, L.L., Hughes, W.T., Stagno, S., et al., *Pneumocystis carinii* infection: evidence for high prevalence in normal and immunosuppressed children. J Pediatr 82:404-415 (1973)

46. Kovacs, J.A., Gill, V., Swan, J.C., et al., Prospective evaluation of a monoclonal antibody for diagnosing *Pneumocystis carinii* pneumonia. Lancet 2:1-3 (1986)

47. Venet, A., Dennewald, G., Sandron, D., et al., Bronchoalveolar lavage in the acquired immune deficiency syndrome. Lancet 2:53 (1983)

48. Wallace, J.M., Barbers, R.G., Oishi, J.S., et al., Cellular and T-lymphocyte subpopulation profiles in bronchoalveolar lavage fluid from patients with acquired immune deficiency syndrome and pneumonitis. Am Rev Respir Dis 130:786-790 (1984)

49. Young, K.R., Jr., Rankin, J.A., Naegel, G.P., et al., Bronchoalveolar lavage cells and proteins in patients with the acquired immune deficiency syndrome. Ann Intern Med 103: 522-533 (1985)

50. White, D.A., Gellene, R.A., Gupta., S., et al., Pulmonary cell populations in the immunosuppressed patient: bronchoalveolar lavage findings during episodes of pneumonitis. Chest 88:352-359 (1985)

51. Yoneda, K., Walzer, P.D., Attachment of *Pneumocystis carinii* to type 1 alveolar cells studied by freeze-fracture electron microscopy. Infect Immun 40:812-815 (1983)

52. Henshaw, N.G., Carson, J.L., Collier, A.M., Ultrastructural observations of *Pneumocystis carinii* attachment to rat lung. J Infect Dis 151:181-186 (1985)

53. Yoneda, K., Walzer, P.D., Mechanism of pulmonary alveolar injury in experimental *Pneumocystis carinii* pneumonia in the rat. Br J Exp Path 62:339-346 (1981)

54. Kernbaum, S., Masliah, J., Alcindor, L.G., et al., Phospholipase activities of bronchoalveolar lavage fluid in rat *Pneumocystis carinii* pneumonia. Br J Exp Path 64:75-80 (1983)

55. Stokes, D.C., Hughes, W.T., King, R.E., Rat model of *Pneumocystis carinii* pneumonia: changes in lung compliance. Am Rev Respir Dis 123:S163 (1981)

56. Katzenstein, A.L.A., Askin, F.B., Surgical Pathology of Non-neoplastic Lung Disease. W.B. Saunders, Philadelphia, p 9-42, 241-252 (1982)

57. Price, R.A., Hughes, W.T., Histopathology of *Pneumocystis carinii* infestation and infection in malignant disease in childhood. Hum Pathol 5:737-752 (1974)

58. Weber, W.R., Askin, F.B., Dehner, L.P., Lung biopsy in *Pneumocystis carinii* pneumonia: a histopathologic study of typical and atypical features. Am J Clin Pathol 67:11-19 (1977)

59. Askin, F.B., Katzenstein, A.L.A., Pneumocystis infection masquerading as diffuse alveolar damage: a potential source of diagnostic error. Chest 79:420-422 (1981)

60. Nash, G., Fligiel, S., Pathologic features of the lung in the acquired immune deficiency syndrome: an autopsy study of seventeen homosexual males. Am J Clin Pathol 81: 6-12 (1984)

61. Hughes, W.T., Feldman, S., Aur, R.J.A., et al., Intensity of immunosuppressive therapy and the incidence of *Pneumocystis carinii* pneumonitis. Cancer 36:2004-2009 (1975)

62. Singer, C., Armstrong, D., Rosen, P.P., et al., *Pneumocystis carinii* pneumonia: a cluster of eleven cases. Ann Intern Med 82:772-777 (1975)

63. Hardy, A.M., Wajszczuk, C.P., Suffredini, A.F., et al., Pneumocystis pneumonia in renal transplant recipients treated with cyclosporin and steroids. J Infect Dis 149:143-147 (1984)

64. Hughes, W.T., Johnson, W.W., Recurrent *Pneumocystis carinii* pneumonia following apparent recovery. J Ped 79:755-759 (1971)

65. Ryning, F.W., Mills, J., *Pneumocystis carinii, Toxoplasma gondii* cytomegalovirus and the compromised host. West J Med 130: 18-34 (1979)

66. Coleman, D.L., Luce, J.M., Wilber, J.C., et al., Antibody to the retrovirus associated with the acquired immunodeficiency syndrome (AIDS): presence in presumably healthy San Franciscans who die unexpectantly. Arch Intern Med 146:713-715 (1986)

67. Rosen, M.J., Tow, T.W.Y., Chuang, M.T., et al., Prognosis of *Pneumocystis carinii* pneumonia in the acquired immunodeficiency syndrome. Ann Intern Med 101:276 (1984)

68. McCullough, P., Cole, R.P., Prognostic indicators in patients with the acquired immune deficiency syndrome and respiratory failure. Am Rev Respir Dis 131:A220 (1985)

69. Curtis, J., Goodman, P., Hopewell, P., Noninvasive tests in the diagnostic evaluation for *P. carinii* pneumonia in patients with or suspected of having AIDS. Am Rev Respir Dis 133:A182 (1986)

70. Doppman, J.L., Geelhoed, G.W., Atypical radiographic features in *Pneumocystis carinii* pneumonia. In: Symposium on Pneumocystis Carinii Infection NCI Monograph #43 (Robbins, J.B., DeVita, V.T., Dutz, W., eds), National Cancer Institute, Washington, DC, p 89-91 (1973)

71. Sirotzky, L., Memoli, V., Roberts, J.L., et al., Recurrent pneumocystis pneumonia with normal chest roentgenograms. JAMA 240:1513-1515 (1978)

72. DeLorenzo, L.J., Huang, C.T., Maguire, G.P., et al., Roentgenographic patterns of *Pneumocystis carinii* pneumonia in 104 patients with the acquired immunodeficiency syndrome. Am Rev Respir Dis 133:A181 (1986)

73. Goodman, J.L., Tashkin, D.P., Pneumocystis with normal chest x-ray film and arterial oxygen tension: early diagnosis in a patient with the acquired immune deficiency syndrome. Arch Intern Med 143:1981-1982 (1983)

74. Cohen, B.A., Pomeranz, S., Rabinowitz, J.G., et al., Pulmonary complications of AIDS: radiologic features. Am J Roentgen 143:115-122 (1984)

75. Barron, T.F., Birnbaum, N.S., Shane, L.B., et al., *Pneumocystis carinii* pneumonia studied by gallium-67 scanning. Radiology 154:791-793 (1985)

76. Coleman, D.L., Hattner, R.S., Luce, J.M., et al., Correlation between gallium lung scans and fiberoptic bronchoscopy in patients with suspected *Pneumocystis carinii* pneumonia and the acquired immune deficiency syndrome. Am Rev Respir Dis 130:1166-1169 (1984)

77. Tuazon, C.U., Delaney, M.D., Simon, G.L., et al., Utility of gallium-67 scintigraphy and bronchial washings in the diagnosis and treatment of *Pneumocystis carinii* pneumonia in patients with the acquired immune deficiency syndrome. Am Rev Respir Dis 132:1087-1092 (1985)

78. Mason, G.R., Mena, I., Effros, R.M., 99mTc-DTPA aerosol clearance in patients with pneumocystis pneumonia and AIDS. Am Rev Respir Dis 133:A18 (1986)

79. Meignan, M., Touboul, J.L., Rosso, J., et al., Early detection of opportunistic lung infection in patients with AIDS by measuring the lung clearance of 99m Tc DTPA aerosol. International Conference on Acquired Immunodeficiency Syndrome (AIDS), Paris, France (1986)

80. Hopewell, P.C., Luce, J.M., Pulmonary involvement in the acquired immune deficiency syndrome. Chest 87:104-112 (1985)

81. Gosey, L.L., Howard, R.M., Witebsky, F.G., et al., Advantages of a modified toluidine blue O stain and bronchoalveolar lavage for the diagnosis of *Pneumocystis carinii* pneumonia. J Clin Micro 22:803-807 (1985)

82. Macher, A.M., Shelhamer, J., Maclowery, J., et al., *Pneumocystis carinii* identified by gram stain of lung imprints. Ann Intern Med 99:484-485 (1983)

83. Rorat, E., Garcia, R.L., Skolom, J., Diagnosis of *Pneumocystis carinii* pneumonia by cytologic examination of bronchial washings. JAMA 254:1950-1951 (1985)

84. Ghali, V.S., Garcia, R.L., Skolom, J., Fluoresence of *Pneumocystis carinii* in Papanicolaou smears. Hum Pathol 15:907-909 (1984)

85. Lau, W.K., Young, L.S., Remington, J.S., *Pneumocystis carinii* pneumonia: diagnosis by examination of pulmonary secretions. JAMA 236:2399-2402 (1976)

86. Pitchenik, A.E., Ganjei, P., Torres, A., et al., Sputum examination for the diagnosis of *Pneumocystis carinii* pneumonia in the acquired immunodeficiency syndrome. Am Rev Respir Dis 133:226-229 (1986)

87. Bigby, T.D., Margolskee, D., Curtis, J.L., et al., The usefulness of induced sputum in the diagnosis of *Pneumocystis carinii* pneumonia in patients with the acquired immunodeficiency syndrome. Am Rev Respir Dis 133:515-518 (1986)

88. Markowitz, S., Leiman, G., Cytologic detection of *Pneumocystis carinii* by ultraviolet light examination of Papanicolaou-stained sputum specimens. Acta Cytol 30:79-80 (1986)

89. Coleman, D.L., Dodek, P.M., Luce, J.M., et al., Diagnostic utility of fiberoptic bronchoscopy in patients with *Pneumocystis carinii* pneumonia and the acquired immune deficiency syndrome. Am Rev Respir Dis 128:795-799 (1983)

90. Ognibene, F.P., Shelhamer, J., Gill, V., et al., The diagnosis of *Pneumocystis carinii* pneumonia in patients with the acquired immundeficiency syndrome using subsegmental bronchoalveolar lavage. Am Rev Respir Dis 129:929-932 (1984)

91. Stover, D.E., White, D.A., Romano, P.A., et al., Diagnosis of pulmonary disease in acquired immune deficiency syndrome (AIDS): role of bronchoscopy and bronchoalveolar lavage. Am Rev Respir Dis 130:659-662 (1984)

92. Broaddus, C., Dake, M.D., Stulbarg, M.S., et al., Bronchoalveolar lavage and transbronchial biopsy for the diagnosis of pulmonary infections in the acquired immunodeficiency syndrome. Ann Intern Med 102:747-752 (1985)

93. Caughey, G., Wong, H., Gamsu, G., et al., Nonbronchoscopic bronchoalveolar lavage for the diagnosis for *Pneumocystis carinii* pneumonia in the acquired immune deficiency syndrome. Chest 88:659-662 (1985)

94. Mann, J.M., Altus, C., Ligorski, M., et al., Non-bronchoscopic lung lavage for the diagnosis of opportunistic infections in acquired immunodeficiency syndrome. Am Rev Respir Dis 133:A181 (1986)

95. Karpel, J.P., Prezant, D., Appel, D., et al., Endotracheal lavage for the diagnosis of *Pneumocystis carinii* pneumonia in intubated patients with acquired immune deficiency syndrome. Crit Care Med 14:741 (1986)

96. Zackson, H.J., Cole, R.P., A simple technique for diagnosing *Pneumocystis carinii* pneumonia in intubated patients. Am Rev Respir Dis 133:A181 (1986)

97. Wallace, J.M., Batra, P., Gong, H., et al., Percutaneous needle lung aspiration for diagnosing pneumonitis in the patient with acquired immunodeficiency syndrome (AIDS). Am Rev Respir Dis 131:389-392 (1985)

98. Pass, H.I., Potter, D., Shelhammer, J., et al., Indications for and diagnostic efficacy of open-lung biopsy in the patient with acquired immunodeficiency syndrome (AIDS). Ann Thor Surg 41:307-312 (1986)

99. Ognibene, F.P., Suffredini, A.F., Shelhammer, J.H., et al., Nonspecific interstitial pneumonitis is a frequent cause of pneumonia in the acquried immunodeficiency syndrome. International Conference on Acquired Immunodeficiency Syndrome (AIDS), Paris, France (1986)

100. Katzenstein, A.L.A., Askin, F.B., Interpretation and significance of pathologic findings in transbronchial lung biopsy. Am J Surg Pathol 4:223-234 (1980)

101. Nash, G., Pathologic features of the lung in the immunocompromised host. Hum Pathol 13:841-858 (1982)

102. Hughes, W.T., Trimethoprim-sulfamethoxazole therapy for *Pneumocystis carinii* pneumonitis in children. Rev Infect Dis 2:602-607 (1982)

103. Young, L.S., Trimethoprim-sulfamethoxazole in the treatment of adults with pneumonia due to *Pneumocystis carinii*. Rev Infect Dis 2:608-613 (1982)

104. Sattler, F.R., Remington, J.S., Intravenous trimethoprim-sulfamethoxazole therapy for *Pneumocystis carinii* pneumonia. Am J Med 70:1215-1221 (1981)

105. Haverkos, H.W., Assessment of therapy for *Pneumocystis carinii* pneumonia: PCP therapy project group. Am J Med 76:501-508 (1984)

106 Engelberg, L.A., Lerner, C.W., Tapper, M.L., Clinical features of *Pneumocystis carinii* pneumonia in the acquired immune deficiency syndrome. Am Rev Respir Dis 130:689-694 (1984)

107. Small, C.B., Harris, C.A., Friedland, G.H., et al., The treatment of *Pneumocystis carinii* pneumonia in the acquired immunodeficiency syndrome. Arch Intern Med 145: 837-840 (1985)

108. Winston, D.J., Lau, W.K., Gale, R.P., et al., Trimethoprim-sulfamethoxazole for the treatment of *Pneumocystis carinii* pneumonia. Ann Intern Med 92:762-769 (1980)

109. Mitsuyasu, R., Groopman, J., Volberding, P., Cutaneous reaction to trimethoprim-sulfamethoxazole in patients with AIDS and Kaposi's sarcoma. N Engl J Med 308:1535-1536 (1983)

110. Jaffe, H.S., Abrams, D.I., Ammann, A.J., et al., Complications of co-trimoxazole in treatment of AIDS-associated *Pneumocystis carinii* pneumonia in homosexual men. Lancet 2:1109-1111 (1983)

111. Kinzie, B.J., Taylor, J.W., Trimethoprim and folinic acid. Ann Intern Med 101:565 (1984)

112. D'Antonio, R.G., Johnson, D.B., Winn, R.E., et al., Effect of folinic acid on the capacity of trimethoprim-sulfamethoxazole to prevent and treat *Pneumocystis carinii* pneumonia in rats. Antimicrob Agents Chemother 29:327-329 (1986)

113. Pearson, R.D., Hewlett, E.L., Pentamidine for the treatment of *Pneumocystis carinii* pneumonia and other protozoal diseases. Ann Intern Med 103:782-786 (1985)

114. Siegal, S.E., Wolff, L.J., Baehner, R.L., et al., Pentamidine for the treatment of *Pneumocystis carinii* pneumonitis: a comparative trial of sulfamethoxazole-trimethoprim vs. pentamidine in pediatric patients with cancer: report from the childrens cancer study group. Am J Dis Child 138:1051-1054 (1984)

115. Klein, N.C., Duncanson, F.P., Lenox, T.H., et al., Prospective randomized treatment for *Pneumocystis carinii* pneumonia in AIDS patients. International Conference on Acquired Immunodeficiency Syndrome (AIDS), Paris, France (1986)

116. Navin, T.R., Fontaine, R.E., Intravenous versus intramuscular administration of pentamidine. N Engl J Med 311:1701-1702 (1984)

117. Mallory, D.L., Parrillo, J.E., Lane, H.C., et al., The hemodynamics and safety of intravenous pentamidine. Crit Care Med 14:395 (1986)

118. Donnelly, H., Bernard, E.M., Rothkotter, H.E., et al., Distribution of pentamidine in humans. 26th Interscience Conference on Antimicrobial Agents and Chemotherapy, New Orleans, Louisana (1986)

119. Debs, R., Blumenfeld, W., Brunette, E., et al., Successful treatment of *Pneumocystis carinii* pneumonia in rats with aerosolized pentamidine. International Conference on Acquired Immunodeficiency Syndrome (AIDS), Paris, France (1986)

120. Golden, J.A., Sjoerdsma, A., Santi, D.V., *Pneumocystis carinii* pneumonia treated with alpha-difluoromethylornithine: a prospective study among patients with the acquired immunodeficiency syndrome. West J Med 141:613-623 (1984)

121. Dieterich, D.D., Chachova, A., Greene, J., et al., Eflornithine treatment of resistant *Pneumocystis carinii* pneumonia in AIDS patients. International Conference on Acquired Immunodeficiency Syndrome (AIDS), Paris, France (1986)

122. Neibart, E., Sacks, H.S., Hammer, G., et al., Difluromethylornithine in the treatment of *Pneumocystis carinii* pneumonia. 26th Interscience Conference on Antimicrobial Agents and Chemotherapy, New Orleans, Louisiana (1986)

123. Paulson, Y.J., Gilman, T.M., Boylen, C.T., et al., Eflornithine treatment of *Pneumocystis carinii* pneumonia in patients failing other therapy. 26th Interscience Conference on Antimicrobial Agents and Chemotherapy, New Orleans, Louisiana. (1986)

124. Barlow, J.L.R., Roberts, N.E., Sjoerdsma, A., Eflornithine hydrochloride in the treatment of *Pneumocystis carinii* pneumonia in patients with the acquired immune deficiency syndrome. International Conference on Acquired Immunodeficiency Syndrome (AIDS), Paris, France (1986)

125. Hughes, W.T., Smith, B.L., Efficacy of diaminodiphenylsulfone and other drugs in murine *Pneumocystis carinii* pneumonitis. Antimicrob Agents Chemother 26:436-440 (1984)

126. Mills, J., Leoung, G., Medina, I., et al., Dapsone is less effective than standard therapy for pneumocystis pneumonia in AIDS patients. Am Rev Respir Dis 133:A184 (1986)

127. Leoung, G.S., Mills, J., Hopewell, P.C., et al., Dapsone-trimethoprim for *Pneumocystis carinii* pneumonia in the acquired immunodeficiency syndrome. Ann Intern Med 105:45-48 (1986)

128. Hughes, W.T., Smith, B.L., Jacobus, D.P., Successful treatment and prevention of murine *Pneumocystis carinii* pneumonitis with 4',4'-sulfonylbisformanilide. Antimicrob Agents Chemother 29:509-510 (1986)

129. Allegra, C.J., Drake, J., Swan, J., et al., Preliminary results of a phase I-II trial for the treatment of *Pneumocystis carinii* pneumonia using a potent lipid-soluble dihydrofolate reductase inhibitor, trimetrexate. 26th Interscience Conference on Antimicrobial Agents and Chemotherapy, New Orleans, Louisiana (1986)

130. Hughes, W.T., Smith-McCain, B.L., Effects of sulfonylurea compounds on *Pneumocystis carinii.* J Infect Dis 153: 944-947 (1986)

131. Kluge, R.M., Spaulding, D.M., Spain, A.J., Combination of pentamidine and trimethoprim-sulfamethoxazole in the therapy of *Pneumocystis carinii* pneumonia in rats. Antimicrob Agents Chemother 13:975-978 (1978)

132. DeLorenzo, L.J., Maguire, G.P., Wormser, G.P., et al., Persistence of *Pneumocystis carinii* pneumonia in the acquired immune deficiency syndrome: evaluation of therapy by follow-up transbronchial lung biopsy. Chest 88:79-83 (1985)

133. Hughes, W.T., Persistence of pneumocystis. Chest 88:4-5 (1985)

134. Hughes, W.T., Kuhn, S., Chaudhary, S., et al., Successful chemoprophylaxis for *Pneumocystis carinii* pneumonitis. N Engl J Med 297:1419-1426 (1977)

135. Busch, D.F., Follansbee, S.E., Continuation of therapy with pentamidine isethionate for prevention of relapse of *Pneumocystis carinii* pneumonia in AIDS. International Conference on Acquired Immunodeficiency Syndrome (AIDS), Paris, France (1986)

136. Karaffa, C., Rehm, S., Calabrese, L., Efficacy of monthly pentamidine infusions in preventing recurrent *Pneumocystis carinii* pneumonia in AIDS patients. 26th Interscience Conference on Antimicrobial Agents and Chemotherapy, New Orleans, Louisiana (1986)

137. Gottlieb, M.S., Knight, S., Mitsuyasu, R., et al., Prophylaxis of *Pneumocystis carinii* infection in AIDS with pyrimethamine-sulfadoxine. Lancet 2:398-399 (1984)

138. Madoff, L.C., Scavuzzo, D., Roberts, R.B., Fansidar secondary prophylaxis of *Pneumocystis carinii* pneumonia in AIDS patients. Clin Res 34:524A (1986)

139. Navin, T.R., Miller, K.D., Satriale, R.F., et al., Adverse reactions associated with pyrimethamine-sulfadoxine prophylaxis for *Pneumocystis carinii* infections in man. Lancet 1:1332 (1985)

140. Rosen, M.J., Cucco, R.A., Teirstein, A.S., Outcome of intensive care in patients with the acquired immunodeficiency syndrome. J Int Care Med 1:55-60 (1986)

141. Wachter, R.M., Luce, J.M., Turner, J., et al., Intensive care of patients with the acquired immunodeficiency syndrome: outcome and changing pattern of utilization. Am Rev Respir Dis 134:891-896 (1986)

142. Parker, M.M., Shelhamer, J.H., Ognibene, F.P., et al., Pneumocystis pneumonia and bacterial pneumonia produce similar hemodynamic abnormalities. Clin Res 32:252A (1984)

143. Garay, S., Respiratory failure in AIDS. Am Rev Respir Dis 133:A344 (1986)

144. Foltzer, M.A., Hannan, S.E., Kozak, A.J., Pneumocystis pneumonia: response to corticosteroids. JAMA 253:979 (1985)

145. Rankin, J.A., Walzer, P.D., Dwyer, J.M., et al., Immunologic alterations in bronchoalveolar lavage fluid in the acquired immunodeficiency syndrome (AIDS). Am Rev Respir Dis 128:189-194 (1983)

146. Walmsey, S., Salit, I.E., Brunton, J., Corticosteroid therapy for pneumocystis pneumonia in AIDS. 26th Interscience Conference on Antimicrobial Agents and Chemotherapy, New Orleans, Louisiana (1986)

147. Rivin, B.E., Monroe, J.M., Hubschman, B.P., et al., AIDS outcome: A first follow-up. N Engl J Med 311:857 (1984)

148. Steinbrook, R., Lo, B., Tirpack, J., et al., Ethical dilemmas in caring for patients with the acquired immunodeficiency syndrome. Ann Intern Med 103:787-790 (1985)

149. Health and Public Policy Committee, American College of Physicians, and The Infectious Diseases Society of America. Acquired immunodeficiency syndrome. Ann Intern Med 104:575-581 (1986)

150. Steinbrook, R., Lo, B., Moulton, J., et al., Preferences of homosexual men with AIDS for life-sustaining treatment. N Engl J Med 314:457-460 (1986)

24
Cytomegalovirus Infections in AIDS

Robert L. Yarrish

Many of the first reports of what was to become known as the acquired immune deficiency syndrome (AIDS) noted a remarkable frequency and severity of cytomegalovirus (CMV) infection among the affected individuals (1)-(5). Based on these experiences, plus the known "immunosuppressive" properties of CMV (6),(7) and the extremely high prevalence of CMV infection among homosexual men (8), there was much speculation on the possibility that this virus caused the new syndrome. Since discovery of human immunodeficiency virus (HIV), most such speculation has ceased; but recent autopsy series (9)-(13) leave no doubt that CMV infection remains one of the most common and devastating infections of AIDS patients. These patients also continue to teach us new lessons about the pathogenic potential of CMV and to remind us of the need for effective weapons to combat this virus. It is almost certainly no coincidence that the greatest strides in anti-CMV chemotherapy have been made only since the appearance of AIDS.

THE VIRUS

Human CMV belongs taxonomically to the *Herpesviridae* and has the same basic structure as other members of this family. The complete enveloped virion ranges in size from 180 to 250 nm. in diameter, making it second in size only to the poxviruses among human viral pathogens. The large CMV genome - ca. 150 x 10^6 daltons - is sufficient to code for over 30 proteins and imparts great genetic and antigenic complexity to the virus. One consequence of this seems to be the variability found among CMV strains. Although all appear to share at least 80% DNA homology (14), it is uncommon to find two strains with identical nucleic acid composition, as demonstrated by restriction endonuclease analysis (15). Strains also seem to vary somewhat with respect to their antigenicity (16),(17) and their cytopathic effects in tissue culture (18); but these differences have been difficult to classify, and no serotyping or biotyping system for human CMV presently exists.

Although it is morphologically indistinguishable from other herpesviruses, human CMV shares no cross-reactive antigens with any of them and has enough biological peculiarities to set it apart as a prototype of its own subfamily, the *Betaherpesvirinae*. Other members of this group include the cytomegaloviruses of mice, guinea pigs, and swine, and all share properties of slow, focal growth in culture and narrow host range. Human CMV, in fact, causes in vivo infection only in man and in vitro infection only in human fibroblasts. The characteristic features of infected cells are enlargement, or cytomegaly, and the formation of both nuclear and cytoplasmic inclusion bodies. Although these inclusions largely consist of virions and aggregates of viral proteins (19), it is likely that much of the observed cytomegaly stems from stimulation of host cell nucleic acid and protein synthesis which accompanies CMV infection (20),(21).

An important property which CMV shares with other herpesviruses is that of latency; i.e., the ability of virus to persist indefinitely in the infected host in a quiescent form, subject to reactivation by appropriate stimuli. Unlike the other human herpesviruses, CMV has no clearly identified site of latency, although transmission of CMV infection by transfusions of blood and blood components (22) and renal allografts (23),(24) suggest that at least some white blood cells and some cells in the kidney may harbor latent virus. Spontaneous reactivation of CMV infection in the healthy individual, such as that seen commonly with *Herpes simplex* and varicella-zoster infections, is not well documented; but reactivation does occur reliably when cytotoxic immunosuppressive therapy is instituted after organ transplantation (23),(25),(26). This, along with the observation that fulminant CMV infections most often occur in the setting of profound depression of cell-mediated immunity (e.g., AIDS, bone marrow transplantation), is generally interpreted to indicate that cell-mediated immunity is the host's main defense against the virus. That such infections frequently run a malignant course despite the presence of neutralizing antibody has been cited as evidence that humoral immunity plays little role in CMV infection; but antibodies may in fact benefit the host in certain situations. One study of premature infants who acquired CMV via blood transfusions strongly suggests that although maternal antibodies may not prevent infection, they almost certainly modulate its severity (27). Similar conclusions about the role of humoral immunity may be drawn from several studies showing that administration of CMV hyperimmune plasma, hyperimmune globulin, or even commercially-available intravenous immunoglobulin may substantially lower morbidity from CMV infection when administered prophylactically to bone marrow transplant recipients (28)-(30).

EPIDEMIOLOGY

Cytomegalovirus infection appears to be exceedingly common throughout the world. Since CMV leads to latent infection which appears to persist for the life of the host, the presence of antibody to the virus is considered a reliable indicator of infection. The prevalence of CMV infection in a population can, therefore, be assessed by seroepidemiologic means. One of the most comprehensive studies of this kind surveyed the distribution of CMV complement-fixing antibodies among healthy blood donors from 25 cities in different parts of the world and found that seropositivity rates generally ranged from 40 to 60% in Europe, North America, and Australia and from 80 to 100% in South America, Asia, and Africa (31). While clearly demonstrating the almost universal occurrence of CMV infection among populations in developing nations, there is reason to believe that this study underestimated the probability of eventual infection for inhabitants of the industrialized world. It is well known that children in developing nations tend to acquire their CMV infections early in life (32), with almost universal infection, and hence, a flat age-specific prevalence curve, by the end of childhood. In the developed countries, however, infections occur less predictably throughout life, with the age-specific prevalence continuing to rise throughout life and actually showing the most rapid increase in infections among young adults (33),(34). Thus, a survey of seropositivity among healthy, young European or American blood donors is likely to be sampling a few points on a curve which is rising; in Asia and Africa, the same study is working on a flat curve. It should also be noted that the complement fixation test used in most studies of CMV prevalence is not highly sensitive (35). For example, when we recently tested sera from over 400 adults (mean age 60 yr.) in Philadelphia for CMV antibodies, the complement fixation test showed a prevalence of 66%, while the highly sensitive immunofluorescence test indicated that 95% of those tested were seropositive (unpublished data). Thus, it seems likely that CMV infection is an almost inescapable fact of life for people throughout the world.

As might be expected for a virus of such ubiquity, there are many ways in which CMV is known or suspected to be transmitted. Transmission via blood transfusions (23),(24) and renal allografts (22) are well documented but obviously account for a very small proportion of infections. Vertical transmission - i.e., from mother to child - is certainly a much more significant factor, especially in the Third World where the prevalence of infection among young mothers is very high. Transplacental transmission leading to congenital infection occurs in approximately 0.5 to 2.5% of live births, varying little from study to study (36). Intrapartum transmission via infected cervical secretions (37), (38) and postpartum transmission via breast milk (39) are, however, probably much more common routes of transmission from mother to child. For the infant who avoids vertical CMV transmission, opportunities for horizontally-transmitted infection exist, especially for children cared for in group settings. Unusually high rates of infection have been observed in day care centers and Israeli kibbutz nurseries (40)-(42), and although the route of transmission here is not definitely known, transfer of virus via saliva on toys and hands is most likely (40)-(43).

Acquisition of CMV by older children and adults is common in the developed countries but more difficult to explain than infection in early childhood. The apparent acceleration in the rate of CMV infection seen in early adulthood has two likely explanations. One is transmission via urine and saliva from young children to their parents (44). The other likely mode of CMV acquisition by young adults, and the one which is certainly more relevant to the majority of AIDS patients, is venereal transmission. The presence of CMV in cervical secretions is not peculiar to pregnant women; positive cervical cultures have been obtained from up to 13% of women attending venereal disease clinics in England and America (45),(46). Likewise, CMV may be present in semen, sometimes in large quantities (47); but this appears to be uncommon in the general population. In two studies from the U.S.A. and Canada, semen specimens from several hundred men, including college students, prison inmates, professional blood donors, venereal disease patients, and fertility clinic patients, were cultured for CMV, and between 0.6 and 10% of specimens from the different groups were positive (48),(49). Excretion of CMV in the semen of homosexual men may be much more common, however, as suggested by three studies in which over one-third of semen samples from a total of 80 homosexuals were CMV-positive (49)-(51).

Evidence that such virus-bearing fluids actually transmit CMV during sexual intercourse is circumstantial but worth consideration. In developed nations, the age at which individuals contract CMV infection most frequently does seem to coincide with the age of peak sexual activity, and several studies have noted a strong correlation between CMV infection and other sexually-transmitted diseases (45),(46),(52). There is also a report of an outbreak of CMV mononucleosis in a group of college students where sex partners were involved, while roommates were spared (53). The best evidence for venereal transmission of CMV is a recent study of women attending a venereal disease clinic in Seattle and their sex partners (54). CMV was cultured from the cervix in 46 (13.3%) of 347 women, and 64% of the women tested were seropositive for CMV. Testing of 58 male sex partners showed that 74% of partners of CMV-seropositive women were seropositive themselves, as opposed to only 31% of partners of seronegative women. In addition, restriction endonuclease analysis of CMV isolates from three pairs of sex partners showed that in two pairs, both partners were infected by the same CMV strain, almost certainly a result of transmission of the virus from one partner to the other.

If CMV is in fact sexually transmitted, as the above data suggest, it might explain the unusual epidemiology of CMV infection in homosexual men. Studies of this group regularly show CMV seropositivity rates of 90% and more, always significantly higher than the rates of 40-70% seen in age-matched controls (8),(51), (55). In addition, sexually active homosexuals not already infected seem likely to become so in a very short time. One study of such men found that 71% of those who where initially seronegative had become infected during nine months of follow-up (50), suggesting an extraordinary intensity of CMV transmission among the study population. This would be consistent with the observation that homosexual men are much more likely than controls to have CMV IgM antibody (55),(56). This antibody is most commonly found in recent infections (57) and might be expected to occur more often in a setting of frequent infection and reinfection. In this regard, it is also of note that the first documented instances of simultaneous active infection with more than one strain of CMV were recently observed in homosexual men with AIDS (58),(59). One group's data suggest that the most likely route of CMV transmission among homosexual men is anal-genital intercourse, with the receptive partner most at risk (50), a finding wholly consistent with the high rate of seminal CMV excretion observed in homosexuals.

Epidemiologic data on CMV infection for other AIDS risk groups is less abundant. One would expect intravenous drug abusers and Haitian immigrants to have a high prevalence of CMV infection - the former because of their usually low socioeconomic status, and the latter because of their Third World origins - but not to have frequent primary infections and reinfections during adulthood. This expectation is supported somewhat by a small study of AIDS patients in which these two groups showed respectively an 80% and 100% prevalence of CMV seropositivity yet had mean CMV antibody titers which were significantly lower than those of homosexual men (60). Differences in recentness and intensity of infection may also explain why AIDS patients from the intravenous drug abuser subgroup appear to have less morbidity from CMV infections than do patients who are homosexuals (61) (Stahl, R.E., unpublished data).

The epidemiology of CMV infection in hemophiliacs, a much smaller AIDS risk group, is also not well documented but probably follows a pattern similar to that of the general population. Two studies involving over 170 American hemophiliacs showed an age-specific prevalence of CMV infection similar to that of the general population (62),(63), and another smaller study found no significant differences between hemophiliacs and controls in terms of CMV seropositivity and antibody titers (64). These data strongly suggest that unlike hepatitis B and HIV, CMV is not transmitted efficiently by factor VIII concentrate or cryoprecipitate. One might also infer from these studies that because of a lower prevalence of infection, hemophiliac AIDS patients would suffer less morbidity from CMV than would members of other AIDS risk groups, and one recent review suggests that this may, in fact, be the case (61).

MANIFESTATIONS OF CMV INFECTION

The most common manifestation of CMV infection is no disease at all. There is no syndrome associated with the latent infections which prevail among most people, and the primary infections which precede them appear, in the vast majority of cases, either to be completely asymptomatic or to pass unrecognized in the succession of "benign viral illnesses" which punctuate everyone's medical history. The only indication that such infections have occurred is the presence of a positive CMV antibody test. The syndromes associated with the minority of cases which are symptomatic have been well described in several excellent reviews (65)-(68) and include: congenital CMV infections (cytomegalic inclusion disease) (69)-(72) and CMV mononucleosis (73).

An illness similar to spontaneous CMV mononucleosis has also been noted in patients one to two months after cardiac surgery and labeled the "postperfusion syndrome" (74). It has since been observed in other types of multiply-transfused patients and is felt to result from CMV transmission by blood. The exact cell which carries the virus is unknown but is probably some type of leukocyte. Transfusion of leukocytes from CMV-seropositive donors appears to transmit CMV infection to bone marrow transplant recipients (75),(76), and, conversely, use of only frozen deglycerolized red cells seems to carry less risk of transmission than the use of whole blood (77). Although the postperfusion syndrome, like CMV mononucleosis, is a benign, self-limited illness in most cases, certain patients, such as severely immunosuppressed transplant recipients (66) and seronegative premature neonates (27), may suffer severe morbidity from transfusion-related CMV infections. Some have, therefore, proposed that only blood products from CMV-seronegative donors be used for transfusions in such cases. Such a policy might also benefit the rare CMV-seronegative AIDS patient, but this has yet to be documented.

Primary CMV infection in the immunocompetent host, when symtomatic at all, is usually a generalized illness with diffuse, poorly localized symptoms. Clinical involvement of specific organs is not uncommon, however. Some degree of hepatitis is seen in the majority of cases of CMV mononucleosis, but it also occurs independently of the rest of the syndrome. Hepatitis caused by CMV is frequently accompanied by selective elevation of the serum alkaline phosphatase and may show granulomata on histopathology, both unusual findings for a viral hepatitis (78),(79). Liver failure and significant jaundice fortunately, are rare. A recent review also noted that skin rashes occur in approximately one-third of CMV mononucleosis cases, but most other types of organ-specific CMV involvement - e.g., encephalitis, myo- and pericarditis, pneumonia, retinitis, and gastrointestinal ulceration - are distinctly uncommon in the normal host (68). One condition which may deserve special mention is the Guillain-Barre syndrome, a type of polyneuritis which occurs sporadically and is usually idiopathic. Various series have used viral cultures and serology to implicate CMV in between 10 and 25% of cases, making this virus one of the best documented pathogens in this poorly-understood disease (80),(81).

Despite its benign behavior in the vast majority of infected individuals, CMV is well established as a cause of serious and frequently lethal disease in the host with impaired cell-mediated immunity. The pathology of CMV infection in AIDS patients exemplifies this perfectly, but the AIDS epidemic certainly has not provided our first opportunity to observe the full pathologic potential of this virus. By the early 1960's it was known that CMV induced lesions could be found at autopsy in patients with various types of malignancies (82),(83). Both localized and disseminated disease were seen, the former most commonly involving the gastrointestinal tract with ulceration, diarrhea, and hemorrhage, and the latter affecting most often the lungs, adrenals, and liver. The spleen, pancreas, kidneys, and myocardium were also occasionally involved, suggesting that in an appropriately compromised host, CMV was capable of causing disease in almost any organ. CMV infections super-imposed on malignancy initially appeared to be quite rare (84),(85), but subsequently seem to be increasing in frequency, perhaps coincident with the use of more immunosuppressive chemotherapy regimens, especially in the treatment of lymphomas (86).

Since the late 1960's, CMV has also emerged as one of the major problems of renal transplant patients, and this group in particular has taught us some invaluable lessons about CMV latency and the biology of CMV infection. CMV latency and its propensity to reactivate during immunosuppression with cytotoxic drugs, were first convincingly demonstrated in renal transplant patients (87). In this setting it also became clear that the virus could be transmitted even while in its latent phase, as is the case when a kidney allograft from a healthy donor is followed by active infection in the graft recipient (23). Surprisingly, most infections in this group are asymptomatic, and the most common CMV-related illness is a non-specific febrile syndrome occurring one to two months after transplantation and sharing many clinical features with CMV mononucleosis in the normal host (66). Unfortunately, it sometimes occurs with severe leukopenia, which may lead to serious bacterial or fungal superinfection (88). Next most common is an interstitial pneumonia which typically involves both lungs and is usually fatal. A problem peculiar to renal transplant patients is a form of glomerulopathy which affects the allograft and is characterized by necrosis and enlargement of endothelial cells and accumulation of mononuclear cells in glomerular capillaries (89). Clinically, it is difficult to distinguish from allograft rejection, but unlike rejection, it responds to decreased immunosuppression.

A significant finding in renal transplant patients has been that primary CMV infections, i.e., those occurring in a patient with no evidence of previous infection, are much more likely to cause symptoms and serious disease than are latent infections which are reactivated (90),(91). This strongly suggests that pre-existing immunity may help to moderate infection, even during immunosuppression. However, after allogeneic bone marrow transplantation, where ablation of the patient's immune system is necessary to insure survival of the engrafted marrow cells, CMV immunity prior to transplantation does not appear to moderate the course of post-transplant CMV infection (76),(92). Perhaps due to the profound nature of their immunosuppression, bone marrow transplant recipients appear to be more vulnerable to severe morbidity from CMV infection than are other transplant patients. CMV is, in fact, the most common infectious cause of death following allogeneic marrow transplantation (93). Most of the mortality results from CMV pneumonia, which occurs in approximately 15% of patients and has a case fatality rate around 90%. Other CMV-associated problems in these patients include serious ulcerative disease which may occur throughout the gastrointestinal tract, hepatitis, arthritis and arthralgias, retinitis, leukopenia, and prolonged fevers. It is interesting to note that most of these same problems, which were first widely seen as complications of marrow transplantation, are now encountered relatively commonly in AIDS patients, and that these two groups of patients show striking similarities in terms of their response to CMV infection.

CMV AS A CAUSE OF IMMUNOSUPPRESSION

As the above discussion is meant to suggest, the most malignant forms of CMV infection in adults occur almost exclusively in patients with impaired cell-mediated immunity, presumably due to their inability to control viral replication and spread. This strong association between CMV and immunosuppression was first observed in cancer patients over twenty years ago, and it has since been confirmed through experience with transplant recipients and AIDS patients. That CMV itself may cause significant immunosuppression, and thereby render some of these already vulnerable individuals even more susceptible to opportunistic pathogens, is a more recent idea. While it has received some support from laboratory and clinical studies over the past decade, it remains somewhat speculative.

The first investigations into CMV immunosuppression were to some extent prompted by earlier studies which suggested impairment of cell-mediated immunity in mice infected with murine cytomegalovirus (94). Hirsch and co-workers subsequently found that lymphocytes from patients with CMV mononucleosis showed decreased responsiveness to mitogens (95) and various herpesvirus antigens (6). This phenomenon correlated with increased suppressor activity which appeared to be mediated by monocytes and T lymphocytes (7),(96). The same group later demonstrated that in the acute phases of CMV mononucleosis, patients show a reversal of the normal helper/suppressor T-cell ratio, with both decreased numbers of helper cells and increased numbers of suppressor cells (97).

The basis for the changes in lymphocyte function observed during CMV mononucleosis is still poorly understood, but the excessive numbers of suppressor cells generated are probably at least partly responsible. Carney et al. found that when cultures of mononuclear cells from CMV mononucleosis patients were depleted of OKT8$^+$ lymphocytes, proliferative and cytotoxic functions of the remaining cells increased significantly (98). A direct effect of CMV on lymphocyte function is also possible, however. It was recently shown that human lymphocytes and monocytes can be infected with CMV in vitro, resulting in expression of some viral proteins but without production of whole virions in the infected cells (99). Monocytes which are so infected appear to be normal in terms of their ability to activate immune lymphocytes by presenting CMV antigens to them (100). Infected lymphocytes are, however, less responsive to mitogens than are uninfected cells (100).

As provocative as these in vitro studies are, evidence that CMV causes clinically significant immunosuppression in patients has been difficult to find. Despite the abnormal performance of their lymphocytes in vitro, CMV mononucleosis patients seem to have no special susceptibility to opportunistic infections. Patients with more serious forms of CMV infection, on the other hand, are usually already immunosuppressed to some degree, and it has been very difficult to demonstrate that the virus makes their immune function any worse. In an attempt to do so, Chatterjee et al. followed 35 renal allograft recipients in the post-transplant period and found that mortality and severe morbidity from opportunistic fungal infections was limited to those patients who were CMV-seronegative prior to transplantation (101). Of the four patients who died of fungal infections, three had documented active CMV infections. The authors concluded that primary CMV infections in the post-transplant period render patients more susceptible to opportunistic fungal infections, while reactivated CMV infections appear to have no such effect. In another study, Schooley et al. found that among 18 recipients of cadaveric kidney grafts, both primary and reactivated CMV infections occurring in the first three months after transplantation were invariably followed by inversions of the helper/suppressor T-cell ratio similar to those observed in CMV mononucleosis patients (102). Among 10 patients who received kidneys from living related donors, and were, therefore, less heavily immunosuppressed than the cadaver kidney recipients, T-cell subset inversions also occurred, but only in the presence of symptomatic CMV infection. In both groups, CMV-related inversions of the helper/suppressor ratio were associated with an increased frequency of opportunistic infections.

Although they involve a relatively small number of patients, these two prospective studies provide some evidence that CMV infection leads to clinically significant immunosuppression in patients who are receiving immunosuppressive therapy after organ transplantation. Although it remains to be proven, a similar scenario may occur in patients who are immunosuppressed as a result of HIV infection. The presence or absence of active CMV infection might then be one of the factors which determine why some AIDS patients seem less vulnerable to opportunistic infections and respond well to antimicrobial therapy while others quickly succumb despite appropriate treatment.

It has also been suggested that CMV may act as a cofactor with HIV in the development of AIDS, since several studies indicate that nearly all patients with AIDS and AIDS related complex (ARC) show either serologic or virologic evidence of CMV infection (103)-(105). In a group of over 100 homosexual men in the San Francisco Bay area, Drew et al. found that nearly one-half of those who were CMV-seropositive had helper/suppressor T-cell ratios of 1 or less, while less than 5% of those who were seronegative had inverted ratios (106). In a subgroup of seronegative men who were followed prospectively, all 12 who acquired new CMV infections also developed inversions of the helper/suppressor ratio which lasted for up to 15 months. Notably, none of the men in this study were HIV seropositive and none had clinical findings of AIDS or ARC. If these observed alterations in lymphocyte subsets are accompanied by some degree of immunosuppression, it is conceivable that CMV infection might facilitate the growth and spread of an agent such as HIV and thereby promote the development of AIDS.

Even though HIV has now been convincingly established as the causative agent of AIDS, the idea of a secondary cofactor remains attractive as a means of explaining why most individuals remain well after HIV infection while others go on to develop ARC and AIDS. As a virus which infects nearly all AIDS patients and almost certainly has some immunosuppressive capability, CMV must still be regarded seriously as one of the most likely potential cofactors.

CMV INFECTION IN AIDS PATIENTS

Whether or not CMV has any role in the pathogenesis of AIDS, its significance as a major cause of morbidity and mortality among AIDS patients is undeniable. Defining the frequency of CMV infections and their complications during the course of AIDS, however, is extremely difficult. Signs and symptoms of CMV infection are often non-specific and subtle, and most infections probably go undiagnosed during the life of the patient (10),(11),(13). As a result, data based on clinical case reporting may severely underestimate the importance of CMV in AIDS. A recent update from the Centers for Disease Control, for instance, reports CMV infection in only 7% of AIDS cases (107). Autopsy studies, on the other hand, typically find the inclusion-bearing cells of CMV infection in well over 50% of patients dying with AIDS, making this virus by far the most common opportunistic pathogen associated with AIDS at death (10)-(13),(108). These studies also reveal that AIDS-related CMV infections tend to be disseminated and may, on occasion, involve virtually all organs (10).

Pathology caused by CMV in AIDS patients ranges from occasional scattered cytomegalic cells with little or no surrounding inflammation to large areas of necrosis with a prominent neutrophilic or mononuclear cell response. The pattern and severity of involvement vary widely from patient to patient, and even from organ to organ in the same patient (12). Clinical manifestations of these infections do not always correlate well with histopathology and range from no apparent disease to life-threatening dysfunction of major organ systems. It is quite likely that CMV is also a frequent cause of non-specific febrile illness in AIDS, but this has been difficult to document since these patients so commonly have several different active infections at once.

Table 1 presents a list of manifestations of CMV infection which have been described in connection with AIDS. As can be seen, the virus may attack virtually any organ, but not all the lesions which have been found on histopathology have definite clinical significance. The most important ones merit individual attention and will be discussed below.

Pneumonitis

Cytomegalovirus pneumonitis is the most common, and probably the most serious, manifestation of CMV infection in AIDS. In autopsy studies of AIDS patients, it is almost always the most common pulmonary infection, with lesions being found in 50-90% of cases (10),(11,(13),(109),(110). In clinical studies, it is diagnosed much less frequently but still ranks second, behind *Pneumocystis carinii* pneumonia (PCP), as a cause of lung pathology (111)-(113). The reason for the discrepancy is probably the relative difficulty of diagnosing CMV pneumonia. While PCP can almost always be diagnosed from microscopic examination of bronchoalveolar lavage fluid or transbronchial lung biopsies (114), (115), the cytomegalic cells, which are the most reliable indicators of CMV infection, are often so sparse as not to be detected in these specimens. The fact that CMV pneumonia is found more often in open lung biopsies and at autopsy suggests that a relatively large tissue specimen may be required for reliable diagnosis. CMV can easily be cultured from bronchoalveolar lavage fluids of many AIDS patients, but a positive viral culture alone is probably not a good indicator of clinically significant pneumonia. At Westchester County Medical Center we performed viral cultures on bronchoalveolar lavage specimens from 31 consecutive AIDS patients undergoing bronchoscopy for the diagnosis of pneumonia, and 39% were positive for CMV. Most of these patients had concurrent PCP, however, and their clinical response to trimethoprim-sulfamethoxazole or pentamidine was similar to that of the patients with negative viral cultures (unpublished data). Significant lung disease secondary to CMV was, therefore, felt to be unlikely. Lung biopsy cultures are felt by some to be more helpful, but they also should be interpreted with caution since CMV viremia is not uncommon in AIDS patients (108), and contamination of a biopsy specimen with blood could yield a positive culture even in the absence of significant viral disease in the lung tissue.

The pathology of AIDS-related CMV pneumonitis, as described in several reports, is similar to that seen in transplant patients. Nuclear and cytoplasmic inclusions typical of CMV can be found in endothelial, epithelial, and pulmonary parenchymal cells, and even in pulmonary macrophages, but some have found endothelial cell involvement to be the predominant lesion (12). Alveolar septal thickening and hemorrhage are common. As with other CMV

Table 1. Sites of CMV Infection in AIDS Patients

Sites of CMV Infection
Established Clinical Significance
Disseminated infection
Lungs
Colon
Esophagus
Small bowel
Gallbladder
Brain
Spinal cord
Retina
Perianal skin
Probable Clinical Significance
Adrenal glands
Stomach
Epididymis
Questionable Clinical Significance
Liver
Kidneys
Spleen
Lymph nodes
Heart
Testes
Prostate
Thyroid gland
Parathyroid glands
Pituitary gland
Pancreas (islets and acini)
Skin

lesions in AIDS, the severity of CMV pneumonitis varies widely from only scattered inclusion-bearing cells to diffuse alveolar damage. A peculiar feature of CMV pneumonia in AIDS patients is the frequency with which it occurs as one component of a mixed infection. Mixed CMV-*Pneumocystis carinii* pneumonia is a common finding on histopathology, but combinations with *Mycobacterium avium-intracellulare* and *Cryptococcus neoformans* are occasionally reported as well (110),(112),(113).

The cardinal symptoms of CMV pneumonitis are non-productive cough and dyspnea; hemoptysis is rare (113). The onset of illness tends to be insidious, and symptoms may be present for weeks to months before the diagnosis is made. One series describes a more fulminant course for mixed CMV-pneumocystis pneumonias, however (113). The majority of patients have diffuse infiltrates on chest roentgenograms, but chest radiographs may be normal in up to 10% of patients (113).

The small amount of published data available suggests that the prognosis of CMV pneumonia in AIDS is extremely grave. The mortality among 21 patients with AIDS and CMV pneumonia studied by Stover et al. at Memorial Sloan-Kettering Cancer Center was 86% (113). The majority of these patients actually had mixed CMV-pneumocystis pneumonia, and when considered as a separate group, the mortality of the mixed pneumonias was even higher, at 92%. The eight patients with pure CMV pneumonia, despite the less fulminant nature of their disease, ultimately experienced a 75% mortality (113). A few patients in this series were treated with unspecified experimental antiviral therapy, but no benefit was apparent. Otherwise promising studies with the new antiviral agent (dihydroxypropoxymethyl) guanine (DHPG) similarly suggest that CMV pneumonia may be more refractory to treatment than some of the other manifestations of CMV infection (116).

Adrenalitis

After the lungs, the organ most commonly affected by CMV in AIDS patients is the adrenal gland. CMV adrenalitis has been reported in 40-90% of AIDS patients coming to autopsy (10),(12), (109),(117), and some suggest that it may be a special feature of AIDS since it seems to occur much more commonly in this condition than in other immunodeficiency states (118). It has also been noted that adrenal necrosis caused by CMV in AIDS patients is often disproportionate to damage caused by the virus in other organs (109), suggesting that the adrenals may be especially vulnerable to attack by CMV in AIDS.

The pathology of CMV adrenalitis in AIDS patients has been well described. Nuclear and cytoplasmic inclusions may be seen in endothelial, medullary, and cortical epithelial cells; but disease tends to be worst in the medulla and in many cases is entirely limited to this part of the gland (109),(117). Degree of involvement varies from focal single-cell necrosis in the medulla to hemorrhagic infarction of the entire gland (108). In most cases, however, cortical destruction is less than 50% (117). Cellular infiltration appears to differ according to the extent of necrosis, with lymphocytes and plasma cells in areas of scattered single-cell involvement, but with neutrophils predominating in zones of confluent necrosis.

The clinical significance of CMV adrenalitis in AIDS has not yet been convincingly established. Hypoadrenalism has been documented in AIDS patients but not definitely linked to any well-defined adrenal pathology (119). Conversely, other studies note that patients in whom subtotal adrenal cortical necrosis was found at autopsy showed no obvious findings of hypoadrenalism during life (12),(117). It is likely that in the great majority of cases of adrenalitis, enough functional cortex remains to avoid frank adrenal insufficiency; but this is obviously not the case in patients with bilateral total adrenal necrosis. Especially in the terminal phases of AIDS, many patients do, in fact, exhibit fever, hypotension, hyponatremia, and other non-specific abnormalities which are consistent with hypoadrenalism; but corticotrophin stimulation tests which would allow a definitive diagnosis are almost never performed. Physicians caring for these patients should at least be alert to the possibility of hypoadrenalism and perhaps be more aggressive in testing adrenal function so that steroid replacement therapy can be undertaken on a more timely and rational basis.

Other Endocrine Disease

CMV disease of the thyroid, parathyroid, and pituitary glands, as well as pancreatic islet cells, has been found at autopsy in up to 25% of AIDS patients. Involvement is generally limited to scattered inclusion-bearing cells, however, without the prominent necrosis seen in the adrenals (10),(12). Thus far, other endocrine dysfunction secondary to CMV has not been reported.

Gastrointestinal Ulceration

Autopsy studies of AIDS patients generally report CMV involvement of the gastrointestinal tract with a frequency only slightly lower than that of adrenalitis. Unlike adrenalitis, however, CMV gastrointestinal disease is a well known complication of immunodeficiency states other than AIDS, and its clinical consequences are often quite obvious and occasionally life-threatening.

The colon and terminal ileum seem to be the gastrointestinal sites most commonly affected by CMV. In the mildest form of disease, viral inclusions are found in epithelial, endothelial, and mesenchymal cells of the gut with little or no inflammatory response. Such lesions are often found in patients with no history of gastrointestinal symptoms, and it is difficult to determine if they are ever clinically significant (118). More advanced disease involves mucosal ulceration which may be extensive and often shows bacterial and fungal super-infection (12),(109). This stage is frequently severely symptomatic, with chronic, watery diarrhea which is clinically indistinguishable from the bacterial, mycobacterial and cryptosporidial diarrheas which so commonly affect AIDS patients. Weight loss and wasting may be severe, and some patients eventually die from refractory diarrhea (12),(118),(120). In its most severe form, CMV infection may lead to focal or extensive hemorrhagic necrosis in the terminal ileum, colon, or rectum. The underlying lesion in such cases appears to be vasculitis of the bowel caused by CMV (12),(121), and reported outcomes include bowel perforation, peritonitis, and severe hemorrhage; emergency colectomy may be necessary (10),(122).

Both roentgenographic and endoscopic findings are quite nonspecific in CMV enterocolitis. Barium enema shows mucosal granularity, superficial erosions, and effacement of haustral markings resembling, to a great extent, ulcerative colitis (123), and lesions seen on colonoscopy may also be confused with inflammatory bowel disease (120), pseudomembranous colitis (122), or even Kaposi's sarcoma (123). Diagnosis, therefore, rests on histopathology of biopsies taken from suspicious lesions, with viral culture of biopsy tissue sometimes providing helpful confirmation of the presence of CMV.

CMV involvement of the upper gastrointestinal tract is also described in connection with AIDS, but it appears to be much less common than colonic disease. Several cases are described in which patients presented with odynophagia and dysphagia and were subsequently found to have CMV esophagitis (124)-(126). The patterns of involvement seen included focal ulceration of the distal esophagus, complete mucosal erosion in the distal three-fourths of the esophagus, and a giant ulcer of the mid-esophagus. In this last case, the underlying pathology was clearly CMV vasculitis (124). CMV-related ulcerations have also been reported in the gastric fundus and antrum and in the duodenum (120),(126). Most of these lesions appear to have been clinically silent, but one patient with involvement of the distal stomach did experience postprandial vomiting and epigastric pain (126). CMV lesions of the upper gastrointestinal tract, like those of the colon, have no specific radiographic or endoscopic features, and diagnosis requires biopsy for microscopic examination.

Hepatobiliary Disease

Although hepatitis is a common feature of CMV mononucleosis in normal hosts, it is rarely reported in AIDS-related CMV infections. In the one autopsy study which concentrated specifically on hepatic pathology, over 80% of cases had systemic CMV infection, but only 6% of these showed any evidence of liver involvement (127). This was limited to scattered intranuclear and intracytoplasmic inclusions present mainly in Kupffer cells, but also in some hepatocytes, endothelial cells, and biliary epithelial cells. Several small series describe similar findings in a somewhat higher percentage of cases, but in none of them does CMV hepatitis appear to be a clinically important entity (9),(13), (109).

One of the most surprising lesions associated with CMV infection in AIDS is acalculous cholecystitis, which has been reported in three patients (128),(129). All three underwent laparotomy for severe, progressive abdominal pain, which in two patients had been present for several months. Gallbladder disease was suspected preoperatively in each case because of findings such as right upper quadrant tenderness, abnormal oral cholecystogram, and elevated alkaline phosphatase; and in one case each, ultrasonography and computed tomography strongly suggested a diagnosis of acalculous cholecystitis. Cholecystectomy was performed on all three; and gallbladder histopathology showed extensive mucosal ulceration and, in one case, areas of transmural necrosis. Numerous CMV inclusions were found in epithelial cells of all three gallbladders, and two also showed endothelial involvement. In one case, all pathology was apparently due to CMV; and when the patient died of pneumonia several months later, severe necrotizing cholangitis due to CMV was found in the common bile duct and major intrahepatic ducts. Simultaneous infections with *Candida albicans* and cryptosporidium in the other cases make the role of CMV in the etiology of cholecystitis difficult to determine. In any case, it is probably important for clinicians to be aware of the syndrome of acalculous cholecystitis in AIDS since timely surgery in this condition may relieve the patient's pain and avoid eventual rupture of the gallbladder.

Encephalitis and Myelitis

Unlike congenital CMV infections, acquired infections rarely involve the central nervous system (130). This then appears to be another area in which AIDS diverges from other immunodeficiency states, since autopsy studies report CMV encephalitis in 8 to 28% of AIDS patients with CMV infection (10),(12),(109). In one study, in fact, CMV encephalitis was considered the third most common cause of death, behind CMV pneumonia and *Pneumocystis carinii* pneumonia (12).

The characteristic lesion of CMV encephalitis and myelitis is the glial nodule, a focal dense collection of microglial cells in the cortical or spinal gray matter (130). Usually there is little accompanying inflammation or necrosis, and occasional nodules will contain one or two CMV inclusion cells. The origin of these cytomegalic cells is not always clear; most seem to be glial cells, but neurons also may be so involved (13). Extensive necrotizing lesions of the brain (12) and focal areas of demyelination in the brain and spinal cord featuring foamy macrophages and numerous CMV giant cells have also been described (131). In one AIDS case which terminated in massive subarachnoid hemorrhage, CMV vasculitis of the brain seems to have been the predominant lesion (132).

Relating the lesions of CMV encephalitis found in histopathology to signs and symptoms is difficult since autopsy studies and reports which stress pathologic findings rarely detail the patients' clinical presentations. In a large study of the neurologic complications of AIDS, Snider et al. describe a syndrome involving slowly progressive cognitive changes, lethargy, and psychomotor retardation, and terminating in severe dementia (133). In eight of nine brains from patients with this syndrome which were examined postmortem, microglial nodules were found, and there were typical CMV inclusion cells in four of these. The authors, therefore, attributed this syndrome, which they called subacute encephalitis, to CMV, but this attribution probably deserves re-examination in light of more recent findings of the neurotropic and neuropathic properties of HIV itself (134). The demyelinating lesions described and attributed to CMV by Moskowitz et al. (131) were associated with progressive motor weakness in the extremities; but the disease described does not appear clinically distinguishable from the syndrome of vacuolar myelopathy in AIDS, which is probably due to HIV involvement of the spinal cord (135).

There is also one report of an AIDS patient who presented with headache and photophobia and who had a mononuclear pleocytosis in the cerebrospinal fluid (136). CMV was isolated from centrifuged CSF cells, and the patient is described as having CMV meningoencephalitis. Such an entity may, in fact, affect AIDS patients, but in the CNS, as elsewhere, diagnosis of CMV-related disease, as opposed to CMV infection, should probably rest on tissue histopathology rather than culture of body fluids. CMV may on occasion be cultured from the CSF of patients who subsequently show no CMV disease on postmortem examination of the brain and spinal cord (137).

Retinitis

CMV retinitis is probably the major cause of visual loss in AIDS. Although some autopsy series scarcely mention it, other sources find it in 10-40% of patients with CMV infection at other sites (13),(138),(139). Because its cardinal symptom - visual loss - is so distressing and its physical findings are so distinctive, it is not unusual for CMV retinitis to be the first clinical sign of disseminated CMV infection (138),(140).

The affected eye in CMV retinitis is neither red nor painful, and the patient generally presents because of blurred vision or visual field loss. The initial lesions seen on fundoscopy usually appear as small, multifocal yellow-white patches on the retina which may have associated hemorrhage and may be confused with cotton-wool spots (141). The gradual progression of hemorrhagic necrosis of the retina along vascular arcades, with associated vascular sheathing, however, is distinctly characteristic of CMV infection. Some inflammatory cells are usually present in the vitreous, but these generally fade in the late stages of the disease as the retina becomes completely atrophic. Visual acuity may be maintained as long as the macula is spared, but most patients eventually experience severe loss of acuity (139). If not treated, the disease generally runs its course over three to six months. While often unilateral in the early stages, CMV retinitis will eventually involve both eyes in most patients (139).

Histopathology of involved eyes varies with the stage of the disease. In the active stage there is focal necrosis, with the retina itself being more severely involved than adjacent tissues. CMV inclusions can be found in retinal and choroidal cells, and small to moderate numbers of mononuclear inflammatory cells are often present. In the late stages, there is retinal atrophy, with mainly glial cells remaining (139).

Of all CMV-related lesions, CMV retinitis is probably the most responsive to experimental antiviral therapy. Making the correct diagnosis is, therefore, important, and fortunately, this can be done without biopsy. The characteristic ophthalmoscopic findings, along with a positive CMV culture from any body fluid or a positive CMV serology, are generally considered adequate indications for starting therapy.

Other Sites

As previously mentioned, evidence of CMV infection has been found in AIDS patients at many body sites other than those discussed here in detail. A few of these "other sites" should probably be mentioned briefly either because they have already presented interesting clinical problems or it is anticipated that they will as the number of AIDS cases grows.

CMV-related lesions of the kidneys are mentioned in several studies and are probably not uncommon (10),(11),(109). In one study, it is further noted that the glomeruli seem to be most affected, raising the question of whether a clinically significant CMV-related glomerulopathy, perhaps analogous to that already described in renal transplant recipients (142), may eventually be recognized in AIDS. Elsewhere in the urinary tract, symptomatic epididymitis due to CMV has been described in one AIDS patient (109), and this diagnosis is worth considering in the AIDS patient with clinical epididymitis who has a negative urine culture or seems not to benefit from antibiotic therapy.

One study noted four AIDS cases in which CMV caused focal necrosis in the myocardium (12). Although congestive heart failure, arrhythmias, and electrocardiographic changes were not detected in these patients, there is no reason to doubt that clinically significant cardiomyopathy will occur in more severe cases, and physicians should remain alert to this possibility.

Finally, a recent case report describes an AIDS patient with violaceous skin lesions which were presumed to be Kaposi's sarcoma until biopsy showed a cutaneous vasculitis due mainly to CMV (143). The lesson is clear; skin lesions in AIDS patients may have many etiologies and must be biopsied to avoid serious diagnostic errors.

IMPACT ON MORTALITY

The manifestations of CMV infection in AIDS are numerous, and their consequences for patients may be extremely serious. Perhaps the ultimate measure of the importance of any opportunistic pathogen in AIDS, however, is its impact on mortality. Because several severe infections are often present simultaneously in the later stages of AIDS, the cause of a patient's death cannot always be determined unequivocally; but several autopsy studies have attempted to do so (10)-(13),(109), and their results with respect to CMV are summarized in Table 2. Some caution must be exercised in generalizing from these data since they are based on findings in less than 1% of the AIDS patients diagnosed thus far in the U.S. All of these studies also deal mainly with homosexual patients, who may have a higher frequency of CMV-related complications than members of the smaller AIDS risk groups. Even with these caveats in mind, however, the data are impressive. CMV was the most common pathogen in all series, being found in 56 and 90% of all patients. Either alone or in combination with some other infection, CMV was also determined to be the most frequent immediate cause of death in all series except that of Moskowitz et al. (11) where PCP and toxoplasma encephalitis were slightly more frequent. The most lethal form of CMV infection was pneumonitis, with colitis and encephalitis also contributing significantly to mortality.

Table 2. CMV Infection as the Immediate Cause of Death (ICOD) in AIDS Patients

Autopsy study (ref. no.)	Total No. of Cases	No. With CMV Infections (%)	No. With CMV as ICOD (%)
Reichert et al., 1983 (109)	10	9 (90%)	4 (40%)
Welch et al., 1984 (10)	36	25 (69%)	18 (50%)
Mobley et al., 1985 (13)	12	10 (83%)	6 (50%)
Moskowitz et al., 1985 (11)	54	30 (56%)	10 (19%)
Niedt et al., 1985 (12)	56	43 (77%)	30 (54%)

CMV AND KAPOSI'S SARCOMA

Like CMV infection, Kaposi's sarcoma (KS) occurs with an unexpectedly high frequency in homosexual men with AIDS. This association may be coincidental, but there is a small body of evidence which suggests that it is not. The peculiar epidemiology of Kaposi's sarcoma in parts of Africa would seem to suggest an infectious etiology; and almost a decade before the arrival of the AIDS epidemic, Giraldo et al. demonstrated herpes-type viral particles in tissue culture lines derived from several African KS cases (144). When a virus was eventually isolated from one of these lines, it appeared to be a strain of CMV (145). In the seroepidemiologic studies which followed these virologic observations, it was noted that mean anti-CMV antibody titers of European and American KS patients were significantly higher than those of age-matched melanoma patients and healthy adults, while titers of antibodies to other herpesviruses were similar in KS patients and control subjects (146),(147). The form of KS which was most commonly seen in Europe and North America at that time was an indolent disease of elderly men. Among Africans, who develop a highly malignant form of KS which is very similar to that now being seen in AIDS patients, these studies found no difference between KS patients and controls in terms of anti-CMV antibody titers. The same group later demonstrated, however, that between one-fourth and one-half of tissue specimens and cell lines from African KS tumors contain CMV DNA sequences and express some CMV antigens (148),(149).

Thus, as the AIDS era dawned, there was evidence from one group of researchers of a relationship between CMV and both the African and non-African forms of KS. In the meantime, others had independently noticed a much higher than expected incidence of KS among renal transplant recipients (150), strongly suggesting that immunosuppression may be a risk factor in the development of at least some cases of KS. The high frequency of CMV infection among transplant patients also seemed compatible with theories giving CMV a major role in the pathogenesis of KS. In addition, some of the biological properties of the virus lend plausibility to the idea of CMV oncogenesis. These include CMV's ability to establish latency, its stimulation of host cell DNA synthesis, and its ability to cause malignant transformation of cells in vitro (151).

When AIDS first appeared, the association in these patients between severe CMV infections and KS was immediately noticed (4). CMV RNA and CMV antigens have also been found in most of the KS specimens from AIDS patients tested thus far (152). Thus, the close association between CMV and KS is confirmed in AIDS, but the nature of that association is still uncertain. CMV may initially cause the cellular transformation which leads to KS; or alternatively, KS tumors may be caused by another virus but at the same time be permissive for an abortive type of CMV infection. Only the elucidation of the molecular mechanisms of KS pathogenesis is likely to clarify the matter.

DIAGNOSIS OF CMV INFECTION

The diagnosis of CMV infection is more complicated in AIDS than it is in most other settings. Serodiagnosis, which is extremely useful in normal hosts, is, in most respects, useless in AIDS patients. Nearly all AIDS patients appear to have complement fixing IgG anti-CMV antibodies, frequently at high titers (104),(105), and fourfold increases in titer may occur in the absence of clinical disease (104). Thus, IgG serologies have no discriminative value for identifying significant CMV infections in this group. Likewise, IgM anti-CMV antibody, which is a helpful indicator of acute infection in normal hosts (57),(153), may be present in the asymptomatic AIDS patient or absent in patients with serious CMV-related disease (104). A positive IgG or IgM CMV antibody test confirms the possibility of CMV infection, but a negative test probably does not rule it out. In addition to the complement fixation procedure, indirect immunofluorescence, enzyme immunoassay, indirect hemagglutination, and latex agglutination tests for detecting CMV antibodies are commercially available. All seem to have good sensitivity and specificity (35), but the recently developed latex agglutination test requires the least specialized equipment and may be the easiest test to perform in most laboratories (154).

Compared with serologic tests, tissue culture for CMV is a much more expensive and technically demanding means of documenting CMV infection. However, this procedure provides little additional information in terms of diagnosing clinically significant infection, since such a high proportion of AIDS patients persistently shed CMV in body fluids. Many, in fact, are persistently viremic, even when no apparent serious CMV-related disease is present (104),(155). CMV cultures are nonetheless occasionally helpful to fulfill criteria for anti-viral therapy protocols or to suggest a diagnosis when a biopsy cannot be performed or when biopsy results are equivocal. Because of the slow growth of this virus in tissue culture, virologic confirmation of CMV infection has traditionally required up to three weeks. It has recently become possible to detect CMV in cultures of body fluids between 16 and 48 hours after inoculation, however, by using a commercially-available monoclonal antibody against the 72,000 dalton CMV early protein. Infected fibroblasts in these early cultures can be visualized using immunofluorescence or immunoperoxidase techniques, and in either case, the sensitivity and specificity are over 90% when compared with conventional culture techniques (156),(157). An alternative for rapid detection of CMV does not use tissue culture at all, but instead relies on hybridization of radiolabeled cloned fragments of CMV DNA with viral DNA from a clinical specimen (158). This technique has been applied to urine for detection of CMV with a sensitivity of 92% (159), but its requirement for the use of an ultracentrifuge and radioactive material may make it inconvenient for many clinical laboratories.

As previously stressed, however, definitive diagnosis of CMV-related disease of any organ in an AIDS patient can be made only by finding typical CMV cytopathology in that organ. The characteristic "owl's eye" cell of CMV infection is markedly enlarged (cytomegaly) with a large, ovoid eosinophilic inclusion, surrounded by a clear halo, seeming to occupy most of the nucleus. Cells also often show a large globular cytoplasmic inclusion or dense cytoplasmic granules. To detect CMV sooner than the two days generally required for preparing and staining tissue sections, touch preparations can be made from large biopsy specimens, Giemsa-stained and inspected for cytomegalic cells, with a sensitivity of around 50% when compared with standard histologic diagnosis (160). Another rapid diagnostic procedure involves immunofluorescent staining of frozen sections of biopsy specimens with an anti-CMV monoclonal antibody. This procedure appears to be even more sensitive for diagnosing CMV pneumonia than standard histology, but its specificity requires better definition (161).

Unfortunately, lung biopsy cannot be safely performed in all AIDS patients with interstitial pneumonia; bronchoalveolar lavage (BAL) has recently emerged as an extremely helpful diagnostic aid in such cases. Most useful in diagnosing PCP, BAL may have diagnostic potential in CMV pneumonia as well. In one small study, inspection of Papanicolau-stained smears of BAL cells for CMV-type inclusions was quite specific and had a sensitivity of 58% (162). Staining such smears with anti-CMV monoclonal antibodies greatly increases the sensitivity for detecting CMV infection, but apparently at the expense of specificity for pneumonia (163),(164). If fluorescent cells are quantitated as a percentage of total cells, however, it appears that specificity is regained (163). Thus BAL may eventually play a more important role in the diagnosis of CMV pneumonia in AIDS patients.

ANTIVIRAL CHEMOTHERAPY

Although the past decade has seen great progress in the control of other herpesvirus infections in compromised hosts, there has until quite recently been no similar success against CMV and little reason to anticipate any in the immediate future. Vidarabine and acyclovir, which have proven so effective in the systemic therapy of *Herpes simplex* and varicella-zoster virus infections, are both active against CMV in vitro, but only at concentrations which would be toxic in patients (165),(166). In the case of acyclovir, the reason for this seems clear, since activation of the drug in infected cells is largely dependent on the presence of a viral thymidine kinase (167). Both *Herpes simplex* and varicella-zoster virus have genes which code for such an enzyme; CMV does not. Thus, it is not surprising that whether used alone or in combination with alpha or beta interferon, acyclovir has shown no efficacy in the therapy of CMV pneumonia in bone marrow transplant patients (168)-(170). Vidarabine has proven similarly ineffective for serious CMV infections in both kidney and bone marrow transplant patients, and in the former it appeared to be associated with significant neurotoxicity as well (171),(172). Vidarabine, acyclovir, and alpha-interferon have also been used in small numbers of AIDS patients to treat CMV retinitis without any apparent effect on disease activity (139),(173). The most encouraging report involving any of the above mentioned agents was one showing that alpha-interferon given two or three times weekly by intramuscular injection to renal transplant recipients appeared to prevent the development of serious CMV infections (174).

Prospects for anti-CMV chemotherapy began to improve in 1983 when two groups demonstrated significant in vitro anti-CMV activity with a new purine analogue known as 9-(1,3-dihydroxy-2-propoxymethyl)guanine, or DHPG (175),(176). Despite its structural similarity to acyclovir, this agent does not depend on thymidine kinase for phosphorylation, and is presumably activated by one or more of the cellular kinases induced by CMV infection. In any case, much higher levels of the active DHPG triphosphate are found in infected cells than in uninfected cells, so the drug has some measure of selectivity (177). In its active form, DHPG appears to block viral DNA synthesis by inhibiting the binding of deoxyguanosine triphosphate to DNA polymerase.

Human studies with DHPG were begun in 1984, and initial results were mixed. At doses of 7.5 and 15 mg/kg/day, the drug was effective in eliminating CMV from blood, urine, and sputum of bone marrow transplant recipients with CMV pneumonia but nine of the 10 patients so treated died of respiratory failure (178). In addition, therapy had to be discontinued in three cases because of severe neutropenia. At the same time, two other groups reported much better results in the treatment of five AIDS patients with CMV retinitis (179),(180). Patients received 7.5 or 15 mg/kg/day of DHPG for 20 to 30 days, and all had dramatic improvement in fundoscopic examination and visual acuity. When the drug was stopped, all patients experienced worsening of retinitis within weeks but responded to a daily maintenance dose of DHPG therapy. Serious toxicity was not noted in these patients. More recently 13 AIDS patients with CMV retinitis had a similarly favorable response to DHPG but five developed neutropenia (181), (182). These studies found 7.5 mg/kg/day of DHPG to be the minimum effective dose. DHPG response in 18 AIDS patients with several types of CMV infection was also assessed in a collaborative study (183). Eleven of 14 patients with retinitis improved, as did five of 8 patients with colitis. Among seven patients with pneumonia, however, four died before completing two weeks of therapy, and the other three died later of respiratory failure. As in prior studies, patients showed a tendency to relapse when therapy was discontinued, and rapidly reversible neutropenia was the major toxicity.

Thus, DHPG shows great promise in the treatment of CMV retinitis in AIDS, and it appears to be able to prevent blindness if given indefinitely in a maintenance therapy regime. Its palliative effect in CMV colitis is somewhat less reliable; and it seems to be of very little benefit in CMV pneumonia. While it may not be the panacea for CMV infection in AIDS, it is quite likely that the full therapeutic potential of DHPG has not yet been realized. The synergy observed in vitro between DHPG and interferon (184), for instance, has not yet been investigated clinically. There are also other agents such as phosphonoformate (185) and several new nucleoside analogs (186) which are active against CMV in vitro but whose mechanisms of action are not identical to that of DHPG. These drugs then may also prove to be interesting candidates for use in combination with DHPG. It is not possible at this time to predict what will eventually emerge as the optimal therapy for CMV infection, but it is almost certain that research in this area will continue at a rapid pace in order to meet the urgent demand of CMV morbidity and mortality in the AIDS epidemic.

SUMMARY

Infection with human cytomegalovirus is extremely common in all populations, but transmission of infection seems to be particularly intense among sexually active homosexual men. In immunocompetent individuals, CMV may cause a form of mononucleosis but is most often asymptomatic. In patients with impaired cell-mediated immunity, however, CMV frequently causes severe and even life-threatening disease. There are also some data which suggest that CMV infection itself may have an immunosuppressive effect.

CMV infection is the most common opportunistic infection and one of the most frequent causes of death in AIDS patients. Manifestations include interstitial pneumonitis, necrotizing adrenalitis, gastrointestinal ulceration, encephalomyelitis, retinitis, and less serious disease at numerous other sites. Diagnosis of significant CMV infection in AIDS patients rests on demonstration of the characteristic cytomegalic cells in tissues, but virus culture is sometimes helpful, especially when used with new rapid detection techniques. DHPG, a new antiviral agent, has produced good results in the treatment of CMV retinitis and gastrointestinal disease in AIDS patients, but effective therapy for CMV pneumonitis has yet to be developed.

ACKNOWLEDGMENTS

The author wishes to thank Dr. Gary P. Wormser for inspiration and Lynda Mack, R.N., for help with numerous aspects of the preparation of this manuscript.

REFERENCES

1. Gottlieb, M.S., Schroff, R., Schanker, H.M., et al., *Pneumocystis carinii* pneumonia and mucosal candidiasis in previously healthy homosexual men. N Engl J Med 305:1425-1431 (1981)

2. Masur, H., Michelis, M.A., Greene, J.B., et al., An outbreak of community-acquired *Pneumocystis carinii* pneumonia: initial manifestation of cellular immune dysfunction. N Engl J Med 305:1431-1438 (1981)

3. Siegal, F.P., Lopez, C., Hammer, G.S., et al., Severe acquired immunodeficiency in male homosexuals manifested by chronic perianal ulcerative *Herpes simplex* lesions. N Engl J Med 305:1439-1444 (1981)

4. Urmacher, C., Myskowski, P., Ochoa, M., et al., Outbreak of Kaposi's sarcoma and cytomegalovirus infection in young homosexual men. Am J Med 72:569-575 (1982)

5. Mildvan, D., Mathur, U., Enlow, R.W., et al., Opportunistic infections and immune deficiency in homosexual men. Ann Intern Med 96:700-704 (1982)

6. Levin, M.J., Rinaldo, C.R., Leary, P.L., et al., Immune response to herpesvirus antigens in adults with acute cytomegalovirus mononucleosis. J Infect Dis 140:851-857 (1979)

7. Rinaldo, C.R., Carney, W.P., Richter, B.S., et al., Mechanisms of immunosuppression in cytomegaloviral mononucleosis. J Infect Dis 141:488-495 (1980)

8. Drew, L.W., Mintz, L., Miner, R.C., et al., Prevalence of cytomegalovirus infection in homosexual men. J Infect Dis 143:188-192 (1981)

9. Guarda, L.A., Luna, M.A., Smith, J.L., et al., Acquired immune deficiency syndrome: postmortem findings. Am J Clin Pathol 81:549-557 (1984)

10. Welch, K., Finkbeiner, W., Alpers, C.E., et al., Autopsy findings in the acquired immune deficiency syndrome. JAMA 252:1152-1159 (1984)

11. Moskowitz, L., Hensley, G.T., Chan, J.C., et al., Immediate causes of death in acquired immunodeficiency syndrome. Arch Pathol Lab Med 109:735-738 (1985)

12. Niedt, G.W., Schinella, R.A., Acquired immunodeficiency syndrome: clinicopathologic study of 56 autopsies. Arch Pathol Lab Med 109:727-734 (1985)

13. Mobley, K., Rotterdam, H.Z., Lerner, C.W., et al., Autopsy findings in the acquired immune deficiency syndrome. Pathol Annual 20:45-65 (1985)

14. Huang, E.-S., Kilpatrick, B.A., Huang, Y-T., et al., Detection of human cytomegalovirus and analysis of strain variation. Yale J Biol Med 49:29-43 (1976)

15. Huang, E.-S., Huang, S-M., Tegtmeier, G.E., et al., Cytomega- lovirus: genetic variation of viral genomes. Ann NY Acad Sci 354:332-346 (1980)

16. Beutner, K.R., Morag, A., Deibel, R., et al., Strain-specific local and systemic cell-mediated immune responses to cytomegalovirus in humans. Infect Immun 20:82-87 (1978)

17. Waner, J.L., Weller, T.H., Analysis of antigenic diversity among human cytomegaloviruses by kinetic neutralization tests with high-titered rabbit antisera. Infect Immun 21: 151-157 (1978)

18. Albrecht, T., Weller, T.H., Heterogeneous morphologic features of plaques induced by five strains of human cytomegalovirus. Am J Clin Pathol 73:648-654 (1980)

19. Kanich, R.E., Craighead, J.E., Human cytomegalovirus infection of cultured fibroblasts. I. Cytopathologic effects induced by an adapted and a wild strain. Lab Invest 27:263-272 (1972)

20. St. Jeor, S.C., Albrecht, T.B., Funk, R.D., et al., Stimulation of cellular DNA synthesis by human cytomegalovirus. J Virol 13:353-362 (1974)

21. Stinski, M.F., Sequence of protein synthesis in cells infected by human cytomegalovirus: early and late virus-induced polypeptides. J Virol 26:686-701 (1978)

22. Adler, S.P., Transfusion-associated cytomegalovirus infections. Rev Infect Dis 6:979-993 (1985)

23. Betts, R.F., Freeman, R.B., Douglas, R.G., et al., Transmission of cytomegalovirus infection with renal allograft. Kidney Int 8:387-394 (1975)

24. Chou, S., Acquisition of donor strains of cytomegalovirus by renal-transplant recipients. N Engl J Med 314:1418-1423 (1986)

25. Marker, S.C., Howard, R.J., Simmons, R.L., et al., Cytomegalovirus infection: a quantitative prospective study of 320 consecutive renal transplants. Surgery 89:660-671 (1981)

26. Pollard, R.B., Rand, K.H., Arvin, A.M., et al., Cell-mediated immunity to cytomegalovirus infection in normal subjects and cardiac transplant patients. J Infect Dis 137: 541-549 (1978)

27. Yeager, A.S., Grumet, F.C., Hafleigh, E.B., et al., Prevention of transfusion-acquired cytomegalovirus infections in newborn infants. J Pediatr 98:281-287 (1981)

28. Winston, D.J., Pollard, R.B., Ho., W.G., et al., Cytomegalovirus immune plasma in bone marrow transplant recipients. Ann Intern Med 97:11-18 (1982)

29. O'Reilly, R.J., Reich, L., Gold, J., et al., A randomized trial of intravenous hyperimmune globulin for the prevention of cytomegalovirus (CMV) infections following bone marrow transplantation: preliminary results. Transplant Proc 15: 1405-1411 (1983)

30. Winston, D.J., Ho, W.G., Lin, C.-H., et al., Intravenous immunoglobulin for modification of cytomegalovirus infections associated with bone marrow transplantation. Am J Med 76 (3A):128-133 (1984)

31. Krech, U., Complement-fixing antibodies against cytomegalovirus antibodies in different parts of the world. Bull WHO 49:103-106 (1973)

32. Krech, U., Tobin, J., A collaborative study of cytomegalovirus antibodies in mothers of young children in 19 countries. Bull WHO 59:605-610 (1981)

33. Carlstrom, G., Jalling, B., Cytomegalovirus infection in different groups of pediatric patients. Acta Paediatr Scand 59:303-309 (1970)

34. Wentworth, B.B., Alexander, E.R., Seroepidemiology of infections due to members of the herpesvirus group. Am J Epidemiol 94:496-507 (1971)

35. Horodniceanu, F., Michelson, S., Assessment of cytomegalovirus antibody detection techniques. Arch Virol 64:287-301 (1980)

36. Hanshaw, J.B., Dudgeon, J.A., Marshall, W.C., Viral Diseases of the Fetus and Newborn, W.B., Saunders, Co., Philadelphia (1985)

37. Reynolds, D.W., Stagno, S., Hosty, T.S., et al., Maternal cytomegalovirus excretion and perinatal infection N Engl J Med 289:1-5 (1973)

38. Montgomery, R., Youngblood, L., Medearis, D.N., Recovery of cytomegalovirus from the cervix in pregnancy. Pediatrics 49:524-531 (1972)

39. Stagno, S., Reynolds, D.W., Pass, R.F., et al., Breast milk and the risk of cytomegalovirus infection. N Engl J Med 302:1073-1076 (1980)

40. Pass, R.F., August, A.M., Dworsky, M., et al., Cytomegalovirus infection in a day-care center. N Engl J Med 307:477-479 (1982)

41. Hutto, C., Ricks, R., Garvie, M., et al., Epidemiology of cytomegalovirus infection in young children: day care vs. home care. Pediatr Infect Dis 4:149-152 (1985)

42. Sarov, B., Naggan, L., Rosenzveig, R., et al., Prevalence of antibodies to human cytomegalovirus in urban, kibbutz, and Bedouin children in southern Israel. J Med Virol 10:195-201 (1982)

43. Faix, R.G., Survival of cytomegalovirus on environmental surfaces. J Pediatr 106:649-652 (1985)

44. Yeager, A.S., Transmission of cytomegalovirus to mothers by infected infants: another reason to prevent transfusion-acquired infections. Pediatr Infect Dis 2:295-297 (1983)

45. Jordan, M.C., Rousseau, W.E., Noble, G.R., et al., Association of cervical cytomegaloviruses with venereal disease. N Engl J Med 288:932-934 (1973)

46. Wilmott, F.E., Cytomegalovirus in female patients attending a VD clinic. Br J Vener Dis 51:278-280 (1975)

47. Lang, D.J., Kummer, J.F., Hartley, D.P., Cytomegalovirus in semen: persistence and demonstration in extracellular fluids. N Engl J Med 291:121-123 (1974)

48. Lang, D.J., Kummer, J.F., Cytomegalovirus in semen: observations in selected populations. J Infect Dis 132:472-473 (1975)

49. Embil, J.A., Manuel, F.R., Garner, J.B., et al., Cytomegalovirus in the semen. Can Med Assoc J 126:391-392 (1982)

50. Mintz, L., Drew, W.L., Miner, R.C., et al., Cytomegalovirus infections in homosexual men: an epidemiological study. Ann Intern Med 99:326-329 (1983)

51. Lange, M., Klein, E.B., Kornfield, H., et al., Cytomegalovirus isolation from healthy homosexual men. JAMA 252:1908-1910 (1984)

52. Chandler, S.H., Alexander, E.R., Holmes, K.K., Epidemiology of cytomegaloviral infection in a heterogeneous population of pregnant women. J Infect Dis 152:249-256 (1985)

53. Chretien, J.H., McGinniss, C.G., Muller, A., Venereal causes of cytomegalovirus mononucleosis. JAMA 238:1644-1645 (1977)

54. Handsfield, H.H., Chandler, S.H., Caine, V.A., et al., Cytomegalovirus infection in sex partners: evidence for sexual transmission. J Infect Dis 151:344-348 (1985)

55. Kryger, P., Gerstoft, J., Pedersen, N.S., et al., Increased prevalence of cytomegalovirus antibodies in homosexual men with syphilis: relation to sexual behavior. Scand J Infect Dis 16:381-384 (1984)

56. Buimovici-Klien, E., Tinker, M.K., O'Beirne, A.J., et al., IgM detection by ELISA in the diagnosis of cytomegalovirus infections in homosexual and heterosexual immunosuppressed patients. Arch Virol 78:203-212 (1983)

57. Langenhuysen, M.M.A.C., The, T.H., Nieweg, H.O., et al., Demonstration of IgM cytomegalovirus antibodies as an aid to early diagnosis in adults. Clin Exp Immunol 6:387-393 (1970)

58. Drew, W.L., Sweet, E.S., Miner, R.C., et al., Multiple infections by cytomegalovirus in patients with acquired immunodeficiency syndrome: documentation by Southern blot hybridization. J Infect Dis 150:952-953 (1984)

59. Spector, S.A., Hirata, K.K., Neuman, T.R., Identification of multiple cytomegalovirus strains in homosexual men with acquired immunodeficiency syndrome. J Infect Dis 150:953-955 (1984)

60. Guinan, M.E., Thomas, P.A., Pinsky, P.F., et al., Heterosexual and homosexual patients with the acquired immunodeficiency syndrome. Ann Intern Med 100:213-218 (1984)

61. Blaser, M.J., Cohen, D.L., Opportunistic infections in patients with AIDS: clues to the epidemiology of AIDS and the relative virulence of pathogens. Rev Infect Dis 8:21-30 (1986)

62. Enck, R.E., Betts, R.F., Brown, M.R., et al., Viral serology (hepatitis B virus, cytomegalovirus, Epstein-Barr virus) and abnormal liver function tests in transfused patients with hereditary hemorrhagic diseases. Transfusion 19:32-38 (1979)

63. Cheeseman, S.H., Sullivan, J.L., Brettler, D.B., et al., Analysis of cytomegalovirus and Epstein-Barr virus antibody responses in treated hemophiliacs: implications for the study of acquired immune deficiency syndrome. JAMA 252: 83-85 (1984)

64. Landay, A., Poon, M-C., Abo, T., et al., Immunologic studies in asymptomatic hemophilia patients: relationship to acquired immune deficiency syndrome (AIDS). J Clin Invest 71: 1500-1504 (1983)

65. Betts, R.F., Syndromes of cytomegalovirus infection. Advances Intern Med 26:447-466 (1980)

66. Ho., M., Dowling, J.N., Cytomegalovirus infections in transplant and cancer patients. Current Clinical Topics in Infectious Diseases 1:45-67 (1980)

67. Panjvani, Z.F.K., Hanshaw, J.B., Cytomegalovirus in the perinatal period. J Dis Children 135:56-60 (1981)

68. Cohen, J.I., Corey, G.R., Cytomegalovirus infection in the normal host. Medicine 64:100-114 (1985)

69. Weller, T.H., Hanshaw, J.B., Scott, D.E., Serologic differentiation of viruses responsible for cytomegalic inclusion disease. Virology 12:130-132 (1960)

70. Berenberg, W., Nankervis, G., Long-term follow-up of cytomegalic inclusion disease of infancy. Pediatrics 46:403-410 (1970)

71. Pass, R.F., Stagno, S., Myers, G.J., et al., Outcome of symptomatic congenital cytomegalovirus infection: results of long-term longitudinal follow-up. Pediatrics 66:758-762 (1980)

72. Hanshaw, J.B., Scheiner, A.P., Moxley, A.W., et al., School failure and deafness after "silent" congenital cytomegalovirus infection. N Engl J Med 295:468-470 (1976)

73. Evans, A.S., Infectious mononucleosis and related syndromes. Am J Med Sci 276:325-338 (1978)

74. Lang, D.J., Scolnik, E.M., Willerson, J.T., Association of cytomegalovirus infection with the postperfusion syndrome. N Engl J Med 278:1147-1149 (1968)

75. Winston, D.J., Ho, W.G., Howell, C.L., et al., Cytomegalovirus infections associated with leukocyte transfusions. Ann Intern Med 93:671-675 (1980)

76. Hersman, J., Meyers, J.D., Thomas, E.D., et al., The effect of granulocyte transfusions on the incidence of cytomegalovirus infection after allogeneic marrow transplantation. Ann Intern Med 96:149-152 (1982)

77. Bayer, W.E., The effect of frozen blood on the relationship of cytomegalovirus and hepatitis virus to infection and disease, in: Clinical and Practical Aspects of the Use of Frozen Blood (Dawson, R.B., Barnes, A., eds), American Association of Blood Banks, Washington, D.C. p 133-147 (1977)

78. Bonkowski, H.L., Lee, R.V., Klatskin, G., Acute granulomatous hepatitis: occurrence in cytomegalovirus mononucleosis. JAMA 233:1284-1288 (1975)

79. Clarke, J., Craig, R.M., Saffro, R., et al., Cytomegalovirus granulomatous hepatitis. Am J Med 66:264-269 (1979)

80. Leonard, J.C., Tobin, J.O., A report from various centers: polyneuritis associated with cytomegalovirus infection. Q J Med 40:435-442 (1971)

81. Dowling, P., Menonna, J., Cook, S., Cytomegalovirus complement fixation antibody in Guillain-Barre syndrome. Neurology 27:1153-1156 (1977)

82. Wong, T.W., Warner, N.E., Cytomegalic inclusion disease in adults. Report of 14 cases with review of literature. Arch Pathol 74:403-421 (1962)

83. Gottman, A.W., Beatty, E.C., Cytomegalic inclusion disease in children with leukemia or lymphosarcoma. Am J Dis Child 21:415-425 (1962)

84. Bodey, G.P., Wertlake, P.T., Douglas, G., et al., Cytomegalic inclusion disease in patients with acute leukemia. Ann Intern Med 62:899-906 (1965)

85. Rosen, P., Hadju, S., Cytomegalovirus inclusion disease at autopsy of patients with cancer. Am J Clin Pathol 55:749-756 (1971)

86. Armstrong, D., Rosen, P., Cytomegalovirus and *Herpes simplex* pneumonia complicating neoplastic disease, In: Pathogenic Microorganisms from Atypical Clinical Sources (von-Graevenitz, A., Sall, T., eds), Marcel Dekker, New York, p 89-99 (1975)

87. Craighead, J.E., Henshaw, J.B., Carpenter, C.B., Cytomegalovirus infection after renal allotransplantation. JAMA 201: 725-728 (1967)

88. Rubin, R.H., Cosimi, A.B., Tolkoff-Rubin, N.E., et al., Infectious disease syndromes attributable to cytomegalovirus and their significance among renal transplant recipients. Transplantation 24:458-464 (1977)

89. Richardson, W.P., Colvin, R.B., Cheeseman, S.H., et al., Glomerulopathy associated with cytomegalovirus viremia in renal allografts. N Engl J Med 305:57-63 (1981)

90. Suwansirikul, S., Rao, N., Dowling, J.N., et al., Primary and secondary cytomegalovirus infection: clinical manifestations after renal transplantation. Arch Intern Med 137:1026-1029 (1977)

91. Betts, R.F., Freeman, R.B., Douglas, R.G., et al., Clinical manifestations of renal allograft derived primary cytomegalovirus infection. Am J Dis Child 131:759-763 (1977)

92. Peterson, P.K., McGlave, P., Ramsay, N.K.C., et al., A prospective study of infectious diseases following bone marrow transplantation: emergence of aspergillus and cytomegalovirus as the major causes of mortality. Infect Control 4:81-89 (1983)

93. Meyers, J.D., Flournoy, N., Thomas, E.D., Risk factors for cytomegalovirus infection after human marrow transplantation. J Infect Dis 153:478-488 (1986)

94. Howard, R.J., Miller, J., Najarian, J.S., Cytomegalovirus induced immune suppression. II. Cell-mediated immunity. Clin Exp Immunol 18:119-126 (1974)

95. Rinaldo, C.R., Black, P.H., Hirsch, M.S., Interaction of cytomegalovirus with leukocytes from patients with mononucleosis due to cytomegalovirus. J Infect Dis 136:667-677 (1977)

96. Carney, W.P., Hirsch, M.S., Mechanisms of immunosuppression in cytomegalovirus mononucleosis. II. Virus-monocyte interactions. J Infect Dis 144:47-54 (1981)

97. Carney, W.P., Rubin, R.H., Hoffman, R.A., et al., Analysis of T lymphocyte subsets in cytomegalovirus mononucleosis. J Immunol 126:2114-2116 (1981)

98. Carney, W.P., Iacoviello, V., Hirsch, M.S., Functional properties of T lymphocytes and their subsets in cytomegalovirus mononucleosis. J Immunol 130:390-393 (1983)

99. Rice, G.P.A., Schrier, R.D., Oldstone, M.B.A., Cytomegalovirus infects human lymphocytes and monocytes: virus expression is limited to immediate-early gene products. Proc Nat Acad Sci USA 81:6134-6138 (1984)

100. Wahren, B., Ljungman, P., Paulin, T., et al., Enhancive and suppressive effects of cytomegalovirus on human lymphocyte responses in vitro. J Virol 58:909-913 (1986)

101. Chatterjee, S.N., Fiala, M., Weiner, J., et al., Primary cytomegalovirus and opportunistic infections: incidence in renal transplant recipients. JAMA 240:2446-2449 (1978)

102. Schooley, R.T., Hirsch, M.S., Colvin, R.B., et al., Association of herpesvirus infections with T-lymphocyte subset alterations, glomerulopathy, and opportunistic infections after renal transplantation. N Engl J Med 308:307-313 (1983)

103. Drew, W.L., Mintz, L., What is the role of cytomegalovirus in AIDS? Ann NY Acad Sci 437:320-324 (1984)

104. Quinnan, G.V., Masur, H., Rook, A.H., et al., Herpesvirus infections in the acquired immune deficiency syndrome. JAMA 252:72-77 (1984)

105. Halbert, S.P., Kiefer, D.J., Friedman, A.E., et al., Antibody levels of cytomegalovirus, *Herpes simplex* virus, and rubella in patients with acquired immune deficiency syndrome. J Clin Microbiol 23:318-321 (1986)

106. Drew, W.L., Mills, J., Levy, J., et al., Cytomegalovirus infection and abnormal T-lymphocyte subset ratios in homosexual men. Ann Intern Med 103:61-63 (1985)

107. CDC., Update: acquired immunodeficiency syndrome - United States. MMWR 35:17-21 (1986)

108. Macher, A.M., Reichert, C.M., Straus, S.E., et al., Death in the AIDS patient. N Engl J Med 309:1454 (1983)

109. Reichert, C.M., O'Leary, T.J., Levens, D.L., et al., Autopsy pathology in the acquired immune deficiency syndrome. Am J Pathol 112:357-382 (1983)

110. Nash, G., Fligiel, S., Pathologic features of the lung in the acquired immune deficiency syndrome (AIDS): an autopsy study of seventeen homosexual males. Amer J Clin Pathol 81:6-12 (1984)

111. Lerner, C.W., Tapper, M.L., Opportunistic infection complicating acquired immune deficiency syndrome: clinical features of 25 cases. Medicine 63:155-164 (1984)

112. Murray, J.F., Felton, C.P., Garay, S.M., et al., Pulmonary complications of the acquired immunodeficiency syndrome: report of a National Heart, Lung, and Blood Institute workshop. N Engl J Med 310:1682-1688 (1984)

113. Stover, D.E., White, D.A., Romano, P., et al., Spectrum of pulmonary diseases associated with the acquired immune deficiency syndrome. Am J Med 78:429-437 (1985)

114. Blumenfeld, W., Wagar, E., Hadley, W.K., Use of transbronchial biopsy for diagnosis of opportunistic pulmonary infections in acquired immune deficiency syndrome (AIDS). Am J Clin Pathol 81:1-5 (1983)

115. Broaddus, C., Dake, M., Stulbarg, M.S., et al., Bronchoalveolar lavage and transbronchial biopsy for the diagnosis of pulmonary infections in the acquired immunodeficiency syndrome. Ann Intern Med 102:747-752 (1985)

116. Collaborative DHPG Treatment Study Group, Treatment of serious cytomegalovirus infections with 9-(1, 3-dihydroxy-2-propoxy-methyl)guanine in patients with AIDS and other immunodeficiencies. N Engl J Med 314:801-805 (1986)

117. Glasgow, B.J., Steinsapir, K.D., Anders, K., et al., Adrenal pathology in the acquired immune deficiency syndrome. Am J Clin Path 84:594-597 (1985)

118. Tapper, M.L., Rotterdam, H.Z., Lerner, C.W., et al., Adrenal necrosis in the acquired immunodeficiency syndrome. Ann Intern Med 100:239-241 (1984)

119. Greene, L.W., Cole, W., Greene, J.B., et al., Adrenal insufficiency as a complication of the acquired immunodeficiency syndrome. Ann Intern Med 101:497-498 (1984)

120. Knapp, A.B., Horst, D.A., Eliopoulos, G., et al., Widespread cytomegalovirus gastroenterocolitis in a patient with acquired immunodeficiency syndrome. Gastroenterology 85:1399-1402 (1983)

121. Frank, D., Raicht, R.F., Intestinal perforation associated with cytomegalovirus infection in patients with acquired immunodeficiency syndrome. Am J Gastro 79:201-205 (1984)

122. Meiselman, M.S., Cello, J.P., Margareten, W., Cytomegalovirus colitis: report of clinical, endoscopic, and pathologic findings in two patients with the acquired immune deficiency syndrome. Gastroenterology 88:171-175 (1985)

123. Balthazar, E.J., Megibow, A.J., Frazzini, E., et al., Cytomegalovirus colitis in AIDS: radiographic findings in 11 patients. Radiology 155:585-589 (1985)

124. St. Onge, G., Bezahler, G.H., Giant esophageal ulcer associated with cytomegalovirus. Gastroenterology 83:127-130 (1982)

125. Gertler, S.L., Pressman, J., Price, P., et al., Gastrointestinal cytomegalovirus infection in a homosexual man with severe acquired immunodeficiency syndrome. Gastroenterology 85:1403-1406 (1983)

126. Balthazar, E.J., Megibow, A.J., Hulnick, D.H., Cytomegalovirus esophagitis and gastritis in AIDS. Am J Radiol 144:1201-1204 (1985)

127. Glasgow, B.J., Anders, K., Layfield, L.J., et al., Clinical and pathologic findings of the liver in the acquired immune deficiency syndrome. Am J Clin Pathol 83:582-588 (1985)

128. Blumberg, R.S., Kelsey, P., Perrone, T., et al., Cytomegalovirus- and cryptosporidium-associated acalculous cholecystitis. Am J Med 76:1118-1123 (1984)

129. Kavin, H., Jonas, R.B., Chowdhury, L., et al., Acalculous cholecystitis and cytomegalovirus infection in the acquired immunodeficiency syndrome. Ann Intern Med 104:53-54 (1986)

130. Bales, J.F., Human cytomegalovirus infection and disorders of the nervous system. Arch Neurol 41:310-320 (1984)

131. Moskowitz, L.B., Gregorios, J.B., Hensley, G.T., et al., Cytomegalovirus induced demyelination associated with acquired immune deficiency syndrome. Arch Pathol Lab Med 180:873-877 (1984)

132. Hawley, D.A., Schaefer, J.F., Schulz, D.M., et al., Cytomegalovirus encephalitis in acquired immunodeficiency syndrome. Am J Clin Pathol 80:874-877 (1983)

133. Snider, W.D., Simpson, D.M., Nielsen, S., et al., Neurological complications of acquired immune deficiency syndrome: analysis of 50 patients. Ann Neurol 14:403-418 (1983)

134. Shaw, G.M., Harper, M.E., Hahn, B.H., et al., HTLV-III infection in brains of children and adults with AIDS encephalopathy. Science 227:177-181 (1985)

135. Petito, C.K., Navia, B.A., Cho, E-S., et al., Vacuolar myelopathy pathologically resembling subacute combined degeneration in patients with the acquired immune deficiency syndrome. N Engl J Med 312:874-879 (1985)

136. Edwards, R.H., Messing, R., McKendall, R.R., Cytomegalovirus meningoencephalitis in a homosexual man with Kaposi's sarcoma: isolation of CMV from CSF cells. Neurology 35:560-562 (1985)

137. Singh, B., Levine, S., Yarrish, R.L., et al., Spinal cord syndromes in the acquired immune deficiency syndrome. Acta Neurol Scand 73:590-598 (1986)

138. Freeman, W.R., Lerner, C.R., Mines, J.A., et al., A prospective study of the ophthalmologic findings in the acquired immune deficiency syndrome. Am J Ophthalmol 97:133-142 (1984)

139. Palestine, A.G., Rodrigues, M.M., Macher, A.M., et al., Ophthalmic involvement in acquired immunodeficiency syndrome. Ophthalmology 91:1092-1099 (1984)

140. Khadem, M., Kalish, S.B., Goldsmith, J., et al., Ophthalmologic findings in acquired immune deficiency syndrome. Arch Ophthalmol 102:201-206 (1984)

141. Teich, S., Orellana, J., Retinal lesions in cytomegalovirus infection. Ann Intern Med 104:132 (1986)

142. Richardson, W.P., Colvin, R.B., Cheeseman, S.H., et al., Glomerulopathy associated with cytomegalovirus infection in renal allografts. N Engl J Med 305:57-63 (1981)

143. Kwan, T.H., Kaufman, H.W., Acid-fast bacilli with cytomegalovirus and herpesvirus inclusions in the skin of an AIDS patient. Am J Clin Pathol 85:236-238 (1986)

144. Giraldo, G., Beth, E., Haguenau, F., Herpes-type virus particles in tissue culture of Kaposi's sarcoma from different geographic regions. J Natl Cancer Inst 49:1509-1526 (1972)

145. Glaser, R., Geder, L., St. Jeor, S., et al., Partial characterization of a herpes-type virus (K9V) derived from Kaposi's sarcoma. J Natl Cancer Inst 59:55-60 (1977)

146. Giraldo, G., Beth, E., Kourilsky, F.M., et al., Antibody patterns to herpesviruses in Kaposi's sarcoma: serological association of European Kaposi's sarcoma with cytomegalovirus. Int J Cancer 15:839-848 (1975)

147. Giraldo, G., Beth, E., Henle, W., et al., Antibody patterns to herpesviruses in Kaposi's sarcoma. II. Serological association of American Kaposi's sarcoma with cytomegalovirus. Int J Cancer 22:126-131 (1978)

148. Giraldo, G., Beth, E., and Huang, E.-S., Kaposi's sarcoma and its relationship to cytomegalovirus (CMV). III. CMV DNA and CMV early antigens in Kaposi's sarcoma. Int J Cancer 26:23-29 (1980)

149. Boldogh, I., Beth, E., Huang, E.-S., et al., Kaposi's sarcoma. IV. Detection of CMV DNA, CMV RNA, and CMNA in tumor biopsies. Int J Cancer 28:469-474 (1981)

150. Penn, I., Kaposi's sarcoma in organ transplant recipients. Transplantation 27:8-11 (1979)

151. Geder, L., Lausch, R., O'Neill, F., et al., Oncogenic transformation of human embryo lung cells by human cytomegalovirus. Science 192:1134-1137 (1976)

152. Drew, W.L., Miner, R.C., Ziegler, J.L., et al., Cytomegalovirus and Kaposi's sarcoma in young homosexual men. Lancet 2:125-127 (1982)

153. Griffiths, P.D., Stagno, S., Pass, R.F., et al., Cytomegalovirus infection during pregnancy: specific IgM antibodies as a marker of recent primary infection. J Infect Dis 145:647-653 (1982)

154. McHugh, T.M., Casavant, C., Wilber, J.C., et al., Comparison of six methods for the detection of antibody to cytomegalovirus. J Clin Microbiol 22:1014-1019 (1985)

155. Epstein, J.S., Frederich, W.R., Rook, A.H., et al., Selective defects in cytomegalovirus- and mitogen-induced lymphocyte proliferation and interferon release in patients with acquired immunodeficiency syndrome. J Infect Dis 152:727-733 (1985)

156. Shuster, E.A., Beneke, J.S., Tegtmeier, G.E., et al., Monoclonal antibody for rapid laboratory detection of cytomegalovirus infections: characterization and diagnostic application. Mayo Clinic Proc 60:577-585 (1985)

157. Swenson, P.D., Kaplan, M.H., Rapid detection of cytomegalovirus in cell culture by indirect immunoperoxidase staining with monoclonal antibody to an early nuclear antigen. J Clin Microbiol 21: 669-673 (1985)

158. Chou, S., Merigan, T.C., Rapid detection and quantitation of human cytomegalovirus in urine through DNA hybridization. N Engl J Med 308:921-925 (1983)

159. Schuster, V., Matz, B., Wiegand, H., et al., Detection of human cytomegalovirus in urine by DNA-DNA and RNA-DNA hybridization. J Infect Dis 154:309-314 (1986)

160. Shulman, H.M., Hackman, R.C., Sale, G.E., et al., Rapid cytologic diagnosis of cytomegalovirus interstitial pneumonia on touch imprints from open-lung biopsy. Am J Clin Pathol 77:90-94 (1982)

161. Hackman, R.C., Meyerson, D., Meyers, J.D., et al., Rapid diagnosis of cytomegaloviral pneumonia by tissue immunofluorescence with a murine monoclonal antibody. J Infect Dis 151:325-329 (1985)

162. Stover, D.E., Zaman, M.B., Hajdu, S.I., et al., Bronchoalveolar lavage in the diagnosis of diffuse pulmonary infiltrates in the immunosuppressed host. Ann Intern Med 101:1-7 (1984)

163. Emanuel, D., Peppard, J., Stover, D.E., et al., Rapid diagnosis of cytomegalovirus pneumonia by bronchoalveolar lavage using human and murine monoclonal antibodies. Ann Intern Med 104:476-481 (1986)

164. Martin, W.J., Smith, T.F., Rapid detection of cytomegalovirus in bronchoalveolar lavage specimens by a monoclonal antibody method. J Clin Microbiol 23:1006-1008 (1986)

165. Tyms, A.S., Seamans, E.M., Naim, H.M., The in vitro activity of acyclovir and related compounds against cytomegalovirus infections. J Antimicrob Chemother 8:65-72 (1981)

166. Spector, S.A., Kelley, E., Inhibition of human cytomegalovirus by combined acyclovir and vidarabine. Antimicrob Agents Chemother 27:600-604 (1985)

167. Elion, G.B., Furman, P.A., Fyfe, J.A., et al., Selectivity of action of an antiherpetic agent, 9- (2'-hydroxyethoxymethyl) guanine. Proc Natl Acad Sci USA 74:5716-5720 (1977)

168. Wade, J.C., Hintz, M., McGuffin, R.W., et al., Treatment of cytomegalovirus pneumonia with high-dose acyclovir. Am J Med 73:249-256 (1982)

169. Wade, J.C., McGuffin, R.W., Springmeyer, S.C., et al., Treatment of cytomegaloviral pneumonia with high-dose acyclovir and human leukocyte interferon. J Infect Dis 148:557-562 (1983)

170. Shepp, D.H., Newton, B.A., Meyers, J.D., Intravenous lymphoblastoid interferon and acyclovir for treatment of cytomegaloviral pneumonia. J Infect Dis 150:776-777 (1984)

171. Marker, S.C., Howard, R.J., Groth, K.E., et al., A trial of vidarabine for cytomegalovirus infection in renal transplant patients. Arch Intern Med 140:1441-1444 (1980)

172. Meyers, J.D., McGuffin, R.W., Bryson, Y.J., et al., Treatment of cytomegalovirus pneumonia after marrow transplant with combined vidarabine and human leukocyte interferon. J Infect Dis 146:80-84 (1982)

173. Chou, S., Dylewski, J.S., Gaynon, M.W., et al., Alpha-interferon administration in cytomegalovirus retinitis. Antimicrob Agents Chemother 25:25-28 (1984)

174. Hirsch, M.S., Schooley, R.T., Cosimi, A.B., et al., Effects of interferon-alpha on cytomegalovirus reactivation syndromes in renal-transplant recipients. New Engl J Med 308: 1489-1493 (1983)

175. Smee, D.F., Martin, J.C., Verheyden, J.P.H., et al., Anti-herpesvirus activity of the acyclic nucleoside 9-(1, 3-dihydroxypropoxymethyl) guanine. Antimicrob Agents Chemother 23:676-682 (1983)

176. Mar, E.C., Cheng, Y.C., Huang, E.-S., Effect of 9-(1,3-dihydroxy-2-propoxymethyl)guanine on human cytomegalovirus replication in vitro. Antimicrob Agents Chemother 24:518-521 (1983)

177. Freitas, V.R., Smee, D.F., Chernow, M., et al., Activity of 9-(1,3-dihydroxy-2-propoxymethyl)guanine compared with that of acyclovir against human, monkey, and rodent cytomegalovirus. Antimicrob Agents Chemother 28:240-245 (1985)

178. Shepp, D.H., Dandliker, P.S., de Miranda, P., et al., Activity of 9-[2-hydroxy-1-(hydroxymethyl)ethoxymethyl] guanine in the treatment of cytomegalovirus pneumonia. Ann Intern Med 103:368-373 (1985)

179. Felsenstein, D., D'Amico, D.J., Hirsh, M.S., et al., Treatment of cytomegalovirus retinitis with 9-[2-hydroxy-1-(hydroxymethyl)ethoxymethyl]guanine. Ann Intern Med 103:377-380 (1985)

180. Bach, M.C., Bagwell, S.P., Knapp, N.P., et al., 9-(1,3-dihydroxy-2-propoxymethyl)guanine for cytomegalovirus infections in patients with the acquired immunodeficiency syndrome. Ann Intern Med 103:381-382 (1985)

181. Masur, H., Lane, H.C., Palestine, A., et al., Effect of 9-(1,3-dihydroxy-2-propoxymethyl)guanine on serious cytomegalovirus disease in eight immunosuppressed homosexual men. Ann Intern Med 104:41-44 (1986)

182. Rosecan, L.R., Stahl-Bayliss, C.M., Kalman, C.M., et al., Antiviral therapy for cytomegalovirus retinitis in AIDS with dihydroxy propoxymethyl guanine. Am J Ophthamol 101:405-418 (1986)

183. Collaborative DHPG Treatment Study Group., Treatment of serious cytomegalovirus infections with 9-(1, 3-dihydroxy-2-propoxymethyl)guanine in patients with AIDS and other immunodeficiencies. N Engl J Med 314:801-805 (1986)

184. Rasmussen, L., Chen, P.T., Mullenax, J.G., et al., Inhibition of human cytomegalovirus replication by 9-(1,3-dihydroxy-2-propoxymethyl)guanine alone and in combination with human interferons. Antimicrob Agents Chemother 26:441-445 (1984)

185. Wahren, B., Oberg, B., Reversible inhibition of cytomegalovirus replication by phosphonoformate. Intervirology 14:7-15 (1980)

186. Colacino, J.M., Lopez, C., Efficacy and selectivity of some nucleoside analogs as anti-human cytomegalovirus agents. Antimicrob Agents Chemother 24:505-508 (1983)

25
Bacterial Infections in Patients with AIDS

Michael S. Simberkoff, Abigail Zuger

A variety of specific and non-specific host defense mechanisms are essential for the prevention of bacterial infection. These include immunoglobulins, phagocytic cells, and the integrity of the skin and mucous membranes. Each of these defenses may be compromised in patients with the acquired immunodeficiency syndrome (AIDS), predisposing them to infections with pyogenic bacteria.

ABNORMALITIES OF HOST DEFENSES AGAINST BACTERIAL INFECTION

Immunoglobulin abnormalities are very common among patients with AIDS. Although concentrations of serum immunoglobulins are usually elevated, patients have been found to have paradoxically hypoactive B cell function. B cells from patients with AIDS respond poorly to new antigenic stimuli, including protein (keyhole-limpet hemocyanin) and polysaccharide (pneumococcal) antigens in vitro and in vivo (1),(2). In addition, their lymphocytes respond poorly to a variety of mitogens in vitro including phytohemagglutinin (T-cell), pokeweed (T and B cell) and formalinized *Staphylococcus aureus* Cowan (B-cell) (2),(3). Clinically, these observations have several implications. First, it has been noted that infections caused by organisms such as cytomegalovirus and *Toxoplasma gondii*, for which antibody titers are usually valuable diagnostic tools, infrequently provoke significant antibody titers in patients with AIDS. Second, it has been observed that patients with AIDS may fail to form adequate antibodies following exposure to standard vaccines (4). Thus, they may be susceptible to infection despite active efforts at immunization, and they may suffer recurrent infections with the same pyogenic pathogen.

Granulocytopenia may occur both as a primary abnormality in AIDS and as a result of drug therapy and toxicity. Bone marrow dysfunction is commonly observed in these patients (5). Though anemia and thrombocytopenia predominate, mild to moderate granulocytopenia also may occur. Granulocytopenia can result from cytotoxic agents used to treat the malignancies associated with AIDS, as well as from antimicrobial agents such as trimethoprim-sulfamethoxazole (TMP-SMX) (6) and dihydroxypropoxymethyl guanine (DHPG) (7), which are used in the treatment of opportunistic infections.

Granulocyte dysfunction also may occur in AIDS. Ras et al. have demonstrated abnormal granulocyte chemotaxis in incubation mixtures containing AIDS serum and cells (8). Normal granulocytes incubated with AIDS serum demonstrated the same defect (9). These data suggest that an inhibitor of membrane receptors for leuko-attractants might be present in AIDS sera. In addition, we have found evidence of an opsonic deficiency against *Klebsiella pneumoniae* and *Pseudomonas aeruginosa* in AIDS sera (Zuger, A., Simberkoff, M., unpublished data). In most instances, the opsonic defect was corrected by addition of normal serum, but in one instance, an inhibitor of bacterial opsonization was demonstrated. Further characterization of that inhibitor is now in progress.

Finally, the skin and mucous membranes of patients with AIDS are often affected by disease processes or therapeutic interventions which lead to secondary pyogenic infections. Kaposi's sarcoma is present as the initial manifestation of AIDS in 24-30% of patients (10),(11). The tumor may be confined to the skin, it may involve mucous membranes with or without lymph node involvement, or it may disseminate viscerally (12),(13). The lesions on the skin and in the oral and gastrointestinal mucosa may be very numerous and coalesce (14). They can erode or bleed, and serve as foci of infection by the microbial flora of the surface involved. The gingival mucosa is most frequently the site of superinfected Kaposi's sarcoma lesions. However, bacterial pneumonia has also been reported as a complication of pulmonary Kaposi's sarcoma (15),(16), and *Clostridium perfringens* (16) and *Streptococcus bovis* (see below) bacteremias have occurred in patients with gastrointestinal lesions.

Similarly, the characteristic opportunistic infections of skin and mucous membranes seen in patients with AIDS can in turn become superinfected with pyogenic organisms. Cytomegalovirus infections of the lung, esophagus, colon and gallbladder may lead to secondary bacterial infections: intestinal perforation with peritonitis and/or bacteremia may occur (17) and secondary bacterial infection of cytomegalovirus cholecystitis has also been reported (18). Chronic oral and perianal infections due to *Herpes simplex*, and seborrheic dermatitis, tinea faciale and a variety of other dermatophyte infections also are common in these patients, and may become secondarily infected by bacterial pathogens (19),(20). Furunculosis and impetigo can serve as sources of persistent infection and bacteremia. Additionally, *Candida species* are a common cause of pharyngitis and esophagitis in patients with AIDS (21),(22), although to our knowledge bacterial superinfection of these lesions and resultant bacteremias have not been reported.

Iatrogenic intervention, such as the use of cytotoxic agents for malignancies, also frequently impairs the integrity of the mucocutaneous barrier in AIDS and may lead to mucosal ulcerations. Hospitalized AIDS patients frequently require intravenous catheters which can serve as conduits for bacterial invasion of the vascular system. Catheter-related infections have been documented to be a prominent source of the *Staphylococcus aureus* and Gram-negative bacillary bacteremias seen in these patients (16). In addition, we have noted that patients with AIDS appear to have significantly impaired abilities to heal even minor iatrogenic trauma to skin and mucous membranes: for example, the tongue biopsy on one of our patients with a lesion suggestive of hairy leukoplakia resulted in a painful purulent ulcer which required six weeks of parenteral antibiotics for resolution.

BACTERIAL PNEUMONIA

The early clinical experience with AIDS suggested that opportunistic pathogens were responsible for virtually all the pulmonary infections seen in the syndrome. However, it has become evident that although opportunistic pulmonary infections do predominate in AIDS, "classic" respiratory tract pathogens also cause significant disease among these patients.

Estimates of the prevalence of pyogenic pneumonia among AIDS patients have varied considerably. In one of the first clinical discussions of *Pneumocystis carinii* pneumonia (PCP), three or 27% of 11 patients developed a nosocomial gram-negative pneumonia during or after treatment for PCP (23). Two other patients in this group had bacterial sepsis. At the other extreme is a report of a National Heart, Lung and Blood Institute Workshop on the pulmonary complications of AIDS, which pooled data from six institutions (24). Four hundred and forty-one of the reported 1067 patients with AIDS developed pulmonary infections or malignancies; 11 of these infections were caused by pyogenic bacteria and an additional 10 by Legionella, a prevalence of less than 2%.

Several more recent reports cite figures somewhere between these two extremes. Of 130 patients with AIDS seen by Stover et al. during a four year period, nine cases of bacterial pneumonia occurred in four patients (25). *Hemophilus influenzae* or *Streptococcus pneumoniae* were recovered from sputum cultures in five of these cases; in the remainder, Gram stains suggested bacterial pneumonia but pathogens were not recovered. In 336 patients seen over six years by Polsky and colleagues, 18 episodes of community-acquired bacterial pneumonia occurred in 13 patients (15). In our own experience at the New York Veterans Administration Medical Center with 220 AIDS patients seen over a five year period, there were 30 episodes bacterial pneumonia in 28 patients, a prevalence of 14.5%.

In contrast to the array of exotic opportunistic pathogens which can infect the respiratory tract in patients with AIDS, the number of pyogenic organisms associated with significant disease is fairly small. *Streptococcus pneumoniae* (4),(15),(25) and *Hemophilus influenzae* (15),(25) have been responsible for the majority of significant community acquired bacterial pneumonias reported. There have been occasional case reports of significant Klebsiella (23),(26), group B streptococcus and *Branhamella catarrhalis* pneumonia (15) in patients with AIDS. A clustering of Legionella infections was noted early in the epidemic in New York City (24), although details of these cases, their clinical manifestations and their responses to therapy have not been published. We have encountered four cases of community-acquired *Pseudomonas aeruginosa* pneumonia among three of our patients, two cases of Legionella pneumonia, and several cases of nosocomial Gram negative infections which complicated treatment of PCP.

It has been our experience, as well as that of others, that the clinical presentation of a classic bacterial infection in a patient with AIDS is seldom "classic". It is frequently difficult to distinguish pyogenic from opportunistic infection by clinical criteria alone. Both are generally accompanied by fever, and the presence or absence of leukocytosis has not been a reliable clue. Similarly, the appearance of the chest roentgenogram is surprisingly unhelpful in distinguishing pyogenic from opportunistic infection. On the one hand, it has been repeatedly noted that the classic diffuse interstitial infiltrate of PCP may actually be present in a minority of patients with this infection (26),(27). On the other hand, it is by no means infrequent for bacterial pneumonia in this group to present with a diffuse or patchy pulmonary infiltrate, rather than the more typical lobar consolidation. This overlap of radiologic appearances has led at least one group to add antibacterial coverage to all empiric treatment regimens of pneumonia in patients with AIDS, ensuring that the pyogenic pathogens are not overlooked while a diagnosis is being made (15).

The presence of purulent sputum which is microscopically consistent with a bacterial infection, is probably the most important indicator of a bacterial infection of the respiratory tract. However, polymicrobial infections are the rule rather than the exception in patients with AIDS, and the presence of a bacterial infection in the lung does not exclude the simultaneous occurrence of one or more opportunistic infections. While there are no statistics regarding the frequency with which bacterial respiratory infections in patients with AIDS are associated with underlying, perhaps more chronic, opportunistic infections, the phenomenon is not uncommon. Following one memorable case in which pneumococcal pneumonia with bacteremia, PCP, and Legionella pneumonia, appeared simultaneously in one patient (4), we usually presume the coexistence of PCP until diagnostic tests or response to therapy satisfy us that only the bacterial infection is present.

Pyogenic respiratory infections among patients with AIDS frequently respond well to appropriate therapy. In Polsky and colleagues' series of 18 episodes of community-acquired bacterial pneumonias in 13 patients, 16 of 18 episodes were cured (15). Other authors have described cures of patients with immunologic abnormalities suggestive of human immunodeficiency virus (HIV) infection and life-threatening bacterial pneumonia (28),(29). On the other hand, two of the three episodes of nosocomial Gram-negative pneumonia mentioned in Masur's early series were fatal (23), as has been the case in several anecdotal reports of overwhelming bacterial pneumonias in patients with previously diagnosed AIDS , (15),(29a). Thus, the most important factor affecting immediate prognosis of severe bacterial pulmonary infection appears to be the patient's overall clinical condition. Patients who have not been weakened by long hospitalizations or bouts with other infections tend to respond well to appropriate therapy.

An issue which has been repeatedly raised in discussions of pyogenic pneumonias in patients with AIDS has been the utility of prophylaxis of pneumococcal infections with the pneumococcal vaccine. The incidence of significant pneumococcal infections in this population appears to exceed substantially that seen in the general US population as a whole. Polsky et al. (15) contrasted an attack rate of pneumococcal pneumonia of 17.9/1000/year among AIDS patients with an estimated incidence in the general population of 2.6/1000/year (P=0.001). Among our patients at the New York Veterans Administration Medical Center, we have seen an incidence of pneumococcal bacteremias in AIDS patients of 5.7/100/year contrasted with an incidence in other medical patients of 0.35/100/year, again a highly significant difference (4). These data suggest that patients with AIDS should be candidates for routine immunization with the polyvalent pneumococcal vaccine.

Results of immunization in this population, however, have been extremely variable. Some reports (23),(30) have documented adequate antibody responses to the pneumococcal vaccine, with the suggestion that active immunization against pneumococcal disease in AIDS patients is a feasible proposition. Others (1),(2),(4) have documented a wholly inadequate antibody response, citing the now well-recognized phenomenon of B-cell dysfunction among these patients (vide supra). We have reported one frank clinical failure of the pneumococcal vaccine, in which bacteremia with a vaccine-type pneumococcus occurred six months after the vaccine was administered (4). Thus, it is evident that active immunization, although possibly of value in individual patients, is not the solution to the problem of bacterial infections in the AIDS population as a whole.

BACTEREMIA

Whimbey et al. recently reviewed 38 episodes of bacteremia occurring among 336 patients with AIDS followed at the Memorial Sloan-Kettering Cancer Center in New York City (16). Nine of these were nosocomial infections, of which seven were associated with vascular catheters. An additional four vascular catheter-associated episodes were caused by *Candida albicans.* Two episodes of *Pseudomonas aeruginosa* bacteremia were observed. Both of these were associated with pneumonia and one of the patients was neutropenic. Two other episodes of bacteremia occurred in neutropenic patients. One was caused by *Staphylococcus epidermidis* and the other by *Streptococcus faecalis.* There were 10 episodes of *Staphylococcus aureus* bacteremia, nine community acquired and one nosocomial. The latter was associated with a vascular catheter and a mixed bacteremia (group G streptococcus).

In our own series of 220 patients with AIDS, we have observed bacteremias in 40 patients, a significantly higher prevalence than that observed at the Memorial Sloan-Kettering Cancer Center ($P<0.05$ by chi-square test.) There have been 15 episodes of *Staphylococcus aureus* bacteremia occurring among 13 patients, nine with *Pseudomonas aeruginosa*, seven with *Streptococcus pneumoniae*, four with Klebsiella, three with Salmonella, two with *Enterobacter species*, and two with *Hemophilus influenzae.* In addition, there were two episodes of *Candida albicans* fungemia.

The explanation of the higher prevalence of bacteremia among our patients is not immediately apparent. The difference may be related to the different patient populations of the two hospitals: only 21.6% of our patients have had Kaposi's sarcoma compared to 73% of the patients at the Memorial Sloan-Kettering Cancer Center, and almost 90% of our patients have had opportunistic infections during their treatment. In vitro studies (31), (32) have indicated that AIDS patients with opportunistic infections have fewer circulating B cells than those with Kaposi's sarcoma alone, as well as poorer mitogen responses of both T and B cells. It may be that our patients are more profoundly immunodeficient than those at Memorial Sloan-Kettering, and, therefore, more vulnerable to pyogenic as well as opportunistic infections.

Other organisms have caused bacteremia in patients with AIDS. There are reports of *Listeria monocytogenes* bacteremia in several male patients with AIDS, including one with small cell carcinoma of the rectum (33),(34). An additional fatal case of Listeria bacteremia occurred in a postpartum 27 year-old Haitian immigrant (35), in whom AIDS was diagnosed when skin lesions noted on admission proved to be an inflammatory variant of Kaposi's sarcoma (36). *Streptococcus bovis* bacteremia was observed in a 33 year-old Haitian male with gastrointestinal Kaposi's sarcoma (37). This organism has previously been associated with gastrointestinal diseases including malignancies (38),(39). *Clostridium perfringens* bacteremia has also been observed in a patient with gastrointestinal Kaposi's sarcoma (16).

We have found that response to treatment for bacteremia, as for pneumonia, tends to parallel the patient's overall clinical condition. Patients not weakened by chronic infections or malignancies respond well, while bacteremia is frequently the modus exitus of terminal patients. Exceptions to this generalization have been patients with Salmonella bacteremia. In an experience paralleling that reported in the literature (40)-(42), two of our three patients with Salmonella bacteremia responded well to treatment, but invariably relapsed weeks to months after the treatment was stopped; in both cases cytopenia on TMP-SMX and resistance of the organism to ampicillin prevented use of chronic prophylactic treatment which has been advocated elsewhere (41).

PEDIATRIC INFECTIONS

A total of 231 cases of AIDS were reported in children under 13 years old in the United States between January 1981 and January 13, 1986 (11).

As in adult patients, cell mediated immunity is depressed in children with AIDS, T helper cell numbers are reduced and T cell ratios are reversed (43). Humoral immunity also is affected in these children. Bernstein et al. showed that the primary and secondary responses to bacteriophage antigens, tetanus toxoid and pneumococcal vaccine were profoundly depressed in pediatric AIDS patients (44).

The clinical manifestations of AIDS in children and adults are frequently similar. Like adults, children become cachectic and may suffer from chronic diarrhea. Opportunistic infections are common, as is an interstitial pneumonia with a unique histologic pattern, lymphoid interstitial pneumonia, which is rarely seen in adults (45). It is noteworthy that the malignancies commonly seen in adult patients with AIDS are far less frequent in children with this syndrome. For example, Kaposi's sarcoma has been reported in 24-30% of adults with AIDS, but in only 4% of children (11).

In addition, a striking feature of AIDS in children is the high incidence of bacterial infections, including bacteremia. For example, five or seven patients reported by Rubinstein et al. (45), five of eight cases reported by Oleske et al. (46), and 10 of 14 reported by Scott et al. (47) had infections with classic pathogens, including *Staphylococcus aureus*, *Streptococcus pneumoniae*, *Escherichia coli* or other Gram-negative bacilli. Recurrent infections with the same bacterial pathogen are very common among these patients. We observed a child with four episodes of type 6A *Streptococcus pneumoniae* bacteremia at Bellevue Hospital.

The causes of frequent bacterial infections among children with AIDS have not been clearly established. It has been postulated that the relative immaturity of humoral immunity in patients at the time of initial HIV infection results in more profound defects in defenses against pyogenic organisms (1), (44)-(48). Indeed, monthly administration of parenteral immunoglobulins has been recommended to limit the number of these infections in children (48).

CONCLUSIONS

It is becoming evident that bacterial infection, although less common than opportunistic infection among patients with AIDS, causes a significant amount of morbidity and mortality in this population. AIDS patients particularly at risk for bacterial infections include children, as well as adults whose overall clinical condition has been affected by long hospitalizations or bouts with other AIDS-related infections or malignancies. The causes of pyogenic infection include alterations in the cutaneous and mucosal barriers against these organisms, B-cell dysfunction and decreases in phagocytic cell number and function. The clinician must be aware of the increased risk of these infections and be prepared to initiate appropriate diagnostic studies and therapies promptly.

REFERENCES

1. Ammann, A.J., Schiffman, G., Abrams, D., et al., B-cell immunodeficiency in acquired immunodeficiency syndrome. JAMA 251:1447-1449 (1984)

2. Lane, H.C., Masur, H., Edgar, L.C., et al., Abnormalities of B-cell activation in patients with the acquired immunodeficiency syndrome. N Engl J Med 309:453-458 (1983)

3. Stahl, R.E., Friedman-Kien, A., Dubin, R., et al., Immunologic abnormalities in homosexual men: Relationship to Kaposi's sarcoma. Am J Med 73:171-178 (1982)

4. Simberkoff, M.S., El-Sadr, W., Schiffman, G., et al., *Streptococcus pneumoniae* infections and bacteremia in patients with the acquired immune deficiency syndrome, with report of a pneumococcal vaccine failure. Am Rev Resp Dis 130:1174-1176 (1984)

5. Spivak, J.L., Bender, B.S., Quinn, T.C., Hematologic abnormalities in the acquired immune deficiency syndrome. Am J Med 77:224-228 (1984)

6. Gordin, F.M., Simon, G.L., Wofsy, C.B., et al., Adverse reactions to trimethoprim-sulfamethoxazole in patients with the acquired immunodeficiency syndrome. Ann Intern Med 100: 495-499, (1984)

7. Masur, H., Lane, H.C., Palestine, A., et al., Effect of 9-(1,3-dihydroxy-2-propoxymethyl) guanine on serious cytomegalovirus disease in eight immunosuppressed homosexual men. Ann Intern Med 104:41-44 (1986)

8. Ras, G.J., Anderson, R., Lecatus, G., et al., Acquired neutrophil dysfunction in male homosexuals with the acquired immunodeficiency syndrome. S African Med J 65:873-74 (1984)

9. Ras, G.J., Anderson, R., Lukey, P.T., Defective polymorphonuclear leukocyte migration in AIDS. S African Med J 68:292-293 (1985)

10. Safai, B., Johnson, K.G., Myskowski, P.L., et al., The natural history of Kaposi's sarcoma in the acquired immunodeficiency syndrome. Ann Intern Med 103:744-750 (1985)

11. CDC., Update: Acquired immunodeficiency syndrome - United States. MMWR 35:17-21 (1986)

12. Krigel, R.L., Laubenstein, L.J., Muggia, F.M., Kaposi's sarcoma: A new staging classification. Canc Treat Rep 367: 531-534 (1983)

13. Laubenstein, L., Staging and treatment of Kaposi's sarcoma in patients with AIDS. In: AIDS: The Epidemic of Kaposi's Sarcoma and Opportunistic Infection (Friedman-Kien, A.E., Laubenstein, L.J., eds) Masson Publishing USA, Inc., New York, p 51-55 (1984)

14. Friedman-Kien, A.E., Ostreicher, R., Overview of classical and epidemic Kaposi's sarcoma. In: AIDS: The Epidemic of Kaposi's Sarcoma and Opportunistic Infection. (Friedman-Kien, A.E., Laubenstein, L.J., eds) Masson Publishing USA, Inc., New York, p. 23-34 (1984)

15. Polsky, B., Gold, J.W.M., Whimbey, E., et al., Bacterial pneumonia in patients with the acquired immunodeficiency syndrome. Ann Intern Med 104:38-41 (1986)

16. Whimbey, E., Gold, J.W.M., Polsky, B., et al., Bacteremia and fungemia in patients with the acquired immunodeficiency syndrome. Ann Intern Med 104:511-514 (1986)

17. Horowitz, L., Stern, J.O., Segarra, S., Gastrointestinal manifestations of Kaposi's sarcoma and AIDS. In: AIDS: The Epidemic of Kaposi's Sarcoma and Opportunistic Infection (Friedman-Kien, A.E., Laubenstein, L.J., eds) Masson Publishing, New York, p 235-240 (1984)

18. Kavin, H., Jonas, R.B., Chowdhury, L., et al., Acalculous cholecystitis and cytomegalovirus in the acquired immunodeficiency syndrome. Ann Intern Med 104:53-54 (1986)

19. Eisenstat, B.A., Wormser, G.P., Seborrheic dermatitis and butterfly rash in AIDS. N Engl J Med 311:189 (1984)

20. Hatcher, V.A., Mucocutaneous infections in acquired immune deficiency syndrome. In: AIDS: The Epidemic of Kaposi's Sarcoma and Opportunistic Infection. (Friedman-Kien, A.E., Laubenstein, L.J. eds) Masson Publishing USA, Inc., New York, p 245-251 (1984)

21. Klein, R.S., Harris, C.A., Small, C.B., et al., Oral candidiasis in high-risk patients as the initial manifestation of the acquired immunodeficiency syndrome. N Engl J Med 311: 354-358 (1984)

22. Tavitian, A., Raufman, J.P., Rosenthal, L.E., Oral candidiasis as a marker for esophageal candidiasis in the acquired immunodeficiency syndrome. Ann Intern Med 104:54-55 (1986)

23. Masur, H., Michelis, M.A., Greene, S.B., et al., An outbreak of community-acquired *Pneumocystis carinii* pneumonia. Initial manifestations of cellular immune dysfunction. N Engl J Med 305:1431-1438 (1981)

24. Murray, J.F., Felton, C.P., Garay, S.M., et al., Pulmonary complications of acquired immunodeficiency syndrome: Report of a National Heart, Lung and Blood Institute Workshop. N Engl J Med 310:1682-1686 (1984)

25. Stover, D.E., White, D.A., Romano, P.A., et al., Spectrum of pulmonary diseases associated with the acquired immune deficiency syndrome. Am J Med 78:429-437 (1985)

26. Wollschlanger, C.M., Khan, F.A., Chitkara, R.K., et al., Pulmonary manifestations of the acquired immunodeficiency syndrome (AIDS). Chest 85:197-202 (1984)

27. Hopewell, P.C., Luce, J.M., Pulmonary involvement in the acquired immunodeficiency syndrome. Chest 87:104-112 (1985)

28. White, S., Tsou, E., Waldhorn, R.E., et al., Life-threatening bacterial pneumonia in male homosexuals with laboratory features of the acquired immunodeficiency syndrome. Chest 87:486-488 (1985)

29. Promisloff, R.A., Lenchner, G.S., Virulent course of bacterial pneumonia in a male homosexual. Chest 88:935 (1985)

29a. Turck, M., An AIDS patient who died too soon. Hosp Pract 20:77-80 (1985)

30. Mildvan, D., Mathur, U., Enlow, R.W., et al., Opportunistic infections and immune deficiency in homosexual men. Ann Intern Med 96:700-704 (1982)

31. Lane, H.C., Masur, H., Gelmann, E.P., et al., Correlation between immunologic function and clinical subpopulations of patients with the acquired immune deficiency syndrome. Am J Med 78:417-422 (1985)

32. Zolla-Pazner, S., Immunologic abnormalities in HTLV-III/LAV infection. Laboratory Medicine 17:685-689 (1986)

33. Real, F.X., Gold, J.W.M., Krown, S.E., et al., *Listeria monocytogenes* bacteremia in the acquired immunodeficiency syndrome. Ann Intern Med 101:883-884 (1984)

34. Read, E.J., Orenstein, J.M., Chorba, T.L., et al., *Listeria monocytogenes* sepsis and small cell carcinoma of the rectum: An unusual presentation of the acquired immunodeficiency syndrome. Am J Clin Path 83:385-389 (1985)

35. Wetli, C.V., Roldan, E.O., Fojaco, R.M., Listeriosis as a cause of maternal death: An obstetric complication of the acquired immunodeficiency syndrome (AIDS). Am J Obstet Gynec 147:7-9 (1983)

36. Wetli, C.V., Roldan, E.O., Fojaco, R.M., Reply to letter. Am J Obstet Gynec 147:805-806 (1983)

37. Glaser, J.B., Landesman, S.H., *Streptococcus bovis* bacteremia and acquired immunodeficiency syndrome. Ann Intern Med 99:878 (1983)

38. Klein, R.S., Recco, R.A., Catalano, M.T., et al., Association of *Streptococcus bovis* with carcinoma of the colon. N Engl J Med 297:800-802 (1977)

39. Murray, H.W., Roberts, R.B., *Streptococcus bovis* bacteremia and underlying gastrointestinal disease. Arch Intern Med 138:1097-1099 (1978)

40. Smith, P.D., Macher, A.M., Bookman, M.A., et al., *Salmonella typhimurium* enteritis and bacteremia in the acquired immunodeficiency syndrome. Ann Intern Med 102:207-209 (1985)

41. Jacobs, J.L., Gold, J.W.M., Murray, H.W., et al., Salmonella infections in patients with the acquired immunodeficiency syndrome. Ann Intern Med 102:186-188 (1985)

42. Glaser, J.B., Morton-Kute, L., Berger, S.R., et al., Recurrent *Salmonella typhimurium* bacteremia associated with the acquired immunodeficiency syndrome. Ann Intern Med 102:189-193 (1985)

43. Rubinstein, A., Sicklick, M., Gupta., A., et al., Acquired immunodeficiency with reversed T4/T8 ratios in infants born to promiscuous and drug-addicted mothers. JAMA 249:2350-2356 (1983)

44. Bernstein, L.J., Ochs, H.D., Wedgewood, R.T., et al., Defective humoral immunity in pediatric acquired immune deficiency syndrome. J Ped 107:352-357 (1985)

45. CDC., Revision of the case definition of acquired immunodeficiency syndrome for national reporting - United States. MMWR 34:373-375 (1985)

46. Oleske, J., Minnefor, A., Cooper, R., et al., Immune deficiency in children. JAMA 249:2345-2349 (1983)

47. Scott, G.B., Buck, B.E., Leterman, J.G., et al., Acquired immunodeficiency in infants. N Engl J Med 310:76-81 (1984)

48. Shannon, K.M., Ammann, A.J., Acquired immune deficiency syndrome in childhood. J Ped 106:332-342 (1985)

26
Tuberculosis in AIDS

Frederick P. Duncanson, Natalie C. Klein

Tuberculosis is an infectious disease that has been known since the time of Hippocrates. Tuberculosis has been regarded primarily as a pulmonary infection associated with fever, night sweats, chills, cough (which is usually productive of varying amounts of sputum), and weight loss, which can be substantial. Extrapulmonary and disseminated tuberculosis have been uncommon and often require tissue biopsies with positive culture results in order to establish the diagnosis. In 1979, Millar and Horne showed that the disseminated form of tuberculosis was frequent in patients with underlying immunosuppression (1). Since human immunodeficiency virus (HIV) infection severely diminishes the number and function of helper T-lymphocytes, it is not surprising that the most common infections acquired by acquired immunodeficiency syndrome (AIDS) patients, *Pneumocystis carinii* pneumonia, cryptococcal meningitis, disseminated cytomegalovirus infection, and disseminated *Mycobacterium avium-intracellulare* infection, are those which are normally contained by the cell mediated immune system. Cell-mediated immunity is also the major host defense against *Mycobacterium tuberculosis*. Although *M. tuberculosis* is not considered to be an opportunistic pathogen, patients with AIDS, nevertheless, appear to have a higher incidence of tuberculosis and, often, a different presentation from immunocompetent hosts.

EPIDEMIOLOGY

Except for the years 1978-1981 and 1985, there has been a steady average annual decrease in reported tuberculosis cases of more than 5.7% per year in the United States since 1975 (2). The average decline of only 1.4% per year in 1978-1981 was felt to be due to the influx of refugees from Southeast Asia (3). The current decline of only 2.0% in 1985 is unexplained, but concern has been raised that an increased number of cases of tuberculosis in patients with AIDS, or in members of certain high risk groups for AIDS, may account for the lower than expected drop in cases (4). In support of the relationship between HIV infection and the change in the rate of decline in incidence of tuberculosis is the observation that in 1985, some of the areas with the highest incidence rates of AIDS such as New York City, California, Florida, and Texas, reported increasing numbers of patients with tuberculosis (2).

Although the national prevalence of tuberculosis among AIDS patients is not known, some data are available from Dade County, Florida and New York City. In Dade County, where there is a large population of Haitian immigrants, 10% of the AIDS patients reported up to December 31, 1985 had tuberculosis (2). This is a fifteen fold higher prevalence rate than that found for all recent Haitian immigrants in Dade County and four hundred fold higher than the estimated overall prevalence rate of tuberculosis in the United States (5),(6). In New York City, the rate of tuberculosis in AIDS patients is also much higher than the overall national prevalence. Between 1981-1984, 5.4% of all reported New York City AIDS patients had tuberculosis (4).

At Lincoln and Metropolitan Hospitals in New York City and at the Westchester County Medical Center in Valhalla, NY, hospitals which serve large narcotic addict populations, 14 of 129 AIDS patients who were diagnosed between March 1982 and March 1984, had a culture proven *M. tuberculosis* infection, for an overall incidence of 11% (7). This contrasts sharply with the .023% reported incidence of tuberculosis in the general New York City population (8). These data suggest that *M. tuberculosis* is a relatively common pathogen in certain patients with HIV infection. Physicians in areas where both diseases are endemic need to be vigilant for this pathogen among patients with AIDS.

PATHOGENESIS

It is unclear what proportion of tuberculosis cases among AIDS patients is the result of primary infection versus reactivation of a latent tuberculous focus but probably either pathogenesis can occur. Since tuberculosis is a common infectious disease in Haiti, one may presume that Haitian AIDS patients were initially infected in Haiti, and as their HIV infection progressively suppressed cellular immunity, tuberculosis was reactivated (5),(6). However, in one report of Haitian AIDS patients with pulmonary tuberculosis, the chest roentgenograms were often atypical for reactivation disease, showing lower lobe infiltrates or hilar adenopathy, findings more commonly associated with primary infection (9).

Since *M. tuberculosis* is a more virulent pathogen than the opportunistic organisms that infect AIDS patients, it may be theorized that this organism would cause clinical disease at an earlier stage of immune dysfunction (6). In fact, clinical observations have shown that tuberculosis commonly precedes opportunistic infections and/or Kaposi's sarcoma by weeks to months (6),(7),(9),(10).

While pulmonary tuberculosis is the predominant form of disease in normal hosts (11),(12), in AIDS patients disseminated and other forms of extrapulmonary tuberculosis are much more common (7),(10),(13)-(23). Only 14.9% of newly diagnosed cases of tuberculosis in the United States in 1979 were extrapulmonary (11), in contrast to a rate of 80% among 70 reported AIDS patients with tuberculosis (Table 1) (7),(10),(13)-(23). Although there is also a higher prevalence rate of extrapulmonary tuberculosis in other immunosuppressed patients who do not have AIDS compared to the general population, the rate does not appear to be as high as in AIDS patients. For example, in one series of 11 patients with tuberculosis who were receiving long term immunosuppressive drug therapy, 45% had extrapulmonary involvement (1). The apparent greater propensity for extrapulmonary tuberculosis, especially the disseminated forms, in AIDS patients may be a result of their more severely compromised cellular immune system.

Table 1. Clinical Presentation of Tuberculosis in AIDS Patients Compared to Non-AIDS Patients

Presentation of Tuberculosis	General Population U.S.A. 1979 (11)*	General Population New York City 1983 (8)	70 AIDS Patients (based on a compilation of studies) (7),(10,(13)-(23)
Pulmonary	85.1%	81%	20%
Extra-Pulmonary	14.9%	19%	80%

* References shown in parentheses.

CLINICAL PRESENTATIONS

Disseminated tuberculosis in AIDS patients is associated with a constellation of non-specific constitutional symptoms, often inseparable from HIV infection alone (7). Patients most often present with the insidious onset of fever, night sweats, chills, anorexia, weight loss (usually greater than 15% of body weight), and/or profound cachexia (7),(10),(15)-(17),(23). Pulmonary complaints and abnormalities on chest radiograph are common, but the classic miliary roentgenographic pattern is unusual. Generalized lymphadenopathy with evidence of tuberculous infection of lymph nodes is also very frequent (see below).

Thoracic manifestations of tuberculosis in AIDS patients can differ considerably from those found in the immunocompetent host (Table 2). In a recent review of chest radiographic findings in 17 Haitian immigrants with AIDS who had a positive culture of sputum or bronchial washings, 59% had hilar and/or mediastinal lymphadenopathy and 29% had lower lobe or middle lobe infiltrates, roentgenographic findings resembling that of primary tuberculosis (9). Only 18% had upper lobe infiltrates and none had cavities. In contrast, in a control group of 30 age and sex matched non-AIDS Haitian patients with tuberculosis, 97% had upper lobe infiltrates and 67% had cavities, while hilar/mediastinal adenopathy or lower/middle lobe infiltrates were each present in only 3% of patients (9). Scar formation was not observed in any of the Haitian AIDS patients during or after resolution of the tuberculous infection (9). Similarly, among 11 of our AIDS patients with pulmonary tuberculosis, 45% had hilar lymphadenopathy and 18% had lower lobe infiltrates (7). One of our patients, however, did have an upper lobe cavitary lesion.

Table 2. Comparison of Roentgenographic Findings in AIDS Patients with Pulmonary Tuberculosis with Those of Non-AIDS Patients

Roentgenographic Findings	Duncanson, et al.(Ref 7) AIDS N = 11	Pitchenik, et al. (Ref 9) AIDS N = 17	Controls* N = 30
Hilar/Mediastinal adenopathy	45%	59%	3%
Middle or lower lobe infiltrate	18%	29%	3%
Upper lobe infiltrate	9%	18%	97%
Miliary pattern	0%	6%	0%
Linear, interstitial infiltrate	18%	12%	0%
Cavity	9%	0%	67%
Pleural effusion	9%	12%	7%
No infiltrates	45%	35%	0%
Normal	9%	12%	0%

* Age and sex matched non-AIDS Haitian patients with tuberculosis from Pitchenik et al. (9).

A particularly common and important manifestation of tuberculosis in AIDS patients is tuberculous lymphadenitis. In 1979, the Centers for Disease Control reported that tuberculous lymphadenitis comprised 3.7% of all tuberculosis cases (11). In 1983, the New York City Department of Health reported that 5.9% of all tuberculosis cases had tuberculous lymphadenitis (25). In contrast, at least 26 (37%) of 70 AIDS patients with tuberculosis had *M. tuberculosis* cultured from lymph nodes (7),(10),(14)-(18),(22)-(23). Patients with AIDS related complex (ARC) also have an increased prevalence of tuberculous lymphadenitis. Sherer and Sable found that the cause of generalized lymphadenopathy in five (14%) of 35 ARC patients was *M. tuberculosis* (24). Hewlett et al. (25) demonstrated that tuberculosis was the most common cause of generalized lymphadenopathy among parenteral drug abusers with constitutional symptoms from an inner city section of the Bronx, New York. Hewlett et al. emphasized the importance of biopsy and culture of lymph nodes for mycobacteria in patient populations where AIDS and tuberculosis are both common and the potential disservice of assuming that histologic findings and culture results will be non-specific (25).

Less common manifestations of tuberculosis reported in AIDS patients have included tuberculous brain abscesses, granulomatous hepatitis, intestinal lesions, and skin lesions (14),(15),(17),(20)-(22).

PATHOLOGY

The classic pathologic findings of caseating granulomas with Langhans giant cells are also often seen in tissue biopsies from AIDS patients. However, some AIDS patients fail to develop granulomas and show minimal inflammatory response. In one series of AIDS patients, granulomas ranged from few to multiple, small to large, with mostly loose aggregates of epitheloid histiocytes and macrophages and minimal lymphocytic cuffing (26). Necrosis was found most often in granulomas present in lymph nodes but was also seen in granulomas in bone marrow. Acid fast bacilli may be demonstrated in granulomas in some, but not all patients. In our own experience with 12 intravenous drug abusers from New York City with tuberculous lymphadenitis, caseating granulomas were seen in eight patients, four of whom had positive acid fast smears (25). In a series of 14 AIDS patients with proven tuberculosis, of the 19 tissue biopsies performed (seven bone marrow, four lymph node, four lung, three liver, one pleural) eight had no granulomas, six had non-caseating granulomas, five had caseating granulomas, and only three had acid fast bacilli present; mycobacterial cultures grew *M. tuberculosis* from nine (7).

DIAGNOSIS

The diagnosis of tuberculosis should be considered in an AIDS patient with any of the previously mentioned clinical presentations. The PPD skin test is of minimal value, since HIV infection usually results in anergy. Definitive diagnosis is made by culturing *M. tuberculosis* from the patient. Repetitive culturing of sputum, body fluids (including blood), and available tissue samples is essential even if acid fast smears are negative and/or if histologic evaluation does not show granulomas. Sputum, bone marrow, and lymph nodes appear to have the highest yield on culture (7),(10),(14)-(19),(22),(23).

THERAPY AND OUTLOOK

Choice of therapy for *M. tuberculosis* infection in AIDS patients is the same as in non-AIDS patients, usually isoniazid and rifampin. We would, however, be reluctant to recommend the now standard abbreviated treatment course of nine months and prefer to extend therapy for at least 18 months. If the patient is Haitian or originates from another area where drug resistance is a problem, initial therapy should include at least three anti-tuberculous agents.

A one year course of isoniazid prophylaxis is recommended for members of risk groups who are HIV positive and have, or are known to have had, a positive tuberculin skin test (27).

In contrast to experience with the usual serious opportunistic infections that AIDS patients acquire, tuberculosis typically responds favorably to standard therapy, although initial response may be somewhat slower (6),(7),(10),(14),(21),(25). Mortality in AIDS patients with tuberculosis is high, however, but is generally due to an opportunistic infection rather than to tuberculosis (6),(7),(10),(13)-(16),(22),(23).

REFERENCES

1. Millar, J.W., Horne, N.W., Tuberculosis in immunosuppressed patients. Lancet 1:1176-1178 (1979)

2. CDC., Tuberculosis - United States, 1985 - and the possible impact of human T-lymphotropic virus type III/lymphadenopathy associated virus. MMWR 35:74-76 (1986)

3. CDC., Tuberculosis - United States, 1982. MMWR 32:478-480 (1983)

4. Stoneburner, R.L., Kristal, A., Increasing tuberculosis incidence and its relationship to acquired immunodeficiency syndrome in New York City. International Conference on Acquired Immunodeficiency Syndrome (AIDS), Atlanta, GA (1985)

5. Pitchenik, A.E., Russell, B.W., Cleary, T., et al., The prevalence of tuberculosis and drug resistance among Haitians. N Engl J Med 307:162-165 (1982)

6. Pitchenik, A.E., Cole, C., Russell, B.W., et al., Tuberculosis, atypical mycobacteriosis, and the acquired immunodeficiency syndrome among Haitian and non-Haitian patients in South Florida. Ann Intern Med 101:641-645 (1984)

7. Duncanson, F.P., Hewlett, D., Maayan, S., et al., *Mycobacterium tuberculosis* infection in the acquired immunodeficiency syndrome. A review of 14 patients. Tubercle (In Press)

8. New York City Department of Health, Tuberculosis in New York City 1979-1984, Special Supplement, New York Lung Association, New York (1985)

9. Pitchenik, A.E., Rubinson, H.A., The radiographic appearance of tuberculosis in patients with the acquired immune deficiency syndrome (AIDS) and pre-AIDS. Am Rev Respir Dis 131: 393-396 (1985)

10. Vieira, J., Frank, E., Spira, T.J., et al., Acquired immune deficiency in Haitians. Opportunistic infections in previously healthy Haitian immigrants. N Engl J Med 308:125-129 (1983)

11. CDC., Tuberculosis in the United States - 1979, U.S. Public Health Service, Atlanta, p 10, (1981)

12. New York City Department of Health, Tuberculosis in New York City, 1983, New York Lung Association, New York (1985)

13. Goedert, J.J., Weiss, S.H., Biggar, R.J., et al., Lesser AIDS and tuberculosis. Lancet 2:52 (1985)

14. Louie, E., Rice, L.B., Holzman, R.S., *Mycobacterium tuberculosis* infection in patients with AIDS. International Conference on Acquired Immunodeficiency Syndrome (AIDS), Atlanta, GA (1985)

15. Pitchenik, A.E., Fischl, M.A., Dickinson, G.M., et al., Opportunistic infections and Kaposi's sarcoma among Haitians: evidence of a new acquired immunodeficiency state. Ann Intern Med 98:277-284 (1983)

16. Clumeck, N., Sonnet, J., Taelman, H., et al., Acquired immunodeficiency syndrome in African patients. N Engl J Med 310:492-497 (1984)

17. De la Loma, A., Manrique, A., Rubio, R., et al., Generalized tuberculosis in a patient with acquired immunodeficiency syndrome. J Infect 10:57-59 (1985)

18. Mess, T.P., Hadley, W.K., Wofsy, C.B., Bacteremia due to *Mycobacterium tuberculosis* and *Mycobacterium avium-intracellulare* in homosexual males. International Conference on Acquired Immunodeficiency Syndrome (AIDS), Atlanta, GA (1985)

19. Frank E., Siegal, F.P., Siegal, M., et al., T-cell subsets in Haitians with tuberculosis: Predictive value for acquired immune deficiency syndrome. Twenty-Third Interscience Conference on Antimicrobial Agents and Chemotherapy, Washington, D.C. (1983).

20. Moskowitz, L.B., Hensley, G.T., Chan, J.C., et al., Brain biopsies in patients with acquired immune deficiency syndrome. Arch Pathol Lab Med 108:368-371 (1984)

21. Kahn, S., Saltzman, B., Brandt, L.S., et al., Granulomatous hepatitis in AIDS patients. International Conference on Acquired Immunodeficiency Syndrome (AIDS), Atlanta, GA (1985)

22. Schroeder, H.W., Yarrish, R.L., Perkins, T.F., et al., Sequential disseminated tuberculosis and toxoplasmosis in a Haitian refugee. South Med J 77:533-534 (1984)

23. Offenstadt, G., Pinta, P., Hericord, P., et al., Multiple opportunistic infections due to AIDS in a previously healthy Black woman from Zaire. N Engl J Med 308:775 (1983)

24. Sherer, R., Sable, R., The evaluation of unexplained generalized lymphadenopathy in the AIDS-related complex. International Conference on Acquired Immunodeficiency Syndrome (AIDS), Atlanta, GA (1985)

25. Hewlett, D., Duncanson, F., Jagadha, V., et al., Lymphadenopathy in an inner city population consisting principally of intravenous drug abusers with suspected AIDS (manuscript submitted)

26. Jagadha, V., Andavolu, R.H., Huang, C.T., Granulomatous inflammation in the acquired immune deficiency syndrome. Am J Clin Pathol 84:598-602 (1985)

27. Pitchenik, A.E., Burr, J., Cole, C.H., Tuberculin testing for persons with positive serologic studies for HTLV-III. N Engl J Med 314:447 (1986)

27
Mycobacterium avium-intracellulare Infections in AIDS

Natalie C. Klein, Frederick P. Duncanson, Beca Damsker

The *Mycobacterium avium-intracellulare* complex (MAI) includes the organisms *Mycobacterium avium* and *Mycobacterium intracellulare*, members of Runyon's group III nonchromogenic mycobacteria. Until the onset of the acquired immunodeficiency syndrome (AIDS) epidemic, infections due to MAI were primarily limited to the lungs in patients with underlying pulmonary disease. Other less frequent manifestations of infection with MAI included lymphadenitis, bone and joint infections, and genitourinary tract disease. Disseminated MAI infections were rarely reported prior to 1981. In fact, from 1940 to 1984, only 37 cases of disseminated MAI were described in non-AIDS patients (1).

With the increasing incidence of AIDS, disseminated MAI infection has become common. Autopsy findings at Memorial Sloan-Kettering Cancer Center revealed disseminated MAI infection in more than 60 percent of their AIDS patients (2). It is, therefore, important for physicians caring for patients with AIDS to be familiar with the epidemiology, bacteriology, methods of diagnosis, clinical manifestations, and therapy of MAI.

EPIDEMIOLOGY

MAI is the most ubiquitous non-tuberculous mycobacterium in the environment (3) and has been isolated from a variety of sources including soil, water, dust, avians, mammals and their excretions (4),(5). The route of acquiring MAI infections is unknown, but there is minimal evidence to suggest person to person transmission. It is generally believed that MAI is acquired from the environment. Although MAI produces disease in poultry and swine, animal reservoirs are not thought to be an important source for human infection (6). The isolation of MAI from 25 percent of water samples taken from the South Carolina-Georgia coast and the demonstration of MAI in aerosol specimens lends support to the hypothesis that pulmonary infection in man is acquired by inhalation of aerosolized droplets containing MAI (7). However, in patients with AIDS, MAI involvement of the bowel is often extensive suggesting that the gastrointestinal tract may be the site of initial infection with dissemination to other organs occurring thereafter.

Serotyping of isolates of MAI has been useful in epidemiologic studies (8). Three serovars of *M. avium* and 25 serovars of *M. intracellulare* have been identified. Serotype 8 was the serotype most commonly isolated from patients with localized pulmonary disease in the United States from 1976 to 1978 (9). No predominant serotype has been associated with disseminated MAI disease in non-AIDS patients, although more than half the cases were caused by avian serotypes 1, 2, or 3 (1). Interestingly, in one group of AIDS patients in New York City with disseminated MAI, 78 percent of 23 strains were serotype 4 (10). The unusually high frequency of serotype 4 among this group of AIDS patients may be due to a common source of infection (10), or perhaps to a seasonal or geographical predominance of this serotype. In this group of AIDS patients with disseminated mycobacterial disease, many isolates had a yellow pigmentation on primary isolation, rather than the usual buff color (10). However, we have observed both pigmented and non-pigmented isolates from AIDS and non-AIDS patients with disseminated disease.

PATHOGENESIS

Although the pathogenesis of MAI infection is unknown, it is likely that colonization precedes the development of disease. Colonization occurs as the result of exposure to the pathogen in the environment. Possible routes of acquisition include inhalation of the organism, ingestion of the organism, or acquisition through sexual contact (11).

The length of time from colonization to development of infection is unknown. Most people who are colonized with MAI remain healthy. Infection is produced by a coincidence of two factors: a transient or permanent, localized or generalized impairment of immune defenses, and colonization with a large number of mycobacteria (12).

Disseminated MAI infection occurs when the organism invades the bloodstream, an event which occurs more commonly in immunocompromised patients, but can also occur in immunocompetent hosts. In a recent review of disseminated MAI infections in non-AIDS patients, approximately one-half occurred in immunocompetent individuals (1). Disseminated disease is the rule for MAI infection in patients with AIDS (13)-(21). In one series, of 13 AIDS patients with MAI isolated from tissues and body fluids, 10

(77 percent) had evidence of disseminated infection (13). This high prevalence of disseminated MAI infection in AIDS patients contrasts strikingly with the five percent prevalence of disseminated MAI infection in non-AIDS patients (1).

BACTERIOLOGY AND METHODS OF DIAGNOSIS

Disseminated infection is definitively diagnosed on the basis of isolation of MAI from blood or bone marrow. However, isolation of MAI from any two body sites in an AIDS patient is strongly suggestive of disseminated disease. Recent improvements in techniques for culturing mycobacteria from blood have been exceedingly useful in diagnosing disseminated disease in AIDS patients. In one series of 47 AIDS patients with disseminated infection, 96 percent had a positive blood culture for MAI (2). Buffy coat smears for acid fast bacilli are also sometimes useful in diagnosing disseminated mycobacteremia (22). The mycobacteremia in AIDS patients appears to be high grade and sustained, and, therefore, serial quantitative blood cultures may provide a parameter for monitoring progression of disease or efficacy of therapy (23).

Other normally sterile sites which may be culture positive for MAI include bone marrow, lung parenchyma, lymph nodes, liver, spleen, kidney, pleural and pericardial fluids, urine, and, very rarely, cerebrospinal fluid. Non-sterile sites with a high yield for MAI include sputum and stool (11). In one series of 12 patients with disseminated disease who had cultures of stool, all specimens were positive on both acid fast smear and culture (2),(10). The culture yield for MAI from various sites in AIDS patients with disseminated disease is shown in Table 1. In AIDS patients in whom disseminated MAI disease is suspected, specimens of blood, stool, and bone marrow should be obtained for mycobacterial microscopy and culture. In addition, specimens from visceral sites should be cultured, if obtainable, and if the patient dies, autopsy specimens should be collected.

PATHOLOGY

The pathological findings in AIDS patients with disseminated MAI are variable. Most often the inflammatory reaction is minimal. Granulomas are frequently poorly formed or may be entirely absent (14). Occasionally, however, the pathology may resemble that of tuberculosis with the presence of caseating granulomas (15). Acid fast staining of pathologic specimens usually reveals large numbers of bacilli, and should be performed on all specimens from patients with suspected disseminated MAI infection (even in the absence of granulomas or abnormal histologic appearance). Small bowel and colonic biopsies of AIDS patients with disseminated MAI frequently reveal the presence of foamy macrophages filled with acid fast bacilli (24)-(27).

TABLE 1. Percent Yield of Specimens in AIDS Patients with Disseminated MAI Infection

Reference	Specimen	No Patients Cultured	Percent Yield
Kiehn et al. (10)	Stool	12	100
Damsker and Bottone (11)		6	83
Whimbey et al. (2)	Blood	47	96
Macher et al. (15)		10	70
Iseman et al. (6)		149 *	23
Iseman et al. (6)	Bone Marrow	149 *	54
Iseman et al. (6)	Sputum/Lung	149 *	46
Iseman et al. (6)	Lymph node	149 *	14
Iseman et al. (6)	Gastro-intestinal tract	149 *	14
Damsker and Bottone (11)		4	75
Whimbey et al. (2)	CSF	19	11

* It is not clear whether all patients in this series were cultured.

CLINICAL MANIFESTATIONS

Patients with AIDS frequently have multiple simultaneous opportunistic infections. Therefore, it is difficult to determine precisely which symptoms can be specifically attributed to infection with MAI. Persistent fever, diarrhea, and weight loss appear to be the most common presenting symptoms in AIDS patients with disseminated MAI. Fever is almost universally present and may be the only symptom. Often the patient will present with fever of unknown origin. Night sweats are also commonly seen. Diarrhea can vary in volume, consistency, and frequency. The most frequent presentation is a watery, non-bloody diarrhea (25) but MAI can also cause a full-blown colitis (26) as well as a malabsorption syndrome resembling Whipple's disease (24). Weight loss can be dramatic with loss of more than 15 percent of body weight over several weeks. Patients presenting with a wasting syndrome should be evaluated for the presence of disseminated mycobacterial infection. Other less frequent manifestations include lymphadenopathy, hepatomegaly, splenomegaly, and cutaneous and oral lesions. Generalized lymphadenopathy in AIDS patients is quite common and can be attributed to a variety of potential pathogens, including MAI (14). In one series of 17 AIDS patients with documented MAI infections, 82 percent were found to have multiple large retroperitoneal and mesenteric lymph nodes (27). Ulcerated mucosal lesions on the palate and gingiva have been described as a manifestation of disseminated MAI disease (28). Although MAI is frequently isolated from the sputum of AIDS patients, pulmonary manifestations are difficult to assess because of the high frequency of concurrent infection with *Pneumocystis carinii.* The role of MAI in AIDS patients with neurological complications is unknown, but MAI has been isolated from brain and cerebrospinal fluid in patients with disseminated disease (29).

THERAPY

In the past, a combination of five or six antituberculous drugs was used in the treatment of pulmonary and disseminated MAI infection in non-AIDS patients. The most active agents were rifampin, ethambutol, ethionamide, cycloserine, kanamycin, and streptomycin (5). Unfortunately, these agents are not very effective in treating MAI in AIDS. Of the currently available drugs, the most active against MAI in vitro are ansamycin LM427 (rifabutin) and clofazimine, both investigational agents.

Ansamycin is a spiropiperidyl derivative of rifamycin-S with excellent in vitro activity against MAI. It has also been found to inhibit all rifampin-sensitive strains and one-third of rifampin-resistant strains of *Mycobacterium tuberculosis* (30). Eight-five percent of strains of MAI tested by the Centers for Disease Control were sensitive to ansamycin at a concentration of 2 micrograms/ml (6). The adverse side effects are similar to rifampin. One-third of a group of New York City AIDS patients receiving this medication had mild elevations of liver enzymes (30). Occasionally, bone marrow suppression can occur which is gradually reversible after discontinuing therapy (30). Transient thrombocytopenia has also been observed (30). Since ansamycin is excreted in the urine, the dose must be lowered in patients with renal insufficiency, a noteworthy difference from the related drug, rifampin, which does not need dosage adjustment. Patients with neutropenia or hepatic dysfunction should also receive a lowered dose. The standard dose is now considered to be 300 mg p.o daily. The drug is available from the Centers for Disease Control in Atlanta, Georgia.

Clofazimine, a phenazine dye used in the therapy of leprosy, is bacteriocidal against most strains of MAI at concentrations varying from 1 to 5 micrograms/ml (2),(14). Clofazimine distributes particularly well into epithelium, bone marrow, and the reticuloendothelial system, achieving higher drug levels than in serum or pulmonary tissue (6). The most common adverse effect is a gradual, dose-related, pink to brownish-black skin discoloration which is slowly reversible when the drug is stopped. Occasional gastrointestinal symptoms including nausea, vomiting, abdominal pain, diarrhea, and anorexia are probably related to drug deposition in the intestinal wall with accompanying bowel wall edema (31). Rarely bowel obstruction or perforation can occur. The usual dose of clofazimine is 100 mg orally three times a day given with meals to minimize gastrointestinal complaints. At present, clofazimine can be obtained from the Ciba-Geigy Corporation in Summit, New Jersey.

Other drugs which show some in vitro activity against MAI include thienamycin, amikacin, dapsone, trimethoprim-sulfamethoxazole, and several cephalosporins (2),(32). There is minimal clinical experience, however, with the use of these agents for treating MAI infections in AIDS patients.

We generally initiate therapy of suspected MAI infections in AIDS patients with a combination of drugs including ansamycin, clofazimine, ethambutol, and isoniazid. This regimen includes agents active against *M. tuberculosis* as well as MAI. Some clinicians also add ethionamide and streptomycin. Whether inclusion of the investigational agents, ansamycin and clofazimine, enhances therapeutic efficacy over a "standard" multi-drug regimen is unknown. The role of conventional single-drug in vitro susceptibility testing in selection of therapeutic agents is unclear.

Despite in vitro activity of some medications, unfortunately, there is at present no effective therapy for disseminated MAI infection in AIDS patients. In one series, treatment reduced the magnitude of mycobacteremia (23). However, at autopsy, MAI could still be cultured from all patients despite on-going anti-mycobacterial treatment (33).

REFERENCES

1. Horsburgh, C.R., Mason, U.G., Farhi, D.C., et al., Disseminated infections with *Mycobacterium avium-intracellulare.* Medicine 64: 36-48 (1985)

2. Whimbey, E., Kiehn, T.E., Armstrong, D., Disseminated *Mycobacterium avium-intracellulare* disease: diagnosis and therapy; in: Current Clinical Topics in Infectious Diseases (Remington, J.S., Swartz, M.N., eds.), Mc-Graw Hill, New York, Vol 7: 112-133, (1986)

3. Good, R.C., Snider, D.E., Isolation of nontuberculous mycobacteria in the United States. J Infect Dis 146: 829-833 (1982)

4 Wolinsky, E., Nontuberculous mycobacteria and associated diseases. Am Rev Resp Dis 119: 107-159 (1979)

5. Songer, J.C., Environmental sources of *Mycobacterium avium* for infection of animals and man. Proc Ann Meeting US Anim Health Assoc 84: 528-535 (1980)

6. Iseman, M.D., Corpe, R.F., O'Brien, R.J., et al., Disease due to *Mycobacterium avium-intracellulare.* Chest 87(S):139-149 (1985)

7. Gruft, H., Falkinham, J.O. Parker, B.C., Recent experience in the epidemiology of disease caused by atypical mycobacteria. Rev Infect Dis 3: 990-996 (1981)

8. Schaefer, W.B., Serologic identification and classification of the atypical mycobacteria by their agglutination. Am Rev Resp Dis 92: 85-93 (1965)

9. McGlatchy, J.K., The seroagglutination test in the study of non-tuberculous mycobacteria. Rev Infect Dis 3: 867-870 (1981)

10. Kiehn, T.E., Edwards, F.P., Brannon, P., et al., Infections caused by *Mycobacterium avium* complex in immunocompromised patients: Diagnosis by blood culture and fecal examination, antimicrobial susceptibility tests, and morphological and seroagglutination characteristics. J Clin Micro 21:168-173 (1985)

11. Damsker, B., Bottone, E.J., *Mycobacterium avium-Mycobacterium intracellulare* from the intestinal tracts of patients with the acquired immunodeficiency syndrome: Concepts regarding acquisition and pathogenesis. J Infect Dis 151:179-181 (1985)

12. Chapman, J.S., The Atypical Mycobacteria and Human Mycobacteriosis, Plenum Medical Book Co., New York and London (1977)

13. Berlin, O.G.W., Zakowski, P., Bruchner, D.A. et al., *Mycobacterium avium*: A pathogen of patients with acquired immunodeficiency syndrome. Diagn Microbiol Infect Dis 2: 213-218 (1984)

14. Green, J.B., Sidhu, G.S., Lewin, S., et al., *Mycobacterium avium-intracellulare*: A cause of disseminated life-threatening infection in homosexuals and drug abusers. Ann Intern Med 97:539-546 (1982)

15. Macher, A.B., Kovacs, J.A., Gill, V., et al., Bacteremia due to *Mycobacterium avium-intracellulare* in the acquired immunodeficiency syndrome. Ann Intern Med 99: 782-785 (1983)

16. Masur, H., Michelis, M.A., Wormser, G.P., et al., Opportunistic infection in previously healthy women. Ann Intern Med 97:533-539 (1982)

17. Elliott, J.L., Hoppes, W.L., Platt, M.S., et al., The acquired immunodeficiency syndrome and *Mycobacterium avium-intracellulare* bacteremia in a patient with hemophilia. Ann Intern Med 98:290-293 (1983)

18. Zakowski, P., Fligiel, S., Berlin, G.W., et al., Disseminated *Mycobacterium avium-intracellulare* infection in homosexual men dying of acquired immunodeficiency. JAMA 248:2980-2982 (1982)

19. Poon, M., Landay, A., Prasthofer, E.F., et al., Acquired immuno-deficiency syndrome with *Pneumocystis carinii* pneumonia and *Mycobacterium avium-intracellulare* infection in a previously healthy patient with classic hemophilia. Ann Intern Med 98: 287-290 (1983)

20. Waxman, J.S., Subietas, A., Malowany, M., et al., Overwhelming mycobacteriosis in an immunodeficient homosexual. Mount Sinai J Med 50: 19-21 (1983)

21. Sohn, C.C., Schroff, R.W., Kliewer, K.E., et al., Disseminated *Mycobacterium avium-intracellulare* infection in homosexual men with acquired cell-mediated immunodeficiency: A histologic and immunologic study of two cases. Am J Clin Pathol 79: 247-252 (1983)

22. Graham, B.S., Hinson, M.V., Bennett, S.R., et al., Acid fast bacilli on buffy coat smears in the acquired immunodeficiency syndrome: A lesson from Hansen's bacillus. South Med J 77: 246-248 (1984)

23. Wong, B., Edwards, F.F., Kiehn, T.E., et al., Continuous high-grade *Mycobacterium avium-intracellulare* bacteremia in patients with the acquired immune deficiency syndrome. Am J Med 78: 35-40 (1985)

24. Strom, R.L., Gruninger, R.P., AIDS with *Mycobacterium avium-intracellulare* lesions resembling those of Whipple's disease. N Engl J Med 309: 1323-1324 (1983)

25. Gillin, J.S., Urmacher, C., West, R., et al., Disseminated *Mycobacterium avium-intracellulare* infection in acquired immunodeficiency syndrome mimicking Whipple's disease. Gastroenterology 85: 1187-1191 (1983)

26. Wolke, A., Meyers, S., Adelsberg, B.R., et al., *Mycobacterium avium-intracellulare*-associated colitis in a patient with the acquired immunodeficiency syndrome. J Clin Gastro 6: 225-229 (1984)

27. Nyberg, D.A., Federle, M.P., Jeffrey, R.B., et al., Abdominal CT findings of disseminated *Mycobacterium avium-intracellulare* in AIDS. AJR 145: 297-299 (1985)

28. Volpe, F., Schwimmer, A., Barr, C., Oral manifestation of disseminated *Mycobacterium avium-intracellulare* in a patient with AIDS. Oral Surg 60: 567-570 (1985)

29. Snider, W.D., Simpson, D.M., Nielsen, S., et al., Neurological complications of acquired immune deficiency syndrome: Analysis of 50 patients. Ann Neurol 14: 403-418 (1983)

30. Centers for Disease Control. Rifabutin (ansamycin LM 427) - informational material for physicians (1986)

31. Fact sheet on clofazimine. U.S. Public Health Service Hospital, Carville, Louisiana. March 21, 1979, Fourth Revision

32. Baron, E.J. Berlin, O.G.W., Bruckner, D.A., et al., Antimicrobial combinations with N-formimidoyl thienamycin and amikacin inhibit *Mycobacterium avium-intracellulare*, International Conference on Acquired Immunodeficiency Syndrome (AIDS), Atlanta, GA (1985)

33. Hawkins, C., Kiehn, T.E., Whimbey, E., et al., Treatment of *Mycobacterium avium-intracellulare* infection in AIDS, International Conference on Acquired Immunodeficiency Syndrome (AIDS), Atlanta, GA (1985)

28
Neurological Complications of HIV Infection: An Overview

Barbara S. Koppel

Neurological complications are common in the acquired immunodeficiency syndrome (AIDS). Central nervous system (CNS) involvement is reported in 80-95% of autopsied cases (1), (2) and 40% of AIDS patients have symptoms during life (3). Neurological complaints are the initial manifestation of the disease in at least 10% of patients (3), (4) and may precede diagnosis by up to one year (5). The relative risk of different complications varies with the age of the patient (6), geographic origin or travel history, duration of HIV infection, and AIDS risk category.

Presently, the neurologist's role is to diagnose and document nervous system involvement and to assist in recognizing treatable infective and neoplastic complications. In addition, expertise is often required for advice regarding nonspecific supportive measures, such as for controlling seizures, pain, psychotic symptoms or other behavioral problems. As better anti-HIV treatment regimens become available, it may become more essential to detect CNS symptoms early to preserve normal neurological status.

PATHOPHYSIOLOGICAL CONSIDERATIONS

Neurological complications have now been reported from a number of different centers (Table 1) (1),(3),(4),(7)-(20). In some series (3),(7),(16),(17), the main groups at risk have been male homosexuals, whereas intravenous drug abusers (4),(8),(11),(12),(18),(19), Haitians (10),(13),(15),(20), and children of drug abusers (21) are prominently represented in others. In the

Table 1. Comparison of Neurologic Findings in Patients with AIDS from Published Series

Series (Ref. No.)	7	8	9#	10	11	12	13	14	15#	16#	17#	1#	4	3	18	19#	20
Number of Cases																	
AIDS Total	160					52		31	39	36	40		121	318	100		
AIDS with CNS	50	19	10	10	15	15	16	7	25	26	31	104	28	124	33	8	51
INFECTIONS																	
Chronic Encephalitis*	18	1	1			1		1	5	10	19	69	7	39	13		1
Herpes Species							1	1						12			
Presumed CMV			1		6			1	2	2		28			7	1	5
Toxoplasmosis	5	7	1	2	1	8	15	2	16		5	13	9	19		4	31
Cryptococcosis	2	9	3	3	4	5	1		1	3		2	7	16		1	10
Mycobacteria	3			1	4	1	2		2				1	1		1	1
Candidiasis	1		1					1				2	1	1			3
PML##	2	1	1				1		2		1	2	1	2			3
Aseptic Meningitis	4			2										17			
NEOPLASMS																	
1° CNS Lymphoma	3	1		1				1	1	2	3	5	3	10	1		2
2° CNS Lymphoma (includes meninges)	4		1	1						1		3		2			
Other Tumors**	2									2				2			
VASCULAR PATHOLOGY																	
Infarction	3								7	2	2			2		1	
Hemorrhage									3						2		1
OTHER (and undiagnosed)	3	1	2					1	2	1	1			10		2	3

* Presumed HIV Infection
** Kaposi's sarcoma, plasmacytoma, lymphoma of spinal cord
# Post mortem series
Progressive Multifocal Leukoencephalopathy

homosexual population and in children with HIV infection, a subacute encephalitis, thought to be due to HIV infection itself, is the most commonly encountered syndrome. In intravenous drug users and Haitian patients, opportunistic infections predominate. One hypothesis for this difference is that homosexuals, often coming from middle and upper class social strata, have better baseline health and nutritional status which offers them some resistance to opportunistic organisms (19),(22)-(24). This advantage favors increased longevity which may be necessary in some cases for the pathological and clinical features of the subacute encephalitis to become apparent. Alternatively, the exposure history of risk groups other than homosexual men may simply place them at greater risk to develop common opportunistic infections of the central nervous system such as toxoplasmosis and cryptococcosis.

Receptors for HIV, similar to those identified on T4 lymphocytes, have been found on cellular membranes from normal brain, especially in tissue from temporal lobe, cingulate gyrus and hippocampus (25). A transient aseptic meningitis may correspond to the time of seroconversion and viral entry into the CNS (3), (7),(26)-(28). Clinical symptoms include headache, fever, photophobia, stiff neck and, occasionally, cranial neuropathies (3), (7),(26). In some patients, an inflammatory neuropathy or polyradiculopathy has preceded the development of AIDS by one to six months and similarly may be a marker of initial infection (3), (29),(30). Plasmapheresis-lymphopheresis seemed to benefit some of the latter patients including eight of nine in whom AIDS had not yet been diagnosed (29),(30). Herpes zoster radiculitis (shingles) has preceded AIDS by as much as three years (3),(5), (31), as has zoster ophthalmicus (32),(33). These early syndromes should be watched for as valuable warning signs in any member of an AIDS risk group.

CLINICAL SYNDROMES

Three major clinical syndromes are regularly encountered in patients with neurological complications: subacute encephalitis, focal cerebral syndromes, and meningitis.

Subacute Encephalitis

The clinical picture is of a slowly evolving encephalopathy marked by gradual loss of normal cognitive functions. The onset is often insidious with decreased interest in work or leisure activities, loss of libido and social withdrawal. Overt depression and personality change are also common. Patients report difficulty concentrating and having problems with fine motor control. A professional pianist, for instance, could no longer play with his former accuracy (B. Koppel, personal observation). Hallucinations and visual blurring may occur (2),(4),(7) and seizures are eventually seen in 50% of this group (4),(7). Headache is rare (3), and significant focal findings are uncommon. When present, focal findings usually indicate brainstem involvement and include ataxia, diplopia, dysarthria and patchy numbness (2),(4),(7),(34). Mental status testing initially reveals accurate but delayed responses complicated by a poor attention span and variable cooperation. The patient becomes increasingly apathetic, and signs of hypothalamic dysfunction including inappropriate ADH secretion, unexplained fever and wasting can be present (3),(4). Tremor, myoclonus and asterixis may appear, and coma ensues preterminally (2),(4),(7).

In one-half of these patients, a spinal cord syndrome develops with spastic paraparesis or quadriparesis, bladder and bowel incontinence and muscle wasting (1),(2),(35)-(37). There is often an associated painful sensory neuropathy (7), but back or radicular pain is infrequent.

In children, HIV brain infection may occur as early as the first trimester of pregnancy (6) and may be manifested by developmental delay in addition to progressive dementia (21).

Laboratory tests are usually nonspecifically abnormal. Computed tomography (CT) reveals diffuse cerebral atrophy, and magnetic resonance imaging (MRI) demonstrates signal attenuation in the frontal white matter. The electroencephalogram (EEG) shows mild diffuse, relatively symmetric slowing of background rhythms. The cerebrospinal fluid (CSF) is either normal or marked only by slight protein elevation and a mild monocytic pleocytosis.

Neuropathologic findings include glial and microglial nodules (3),(19),(21), bizarre multinucleated giant cells (38), demyelination, gemistocytic astrocytosis, perivascular inflammation, and occasional mineralization (21). There are vacuolar changes in the posterior columns of the spinal cord and white matter of the brain (Figure 1) (2),(19),(21),(36),(37),(39). Current evidence suggests that most cases of subacute encephalitis are caused by brain infection with HIV (2),(27),(28),(39)-(41), with a few cases probably due to cytomegalovirus (CMV) infection (1),(3),(9), (11),(13)-(17),(42),(43). HIV has been grown from CSF (27),(28), and specific antiviral antibodies have recently been demonstrated in spinal fluid (40).

Focal Cerebral Syndromes

A neurological picture marked by headache and focal signs is most often due to opportunistic infections or tumors affecting the brain parenchyma. Other causes of focal brain disease are much less common. Vascular syndromes include cerebral infarction or hemorrhage (3),(7),(15)-(19),(44),(45). Pituitary infarction has been reported in three patients (3),(7). Infarcts have occurred in a case of progressive multifocal leukoencephalopathy near an area of demyelination (19), with CMV infection (46), and as a result of herpes zoster arteritis in a patient with Ramsey-Hunt syndrome (7). Hemorrhage has occurred into lymphoma and metastatic Kaposi's sarcoma (3),(7),(20). In other patients with intracranial bleeding, systemic factors have been implicated including disseminated intravascular coagulopathy (15), nonbacterial thrombotic endocarditis (3),(15),(45) and thrombocytopenia (3).

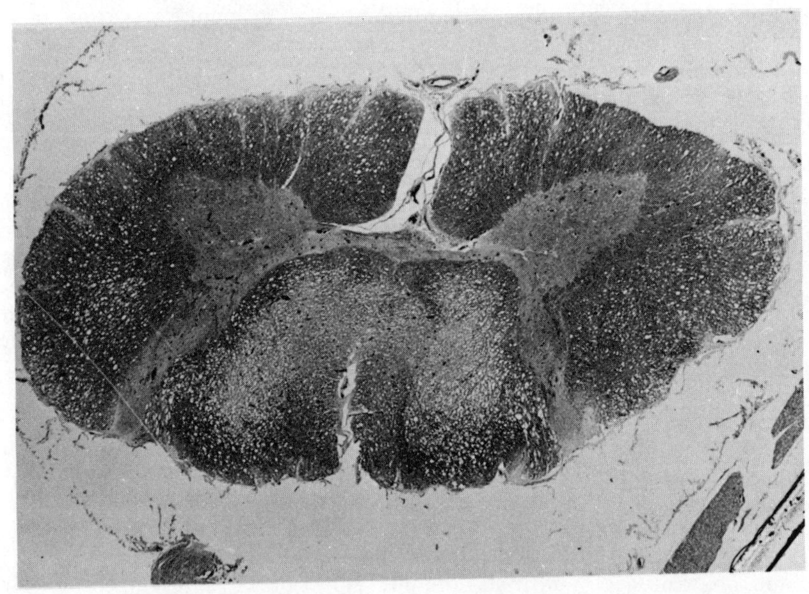

Figure 1. Vacuolar degeneration of the posterior and lateral columns of the spinal cord. Cross section of spinal cord stained with hematoxylin-eosin and luxol fast blue for myelin. Courtesy of Dr. Seymour Levine, New York Medical College.

Clinical signs include aphasia, lateralized changes in tone or muscle strength, hemisensory loss, gaze preference or palsy, visual field deficit, diplopia, deafness, blindness, ataxia, dysarthria or dysphagia, asymmetric stretch reflexes, and unilateral grasp reflex or Babinski response. Focal or secondarily generalized seizures are common. Sometimes, the focal signature must be carefully looked for as the clinical picture may be dominated by evidence of more global cerebral dysfunction due to multiple lesions, increased intracranial pressure or involvement of the reticular activating system in the brainstem (3),(4),(7),(39),(47). Despite the frequency with which the basal ganglia are involved (with toxoplasmosis, for example), classical extrapyramidal signs such as resting tremor or other adventitious movements, bradykinesia and rigidity are rare. Fever may occur with either tumor or infection, and is not often helpful diagnostically.

It is usually impossible to determine clinically the nature of the specific pathogen or even whether a focal lesion is due to infection or tumor. Although it is often said that the deterioration due to tumor occurs more rapidly than that caused by infection, this dictum is completely unreliable in the immunodeficient patient.

Meningitis

A meningeal syndrome is the third major manifestation of CNS disease. Headache, fever and photophobia are the most prominent symptoms, but stiff neck, cranial neuropathies, altered mentation, increased intracranial pressure with vomiting and papilledema, blindness and seizures occur frequently. In neoplastic meningitis especially, back pain, areflexia, radicular pain or segmental sensory loss may occur (48).

Cryptococcus neoformans is the most common pathogen causing this condition, but other fungi including candida and aspergillus (49), mycobacterial strains (4),(7),(12),(50), viruses (51),(52), treponema (3),(53), bacteria (9),(15),(16),(20),(54), (55) and cancer (1),(7),(9) have been cited as etiologies.

As indicated above, early in HIV infection, a less severe aseptic meningitis picture may occur, presumably caused by entry of HIV into the CNS (3),(7),(26),(28).

CSF findings may be valuable in establishing a specific diagnosis. Most helpful is the discovery of a low glucose content (less than two-thirds that of serum). Pleocytosis and elevated protein are common, and the pressure may be elevated. CSF changes specific to individual infections will be discussed in subsequent sections. CT scans in chronic meningitis characteristically show large ventricles, presumably consequent to poor CSF absorption by arachnoid villi clogged with inflammatory cellular debris.

Miscellaneous Syndromes

Motor neuron disease with the clinical picture of amyotrophic lateral sclerosis has been reported in one patient (56). Isolated cranial mononeuropathies, especially "Bell's palsy", have been described, but these are usually due to undiagnosed aseptic or neoplastic meningitis (57), brainstem encephalitis (44) or tumor (58). Since lymphoma and Kaposi's sarcoma may involve the nasopharynx (59),(60), direct extension to the base of the skull with involvement of cranial nerves should be anticipated, although this has not yet been reported in AIDS patients.

Metabolic encephalopathy can be anticipated in patients with kidney or liver failure, malnutrition, hypoxia and fever, all of which are frequent problems in AIDS patients (4),(15),(17),(53). Minor metabolic derangements may "unmask" subacute encephalitis (2). Since respiratory failure is a frequent terminal event in these patients, postmortem examination of the brain oftens shows changes consistent with hypoxic damage (15)-(17). In one patient without documented hyponatremia, central pontine myelinolysis was an unexpected autopsy finding (19).

In addition to the aforementioned vacuolar myelopathy, the spinal cord may be involved in other ways. Rapid rostral progression of spinal cord symptoms and findings suggests a viral infection, usually due to one of the herpes group (51),(61), (62). Metastatic tumor with epidural cord compression produces segmental symptoms at one level, including pain which is often midthoracic, and paralysis or sensory loss below that (7),(63),(64). Neoplastic meningitis may involve multiple nerve roots resulting in signs referable to many levels (3),(7),(9),(48).

The peripheral nervous system is also involved in AIDS. Brachial plexopathy due to Kaposi's sarcoma (3) and radiculitis secondary to varicella-zoster (3),(5),(7) have been reported. As already mentioned, an inflammatory polyneuropathy or mononeuritis multiplex may occur, sometimes before AIDS has developed (29),(65). A subacute peripheral neuropathy causing stocking-glove numbness and less often weakness and atrophy is common in patients with subacute encephalitis (3),(5),(7). Drug-induced neuropathy occurs especially in patients with Kaposi's sarcoma treated with vincristine, but may also be seen in patients receiving isoniazid without pyridoxine supplementation (35). Kimbrough (66) has speculated that cleansing solutions such as hexachlorophene may be neurotoxic when absorbed through decubiti. Guillain-Barre syndrome, or acute postinfectious polyradiculopathy, has occurred in several patients (3),(5),(30),(37). CMV was identified in one case (37), but usually the syndrome is attributed to an autoimmune reaction triggered by an unknown antecedent viral infection. Myositis and myopathy have caused muscle weakness, cramps and atrophy (3),(7),(53),(67). Toxoplasma infection has been suspected, but to date pathological confirmation has not been demonstrated. In one patient, systemic infection due to *Mycobacterium tuberculosis* masqueraded as polymyalgia rheumatica (68).

DIAGNOSTIC EVALUATION

Aggressive, but appropriate, diagnostic studies in this population are aimed at early diagnosis of opportunistic infections and malignancies and prevention of complications. Ideally, baseline data including skin tests for mycobacteria (69) and toxoplasma serology (13) should be obtained in patients at risk before immunodeficiency is complete. This may be especially important in Haitian patients and intravenous drug abusers in whom these infections are particularly common. It may be wise to perform neuropsychological testing at the time of first visit and then to repeat the assessment periodically (2). This seems to be especially important in children where test results may play a role in deciding issues of public safety related to continued school attendance.

Computed Tomography

There can be little question that in this population the most important diagnostic tool in the detection of structural brain disease is computed tomography (CT). Three major groups of findings have been reported (8),(10),(18),(20),(70)-(73): diffuse cortical atrophy with nonfocal decreased density of white matter in patients with subacute encephalitis; ventricular dilation in chronic meningitis; and low density mass lesions with variable degrees of contrast enhancement, with or without mass effect and edema of the surrounding tissue, in brain abscesses and tumors. The general features of common pathological findings are tabulated in Table 2.

Brain abscesses usually arise in an area of ischemic brain if the organism is blood-born, near the cortical surface in patients with meningitis, or adjacent to a focus of infection such as otitis media or sinusitis (20),(74),(75). In the initial stage of cerebritis, CT may demonstrate a poorly defined area of uneven density and mottled enhancement producing edema and, depending upon location, ventricular compression. Subsequent steps in abscess formation are affected by the patient's immune status, and the CT picture correspondingly differs in immunocompromised hosts from that seen classically in immunocompetent individuals. In the AIDS patient, capsule formation is limited, or lacking altogether, due to poor macrophage and fibroblast recruitment. As a result, the expected enhancing ring does not always develop despite evidence pathologically of extensive inflammation and necrosis (8),(10),(23),(76),(77). If some immunity is preserved, a defective capsule is formed that may show some enhancement (10). Relatively homogeneous enhancement sometimes occurs with toxoplasmosis, presumably due to extensive breakdown locally of the blood-brain barrier. Cerebral lymphomas enhance both because of local alteration in the blood-brain barrier and because of neoplastic blood vessel formation. Thus, similar CT abnormalities may be seen with different infections (Figure 2), or with infections and tumors (4),(8),(10),(17),(18),(78)-(80). Even viral infections may rarely present as a focally enhancing lesion (3),(73).

Double-dose contrast injection with delayed imaging improves visualization of less intensely enhancing lesions (8),(20),(73),(81), but use of this technique is often limited by the patient's renal function (18),(20). When serial studies are performed in the same patient, it is important to use consistent amounts of contrast on each occasion to facilitate meaningful comparisons. Even with optimal use of current CT techniques, however, the extent of brain pathology is almost always underrepresented.

Demonstration of ring enhancement around an infective lesion is associated with a somewhat better prognosis because it implies host capability to produce a capsule. Conversely, disappearance of enhancement may represent deterioration rather than response to treatment. Corticosteroids may decrease enhancement because of their salutary effect on restoring the blood-brain barrier. In such circumstances, degree of enhancement is not a reliable indicator of lesion status, and a better measure of disease progression or response to treatment is a change in the number and size of the lesions (20). Calcification of lesions implies chronicity as in immunocompetent hosts (20),(82), but it should not be taken as evidence of inactive disease. In toxoplasma encephalitis, for example, some calcified lesions continue to enhance (20). Meningitis or ependymitis can result in diffuse enhancement of the meninges or ventricular lining (8),(18),(83), but the CT is frequently normal with meningeal lymphoma (84). Chronic meningitis

Table 2. CT Scan Findings in AIDS Patients

Pathology	Typical Location	Enhancement	Atrophy
Toxoplasma abscesses	Deep (basal ganglia, thalamus) corticomedullary	Variable ring, homogeneous, or none	After treatment
Cryptococcoma	Unknown	Variable	-
Fungal* brain lesion	Cortical or near sinuses	+	-
Mycobacterial brain lesion	Cortical	++ Ring or solid	-
Subacute encephalitis#	White matter, especially frontal	Rarely	++ Progressive
PML=	White matter, can be posterior fossa	-	-
Chronic meningitis@	-	Meninges, ependyma of ventricles	+
Lymphoma and other tumors	Periventricular, rarely cortical	++	-

Scale: - = absent; + = present; ++ = prominent

* Candida, aspergillus (may be hemorrhagic), also nocardia (which is not a fungus)
\# due to HIV or cytomegalovirus infection
= Progressive multifocal leukoencephalopathy due to JC papova virus
@ Due to toxoplasma, cryptococcus, mycobacterial species, or tumor. May see infarctions as well.

Table 2. CT Scan Findings in AIDS Patients (Continued)

Pathology	Hydrocephalus	Edema or Mass Effect	Multiple Sites
Toxoplasma abscesses	Rare, with meningitis	Usually	Usually
Cryptococcoma	Rare	Usually	Rarely
Fungal* brain lesion	-	+	Occasionally
Mycobacterial brain lesion	++, after meningitis	+	Rarely
Subacute encephalitis#	+	-	-
PML=	-	-	Occasionally (Increased number over time)
Chronic meningitis@	+	-	-
Lymphoma and other tumors	-	++	+

Scale: - = absent; + = present; ++ = prominent

* Candida, aspergillus (may be hemorrhagic), also nocardia (which is not a fungus)
\# due to HIV or cytomegalovirus infection
= Progressive multifocal leukoencephalopathy due to JC papova virus
@ Due to toxoplasma, cryptococcus, mycobacterial species, or tumor. May see infarctions as well.

leads to subependymal gliosis, hydrocephalus and enlargement of the basal cisterns (10),(74),(85).

Because of the importance of early detection of opportunistic brain infection and tumor (86), some investigators have recommended regular CT scans even in asymptomatic patients (87).

Magnetic Resonance Imaging (MRI)

MRI is complementary to CT, especially when white matter is involved, in accurately depicting the number and extent of focal lesions and in demonstrating edema (3),(73). MRI has also been used successfully to guide stereotaxic brain biopsy. MRI findings in toxoplasmosis have been described (3),(81),(88), and alterations in cerebral white matter, especially of the frontal lobes, have been reported in subacute encephalitis (3),(73). Using the contrast agent gadolimium DTPA, alteration in blood-brain barrier and abnormal perfusion can be detected (73). It is likely that in the future MRI will play an important role in establishing the presence of HIV infection in the brain and spinal cord.

Positron Emission Tomography

Use of positron emission tomography (PET) in AIDS patients has been limited. Navia et al. (89) described decreased glucose utilization in the mesial temporal lobes of two patients with subacute encephalitis.

Electroencephalography and Evoked Potentials

Electroencephalography is rarely of specific help, but diffuse abnormalities of background rhythms may assist in documenting organic cerebral dysfunction in patients with equivocal mental or psychological symptoms. In one German survey (90), 50% of 26 patients with AIDS or progressive generalized lymphadenopathy had slowing of mean alpha frequency. Persistence of this slowing over time correlated with development of a chronic encephalopathy. In rare cases, confusion, bizarre behavior or unresponsiveness may be due to unsuspected nonconvulsive status epilepticus. A triphasic wave pattern may help diagnose a metabolic encephalopathy.

Somatosensory evoked potentials may help document sites of abnormal central conduction and establish a wider extent of disability than is apparent from clinical examination alone.

Cerebrospinal Fluid

Analysis of CSF is essential in establishing a diagnosis of meningitis and should be performed whenever this is suspected. CSF studies may also contribute to the diagnosis of parenchymal brain disease as well. IgG specific for HIV is synthesized within the blood brain barrier (40) and HIV virus has been isolated from CSF (27),(28). It is, therefore, necessary to take appropriate precautions when handling samples. At least 20 ml should be obtained where possible in order to carry out the necessary battery of tests.

Routine studies include determination of opening and closing pressures, cell counts, protein and glucose levels, Gram stain and bacterial cultures. Blood should always be obtained simultaneously for comparison glucose measurements.

In addition, other analyses directed to the special problems presented by the AIDS patient must be carried out. These include an India ink preparation for cryptococcus, a test for cryptococcal antigen, a test for syphilis, a Ziehl-Neelsen stain, and appropriate cultures for mycobacteria and fungi. Cytologic examination of the sediment from at least 3 ml of CSF should be done to detect malignant cells. When the clinical suspicion of intracranial or spinal neoplastic disease is high, this may need to be repeated several times. Measurement of myelin basic protein may be of interest in quantifying the extent of ongoing demyelination. Atypical oligoclonal band patterns occur as a nonspecific consequence of viral infection (91) or acute destructive processes and thus are usually not helpful. Serologic studies on serum for specific viruses as well as for syphilitic, fungal (*Cryptococcus neoformans*) and protozoan organisms (*Toxoplasma gondii*) may be helpful with both meningeal and parenchymal infections.

Myelography

Except where MRI is readily available, myelography is required to diagnose spinal cord compression caused by extrinsic lesions such as tumor or epidural abscess. Although most AIDS patients with myelopathy have vacuolar degeneration due to HIV infection or a viral myelitis, clinical differentiation between these entities and a treatable compressive lesion is often not possible. Because of the disastrous consequences of missing spinal cord compression, early myelography (or spinal MRI) is recommended in appropriate cases to settle this point unequivocally.

Brain Biopsy

Because of the similarity in clinical and CT presentations of etiologically different neurological complications, brain biopsy is often crucial for accurate diagnosis (70),(72),(92). Which patients to biopsy, and when, remains controversial. Morbidity associated with brain biopsy is probably higher in AIDS patients than in other groups for several reasons. First, systemic factors are frequently present that predispose to hemorrhage, such as thrombocytopenia or liver dysfunction with clotting abnormalities (4),(7),(15),(20),(46). Second, the deep location of many lesions requires violation of normal brain.

Even with brain biopsy specimens, it is often not possible to make a definitive diagnosis, either because the amount of tissue is inadequate or because the sample is obtained from a part of the lesion not containing diagnostic pathology (3),(8),(10),(15),(48),(81). An additional problem is that sections stained with hematoxylin and eosin may appear normal even in the presence of infection (86),(93). Thus, special stains and cultures are always necessary and these cannot be neglected. It is also important to recognize that multiple infectious agents may be present simultaneously (1),(3),(4),(9),(15),(19),(46),(94), or that different pathologic processes may coexist, such as cryptococcosis or toxoplasmosis with lymphoma (3),(8),(9),(19),(20). Further, the histopathology may be atypical in the immunodeficient host. For example, toxoplasma tachyzoites may be round rather than crescentic (72), microglial nodules may be seen with infections other than CMV and HIV (19), and the capsule of the cryptococcal yeast organisms may appear unusually small (95).

Awareness of these problems can reduce their influence on the outcome. Chance of hemorrhage can be minimized by replacing deficient clotting factors and platelets. Stereotactic localization using CT or MRI guidance is helpful but time-consuming (3),(70),(73); progress has been made using intraoperative realtime ultrasound (96). At our center, realtime ultrasound guidance has been used in 20 biopsy procedures, and an unambiguous diagnosis was made in 10 (Dr. J. Mangiardi, personal communication) (Figure 3b). Also, this technique allowed prompt detection of a hemorrhagic complication which was effectively treated. A frozen section should be done to ensure that the surgeon has obtained an appropriate sample. When the tissue is processed, all relevant modalities should be employed including electron microscopy (97). Detection of toxoplasmosis may be improved by use of a peroxidase-antiperoxidase method (98),(99). Cultures for bacteria, mycobacteria, and fungi should be routine (19),(94),(100). Viral cultures, especially for herpes viruses, may be useful in selected patients.

SPECIFIC CNS INFECTIONS

Cytomegalovirus (CMV) Infection

CMV was originally believed to be the causative agent in subacute encephalitis, but the evidence for this was inconclusive. It is now recognized, for example, that most of the pathological findings considered "typical" of CMV encephalitis are equally characteristic of HIV infection. Nonetheless, in a few AIDS patients with a subacute encephalopathy similar to that described in transplant patients, good evidence for CMV infection was present. This evidence included positive CSF cultures for CMV (52), characteristic findings on electron microscopy (37),(43),(101),(102), and positive results from various molecular probes and immunohistochemical techniques for CMV (42),(44),(52),(101). CMV has also been isolated from blood, urine and CSF from individual patients with myelitis (61), chorio-retinitis (103) and an illness resembling Guillain-Barre syndrome (37),(104).

CMV seems to gain access to the nervous system by passing through capillary endothelium (43) or the ependymal lining of ventricles (42),(44). It then produces an arteritis and demyelination (37),(44),(104). CMV, along with other herpes group viruses, may play a causative role in the development of Kaposi's sarcoma (23),(24) which occasionally involves the nervous system.

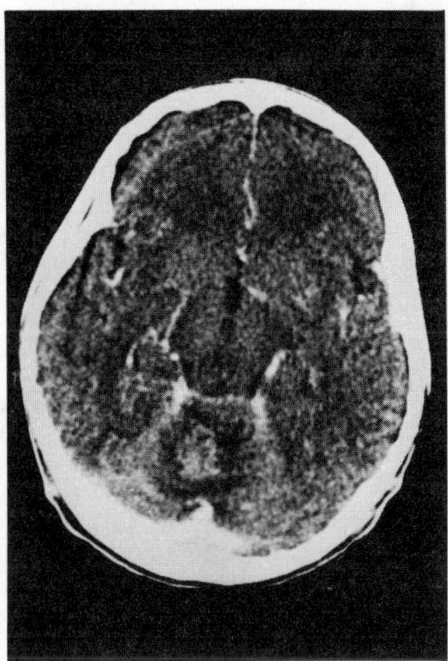

Figure 2a. Transaxial brain CT showing contrast-enhancing round nodule in the cerebellar vermis associated with moderate edema.

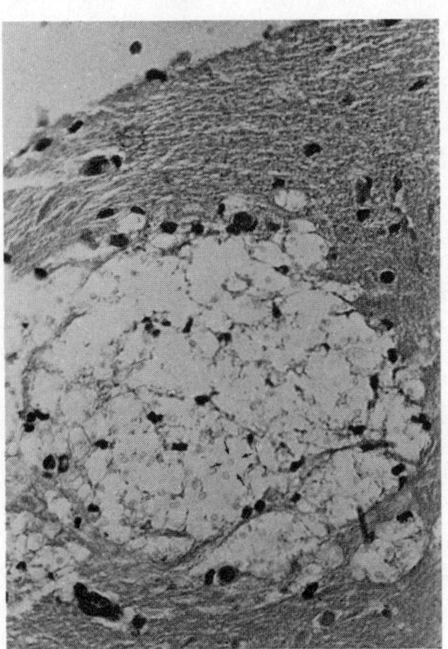

Figure 2b. Biopsy specimen of lesion in Figure 2a showing cryptococcal yeast forms (arrow) surrounded by blank space containing nonstaining capsular material. (Hematoxylin-eosin stain. Courtesy of Dr. Tung Pui Poon, New York Medical College.)

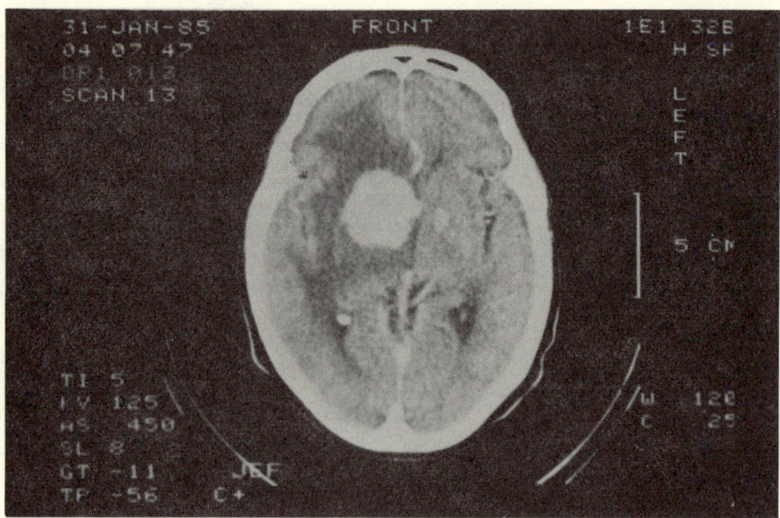

Figure 3a. Transaxial brain CT showing dense homogenously enhancing nodular tumor mass in the right frontal lobe surrounded by marked edema.

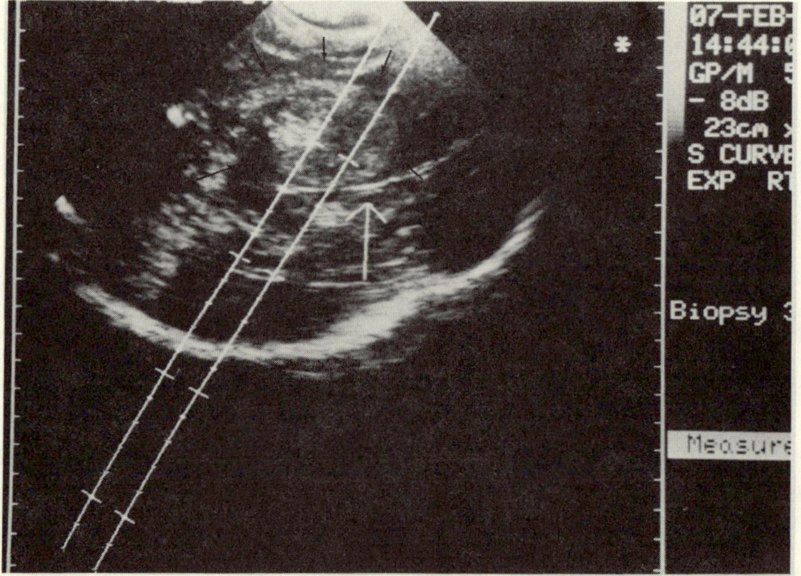

Figure 3b. Real time intraoperative ultrasonography with trajectory for biopsy needle in the center of the lesion shown in Figure 3a. (Courtesy of Dr. John Mangiardi, New York Medical College.)

Treatment of CMV infection using interferon alpha and acyclovir has been unsuccessful (44),(103),(105). Some benefit may have accrued to three patients treated with immunoglobulin preparations (106), and dihydroxypropoxymethylguanine (DHPG) has been beneficial in chorioretinitis (107), although relapses are frequent when the drug is discontinued.

Other Herpes Infections

Herpes viruses have caused myelitis (*Herpes simplex 2*) (3),(61),(62), and encephalitis (*Herpes simplex 1 and 2* and varicella/zoster) (1),(3),(14),(108)-(112) in AIDS patients. The clinical course is often less fulminant than in the case of sporadic infections in the immunocompetent patient (3), and CT changes are correspondingly innocuous. MRI may show a bifrontal leukoencephalopathy (3). Treatment with intravenous acyclovir is recommended (113). One patient with herpes ophthalmicus which progressed to encephalitis responded to vidarabine (33).

Adenovirus Infection

Adenovirus type 31 was cultured from the spinal fluid of one patient with subacute encephalopathy (51), but proof of a pathogenic relationship was lacking.

Progressive Multifocal Leukoencephalopathy (PML)

PML is due to infection with JC papova virus and occurs with some frequency in patients with AIDS (19),(76),(114)-(117), up to 4% in one study (117). Initial symptoms are usually mental changes, weakness or visual loss. A posterior fossa presentation is also described (91). It is not unusual for the patient to appear sicker than the CT changes would seem to indicate (117). Oligoclonal bands were reported in one patient (91), but this is exceptional. The EEG demonstrates moderate to severe focal or multifocal slowing early (76),(114),(115),(117) with diffuse changes appearing later (117). To date, antiviral treatment including acyclovir (76), cytosine arabinoside (117) and vidarabine (91) has been ineffective.

Toxoplasmosis

Toxoplasmosis is the most common opportunistic infection of the central nervous system reported among AIDS patients (7),(15), (77),(81),(98),(99),(118)-(122). The clinical presentation of brain involvement may be that of a mass lesion, lethargy and personality change, non-specific symptoms of increased intracranial pressure, or, less frequently, meningitis and panhypopituitarism (123). Toxoplasmosis is uncommon in children with AIDS, probably because its occurrence usually depends upon reactivation of latent infection and children may not yet have been exposed. Children and AIDS patients with negative serology should be warned of the usual routes of transmission through accidental ingestion of infected cat feces or by consumption of undercooked infected meat (124).

Neuropathological findings include necrotizing abscesses with vascular proliferation, chronic inflammatory cells and microglial nodules (19),(72),(81). Occasionally, thrombosed blood vessels and petechial hemorrhages are seen (72),(124). Special techniques for processing brain biopsy specimens are often necessary (see Brain Biopsy Section). Differentiation from lymphoma may be especially difficult when the organism is not visualized (4),(7),(8),(10).

Presumptive clinical diagnosis is made by finding multiple enhancing hypodense or nodular lesions on CT combined with a positive serum serology. Since most patients with toxoplasmosis have persistently low titers (81) without either an IgM antibody response or a four fold rise in titer, brain biopsy is often necessary to confirm the diagnosis. An alternative practical approach is to treat empirically for two weeks, gauging clinical and CT response. Biopsy becomes imperative, however, in patients with a rapidly deteriorating clinical course or when there is no evidence of clinical or radiographic response to therapy. In affected Haitians and parenteral drug abusers where the incidence of toxoplasmosis is especially high, empiric drug treatment is more likely to succeed (13),(15),(119),(122).

Standard treatment is with pyrimethamine and a sulfonamide, but in patients who fail to respond, or who develop a medication allergy, clindamycin or spiramycin has been used (87),(125). Successful desensitization to sulfadiazine has been accomplished using dexamethasone and a gradually increasing sulfonamide dosage (126). In a series of 27 patients reported by Navia et al. (81), 18 responded favorably to treatment, but four relapsed on pyrimethamine alone. Since the organism appears to persist despite an apparent therapeutic response, lifelong treatment is recommended (81),(82),(122).

Mycobacterial Infection

Disseminated mycobacterial infections of all types are seen in AIDS patients, especially Haitians (69) and intravenous drug abusers (127). Despite the high incidence of systemic mycobacterial infection, CNS involvement is uncommon and usually takes the form of abscesses (3),(10),(13),(19),(20),(72),(100), although meningitis due to *Mycobacterium tuberculosis* (12),(100),(112),(128), *M. avium-intracellulare* (7),(50) and *M. kansasii* (4) has been reported. Coinfection with toxoplasma (3),(13),(15),(19),(20), and cryptococcus (11) may also occur. *M. tuberculosis* infections are usually responsive to therapy while atypical mycobacteria may be resistant to antituberculous drugs and often persist during drug treatment (11),(15),(100),(128).

Bacterial Infection

As in other settings in which acquired immunosuppression occurs, such as following transplantation, bacterial infections of the CNS are uncommon in AIDS. However meningitis caused by *Escherichia coli* (15),(16),(20),(54) or *Hemophilus influenzae* (55), and abscesses due to salmonella (19), *Staphylococcus epidermidis* (94), *Streptococcus mitis* (9) and *Streptococcus pneumoniae* (112) have been reported. Gram-negative organisms are especially prevalent in children (112). Bacterial infection complicating brain tumor or opportunistic infections has been found at postmortem examination but is usually not diagnosed during life (4),(19,(46),(92),(94), (129).

Fungal Infection

The majority of CNS fungal infections are due to *Cryptococcus neoformans* which usually causes meningitis (3),(4),(7),(8),(10)-(14),(20),(98),(109). Occasionally, cryptococcal brain involvement is associated with the formation of cryptococcomas (4),(8),(46) (Figure 2). Cryptococcal infection responds variably to treatment with amphotericin B with or without the addition of 5-flucytosine, but organisms are rarely eradicated completely. Consequently, treatment should be continued indefinitely .

Coccidioidomycosis was discovered in the brain of one patient at autopsy (3), and an agent of mucormycosis was grown from two cerebral lesions (130). Candida may result in abscess formation (1),(3),(4),(7),(10),(92),(94),(131), and candida meningitis has occurred in two children (54),(132). There are rare reports of aspergillus infection (49),(53),(133), and nocardia was described once (19).

TUMOR

Primary brain lymphoma occurs with increased frequency in AIDS patients (17),(60),(78) but not as frequently as has been observed in transplant recipients (124). This difference may result from: 1) the shorter life span of AIDS patients; 2) the relative lack of B cell stimulation in the absence of a donated organ; or 3) the overall lower incidence of oncogenic viral infection in AIDS patients (124). Nonetheless, brain tumor occurs sufficiently often in AIDS patients to warrant a high index of suspicion in appropriate cases.

Nervous system involvement by malignancy presents as headache and confusion, seizures, cranial neuropathies, radiculopathy or plexopathy. Tumor may be primary or metastatic, and may involve the brain parenchyma, meninges or paraspinal areas (3),(4),(7),(18),(57),(58),(60),(78)-(80),(134),(135). CT scans demonstrate isodense or slightly hyperdense lesions which enhance substantially (84),(136) (Figure 3). Mass effect is usually evident. CNS lymphoma is treated with whole brain irradiation using a total dose of 3500-4000 Gy (136). Intrathecal methotrexate or cytosine arabinoside has had limited success with meningeal disease (57),(60),(136), and drug-related necrotizing leukoencephalopathy caused death in one case.

Kaposi's sarcoma only rarely metastasizes to brain and responds poorly to radiation (3),(10),(73),(137). Metastatic rhabdomyosarcoma has also been reported (138). Epidural spinal cord compression caused by sarcoma (7) and plasmacytoma (64) has been treated by surgical decompression and radiation.

DRUG REACTIONS AND TOXICITY

Chemotherapy may cause or contribute to peripheral neuropathy, especially when vincristine is used. Isoniazid is neurotoxic, especially if supplemental pyridoxine is omitted (35). Hexachlorophene may be related to vacuolar myelopathy in some patients (66). Other pertinent toxic effects from medications that have been reported include orofacial dyskinesias from phenytoin (4), pentamidine-induced hypoglycemia (139), and probable malignant neuroleptic syndrome (67).

SUMMARY

The nervous system is commonly involved in patients with AIDS, and vigilance in looking for early signs and symptoms should facilitate diagnosis at a time when specific treatment for opportunistic infections may be of benefit. Nevertheless, the ultimate prognosis remains poor in the face of the overwhelming immunodeficiency. Ultimately, prevention of HIV infection altogether or eradication of the virus before it has become entrenched may be the most meaningful approaches to management. To achieve these goals, there must be awareness of the special status of the brain, especially regarding its early involvement in HIV infections, and the special therapeutic problems caused by the blood-brain barrier.

REFERENCES

1. Lemann, W., Cho, E-S., Nielsen, S., et al., Neuropathologic (NP) findings in 104 cases of acquired immune deficiency syndrome (AIDS): an autopsy study. J Neuropath Exp Neurol 44:349 (1985)

2. Price, R.W., Navia, B.A., Cho, E-S., AIDS encephalopathy. Neurol Clinics 4:285-301 (1986)

3. Levy, R.M., Bredesen, D.E., Rosenblum ML. Neurological manifestations of the acquired immunodeficiency syndrome (AIDS): experience at UCSF and review of the literature. J Neurosurg 62:475-495 (1985)

4. Koppel, B.S., Wormser, G.P., Tuchman, A.J., et al., Central nervous system involvement in patients with acquired immune deficiency syndrome (AIDS). Acta Neurol Scand 71:337-353 (1985)

5. Bredesen, D.E., Messing, R., Neurological syndromes heralding the acquired immune deficiency syndrome. Ann Neurol 14:141 (1983)

6. Marion, R., Wisnic, A., Hutcheon, R.G., et al., The AIDS embyropathy; a new dysmorphic syndrome in children with AIDS. Ped Res 20 (4): 339 (1986)

7. Snider, W.D., Simpson, D.M., Nielsen, S., et al., Neurological complications of acquired immune deficiency syndrome: analysis of 50 patients. Ann Neurol 14:403-418 (1983)

8. Whelan, M., Kricheff, I., Handler, M., et al., Acquired immunodeficiency syndrome: cerebral computed tomographic manifestations. Radiology 149:477-484 (1983)

9. Reichert, C.M., O'Leary, T.J., Levens, D.L., et al., Autopsy pathology in the acquired immune deficiency syndrome. Am J Pathol 112:357-382 (1983).

10. Kelly, W.M., Brant-Zawadzki, M., Acquired immunodeficiency syndrome: neuroradiologic findings. Radiology 149: 485-491 (1983)

11. Gopinathan, G., Laubenstein, L., Mondale, B., CNS manifestations of the acquired immunodeficiency syndrome in homosexual men. Neurology 33:105 (1983)

12. Grenell, S.L., Small, C.B., Harris, C.A., et al., Central nervous system (CNS) infections in acquired immune deficiency syndrome (AIDS). Interscience Conference on Antimicrobial Agents and Chemotherapy, Las Vegas, Nevada (1983)

13. Pitchenik, A., Fischl, M., Walls, K., Evaluation of cerebral mass lesions in acquired immunodeficiency syndrome. N Engl J Med 308:1099 (1983)

14. Pitlik, S.D., Fainstein, V., Bolivan, R., et al., Spectrum of central nervous system complications in homosexual men with acquired immune deficiency syndrome. J Infect Dis 148:771-772 (1983)

15. Moskowitz, L.B., Hensley, G.T., Chan, J.C., et al., The neuropathology of acquired immune deficiency syndrome. Arch Pathol Lab Med 108: 867-872 (1984)

16. Welch, K., Finkbeiner, W., Alpers, C.E., et al., Autopsy findings in the acquired immune deficiency syndrome. JAMA 252:1152-1159 (1984)

17. Urmacher, C., Nielsen, S., The histopathology of the acquired immune deficiency syndrome. Pathol Annu 20:197-220 (1985)

18. Elkin, C.M., Leon, E., Grenell, S.L., et al., Intracranial lesions in the acquired immunodeficiency syndrome. Radiological (computed tomographic) features. JAMA 253:393-396 (1985)

19. Sharer, L.R., Kapila, R., Neuropathologic observations in acquired immunedeficiency syndrome (AIDS). Acta Neuropathol (Berl) 66:188-198 (1985)

20. Post, M.J.D., Kursunoglu, S.J., Hensley, G.T., et al., Cranial CT in acquired immunodeficiency syndrome: spectrum of diseases and optimal contrast enhancement technique. Am J Roentgen 145: 929-940 (1985)

21. Sharer, L.R., Epstein, L.G., Joshi, V.V., et al., Neuropathological observations in children with acquired immune deficiency syndrome and with HTLV-III infection of brain. J Neuropathol Exp Neurol 44:350 (1985)

22. DeJarlais, D.C., Marmor, M., Thomas, P., et al., Kaposi's sarcoma among four different AIDS risk groups. N Engl J Med 310:119 (1984)

23. Quinnan, G.V., Jr, Masur, H., Rook, A.H., et al., Herpesvirus infections in the acquired immune deficiency syndrome. JAMA 252:72-79 (1984)

24. Drew, W.L., Miner, R.C., Ziegler, J.L., et al., CMV and Kaposi's sarcoma in young homosexual men. Lancet 2:125-127 (1982)

25. Hill, J.M., Farrar, W.L., Pert, C.B., Localization of the T4 antigen/AIDS virus receptor in monkey and rat brain: prominence in cortical regions. Psychopharmacol Bull 22 (In press)

26. Bredesen, D.E., Lipkin, W.I., Messing R. Prolonged, recurrent aseptic meningitis with prominent cranial nerve abnormalities: a new epidemic in gay men? Neurology 33 (Suppl 2):85 (1983)

27. Levy, J.A., Hollander, H., Shimabukuro, J., et al., Isolation of AIDS-associated retroviruses from cerebrospinal fluid and brain of patients with neurological symptoms. Lancet 2:586-588 (1985)

28. Ho, D.D., Roth, T.R., Schooley, R.T., et al., Isolation of HTLV-III from cerebrospinal fluid and neural tissues of patients with neurologic symptoms related to the acquired immunodeficiency syndrome. N Engl J Med 313:1493-1498 (1985)

29. Lipkin, W.I., Parry, G.J., Subacute polyneuropathy in homosexual males. Neurology 34 (Suppl 1): 135 (1984)

30. Cornbath, D.R., McArthur, J.C., Griffin, J.W., Inflammatory demyelinating polyneuropathies associated with AIDS-related virus (ARV) infection. Neurology (Supp 1) 36: 206 (1986)

31. Cone, L.A., Schiffman, M.A., Herpes zoster and the acquired immune deficiency syndrome. Ann Intern Med 100:426 (1984)

32. Sandor, E., Croxson, T.S., Millman, A., et al., Herpes zoster ophthalmicus in patients at risk for AIDS. N Engl J Med 310: 118-119 (1984)

33. Cole, L.E., Meisler, D.M., Calabrese, L.H., et al., Herpes zoster ophthalmicus and acquired immune deficiency syndrome. Arch Ophthamol 102:1027-1029 (1984)

34. Jordan, B.A., Posner, J.B., "Subacute encephalitis" in acquired immune deficiency syndrome (AIDS): clinical findings in 18 patients. Neurology 34 (Suppl 1):135 (1984)

35. Goldstick, L., Mandybur, T.I., Bode, R., Spinal cord degeneration in AIDS. Neurology 35: 103-106 (1985)

36. Petito, C.K., Navia, B.A., Cho, E-S., et al., Vacuolar myelopathy pathologically resembling subacute combined degeneration in patients with the acquired immunodeficiency syndrome. N Engl J Med 312:874-879 (1985)

37. Singh, B.M., Levine, S., Yarrish, R.L., et al., Spinal cord syndromes in the acquired immune deficiency syndrome. Acta Neurol Scand 73:590-598 (1986)

38. Sharer, L.R., Cho, E-S., Epstein, L.G., Multinucleated giant cells and HTLV-III in AIDS encephalopathy. Hum Pathol 16:760 (1985)

39. Shaw, G.M., Harper, M.E., Hahn, B.H., et al., HTLV-III infection in brains of children and adults with AIDS encephalopathy. Science 227:177-181 (1985)

40. Resnick, L., DiMarzo-Veronese, F., Schuphean, V., et al., Intra-blood-brain-barrier synthesis of HTLV-III specific IgG in patients with neurologic symptoms associated with AIDS or AIDS-related complex. N Engl J Med 313:1498-1504 (1985)

41. Mirra, S.S., Anand, R., Spira, T.J., HTLV-III/LAV infection of the central nervous system in a 57-year-old man with progressive dementia of unknown cause. N Engl J Med 314:1191-1192 (1986)

42. Wiley, C.A., Schrier, R.D., Denaro, F.J., et al., Localization within the CNS of cytomegalovirus proteins and genome during fulminant infection in an AIDS patient. J Neuropathol Exp Neurol 44:350 (1985)

43. Morgello, S., Cho, L., Nielsen, S., et al., The pathology of cytomegalovirus (CMV) encephalitis: a review of 30 autopsy cases. J Neuropathol Exp Neurol 44:350 (1985)

44. Hawley, D.A., Schaefer, J.S., Schulz, D.M., et al., Cytomegalovirus encephalitis in acquired immunodeficiency syndrome. Am J Clin Pathol 80:874-877 (1983)

45. Garcia, I., Fainstein, V., Rios, A., et al., Nonbacterial thrombotic endocarditis in a male homosexual with Kaposi's sarcoma. Arch Intern Med 143:1243-1244 (1983)

46. Mobley, K., Rotterdam, H.Z., Lerner, C.W., et al., Autopsy findings in the acquired immune deficiency syndrome. Pathol Annu 20:45-65 (1985)

47. Navia, B.A., Jordan, B.D., Cho, E-S., et al., Acquired immune deficiency syndrome dementia: clinicopathological analysis. Neurology 35 (Suppl 1): 145 (1985)

48. Britton, C.B., Miller, J.R., Neurologic complications in acquired immunodeficiency syndrome (AIDS). Neurol Clinics 2: 315-339 (1984)

49. Gapen, P., Neurological complications now characterizing many AIDS victims. JAMA 248:2941-2942 (1982)

50. Zakowski, P., Fligiel, S., Berlin, G.W., et al., Disseminated *Mycobacterium avium-intracellulare* infection in homosexual men dying of acquired immunodeficiency. JAMA 248:2980-2982 (1982)

51. Horoupian, D.S., Pick, D., Spigland, I., et al., Acquired immune deficiency syndrome and multiple tract degeneration in a homosexual man. Ann Neurol 15:502-505 (1984)

52. Edwards, R.H., Messing, R., McKendall, R.R., Cytomegalovirus meningoencephalitis in a homosexual man with Kaposi's sarcoma: isolation of CMV from CSF cells. Neurology 35:560-562 (1985)

53. Berger, J.R., Moskowitz, L., Fischl, M., et al., The neurologic complications of AIDS: frequently the initial manifestation. Neurology 34 (Supp 1):134 (1984)

54. Belman, A.L., Ultmann, M.H., Horoupian, D., et al., Neurological complications in infants and children with acquired immune deficiency syndrome. Ann Neurol 18: 560-566 (1985)

55. Epstein, L.G., Sharer, L.R., Joshi, V.V., et al., Progressive encephalopathy in children with acquired immune deficiency syndrome. Ann Neurol 17:488-496 (1985)

56. Hoffman, P.M., Festoff, B.W., Giron, L.T., Jr., et al., Isolation of LAV/HTLV-III from a patient with amyotrophic lateral syndrome. N Engl J Med 313:324-325 (1985)

57. Jack, M.K., Smith, T., Collier, A.C., Oculomotor cranial nerve palsy associated with acquired immunodeficiency syndrome. Ann Ophthalmol 16:460-462 (1984)

58. CPC 32-1983. A 31-year-old man with persistent fever and cranial nerve defects. N Engl J Med 309:359-369 (1983)

59. Lozada, F., Silverman, Jr. S., Conant, M., New outbreak of oral tumors, malignancies and infectious diseases strikes young male homosexuals. J Canad Dent Assoc 19:39-42 (1982)

60. Ziegler, J.L., Beckstend, J.A., Vodberdin, P.A., et al., Non-Hodgkin's lymphoma in 90 homosexual men. N Engl J Med 311: 565-570 (1984)

61. Tucker, T., Dix, R.D., Katzen, C., et al., Cytomegalovirus and *Herpes simplex* virus ascending myelitis in a patient with acquired immune deficiency syndrome. Ann Neurol 18:74-79 (1985)

62. Britton, C.B., Mesa-Tejada, R., Fenoglio, C.M., et al., A new complication of AIDS: thoracic myelitis caused by *Herpes simplex* virus. Neurology 35:1071-1074 (1985)

63. Herman, P., Neurologic complications of AIDS. Neurology 33: 105 (1983)

64. Israel, A.M., Koziner, B., Straus, D.J., Plasmacytoma and the acquired immunodeficiency syndrome. Ann Intern Med 99:635-636 (1983)

65. Miller, R.G., Parry, G., Lang, W., et al., AIDS-related inflammatory polyradiculoneuropathy: successful therapy with plasma exchange. Neurology 36 (Suppl 1):206 (1986)

66. Kimbrough, R.D., Vacuolar myelopathy in patients with the acquired immunodeficiency syndrome. N Engl J Med 313:827 (1985)

67. Britton, C.B., Marquardt, M.D., Koppel, B., et al., Neurological complications of the gay immunosuppressed syndrome. Clinical and pathological features. Ann Neurol 12:80 (1982)

68. CPC 2-1986. A 58-year-old woman with fever and nodular pulmonary infiltrates. N Engl J Med 314:167-174 (1986)

69. Pitchenik, A.E., Burr, J., Cole, C.H., Tuberculin testing for persons with positive serologic studies for HTLV-III. N Engl J Med 314:447 (1986)

70. Denton, I.C., Jr, Stevens, E.A., Seidenfeld, S.M., et al., The diagnosis of intracranial lesions in AIDS. JAMA 253:3398 (1985)

71. Bursztyn, E.M., Lee, B.C., Bauman, J., CT of acquired immunodeficiency syndrome. AJNR 5:711-714 (1984)

72. Moskowitz, L.B., Hensley, G.T., Chan, J.C., et al., Brain biopsies in patients with acquired immune deficiency syndrome. Arch Pathol Lab Med 108:368-371 (1984)

73. Post, M.J.D., Sheldon, J.J., Hensley, G.T., et al., Central nervous system disease in acquired immunodeficiency syndrome: prospective correlation using CT, MR imaging and pathologic studies. Radiology 158:141-148 (1986)

74. Zimmerman, R.A., Patel, S., Bilanink, L., Demonstration of purulent bacterial intracranial infections by computed tomography. Am J Roentgen 127:155-165 (1976)

75. Enzmann, D.R., Brant-Zawadzki, M., Britt, R.L.T., Computed tomography of CNS infections in immunocompromised patients. Am J Roentgen 135:263-267 (1980)

76. Bedri, J., Weinstein, W., DeGregorio, P., et al., Progressive multifocal leukoencephalopathy in acquired immunodeficiency syndrome. N Engl J Med 309:492-493 (1983)

77. Alonso, R., Heiman-Patterson, T., Mancall, E.L., Cerebral toxoplasmosis in acquired immune deficiency syndrome. Arch Neurol 41:321-323 (1984)

78. Snider, W.D., Simpson, D.M., Aronyk, K.E., et al., Primary lymphoma of the nervous system associated with acquired immune-deficiency syndrome. N Engl J Med 308:45 (1983)

79. Reyes, C.V., Primary malignant lymphoma of the brain in acquired immune deficiency syndrome. Acta Cytologica 29: 85-86 (1985)

80. Shiach, C.R., Burt, A.D., Isles, C.G., et al., Pyrexia of undetermined origin, diarrhoea, and primary cerebral lymphoma associated with acquired immunodeficiency. Br Med J 288:449-450 (1984)

81. Navia, B.A., Petito, C.K., Gold, J.W.M., et al., Cerebral toxoplasmosis complicating the acquired immune deficiency syndrome: clinical and neuropathological findings in 27 patients. Ann Neurol 19:224-238 (1986)

82. Emerson, R.G., Jardine, D.S., Milvenan, E.S., et al., Toxoplasmosis: a treatable neurologic disease in the immunologically compromised patients. Pediatrics 67:653-655 (1981)

83. Cohen, W., Koslow, M., An unusual CT presentation of cerebral toxoplasmosis. J Computed Assist Tomogr 9:384-386 (1985)

84. Brant-Zawadzki, M., Enzmann, D.R., Computed tomographic brain scanning in patients with lymphoma. Radiology 129:67-71 (1978)

85. Trautmann, M., Kluge, W., Otto, H-S., et al., Computed tomography in CNS tuberculosis. Eur Neurol 25:91-97 (1986)

86. Wormser, G.P., Multiple opportunistic infections and neoplasms in the acquired immunodeficiency syndrome. JAMA 253: 3441-3442 (1985)

87. Roue, R., Debord, T., Denamur, E., et al., Diagnosis of toxoplasma encephalitis in absence of neurologic signs by early computed tomographic scanning in patients with AIDS. Lancet 2:1472 (1984)

88. Zee, C-S., Segall, H.D., Rogers, C., et al., Imaging of cerebral toxoplasmosis: correlation of computed tomography and pathology. J Computed Assist Tomogr 9:797-799 (1985)

89. Navia, B.A., Rottenberg, D.A., Sidkis, J., et al., Regional cerebral glucose metabolism in AIDS dementia. Neurology 35 (Suppl 1): 233-234 (1985)

90. Enzensberger, W., Fischer, P-A., Helm, E.B., et al., Value of electroencephalography in AIDS. Lancet 1:1047-1048 (1985)

91. Miller, J., Barrett, R., Britton, C.B., et al., Progressive multifocal leukoencephalopathy in a male homosexual with T-cell immune deficiency. N Engl J Med 307:1436-1438 (1982)

92. Levy, R.M., Pons, V.G., Rosenblum, M.L., Central nervous system mass lesions in the acquired immunodeficiency syndrome (AIDS). J Neurosurg 61:9-16 (1984)

93. Stahl, R.E., Omar, R.A., Wormser, G.P., Fungal stains in the acquired immunodeficiency syndrome. Ann Intern Med 102:413 (1985)

94. Pitlik, S.D, Rios, A., Hersh, E.M., et al., Polymicrobial brain abscess in a homosexual man with Kaposi's sarcoma. South Med J 77:271-272 (1984)

95. Bottone, E.J., Toma, M., Johansson, B.E., et al., Capsule-deficient *Cryptococcus neoformans* in AIDS patients. Lancet 1:400 (1985)

96. Chandler, W.F, Knake, J.E., McGillicuddy, J.E., et al., Intraoperative use of real-time ultrasonography in neurosurgery. J Neurosurg 57:157-163 (1982)

97. Cerezo, L., Alvarez, M., Price, G., Electron microscopic diagnosis of cerebral toxoplasmosis. J Neurosurg 63:470-472 (1985)

98. Luft, B.J., Brooks, R.G., Conley, F.K., et al., Toxoplasmic encephalitis in patients with acquired immune deficiency syndrome. JAMA 252:913-917 (1984)

99. Hauser, W., Luft, B., Conley, F., et al., Central nervous system toxoplasmosis in homosexual and heterosexual adults. N Engl J Med 307:498-499 (1982)

100. Fischl, M.A., Pitchenik, A.E., Spira, T.A., Tuberculous brain abscess and toxoplasma encephalitis in a patient with the acquired immunodeficiency syndrome. JAMA 253:3428-3430 (1985)

101. Nielson, S.L., Petito, C.K., Urmacher, C.D., et al., Subacute encephalitis in acquired immune deficiency syndrome: a postmortem study. Am J Clin Pathol 82:678-682 (1984)

102. Munoz-Garcia, D., Pendlebury, W., Perl, D.P., et al., Subacute encephalitis in AIDS: ultrastructural demonstration of cytomegalovirus in brain. J Neuropathol Exp Neurol 44:349 (1985)

103. Chou, S.W., Dylewski, J.S., Gaynon, M.W., et al., Alpha-interferon administration in cytomegalovirus retinitis. Antimicrob Agents Chemother 25:25-28 (1984)

104. Moskowitz, L.B., Gregorios, J.B., Hensley, G.T., et al., Cytomegalovirus: induced demyelination associated with acquired immune deficiency syndrome. Arch Pathol Lab Med 108:873-877 (1984)

105. Lane, H.C., Masur, H., Longo, D.L., et al., Partial immune reconstitution in a patient with the acquired immunodeficiency syndrome. N Engl J Med 311:1099-1103 (1984)

106. Jordan, W.C., Hepatitis B immune globulin as treatment of CMV infections in patients with AIDS. J Natl Med Assoc 78:61-62 (1986)

107. Collaborative DHPG Treatment Study Group, Treatment of serious cytomegalovirus infections with 9-(1,3-dihydroxy-2-propoxymethyl) guanine in patients with AIDS and other immunodeficiencies. N Engl J Med 314:801-805 (1986)

108. Dix, R.D., Waitzman, D.M., Follansbee, S., et al., *Herpes simplex* virus type 2 encephalitis in two homosexual men with persistent lymphadenopathy. Ann Neurol 17:203-206 (1985)

109. Follansbee, S.E., Busch, D.F., Wofsy, C.B., et al., An outbreak of *Pneumocystis carinii* pneumonia in homosexual men. Ann Intern Med 96:705-713 (1982)

110. Siegal, F.P., Lopez, C., Hammer, G.S., Severe acquired immunodeficiency in male homosexuals, manifested by chronic perianal ulcerative *Herpes simplex* lesions. N Engl J Med 305:1439-1444 (1981)

111. Ryder, J.W., Croen, K., Kleinschmidt-DeMasters, B.K., et al., Progressive encephalitis three months after resolution of cutaneous zoster in a patient with AIDS. Ann Neurol 19:182-188 (1986)

112. Scott, G.B., Buck, B.E., Leterman, J.G., et al., Acquired immunodeficiency syndrome in infants. N Engl J Med 310:76-81 (1984)

113. Whitley, R.J., Alford, C.A., Hirsch, M.S., et al., Vidarabine versus acyclovir therapy in *Herpes simplex* encephalitis. N Engl J Med 314:144-149 (1986)

114. Bernick, C., Gregorios, J.B., Progressive multifocal leukoencephalopathy in a patient with acquired immune deficiency syndrome. Arch Neurol 41:780-782 (1984)

115. Blum, L.W., Chambers, R.A., Schwartzman, R.J., et al., Progressive multifocal leukoencephalopathy in acquired immune deficiency syndrome. Arch Neurol 42:137-139 (1985)

116. Ho, J.L., Poldre, P.A., McEniry, D., et al., Acquired immunodeficiency syndrome with progressive multifocal leukoencephalopathy and monoclonal B-cell proliferation. Ann Intern Med 100:693-696 (1984)

117. Krupp, L.B., Lipton, R.B., Swerdlow, M.L., et al., Progressive multifocal leukoencephalopathy: clinical and radiographic features. Ann Neurol 17:344-349 (1985)

118. Handler, M., Ho., V., Whelan, M., et al., Intracerebral toxoplasmosis in patients with acquired immune deficiency syndrome. J Neurosurg 59:994-1001 (1983)

119. Post, M.J.D., Chan, J.C., Hensley, G.T., et al., Toxoplasma encephalitis in Haitian adults with acquired immunodeficiency syndrome: a clinico-pathological-CT correlation. Am J Roentgen 140:861-868 (1983)

120. Horowitz, S.L., Bentson, J.R., Benson, D.F., et al., CNS toxoplasmosis in acquired immunodeficiency syndrome. Arch Neurol 40:649-652 (1983)

121. Moskopp, D., AIDS with central nervous system toxoplasmosis. J Neurosurg 62:459-460 (1985)

122. Wong, B., Gold, J.W.M., Brown, A.E., et al., Central nervous system toxoplasmosis in homosexual men and parenteral drug abusers. Ann Intern Med 100:36-42 (1984)

123. Milligan, S.A., Katz, M.S., Craven, P.C., et al., Toxoplasmosis presenting as panhypopituitarism in a patient with the acquired immune deficiency syndrome. Am J Med 77:760-764 (1984)

124. Millard, P.R., AIDS: histopathologic aspects. J Pathol 143: 223-239 (1984)

125. Editor. Drugs for parasitic infections. Med Letter 28:9-16 (1986)

126. Bell, E.T., Tapper, M.L., Pollack, A.A., Sulphadiazine desensitization in AIDS patients. Lancet 1:163 (1985)

127. Maayan, S., Wormser, G.P., Hewlett, D., et al., Acquired immunodeficiency syndrome (AIDS) in an economically disadvantaged population. Arch Intern Med 145:1607-1612 (1985)

128. Duncanson, F.P., Hewlett, D., Maayan, S., et al., *Mycobacterium tuberculosis* infection in the acquired immunodeficiency syndrome. A review of 14 patients. Tubercle (In press)

129. Hui, A.N., Koss, M.N., Meyer, P.R., Necropsy findings in acquired immune deficiency syndrome: a comparison of premortem diagnoses with postmortem findings. Hum Pathol 15:670-676 (1984)

130. Micozzi, M.S., Wetli, C.V., Intravenous amphetamine abuse, primary cerebral mucormycosis, and acquired immunodeficiency. J Forensic Sci 30:504-510 (1985)

131. Burkes, R.L., Gal, A.A., Stewart, M.L., et al., Simultaneous occurrence of *Pneumocystis carinii* pneumonia, cytomegalovirus infection, Kaposi's sarcoma and B-immunoblastic sarcoma in homosexual men. JAMA 253:3425-3428 (1985)

132. Oleske, J., Minnefor, A., Cooper, R., Jr., et al., Immune deficiency syndrome in children. JAMA 249:2345-2349 (1983)

133. Lissen, E., Wichmann, I., Jiminez, J.M., AIDS in hemophilia patients in Spain. Lancet 1:992-993 (1983)

134. Payan, M.J., Gambarelli, D., Routy, J.P., et al., Primary lymphoma of the brain associated with AIDS. Acta Neuropathol (Berl) 64:78-80 (1984)

135. Bates, S., McKeever, P., Masur, H., et al., Myelopathy following intrathecal chemotherapy in a patient with extensive Burkitt's lymphoma and altered immune status. Am J Med 78:697-702 (1985)

136. Kawakami, Y., Tabuchi, K., Ohnishi, R., et al., Primary central nervous system lymphoma. J Neurosurg 62:522-527 (1985)

137. Gorin, F.A., Bale, J.F., Halks-Miller, M., et al., Kaposi's sarcoma metastatic to the CNS. Arch Neurol 42:162-165 (1985)

138. CPC 9-1986. A 40 month-old girl with the acquired immunodeficiency syndrome and spinal cord compression. N Engl J Med 314:629-640 (1986)

139. Sands, M., Kron, M.A., Brown, R.B., Pentamidine: a review. Rev Infect Dis 7:625-634 (1985)

29
Psychiatric Aspects of AIDS: A Biopsychosocial Approach

Mary Ann Adler Cohen

The acquired immunodeficiency syndrome (AIDS) may be thought of as a paradigm of a medical problem that requires a coordinated, humane, comprehensive, holistic, and biopsychosocial approach (1)-(4). AIDS has created a multidimensional crisis affecting not only persons with AIDS, but also their loved ones, caregivers, and communities. The crisis is one of fear, anxiety and uncertainty. Persons with AIDS are overwhelmed by devastating illnesses that result in profound emaciation, weakness, depression, confusion, pain, disfigurement and, ultimately, death (5). Persons with AIDS have a disease that, until now, is considered to be uniformly fatal, with a mean survival time of less than eight months after hospitalization for an opportunistic infection, even with optimal treatment (6). There is no effective therapy for the underlying immunodeficiency (7) or for the retrovirus identified as the causative organism for AIDS, human immunodeficiency virus (HIV) (8)-(13). The outlook for an AIDS vaccine is uncertain (14),(15). It has been estimated that almost 1.8 million United States' residents may be infected with HIV (16). In 1986 alone, it is predicted that 16,000 new AIDS cases will be diagnosed (17). This number is approximately equal to the number of persons diagnosed from 1978 until 1985 (18)-(22).

Most AIDS victims are members of risk groups such as gay or bisexual men and intravenous drug users. Many of them may have felt alienated from society even before developing AIDS because of the homophobia, discrimination and cruelty that they may have experienced. The diagnosis of AIDS leads to further alienation since families, loved ones, friends and even health professionals may be frightened of contagion.

Both health care personnel and patients are often overwhelmed by the sheer magnitude of problems as well as the psychological reactions encountered. The nature and severity of the illnesses that comprise AIDS diminish the individual's capacity to cope. Severe and multiple illnesses often involving many organ systems may overwhelm the patient. Caregivers are also overwhelmed by the multiplicity and severity of their patient's medical, psychological and social problems. Caregivers are also faced with the lack of adequate and available medical treatments, social support systems and community resources for on-going care. This may result in a crisis of shared hopelessness, helplessness and despair. There is a need for a biopsychosocial approach to understand the crisis of AIDS and to develop new coping strategies.

COPING WITH AIDS

Serious illness can be understood as a life crisis. Any severe physical illness, especially a life-threatening illness, has a profound impact on its victims.

> "A person may face separation from family and friends, the loss of key roles in his or her life, permanent changes in appearance or in bodily functions, assaults on self-image and self-esteem, distressing feelings of anxiety, guilt, anger or helplessness and an uncertain unpredictable future." (23)

Although these words were written prior to the AIDS epidemic, they apply only too well to the crisis of AIDS. People with AIDS are overwhelmed with severe and multiple illnesses, decreased cognitive functioning, devastating weakness, weight loss, fevers, cancers, opportunistic infections, disfigurement, pain and psychiatric disorders (24). Upon learning the diagnosis of AIDS, each person is faced with severe anxiety, fears of unknown illnesses, unknown treatments, unlikely cure and early death. Any severe illness constitutes a loss of health and the usual reaction to loss is grief or bereavement.

Coping with the crisis presented by severe life-threatening illness depends on several important adaptive tasks. The first and most crucial step is a cognitive appraisal of the crisis. It is the cognitive appraisal, or the perception of adaptive tasks and selection of appropriate coping skills, that determines the outcome of the crisis. In AIDS, even the initial step, the cognitive appraisal of the significance of the illness, may be hampered because of the diminished cognitive capacities (25)-(29) associated with the illnesses that comprise the syndrome as well as the affinity of HIV for brain tissue (30)-(32). The following case illustrates this problem.

Case 1: The patient was a 32 year old separated, unemployed former waitress who was an intravenous drug user diagnosed as having AIDS on the basis of *Pneumocystis* *carinii* pneumonia. She had difficulty accepting her diagnosis and was found to have impairment of memory and immediate recall. Her cognitive deficits combined with use of massive denial resulted in difficulties in adherence to medical regimen and plans for on-going care following her initial illness and treatments. She was readmitted later for subacute bacterial endocarditis. During her second admission, she denied ever having been told that she had AIDS. She stated that if her doctors had informed her of her diagnosis she would have abstained from needle-sharing. The patient agreed to return for follow up as an out-patient, but returned in respiratory distress. On her third, and last admission, the patient was suspected of having *P. carinii* pneumonia. She was seen prior to intubation. She was still unaware of her diagnosis. She died on the night of this admission.

This clinical vignette illustrates the problem of cognitive appraisal when there is a diminution of cognitive capacity. The patient reacted with shock, disbelief, denial and anger that "no one told me, until now" during each of her admissions. She could not adhere to suggestions for follow-up care, safe sex or abstinence from intravenous drug use. Her illness was complicated by the psychiatric diagnoses of delirium and dementia as well as denial and anosognosia (the inability to recognize disease or physical disability). Her follow-up was further complicated by her fugitive status and her reluctance to give information about the whereabouts of her family.

The special adaptations required by the AIDS crisis have been described (33) as:

Initial crisis - catastrophic effect
Transitional state
Deficiency state
Preparation for death

Initial Crisis

This stage is characterized by catastrophic effects on patients and on their loved ones, as in any severe, life-threatening illness. Patients may react with denial alternating with intense anxiety (34)-(36). They may move rapidly from shock and denial to guilt, fear, sadness, anger, bargaining and acceptance (37),(38). Families and loved ones go through very similar reactions. However, with AIDS, the reactions may be more intense and more negative because of fear of transmission as well as discrimination, homophobia and sexual taboos.

Intravenous drug users may be depressed and self-destructive individuals who have effectively severed the bond that linked them with their families and communities. Because of their antisocial behavior, they may have incurred the anger of their loved ones and may have spent time in prison for crimes associated with buying or selling drugs. They may perceive that they are unwanted and expendable. This perception may indeed be confirmed by their families and friends. In some situations it is possible to intervene and reunite a family after many years of separation. In others, the bonds have been severed and intervention may not be effective. The following case vignette illustrates an example of a successful intervention.

> **Case 2:** The patient was a 29 year old gay gymnastics instructor who was diagnosed as having AIDS on the basis of Kaposi's sarcoma. The patient's parents were unaware of his homosexuality. With support from his caregivers, the patient informed his parents of his diagnosis and his homosexuality. They were supportive and accepting. The family mobilized rapidly and lovingly divided tasks. They cooked his favorite foods and brought him objects from home. He was surrounded by his family every day he was in the hospital. The family made plans to care for him upon his discharge and provided him with the love, support and acceptance he desperately needed.

It is obvious that intervention is not always successful. However, when it is effective, the support from family and loved ones can make the difference between dying with despair and dying with dignity and love. The fact that it does not always work is never a reason not to try. The support and caring that comes from the staff even when there is an unsuccessful intervention can help the patient by increasing his or her self-respect.

The initial crisis period is an ideal time to begin to provide education, support, and therapy as well as whatever legal and financial assistance that may be needed. Often, when families and patients are reassured that AIDS is not transmissible by casual contact, they are able to provide the patient with the care and support needed.

Transitional State

Individuals with AIDS may experience feelings of anger, guilt, self-pity and anxiety. In reviewing the past, they may go through a period of distress, confusion and self-devaluation. During this time, lowered self-esteem, alterations in sense of identity and values as well as estrangement and alienation from families and loved ones may lead to suicidal ideas. Anger may be turned against the self accompanied by withdrawal, depression and suicide attempts. Anger may be projected or displaced onto family, loved ones and caregivers. It may result in acting out sexually or through increased use of drugs in intravenous drug users. The transition from being a healthy individual to acceptance of the illness role may be stormy. Once again, this is a time that crisis intervention, communication and support are crucial. A clinical vignette illustrates a transition made by a gay man who reacted to his growing understanding of his illness with a resurgence of homophobia, rage, shame and renunciation of his sexuality.

Case 3: The patient was a 35 year-old gay factory worker who was diagnosed as having AIDS on the basis of Kaposi's sarcoma. When he was hospitalized for the first time, he was found to have cryptococcal meningitis. He had been in a long-term monogamous relationship until his lover left him six years prior to his illness. For several years after that loss the patient had multiple partners, making certain not to become attached for fear of rejection. Upon learning the diagnosis, he reacted with initial shock and denial. Later, with support, he began to verbalize his feelings. As denial diminished, he began to express guilt over his homosexuality and swore to abstinence. He reviewed his religious feelings and became more interested in the Catholic religion. A resurgence of spiritual feelings led to a consultation with a spiritual healer. He renounced sexuality in any form and sought consolation from his religion and family.

Deficiency State - Acceptance

Nichols (33) has described this as the formation of a new, stable identity with acceptance of AIDS, and its limitations, accompanied by a conscious effort to live each day fully with a reassessment of the values of courage, commitment, concern for others, and appreciation of quality rather than quantity in living. Often this period is accompanied by a resurgence of spirituality. Individuals begin to feel less victimized by life and less egocentric, deriving satisfaction from altruistic and community activities. They may take an active and responsible role in maintaining health, may experiment with holistic medical practices and may begin to have a fighting spirit toward the illness and physicians.

The following vignette illustrates these issues.

Case 4: The patient was a 40 year-old divorced, social worker and former intravenous drug user. She was the mother of four children and was found to have AIDS on the basis of *P. carinii* pneumonia. She was seen on an on-going basis from the day that her diagnosis was made. She reacted initially with shock and denial. She progressed rapidly to anger and then gradually to acceptance. Within two months after her diagnosis she stated that she felt thankful for her illness. She stated, "I'm grateful to the disease. I know you'll think this is crazy because the disease is terrible, it's worse than leprosy, but I'm actually thankful for the disease.... Before the disease I lived an empty, banal sort of existence.... But since I have the disease, it has made me appreciate the smallest thing." The patient insisted that she found life, her self and her relationships all more meaningful after she developed AIDS. During her hospital course, she developed many relationships with other patients. She attempted to encourage other persons with AIDS to comply with their treatments and to fight their disease.

Preparation for Death

Preparation for death should begin early while individuals have adequate cognitive capacities and ego strengths. Persons with AIDS are confronted, from the day of diagnosis, with anticipation of death. It is common for people to react to learning their diagnosis with an immediate statement indicating their awareness of the fatal prognosis. "If I have AIDS - then let me die now" (39), which is also the title of an article, has been heard by those of us who work with persons with AIDS shortly after diagnosis. Persons with AIDS need to be helped to complete unfinished business, get their affairs in order, write a will, and provide their families and physicians with plans or wishes for their care when they may be too ill to make plans for themselves. They may be encouraged to make plans for a living will and for their funerals. They need to be able to discuss openly feelings and fears of death and dying and of becoming dependent on others for care.

The stages that have been described do not occur in any necessary order, nor do they fit specific time frames. Persons with AIDS, as with any severe illness, move back and forth between stages. Physicians and caregivers can help facilitate transitions for patients and families and enable people to cope better with the devastating process. However, it is important to recognize that AIDS and AIDS-related complex (ARC) are also associated with issues, taboos and prejudices that make coping much more difficult.

Persons with AIDS are confronted with crises of uncertainty, pain, weakness, disfigurement and multiple losses. Losses may include health, fitness, attractiveness, strength, independence, friends, lovers, jobs, homes, money, and ultimately life itself. These stresses and losses are profound and devastating and they are compounded further by societal stigmatization resulting in a sense of alienation and expendability.

Alienation, Expendability and Discrimination

The individual who is faced with a diagnosis of AIDS may be in a crisis of alienation and expendability. Expendability is defined as "designating equipment or men considered replaceable and therefore worth sacrificing to gain an objective" (40). Alienation is defined as "a withdrawing or estrangement, as of the heart or affections" (40). The diagnosis of AIDS leads to alienation since families, friends, loved ones, employers, landlords and even health professionals may be frightened of developing AIDS. Many persons with AIDS have been given both overt and covert messages by families, employers, landlords and communities that they are unwanted. Many had isolated themselves and felt unloved, unwanted and expendable even before developing AIDS. Some were subjected to discrimination because they were members of risk groups initially associated with AIDS.

Case 5: The patient was a 44 year old gay journalist who had Kaposi's sarcoma and AIDS. Prior to his hospital admission, his landlord had attempted to evict him from the apartment where he had lived for 15 years. He sought and obtained legal help and testified from his bedside on his own behalf. The legal battle continued during the course of his hospitalization, providing yet another stress to an individual who was coping with multiple losses.

Many individuals who develop AIDS may be undomiciled. Some individuals have lost their homes and reside at shelters for the homeless. Once a diagnosis of AIDS is confirmed, they are no longer eligible for shelters and have no place to go at all. Some chronic facilities such as nursing homes, chronic care hospitals and homes for the terminally ill, do not accept persons with AIDS. Funeral homes may refuse to provide services. The attitudes of families, landlords, employers, chronic care facilities, health professionals and funeral directors are compounded by discrimination as well as fears and anxieties about the possibility of contagion. As a result, persons with AIDS have problems obtaining health care, finding a place to live while they can still care for themselves, finding a chronic care facility or even a place to die.

Cassens (41) delineates the special social consequences of AIDS for gay men. He states, "In a society that scarcely accepts sexuality, even heterosexuality, the guilt associated with homosexuality and AIDS is crippling.... Persons with anxiety about AIDS frequently respond that they would be embarrassed by the diagnosis.... Guilt further magnifies the sense of isolation and estrangement that many gay men have experienced throughout their lives." He points out that coping is made far more difficult because of the forced disclosure of sexual orientation with secrecy about homosexuality an "impossible luxury". He states, "Landlords evict tenants suspected of carrying the illness, hospital unions seek to exclude persons with AIDS from medical care, and morticians refuse to handle the bodies of those who die of the disease. Even lepers were provided with shelters and support" (41). And Nichols states, "Medicine and its allied professions can help marshal intelligent responses to regressive societal forces unleased by the AIDS dilemma as well as help patients stave off senses of impending doom and hopelessness and accept the losses imposed on them by the disease" (33).

Coping with AIDS, as with any severe illness, can be adaptive or maladaptive. The caregiver can be influential in providing an atmosphere of concern, comfort and support for persons with AIDS and their loved ones. Coping with AIDS is, at times, complicated by the profound psychological reactions associated with AIDS. Recognition of specific psychiatric disorders frequently associated with AIDS is important to provide not only greater understanding of the behavior of persons with AIDS, but also for early recognition and diagnosis of AIDS and for increasing adherence to a medical regimen as well as risk-reduction guidelines.

PSYCHIATRIC DISORDERS ASSOCIATED WITH AIDS

Since HIV has a special affinity for brain and neural tissues (30), it is understandable that early diagnosis and recognition of the syndrome may be made possible through an understanding of the psychopathology associated with AIDS. It is of significance that organic brain syndromes have been described in persons with ARC as well as AIDS (25), (31). Psychiatric diagnoses associated with AIDS are shown in Table 1 (26),(28),(29),(42)-(44). Definitions of psychopathologic disorders associated with AIDS can be found in the Diagnostic and Statistical Manual of Mental Disorders (DSM III) (45).

Psychopathology associated with AIDS may be understood as having several roles in the process of the syndrome. Persons at risk for AIDS, include intravenous drug users. With intravenous drug users who develop AIDS, it can be postulated that psychopathology plays the following roles in the initiation, onset and course of AIDS. The Affective Disorders may play a major role in the initiation of substance abuse. Khantzian has proposed (46) that intravenous drug users are depressed individuals who seek drugs in order to medicate their depression. He and others have proposed the "self-medication" and "drug-of-choice" theories to explain use of intravenous drugs. The association of depression and use of intravenous drugs, as well as the high incidence of suicide in Major Depression and Substance Abuse Disorders, place these individuals at an increased risk for suicide. Easy access to drugs as well as other weapons makes suicide a relatively accessible alternative.

Substance Abuse Disorders entail the use of intravenous drugs and, because of sharing of contaminated needles, play a major part in the transmission of AIDS. Since intravenous drug users may also transmit the disease sexually, and since women may be intravenous drug users, the Substance Abuse Disorders indirectly play a major role in transmission of AIDS to children. The majority of infants and children with AIDS are the offspring of intravenous drug users or of mothers whose partners are intravenous drug users.

The Antisocial Personality Disorder is associated with the buying and selling of illegal drugs. Hence, this disorder may perpetuate the spread of AIDS. The acting out behaviors associated with this disorder may contribute to difficulties with management, disruptive behavior and problems with adherence to a medical regimen. Because of the difficulties, these patients may require special approaches in order to work toward risk-reduction.

The Organic Brain Syndromes associated with intoxication and long-term drug use may also contribute to and confuse the pictures of cognitive dysfunction association with AIDS and ARC. Cognitive dysfunction is a major factor interfering with understanding, coping and adapting to AIDS and ARC and may prevent individuals from learning risk-reduction measures or complying with care.

The psychiatric disorders described above are only the major

Table 1. Psychiatric Disorders Associated with AIDS

Organic Brain Syndromes
- Delirium
- Dementia
- Organic affective syndrome
- Organic delusional syndrome

Affective Disorders
- Major depression
- Dysthymic disorder

Adjustment Disorder
- With depressed mood
- With anxious mood

Substance Abuse Disorders

Anxiety Disorders

Personality Disorders
- Antisocial personality disorder
- Borderline personality disorder

Uncomplicated Bereavement

ones most frequently seen in intravenous drug users, but these serve to provide a profile of how psychopathology may contribute to the etiology and course of AIDS. Furthermore, there is need for further research into the area of psychological co-factors in the cause of AIDS. The effect of separation, loss, depression or stress upon the immune system have been explored by Spitz (47), (48), Engel (49), Schmale (50), Hofer (51), Holmes (52), Rahe (53), and Weiner (54). Silberstein (55) has proposed that the association of stress and depression with alterations of cell-mediated immunity may play a role as a co-factor in the cause of AIDS.

Although it is clear that persons with AIDS and ARC may have no specific psychopathology or any one of the full range of disorders in DSM III, the diagnoses that are of most significance in the care of persons with AIDS will be described in detail. These include certain organic brain syndromes, major depression and uncomplicated bereavement.

Organic Brain Syndromes

Despite the frequent occurrence of organic brain syndromes in general hospital patient populations, they are frequently undiagnosed (56). Even delirium, which has a high mortality rate, is frequently misdiagnosed. The organic brain syndromes associated with AIDS are evidently even more elusive. It is probably difficult for physicians to associate aberrant behavior, mood swings or treatment refusal with the dementias and deliria associated with AIDS.

Organic brain syndromes occur frequently in persons with AIDS. They may or may not be associated with other neurological findings. The presence of central nervous system involvement with *Toxoplasma gondii, Cryptococcus neoformans*, HIV or cerebral lymphoma may or may not be indicators of associated cognitive dysfunction. Although cerebral atrophy is often associated with AIDS dementia, the degree of atrophy may not correlate with the severity of dementia.

Delirium

Delirium is the most frequently encountered organic brain syndrome. Lipowski (57),(58) describes delirium as a disorder of cognition including global cognitive impairment with concurrent disorders of memory, thinking, orientation, perception, disturbances of the sleep-wake cycle and a characteristic course marked by rapid onset, relatively brief duration, and fluctuations in the severity of the disturbance over the course of a day.

There is impaired ability to extract, process, retain, retrieve and apply information about the environment, body and self. The patient's level of awareness is reduced. Thinking, perceiving and remembering are all impaired in delirium. Etiologic factors for delirium in patients with AIDS are shown in Table 2. The most frequent causes of delirium are: hypoxia, for example, from *P. carinii* pneumonia; cerebral infections, for example, HIV encephalopathy or cryptococcal meningitis; systemic infections such as staphylococcal bacteremia; space occupying lesions of the brain, such as brain abscesses due to toxoplasmosis or cerebral lymphoma; and drugs such as opiates, sedatives and various therapeutic agents.

Diagnosis of Delirium

Diagnostic criteria for delirium are (45):

A. Clouding of consciousness (reduced clarity of awareness of the environment) with reduced capacity to shift, focus and sustain attention to environmental stimuli.

B. At least two of the following:

1. Perceptual disturbance: misinterpretations, illusions or

Table 2. Etiology of Delirium in AIDS

I. Predisposing Factors

- A. Addiction to alcohol or drugs
- B. Brain damage
- C. Chronic illness

II. Facilitating Factors

- A. Psychological stress
- B. Sleep deprivation
- C. Sensory deprivation with immobilization
- D. Sensory overload with intensive care unit admission

III. Organic factors

- A. Intoxication
  1. Drugs: antibiotics, anticonvulsants, sedative-hypnotics, opiates, phencyclidine, antineoplastic drugs, anticholinergic agents
  2. Alcohol
- B. Alcohol or drug withdrawal
  1. Alcohol
  2. Opiates
  3. Sedative - hypnotics
- C. Metabolic encephalopathies
  1. Hypoxia
  2. Hepatic, renal, pulmonary
  3. Hypoglycemia
  4. Disorders of fluid, electrolyte and acid-base balance
  5. Endocrine disorders
- D. Infections
  1. Systemic
  2. Intracranial
- E. Epilepsy
- F. Head trauma
- G. Space-occupying lesions of brain
- H. Severe anemia

other perceptual hallucinations.

2. Speech that is at times incoherent.

3. Disturbance of the sleep-wake cycle, with insomnia or daytime drowsiness.

4. Increased or decreased psychomotor activity.

   a) Increased psychomotor activity is often associated with delirium.

      1) Carphologia - picking up of small pieces of thread or twigs from the air.

      2) Crocidismus - picking of threads or wool from blankets or bed clothes.

   b) Decreased psychomotor activity is less commonly seen.

C. Disorientation and memory impairment (if testable).

D. Clinical features that develop over a short period of time (usually hours to days) and tend to fluctuate over the course of a day.

E. Evidence from the history, physical examination or laboratory tests of a specific organic factor judged to be etiologically related to the disturbance.

Several standardized tests have been developed including the Short Portable Mental Status Questionnaire (59), the Mini-Mental State Examination (60), and the Cognitive Capacity Screening Examination (61). These are all screening tests for cognitive dysfunction and do not detect subtle signs or mild degrees of impairment. These require careful psychiatric examination and neuropsychological assessment.

Romano and Engel (62), Pro and Wells (63), and Obrecht (64) have stressed the usefulness of the electroencephalogram (EEG) in helping to support a diagnosis of delirium. Decrease in frequency of the EEG background activity is indicative of delirium, possibly as a result of a reduction of brain metabolism. EEG changes virtually always accompany delirium and make the electroencephalogram a useful diagnostic tool in persons with AIDS who manifest a change in mental status (25),(29),(65).

Treatment of delirium consists first of treating the underlying cause, maintaining fluid and electrolyte balance and nutrition. In addition, it is important to provide an optimal environment for the patient: a quiet, well-lit room with a dim light at night, radio or television, a calendar, clock, photographs and familiar objects and, if possible, visits from familiar people. Medical and nursing support should be directed toward re-orientation and companionship as well as adequate sleep and sedation.

Haloperidol may be recommended as a standing order for sleep until identification and treatment of the underlying cause has been accomplished.

Dementia

Dementia is an organic brain syndrome characterized by loss of intellectual abilities that is sufficiently severe to interfere with the individual's social or occupational functioning or both (45). Dementia (66) may be regarded as a global disorder of cognition, in the sense that several cognitive functions are impaired concurrently. They include memory, judgement and abstract thinking which are decreased in function relative to the individual's premorbid level of performance. Apraxia, agnosia, constructional difficulty as well as anosognosia may be present. Anosognosia, in particular, when coupled with denial and impaired memory and abstraction, make it difficult for some patients to comprehend a diagnosis such as AIDS. Personality changes include alteration of the characteristic personality or accentuation of personality traits. Loss of cortical inhibitions may lead to promiscuity, assaultive behavior, or lack of awareness of social amenities. There may be use of obscenities in individuals who were not known to use them. A patient may be unaware that he or she is not adequately clothed or that breasts or genitalia are exposed. These changes have a profound impact on family members, loved ones and caregivers who might expect to see such changes in the elderly, but not in young adults.

Other features include depression, psychosis and anxiety. Delusions of persecution or jealousy are common. When a patient is confronted with a difficult series of tasks, such as during a careful psychiatric examination or neuropsychological testing, a "catastrophic reaction" (67) may result. This is manifested by a full-blown anxiety attack and can be averted by the examiner's awareness and the use of a supportive approach during evaluation of cognitive capacities.

The most frequent cause of dementia in AIDS and ARC is HIV encephalopathy (Table 3).

Diagnosis of Dementia

The diagnostic criteria for dementia are as follows (45):

A. A loss of intellectual abilities of sufficient severity to interfere with social or occupational functioning.

B. Memory impairment.

C. At least one of the following:

1. Impairment of abstract thinking as manifested by concrete interpretation of proverbs, inability to find similarities and differences between related words, difficulty in defining words and concepts and other similar

tasks.

2. Impaired judgement.

3. Other disturbances of higher cortical function such as aphasia (disorder of language due to brain dysfunction), apraxia (inability to carry out motor activities despite intact comprehension and motor function), agnosia (failure to recognize or identify objects despite intact sensory function), "constructional difficulty" (inability to copy three-dimentional figures, assemble blocks or arrange sticks in specific designs).

Table 3. Causes of Dementia in AIDS

Brain Involvement

- Tumors
  - Primary cerebral lymphoma
  - Kaposi's sarcoma
- Infections
  - Viral
    - HIV
    - *Herpes simplex*
    - Herpes zoster
    - Cytomegalovirus
    - Papovavirus (progressive multifocal leukoencephalopathy)
  - Fungal
    - Cryptococcosis
    - Candida abscesses
  - Protozoal
    - Toxoplasmosis
  - Bacterial
    - *Mycobacterium avium-intracellulare*

Systemic Involvement

- Metabolic
  - Hypoxic or anoxic encephalopathy
- Toxic substances
  - Chronic abuse of drugs

4. Personality change, i.e., alteration or accentuation of premorbid traits.

D. State of consciousness not clouded (i.e., does not meet criteria for delirium or intoxication, although these may be superimposed).

E. Either (1) or (2):

(1) Evidence from the history, physical examination or laboratory tests of a specific organic factor that is judged to be etiologically related to the disturbance.

(2) In the absence of such evidence, an organic factor can be presumed if conditions other than organic mental disorders have been reasonably excluded and if the behavior change represents cognitive impairment in a variety of areas.

In general, differentiation of delirium from dementia may be based on the normal state of consciousness in dementia versus the rapidly fluctuating course in delirium, and the EEG slowing in delirium. Although delirium may be superimposed on dementia in AIDS, it is worthwhile understanding how to distinguish the two (Table 4).

Dementia may be associated with specific personality or behavorial manifestations if there is invasion of certain brain areas by the infectious agents or tumors associated with AIDS. For example, if the frontal lobes are involved, then the characteristic picture may include reduced drive, diminished self-concern, inability to delay gratification, impulsivity, lack of judgement, shallow or blunted affect, perseveration, concrete thinking and inability to change mental set quickly (68).

It is important to provide the necessary support, psychotherapy and family therapy for AIDS-associated dementia. Persons with dementia may benefit from on-going therapy and may have a less precipitous course. Therapy is primarily supportive. Haloperidol may be of help in reducing anxiety and agitation as well as psychotic symptomatology. Therapy should also include the family and should provide caregivers with enough information about dementia so that they will be able to understand the patient's behavior and help to orient and educate as much as possible.

The treatment of dementia is similar to that of delirium. Although not all AIDS-related dementias are reversible at the present time, it is important to make an effort to identify and treat underlying causes.

Organic Affective Syndrome

Organic affective syndrome is a disorder in which there is a disturbance of mood with symptoms of a major depressive or manic episode (45). There is an underlying organic cause for the disturbance of mood, but no evidence of either delirium or dementia.

Table 4. Differentiation of Delirium and Dementia in AIDS[a]

	Delirium	Dementia
EEG background slowing	+	-
Fluctuation of symptoms	+	-
Drowsiness	+	-
Illusions	+	-
Hallucinations	+	-
Confusion	+	-
Carphologia	+	-
Insomnia	+	+
Impaired attention	+	+
Impaired concentration	+	+
Slow speech	-	+
Slow motor responses	-	+
Delusions	-	+
Ataxia	-	+
Leg weakness	-	+

a Please note that the differentiation is not absolute and there is occasional overlap of symptoms and frequent appearance of delirium superimposed on pre-existing dementia in AIDS.

The following example illustrates organic affective syndrome in a person with AIDS.

Case 6: The patient was a 30 year old gay artist who was admitted to the psychiatric unit because of depression with suicidal ideation. History revealed that he had been hospitalized twice within the year prior to admission because of depression. There was no family history of affective disorder and no history of substance abuse in either patient or family. The patient was found to have major depression, recurrent. He was treated with antidepressants and psychotherapy but did not respond. He was treated with electroshock therapy and continued to remain depressed and withdrawn with anorexia, weight loss and suicidal ideation. He developed a fever and was found to have cryptococcal pneumonia and AIDS was diagnosed. He was treated with amphotericin B and responded well. He was evaluated and found to have organic affective syndrome with depression. He responded well to psychotherapy and anti-depressants and was discharged and lost to follow up for a period of one year. At the end of that year, he was hospitalized at another hospital where he was described as acting aggressively and bizarrely. He was ultimately brought to our hospital. He was then found to be alert and oriented, talkative, with pressure of speech, tangentiality, and euphoric mood. He was grandiose, with mood-congruent delusions. He was extremely agitated at times. He was treated with psychotherapy and trifluoperazine, to which he responded well. He was found to have cryptococcal meningitis and disseminated *Mycobacterium avium-intracellulare* infection. He deteriorated rapidly, became depressed and died during this admission. His psychiatric diagnosis was organic affective syndrome with recurrent manic and depressive episodes probably associated with AIDS and cryptococcal disease.

The treatment of organic affective syndrome includes individual psychotherapy and, at times, use of psychotropic medication. The tricyclic antidepressants, such as imipramine, may be used in doses as low as 10-25mg or up to 75mg-200mg at bedtime. Neuroleptics may be used in low doses, when necessary. Haloperidol 0.5 - 10mg at bedtime or trifluoperazine 1mg to 30mg daily may be recommended.

Organic Delusional Syndrome

Diagnostic criteria for organic delusional syndrome are as follows (45):

A. Delusions are the predominant clinical feature.

B. There is no clouding of consciousness, as in delirium; there is no significant loss of intellectual abilities, as in dementia; there are no prominent hallucinations, as in organic hallucinosis.

C. There is evidence, from the history, physical examination, or laboratory tests, of a specific organic factor that is judged to be etiologically related to the disturbance.

Case 7: The patient was a 35 year-old married mother of three teenage children and grandmother of an eight month old. She was brought to the emergency room of another hospital because of a one week history of bizarre behavior. This consisted of staring, mumbling incoherently, and saying that she had killed her daughter and grandson. She had two prior admissions to that hospital at age 34 years, followed by several emergency room visits. Her diagnosis on her previous admission was atypical psychosis and on her emergency room visits, schizophrenia, paranoid type. There was no prior psychiatric history before age 34, nor family history of psychiatric disorder or substance abuse. Her history of intravenous drug use was not obtained until later, although history of alcohol use was elicited. She was unresponsive to treatment with a neuroleptic and was transferred to our hospital. She was angry and depressed with bizarre delusions. Diagnosis of major depression was made. The patient did not respond to haloperidol, but developed fever and lethargy. She was found to have anemia, dehydration, a fever of 101°F and delirium. Ultimately, candida esophagitis, *P. carinii* pneumonia and AIDS were diagnosed. She was found to have dementia with superimposed delirium and died two years after her psychiatric admission. It is likely that her initial psychiatric hospitalizations and emergency room visits were a result of organic delusional syndrome associated with HIV encephalopathy.

Treatment of organic delusional syndrome includes psychotherapy and neuroleptic medication.

Major Depression

Major depression is a disorder characterized by depressed mood, guilt, loss of interest in most activities (anhedonia) and hopelessness (45). There is evidence of anorexia and weight loss (difficult to assess significance in persons with AIDS). There can be insomnia or hypersomnia and psychomotor retardation or agitation. There is diminution of self-esteem, worthlessness and hopelessness and there may also be evidence of diminished ability to think or concentrate. The patient may be preoccupied with suicidal thoughts.

Treatment for major depression includes individual and family therapy. Antidepressants may be recommended in low doses with gradual build-up to therapeutic levels.

Uncomplicated Bereavement

Although uncomplicated bereavement is defined in relationship to the loss of a loved one, in AIDS, as in other severe illnesses, the losses of health, functioning, body integrity and anticipatory loss of life may result in the same reaction (45). Additionally, many persons with AIDS have also suffered the loss of their loved ones, or of friends who may have died of AIDS.

A full depressive syndrome frequently is a normal reaction to such a loss, with feelings of depression and such associated symptoms as poor appetite, weight loss, and insomnia. However, morbid preoccupation with worthlessness, prolonged and marked functional impairment, and marked psychomotor retardation are uncommon and suggest that the bereavement is complicated by the development of a major depression. See Table 5 for differentiation of major depression and bereavement.

In uncomplicated bereavement, guilt, if present, is chiefly about things done or not done at the time of the death by the survivor; thoughts of death are usually limited to the individual's thinking that he or she would be better off dead or that he or she should have died with the person who died. The individual

Table 5. Differentiation of Major Depression and Bereavement

	Uncompleted Bereavement	Major Depression
General	exhaustion, lack of strength, restlessness, inability to sit still, aimless moving, decreased capacity for organized living, "going through the motions," insomnia	insomnia, psychomotor retardation or agitation, diminished ability to function, decreased libido, headache, backache
Gastrointestinal	empty feeling in abdomen, anorexia, tightness in throat, dysphagia, constipation	somatic delusions ("my insides are rotting away"), anorexia, weight loss, constipation
Respiratory	sighing respirations, dyspnea	
Emotional	sorrow, sadness, guilt over survival, loss of warmth in other relations, hostility, preoccupation with image of deceased	sadness, depressed, worthlessness, hopelessness, helplessness, decreased self-esteem, suicidal thoughts or acts
Course	self-limiting	requires intervention
Treatment	working through of ambivalent feelings to achieve freedom from bondage to the deceased, readjustment to environment without the deceased, formation of new relationships; no medication	psychotherapy, antidepressants

with uncomplicated bereavement generally regards the feeling of depressed mood as "normal," although he or she may seek professional help for relief of such associated symptoms as insomnia and anorexia.

The reaction to the loss may be immediate, but rarely occurs after the first two or three months. The duration of "normal" bereavement varies considerably among different subcultural groups.

The treatment is to provide support, and if possible, encourage communication with family, loved ones and friends.

Table 6. Services Offered by the Gay Men's Health Crisis in New York City

- Crisis Intervention Counseling
- AIDS Therapy Groups
- Care Partners' Groups
- Parents' Support Groups
- Social Activities
- Buddy Support System
- Religious Counseling
- Financial Advocacy Program
- Psychiatric Consultation
- "Worried Well" Groups

TREATMENT APPROACHES TO PERSONS WITH AIDS, ARC, HIV SEROPOSITIVITY AND THE "WORRIED WELL"

The anxiety, fear, problems in coping, psychological reactions and psychopathology associated with AIDS all indicate a need for intervention. There are many levels and kinds of intervention and each needs to be tailored to the needs of the individual or group involved.

One of the most important resources for persons with AIDS has been the programs provided by the gay community. Even before AIDS was described in the medical literature, a group of gay men in New York City began to meet to discuss the recent deaths of some of their close friends (69). These meetings resulted in the formation of the Gay Men's Health Crisis (G.M.H.C.). Similar organizations have formed throughout the United States. They offer services (Table 6) to any person with AIDS or ARC or individuals with AIDS-related concerns. Services are not limited to gay or bisexual men. GMHC and other similar organizations have also provided leadership in education for risk-reduction.

Psychiatrists and other mental health professionals can provide services in hospitals, out-patient clinics and private offices. Persons with AIDS and ARC are responsive to therapy and are rewarding to work with. The needs of persons with AIDS and the anxieties of persons with ARC and the "worried well" have been recognized (42),(43),(70),(71). There is a need for a relationship because of loneliness or losses. There is a sense of time urgency, an existential anxiety that makes for less resistance. There is a tendency to review life's experiences and past relationships. All of these factors make persons with AIDS good candidates for therapy.

The models for treatment include all forms of therapy and should also incorporate the services of programs such as GMHC.

Crisis intervention may be indicated when an individual and loved ones first learn of the diagnosis. Crisis intervention is also effective during initial stages and if suicidal ideation develops. It is also helpful for both patients and families at the time of death and afterward, during the period of mourning. Crisis intervention should be available to persons with AIDS.

Supportive therapy and group therapy (72),(73) are extremely effective for persons with AIDS.

Individual therapy directed toward treatment of specific psychiatric problems or resolution of conflicts and bereavement is effective in helping individuals cope and function at the best possible levels.

Family therapy and multiple family groups are extremely effective in resolution of serious family conflicts which often accompany AIDS. Family therapy can help to reconcile issues in families who have rejected a person with AIDS because of their discrimination against intravenous drug users or homophobia.

Finally, psychotropic medications may be effective as adjuncts to therapy when they are indicated for the psychiatric problems described (Tables 1,5). Specific issues in prescribing psychotropic medications include the weight and medical condition of the patient. In particular, concern for the respiratory depressant potential must be recognized. In addition, most psychotropics are detoxified in the liver, so that intact hepatic function is also of importance. In general, use of benzodiazepines is contraindicated because of their depressive and addictive potentials. Benzodiazepines also depress cortical function and may worsen dementia or produce a superimposed delirium.

Medications should be given in the lowest possible doses. The following medications are useful:

Haloperidol	0.5mg to 10mg at bedtime for organic brain syndromes or psychosis
Imipramine	10mg to 75mg at bedtime for major depression (may need up to 200mg)
Trazodone	50mg to 100mg at bedtime for major depression

Other medications include: trifluoperazine for organic mental syndromes or psychosis and desipramine for major depression.

It is best to give psychotropic medications on a routine basis rather than an as needed basis. This is also the case for management of chronic pain associated with AIDS. It is upsetting to be in pain, but it is even more upsetting to be in pain and have to be faced on a regular basis with the humiliation of having to ask for pain medication. Once it is clear that a person with AIDS is experiencing pain, an effective regimen of pain medication should be provided on a round-the-clock basis.

Religious counseling should be available to persons with AIDS throughout the course of the syndrome.

EDUCATION ABOUT AIDS

There is a need for a comprehensive and integrated educational approach for persons with AIDS and ARC, their loved ones and also hospital staff and communities. Education should be geared not only toward giving factual information about AIDS and about risk-reduction, but also toward anxiety reduction. Educators need to be able to be comfortable with discussing the sexual aspects as well as with imparting specific facts about infection control. Educators also need to come to terms with and understand their own feelings about AIDS, fears of contagion and feelings about homosexuality and intravenous drug use.

An organized educational program needs to examine carefully the attitudes of the teachers. These are best discussed in small group settings that give permission to be open with feelings and enable teachers to share feelings without blame, shame or embarrassment. There is no room in the teaching of patient, family, staff, risk group members, or communities for judgmental attitudes. Judgmental attitudes are as detrimental in the educational process as they are in the care of persons with AIDS. It is helpful to attempt to resolve these issues prior to embarking on an educational process.

Educational programs need to address the anxieties and fears of the learners. A well-organized program of training will be forgotten if the anxiety level is too high. Directors of residency training programs are often aware that house officers may remember little from their day of orientation because of the high levels of anxiety on the first day of internship. In AIDS education, the same concept holds and it is helpful to address the anxieties and estimate their levels. Educational programs need to address the biopsychosocial aspects of AIDS as well as stress the importance of risk-reduction. In risk groups such as intravenous drug users, it is necessary to involve the families or loved ones in the educational program.

Education for the community needs to begin with community agencies, centers and community organizations. This education will help to reduce anxiety as well as risk. But the most important program, that of primary prevention, needs to begin in elementary school where systematic programs of sex and health education as well as education about the dangers of substance abuse should begin in kindergarten and continue through high school. The programs can be tailored to the levels of understanding of each age group.

Educational programs about AIDS need to be tailored specifically toward the level of understanding of the learners. In AIDS, as in any illness, it is important to determine the understanding of the illness whether it is for educational programs or direct patient care.

UNDERSTANDING OF THE ILLNESS

A comprehensive approach to AIDS or ARC would not be complete without the concept of determining the patient's understanding of the illness. This is important with all illness, but it becomes more significant in severe and life-threatening illnesses or those around which there is uncertainty. The initial stages of the illness may be frightening to the patient. The person who is a member of a risk group may have severe anxiety about having AIDS even though there is no evidence of signs or symptoms. This anxiety about AIDS may be paralyzing and may cause severe psychiatric symptoms. It may also impair an individual's capacity to function at work or at home.

If a member of a risk group does develop a symptom, the anxiety is also painful and, particularly in those who are aware of the symptoms of AIDS, leads to an immediate assumption that this is the diagnosis, even prior to seeking medical attention. Defenses of denial, suppression or avoidance may delay diagnosis. However, during the period from the onset of the very first symptom of AIDS or ARC, a member of a risk group begins to develop thoughts, worries and fantasies about the syndrome and its impact. Many persons with symptoms begin to mobilize and plan and prepare for death, even when this is premature.

Some may be able to cope as well as possible and mobilize themselves and their families and caregivers. They may cooperate readily and form trusting relationships with their physicians and other caregivers. No matter what the individual's coping capacities, severity of symptoms or psychopathology, the capacity of the physician to elicit the patient's understanding of the illness remains an important factor in communication, development of a supportive relationship and adherence. It is frustrating to physician and patient alike if there are barriers to communication. When a person with AIDS is encouraged to share his or her own perceptions, understanding or theories of the illness, communication proceeds at the appropriate level and pace.

Eliciting an individual's understanding of an illness is not a static event. It is a process that begins from the day of first contact and continues periodically throughout the duration of the illness. The early understanding is important because it gives an opportunity to begin a process of exploration which will result in the education of the patient and physician. The physician learns from the patient what the patient thinks is wrong. Often, the patient may suspect the diagnosis of AIDS. The physician then learns the specific ideas that the patient has about AIDS and what they mean to him or her. The patient may then gradually learn from the physician whether the understanding fits what is actually known about his or her own illness.

Although the concept of eliciting the patient's understanding of the illness is hardly unique to AIDS, AIDS and its victims make the concept even more significant for the following reasons. The societal taboos against openness about sexuality and death and the illicit and illegal nature of intravenous drug use create a climate of discrimination, homophobia and fear. These are heightened by the contagious nature of AIDS and by the specific modes of transmission. Additionally, some of the victims of AIDS and ARC may not have an on-going relationship with a physician. The onset of symptoms may result in the first entry of a young risk group member into the health care system. This may be particularly significant in young intravenous drug users who may have received health care only when emergencies arose. The concept of understanding of illness when applied in the context of a supportive relationship may enhance the development of physician-patient support.

A physician needs to be able to field responses to the question "What is your understanding of your illness?" Patients frequently respond with, "I don't know." or "You're the doctor, you tell me!" A physician may then point out that he or she is interested in learning what the patient thinks, or what ideas or theories that the patient may have about the illness.

Since AIDS is a syndrome whose victims are often in their twenties and thirties, it may be difficult for young physicians not to over-identify with their patients. House officers may be overwhelmed not only with the ethical dilemmas posed by AIDS but also by having to tell a young, previously healthy individual of the diagnosis. Here, the consultation-liaison psychiatrist may provide some support and help a house officer progress from over-identification to understanding and empathic concern. Physicians and other health professionals at all levels may benefit from enabling patients to share with them an ever-evolving understanding of the illness. It is clear that spending time sitting down with the patient, becoming familiar with the patient as a person, and learning the patient's own ideas and perceptions of AIDS or ARC will save time in the long run and improve overall care.

SUICIDE AND AIDS

There are may taboos associated with AIDS. So far, we have touched upon the taboos associated with sexuality and death, as well as the fears associated with contagion. Societal taboos against death are even stronger against death by suicide. The thought of suicide is as universal as its taboo. In persons with AIDS, thoughts of suicide may be universal. Alienation and expendability are consistent themes for persons with AIDS. A natural concomitant of these themes is the thought of, or plan for, suicide.

Persons with AIDS may be members of risk groups who feel isolated, lonely, alienated and expendable even before the diagnosis of AIDS. The suicidal person with AIDS may be thought of as a person in the midst of a crisis in expendability (74),(75). The concept of expendability is conveyed to the suicidal individual in verbal and non-verbal ways. A sense of hopelessness may develop. Once the diagnosis of AIDS is confirmed, the sense of hopelessness, alienation and expendability may be compounded.

Risk factors for suicide in the general population are shown in Table 7 (76)-(78). The diagnosis of AIDS entails all of the usual suicide risk factors and, in addition, adds even more risks. Persons with AIDS are frequently ill and are frequently hospitalized. They are often more alienated and isolated because of the discrimination against persons with AIDS and members of the risk groups associated with AIDS. Hopelessness is further complicated by the high mortality associated with AIDS and the devastating downhill course.

Table 7. Risk Factors for Suicide in the General Population

Hopelessness
Impulsivity
Substance abuse disorder
Recent illness
Recent hospitalization
Recent losses
Depression
Living alone
Inexpressible grief

Further complicating the picture are the symptoms of pain, disfigurement, weakness and depression associated with some of the infections and cancers comprising AIDS. The organic brain syndromes associated with AIDS are often accompanied by impulsivity, impaired judgement and diminution of the individual's capacity to understand and cope with AIDS. Suicidal ideation may be further suggested either consciously or unconsciously by families or loved ones who are unable to deal with AIDS or its social consequences.

Suicidal ideas may be an initial reaction to the diagnosis of AIDS.

> **Case 8:** The patient was a 29 year-old gay man, employed as a salesman, who was admitted with acute respiratory distress. He expressed the wish to hang himself and was found to be depressed. He was diagnosed as having *P. carinii* pneumonia and was treated. He required intubation and a respirator to assist with breathing. While his first episode of *P. carinii* was resolving, he was found to have dementia, probably secondary to hypoxic encephalopathy, as well as depression. His depression gradually responded to psychotherapy.

Case 9: The patient was a 32 year-old unemployed intravenous drug user who stated, upon his admission, that he would kill himself if he were found to have AIDS. A diagnosis of AIDS was made when *P. carinii* pneumonia was diagnosed. The patient was treated with psychotherapy and psychotropic medication and remained on suicide precautions until he was no longer suicidal. A diagnosis of organic affective syndrome with major depression was made.

Although suicidal ideation may be a frequent early reaction to learning the diagnosis of AIDS, suicide may be contemplated at any point during the course of the syndrome. Persons with AIDS have contemplated taking pills, jumping from windows, electrocution and wrist-slashing at various points in their illness. As the illnesses progress and hospitalizations become more frequent, the thought of suicide may be the only way that an individual may have to feel in control of his or her destiny.

The management of the suicidal person with AIDS is a sensitive and complex issue. It is crucial to remember that all suicidal individuals may have mixed feelings about suicide and may move from being preoccupied with hopelessness and suicide to thoughts and plans for the future. No one is suicidal all of the time or in every way. Suicide may be an effort to gain control, to alleviate pain or alienation. Suicide may also be a symptom of major depression or organic affective syndrome. It may be a reaction to a growing realization of loss of health, strength or cognitive capacities.

The caregiver needs to feel comfortable with taking a suicide history and discussing suicide in depth with the person with AIDS. The steps include the following:

1. Establishment of a trusting relationship.

2. Discussion of suicide and death in relation to AIDS, and the patients' philosophies and religious beliefs.

3. Realization of the value of continuity of care and reassurance that the person with AIDS will not be abandoned.

Suicide history-taking includes the following questions:

1. What is it specifically that made you think of suicide?
2. Have you made any plans?
3. What are they?
4. Have you ever tried to kill yourself?
5. Do you feel like killing yourself now?
6. What would you accomplish?
7. Do you plan to rejoin someone who has died?
8. Do you know anyone who committed suicide?

Far from harming the patient, taking a suicide history and being able to speak about suicidal thoughts and feelings is highly relieving. Persons with AIDS may feel isolated and alienated. Their thoughts of suicide, while on the one hand providing some measure of consolation and control, may also be frightening and painful. Sharing suicidal feelings with an empathic listener is not only relieving, but may result in a different perspective.

There is no treatment for AIDS or suicide, only prevention and education. In order to prevent suicide in AIDS, caregivers need to be able to take a suicide history, recognize and treat depression and organic brain syndromes, and provide continuous observation when indicated. In order to resolve a suicidal crisis, it is important to re-establish bonds and provide the patient with a supportive network of family, loved ones, friends and caregivers. Ultimately crisis intervention, network formation, on-going support and family therapy may prevent suicide.

To provide the kind of support, crisis intervention and education that is needed for persons with AIDS, there is a need for a multidisciplinary team approach.

THE MULTIDISCIPLINARY AIDS PROGRAM

There is a need for a comprehensive and coordinated approach to the crisis of AIDS (6). Members of risk groups who are anxious about AIDS (the "worried well"), individuals who are HIV seropositive, and persons with ARC and AIDS are confronted with uncertainty, severe illnesses, profound psychological reactions, discrimination and death. Each individual deserves the best medical and psychological care available, as well as services of other disciplines where indicated. Each person with AIDS may require the care and services of a physician in primary care internal medicine, as well as physicians with specialities in infectious disease, hematology-oncology, consultation-liaison psychiatry, neurology, pulmonary medicine, dermatology, gastroenterology, immunology, gynecology and dentistry. They may need the companionship of a nurse aide during a hospitalization as well as the skills of nursing staff members on medical floors and intensive care units. The nursing care requirements vary, but may become overwhelming as complications such as dementia and paralyses ensue. Besides the depression, regression and dependency needs that often accompany chronic illness, nursing staff is also faced with persons who have frequent diarrhea, may be incontinent and have complicated and unusual treatment regimens that tend to be accompanied by severe side-effects such as even more diarrhea and vomiting.

Persons with AIDS may require the services and care of social workers, psychologists, discharge planners, drug addiction counselors, respiratory therapists, dieticians, chaplains, lawyers, laboratory technicians and community agencies. A multidisciplinary AIDS program can provide a coordinated, humane approach to care and a comprehensive and systematic educational program. The Multidisciplinary AIDS Program at Metropolitan Hospital Center in New York City has been previously described (24),(79). The goals and objectives of the program can be found in the Appendix to this chapter.

The need for improvement in coordination of services for persons with AIDS is well recognized; however, the needs of each hospital and community may differ. Some hospitals may deal with primarily intravenous drug users, while others deal primarily with gay men. The levels of resource community organizations, support and discrimination may vary considerably. And finally, the composition of hospital staff, kind of hospital and resource availability may vary. Each program can be tailored to meet the needs of the patients, their families, the hospital, medical school and community (Appendix).

The multidisciplinary AIDS program at Metropolitan Hospital Center is comprised of physicians with specialities in infectious disease, hematology-oncology, consultation-liaison psychiatry, epidemiology, neurology and employee's health, along with nurses, social workers, discharge planners, a respiratory therapist, a dietician, a psychologist and an administrator. This team has met weekly since 1983. The program has provided help for more than three hundred persons with AIDS and ARC and their loved ones. It has provided medical and psychological care, support, crisis intervention and suicide prevention. It implements educational programs for patients, hospital staff, other hospitals, medical schools and community agencies. At Metropolitan Hospital Center, persons with AIDS are treated on general medical, surgical and pediatric floors and intensive care units with a non-segregated approach. They are seen in ambulatory settings of the medical clinic, chest clinic, psychiatric clinic, dermatology clinic as well as other areas. Persons with AIDS are in two, four and six-bedded rooms with persons with other diagnoses. They are isolated only when they are unable to control secretions, or if respiratory isolation is indicated (80). Although it is clear that there are many approaches and models for the care of persons with AIDS, the sense of isolation and alienation engendered by AIDS and societal responses to AIDS make further isolation in the hospital setting even more unbearable. At least in the hospital, on the in-patient units and in the ambulatory setting, persons with AIDS may find a safe haven where they may be free from discrimination, stigmata and homophobia. Hospital settings are not, however, free from any of these, and work needs to be done in order to help both professional and non-professional staff to overcome societal taboos (44),(81)-(84).

The Multidisciplinary AIDS Program addresses the frustrations and anxieties of staff and campaigns for widespread education, programs of risk reduction, decreased discrimination and increased resources. We regard our program as a model approach for providing humane care for persons with AIDS and helping them and their loved ones and caregivers to cope with the crisis.

The health professionals caring for persons with AIDS have numerous conflicts, fears and concerns (85)-(87). House officers, particularly residents in internal medicine, may be in need of emotional support. The stress of internship and residency training has been recognized (88)-(91). Psychiatric assistance should be available to house officers as a part of residency training (92),(93) in order to alleviate stress and treat depression as well as to prevent some of the tragic consequences such as drug use (94),(95) and suicide (96)-(98). Wachter (99) suggests that the AIDS epidemic has added yet another stress to the stresses of medical residency training. He documents a major impact on workload, education and on the feelings of house officers. A multidisciplinary AIDS program in conjunction with consultation-liaison psychiatry, may provide support for house officers. Nevertheless, there are some ethical issues that are important in the care of persons with AIDS that may leave medical residents and other health professionals with many dilemmas.

ETHICAL ISSUES IN AIDS

The biopsychosocial approach to persons with AIDS and ARC may be implemented through a multidisciplinary AIDS program. This enables persons with AIDS to be treated with love, respect and dignity and provides caregivers and loved ones with the support they need throughout this process. Through educational programs, the painful and tragic societal responses of discrimination and rejection may change. However, in the meanwhile, during this transitional phase, persons with AIDS, ARC and HIV seropositivity, their loved ones and even risk group members are confronted with ethical dilemmas that may range from catastrophic to overwhelming. Their caregivers are confronted with similar dilemmas. Only those ethical issues with practical relevance for a multidisciplinary AIDS program will be raised although there are many other ethical dimensions (100).

Confidentiality

Our patients have taught us, all too poignantly, the importance of confidentiality. An individual who is struggling with as devastating an illness as AIDS, deserves not only humane care, but also confidentiality. This is especially important in a society in which individuals may be discriminated against because they have AIDS. It is crucial that a patient's rights to privacy and confidentiality remain protected in the hospital setting as well as in the community. There are several difficulties with this because of the contagious nature of the illness. Special containers for needles and special red plastic bags are employed in order to help hospital personnel take appropriate precautions. These are also markers for other people who may then guess at the possible diagnosis. The vital importance of confidentiality of all diagnoses must be stressed to all employees during on-going educational programs as well as at orientation. Paradoxically, however, the issue of confidentiality has yet another aspect. The sexual partners of persons with AIDS are at risk for AIDS. Although persons with AIDS should be encouraged to inform partners or potential partners and should be taught methods of risk-reduction, physicians are prevented from informing partners or tracing contacts without the patient's consent. This becomes further complicated when persons with AIDS are illegal aliens or fugitives. In general, most people with AIDS are eager to inform their partners and to take whatever precautions they can to prevent the spread of the illness. Unfortunately, not all persons with AIDS have the courage, wisdom or cognitive capacities to enable them to cooperate in this way. Issues of confidentiality can be exquisitely painful and may not always have answers.

Employees or Students with AIDS, ARC or HIV Seropositivity

Employees or students with AIDS, ARC or HIV seropositivity should be treated in the same way as all other employees. Again, the rights of individuals to confidentiality need to be protected. Persons with AIDS should be allowed to attend school or work until severe illness, incapacitation or death intervenes. The burdens and losses associated with AIDS are painful enough. There is no reason to add more losses. Employees with AIDS within our hospital system have worked for as long as they were able to, and left work only because they chose to do so. This policy was reinforced by the support of both the medical staff and administration. The preservation of a job enables a person with AIDS to continue to support himself or herself financially, to maintain dignity and self-respect and to have a sense of purpose. If the patient is also supporting a family, they too will be protected.

Ethics of HIV Testing

It seems clear that widespread testing of people for HIV seropositivity for purposes of screening is highly discriminatory. HIV testing should not be used to screen prospective employees, insurance applicants or students.

There may be specific indications for HIV testing which need to be defined and clarified. The ethics and meanings of HIV testing are complex and require further definition and clarification.

Orders Not to Resuscitate and the Right to Die

The person with AIDS needs to be able to maintain dignity and humanity from the day of diagnosis until the day of death. Caregivers can discuss issues of heroic measures and resuscitation with persons with AIDS and their loved ones. Since *Pneumocystis carinii* pneumonia is a treatable opportunistic infection, physicians need to explore very carefully the difference between intubation as part of a treatment plan, or as part of heroic attempts to keep a dying person alive. It may be helpful to be very specific with persons with AIDS who have a clear idea of how they want to be cared for once they can no longer care for themselves.

Ask a person who has been intubated or suctioned repeatedly through an endotracheal tube if they would willingly endure the process again. The answer might be "yes," if there was hope for recovery, but if there were none, "what on earth for?"

The following case vignette illustrates an ethical dilemma.

> **Case 10:** The patient was a 38 year-old gay attorney with disseminated Kaposi's sarcoma and cerebral toxoplasmosis who was becoming progressively quadriplegic. The patient, while still aware, alert and with the capacity to make decisions decided with his family that he should have no heroic measures, no intubation and no resuscitation. He became progressively weaker and as his disease progressed, he yearned for human contact. He would perceive most feeling in his right hand, and would ask his psychiatrist to hold his hand for him. He confided that he wished that death would come soon because he hated the complete dependency imposed by his weakness and neurological impairments. When he began to refuse food, the issue of nasogastric intubation arose. By that time, he was lethargic and almost unresponsive, but he made it clear that he did not want to have a nasogastric tube. Since there was no specific instruction, the nasogastric tube was inserted against the patient's will. It was removed shortly thereafter and, ironically, found to have a small but effective knot three inches from its tip. The tube itself had knotted in the process of the struggle. The patient subsequently died, with as little discomfort and as much dignity as was possible.

Persons with AIDS vary in how they approach the process of dying. Some individuals want to be resuscitated and wish for every heroic measure possible (101),(102). Others, like the gentlemen in Case 10 wish to have no heroics. Plans need to be discussed wherever possible so that a person with AIDS can express feelings and explore the process with loved ones and care givers. Plans then can be tailored to fit the individual's wishes and circumstances.

The ethical issues in AIDS demonstrate the importance of humanism and compassion in medical care.

CONCLUSION

"We shall assume that everyone is much more simply human than otherwise... man -- however indistinguished biologically -- as long as he is entitled to the term human personality, will be very much more like every other instance of human personality than he is like anything else in the world. As I have tried to hint before, it is to some extent on this basis that I have become occupied with the science, not of individual differences, but of human identities or parallels, one might say. In other words, I try to study the degrees and patterns of things which I assume to be ubiquitously human."(103) Sullivan's hypothesis about persons with psychopathology and their psychiatrists may apply to persons with AIDS and their caregivers.

AIDS takes a toll on its victims, their loved ones, caregivers and communities. AIDS and AIDS-related disorders are exquisitely painful and may have tragic consequences. We need to work closely together to provide networks of support for victims and caregivers alike in order to cope with the crisis of AIDS. A biopsychosocial approach can provide coordinated, humane care as well as a comprehensive educational program. A multidisciplinary AIDS program addresses the frustrations and anxieties of staff and implements programs of education and risk-reduction. A biopsychosocial approach enables victims, their loved ones and caregivers to meet the challenges of AIDS with optimism and dignity.

REFERENCES

1. Lipowski, Z.J., The holistic approach to medicine. In:Psychosomatic Medicine and Liaison Psychiatry. (Lipowski, Z.J., ed.), Plenum Medical Book Company, New York, p 105-117 (1985)

2. Engel, G.L., The need for a new medical model: A challenge for biomedicine. Science 196:129-136 (1977)

3. Kimball, C. P., The Biopsychosocial Approach to the Patient. Williams and Wilkins, Baltimore (1981)

4. Engel, G.L., The biopsychosocial model and medical education: who are to be the teachers? N Engl J Med 306:802-805 (1982)

5. Cohen, M.A., Weisman, H.W., A biopsychosocial approach to AIDS. Psychosomatics 27:245-249 (1986)

6. Landesman, S.H., Ginzburg, H.M., Weiss, S.H., The AIDS epidemic. N Engl J Med 312:521-525 (1985)

7. Lane, C.H., Fauci, A.S., Immunologic reconstitution in the acquired immunodeficiency syndrome. Ann Intern Med 103:714-718 (1985)

8. Hirsch, M.S., Kaplan, J.C., Prospects of therapy for infections with human T-lymphotropic virus type III. Ann Intern Med 103:750-755 (1985)

9. Montagnier, L., Lymphadenopathy-associated virus: from molecular biology to pathogenicity. Ann Intern Med 103:689-693 (1985)

10. Barre-Sinoussi, F., Chermann, J.C., Rey, R., et al., Isolation of a T-lymphotropic retrovirus from a patient at risk for acquired immunedeficiency syndrome (AIDS). Science 220:868-871 (1983)

11. Gallo, R.C., Salahuddin, S.Z., Popovic, M., et al., Frequent detection and isolation of cytopathic retroviruses (HTLV-III) from patients with AIDS and at risk for AIDS. Science 224: 500-503 (1984)

12. Gallo, R.C., Wong-Staal, F., A human T-lymphotropic retrovirus (HTLV-III) as the cause of the acquired immunodeficiency syndrome. Ann Intern Med 103:679-689 (1985)

13. Montagnier, L., Chermann, J.C., Barre-Sinoussi, F., et al., A new human T-lymphotropic retrovirus: characterization and possible role in lymphadenopathy and acquired immune deficiency syndromes. In: Human T-cell Leukemia/Lymphoma Virus. (Gallo, R.C., Essex, M., Gross, L., eds), Cold Spring Harbor Laboratory Press, Cold Spring Harbor, p 363-370 (1984)

14. Francis, D.P., Petricciani, J.C., The prospects for and pathways toward a vaccine for AIDS. N Engl J Med 313:1586-1590 (1985)

15. Olsen, R.G., Lewis, M., Mathes, L.E., et al., Feline leukemia vaccine: efficacy testing in a large multicat household. Feline Pract 10:13-16 (1980)

16. Sivak, S.L., Wormser, G.P., How common is HTLV-III infection in the United States? N Engl J Med 313:1352 (1985)

17. Curran, J.W., The epidemiology and prevention of the acquired immuno-deficiency syndrome. Ann Intern Med 103:657-662 (1985)

18. CDC., Pneumocystis pneumonia - Los Angeles, MMWR 30:250-252 (1981)

19. CDC., Kaposi's sarcoma and pneumocystis pneumonia among homosexual men - New York City and California. MMWR 30:305-308 (1981)

20. Gottlieb, M.S., Scharoff, R., Schanker, H.M., et al., *Pneumocystis carinii* pneumonia and mucosal candidiasis in previously healthy homosexual men: evidence of a new acquired cellular immunodeficiency. N Engl J Med 305:1425-1431 (1981)

21. Blattner, W.A., Biggar, R.J., Weiss, S.H., et al., Epidemiology of human T-lymphotropic virus type III and the risk of the acquired immunodeficiency syndrome. Ann Intern Med 103: 665-670 (1985)

22. Selik, R.M., Haverkos, H.W., Curran, J.W., Acquired immune deficiency syndrome (AIDS) trends in the United States, 1978-1982. Am J Med 76:493-500 (1984)

23. Moos, R.H., Tsu, V.D., The crisis of physical illness: an overview. In: Coping with Physical Illness. (Moos, R.H., ed) Plenum Medical Book Company, New York, p 7 (1977)

24. Cohen, M.A., Weissman, H.W., A biopsychosocial approach to AIDS. Psychosomatics 27:245-249 (1986)

25. Snider, W.D., Simpson, D.M., Nielson, S., et al., Neurological complications of AIDS: an analysis of 50 patients. Ann Neurol 14:403-408 (1983)

26. Shaw, G.M. Harper, M.E., Hahn, B.H., et al., HTLV-III infection in brains of children and adults with AIDS encephalopathy. Science 227:177-182 (1985)

27. Hoffman, R.S., Neuropsychiatric complications of AIDS. Psychosomatics 25:293-400 (1984)

28. Nurnberg, H.G., Prudic, J., Fiori, M., et al., Psychopathology complicating acquired immune deficiency syndrome. Am J Psychiatry 141:95-96 (1984)

29. Price, W.A., Forejt, J., Neuropsychiatric aspects of AIDS: a case report. Gen Hosp Psychiatry 8:7-10 (1986)

30. Ho, D.D., Rota, T.R., Schooley, R.T., et al., Isolation of HTLV-III from cerebrospinal fluid and neural tissues of patients with neurological syndromes related to the acquired immunodeficiency syndrome. N Engl J Med 313:1493-1497 (1985)

31. Resnik, L., di Marzo-Veronese, F., Schupbach, J., et al., Intra-blood-brain barrier synthesis of HTLV-III-specific IgG in patients with neurologic symptoms associated with AIDS or AIDS-related complex. N Engl J Med 313:1498-1504 (1985)

32. Black, P.H., HTLV III, AIDS and the brain. N Engl J Med 313:1538-1540 (1985)

33. Nichols, S.E., Psychosocial reactions of persons with the acquired immunodeficiency syndrome. Ann Intern Med 103: 765-767 (1985)

34. Hackett, T.P., Cassem, N.H., Psychological reactions to a life-threatening illness. In: Psychological Aspects of Stress. (Abram, H., ed.), Charles C. Thomas, Springfield, IL, p 29-43 (1970)

35. Horowitz, M. T., Stress Responses Syndromes. Jason Aranson, New York (1973)

36. Holtz, H., Dobro, J., Palinkas, R., et al., Psychosocial impact of acquired immune deficiency syndrome. (Letter) JAMA 24:1083-1089 (1983)

37. Kubler-Ross, E., On Death and Dying. Macmillan, New York (1969)

38. Nichols, S.E., Psychiatric aspects of AIDS. Psychosomatics 24:1083-1089 (1983)

39. Vinogradov, S., Thorton, J.E., If I have AIDS, then let me die now! Hasting Cent Rep 14:24-26 (1984)

40. Webster, N., Webster's New Twentieth Century Dictionary of the English Language (Jean McKechnie, ed). The Publisher's Guild, Inc., New York (1958)

41. Cassens, B., Social consequences of the acquired immunodeficiency syndrome. Ann Intern Med 103:768-711 (1985)

42. Perry, S.W, Tross, S., Psychiatric problems of AIDS in patients at the New York Hospital: preliminary report. Pub Health Rep 99:200-205 (1984)

43. Dilley, J.W., Ochitill, H.N., Perl, M., et al., Findings in psychiatric consultations with patients with acquired immune deficiency syndrome. Am J Psych 142:82-86 (1985)

44. Polan, H.J., Hellerstein, D., Amchin, J., Impact of AIDS-related cases on an inpatient therapeutic milieu. Hosp Commun Psych 36:173-176 (1985)

45. Diagnostic and Statistical Manual of Mental Disorders. Third Edition. The American Psychiatric Association. Washington, D.C., (1980).

46. Khantzian, E.J., The self-medication hypothesis of addictive disorders: focus on heroin and cocaine dependence. Am J Psych 142:1259-1264 (1985)

47. Spitz, R.A., Hospitalism, an inquiry into the genesis of psychiatric conditions in early childhood. Psychoanalytic Study of the Child I, p 53-74 (1945)

48. Spitz, R.A., Anaclitic depression. Psychoanalytic Study of the Child II, p 313-342 (1946)

49. Engel, G.L., A life-setting conducive to illness: the giving-up complex. Ann Intern Med 69:293-300 (1968)

50. Schmale, A.H., Relation of separation and depression to disease I. A report on a hospitalized medical population. Psychosomatic Med 20:259-277 (1958)

51. Hofer, M. A., The Roots of Human Behavior. An Introduction to the Psychobiology of Early Development. W.H. Freeman and Company, San Francsico (1981)

52. Holmes, T.H., Rahe, R.H., The social readjustment rating scale. J Psychosom Res 11:213-218 (1967)

53. Rahe, R.H., Meyer, M., Smith, M., et al., Social stress and illness onset. J Psychosom Res 8:35-44 (1964)

54. Weiner, H., Psychobiology and Human Disease. Elsevier North-Holland, New York (1977)

55. Silberstein, C., Psychobiological considerations in the development of acquired immunodeficiency syndrome. Einstein Quarterly J Biol Med 3:136-143 (1985)

56. McEvoy, J.P., Organic brain syndromes. Ann Intern Med 95: 212-220 (1981)

57. Lipowski, Z.J., Delirium (acute confusional state). In: Handbook of Clinical Neurology. Vol 2 (46): Neurobehavioral Disorders. (Fredericks, J.A.M., ed). Elsevier Science Publishers, New York (1985)

58. Lipowski, Z.J., Delirium: Acute Brain Failure in Man. Charles C. Thomas, Springfield (1980)

59. Pfeiffer, E., A short portable mental status questionnaire for the assessment of organic brain deficits in elderly patients. J Am Geriatr Soc 23:433-441 (1975)

60. Folstein, M.F., Folstein, S.E., McHugh, Mini-mental state - a practical method for grading the cognitive state of patients for the clinician. J Psychiatr Res 12:189-198 (1975)

61. Jacobs, J.N., Bernhard, M.R., Delgado, A., et al., Screening for organic mental syndromes in the medically ill. Ann Intern Med 86:40-46 (1944)

62. Romano, J., Engel, G.L., Delirium I. Electroencephalographic data. Arch Neurol Psych 51:227-255 (1944)

63. Pro, J.D., Wells, C.E., The use of the electroencephalogram in the diagnosis of delirium. Dis Nerv Syst 38:807-808 (1977)

64. Obrecht, R., Okhominia, F.O.A., Scott, D.F., Value of EEG in acute confusional states. J Neurol Neurosurg Psych 42:75-77 (1970)

65. Holland, J.C., Tross, S., The psychosocial and neuropsychiatric sequelae of the acquired immunodeficiency syndrome and related disorders. Ann Intern Med 103:760-764 (1985)

66. Lipowski, Z.J., The Concept and Psychopathology of Dementia, In: Psychosomatic Medicine and Liaison Psychiatry. (Lipowski, Z.J., ed), Plenum Medical Book Company, New York, p 307-313 (1985)

67. Goldstein, K., Functional disturbances in brain damage, In: American Handbook of Psychiatry, (Arieti, S., Reiser, M.F., eds) Edition 2, Basic Books, New York, Vol 4, p 182-207, (1975)

68. Loewenstein, R.J., Sharfstein, S.S., Neuropsychiatric aspects of acquired immune deficiency syndrome. Intern J Psych Med 13:255-260 (1984)

69. Taveres, R., Lopez, D.J., Response of the gay community to acquired immune deficiency syndrome, In: Psychiatric Implications of Acquired Immune Deficiency Syndrome, (Nichols, S.E., Ostrow, D.G., eds) American Psychiatric Press, Washington, DC, p 106-110 (1984)

70. Barbuto, J., Psychiatric care of seriously ill patients with acquired immune deficiency syndrome, In: Psychiatric Implications of Acquired Immune Deficiency Syndrome, (Nichols, S.E., Ostrow, D.G., eds) American Psychiatric Press, Washington, DC, p 72-76 (1984)

71. Perry, S., Jacobsen, P., Neuropsychiatric manifestations of AIDS-spectrum disorders. Hospital Commun Psych 37:135-142 (1986)

72. Newmark, D.A., Review of a support group for patients with AIDS. Topics Clin Nurs 6:38-44 (1984)

73. Nichols, S.E., Social and support groups for patients with acquired immune deficiency syndrome, In: Psychiatric Implications of Acquired Immune Deficiency Syndrome, (Nichols, S.E., Ostrow, D.G., eds) American Psychiatric Press, Washington, DC, p 78-82 (1984)

74. Cohen, M.A., Merlino, J.P., The suicidal patient on the surgical ward: a multidisciplinary case conference. Gen Hosp Psych 5:65-71 (1983)

75. Sabbath, J., The suicidal adolescent: the expendable child. J Am Acad Child Psych 8:272-289 (1969)

76. Beck, A.T., Steer, R.A., Kovacs, M., Garrison, B., Hopelessness and eventual suicide. Am J Psychiatry 142:559-563 (1985)

77. Miles, C.P., Conditions predisposing to suicide: a review. J Nerv Ment Dis 164:231-246 (1977)

78. Barraclough, B., Bunch, J., Nelson, B., et al., A hundred cases of suicide: clinical aspects. Br J Psych 125:355-373 (1974)

79. Deuchar, N., AIDS in New York City with particular reference to the psychosocial aspects. Br J Psych 145:612-619 (1984)

80. Conte, J.E., Hadley, W.K., Sande, M., Infection control guidelines for patients with the acquired immunodeficiency syndrome (AIDS). N Engl J Med 309:741-744 (1983)

81. Cox, C., Peer review: face to face with AIDS phobia. Nurs Times 81:22 (1985)

82. Rubinow, D.R., The psychological impact of AIDS. Top Clin Nurs 6:26-30 (1984)

83. Simmons-Alling, S., AIDS: psychosocial needs of the health care worker. Top Clin Nurs 6:31-37 (1984)

84. Lusby, G., AIDS: the impact on the health worker. Front Radiat Ther Onc 19:164-167 (1985)

85. Wellisch, D.K., U.C.L.A. psychological study of AIDS. Front Radiat Ther Onc 19:155-158 (1985)

86. Rosse, R.B., Reactions of psychiatric staff to an AIDS patient. Am J Psych 142:523 (1985)

87. Batten, C.P., Tabor, R., Nursing the patient with AIDS. Can Nurs 79:19-22 (1983)

88. Small, G.W., House officer stress syndrome. Psychosomatics 22:860-869 (1981)

89. Ford, C.V., Emotional distress in internship and residency: a questionaire study. Psych Med 1:143-150 (1983)

90. Valko, R.J., Clayton, P.J., Depression in internship. Dis Nerv Syst 36:26-29 (1975)

91. McCue, J., Distress of internship causes and prevention. N Engl J Med 312:449-452 (1985)

92. Borenstein, D.B., Cook, K., Impairment prevention in the training years. JAMA 247:2700-2703 (1982)

93. Borenstein, D.B., Should physician training centers offer formal psychiatric assistance to house officers? A report on the major findings of a prototype program. Am J Psych 142:1053-1057 (1985)

94. Modlin, H.C., Montes, A., Narcotics addiction in physicians. Am J Psych 121:358-363 (1964)

95. Putnam, P.L., Ellinwood, E.H. Jr., Narcotic addiction among physicians: a ten year follow up. Am J Psych 122:745-748 (1966)

96. Epstein, L.C., Thomas, C.B., Shaffer, J.W., et al., Clinical prediction of physician suicide based on medical student data. J Nerv Ment Dis 156:19-29 (1973)

97. Craig, A.G., Pitts, F.N., Suicide by physicians. Dis Nerv Syst 29:763-772 (1969)

98. Stepphacher, R.C., Mausner, J.S., Suicide in male and female physicians. JAMA 228:323-328 (1974)

99. Wachter, R.M., The impact of the acquired immunodeficiency syndrome on medical residency training. N Engl J Med 314: 177-180 (1986)

100. Steinbrook, R., Lo, B., Tirpack, J., et al., Ethical dilemmas in caring for patients with the acquired immunodeficiency syndrome. Ann Intern Med 103:787-790 (1985)

101. Steinbrook, R., Lo, B., Moulton, J., et al., Preferences of homosexual men with AIDS for life-sustaining treatment. N Engl J Med 314:457-460 (1986)

102. Brown, J.H., Henteleff, P., Barakaf, S., et al., Is it normal for terminally ill patients to desire death? Am J Psych 143:208-211 (1986)

103. Sullivan, H.S., The Interpersonal Theory of Psychiatry, (Perry, H.S., and Garvel, M.L., eds), W.W. Norton and Company Inc., New York, p 32-33,(1953)

APPENDIX

Goals and Objectives of the Multidisciplinary AIDS Program at Metropolitan Hospital Center in New York City.

Goals:

1) To improve the care of the person with AIDS by means of a biopsychosocial approach that maintains a view of each individual as a member of a family and community who deserves a coordinated approach to care and treatment with dignity.

2) To improve communication and diminish alienation and expendability by means of a multidisciplinary team approach.

3) To provide on-going programs of education for persons with AIDS and ARC and their families, for members of risk groups, for hospital staff and community.

4) To provide programs of risk-reduction for members of risk groups and also for schools and community organizations.

Enabling Objectives:

1) Identification of volunteers from all areas of the hospital.

2) Formation of a multidisciplinary team.

3) Development of a comprehensive program.

   a) clinical care of patients
   b) staff education
   c) faculty development
   d) liaison with outside agencies
   e) research

4) Development of methods to provide comprehensive care.

   a) regular rounds on patients with AIDS
   b) special AIDS rounds on a weekly basis to meet with all staff involved
   c) Identification of psychological and social problems frequently encountered in patients with AIDS

5) Development of educational programs for persons with AIDS and ARC and those at risk for AIDS.

   a) regular seminars
   b) special meeting with all members of the team

6) Educational programs of risk-reduction for persons at risk.

   a) special programs for intravenous drug users
   b) methadone maintenance program members
   c) patients in drug detoxification units

7) Community programs of education and risk-reduction.

   a) for schools
   b) for community organizations

8) Integration of inpatient and outpatient care.

   a) home care
   b) home visits
   c) coordination of community services

Terminal Objectives:

1) Heightened awareness of psychological problems encountered in patients with AIDS and their families.

2) Heightened awareness in staff of psychological reactions to patients with AIDS.

3) Improvement in doctor-patient communication.

4) Opening avenues of communication among health professionals dealing with patients with AIDS.

5) Humane approach to patients with AIDS by both professional and nonprofessional hospital staff.

6) Identification and treatment of psychological problems through individual, couple, family, group and psychopharmacological therapy.

7) Abstinence from needle sharing or use of intravenous drugs.

8) Abstinence from exchange of body fluids.

9) Diminution of discrimination against persons with AIDS, ARC or HIV seropositivity.

10) Improvement and increased availability of services for patients with AIDS or ARC.

11) Integration of a comprehensive program of care for persons with AIDS and ARC enabling individuals to remain as functional and healthy as possible and to live as comfortably as possible within the family setting.

12) Primary prevention of AIDS through elementary school education.

Guidelines for Development of a Multidisciplinary AIDS Program

1. Identification of individuals willing to provide organization and leadership.

2. Identification of volunteers from as many areas or specialities as is appropriate.

3. Preliminary meeting to decide on permanent membership of those individuals involved in the care of persons with AIDS.

4. Presentation of the program to the Director of Medicine and the Director of the Hospital and Dean in order to enlist their support or involvement.

5. Organization of a multidisciplinary AIDS program

    a. choice of leadership
    b. review of literature
    c. organization of seminars
    d. invitations to persons experienced in working with persons with AIDS or visits to other centers

6. Scheduling of on-going meetings on a weekly basis.

7. Assessment of programs of surveillance in order to determine the needs of the institution and to design programs to meet those needs.

8. Incorporation of consultation-liaison psychiatry into the program leadership and organization.

    a. provide for psychological care of persons with AIDS and ARC
    b. provide on-going programs of support for staff members
    c. provide for accurate psychiatric diagnosis and treatment

A multidisciplinary AIDS program may be comprised of the following members:

Infectious disease specialists
Consultation-liaison psychiatrists
Oncologists
Pulmonologists
Neurologists
Dermatologists
Gastroenterologists
Gynecologists
Dentists
Nurses
Psychologists
Social Workers
Drug Addiction Counselors
Respiratory Therapists
Dieticians
Chaplains
Discharge Planners
Administrators
House Officers
Community Affairs Representatives

The members may be permanent or rotating with an identified core of permanent members who meet on an on-going basis and provide coordination of clinical, educational and research activities throughout the hospital.

30
HIV Infections of the Nervous System

Dana H. Gabuzda, Joan C. Kaplan, David D. Ho

Human immunodeficiency virus (HIV) is both lymphotropic and neurotropic and appears to be capable of causing neurologic diseases in addition to immunodeficiency. Approximately 40% of patients with the acquired immunodeficiency syndrome (AIDS) have neurologic signs and symptoms (1), while the prevalence of neuropathologic abnormalities is 80-90% in autopsy series (2)-(4). There are many causes of neurologic dysfunction in AIDS (1),(5), but common problems include toxoplasmosis (6), cryptococcosis (7), and lymphoma (8) involving the central nervous system (CNS). Opportunistic viral infections of the CNS have also been documented in patients with AIDS, including cytomegalovirus, *Herpes simplex*, adenovirus, varicella-zoster, and papovavirus (1),(5),(9)-(13). In addition, there are several distinct and previously unexplained neurologic syndromes frequently encountered in AIDS or AIDS-related complex (ARC). These include subacute encephalitis (2), vacuolar myelopathy (14), peripheral neuropathy (15), and atypical aseptic meningitis (1),(16).

Recent findings suggest that HIV is directly involved in the pathogenesis of some of the neurologic syndromes associated with AIDS or ARC. They include the isolation of HIV from neural tissues and cerebrospinal fluid (CSF) of patients with AIDS-related neurologic disorders (16),(17), demonstration of HIV-specific immunoglobulin production in CSF (18), detection of HIV sequences in the brains of patients with AIDS (19), and identification of viral particles consistent with HIV in the brains of patients with AIDS encephalopathy (20),(21). Furthermore, HIV is antigenically related to simian T-lymphotropic virus (STLV-III), which can induce an encephalitis, in addition to immunodeficiency, in macaque monkeys (22)-(24). HIV is also morphologically and genetically similar to visna virus, a non-oncogenic retrovirus (lentivirus) which causes a chronic inflammatory neurodegenerative disease in sheep (25)-(28).

The clinical and pathologic features of neurologic syndromes related to AIDS and evidence that HIV is the etiologic agent of some of these syndromes will be reviewed. The relationship between HIV and other lentiviruses and the possible mechanisms of pathogenesis will also be discussed.

CLINICAL SYNDROMES

The clinical and pathologic features of the dementia, myelopathy, neuropathy, and aseptic meningitis associated with AIDS or ARC are summarized in Table 1. The prevalence of subacute encephalitis, the most common neuropathologic abnormality in these patients, is 70-90% (2)-(4), while vacuolar myelopathy, neuropathy, and aseptic meningitis occur in about 10-20% of patients with AIDS (1),(5),(14),(15). The following case demonstrates several characteristic features of these syndromes.

> **Case 1:** A 28 year-old homosexual male was diagnosed as having AIDS in January, 1985 when he presented with *Pneumocystis carinii* pneumonia, disseminated *Mycobacterium avium-intracellulare*, and oral thrush. He subsequently developed disseminated cytomegalovirus infection. In April 1985, he showed signs of impaired memory and attention and was intermittently confused. He was described as having blunt affect and slurred speech with word-finding difficulties. A lumbar puncture was unremarkable. A CT scan showed cerebral atrophy and an electroencephalogram (EEG) showed diffuse non-specific theta slowing. Over several months he became increasingly demented and developed progressive lower extremity weakness and sensory loss. He reported gait unsteadiness and severe pain and edema of the distal lower extremities. He required narcotics for relief of painful dysesthesias. The patient had a progressively downhill course and expired in February 1986. At autopsy, neuropathologic findings included severe subacute encephalitis with numerous microglial nodules and a striking number of multinucleated giant cells. In addition, there was evidence of vacuolar myelopathy and demyelinating peripheral neuropathy. HIV was isolated from several regions of the brain and spinal cord.

Subacute Encephalitis

Subacute encephalitis is the cause of the progressive dementia in patients with AIDS (3),(29). The clinical spectrum associated with this condition ranges from mild cognitive or behavioral disturbances to severe dementia. Early clinical manifestations may include subtle personality changes, depression, social with-

TABLE 1. Clinical and Pathologic Features of Neurologic Syndromes Associated with AIDS or ARC

Syndrome	Prevalence	Clinical Features	Pathologic Features
Subacute encephalitis	70-90%	Early:impaired memory decreased concentration depression social withdrawal	grey and white matter gliosis microglial nodules foci of necrosis foci of demyelination perivascular inflammation
		Late:cognitive deficits psychomotor retardation severe dementia mutism seizures myoclonus	multinucleated giant cells
Vacuolar myelopathy	20%	gait ataxia progressive paraparesis spasticity incontinence	vacuolar degeneration of lateral and posterior columns
Neuropathy	10%	Type 1:chronic inflammatory demyelinating neuropathy	inflammation and patchy demyelination possibly with axonal degeneration
		Type 2:distal symmetric predominantly sensory neuropathy	patchy demyelination with relative preservation of axons
Aseptic meningitis	5-10%	fever, headache, meningeal signs, often in patients with ARC, usually self-limited, may be chronic or recurrent	

drawal, apathy, and mild impairment of memory and concentration (5),(29). Psychomotor retardation and further deterioration in memory and ability to perform calculations and complex tasks typically occur as the disease slowly progresses, usually over several months. In some cases, psychiatric symptoms such as psychosis, hallucinations, or affective symptoms are particularly prominent (29),(30). In the most severe cases, there is a gradual progression to severe dementia with disorientation, severe global cognitive impairment, mutism, and incontinence. Focal motor signs, frontal release signs, myoclonus, and seizures may also occur late in the course (1),(5),(29). In pediatric cases, common clinical features include loss of developmental milestones, acquired microcephaly, cognitive impairment, and pyramidal tract signs (31),(32). Subacute encephalitis can occasionally be diagnosed prior to the development of AIDS, ARC, or any detectable signs of immunodeficiency (our unpublished observations).

Results of diagnostic studies are generally non-specific. The CSF is abnormal in 60-75% of patients, usually demonstrating a mild elevation in protein (typically 50-100 mg/dL) (1). A mild mononuclear pleocytosis or mild hypoglycorrhachia may also be present (1),(5). The CT scan frequently shows moderate to severe cerebral atrophy in patients with significant dementia but is often normal in patients who are asymptomatic or minimally symptomatic. The EEG usually demonstrates diffuse non-specific theta or delta slowing in patients with dementia, but is often normal in patients who are asymptomatic (unpublished observations). In pediatric cases, the CT scan frequently reveals cerebral atrophy and basal ganglia calcifications and the EEG usually shows diffuse non-specific slowing (31),(32).

The pathologic features of subacute encephalitis suggest a diffuse viral infection of the CNS. Typically, they include grey and white matter gliosis, microglial nodules (Figure 1), foci of demyelination and necrosis, perivascular inflammation, atypical oligodendrocytes, and multinucleated giant cells (Figure 2) (2)-(5). On gross examination, cerebral atrophy is infrequent except in severe cases. The most common histologic findings are gliosis of the white matter (96%) and grey matter (89%), foci of necrosis (81%), and microglial nodules (74%), while multinucleated giant cells are a less common feature (30%) (4). An autopsy study of 30 patients at the Massachusetts General Hospital showed that the regions most frequently involved are the white matter (93%), amygdala (80%), basal ganglia (77%), frontal cortex (58%), and temporal cortex (69%) (4). In some cases, severe white matter damage and long tract degeneration are particularly striking (11),(30). The neuropathologic findings in the pediatric cases show many of the same features, but additional characteristic findings include diminished brain weight, numerous multinucleated giant cells, vascular calcifications, and more prominent inflammatory cell infiltrates (21),(32).

Vacuolar Myelopathy

About 20% of patients with AIDS have evidence of a vacuolar myelopathy at autopsy (14). The clinical syndrome associated with this disorder is a progressive paraparesis often accompanied by ataxia, spasticity, and incontinence. Myelography is usually unremarkable and evoked responses may be abnormal (33). The pathologic findings are vacuolar degeneration of the dorsal and

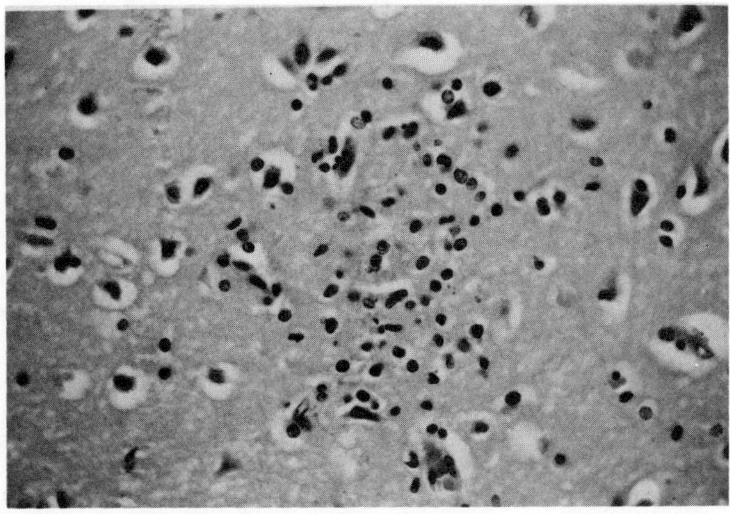

Figure 1. Microglial nodule in putamen. Hematoxylin-eosin. Photograph courtesy of Dr. Suzanne M. de la Monte.

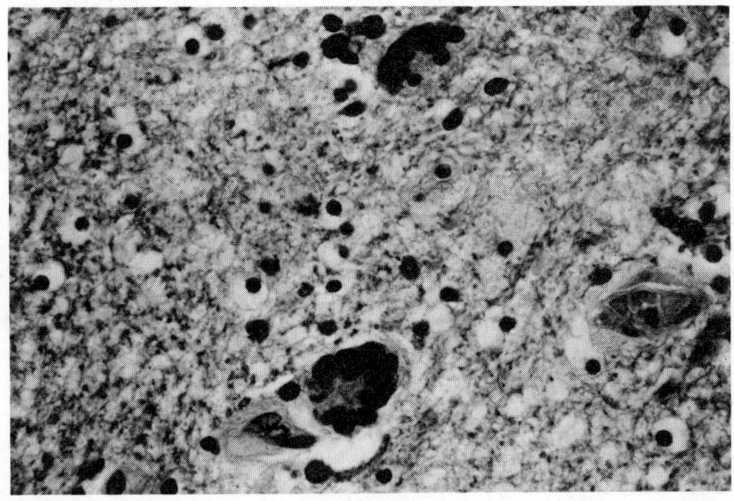

Figure 2. Multinucleated giant cells in frontal white matter. Luxol fast blue-hematoxylin-eosin.

lateral columns resembling subacute combined degeneration (Figure 3). The appearance of these vacuoles suggests that they may result from intramyelin swelling (14).

Neuropathy

Two types of peripheral neuropathy occur in patients with HIV-related disorders (1),(5),(15). The first is a chronic inflammatory demyelinating polyneuropathy which usually occurs in patients with ARC. The clinical features include weakness (particularly of the lower extremities), distal sensory loss, and areflexia. Cranial nerve involvement and features of mononeuropathy multiplex may also occur. Nerve conduction studies suggest demyelinating neuropathy with slowed conduction velocities and, in some cases, axonal damage as well. The CSF usually demonstrates mild pleocytosis and protein elevation. Nerve biopsies showing demyelination and inflammatory cell infiltration (Figure 4) have been reported (15),(16). The symptoms often resolve spontaneously and some cases have responded to plasmaphoresis (1),(15). The case below illustrates typical features of this condition.

> **Case 2:** A 45 year-old homosexual male had unexplained generalized lymphadenopathy since early 1984. In October 1984, he developed numbness and tingling of the hands and feet in a glove-and-stocking distribution and progressive weakness of the upper and lower extremities. Electro-physiologic studies demonstrated slowing of the conduction velocities and evidence of denervation. The CSF showed 15 lymphocytes/mm^3 and a protein of 210 mg/dl. Biopsy of the sural nerve demonstrated demyelination and marked infiltration with inflammatory cells. Cultures of the CSF and sural nerve were positive for HIV.

The second type of neuropathy is a distal symmetric polyneuropathy which usually occurs in patients with AIDS. Sensory symptoms predominate, particularly painful dysesthesias. Examination usually reveals distal sensory loss in a glove-and-stocking distribution and may also show weakness and diminished or absent reflexes. The CSF may show an elevated protein (5). Electrophysiologic studies usually demonstrate slowing of conduction velocities consistent with a demyelinating neuropathy. The nerves may be histopathologically normal or may show mild demyelination with relative preservation of axons (4).

Aseptic Meningitis

Atypical aseptic meningitis usually occurs in patients with ARC and also may be part of the syndrome associated with primary HIV infection. In one series, all 17 patients with this form of atypical aseptic meningitis had ARC but six subsequently developed AIDS or significant immunodeficiency (1). We and others have reported similar cases of acute aseptic meningitis associated with acute (primary) HIV infection (34),(35). The

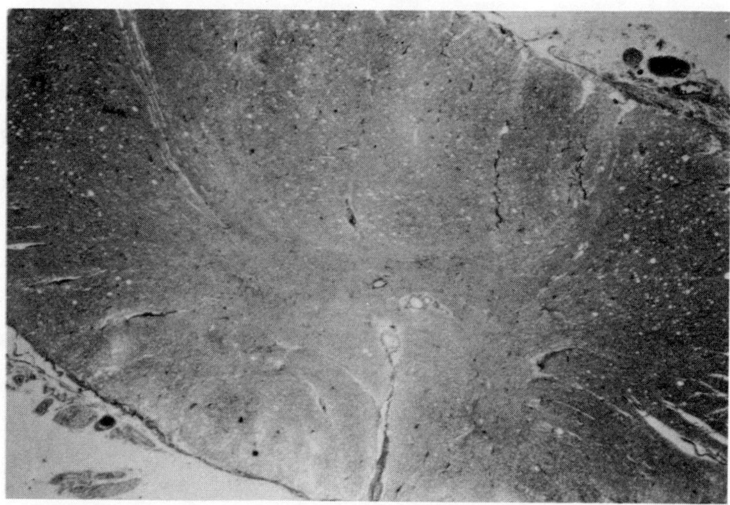

3A. Vacuolar degeneration of the lateral and posterior columns (Luxol fast blue-hematoxylin-eosin, gross specimen).

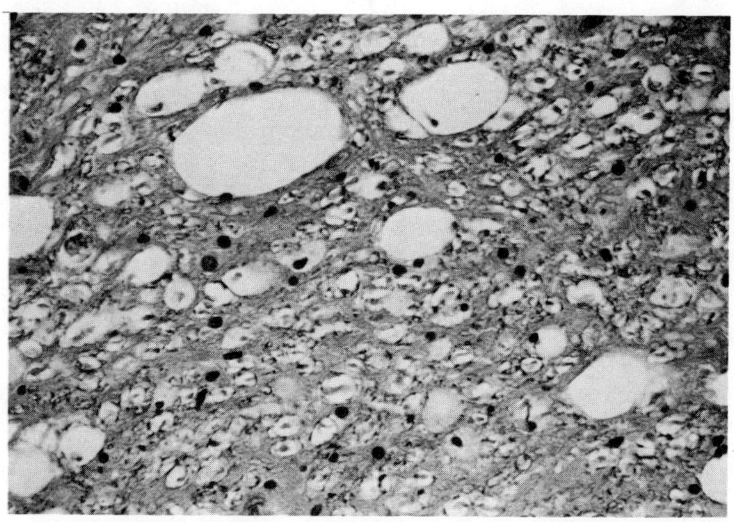

3B. Variable-sized vacuoles and occasional hypertrophic reactive astrocytes and macrophages (Luxol fast blue-hematoxylin-eosin).

Figure 3. Vacuolar myelopathy in thoracic spinal cord.

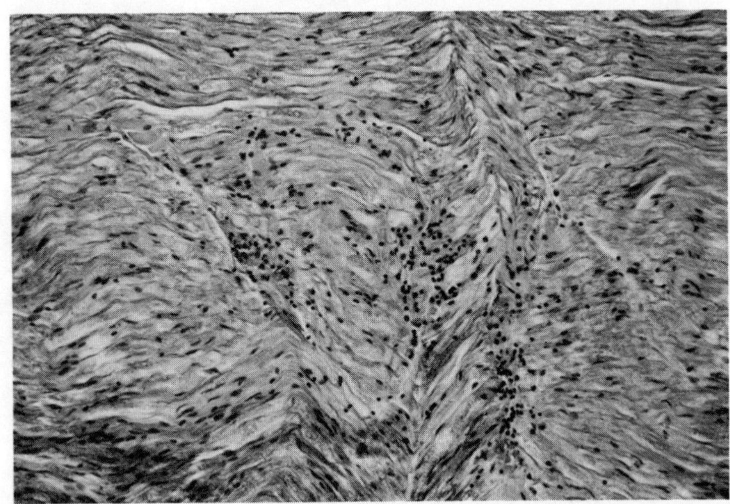

Figure 4. Chronic inflammatory demyelinating neuropathy. Sural nerve with diffuse demyelination and focal mild lymphocytic inflammation (Luxol fast blue-hematoxylin-eosin)

symptoms typically include fever, headache, and meningeal signs and in some cases, cranial nerve palsies (particularly of fifth, seventh and eighth cranial nerves) (1),(5). The course typically lasts two or three weeks and is usually self-limited, but there are some cases which are chronic or recurrent (1),(5),(16). The CSF shows a mononuclear pleocytosis of 20-300 cells/mm^3, elevated protein of 50-100 mg/dL, and occasionally mild hypoglycorrhachia.

Other Neurologic Syndromes

At our institution there have been several cases of unusual neurologic syndromes occurring in patients with risk factors for AIDS who did not have AIDS or immunodeficiency (16),(36). In each case, an extensive evaluation to exclude infectious and non-infectious etiologies was negative, except for evidence of CNS infection with HIV.

Case 3 (36): A 42 year-old homosexual male presented with a one-month history of decline in mental status and episodes of confusion. On admission he was febrile and the CSF showed 329 white cells/mm^3 (97% polymorphonuclear cells), a protein level of 123 mg/dL, and glucose level of 85 mg/dL. On examination there were signs of cognitive impairment, dysmetria, and ataxia. Subsequently, he developed multiple focal neurologic deficits with evidence of cerebral infarcts on CT scan. Angiography showed diffuse segmental narrowing of multiple large and medium-sized cerebral arteries. Systemic blood vessels were uninvolved. Cultures of CSF and brain biopsy were positive for HIV, although the patient was sero-negative for HIV. The patient's focal neurologic deficits and coma did not improve, and he died of bronchopneumonia after a four month hospitalization. At autopsy, neuropathologic findings included granulomatous cerebral angiitis with mononuclear cell infiltrates and multinucleated giant cells involving large and medium-sized arteries and multiple cerebral infarcts. There were rare scattered microglial nodules and multinucleated giant cells. Postmortem brain cultures for HIV were negative.

Case 4: A 38 year-old, HIV-seropositive Haitian male was admitted with a several month history of major depression with psychotic features and mild cognitive difficulties. On examination, he was disoriented and had impairment of memory and ability to perform complex tasks and a right hemiparesis. CT scan revealed enhancing periventricular lesions and nuclear magnetic resonance scan showed large confluent lesions in the white matter and left cingulate gyrus. The CSF was unremarkable except for a protein of 50 mg/dL. The brain biopsy was histopathologically non-diagnostic, but samples of CSF and brain biopsy were positive for HIV on culture.

Case 5: A 38 year-old homosexual male was admitted with a two-week history of headache and progressive left lower extremity weakness. On exam he was disoriented and had decreased memory, evidence of cognitive impairment, and a left hemiparesis. The CSF showed 24 white cells/mm^3 (96% lymphocytes), a protein level of 72 mg/dL, and a glucose level of 70 mg/dL. CT scan revealed a right posterior parietal enhancing lesion. Biopsy of this region showed histopathologic features consistent with progressive multifocal leukoencephalopathy with some unusual features, including prominent perivascular lymphocytic infiltrates. Immunoperoxidase staining was positive for papovavirus antigen. Brain biopsy and CSF cultures for HIV were also positive.

An acute, self-limited encephalopathy associated with seizures has recently been described in individuals at risk for AIDS (37). The syndrome was coincident with HIV seroconversion suggesting that it is a manifestation of primary HIV infection.

EVIDENCE SUPPORTING HIV AS THE ETIOLOGIC AGENT IN AIDS-RELATED NEUROLOGIC SYNDROMES

There is now sufficient evidence to consider HIV as the etiologic agent for subacute encephalitis and aseptic meningitis associated with AIDS or ARC. Shaw et al. first reported the detection of HIV DNA and RNA by Southern blot and in situ hybridization studies in the brains of five of 15 patients with AIDS and subacute encephalitis (19). Direct recovery of infectious HIV from the CNS has also been reported (16),(17). In our investigation, HIV was isolated from CSF or neural tissues in 24/33 patients with AIDS-related neurologic syndromes, including 10/16 patients with subacute encephalitis, one patient with acute aseptic meningitis associated with HIV seroconversion, and six of seven patients with AIDS or ARC and chronic meningitis (16). In addition, HIV was isolated from the CSF and sural nerve of two patients with ARC and peripheral neuropathy and from the spinal cord of two patients with myelopathy (16) (unpublished observations). All of the above CNS specimens were culture-negative for bacteria, fungi, and routinely-cultured viruses. In another clinical study (18), HIV-specific immunoglobulins were demonstrated in CSF from 22/23 patients with AIDS or ARC, the majority of whom were neurologically symptomatic. Furthermore, eight of nine patients demonstrated a higher percentage of HIV-specific IgG in CSF than in serum by enzyme-linked immunosorbent assay, suggesting selective intra-blood-brain-barrier synthesis of antibodies against HIV antigens.

Electron microscopic studies of the brain from patients with AIDS encephalopathy have also demonstrated HIV-like particles in multinucleated giant cells and rarely in astrocytes (20),(21). We recently detected HIV antigens in cells morphologically resembling monocyte/macrophages in brain tissues from five of 13 patients with AIDS-related neurologic syndromes using the immunoperoxidase method with goat anti-HIV serum (38). Additional evidence linking HIV with neurologic diseases includes its similarity to STLV-III, which causes an AIDS-like syndrome and encephalitis in macaque monkeys (22)-(24), and to lentiviruses, which cause chronic neurologic disorders in sheep and goats (25)-(28).

RELATIONSHIP BETWEEN HIV AND OTHER LENTIVIRUSES

Based on morphologic similarity and nucleotide sequence homologies, HIV appears to be related to the lentivirus family of retroviruses, including visna virus, caprine arthritis-encephalitis virus (CAEV), and equine infectious anemia virus (EIAV) (25)-(28). In addition, HIV is morphologically and antigenically related to STLV-III (22)-(24). The recently discovered human T-lymphotropic virus type IV (HTLV-IV) from healthy West Africans from Senegal is closely related to STLV-III and is also antigenically cross-reactive with human T-cell lymphotropic virus type III (HTLV-III) (39). These observations (22),(25)-(28),(39) suggest an evolutionary relationship for retroviruses as depicted in Figure 5.

Visna is an Icelandic term for wasting (40). The disease in sheep was initially reported in 1935, and Sigurdsson was the first to show a transmissible etiology. Approximately 90% of infected sheep are asymptomatic, although they are all persistently virus-positive. Following an incubation period of two to eight years, some animals develop overt disease. The most common manifestation is maedi, an Icelandic term describing interstitial pneumonia. Pathologically, the lungs show intense inflammation with infiltration by mononuclear cells including macrophages.

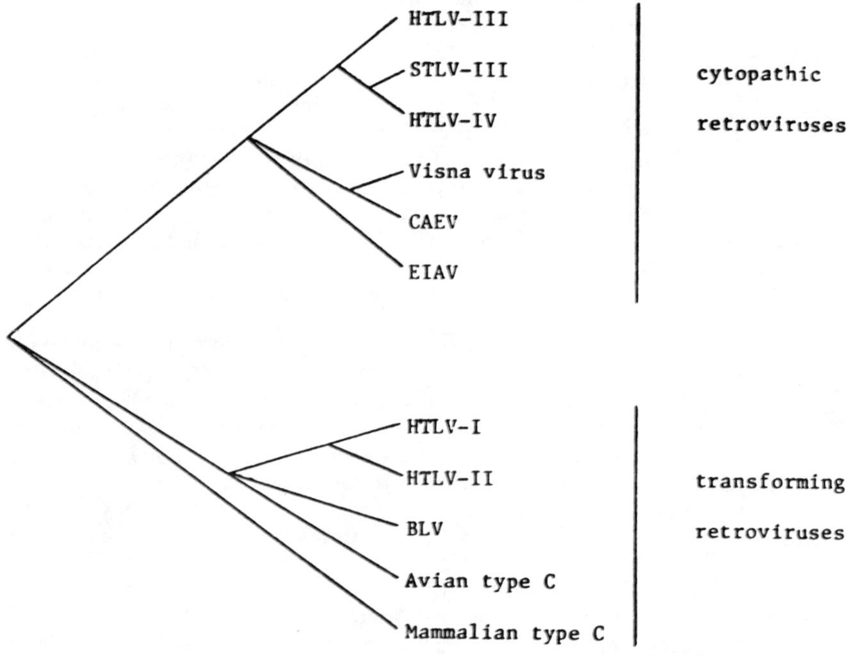

Figure 5. Evolutionary relationship of HTLV-III (HIV) and other retroviruses (References 22-28, 39). HTLV-I and HTLV-II: human T-cell leukemia virus type I and type II; BLV: bovine leukemia virus; CAEV: caprine arthritis-encephalitis virus; EIAV: equine infectious anemia virus.

Only a few of the infected sheep develop visna, a form of encephalomyelitis. This neurologic disease is host and breed dependent; for example, sheep native to Britain do not develop visna. The first neurologic signs of disease are ataxia and a stumbling gait, which gradually worsen, leading to paralysis of hind limbs and occasionally to quadriplegia. The animals remain alert and afebrile, and the CSF typically shows pleocytosis, protein elevation, and increased IgG level. Gliosis, demyelination, and intense mononuclear infiltration are histologically evident in the brain and spinal cord (40). Destruction of neurons is unusual.

CAEV is closely related to visna virus (40). Arthritis, the most common manifestation of infection in adult goats, has an insidious onset and progressive course. Leukoencephalomyelitis is the most frequent clinical expression of CAEV infection in kids and also occurs occasionally in adult goats. Typically, the kids develop weakness of the hindquarters, which gradually progresses to paralysis. Tremors, facial twitching, and other neurologic signs can also develop. The pathologic findings are similar to those described for visna.

EIAV causes a chronic relapsing disease in horses (41). Five to 30 days following virus exposure, a horse develops an acute illness characterized by fever, anemia, and thrombocytopenia. This usually subsides after a few days, although fatal primary forms can occur. The hallmark of equine infectious anemia is periodic recrudescence of disease due to the emergence of viral variants which have altered surface glycoproteins and can temporarily escape host immune surveillance (41), a phenomenon also observed with visna virus and CAEV. Each relapse is accompanied by fever, weight loss, anemia, and depression of the central nervous system. The recurrences decrease in severity and frequency in time, with 90% of the episodes occurring within one year of infection.

Restricted viral gene expression in vivo (27) (42) and persistent infection of monocyte/macrophages (43)-(45) are characteristic features of lentiviral infections. Activation of CAEV gene expression with subsequent viral replication has been demonstrated in vitro during the maturation of monocytes into macrophages (46). It has been postulated that a mobile monocyte population harboring latent virus serves as a vehicle for dissemination of virus to the CNS in encephalomyelitis induced by visna virus and CAEV (27)(45). The terminal differentiation of the monocytes then triggers viral replication, which in turn results in spread of virus to oligodendrocytes and astrocytes, cells in which viral antigens and RNA have been demonstrated (47). The inflammatory lesions and foci of demyelination are thought to be manifestations of a host immunopathologic response to the presence of viral antigen in the CNS (43)(45)(47).

POSSIBLE PATHOGENIC MECHANISMS FOR HIV-RELATED NEUROLOGIC DISEASES

HIV-related neurologic diseases may share common pathophysiologic mechanisms with neurologic diseases caused by other lentiviruses. In this regard, the identification of cell population(s) in the CNS which are infected with HIV is an issue of primary importance. HIV is tropic for cells bearing the T4 molecule (48)-(50), a marker present on helper-inducer T lymphocytes as well as subpopulations of monocytes and macrophages. Ho et al. have shown that HIV can be isolated from blood-derived monocyte/macrophages of infected individuals and that HIV is capable of infecting normal monocyte/macrophages in vitro (51). We have recently detected, by immunohistochemical methods, HIV antigens in cells resembling monocyte/macrophages in brain tissue from patients with AIDS (38). Others have demonstrated HIV RNA in mononucleated and multinucleated macrophages in the brain of patients with AIDS using an in situ hybridization (52). HIV-infected cells of the monocyte/macrophage lineage have been isolated and cultured from brain tissue of a patient with AIDS and subacute encephalitis (53). In addition, viral particles resembling HIV were identified ultrastructurally in mononucleated and multinucleated macrophages in the brains of patients with AIDS (20),(21),(52). Finally, STLV-III viral particles were found by electron microscopy in foamy macrophages in brains of macaque monkeys with STLV-III-induced encephalitis (24). These findings together suggest that monocyte/macrophages are among populations of cells in the CNS infected by HIV and that the pathogenesis of subacute encephalitis and other HIV-related neurologic syndromes may be similar to that of CNS diseases caused by other lentiviruses. HIV may be disseminated to the CNS in infected blood-borne monocytes (Figure 6). It is possible that the maturation of monocytes to macrophages in the target tissue activates HIV replication with subsequent spread of virus to other cell populations. The accumulation of viral antigens then results in a characteristic inflammatory response, which may mediate the destruction in the CNS.

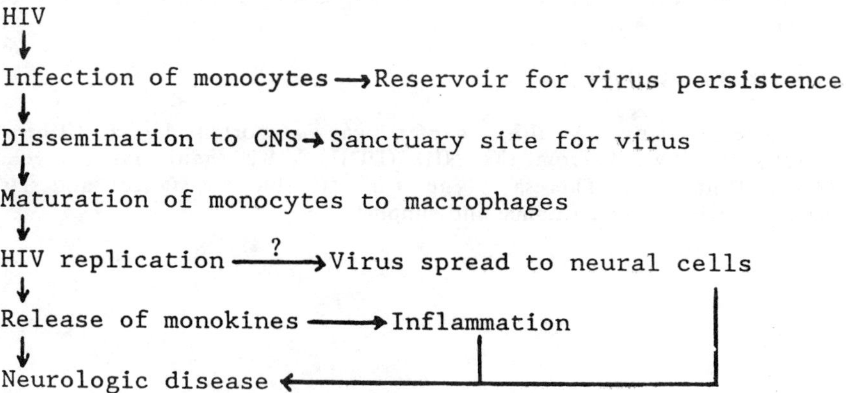

Figure 6. Postulated pathogenic mechanism for HTLV-III (HIV)-related neurologic diseases.

CONCLUSION

HIV is not only lymphotropic but also neurotropic. It is the etiologic agent of subacute encephalitis and aseptic meningitis associated with AIDS and ARC. This neurotropic property implies that the CNS may serve as a sanctuary for the virus so that antiviral therapy, when available, must penetrate the blood-brain-barrier for successful eradication. The cases of acute meningitis and encephalopathy coincident with HIV seroconversion suggest that the virus can enter the nervous system very early in the course of infection. Furthermore, there are examples of HIV-related neurologic diseases which occur without the development of HIV-related immunodeficiency.

The field of HIV-related neurologic disorders is in its infancy and the pathogenic mechanisms need to be defined. In addition, the etiology of vacuolar myelopathy and peripheral neuropathy is still unknown. The unusual neurologic diseases associated with virus recovery from the CNS (cases 3-5) suggest that HIV may cause other neurologic syndromes yet uncharacterized. As the number of cases of HIV infection continues to rise, significant increases in HIV-related CNS disorders should be anticipated.

ACKNOWLEDGMENT

The writing of this chapter was supported by a Clinical Investigator Award from the NIH (DDH). We thank Janet Steele, Teresa Rota, and Theresa Flynn for valuable assistance, and Dr. Martin S. Hirsch for guidance and support.

REFERENCES

1. Levy, R.M., Bredesen, D.E., Rosenblum, M.L., Neurological manifestations of the acquired immunodeficiency syndrome (AIDS): experience at UCSF and review of the literature. J Neurosurg 62:475-495 (1985)

2. Nielson, S., Petito, C.K., Urmacher, C.D., et al., Subacute encephalitis in acquired immune deficiency syndrome: a postmortem study. Am J Clin Pathol 82: 678-682 (1984)

3. Navia, B.A., Cho, E.S., Petito, C.K., et al., The AIDS dementia complex: II. Neuropathology. Ann Neurol 19:525-535 (1986)

4. de la Monte, S.M., Ho, D.D., Schooley, R.T., et al., Subacute encephalomyelitis of AIDS and its relation to HTLV-III infection. Neurology (In press)

5. Snider, W.D., Simpson, D.M. Nielson, S., et. al., Neurological complications of acquired immune deficiency syndrome: analysis of 50 patients. Ann Neurol 14:403-418 (1983)

6. Navia, B.A., Petito, C.K., Gold, J.W.M., et al., Cerebral toxoplasmosis complicating the acquired immune deficiency syndrome: clinical and neuropathological findings in 27 patients. Ann Neurol 19:224-238 (1986)

7. Zuger, A., Louie, E., Holzman, R.S., et al., Cryptococcal disease in patients with the acquired immunodeficiency syndrome. Ann Intern Med 104:234-240 (1986)

8. Gill, P.S., Levine, A.M., Meyer, P.R., et al., Primary central nervous system lymphoma in homosexual men: clinical, immunologic, and pathologic features. Am J Med 78:742-748 (1985)

9. Jordan, B.D., Navia, B.A., Petito, C.K., et al., Neurological syndromes complicating AIDS. Front Radiat Ther Oncol 19:82-87 (1985)

10. Dix, R.D., Waitzman, D.M., Follansbee, S., et al., *Herpes simplex* virus type 2 encephalitis in two homosexual men with persistent lymphadenopathy. Ann Neurol 17:203-206 (1985)

11. Horoupian, D.S., Pick, P., Spigland, T., et al., Acquired immune deficiency syndrome and multiple tract degeneration in a homosexual man. Ann Neurol 15:502-505 (1984)

12. Ryder, J.W., Croen, K., Kleinschmidt-DeMasters, B.K., et al., Progressive encephalitis three months after resolution of cutaneous zoster in a patient with AIDS. Ann Neurol 19:182-188 (1986)

13. Tucker, T., Dix, R.D., Katzen, C., et al., Cytomegalovirus and *Herpes simplex* virus ascending myelitis in a patient with acquired immune deficiency syndrome. Ann Neurol 18:74-79 (1985)

14. Petito, C.K., Navia, B.A., Cho., E-S., et al., Vacuolar myelopathy pathologically resembling subacute combined degeneration in patients with the acquired immunodeficiency syndrome. N Engl J Med 312:874-879 (1985)

15. Lipkin, W.I., Parry, G., Kiprov, D., et al., Inflammatory neuropathy in homosexual men with lymphadenopathy. Neurology 35:1479-1483 (1985)

16. Ho, D.D., Rota, T.R., Schooley, R.T., et al., Isolation of HTLV-III from cerebrospinal fluid and neural tissues of patients with neurologic syndromes related to the acquired immunodeficiency syndrome. N Engl J Med 313:1493-1497 (1985)

17. Levy, J.A., Shimabukuro, J. Hollander, H., et al., Isolation of AIDS-associated retrovirus from cerebrospinal fluid and brain of patients with neurological symptoms. Lancet 2:586-588 (1985)

18. Resnick, L., diMarzo-Veronese, F., Schupbach, J., et al., Intra-blood-brain-barrier synthesis of HTLV-III-specific IgG in patients with neurologic symptoms associated with AIDS or AIDS-related complex. N Engl J Med 313:1498-1504 (1985)

19. Shaw, G.M., Harper, M.E., Hahn, B., et al., HTLV-III infection in brains of children and adults with AIDS encephalopathy. Science 227:177-182 (1985)

20. Epstein, L.G., Sharer, L.R., Cho, E-S., et al., HTLV-III/LAV-like retrovirus particles in the brains of patients with AIDS encephalopathy. AIDS Research 1:447-454 (1984/1985)

21. Sharer, L.R., Epstein, LG., Cho, E-S, et al., Pathologic features of AIDS encephalopathy in children: evidence of LAV/HTLV-III infection of brain. Human Pathol 17:271-284 (1986)

22. Kanki, P.J., McLane, M.F., King, N.W., et al., Serologic identification and characterization of a macaque T-lymphotropic retrovirus closely related to HTLV-III. Science 228:1199-1201 (1985)

23. Daniel, M.D., Letvin, N.L., King, N.W., et al., Isolation of T-cell tropic HTLV-III-like retrovirus from macaques. Science 228:1201-1204 (1985)

24. Letvin, N.L., Daniel, M.D., Sehgal, P.K., et al., Induction of AIDS-like disease in macaque monkeys with T-cell tropic retrovirus STLV-III. Science 230:71-73 (1985)

25. Gonda, M.A., Wong-Staal, F., Gallo, R.C., et al., Sequence homology and morphologic similarity of HTLV-III and visna virus, a pathogenic lentivirus. Science 227:173-177 (1985)

26. Chiu, I-M, Yaniv, A., Dahlberg, J.E., et al., Nucleotide sequence evidence for relationship of AIDS retroviruses to lentiviruses. Nature 317:366-368 (1985)

27. Sonigo, P., Alizon, M., Staskus, K., et al., Nucleotide sequence of the visna lentivirus: relationship to the AIDS virus. Cell 42:369-382 (1985)

28. Stephens, R.M, Casey, J.W., Rice, N.R., et al., Equine infectious anemia virus gag and pol genes: relatedness to visna and AIDS virus. Science 231:589-594 (1986)

29. Navia, B.A., Jordan, B.D., Price, R.W., The AIDS dementia complex: I. Clinical features. Ann Intern Med 19:517-524 (1986)

30. Kleihues, P., Lang, W., Burger, P.C., et al., Progressive diffuse leukoencephalopathy in patients with acquired immune deficiency syndrome. Acta Neuropathol 68:333-339 (1985)

31. Belman, A.L., Ultmann, M.H., Horoupian, S., et al., Neurological complications in infants and children with acquired immune deficiency syndrome. Ann Neurol 18:560-566 (1985)

32. Epstein, L.G., Sharer, L.R., Joshi, V.V., et al., Progressive encephalopathy in children with acquired immune deficiency syndrome. Ann Neurol 17:488-496 (1985)

33. Goldstick, L., Mandybur, T.I., Bode, R., Spinal cord degeneration in AIDS. Neurology 35:103-106 (1985).

34. Ho, D.D., Sarngadharan, M.G., Resnick, L., et al., Primary human T-lymphotropic virus type III infection. Ann Intern Med 103:880-883 (1985)

35. Cooper, D.A., Gold, J., Maclean, P., et al., Acute AIDS retrovirus infection: definition of a clinical illness associated with seroconversion. Lancet 1:537-540 (1985)

36. Yankner, B.A., Skolnik, P.R., Shoukimas, G.M., et al., Cerebral granulomatous angiitis associated with isolation of HTLV-III from the central nervous system. Ann Neurol 20:362-364 (1986)

37. Carne, C.A., Tedder, R.S., Smith, A., et al., Acute encephalopathy coincident with seroconversion for anti-HTLV-III. Lancet 2:1206-1208 (1985)

38. Gabuzda, D.H., Ho, D.D., de la Monte, S.M., et al., Immuno histochemical identification of HTLV-III antigen in brains of patients with AIDS. Ann Neurol 20:289-295 (1986)

39. Kanki, P.J., Barin, F., M'Boup, S., et al., New human T-lymphotropic retrovirus related to simian T-lymphotropic virus type III (STLV-III AGM). Science 232:238-243 (1986)

40. Narayan, O., Cork, L.C., Lentiviral diseases of sheep and goats: chronic pneumonia, leukoencephalomyelitis and arthritis. Rev Infect Dis 7:89-98 (1985)

41. Cheevers, W.P., McGuire, T.C., Equine infectious anemia virus: immunopathogenesis and persistence. Rev Infect Dis 7:83-88 (1985)

42. Haase, A.T., Stowring, L., Narayan, O., et al., Slow persistent infection caused by visna virus: role of host restriction. Science 195:175-177 (1977)

43. Gendelman, H.E., Narayan, O., Molineaux, S., et al., Slow, persistent replication of lentiviruses: role of tissue macrophages and macrophage precursors in bone marrow. Proc Natl Acad Sci 82:7086-7090 (1985)

44. Narayan, O., Wolinsky, J.S., Clements, J.E., et al., Slow virus replication: the role of macrophages in the persistence and expression of visna viruses of sheep and goats. J Gen Virol 59:345-356 (1985)

45. Peluso, R., Haase, A., Stowring, L., et al., A Trojan horse mechanism for the spread of visna virus in monocytes. Virology 147:231-236 (1985)

46. Narayan, O., Kennedy-Sfoskipf, S., Sheffer, D., et al., Activation of caprine arthritis-encephalitis virus expression during maturation of monocytes to macrophages. Infect Immun 41:67-73 (1983)

47. Stowring, L., Haase, A.T., Petursson, G., et al., Detection of visna virus antigens and RNA in glial cells in foci of demyelination. Virology 141:311-318 (1985)

48. Dalgleish, A.G., Beverly, P.C.L., Clapham, P.R., et al., The CD4 (T4) antigen is an essential component of the receptor for the AIDS retrovirus. Nature 312:763-767 (1984)

49. Klatzmann, D.E. Champagne, E., Chamaret, S., et al., T-lymphocyte T4 molecule behaves as the receptor for human retrovirus LAV. Nature 312:767-768 (1984)

50. McDougal, J.S., Mawle, A., Cort, S.P., et al., Cellular tropism of the human retrovirus HTLV-III/LAV. J Immun 135:3151-3162 (1985)

51. Ho, D.D., Rota, T.R., Hirsch, M.S., Infection of monocyte/macrophages by human T-lymphotropic virus type III. J Clin Invest (in press)

52. Koenig, S., Gendelman, H.E., Orenstein, J.R., et al., Detection of AIDS virus in macrophages in brain tissue from AIDS patients with encephalopathy. Science 233:1089-1093 (1986)

53. Gartner, S., Markovits, P., Markovitz, D.M., et al., The role of mononuclear phagocytes in HTLV-III/LAV infection. Science 233:215-219 (1986)

31
Toxoplasmosis in AIDS

Theodore H. Lenox, Harry W. Haverkos

Toxoplasma gondii encephalitis has emerged as an important life-threatening opportunistic infection in patients with the acquired immunodeficiency syndrome (AIDS) (1)-(5). Prior to the AIDS pandemic, central nervous system (CNS) toxoplasmosis was uncommonly reported in adults. However, between June 1981, and July 1, 1986, 710 patients were known to have had CNS toxoplasmosis as a manifestation of their disease (personal communication: Dr. M. Morgan, Surveillance Branch, AIDS Program, CDC). Therefore, it is increasingly important that physicians responsible for the care of AIDS patients be knowledgeable in the epidemiology, clinical manifestations, diagnostic methods and therapy of *Toxoplasma gondii* infections.

PATHOGENESIS

The protozoan *Toxoplasma gondii* is an obligate intracellular parasite which commonly infects animals and man. Most infections are asymptomatic. As determined by serologic studies, human infection is common, although the prevalence rate varies among different populations. Infection rates can be as high as 80% in some groups (6),(7), but these infections are usually benign or asymptomatic if the patient is immunocompetent.

Human infection occurs following either ingestion of tissue cysts (also referred to as zoitocysts, bradyzoites or cystozoites by some parasitologists) in undercooked or raw meat; transplant of tissue cysts in organ transplantation; ingestion of oocysts in fecally contaminated food; transmission of tachyzoites (also referred to as trophozoites, merozoites or endozoites by some parasitologists) from mother to fetus in utero; or, more rarely, by transfusion of granulocytes containing tachyzoites. The organisms enter the lymphatics and blood of infected individuals and disseminate to lymph nodes and other organs of the body where intracellular multiplication occurs with subsequent production of tissue cysts. Distended cells may rupture creating an area of necrosis and releasing tachyzoites to infect other cells.

Primary infection seldom gives rise to clinical illness, but when it does, fatigue and myalgias are the usual symptoms. Rarely fever, lymphadenopathy or lymphocytosis may persist for days to weeks. In the immunocompetent host, with the onset of antibody production following primary infection the parasite generally encysts, causes no further immediate damage, and enters a period of latency. Adult chorioretinitis is generally associated with chronic infection (8). On the other hand, immunocompromised hosts are more likely to experience life-threatening disease, including encephalitis and myocarditis, than immunocompetent patients. Life-threatening disease is believed to result from reactivation of latent tissue cysts during an episode of altered cell-mediated immunity (9)-(11). The most common site of reactivation is the CNS, causing the signs and symptoms characteristic of encephalitis or brain abscess (9),(11),(12). Chorioretinitis and myocarditis are rarely seen in AIDS patients although there are reports of both (4),(13),(14).

EPIDEMIOLOGY

Toxoplasmosis is a world-wide zoonosis. The parasite infects all orders of mammals, some birds, and probably some reptiles. Insects that feed on excrement of cats may also carry the oocysts. The cat is the definitive host of toxoplasma and is the only known animal species in which sexual reproduction of the parasite occurs and oocysts are formed. The oocysts are noninfectious when excreted by the cat. However, within one to five days outside the cat, the oocysts become infectious. Cats are of primary importance in the transmission of toxoplasmosis. However, it is possible that the life cycle of the organism can be perpetuated in the absence of cats through congenital transmission and by eating undercooked, infected meat (15).

Seroprevalence of toxoplasmosis in man varies from population to population and increases with age. However, there are no significant differences by sex. According to seroepidemiologic surveys, there is generally less infection in cold regions, hot and arid areas, and at high elevations (16). Although the reasons for the differences are not completely understood, they possibly reflect differences in cat populations, environmental influences on the viability of oocysts, cultural differences in the areas of personal hygiene, culinary habits and care of pets.

Sixty-three (39%) of 163 homosexual men in New York and

California were positive when tested for toxoplasma antibody (fluoroimmunoassay ≥ 16) in a case control study for AIDS conducted by the CDC (17). This result is slightly higher than the 27% figure reported earlier among 30-40 year old men and women tested by the Sabin-Feldman dye test in Southern California (16).

Although most cases of toxoplasmosis diagnosed in the United States are presumed to be sporadic, outbreaks of acute toxoplasmosis occur. One of the largest reported outbreaks of acute toxoplasmosis in this country occurred among patrons of a riding stable in Georgia in 1977 and was associated with infected cats (18). In that outbreak 29 (38%) of 77 patrons studied developed fever, lymphadenopathy or headache within an eight week period in the fall of 1977. Twenty-eight of the 29 symptomatic individuals had serologic evidence of acute toxoplasmosis. No long term follow-up of infected patrons was reported.

CLINICAL PRESENTATION AMONG IMMUNOSUPPRESSED INDIVIDUALS

Ruskin and Remington (8) reviewed 81 cases of toxoplasmosis in non-AIDS immunocompromised patients who had neoplasia, collagen vascular disorders or had received organ allografts. They noted neurologic syndromes in 45/81 (56%) of their patients consisting of one or more of the following: 1) diffuse encephalopathy, 2) meningoencephalitis, or 3) cerebral mass lesions. More recently, Navia et al. (19) reviewed in detail 27 AIDS patients with cerebral toxoplasmosis. Their patients presented with a subacute picture (progression of symptoms over one to two weeks). Focal neurologic deficits, especially a mild hemiparesis, ataxia and seizures were commonly found. The next most frequent presentations were a global cognitive impairment without decreased arousal and a diffuse encephalopathy characterized by lethargy and confusion. Headache was the major complaint in just over one-half of the patients and was usually bilateral, severe and persistent. The majority of patients had persistent fever with the neurologic symptoms. Only one patient had chorioretinitis.

Haverkos and colleagues (20) organized a Study Group to address clinical questions about cerebral toxoplasmosis by retrospectively reviewing available data from several cooperating medical centers. This study was undertaken to assess the effects of therapy for histologically confirmed cerebral toxoplasmosis among AIDS patients and other immunosuppressed patients. In this survey of 31 medical centers, investigators reported 61 patients who received treatment for cerebral toxoplasmosis. The characteristics of illness in these patients corroborated earlier reports and included focal neurological signs in 59% of cases, most commonly hemiparesis, headache in 44% and seizures in 36%; 44% had various other signs and symptoms (Table 1). Of interest, only 10% reported fever at onset of symptoms of cerebral toxoplasmosis. However, the lack of reports of fever may be due to the way this piece of information was collected, rather than an absence of fever.

Table 1. Central Nervous System Signs and Symptoms Reported at Onset of Toxoplasma Encephalitis in 61 AIDS Patients (Ref.20)

Sign/Symptom	Number (%)
Headache	27 (44)
Seizures	22 (36)
Focal Neurologic Sign	36 (59)
Hemiparesis	19 (31)
Difficulty with vision	7 (11)
Difficulty with speech	4 (7)
Ataxia	4 (7)
Bell's palsy	2 (3)
Numbness	2 (3)
Extra-pyramidal movements	1 (2)
Not specified	2 (5)
Other	27 (44)
Disorientation	23 (38)
Fever	6 (10)
Incontinence	2 (3)
Nuchal rigidity	2 (3)
Dizziness	1 (2)
Generalized weakness	1 (2)
Nausea, vomiting	1 (2)
Psychosis	1 (2)
Syncope	1 (2)
Unknown	1 (2)

Reports of extra-neural involvement with toxoplasmosis are uncommon in AIDS patients. Rash and pneumonitis have been reported in other immunocompromised patients and can precede or occur with neurologic manifestations (21). Recently Parke and Font (13) reported a case of diffuse toxoplasma retinochoroiditis in a patient who subsequently was diagnosed with AIDS. The patient presented with a complaint of mono-ocular loss of vision for 20 days without systemic symptoms, although he was febrile on initial examination. Cases of ocular involvement have been reported by others as well (19),(22).

Recently, Monsuez et al. (14) reported cardiac dysfunction in ten patients with human immunodeficiency virus (HIV) infection. In five of their patients, cardiac involvement was the first manifestation of HIV infection. In one patient, a clinical diagnosis of myocarditis with an associated undescribed neurologic disorder proved fatal. Toxoplasmosis was seen in the myocardium at autopsy in that patient. Other investigators have also reported myocardial toxoplasmosis in AIDS patients (23).

DIAGNOSIS

The diagnosis of toxoplasmosis is not always a simple one, especially in AIDS patients. The clinician must first consider the possibility and then initiate several steps toward confirming this impression. In the AIDS patient, however, no single clinical characteristic, laboratory finding or radiographic feature is diagnostic, aside from examination of a tissue sample. Nonetheless, a highly probable diagnosis can be reached in many instances without a biopsy procedure.

The cerebrospinal fluid (CSF) analysis in patients with toxoplasma encephalitis is usually abnormal but frequently only minimally so, and at times it is totally normal (19),(24). Typically, there are few cells with a mononuclear predominance; a mild to moderate protein elevation is usual and the glucose level is normal or slightly depressed (4),(11),(19),(22)-(24). Only rarely have toxoplasma cysts or trophozoites been found in cerebrospinal fluid.

The Sabin-Feldman dye test is the reference against which other serologic tests for toxoplasmosis are measured (15). It is sensitive and specific in detecting IgG antibodies. Several other tests for IgG and IgM antibodies have been developed and are used to evaluate different stages of infection. In the non-AIDS immunocompromised patient, Carey et al. (12), Armstrong (25) and Hakes et al. (24) have shown that most will exhibit either a high initial titer of IgM, a high initial titer of IgG or a four-fold rise in IgG. Serologic evaluation of toxoplasma infection in AIDS patients has not been as informative. Several studies now indicate that most AIDS patients will have a positive Sabin-Feldman dye test or other test for IgG antibodies although the level of the titer may vary widely (4),(19),(20),(24). On occasion a four-fold rise in titer can be documented (14),(19),(23). Tests for IgM antibodies have been generally less helpful. IgM antibody is rarely detectable and a four-fold rise in titer has not been documented. CSF serology for *Toxoplasma gondii* is reported less frequently but also is usually negative or positive at a low stable titer (4),(19).

The computerized tomographic (CT) scan has proven to be a very important tool in the evaluation of AIDS patients with suspected CNS infections, especially for toxoplasmosis. The most common finding is multiple ring-enhancing lesions (4),(19),(22)-(24),(26), although this is not pathognomonic for any specific infectious process. Cerebral toxoplasmosis has presented as a single ring-enhancing lesion, an area of cerebritis (diffuse enhancement), and as non-enhancing lesions. Sometimes the lesions will be visualized only on subsequent CT examinations after previous studies were negative. The differential diagnosis of cerebral enhancing lesions in AIDS patients includes lymphoma, tuberculosis, cryptococcosis, herpes infection, and candidal abscess. Improved sensitivity of CT has been achieved through a repeat one hour-delay double dose scan (19). At times, lesions not seen on the first scan are noted when the delayed scan is done. Use of magnetic resonance imaging (MRI) has been infrequent but appears promising. MRI appears to be more sensitive than the double dose CT scan (19), but no more specific.

Because clinical and CT scan findings as well as toxoplasma serology are usually non-diagnostic, brain biopsy remains the method of choice for diagnostic confirmation. The principal controversy is when to make use of this invasive technique. Some authorities have advocated early biopsy based on the numerous diagnostic considerations which require different therapeutic approaches, while others favor empiric anti-toxoplasmosis therapy with the biopsy to be done only upon worsening of clinical status and/or of serial CT scans. Recent improvements in stereotactic techniques have, however, diminished the rate of mortality and morbidity from brain biopsy.

Interpreting biopsy specimens may be difficult. Hematoxylin and eosin and Giemsa stains are classically used to demonstrate the cyst and trophozoite forms of *Toxoplasma gondii.* Tang et al. (27) have reported, however, that cysts are less frequently seen in AIDS patients. It is also well known that the amount of cellular debris on most biopsy specimens makes identification of the smaller tachyzoites difficult to all but the most experienced pathologists. One group has emphasized the difficulty in differentiating the histologic findings in brain of toxoplasmosis from lymphoma (28). It has been claimed that immunoperoxidase staining is both an extremely sensitive and specific tool in the identification of *Toxoplasma gondii* (29),(30). However, this technique is not widely available. More recently, electron microscopy has been suggested as being of potential use but further evaluation of this method is needed (27).

THERAPY

The currently recommended therapy for cerebral toxoplasmosis is pyrimethamine (100 mg the first day, then 25 mg daily) and sulfadiazine (4-6 gm daily) with folinic acid (5 mg daily) to prevent bone marrow suppression. With prompt institution of therapy, patients will often show remarkable clinical improvement associated with resolving lesions on CT, usually within two weeks (4),(19).

Relapse of the original infection is a frequent occurrence when therapy is stopped (4),(19),(20),(23). This has prompted most clinicians to treat cerebral toxoplasmosis in AIDS patients indefinitely. Unfortunately, significant toxicity has been attributed to the drug combination pyrimethamine-sulfa (19),(20),(24). In the cerebral toxoplasmosis Study Group, toxicity developed in 61% of cases, requiring discontinuation of therapy in 45% of patients (20) (Table 2). Leukopenia was the most common side effect reported (40%), followed by rash (19%) and fever (11%).

Leukopenia will often occur even with the use of folinic acid. These effects were reversible upon discontinuation of the drugs. Bell et al. (31) have reported successful desensitization to sulfadiazine in three AIDS patients.

Table 2. Toxicity Attributed to Pyrimethamine-Sulfa in 57 AIDS Patients with Toxoplasma Encephalitis* (Ref.20)

Toxicity	Number (%)
Any toxicity	35 (61)
Leukopenia	23 (40)
Rash	11 (19)
Thrombocytopenia	7 (12)
Fever	6 (11)
Stevens-Johnson syndrome	2 (4)
Renal dysfunction	2 (4)
Renal stone	1 (2)
Transaminase elevation	1 (2)
Methemoglobinemia	1 (2)
Hypotension	1 (2)

* One additional patient received initial therapy with pyrimethamine-sulfonamide but follow-up was considered inadequate to assess drug toxicity.

Use of alternative therapeutic modalities is controversial and none has been proven effective. The most commonly used alternative drug is clindamycin; its use in patients who could not continue the sulfonamide for reasons of toxicity has been reported to prevent relapse (19),(32). However, clindamycin does not penetrate well into the CNS so it must be used with caution. Spiramycin is less toxic than the pyrimethamine-sulfa combination. However, CNS penetration is also poor (33). Studies in laboratory animals have demonstrated a poor clinical response in primary infections treated with this drug (33), (34). Spiramycin is readily available outside the United States and can be obtained through Rhone-Poulenc Pharma, Montreal, Quebec, Canada. Given orally, the dose is 2-4 grams daily in two to four divided doses (15). Further study is required to document its efficacy. Trimethoprim-sulfamethoxazole exhibits considerable synergy against *Toxoplasma gondii* in vitro, although this could not be demonstrated in the mouse model (35). Some investigators have reported worsening of lesions while others have reported improvement of clinical status while on trimethoprim-sulfamethoxazole. Until more information is available, we can not recommend its use. Pyrimethamine has been used as a single agent at a higher dose (50 mg daily) (25). However, Navia et al. reported relapse of symptoms while on pyrimethamine alone (19).

For retinochoroiditis, pyrimethamine and sulfa are the agents of choice. However, clindamycin has been used alone or in combination with pyrimethamine-sulfa for this indication with favorable results (36).

The use of corticosteroids remains controversial. The cerebral toxoplasmosis Study Group evaluated the effect of steroid use in 45 patients treated with pyrimethamine-sulfa initially and for whom status was known at 120 days (20). Thirty-four of these patients received corticosteroids and 11 did not. There were no statistically significant differences in survival. However, the number of patients studied was small and the reasons for steroid usage were not made clear in this study. However, cerebral edema is a clear indication for steroid usage and may have contributed to neurologic improvement in some patients (19). On the other hand, there are reports of exacerbation or precipitation of CNS toxoplasmosis by corticosteroids (19).

As the prognosis of AIDS is so poor, it is difficult to separate out the specific impact of cerebral toxoplasmosis on the natural history of patients with both diseases. Wong et al. (4) reported an 80% response to medication, yet all patients died due to causes other than toxoplasmosis. Two had no evidence of toxoplasmosis at autopsy. The cerebral toxoplasmosis Study Group (20) found a median survival time of 121 days, ranging from one week to 18 months. The only characteristic which appeared to affect patient outcome negatively was a depressed mental status at onset of therapy. Investigators reported several concomitant infections, and at autopsy toxoplasmosis was found in 20 of 36 patients.

DISCUSSION

Although much has been learned about toxoplasmosis since the initial descriptions of the organism in animals in 1908 and of neonatal human disease in 1939, several questions remain. The common occurrence of toxoplasma encephalitis in AIDS will likely stimulate investigators to try to understand the pathogenesis of severe life-threatening toxoplasmosis in the immunosuppressed host as the pandemic increases. The reason toxoplasma encephali-

Table 3. Survival of 51 Patients with Toxoplasma Encephalitis Initially Treated With Pyrimethamine-Sulfa by Component of Therapy (Number surviving more than 120 days following initiation of therapy/total*) (Ref.20)

Treatment	Present	Absent	p Value
Pyrimethamine			
Loading dose	22/36	7/13	NS
Daily dose greater than 25 milligrams	6/10	25/41	NS
Sulfadiazine used	24/42	7/9	NS
Sulfonamide levels checked	7/10	22/37	NS
Corticosteroids			
Used	23/34	6/11	NS
Continuous pyrimethamine-sulfa therapy for at least 6 weeks [a]	19/24	12/17	NS

* Patients excluded if details of therapy unknown, of if follow-up less than 120 days.

a All patients who died during the first six weeks of therapy excluded.

tis appears to occur more commonly among AIDS patients than other immunosuppressed patients is unclear. The relative importance of primary exposure to toxoplasma, reexposures, and reactivation of latent tissue cysts in the pathogenesis of disease needs to be clarified. What specific immunologic defects predispose to disease? Some of these questions may be addressed by evaluation of blood samples collected prospectively on individuals at risk for both AIDS and toxoplasma encephalitis in large cohort studies now underway. Hopefully, one may be able to devise effective preventive measures once more is known of the pathogenesis.

Questions remain concerning the diagnosis of toxoplasma encephalitis. We need to improve the diagnostic capabilities of clinicans caring for immunosuppressed patients. Can we improve the predictive value of noninvasive studies in the diagnosis of toxoplasma encephalitis in immunosuppressed patients?

Although pyrimethamine and sulfadiazine appear to be effective in toxoplasma encephalitis in some cases, several questions concerning therapy remain. The role of folinic acid and corticosteroids in the treatment of toxoplasma encephalitis is not known. The optimal dosage regimen and duration of therapy remain to be clarified. What options are there when severe toxicities result from pyrimethamine and/or sulfadiazine? What drug interactions occur when treatments for toxoplasma encephalitis are combined with antiretroviral, antineoplastic, and other drugs? The possibility of developing a vaccine to toxoplasma needs to be explored.

CONCLUSION

In this chapter we have provided background information about toxoplasmosis in AIDS, discussed current diagnostic and therapeutic approaches, and identified areas where knowledge is incomplete. Hopefully, more will be learned about toxoplasmosis as we learn how to prevent and treat the underlying retroviral infection of AIDS.

REFERENCES

1. Luft, J.B., Conley, F., Remington, J.S., Outbreak of CNS toxoplasmosis in Western Europe and North America. Lancet 1:781-783 (1983)

2. Moskowitz, L., Kory, P., Chan, J.C., et al., Unusual causes of death in Haitians residing in Miami. JAMA 250:1187-1191 (1983)

3. Vieira, J., Frank, E., Spira, T.J., et al., Acquired immune deficiency in Haitians: Opportunistic infections in previously healthy Haitian immigrants. N Engl J Med 308:125-129 (1983)

4. Wong, B., Gold, J.W.M., Brown, A.E., et al., Central nervous system toxoplasmosis in homosexual men and parenteral drug abusers. Ann Intern Med 100:36-42 (1984)

5. Luft, B.J., Brooks, R.G., Conley, F.K., et al., Toxoplasmic encephalitis in patients with acquired immune deficiency syndrome. JAMA 252:913-917 (1984)

6. Velimirovic, B., Toxoplasmosis in immunosuppression and AIDS. Infection 12:315-317 (1984)

7. Remington, J.S., Desmonts, G., Toxoplasmosis In: Infectious Diseases of the Fetus and Newborn Infant, Second Ed. (Remington, J.S., Klein, J.O., eds), W.B. Saunders, Philadelphia, 143-263 (1983)

8. Benenson, A.S., (ed), Control of Communicable Diseases in Man, Fourteenth Ed., American Public Health Association, Washington, D.C., p 392-394 (1985)

9. Vietzke, W.M., Gelderman, A.H., Grimley, P.M., et al., Toxoplasmosis complicating malignancy: Experience at the National Cancer Institute. Cancer 21:816-827 (1968)

10. Frenkel, J.K., Effects of cortisone, total body radiation and nitrogen mustard on chronic latent toxoplasmosis. Am J Path 33:618 (1957)

11. Ruskin, J., Remington, J.S., Toxoplasmosis in the compromised host. Ann Intern Med 84:193-199 (1976)

12. Carey, R.M., Kimball, A.C., Armstrong, D., et al., Toxoplasmosis: Clinical experiences in a cancer hospital. Am J Med 54:30-38 (1973)

13. Parke, D.W., Font, R.L., Diffuse toxoplasmic retinochoroiditis in a patient with AIDS. Arch Ophthalmol 104:571-575 (1986)

14. Monsuez, J.J., Vittecoq, D., Rozenbaum, W., et al., Cardiac involvement in AIDS related disorders. International Conference on the Acquired Immunodeficiency Syndrome (AIDS), Paris, France

15. McCabe, R.E., Remington, J.S., *Toxoplasma gondii*, In: Principles and Practice of Infectious Diseases, Second Ed. (Mandell, G.L., Douglas, R.G., Bennett, J.E., eds), John Wiley and Sons, New York, p 1540-1549 (1985)

16. Luft, B.J., Remington, J.S., Toxoplasmosis, In: Infectious Diseases, Third Ed. (Hoeprich, P.D., ed), Harper and Row, Philadelphia, p 1133-1145 (1983)

17. Rogers, M.F., Morens, D.M., Stewart, J.A., et al., National case-control study of Kaposi's sarcoma and *Pneumocystis carinii* pneumonia in homosexual men: Part 2, Laboratory results. Ann Intern Med 99:151-158 (1983)

18. CDC., Toxoplasmosis-Georgia. MMWR 26:409 (1977)

19. Navia, B.A., Petito, C.K., Gold, J.W.M., et al., Cerebral toxoplasmosis complicating the acquired immune deficiency syndrome: Clinical and neuropathological findings in 27 patients. Ann Neurol 19:224-238 (1986)

20. Haverkos, H.W., Remington, J.S., Chan, J.C., et al., Assessment of toxoplasma encephalitis therapy: a cooperative study. International Conference on the Acquired Immunodeficiency Syndrome (AIDS), Paris, France (1986)

21. Luft, B.J., Remington, J.S., Toxoplasmosis of the central nervous system, In: Current Clinical Topics in Infectious Diseases. (Remington, J.S., Swartz, M.N., eds), McGraw-Hill, New York, Vol 6, p 315-358 (1985)

22. Snider, W.D., Simpson, D.M., Nielson, S., et al., Neurological complications of acquired immune deficiency syndrome: Analysis of 50 patients. Ann Neurol 14:403-418 (1983)

23. Koppel, B.S., Wormser, G.P., Tuchman, A.J., et al., Central nervous system involvement in patients with acquired immune deficiency syndrome (AIDS). Acta Neurol Scand 71:337-353 (1985)

24. Hakes, T.B., Armstrong, D., Toxoplasmosis: Problems in diagnosis and treatment. Cancer 52:1535-1540 (1983)

25. Armstrong, D., Central nervous system infections in the immunocompromised host. Infection 12:S58-S62 (1984)

26. Post, M.J.D., Kursunogly, S.J., Hensley, G.T., et al., Cranial CT in acquired immunodeficiency syndrome: Spectrum of diseases and optimal contrast enhancement technique. AJR 145:929-940 (1985)

27. Tang, T.T., Harb, J.M., Dunne, W.M., et al., Cerebral toxoplasmosis in an immunocompromised host: A precise and rapid diagnosis by electron microscopy. Am J Clin Pathol 85:104-110 (1986)

28. Small, C.B., Ahmed, T., Stahl, R.E., et al., Comparison of cerebral toxoplasmosis with primary brain lymphoma in AIDS patients. 25th Interscience Conference on Antimicrobial Agents and Chemotherapy, Minneapolis, MN (1985)

29. Snow, R.B., Lavyne, M.H., Intracranial space-occupying lesions in acquired immune deficiency syndrome patients. Neurosurg 16:148-153 (1985)

30. Conley, F.K., Jenkins, K.A., Remington, J.S., *Toxoplasma gondii* infection of the central nervous system: Use of the peroxidase-antiperoxidase method to demonstrate toxoplasma in formalin-fixed, paraffin embedded tissue specimens. Hum Pathol 12:690-698 (1981)

31. Bell, E.T., Tapper, M.L., Pollock, A.A., Sulphadiazine desensitization in AIDS patients. Lancet 1:163 (1985)

32. Hoy, J., Mansell, P., Rolston, K., Clindamycin in central nervous system toxoplasmosis in patients with AIDS. International Conference on the Acquired Immunodeficiency Syndrome (AIDS), Paris, France (1986)

33. Harper, J.S., London, W.T., Sever, J.L., Five drug regimens for treatment of acute toxoplasmosis in squirrel monkeys. Am J Trop Med Hyg 34:50-57 (1985)

34. Nguyen, B.T., Stadtsbaeder, S., Comparative effects of cotrimoxazole (trimethoprim-sulphamethoxazole), pyrimethamine-sulphadiazine and spiramycin during avirulent infection with *Toxoplasma gondii* (Beverly strain) in mice. Br J Pharmac 79:923-928 (1983)

35. Grossman, P.L., Remington, J.S., The effect of trimethoprim and sulfamethoxazole on *Toxoplasma gondii* in vitro and in vivo. Am J Trop Med Hyg 28:445-455 (1979)

36. Lakhanpal, V., Schocket, S.S., Nirankari, V.S., Clindamycin in the treatment of toxoplasmic retinochoroiditis. Am J Ophthalmol 95:605-613 (1983)

32

Cryptococcus neoformans from AIDS Patients: Mycologic, Animal Virulence, and Epidemiologic Correlates

Edward J. Bottone

Cryptococcus neoformans is a yeast-like fungus first described in 1894 (1). Since its initial description, *C. neoformans* has undergone several nomenclatural changes including: *Saccharomyces neoformans* (1), *Cryptococcus hominis* (2), and *Torula histolytica*, the latter designation being erroneously applied by Stoddard and Cutler (3) who assumed that the clear areas encircling cryptococcal cells in tissue sections were the result of lytic activity.

The genus *Cryptococcus* is presently comprised of at least 15 species of which *C. neoformans*, because of its human pathogenic potential, has served as the principal focus for studies of the organism's basic biology, ecology, epidemiology, pathophysiology, and its interaction with host defense mechanisms. The explosive occurrence of cryptococcosis among patients with the acquired immunodeficiency syndrome (AIDS) (4),(5) has led to a new appreciation of those mycologic, epidemiologic, and pathogenetic attributes underscoring its disease-producing potential. The present work endeavors to place into perspective new information concerning cryptococci isolated from AIDS patients.

Footnote: This chapter is dedicated to Stanley Spector (September 7, 1951 - October 14, 1985), who but for the advent of AIDS, would have been among the 1986 graduating class of The Mount Sinai School of Medicine. In his passage Stan left a legacy of love, of brilliance, of humor and wit, and of courage. All who interacted with him derived a new sense of the human spirit and the belief that we are all entwined in each other's well-being.

PRESENT NOMENCLATURE

In 1975, Kwon-Chung (6) discovered the perfect (sexual) mating state of *C. neoformans* describing the genus *Filobasidiella* and the species *F. neoformans*. Subsequently, in 1976, she described a morphologically and physiologically distinct species *F. bacillispora* (7). *F. neoformans* is obtained when compatible strains of capsular serotypes A and D mate whereas *F. bacillispora* is the perfect stage of mating between serotypes B and C.

Because of the discovery of two morphologically and physiologically distinct perfect states of *C. neoformans*, a decision was made to divide *C. neoformans* into two species, namely *C. neoformans* (serotypes A and D) and *C. bacillisporus* (serotypes B and C) (8). On the basis of additional mycological and pathological characteristics (9), however, *C. bacillisporus* was found to be identical to *C. neoformans var. gattii* (serotypes B and C), a nomenclatural designation already proposed by Vanbreuseghem and Takashio in 1980 (10). Table 1 summarizes some of the characteristics of the two varieties of *C. neoformans.*

Table 1. Characteristics Distinguishing Cryptococcus Neoformans Varieties Neoformans and Gattii

Characteristic	Variety	
	Neoformans	Gattii
Capsular serotype	A and D	B and C
Blastospore (yeast cell) shape	Spherical	Ovoid
Basidiospore shape	Ovoid	Bacillary
Growth at 37°C	Good	Slow - poor
Geographic distribution	Global	Tropical, subtropical
Reservoir in nature	Pigeon droppings, soil	Unknown

CAPSULES

The extracellular polysaccharide capsule of *C. neoformans* has been shown to play a significant role in numerous host-fungus interactions, in diagnosis and prognosis, and in the serotyping of *C. neoformans* strains.

The capsular polysaccharide of *C. neoformans* is a polyvalent anionic gel comprised mainly of uronic acid which surrounds the cryptococcal cell wall. The cell itself is round or oval, measuring from 4-6*u*m in diameter, whereas the surrounding capsule may range from 1 to 30*u*m (11). In rare instances, cells may grow to 20*u*m in diameter and highly encapsulated strains may be encountered in clinical material in which the total cell plus capsule diameter may measure up to 55*um* (12), (13) (Figure 1). On occasion, the presence of the capsule may preclude definitive staining of *C. neoformans* in purulent exudates examined by Gram stain. In such preparations *C. neoformans* may appear as round cells with Gram-positive, stippled granular inclusions (14) (Figure 2).

Although non-encapsulated strains of *C. neoformans* may be occasionally isolated from clinical specimens (15), they abound in natural habitats (16).

The mechanism by which poorly or nonencapsulated *C. neoformans* from environmental sources become encapsulated after entering an animal host, and to what degree, is poorly understood. Certainly, little attention has been paid to the relationship between degree of encapsulation of *C. neoformans* causing human infections and the immune status of the host. Cryptococcosis in different patient populations ranging from normal individuals to those profoundly immunodeficient, as exemplified by AIDS patients, is diagnosed mainly by demonstrating an encapsulated yeast cell in India ink preparations, with little regard paid to the actual size of the capsule, just to its presence.

In our laboratory, we have observed that *C. neoformans* on primary isolation from ten AIDS patients grew as nonmucoid, dry, pasty colonies (Figure 3) and were poorly encapsulated (mean cell plus capsule diameter 4.90*um* to 10.12*um*) (Figure 4) in India ink mounts prepared after 48 hours incubation in 5% CO_2.

In striking contrast, three *C. neoformans* isolates from patients without AIDS produced mucoid colonies (Figure 5) and showed a significantly greater degree of encapsulation (17).

In a follow-up study Bottone and Wormser (18) further demonstrated that *C. neoformans* observed directly in the cerebrospinal fluid of seven AIDS patients consecutively studied were poorly encapsulated; six had a mean capsule plus cell diameter less than 10*um*, while one, was intermediate with a mean total diameter of 15.5*um*. The one non-AIDS patient studied in parallel had cryptococci in cerebrospinal fluid that showed full encapsulation (mean 24.4*um*) (Table 2). Mouse passage of cryptococci from six of these patients, done on the assumption that the poorly encapsulated cryptococci observed in AIDS patients were capable of greater capsule synthesis in normal mice, resulted in a statistically significant ($P<0.05$) (T-test) increase in capsule size over that observed directly in cerebrospinal fluid. In contrast, there was no significant increase in the degree of encapsulation of the non-AIDS isolate after mouse passage (Table 2).

Since publication of these observations, four additional *C. neoformans* isolates from AIDS patients have been studied with identical results. Table 2 shows these data for the original seven AIDS patients (Nos. 1-6, 11), the non-AIDS patient (No. 12) and the four additional AIDS patients (Nos. 7-10) studied. These observations generated the theory that the immunodeficiency state associated with AIDS exerts little host selective pressure on

Table 2. Correlation of C. Neoformans Capsule Plus Cell Size In Fresh Cerebrospinal fluid and After Animal Passage.

Patient	Age	Risk Factors and/or Other Evidence for AIDS	Cryptococcal Capsule Plus Cell Size: CSF Range (mean) μm	Cryptococcal Capsule Plus Cell Size: Animal Passage Range (mean) μm	T-Test
1	44	IV drug abuser, Pneumocystis carinii	2.5 - 12.5 (8.35)	10.0 - 37.5[a] (22.5)	< 0.05
2	28	Homosexual, Kaposi's sarcoma, oral candidiasis	5.0 - 15.0 (9.0)	12.5 - 40[a] (28.8)	< 0.05
3	44	Homosexual, esophageal candidiasis, positive HIV antibody*	5.0 - 12.5 (9.15)	15.0 - 25.0[a] (18.8)	< 0.05
4	37	IV drug abuser, Pneumocystis carinii	5.0 - 25.0 (12.7)	ND	
5	60	Homosexual, oral candidiasis, positive HIV antibody	7.5 - 25.0 (9.1)	12.5 - 25.0[b] (17.7)	< 0.05
6	37	Homosexual, Pneumocystis carinii	5.0 - 15.0 (9.9)	12.5 - 22.5[a] (17.4)	< 0.05
7	27	IV drug abuser, positive HIV antibody	5.0 - 16.25 (9.95)	10.0 - 50.0[a,b] (18.0)	< 0.05
8	35	IV drug abuser, positive HIV antibody	7.5 - 17.5 (10.8)	10.0 - 20.0 (14.0)[a,b]	< 0.05
9	65	Blood transfusion, oral candidiasis positive HIV antibody	2.5 - 20.0 (11.7)	10.0 - 20.0 (16.5)	< 0.05
10	47	Homosexual, Pneumocystis carinii	7.5 - 15.0 (11.7)	7.5 - 20.0 (14.6)[b]	< 0.05
11	30	IV drug abuser, oral candidiasis	8.75 - 25.0 (15.5)	12.5 - 27.5[a] (20.7)	< 0.05
12	20	None (one homosexual experience), negative HIV antibody	15.0 - 40.0 (24.2)	15.0 - 35.0[a] (24.6)	NS

* Abbott ELISA
a Peritoneal cavity
b Brain
HIV = Human immunodeficiency virus

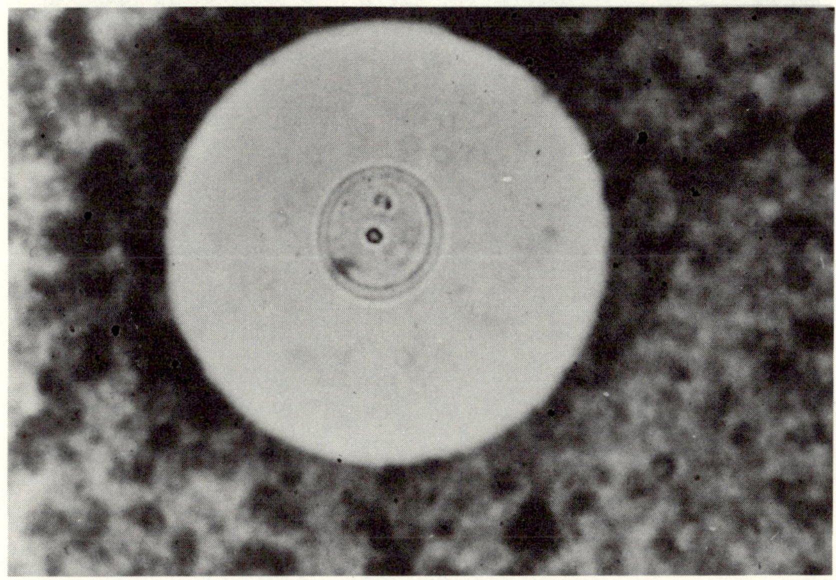

Figure 1. India ink preparation of lung aspirate showing markedly encapsulated yeast cell of *C. neoformans*

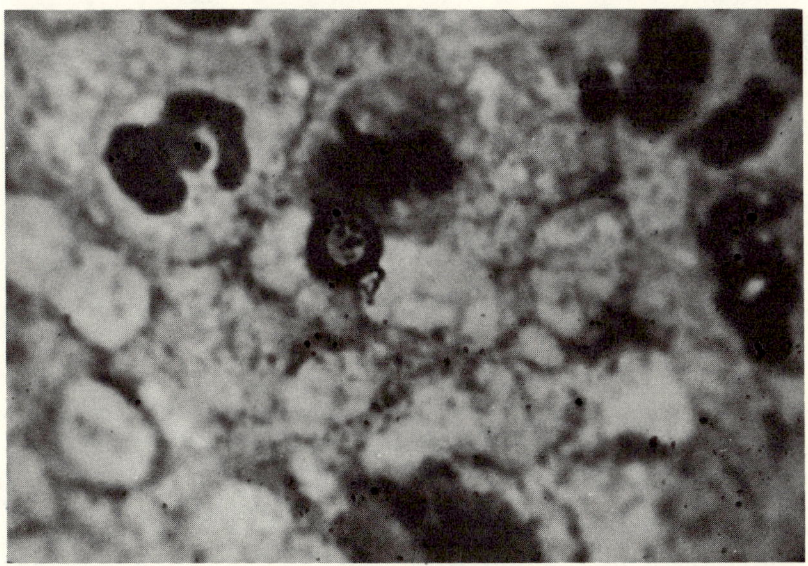

Figure 2. Gram stain smear of purulent exudate from osteomyelitis of rib showing irregularly stained yeast cell of *C. neoformans*

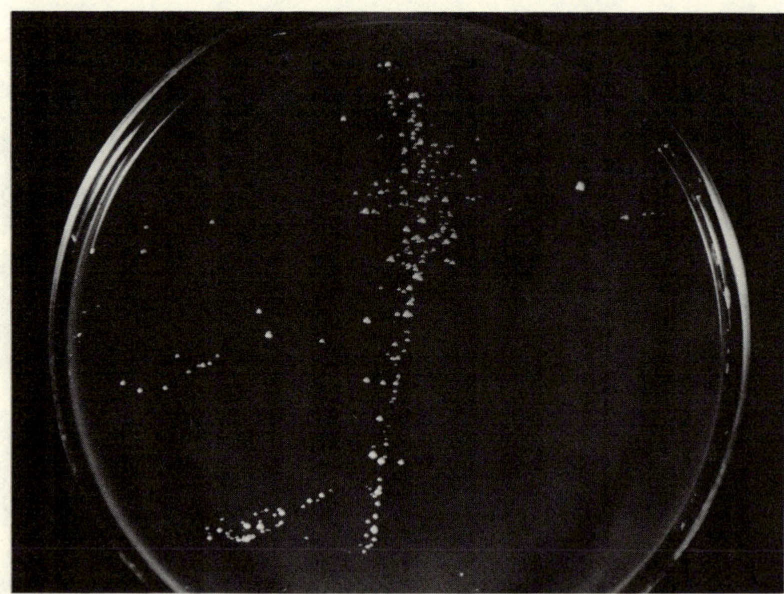

Figure 3. Primary cerebrospinal fluid culture on chocolate agar from an AIDS patient. Dry colonies of *C. neoformans* are seen.

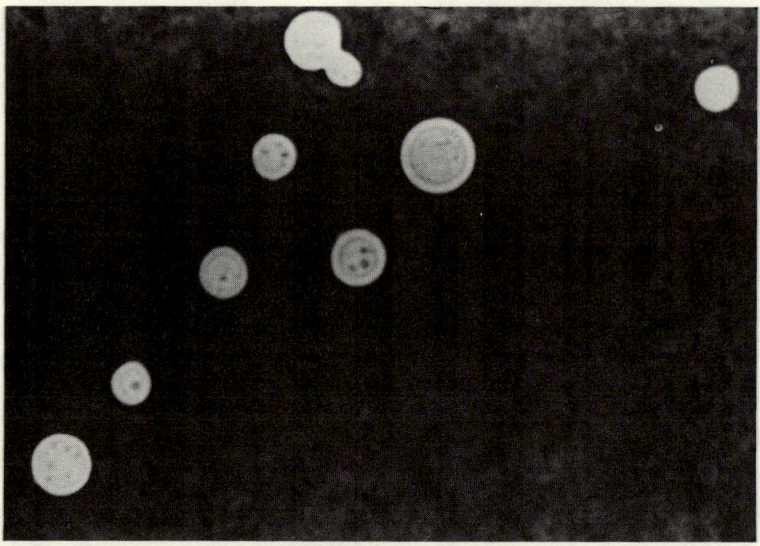

Figure 4. India ink preparation from primary culture of cerebrospinal fluid from an AIDS patient showing poorly encapsulated cells of *C. neoformans*

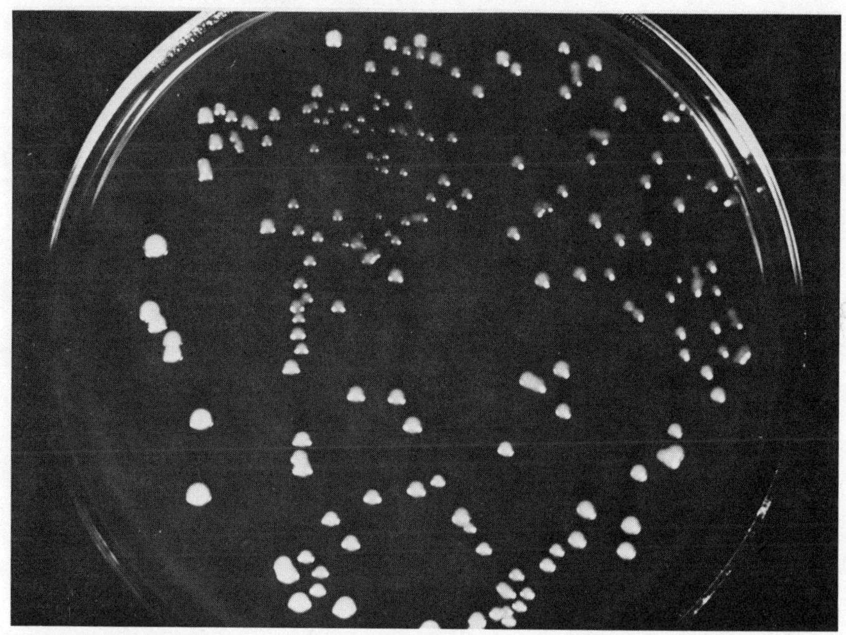

Figure 5. Typical mucoid colonies of *C. neoformans* from non-AIDS patients on sheep blood agar after 48 hours incubation at 37°C.

inhaled poorly encapsulated *C. neoformans*. One may, therefore, envision that cryptococci are maximally encapsulated in normal hosts, with lesser degrees of encapsulation in immunocompromised patients, as an inverse function of the degree of severity of the host's immunodeficiency.

To test this hypothesis, these same investigators compared the size of *C. neoformans* capsules observed directly in cerebrospinal fluid with the helper to suppressor T-lymphocyte ratios of six AIDS and one non-AIDS patient. Interestingly, in this very small sample, there did appear to be a direct correlation between small capsule size and extent of immunodeficiency (as defined by the T-lymphocyte ratio) (Table 3).

Table 3. C. Neoformans Mean Capsule Plus Cell Size As A Function Of T-lymphocyte Helper/Suppressor Ratio.

Patient (Strain)	CSF Cryptococcal Capsule Size(um) Range (mean)	% T lymphocytes Helper Leu 3a	Suppressor Leu 2a	Leu-3a/Leu 2a Ratio*
2(AIDS)	5.0 - 15.0 (9)	3.0	73	0.04
3(AIDS)	5.0 - 12.5 (9.15)	4.0	43.5	0.09
4(AIDS)	5.0 - 25.0 (12.7)	8.4	75.3	0.11
5(AIDS)	7.5 - 25.0 (9.1)	3.5	79.5	0.04
5A(AIDS)	7.5 - 22.5 (13.2)	---	----	0.2
12 (non-AIDS)	15.0 - 40.0 (24.2)	35	24	1.45

* Normal value 1.1 - 3.5

Additional studies are in progress in which capsule dimensions assessed directly in cerebrospinal fluid are compared to that found after animal passage in immunodeficient (nude) and normal mice. As noted in Table 4, in each instance the degree of cryptococcal encapsulation increased after mouse passage from that observed directly in cerebrospinal fluid of AIDS patients; however, there was no significant difference between nude and normal mice. These preliminary studies suggest that either the nude mouse is an inappropriate model for the immunodeficiency state found in AIDS, or that factors other than immunodeficiency per se, are important determinants of in vivo capsule size in the mouse.

The role of cryptococcal encapsulation as a virulence factor has been the subject of numerous studies. To date, several distinct biologic functions have been ascribed to the presence of a capsule surrounding *C. neoformans*. Those attributes of cryptococcal polysaccharide that may impair effective phagocytosis include: 1) the prevention of Fc-mediated attachment to macrophages in the presence of cell wall bound IgG (19); 2) the

Table 4. Correlation Of C. Neoformans Mean Capsule Plus Cell Size Observed Directly In Cerebrospinal Fluid And After Passage Through Nude And Normal Mice.

Strain	Mean Capsule Size (*u*m)			Phenyloxidase	
		Mouse Model			
No.	CSF	Nude	Normal	37°C	30°C
1 (AIDS)	8.4	23.1	22.2	+	+
7 (AIDS)	9.95	18.0	ND	0	+
8 (AIDS)	10.8	13.4	ND	+ (w)	+
9 (AIDS)	11.7	12.8	16.5	+	+
10 (AIDS)	11.7	16.6	14.6*	+ (w)	+
11 (AIDS)	15.5	17.4	19.0	+	+
12 (non-AIDS)	24.2	30.2	24.6	+ (w)	+

* Sacrificed mouse after 90 days ND = Not Done

inhibitory effect of physical size per se in that capsule-deficient cells may be readily phagocytized while well-capsulated cells are more slowly ingested by macrophages (20) and neutrophils (21),(22); and 3) the inhibition of phagocytosis caused by negative surface charge due to the uronic acid content of the capsule. Further support for the role of cryptococcal polysaccharide as an antiphagocytic virulence factor comes from studies of Kozel (23) in which he showed that the addition of purified cryptococcal polysaccharide to non-encapsulated yeast cells restored antiphagocytic activity. The added polysaccharide bound to specific surface receptors on the non-encapsulated cell.

One mechanism by which the cryptococcal capsular polysaccharide inhibits phagocytosis of *C. neoformans* cells appears to be of a passive nature by masking sites or ligands on the cryptococcal surface beneath the capsule. In the absence of specific anticapsular antibody, the capsule presents a surface that is not recognized by the phagocyte (24); phagocytosis will occur, however, in the presence of specific opsonizing antibody directed against capsular determinants (25). Additionally, Ikeda et al. (26) have shown that specific IgG anticapsular antibody is opsonizing for heavily encapsulated cryptococci via activation of the classical complement pathway with C3b deposition on the capsular surface, and that for poorly encapsulated cells, in the non-immune host, the alternative complement pathway plays a major role in opsonization.

ENCAPSULATION, ANIMAL VIRULENCE, AND PHENYLOXIDASE ACTIVITY

While the degree of encapsulation significantly affects phagocytosis by macrophages (20) and neutrophils (21), virulence for white mice appears to be related not to capsule size but rather to the presence or absence of a capsule (27); non-capsulated strains are avirulent (28). Subsequently, Dykstra and colleagues (29) showed that mice inoculated with poorly encapsulated cells (but not completely unencapsulated) began to die before those inoculated with large-encapsulated cells. These investigators attributed these observations to the greater ease with which small-capsulated cells may widely disseminate after intravenous inoculation, whereas the large-capsulated cells became entrapped in the capillary bed of the lungs.

In 1962 Staib (30) showed that *C. neoformans* produced a brown pigment when grown on a medium containing bird manure. He attributed this phenomenon to the assimilation of creatinine present in the bird droppings. With the exception of a rare strain of *C. laurentii*, pigment production on this medium was a property of *C. neoformans*, not shared by other yeast-like organisms. Subsequently, this investigator (31) showed that brown pigmentation could also be elicited by *C. neoformans* grown on media containing the seed of *Guizotia abyssinica* (Niger seed), commonly used in bird feed.

Staib's observation led to the use of pigment production as a diagnostic adjunct for *C. neoformans* and to the development of an isolation medium for *C. neoformans* which incorporated diphenol ($C_6H_5C_6H_5$) (32). Korth and Pulverer (33) additionally showed that pigment formation could ensue in media which incorporated diphenols instead of Niger seed. Shaw and Kapica (34), noting observations made by earlier investigators, reported that the diagnostic pigment was melanin and was produced by the action of phenyloxidase on a variety of diphenols and 3,4-dihydroxyphenylalanine (dopa), and that this pigment was deposited in the yeast cell wall. In some terrestrial fungi, melanin deposition in the cell wall may serve a protective role against enzymatic degradation by other microbial species (35), (36). It is conceivable that melanin serves a similar function in the survival of cryptococci in soil and bird droppings. As melanin is refractory to enzymatic degradation, and apparently non-immunogenic, its deposition in the cell wall of *C. neoformans* may also serve to enhance its survival in the human host after inhalation in the non-encapsulated or poorly encapsulated state found in natural environments (15).

Perhaps the greatest significance of the presence of phenyloxidase activity in *C. neoformans* lies not in its diagnostic potential, but rather in its correlation, along with encapsulation, with animal virulence.

The first in a series of papers associating phenyloxidase activity with virulence in *C. neoformans* was published in 1982 by Polacheck, Hearing, and Kwon-Chung (37). These investigators showed that phenyloxidase is constitutive and membrane bound in *C. neoformans*, two factors which may account for the high uptake of diphenols such as dopamine and norepinephrine, the major catecholamines found in brain tissue. Additionally, these investigators showed that *C. neoformans* can utilize catecholamines especially in the presence of low glucose concentrations, a condition which exists in the brain because of its intensive metabolic activity. In this setting *C. neoformans* may form melanin which in turn enhances its survival and growth in this organ. Low glucose levels and the presence of phenyloxidase substrates such as catecholamines may partially explain the unusual tropism of *C. neoformans* for brain tissue.

Continuing with their studies, Kwon-Chung and colleagues (38) showed that the linked characteristics of growth and melaninogenesis at 37°C may play a major role in *C. neoformans* pathogenicity. Mating a double mutant which was melanin negative (Mel^-) and unable to grow at 37°C (Tem^-) with a wild type *C. neoformans* strain (Mel^+, Tem^+), resulted in progeny (Mel^+ Tem^+, Mel^+ Tem^-, Mel^- Tem^+, Mel^- Tem^-) of which only the Mel^+ Tem^+ phenotype killed mice with an inoculum of 5 x 10^5 cells.

Subsequent to the studies linking phenyloxidase activity to virulence, it seemed logical to assess the effect of encapsulation and melanin synthesis on virulence in *C. neoformans*. Initially, Rhodes and colleagues (39) showed that the presence of a capsule (Cap^+) and ability to grow well at 37°C (Tem^+), and melaninogenesis (Mel^+) resulted in 100% mortality in mice within 30 days after intravenous inoculation of 8 x 10^5 cells. This result contrasted with a greater than 50% survival rate during an eight week observation period in the group of mice inoculated with essentially identical isolates differing only in being Mel^-. Interestingly, Mel^+ revertants (Mel^R) recovered from the brains of dead animals in the latter group were fully virulent on reinoculation into white mice. These data further strengthened the association of phenyloxidase activity in *C. neoformans* and virulence.

Most recently, Kwon-Chung and Rhodes (40) solidified the premise that encapsulation and melanin formation are virulence factors for *C. neoformans*. They showed that *C. neoformans* phenotypes (obtained by mating Cap^- Mel^- and Cap^+ Mel^+ strains) that are Cap^+ Mel^+ were virulent (90-100% fatality within 40 days), whereas Cap^+ Mel^- progeny, produced fatal infection after 40 days with 70-90% of mice surviving for at least 70 days. Cap^+ Mel^+ revertants were recovered from the brains of dead mice. Cap^- Mel^+ and Cap^- Mel^- phenotypes not only failed to produce lethal infection but did not revert in vivo to the Cap^+ Mel^+ phenotype. These results again indicated that both the Cap^+ and Mel^+ phenotype are virulence markers for *C. neoformans.*

Working with nine *C. neoformans* isolates from AIDS and non-AIDS patients, Bottone and colleagues (41) studied the relationships between phenyloxidase production, encapsulation, and mouse virulence. White mice were inoculated either intraperitoneally or intravenously with 0.5 ml of a suspension containing 10^5 cryptococcal cells/ml. In India ink preparations the cryptococcal strains were poorly encapsulated with a mean capsule plus cell diameter of 3.7*u*m to 7.6*u*m.

As shown in Table 5, by the intraperitoneal route, strains 1 to 4 were avirulent during a 90 day observation period.

Table 5. Mouse Virulence Studies

Strain No	Route of inoc*	Capsule + Cell Size Range (mean)*u*m	Antigen Titer (Avg) Day 10	20	40	90	Mouse Virulence[a]	Phenyloxidase 37°C	30°C
1	IP IV	2.5-7.5 (5.1)	250	17	7	0	10/10[b] 5/5	0 (+7day)	0 (+7day)
2	IP IV	2.5-7.5 (5.0)	45	85	20	0	10/10 4/5	0	++
3	IP IV	2.5-5.0 (3.7)	394	128	266	0	10/10 4/5	0	++
4	IP	2.5-10.0 (5.6)	2666	1728	1920	0	5/5	0	+

* Ten mice were inoculated intraperitoneally (IP) and five intravenously (IV) with 0.5 ml of a suspension containing 10^5 cells/ml. For strain no. 4, five mice inoculated IP only.

a Only mice that died had positive brain cultures. All surviving mice were sacrificed and had negative cultures of peritonal cavity, heart blood, brain, lung and liver.

b Number of surviving mice/number inoculated.

In these mice cryptococcal antigen titers rose and declined rapidly and were absent when these mice were sacrificed after 90 days. Postmortem cultures of various organs including the brain of these animals were negative for the inoculated strain. These four strains were subsequently shown to lack phenyloxidase activity at 37°C, a characteristic which, as noted earlier, when present correlates with animal virulence. In the group of animals inoculated intravenously with these four *C. neoformans* isolates, one mouse each out of five inoculated with strains No. 2 and 3 expired 10 and 36 days respectively postinoculation. Serum cryptococcal antigen titers in these mice rose to 1:16,384 just prior to death. Cultures of brain tissue grew *C. neoformans.* As direct plating onto bird seed agar was not performed, we were unable to determine if in vivo reversion to the Mel^+ phenotype occurred which could have accounted for the death of these two animals.

The remaining five strains of *C. neoformans* tested for animal virulence showed an overall correlation between phenyloxidase activity and mouse virulence (Table 6). *C. neoformans* isolates No. 6, 7, 8, which rendered definite brown pigmentation on bird seed agar at 37°C within 48 hours, were rapidly fatal as early as 13 days post-inoculation. Strains that were either weakly phenyloxidase positive (No. 5) or negative (No. 9) appeared less virulent.

The relationship between encapsulation, phenyloxidase activity, and mouse virulence was further delineated by study of two isogenic pairs of *C. neoformans* differing in colony morphology (moist or dry versus mucoid), mean capsule plus cell diameters, and phenyloxidase activity (Table 7).

Neither of the small encapsulated, phenyloxidase negative strains were virulent to white mice within the 90 day observation period, as contrasted to their mucoid, better encapsulated, phenyloxidase positive counterparts which killed white mice as early as five days post-inoculation. Interestingly, two surviving mice inoculated with a phenyloxidase negative variant of one strain both appeared moribund at day 90 when they were sacrificed. In both mice, brain macerates (Figure 6) and cultures revealed numerous cryptococci while culture of the peritoneal cavity was negative for the inoculated strain.

It is noteworthy that this phenomenon of innumerable cryptococci restricted to the brain of sacrificed mice, has been observed in our laboratory on several occasions. Review of data referable to the inoculated strain(s) has revealed them to be encapsulated, phenyloxidase negative at 37°C, but positive at 30°C. While cultures of the brains of these particular mice at the time of sacrifice were not performed on bird seed agar, it has since been observed with animals subsequently that phenyloxidase activity at 37°C has been present in a minority of *C. neoformans* colonies grown from brain cultures (Figure 7).

Perhaps such strain differences may help to explain why some patients with cryptococcal disease are minimally symptomatic with only central nervous system involvement (42), while others have widespread disease and a rapidly fatal downhill course.

Table 6. Mouse Virulence Studies.

Strain No.	Route of Inoc.	Capsule + Cell Size Range (Mean) um	Days to Death (Sacrifice)	Antigen Titer Day 10	20	40	90	Phenyloxidase 37°C	30°C
5	IP (2/3)*	2.5 - 10	30	320,000	320,000	Exp.[a]		+(W)	++
		(6.3)	(90)	320,000	81,920	2560	0		
			(90)	81,920	20,480	1280	0		
6	IP (1/3)	2.5 - 12.5	20	81,920	320,000	Exp.		++	++
		(7.6)	45	20,480	81,920	ND	Exp.		
			(90)	–	20,480	3120	0		
7	IP (2/4)	3.7 - 10	13	160,000	Exp.			+(W)	++
		(5.6)	19	20,480	Exp.				
			(90)	1,280	2,560	80	0		
8	IP (0/2)	3.7 - 8.7	23	1,280	64,000	Exp.		++	++
		(5.6)	30	1,280	32,000	Exp.			
9	IP (3/6)	5.0 - 12.5	19	650,000	Exp.			0	++
		(7.2)	(90)	40,960	2,560	320	0		
			(90)	40,960	5,120	20	0		

* () = Number of survivors/number of mice inoculated.
[a] Exp = Expired

Table 7. Relationship Among Two Isogenic Mutants of C. Neoformans in Degree of Encapsulation, Serum Antigenemia, Mouse Virulence, and Phenyloxidase Acitivity.

Strain No.	Capsule + Cell Size Range (Mean) μm	Days to Death (Sacrifice)	Antigen* Titer Day 10	20	40	90	Phenyloxidase 37°C	30°C
5	3.75-6.25	90[a]	64	2,560	ND	>40,000	0	++
(moist)	(5.1)	90[a]	64	ND	ND	260,000		
5A	7.5-12.5	15[b]	10^5	Exp.			+	++
(mucoid)	(8.5)	21	10^5	327,000	Exp.			
		(90)	10^5	160,000	ND	0		
6	2.5-7.5	(90)	10,240	64,000	2560	0	0	++
(dry)	(4.5)	(90)	10,240	20,480	1280	0		
		(90)	ND	20,480	320	0		
6A	7.2-12.5	5[b]	Exp.				+	++
(mucoid)	(8.5)	62	640,000	131,000	ND	Exp.		
		79	40,960	20,480				

* = by latex agglutination
a = Both mice moribund, brain cultures positive, peritoneal cavity negative.
b = Heart blood, brain, peritoneal cultures positive.
ND = Not done
Exp = Expired

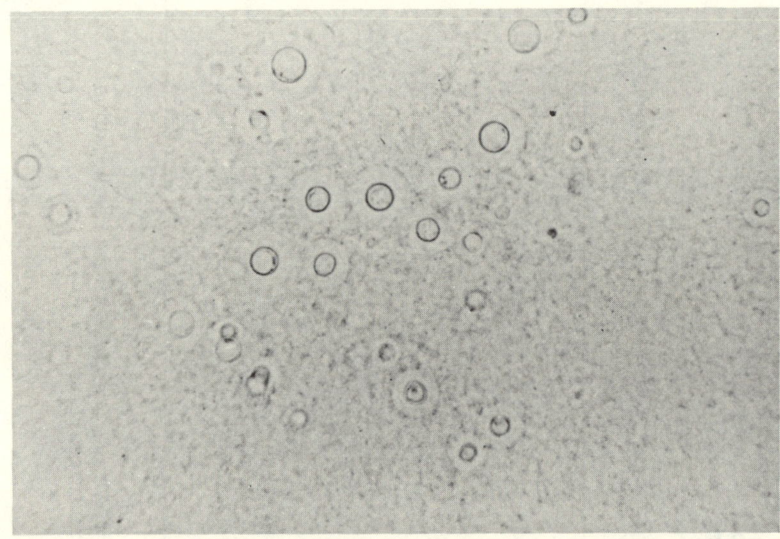

Figure 6. Brain macerate from moribund mouse inoculated intraperitoneally with *C. neoformans* showing numerous encapsulated cells

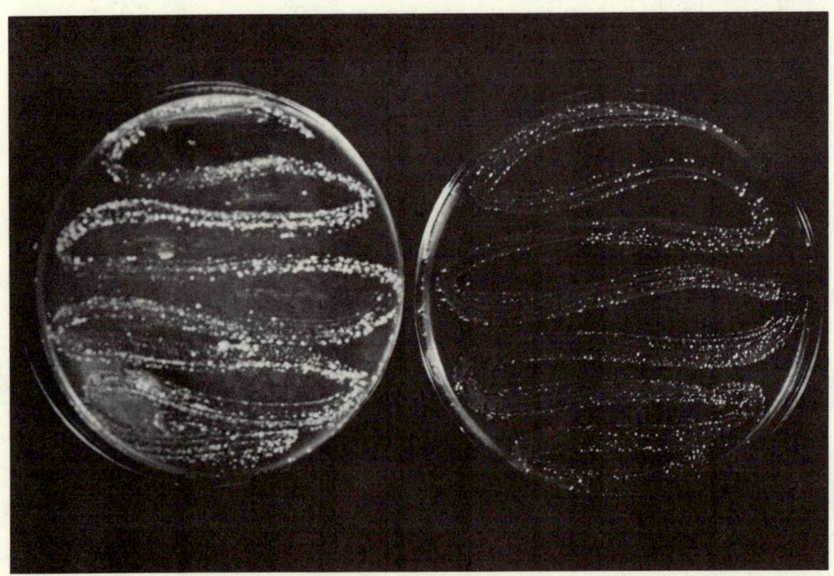

Figure 7. Phenyloxidase activity of *C. neoformans* after direct inoculation of brain macerate on bird seed agar. Left -- lack of phenyloxidase activity at 37°C. Right -- production of brown pigment (melanin) at 30°C by action of phenyloxidase.

SEROTYPE

The antigenic specificity of capsular polysaccharide has enabled the differentiation of *C. neoformans* into four serotypes A,B,C, (43) and D (44). As noted earlier, serotypes A and D are associated with *C. neoformans* var. *neoformans* whereas *C. neoformans* var. *gattii* consists of serotypes B and C (Table 1). Serotypes A and D have been widely encountered in environmental sources, especially pigeon droppings, while serotypes B and C have only been isolated from infected individuals (12) (44)-(46).

Epidemiologically, marked differences in the prevalence of *C. neoformans* serotypes have been noted. Serotype A has a global distribution and is especially prevalent in the United States. Serotype D is rare in the United States and Japan but common in Italy and Germany (47); serotypes B and C are infrequently encountered outside of endemic areas such as southern California, Australia, central Africa, and other tropical and subtropical areas of the world (45),(47). It has been suggested that cryptococcal infections due to serotypes B and C are more refractory to antifungal therapy than those due to serotypes A and D (48).

Bottone and colleagues (49) determined the serogroup of 45 cryptococcal isolates from individual AIDS patients. Of the 45 isolates, 42 were recovered from patients residing in New York State and one each from patients living in San Francisco, CA; New Orleans, LA (courtesy of Dr. Barbara Hanna); and Washington, DC.

Each isolate was serogrouped as either A/D or B/C by its effect on the glycine-cyclohexamide agar (GCA) of Salkin and Hurd (50) and the glycine-canavanine-bromthymol blue agar (GCB) of Kwon-Chung et al. (51). In these media change of GCA from yellow to red and of GCB from light green to blue after three days incubation at 30°C indicates that the isolate is a B/C serotype pair. No color change in both media is indicative of an A/D serotype pair. In this procedure differentiation of serotype pairs B and C from A and D is physiologically based on resistance to cyclohexamide and assimilation of glycine or canavanine as a sole carbon source.

All 45 isolates studied by Bottone et al. were in the A/D serogroup. This finding is consistent with observations reported previously (45) that A and D are the most prevalent serotypes associated with human infections in the United States.

Our observations also confirmed the report of Rinaldi and colleagues (52) who noted that all 28 *C. neoformans* isolates studied from 14 patients with AIDS residing in California (San Francisco) and Texas (San Antonio) were *C. neoformans* var. *neoformans* (serotypes A,D or A/D) (Table 8). Thus, no serotype B or C isolate was present among the 73 isolates studied in total. It would have been of valuable epidemiologic and pathogenetic significance if travel history to endemic areas of the B and C serotype were assessed for these patients. Without this information it is impossible to conclude whether or not the

Table 8. Serogroups of Cryptococcus Neoformans from AIDS Patients

Geographic Location	No of Isolates	Serogroup
New York	42	A/D
San Francisco[a]	28	A/D

[a]Rinaldi et al. (ref 52).

high prevalence rate of the A/D serogroup among AIDS patients represents preferential and/or selective infection with *C. neoformans* var *neoformans*, rather than the *gattii* variety. However, given the reported high prevalence of infection with the B and C serotypes in southern California, e.g., San Francisco southward (44),(45), it seems improbable that travel these areas did not take place among some of the California AIDS subjects studied (52).

Clinically, poor response to antifungal therapy (48) and extensive pulmonary cryptococcomas (12),(53), have been tentatively associated with B/C serogroups, rather than with the A/D serogroups of isolates as found in AIDS patients. A more "virulent" serogroup of *C. neoformans*, therefore, does not appear to account for the marked morbidity and chronicity associated with cryptococcosis in AIDS patients. Further studies will be needed, however, to substantiate this inference.

SUSCEPTIBILITY STUDIES

Cryptococcus neoformans, in the setting of AIDS, has emerged as a significant opportunistic pathogen producing life-threatening infection (4). Few, if any cures have been achieved in AIDS patients with cryptococcal meningitis. Therapeutic failure in patients treated with amphotericin B alone or in combination with 5-fluorocytosine is common, which seems to reflect the severity of the underlying immunodeficiency characterizing AIDS, rather than resistance of the infecting *C. neoformans* strain to the antifungal agents administered. The latter premise, however, is speculative as in vitro antifungal susceptibility of the *C. neoformans* isolates from AIDS patients has not been reported.

Consequently, twenty-six isolates of *C. neoformans* from AIDS patients were tested in our laboratory for susceptibility to amphotericin B, 5-fluorocytosine, ketoconazole, and miconazole (54). Results of this study did not show differences in susceptibility between the 26 AIDS and three additional non-AIDS

Table 9. Comparative Activity of Antifungal Agents Against Cryptococcus Neoformans

Agent		No. Strains Tested	Range (ug/ml)	50%	90%	Achievable Level Serum (ug/ml)	CSF (ug/ml)
Amphotericin B							
	MIC	27	0.25-2	1.0	1.0	0.5-2	0.2-0.3
	MFC	25	0.50-4	2.0	4.0		
5-Fluorocytosine							
	MIC	29	1.0- > 64	8.0	32.0	70-80	45-72
	MFC	27	2.0- > 64	32.0	>64.0		
Ketoconazole							
	MIC	29	0.06-1.0	0.5	0.5	5-9	Minimal
	MFC	29	0.25-16	1.0	4.0		
Miconazole							
	MIC	29	0.06-0.5	0.125	0.25	7.5	0.1-0.78
	MFC	28	0.125- > 2	0.5	2.0		

MIC = Minimum Inhibitory Concentration
MFC = Minimum Fungicidal Concentration

isolates studied in parallel. As noted in Table 9, 90% (MIC_{90}) of all isolates were inhibited by achievable serum levels of amphotericin B (1ug/ml), 5-fluorocytosine (32ug/ml), ketoconazole (0.5ug/ml), and miconazole (0.25ug/ml) (55). The minimum fungicidal concentration (MFC_{90}), however, for amphotericin B (4ug/ml), 5-fluorocytosine (>64ug/ml), ketoconazole (4ug/ml), and miconazole (2ug/ml), exceeded achievable levels in cerebrospinal fluid. These latter data may account for the refractory nature of cryptococcal meningitis in AIDS patients and highlight the potential importance of some preservation of cellular immunity for resolution of cryptococcal meningitis.

The in vitro antifungal susceptibility studies indicate that *C. neoformans* isolated from AIDS patients have a susceptibility pattern to the agents tested that is similar to that reported for non-AIDS isolates by Shadomy and colleagues (56) whose method was used in our studies. It should be pointed out, however, that in our study the *C. neoformans* isolates tested were all recovered from AIDS patients residing in the New York City area. While the serogroup of *C. neoformans* from AIDS patients residing in New York and California are identical, regional differences in antifungal susceptibility may exist.

REFERENCES

1. Sanfelice, F., Sull'azione patogena de blastomiceti como contributo alla etiologia dei tumori maligni. Nota preliminare II. Policlinico, Sez, chir. 2:204-11 (1985)

2. Vuillemin, P., Les blastomycetes pathogenes. Rev Gen Sci 12:732-51 (1901)

3. Stoddard, J.L., Cutler, E.G., Torula infection in man. Rockefeller Institute Med Res Monograph No. 62, p 1-98 (Jan 31) 1916.

4. Kovacs, J.A., Kovacs, A.A., Polis, M., et al., Cryptococcosis in the acquired immunodeficiency syndrome. Ann Intern Med 103:533-8 (1985).

5. Zuger, A., Louie, E., Holzman, R.S., et al., Cryptococcal disease in patients with the acquired immunodeficiency syndrome. Diagnostic features and outcome of treatment. Ann Intern Med 104:234-40 (1986)

6. Kwon-Chung, K.J., A new genus, *Filobasidiella*, the perfect state of *Cryptococcus neoformans*. Mycologia 67: 1197-2000 (1975)

7. Kwon-Chung, K.J., A new species of *Filobasidiella*, the sexual state of *Cryptococcus neoformans* B and C serotypes. Mycologia 68:942-6 (1976)

8. Kwon-Chung, K.J., Bennett, J.E., Theodore, T.S., *Cryptococcus bacillisporus* sp. nov.: serotype B-C of *Cryptococcus neoformans.* Int J Syst Bacteriol 28:616-20 (1978)

9. Kwon-Chung, K.J., Bennett, J.E., Rhodes, J.C., Taxonomic studies of *Filobasidiella species* and their anamorphs. Antonie van Leeuwenkoek J Microbiol Serol 48:25-32 (1982)

10. Vanbreuseghem, R., Takashio, M., An atypical strain of *Cryptococcus neoformans* (San Felice) Vuillemin 1894. II. *Cryptococcus neoformans* var. *gattii* var. nov. Ann Soc Belge Med Trop 50:695-702 (1980)

11. Diamond, R.D., *Cryptococcus neoformans*, In: Principles and Practice of Infectious Diseases (Mandell, G.L., Douglas, R.G., Bennett, J.E., eds.), John Wiley and Sons, New York 1st ed., 2023-2034 (1979)

12. Bottone, E.J., Kirschner, P.A., Salkin, I.F., Isolation of highly encapsulated *Cryptococcus neoformans* serotype B from a patient in New York City. J Clin Microbiol 23:186-8 (1986)

13. Cruickshank, J.G., Cavill, R., Jelbert, M., *Cryptococcus neoformans* of unusual morphology. Appl Microbiol 25:309-12 (1973)

14. Bottone, E.J., *Cryptococcus neoformans*: pitfalls in diagnosis through evaluation of Gram-stained smears of purulent exudates. J Clin Microbiol 12:790-1 (1980)

15. Levenson, D.J., Slicox, D.C., Rippon, J.W., et al., Septic arthritis due to nonencapsulated *Cryptococcus neoformans* with coexisting sarcoidosis. Arth Rheumat 17:1037-47 (1974)

16. Farhi, F., Bulmer, G.S., Tacker, J.R., *Cryptococcus neoformans*. IV. The not-so-encapsulated yeast. Infect Immun 1:526-31 (1970)

17. Bottone, E.J., Toma, M., Johansson, B.E., et al., Poorly encapsulated *Cryptococcus neoformans* from patients with AIDS: I. preliminary observations. AIDS Research 2:211-218 (1986)

18. Bottone, E.J., Wormser, G.P., Poorly encapsulated *Cryptococcus neoformans* from patients with AIDS: II. Correlation of capsule size observed directly in cerebrospinal fluid with that after animal passage. AIDS Research 2:219-225 (1986)

19. McGaw, T.G., Kozel, T.R., Opsonization of *Cryptococcus neoformans* by human immunoglobulin G: masking of immunoglobulin G by cryptococcal polysaccharide. Infect Immun 25:262-7 (1979)

20. Mitchell, T.G., Friedman, L. In vitro phagocytosis and intracellular fate of variously encapsulated strains of *Cryptococcus neoformans*. Infect Immun 5:491-8 (1972)

21. Diamond, R.D., Root, R.K., Bennett, J.E., Factors influencing killing of *Cryptococcus neoformans* by human leukocytes in vitro. J Infect Dis 125:367-76 (1972)

22. Bulmer, G.S., Sans, M.D., *Cryptococcus neoformans*. II. Phagocytosis by human leukocytes. J Bacteriol 94:1480-3 (1967)

23. Kozel, T.R., Non-encapsulated variant of *Cryptococcus neoformans*. II. Surface receptors for cryptococcal polysaccharide and their role in inhibition of phagocytosis by polysaccharide. Infect Immun 16:99-106 (1977)

24. Kozel, T.R., Gotschlich, E.C., The capsule of *Cryptococcus neoformans* passively inhibits phagocytosis of the yeast by macrophages. J Immunol 129:1675-80 (1982)

25. Kozel, T.R., Follette, J.L., Opsonization of encapsulated *Cryptococcus neoformans* by specific anticapsular antibody. Infect Immun 31:978-84 (1981)

26. Ikeda, R., Shinoda, T., Kagaya, K., et al., Role of serum factors in the phagocytosis of weakly or heavily encapsulated *Cryptococcus neoformans* strains by Guinea pig peripheral blood leukocytes. Microbiol Immunol 28:51-61 (1984)

27. Littman, M.L., Tsubura, E., Effect of degree of encapsulation upon virulence of *Cryptococcus neoformans*. Proc Soc Exp Biol Med 101:773-7 (1959)

28. Bulmer, G.S., Sans, M.D., Gunn, C.M., *Cryptococcus neoformans*. 1. Nonencapsulated mutants. J Bacteriol 94:1475-9 (1967)

29. Dykstra, M.A., Friedman, L., Murphy, J.W., Capsule size of *Cryptococcus neoformans*: control and relationship to virulence. Infect Immun 16:129-35 (1977)

30. Staib, F., Vogelkot, ein Nahrsubstrat fur die Gatung *Cryptococcus*. Zentralbl Bakteriol Parasitenkd Infektionskr Hyg Abt 1 Orig. 186:233-47 (1962)

31. Staib, F., *Cryptococcus neoformans* and *Guizotia abyssinica* (syn. *G. oliefera* D.C.). Zentralbl Hyg 148:466-75 (1962)

32. Shields, A.B., Ajello, L., Medium for selective isolation of *Cryptococcus neoformans*. Science 151:208-9 (1966)

33. Korth, H., Pulverer, G., Pigment formation for differentiating *Cryptococcus neoformans* from *Candida albicans*. Appl Microbiol 21:541-2 (1971)

34. Shaw, C.E., Kapica, L., Production of diagnostic pigment by phenoloxidase activity of *Cryptococcus neoformans*. Appl Microbiol 24:824-30 (1972)

35. Bloomfield, B.J., Alexander, M., Melanin and resistance of fungi to lysis. J Bacteriol 93:1276-80 (1966)

36. Kuo, M.J., Alexander, M., Inhibition of lysis of fungi by melanins. J Bacteriol 94:624-9 (1967)

37. Polacheck, I., Hearing V.J., Kwon-Chung, K.J., Biochemical studies of phenyloxidase and utilization of catecholamines in *Cryptococcus neoformans*. J Bacteriol 150:1212-20 (1982)

38. Kwon-Chung, K.J., Polacheck, I., Popkin, T.J., Melanin lacking mutants of *Cryptococcus neoformans* and their virulence for mice. J Bacteriol 150:1414-21 (1982)

39. Rhodes, J.C., Polacheck, I., Kwon-Chung, K.J., Phenyloxidase activity and virulence in isogenic strains of *Cryptococcus neoformans*. Infect Immun 36:1174-84 (1982)

40. Kwon-Chung, K.J., Rhodes, J.C., Encapsulation and melanin formation as indicators of virulence in *Cryptococcus neoformans*. Infect Immun 51:218-23 (1986)

41. Bottone, E.J., Johansson, B.E., Szporn, A., et al., Poorly encapsulated *Cryptococcus neoformans* from AIDS patients: morphologic, cultural, and pathogenic correlates. International Conference on Acquired Immunodeficiency Syndrome, Atlanta, Georgia (1985)

42. Liss, H.P., Rimland, D., Asymptomatic cryptococcal meningitis. Amer Rev Resp Dis 124:88-9 (1981)

43. Evans, E.E., The antigenic composition of *Cryptococcus neoformans*. 1. A serologic classification by means of the capsular and agglutination reactions. J Immunol 64:423-30 (1950)

44. Wilson, D.E., Bennett, J.E., Bailey, J.W., Serologic groupings of *Cryptococcus neoformans*. Proc Soc Exp Biol Med 127:820-3 (1968)

45. Bennett, J.E., Kwon-Chung, K.J., Howard, D.H., Epidemiologic differences among serotypes of *Cryptococcus neoformans*. Amer J Epidemiol 105:582-6 (1977)

46. Fromtling, R.A., Shadomy, S., Shadomy, H.J., et al., Serotype B/C *Cryptococcus neoformans* isolated from patients in nonendemic areas. J Clin Microbiol 16:408-10 (1982)

47. Bhattacharjee, A.K., Bennett, J.E., Glaudemans, C.P.S., Capsular polysaccharides of *Cryptococcus neoformans*. Rev Infect Dis 6:619-24 (1984)

48. Henderson, D.K., Edwards, J.E. Jr., Dismukes, W.E., et al., Meningitis produced by different serotypes of *Cryptococcus neoformans*. Abstr Annu Meet Amer Soc Microbiol F11:p315 (1981)

49. Bottone, E.J., Salkin, I.F., Hurd, N.J., et al., Serogroup of 45 *Cryptococcus neoformans* isolates from AIDS patients. (Submitted)

50. Salkin, I.F., Hurd, N.J., New medium for differentiation of *Cryptococcus neoformans* serotype pairs. J Clin Microbiol 15:169-71 (1982)

51. Kwon-Chung, K.J., Polacheck, I., Bennett, J.E., Improved diagnostic medium for separation of *Cryptococcus neoformans* var *neoformans* (serotypes A and D) and *Cryptococcus neoformans* var *gattii* (serotypes B and C). J Clin Microbiol 15:535-7 (1982)

52. Rinaldi, M.G.., Drutz, D.J., Howell, A., et al., Serotypes of *Cryptococcus neoformans* in patients with AIDS. J Infect Dis 153:642 (1986)

53. Lehmann, P.F., Morgan, R.J. Freimer, E.H., Infection with *Cryptococcus neoformans* var *gattii* leading to pulmonary cryptococcoma and meningitis. J Infect 9:301-6 (1984)

54. Poon, M., Cronin, D.C. II, Wormser, G.P., et al., In vitro susceptibility of *Cryptococcus neoformans* isolates from patients with the acquired immunodeficiency syndrome. (Manuscript submitted for publication.)

55. Sande, M.A., Mandel, G.L., Antimicrobial agents: Antifungal and antiviral agents. In: Goodman and Gilman's The Pharmacological Basis of Therapeutics (Gilman, A.G., Goodman, L.S., Rall, L., S.F. Murads, eds.), 7th ed., Macmillan Publishing Co., New York, p 1219-1229 (1985)

56. Shadomy, S., Espinel-Ingraff, A., Shadomy, H.J., Laboratory studies with antifungal agents: susceptibility tests and bioassays. In: Manual of Clinical Microbiology (Lennette, E.H., Balows, A., Hausler Jr., W.J., Shadomy, H.J., eds.), American Society for Microbiology, Washington, D.C., 4th ed., p 991-999 (1985)

33
Clinical Aspects of Cryptococcosis in AIDS

Joseph R. Masci

Cryptococcal meningitis and disseminated cryptococcosis have become common infections in patients with the acquired immunodeficiency syndrome (AIDS). Clinical features are comparable to those seen in non-AIDS patients with severe immunodeficiency states. However, mortality is greater and relapse rates following therapy are higher in AIDS patients. Improved diagnostic and therapeutic strategies will be necessary for effective management of this fungal infection.

CRYPTOCOCCAL INFECTIONS: EPIDEMIOLOGY AND CLINICAL PATTERNS

Cryptococcus neoformans var *neoformans* is found in environmental sources throughout the world but human infection is relatively uncommon. Although pigeons, whose excreta may harbor large quantities of the organism, have long been thought to have a major role in the epidemiology of cryptococcal infection, recent evidence (1) suggests that *C. neoformans* var *gattii* is not present in this material, implying the existence of additional reservoirs. Human-to-human transmission, however, has not been documented for either variety.

Indirect evidence indicates that the respiratory tract is the most common portal of entry in human infection. Inhalation of yeast cells may be followed by colonization without infection (2), asymptomatic infection (3), symptomatic pulmonary infection, or hematogenous dissemination. Pulmonary infection may take several forms (4) including a mild influenza-like illness, one or more nodules or mass lesions, cavities, or, rarely, a fulminant pneumonia. When pulmonary infection occurs alone, it is often a self-limited process, particularly in the immunologically normal host.

Although hematogenous dissemination can result in involvement of virtually any organ and widespread multiorgan disease is occasionally seen, the organism has a marked predilection for the central nervous system, and basilar meningitis is the most common clinical manifestation of disease. Cryptococcal meningitis may follow an acute or extremely indolent course, but most commonly causes a subacute illness with days to weeks of relatively nonspecific central nervous system signs and symptoms prior to diagnosis (5). Pathologically, the infection often involves the basal ganglia, cerebral white matter, and the cerebellum, as well as the meninges. Extraneural disease may co-exist with meningitis. Dissemination was seen in 25% of patients in a series compiled before the AIDS epidemic (5).

Most cases of progressive cryptococcal infection are associated with diseases or therapies known to cause depression of cellular immunity, including reticuloendothelial malignancy (6), sarcoidosis (7), chronic corticosteroid therapy (8), immunosuppressive therapy following organ transplantation (9) and, most recently, AIDS (10).

Although it is frequently stated that a significant proportion of patients with cryptococcal infection are immunologically normal, recent data suggest that some of these individuals may have a specific inability to mount an appropriate immune response to cryptococcal antigens (11).

HOST IMMUNE RESPONSE AND ORGANISM VIRULENCE IN HUMAN CRYPTOCOCCAL INFECTION

The humoral immune system seems to play a relatively minor role in host defense against cryptococcus. One-third of patients with disease have detectable antibody (a good prognostic sign), but active immunization of mice with capsular polysaccharide is not protective, even when high levels of antibody are produced (12). Specific antibody improves phagocytosis of unencapsulated (13), but not encapsulated (14) organisms in vitro.

Intracellular killing has been studied by Diamond et al. (14) who found that hydrogen peroxide generation as well as myeloperoxidase activity are necessary for effective killing of cryptococci in vitro by human neutrophils from normal volunteers. Although serum was necessary for phagocytosis and killing of encapsulated organisms by both neutrophils and monocytes, specific antibody did not enhance this process, suggesting the presence of other opsonizing elements, perhaps complement, in normal human serum.

However, in studies using unencapsulated organisms (13), McGaw and Kozel found that normal human serum contained opsonizing IgG. However, the addition of exogenous purified capsular polysaccharide to unencapsulated strains with polysaccharide receptors inhibited phagocytosis by macrophages without inhibiting antibody binding to the cell wall. These data suggested that capsular polysaccharide masked IgG bound to the cell wall, blocking Fc-mediated phagocytosis.

The importance of cellular immunity in the host response to cryptococcal infections is largely inferred from the types of patients who are at high risk, including those with underlying diseases or therapy as noted above, as well as those with AIDS. Supporting evidence comes from animal data. Athymic nude mice have a higher mortality in experimentally-induced infection than thymus-bearing or thymus-transplanted animals (15),(16). It has been found that a high percentage of patients, including some who are apparently immunologically normal by standard parameters, have specific defects in skin test reactions and lymphocyte transformation in response to cryptococcal antigen after they have recovered from infection (17)-(19). It is not clear, however, whether this is the cause or the result of the infection since cryptococcal antigen induces suppressor cell proliferation in mice (18).

It has long been thought that the virulence of *C. neoformans* isolates is variable. The size and composition of the organism's polysaccharide capsule have received the most attention as possible virulence factors to account for this variability.

Diamond et al. (14) found that increased capsule size inhibits phagocytosis by neutrophils but not monocytes. Dykstra (20), however, found no correlation between capsule size and virulence in mice, using encapsulated strains.

Capsular composition, in addition to size, has been suggested as a determinant of pathogenicity. Bhattacharjee et al. (21), for example, found that capsular serotypes B and C are associated with relatively low pathogenicity in mice. Human infections with these serotypes, however, generally required longer courses of therapy, suggesting either that the organisms were of increased virulence in humans, or that infection with types B or C is particularly common in the profoundly immunocompromised patient.

Kozel and Cazin (22) found that an unencapsulated variant isolated from a human was less virulent in mice than a normal-capsule variant. When capsular constituents from the encapsulated strain were injected into mice, however, the virulence of the unencapsulated strain was not affected, indicating that capsular polysaccharide is not a virulence factor unless the organism has an intact capsule.

Finally, in in vitro studies, cryptococcal antigen in extremely high concentration has been shown to inhibit phagocytosis by macrophages (23) and by neutrophils (14). Although this effect was demonstrated only at concentrations of antigen generally not seen in human infection, it is possible that it becomes clinically significant at the levels occasionally seen in overwhelming infection (see Case 1).

In regard to AIDS-related cryptococcal infection, Bottone et al. (24) have noted an increased prevalence of small-capsule, rough colony variants among cryptococcal isolates from AIDS patients, suggesting that the immune defect in AIDS is of such a profound nature that poorly encapsulated organisms cause a preponderance of invasive infections. The specificity of this finding for AIDS-related cryptococcal infection has been challenged (25).

CRYPTOCOCCAL INFECTIONS IN THE ACQUIRED IMMUNODEFICIENCY SYNDROME

The incidence of cryptococcal infection was rising prior to the beginning of the AIDS epidemic in 1981, presumably because of the increasing use of immunosuppressive therapy in cancer and organ transplantation patients. AIDS, however, has resulted in an alarming acceleration of this trend. The incidence of cryptococcal meningitis in the United States had been estimated to be 300 cases per year before the advent of AIDS (26). The annual incidence of AIDS-related cases has now surpassed that figure.

According to surveillance through 1985, *C. neoformans* was the initial opportunistic pathogen in 7% of 16,458 AIDS cases reported to the Centers for Disease Control (27). Data for New York City through 1985 were comparable with cryptococcosis occurring in 5% of cases reported (28). Recent data (29) suggest a disproportionately high prevalence among intravenous drug abusers, in comparison to other individuals at risk for AIDS, as well as a relatively higher prevalence among blacks with AIDS, compared to other ethnic groups, even when controlling for use of intravenous drugs.

Clinical Patterns in AIDS Patients

Clinical features of cryptococcal infections in AIDS patients are comparable in many respects to those in non-AIDS patients with profound immunodeficiency states. Although it appears that fulminant infection, extraneural disease and multiorgan involvement may be more common in AIDS patients, this has not been firmly established. Compared to non-AIDS patients, cerebrospinal fluid abnormalities in AIDS patients with cryptococcal meningitis are less severe and may be quite minimal. Cryptococcal antigen levels, however, are generally high (Table 1). Reported response rates to standard therapy are similar in AIDS and non-AIDS populations, but relapse rates appear higher in AIDS (30). As noted earlier, *C. neoformans* with smaller capsule sizes may be associated with infection in AIDS patients.

Central Nervous System Disease

As in non-AIDS patients with cryptococcal infection, the central nervous system (CNS) has been the commonest site of involvement in patients with AIDS. In two recent series (30), (31), with a total of 53 cases of cryptococcal infection in AIDS, 31 patients had CNS involvement alone, 13 had extraneural involvement alone and nine had both. Fever and headache were the most common presenting complaints in patients with CNS infection, each

Table 1. Comparison of Clinical Features of Cryptococcal Meningitis in AIDS and Non-AIDS Patients from Reported Series. (References in parentheses)

	AIDS	Non-AIDS
Laboratory Parameter		
CSF: leukocyte count (per mm^3)	<5: 64% (31)	>180:75% (5)
protein (mg/dL)	>45:69% (31)	>45:95% (5)
glucose (mg/dL)	<50:65% (30)	<50:84% (5)
India ink stain positive	82% (31)	64% (7)
Culture positive	95% (30)(31)	70% (5)
Antigen (reciprocal mean titer)	294 (31)	27.5 (7)
Blood culture positive	35% (31)	21% (7)
Extraneural Infection (coexistent)	17% (30)(31)	25% (5)
Mortality (treated patients)	37% (31)	21% (5)
Relapse rate	40-50% (30)(31)	14% (7)

*CSF = Cerebrospinal fluid

occurring in approximately 90% of cases. Meningismus, photophobia and mental status changes were each seen in more than 10% of patients, while nausea, vomiting or seizures were seen in a few cases. Only three patients had focal neurological deficits.

Cranial nerve palsies and hydrocephalus may occur as sequelae of cryptococcal meningitis in AIDS and in non-AIDS patients. The infection may mimic a number of other processes seen in AIDS patients, including cerebral toxoplasmosis, lymphoma, progressive multifocal leukoencephalopathy and tuberculous meningitis (Table 2).

Non-Central Nervous System Disease

Involvement of sites outside the CNS is relatively common in patients with AIDS, although, as noted above, this is often seen in the presence of active CNS infection.

Autopsy data reported by Welch et al. (32) revealed that three of 36 AIDS patients examined had cryptococcal infection. All of these patients had CNS infection plus extraneural infection at one or more of the following sites: lungs - two patients; lymph nodes - two; kidneys - two; liver - one; and spleen one. None of these patients had cryptococcal infection of the heart, adrenals, thyroid, parathyroids or skin.

In another series by Reichart et al. (33), cryptococcal infection was found in three of 10 patients at postmortem examination. In two of these patients, cryptococcal meningitis was documented premortem. All three had cryptococcal infection of the meninges despite antifungal therapy. In addition, two patients had cryptococcal pneumonitis, one had mediastinal lymph node involvement and one had adrenal involvement.

Little information is available on specific clinical syndromes and laboratory findings of extraneural cryptococcal infection in AIDS patients, in part because it often co-exists with other, more common, opportunistic infections in these patients (Table 2).

In a retrospective series reported by a workshop group of the National Heart, Lung and Blood Institute (34), 441 of 1067 AIDS patients had serious pulmonary abnormalities. Only eight (2%) of these patients had cryptococcal infection of the lungs, in each case coexisting with *Pneumocystis carinii* pneumonia.

This relatively low incidence of pulmonary infection was also observed by Stover et al. (35) who found no cases of cryptococcal infection in the lungs in 61 AIDS patients with respiratory disease over a four-year period. Similarly, Pass et al. (36) found no cases of cryptococcal infection on postmortem examinations of 15 AIDS patients with pulmonary abnormalities.

Several cases of cardiac involvement with cryptococcus have been described including myocarditis (37), with organisms contained within myocytes, and pericarditis (38) diagnosed by culture and cryptococcal antigen determination of pericardial fluid from a high risk-group patient.

Adrenal infection was reported by Glasgow et al. (39) in three patients at postmortem examination. It could not be determined if these patients had manifested functional hypoadrenalism during life.

Several skin lesions have been associated with cryptococcal infection in AIDS patients including chronic ulcers, nodules, herpetiform lesions (40) and papules resembling molluscum contagiosum (41).

DIAGNOSIS

Central Nervous System Disease: Clinical and Laboratory Findings

Central nervous system cryptococcal infection must be ruled

out in patients at risk for AIDS who present with headache, meningismus, photophobia, mental status changes, seizures or focal neurological deficits. The diagnosis should also be considered in patients with unexplained fever in the absence of neurological signs and symptoms. Computerized tomographic findings of hydrocephalus or mass lesions should also prompt a careful evaluation for cryptococcal infection in these patients.

Cerebrospinal fluid (CSF) examination must be performed to exclude the diagnosis. Characteristic findings in patients with AIDS include a mild to moderate lymphocytic pleocytosis, an abnormally elevated protein level, and a depressed glucose level, each found in somewhat more than one-half of cases (30),(31). Variations in this typical profile may include a predominance of polymorphonuclear leukocytes or, in very early or far-advanced cases, completely normal CSF parameters.

India ink examination is positive in 50-80% of cases and should be performed on all CSF specimens from AIDS-risk-group patients. Visualization of organisms by this technique is associated with a poor prognosis in both AIDS (31) and non-AIDS patients (7). Confirmation of a positive India ink examination by culture and serological methods should be done, since lymphocytes or erythrocytes in the CSF, or yeast cells contaminating the India ink, may result in false-positive results.

Detection of cryptococcal antigen, the capsular polysaccharide, by latex agglutination is a highly sensitive and specific means of diagnosis. The test is available in most hospital and commercial laboratories and should be performed on CSF and serum whenever cryptococcal infection is suspected. Patients with positive rheumatoid factor may have false positive tests for cryptococcal antigen by this technique, but if controls are performed, the sensitivity and specificity are both well above 90%. In two recent series, antigen was detected in CSF in 95% and in serum in 75% of AIDS patients with cryptococcal meningitis (30),(31). High titers of antigen in the CSF have been associated with a poor prognosis in AIDS (30) and non-AIDS (42) patients.

Since antigen titers reflect the amount of capsular polysaccharide in the CSF, the recent suggestion that small-capsule variant organisms may be responsible for a disproportionate number of cases of cryptococcal meningitis in AIDS patients (24), raises the possibility that the antigen titers in these patients may, on occasion, be deceptively low and not accurately reflect the severity of the infection. Despite this consideration, it has been noted that antigen titers in these patients generally are quite high and sometimes extraordinarily elevated (see Case 1).

CSF cultures are a reliable means of documenting cryptococcal infection, and are almost always positive in proven cases in AIDS patients. Organisms were isolated from the CSF in 95% of AIDS patients with cryptococcal meningitis in recent series (30),(31). Positive blood cultures are uncommon in non-AIDS patients but have been seen in 50% of AIDS-related cases in our institution. Cryptococcemia is associated with a poor prognosis in both AIDS (31) and non-AIDS (42) patients.

Roentgenographic Findings

Computerized tomographic (CT) patterns have been described in several large series of patients with AIDS and neurological abnormalities. Cryptococcal infection is not consistently associated with specific CT scan abnormalities and rarely produces mass lesions, even when infection is present within the brain substance.

Post et al. (43) conducted a retrospective review of CT scan findings in 51 AIDS patients with documented central nervous system pathology, including 10 with cryptococcal infection. Initial CT scans in these patients were positive in 76%, but the sensitivity was least in the patients with meningitis alone, including nine of the patients with cryptococcal infection. Overall, only two of the 10 patients with CNS cryptococcal infection had a positive scan, in both cases due to the presence of a second process (toxoplasmosis, lymphoma). Among eight patients with negative scans were two in whom perivascular infiltration of the brain with cryptococci was seen at autopsy.

Whelan et al. (44) described 19 AIDS patients with proven CNS pathology. Ten of these patients had structural lesions seen on CT scan including seven with toxoplasmosis, one with lymphoma, one with progressive multifocal leukoencephalopathy and one with nonspecific encephalitis. The other nine patients with no structural lesions had cryptococcal meningitis. CT scans in these patients revealed only mild sulcal prominence and mild ventricular dilatation. As in the series by Post et al. (43), two patients were found to have yeast cells in the brain parenchyma at postmortem examination.

Kelly et al. (45) have reported moderate enlargement of cerebrospinal fluid spaces (ventricles and basal cisternae) in several patients with cryptococcal meningitis. Levy et al. (46) described this same finding, in the absence of mass lesions, in a patient who was found to have multiple cryptococcal brain abscesses at postmortem examination.

Structural lesions apparently due to cryptococcal infection were described by Zuger et al. in three patients (30). Two of these patients demonstrated ring-enhancing lesions on CT scan due to cerebral cryptococcomas, and in one patient a hyperdense region was seen in the temporal lobe and resolved with antifungal therapy.

Non-Central Nervous System Disease

The diagnosis of extraneural cryptococcal infection in AIDS patients is made difficult by the similarity of clinical syndromes with that of more common opportunistic pathogens. Cryptococcal pneumonia, for example, may mimic *Pneumocystis carinii* infection, a far more common process. Similarly, cryptococcal skin lesions may be confused with Kaposi's sarcoma. Widespread dissemination of *C. neoformans* is, in fact, often seen in the setting of multiple, simultaneous opportunistic infections and malignancies.

Cryptococcal antigen determination is of somewhat less value in the diagnosis of extraneural infection than in the diagnosis of cryptococcal meningitis. Antigen determination on serum was negative in four of nine patients with extraneural disease alone in a recent series (31), including one patient with cryptococcemia.

Frequent blood cultures, as well as cultures of CSF, sputum, urine or bone marrow may be helpful, depending on the clinical setting.

Positive serum cryptococcal antigen, as well as positive cultures from any site in patients at risk for AIDS, warrants a thorough search for CNS infection and the institution of aggressive anti-fungal therapy.

Table 2. AIDS-Related Infections and Malignancies Which May Be Mimicked by Cryptococcal Infection

Organ System	Disease
Central Nervous System	Toxoplasmosis
	Lymphoma
	Progressive multifocal leukoencephalopathy
	Tuberculous meningitis
	AIDS encephalopathy
Respiratory	*Pneumocystis carinii* pneumonia
	Cytomegalovirus pneumonia
	Tuberculosis
	Lymphoma
	Kaposi's sarcoma
	Toxoplasmosis
Cardiovascular	Tuberculous pericarditis
Skin	Molluscum contagiosum
	Kaposi's sarcoma
	Mycobacterial infection
	Lymphoma

THERAPY

Prior to the advent of effective anti-fungal therapy, the one-year mortality of cryptococcal meningitis was approximately 75% (47). Amphotericin B used either alone, or in combination with 5-flucytosine (5FC), has become the established mode of therapy for cryptococcal infections and has substantially reduced mortality (48). The toxicity of these agents, however, and the significant relapse rate seen following therapy (49), made the management of cryptococcal infections difficult before the situation was further complicated by the AIDS epidemic.

The sharp rise in incidence of cryptococcal infections that has occurred in AIDS-risk-group populations has not, unfortunately, been accompanied by the development of newer, more effective therapies. The results of initial therapy in these patients seem comparable to those in patients without AIDS, but relapse rates appear to be higher in AIDS patients, most likely reflecting the profound, progressive, and, so far, irreversible nature of the immune defect in AIDS. In addition, the high frequency of refractory leukopenia and thrombocytopenia in AIDS patients has rendered 5-flucytosine difficult to use because of its marrow-depressive effects. Furthermore, the nephrotoxicity of amphotericin B may be potentiated by the chronic renal insufficiency sometimes seen in these patients.

The current management of cryptococcal meningitis has evolved from studies done by Utz et al. (49) and Bennett et al. (48), prior to the beginning of the AIDS epidemic. Utz, in a prospective, uncontrolled study, established that the efficacy of combined regimens of amphotericin B and 5-flucytosine was equal to that of amphotericin B alone, but that such therapy would allow lower doses of amphotericin B and shorter courses of treatment. Bennett et al. in a multicenter, prospective study demonstrated that a regimen of amphotericin B (0.3 mg/kg/day) and 5-flucytosine (150mg/kg/day in four divided doses) achieved a 68% response rate after six weeks of therapy and was comparable to a higher dose, longer course regimen of amphotericin B alone (0.4 mg/kg/day for six weeks followed by 0.9 mg/kg on alternate days for an additional four weeks). Either the combination regimen, or therapy with amphotericin B alone (0.4-0.6 mg/kg/day), represents acceptable therapy, if cultures are shown to revert to negative and cryptococcal antigen becomes negative or the level falls significantly during therapy. Intraventricular amphotericin B is reserved for patients who fail to respond to, or cannot tolerate systemic therapy. At our center, initial response to amphotericin B (0.6 mg/kg/day) has been good in 85% of AIDS patients, but the dose has had to be adjusted often or therapy interrupted because of progressive renal insufficiency. It has not been practical to add 5-flucytosine in our patients because of the almost universal leukopenia. Intraventricular administration of amphotericin B was necessary in one patient because of progressive infection despite systemic therapy with amphotericin B alone.

It has been suggested by several workers that long-term, intermittent, outpatient therapy with intravenous amphotericin B may diminish the relapse rate. In fact, preliminary data on the use of weekly maintenance therapy following standard initial therapy are encouraging (30).

Two additional agents, miconazole and ketoconazole may show in vitro activity against isolates of *C. neoformans*, but data concerning the therapy of human infections with these drugs are extremely limited. Weinstein et al. (50) described a non-AIDS patient with cryptococcal meningitis who was cured with intravenous miconazole after failing to respond to a 40-day course of amphotericin B and 5-flucytosine. Graybill et al. (51) reported a patient who responded to intraventricular miconazole after failing to respond to a five-week course of amphotericin B and 5-flucytosine, this patient was intolerant of intravenous miconazole due to severe thrombophlebitis. It has been pointed out (52) that neither of these patients had received miconazole alone, and that these favorable results have not yet been duplicated in controlled trials.

Dismukes et al. (53) reported seven patients with non-meningeal cryptococcal infection who were treated with ketoconazole. A favorable response to therapy were seen in five, despite the finding that the majority of the isolates were resistant to ketoconazole in vitro. In studies on athymic and thymus-bearing nude mice, Williams et al. (15) showed prolonged survival in animals treated with ketoconazole following challenge with cryptococcus, although cures were seen only in thymus-bearing animals.

ILLUSTRATIVE CASES

The following cases illustrate the variability of clinical syndromes which may be associated with cryptococcal infections in the setting of AIDS.

Case 1. A 41-year-old bisexual, male parenteral drug abuser was admitted to the hospital after being found on the floor of his apartment. He was initially febrile to 104.6F with a blood pressure of 110/70 mm Hg, a heart rate of 100 beats/min and a respiratory rate of 36/min. The patient was unresponsive to stimuli and his eyes were deviated to the right. There was no other focal neurological sign. There was no nuchal rigidity and the remainder of the physical examination was unremarkable except for rales heard in the left lower lung field. Initial laboratory examination included a white blood cell count of 6700/mm^3 with a normal differential and a hemoglobin of 12.3 g/dL. Chest roentgenogram revealed a streaky left lower lobe infiltrate. Cerebrospinal fluid contained no red or white cells, the protein level was 35 mg/dL and the glucose level was 55 mg/dL. India ink examination, however, revealed many encapsulated yeast cells. Computerized tomography of the head was normal. The patient developed progressive hypotension and hypothermia and died within two days of admission despite therapy with amphotericin B and 5-flucytosine. Blood and cerebrospinal fluid cultures were positive for *C. neoformans.* Cryptococcal antigen titer by latex fixation was 1:32 million in the serum and 1:128,000 in the cerebrospinal fluid. At autopsy, cryptococci were found in the lungs, mediastinal and abdominal periaortic lymph nodes, spleen, liver, kidneys, thyroid and myocardium, in addition to the meninges and brain parenchyma. The inflammatory response was minimal or absent in all sites where organisms were found. *Pneumocystis carinii* was also found in the lungs.

Note: This patient manifested overwhelming cryptococcal infection with a clinical picture mimicking bacterial septic shock. It is clear that the complete absence of an inflammatory response in the cerebrospinal fluid was an extremely ominous sign.

Case 2. A 32 year-old black man, who had been a parenteral drug abuser, was admitted to the hospital in June 1984, with a three-day history of fever, headache, nausea and vomiting. The patient, a chronic schizophrenic, had been diagnosed as having AIDS five months earlier when he presented with *Pneumocystis carinii* pneumonia. Physical examination was remarkable only for fever of 102.4F; the patient was without neurological abnormalities. CSF examination was normal but a test for cryptococcal antigen was positive at a titer of 1:40. The patient was treated with amphotericin B (0.6 mg/kg/day) with rapid resolution of his symptoms. Therapy was well-tolerated and was continued for 10 weeks at which time serum and CSF antigen determinations were negative. Over the following 15 months, without further antifungal therapy, the patient was able to return to work. In November 1985, he again-developed fever and headache. Physical examination was notable for a temperature of 101.4F and disorientation to time and place without focal neurological deficits. CSF contained seven white cells/mm^3, all lymphocytes. The protein level was 98 mg/dL and the glucose concentration 40 mg/dL. The India ink examination and culture of CSF were positive for *C. neoformans*, as were cultures of the blood. Cryptococcal antigen titer was 1:640 in both CSF and serum. The patient was again treated with amphotericin B for a total of 10 weeks. His symptoms resolved, but CSF cryptococcal antigen remained positive at 1:10 for the last three weeks of his course of therapy. He refused further therapy. Three months after the completion of therapy and 22 months after cryptococcal meningitis was initially diagnosed, the patient is asymptomatic and has recently returned to work. Off antifungal therapy, there has been no increase in serum cryptococcal antigen and maintenance therapy has not been initiated. Lymphocyte studies done serially throughout his course have consistently shown severe depletion of T helper cells and reversal of the helper-to-suppressor T cell ratio in the range of 0.1 to 0.3.

Note: Despite evidence of profoundly depressed cellular immunity, this patient has survived a relapse of cryptococcal meningitis. Evaluation of the anecdotal reports of maintenance therapy is difficult in light of the fact that reasonably long-term survival may be seen in some patients without continued antifungal therapy. This underscores the fact that more data must be gathered before maintenance therapy with amphotericin B can be recommended for all AIDS patients after initial therapy for cryptococcal meningitis.

SUMMARY

AIDS has accounted for a dramatic increase in cryptococcal infections, already more than doubling the annual incidence. Clinical features of cryptococcal infections in AIDS patients are comparable, or more severe, than those in other profoundly immunocompromised patients. Distinguishing features in AIDS patients include the high frequency of multi-organ involvement, the relatively poor inflammatory response in the cerebrospinal fluid, and the poor prognosis and high relapse rate after therapy.

When cryptococcosis involves extraneural sites, the infection may mimic other, more prevalent AIDS-related opportunistic infections, or malignancies such as *Pneumocystis carinii* pneumonia, lymphoma, and Kaposi's sarcoma. Central nervous system cryptococcal infections in AIDS patients may also simulate other processes including toxoplasmosis, central nervous lymphoma, progressive multifocal leukoencephalopathy, and AIDS encephalopathy. Computerized tomography, however, rarely demonstrates mass lesions or any characteristic abnormality.

The diagnostic approach is the same as in non-AIDS patients making use of the cryptococcal antigen test on CSF which is a highly sensitive and specific technique for detection of cryptococcal meningitis. The sensitivity of a cryptococcal antigen determination on serum for diagnosis of extraneural infection is considerably lower.

Initial therapy with amphotericin B or amphotericin B and 5-flucytosine has been effective in the majority of patients at our center. However, high relapse rates have led to consideration of long-term, maintenance therapy. Too little data are currently available to evaluate this approach fully, but this strategy is sensible and should be considered in patients who respond to initial therapy.

REFERENCES

1. Diamond, R.D., *Cryptococcus neoformans* In: Principles and Practice of Infectious Diseases (Mandell, G.L., Douglas, Jr., R.G., Bennett, J.E., eds) John Wiley & Sons, New York, p 1460-1468 (1985)

2. Duperval, R. Hermans, P.E., Brewer, N.S., et al., Cryptococcosis with emphasis on the significance of isolation of *Cryptococcus neoformans* from the respiratory tract. Chest 72:13-15 (1977)

3. Atkinson, Jr., A.J., Bennett, J.E., Experience with a new skin test antigen prepared from *Cryptococcus neoformans* Am Rev Resp Dis 97:637-639 (1968)

4. Hammerman, K.J., Powell, K.E., Christianson, C.S., et al., Pulmonary cryptococcosis: clinical forms and treatment. Am Rev Resp Dis 108:1116-1123 (1973)

5. Lewis, J.L., Rabinovich, S., The wide spectrum of cryptococcal infections. Am J Med 53:315-322 (1972)

6. Zimmerman, L.E., Rappaport, H., Occurrence of cryptococcosis in patients with malignant disease of the reticuloendothelial system. Am J Clin Path 24:1050-1055 (1954)

7. Diamond, R.D., Bennett, J.E., Prognostic factors in cryptococcal meningitis: a study in 111 cases. Ann Intern Med 80: 176-181 (1974)

8. Bennington, J.L., Haber, S.L., Morgenstern, N.L., Increased susceptibility to cryptococcosis following steroid therapy. Dis Chest 45:262-265 (1964)

9. Schroter, G.P.J., Temple, D.R., Husberg, B.S., et al, Cryptococcosis after renal transplantation. Surgery 79:268-277 (1976)

10. Armstrong, D., Gold, J.W.M., Dryjanski, J., et al., Treatment of infections in patients with the acquired immunodeficiency syndrome. Ann Intern Med 103:738-743 (1985)

11. Diamond, R.D., Bennett, J.E., Disseminated cryptococcosis in man: decreased lymphocyte transformation in response to *Cryptococcus neoformans*. J Infect Dis 127:694-698 (1973)

12. Goren, M.B., Experimental murine cryptococcosis: effect of hyperimmunization to capsular polysaccharide. J Immun 98: 914-922 (1967)

13. McGaw, T.G., Kozel, T.R., Opsonization of *Cryptococcus neoformans* by human immunoglobulin G: masking of immunoglobulin G by cryptococcal polysaccharide. Infect Immun 25: 262-267 (1979)

14. Diamond, R.D., Root, R.K., Bennett, J.E., Factors influencing killing of *Cryptococcus neoformans* by human leukocytes in vitro. J Infect Dis 125:367-376 (1972)

15. Williams, D.M., Graybill, J.R., Drutz, D.J., et al., Suppression of cryptococcosis and histoplasmosis by ketoconazole in athymic nude mice. J Infect Dis 141:76-80 (1980)

16. Graybill, J.R., Mitchell, L., Drutz, D.J., Host defense in cryptococcosis III. Protection of nude mice by thymus transplantation. J Infect Dis 140:546-552 (1979)

17. Henderson, D.K., Bennett, J.E., Huber, M.A., Long-lasting specific immunologic unresponsiveness associated with cryptococcal meningitis. J Clin Invest 69:1185-1190 (1982)

18. Murphy, J.W., Mosley, R.L., Regulation of cell-mediated immunity in cryptococcosis III. Characterization of second-order T suppressor cells (Ts2). J Immunol 134:577-583 (1985)

19. Schimpff, S.C., Bennett, J.E., Abnormalities in cell-mediated immunity in patients with *Cryptococcus neoformans*. J Allergy Clin Immunol 55:430-441 (1975)

20. Dykstra, M.A., Friedman, L., Murphy, J.W., Capsule size of *Cryptococcus neoformans*: control and relationship to virulence. Infect Immunol 16:129-135 (1977)

21. Bhattacharjee, A.K., Bennett, J.E., Glaudemans, C.P.J., Capsular polysaccharides of *Cryptococcus neoformans*. Rev Infect Dis 6:619-624 (1984)

22. Kozel, T.R., Cazin, J., Nonencapsulated variant of *Cryptococcus neoformans*: I. Virulence studies and characterization of soluble polysaccharide. Infect Immunol 3:287-294 (1971)

23. Kozel, T.R., Gotschlich, E.C., The capsule of *Cryptococcus neoformans* passively inhibits phagocytosis of the yeast by macrophages. J Immunol 129:1675-1680 (1982)

24. Bottone, E.J., Toma, M., Johansson, B.E., et al., Capsule-deficient *Cryptococcus neoformans* in AIDS. Lancet 1:400 (1985)

25. Fromtling, R.A., Bulmer, G.S., Capsule-deficient *Cryptococcus neoformans* in AIDS patients. Lancet 1:988 (1985)

26. Hoeprich, P.D., Cryptococcosis. In: Infectious Diseases, Third Ed. (Hoeprich, P.D., ed) Harper & Row, Publishers, Philadelphia, p 1053- 1061 (1983)

27. CDC., Update: Acquired immunodeficiency syndrome--United States. MMWR 35:17-21 (1986)

28. New York City Department of Health: AIDS--surveillance update. January 29, 1986

29. Bottone, E.J., Personal communication (1986)

30. Zuger, A., Louie, E., Holzman, R.S., et al., Cryptococcal disease in patients with the acquired immunodeficiency syndrome: diagnostic features and treatment. Ann Intern Med 104:234-240 (1986)

31. Kovacs, J.A., Kovacs, A.A., Polis, M., et al., Cryptococcosis in the acquired immunodeficiency syndrome. Ann Intern Med 103:533-538 (1985)

32. Welch, K., Finkbeiner, W., Alpers, C.E., et al., Autopsy findings in the acquired immunodeficiency syndrome. JAMA 252:1152-1159 (1984)

33. Reichert, C.M., O'Leary, T.J., Levens, D.L., et al., Autopsy pathology in the acquired immune deficiency syndrome. Am J Pathol 112:357-382 (1982)

34. Murray, J.F., Felton, C.P., Garay, S.M., et al., Pulmonary complications of the acquired immunodeficiency syndrome. N Engl J Med 310:1682-1688 (1984)

35. Stover, D.E., White, D.A., Romano, P.A., et al., Spectrum of pulmonary. diseases associated with the acquired immune deficiency syndrome. Am J Med 78:429-437 (1985)

36. Pass, H.I., Macher, A.M., Shelhammer, J.H., et al., Thoracic manifestations of the acquired immune deficiency syndrome. J Thorac Cardiovasc Surg 88:654-658 (1984)

37. Cammarosano, C., Lewis, W., Cardiac lesions in acquired immune deficiency syndrome (AIDS). J Am Coll Cardiol 5:703-706 (1985)

38. Schuster, M., Valentine, F., Holzman, R., Cryptococcal pericarditis in an intravenous drug abuser. J Infect Dis 152:842 (1985)

39. Glasgow, B.J., Steinsapir, K.D., Anders, K., et al., Adrenal pathology in the acquired immune deficiency syndrome. Am J Clin Pathol 84:594-597 (1985)

40. Borton, L.K., Wintroub, B.U., Disseminated cryptococcosis presenting as herpetiform lesions in a homosexual man with the acquired immunodeficiency. J Am Acad Dermatol 10:387-390 (1984)

41. Rico, M.J., Penneys, N.S., Cutaneous cryptococcosis resembling molluscum contagiosum in a patient with AIDS. Arch Dermatol 121:901-902 (1985)

42. Goodman, J.S., Kauffman, L., Koenig, G.M., Diagnosis of cryptococcal meningitis: value of immunologic detection of cryptococcal antigen. N Engl J Med 285:434-436 (1971)

43. Post, M.J.D., Kursunoglu, S.J., Hensley, G.T., et al., Cranial CT in acquired immunodeficiency syndrome: spectrum of diseases and optimal contrast enhancement technique. Am J Radiol 145:929-949 (1985)

44. Whelan, M.A., Kricheff, I.I., Handler, M., et al., Acquired immunodeficiency syndrome: cerebral computed tomographic manifestations. Radiology 149:477-484 (1983)

45. Kelly, W.M., Brant-Zawadski, M., Acquired immunodeficiency syndrome: neuroradiologic findings. Radiology 149:485-491 (1983)

46. Levy, R.M., Bredesen, D.E., Rosenblum, M.L., Neurological manifestations of the acquired immunodeficiency syndrome (AIDS): Experience at UCSF and review of the literature. J Neurosurg 62:475-495 (1985)

47. Butler, W.T., Alling, D.W., Spickard, A., et al., Diagnostic and prognostic value of clinical and laboratory findings in cryptococcal meningitis. N Engl J Med 70:59-67 (1964)

48. Bennett, J.E., Dismukes, W.E., Duma, R.J., et al., A comparison of amphotericin B alone and combined with flucytosine in the treatment of cryptococcal meningitis. N Engl J Med 301:126-131 (1979)

49. Utz, J.P., Garriques, I.L., Sande, M.A., et al., Therapy of cryptococcosis with a combination of flucytosine and amphotericin B. J Infect Dis 132:368-373 (1975)

50. Weinstein, L., Jacoby, I., Successful treatment of cerebral cryptococcoma and meningitis with miconazole. Ann Intern Med 93:569-571 (1980)

51. Graybill, J.R., Levine, H.B., Successful treatment of cryptococcal meningitis with intraventricular miconazole. Arch Intern Med 138:814-816 (1978)

52. Bennett, J.E., Remington, J.S., Miconazole in cryptococcosis and systemic candidiasis: a word of caution. Ann Intern Med 94:708-709 (1981)

53. Dismukes, W.E., Stamm, A.M., Graybill, J.R., et al., Treatment of systemic mycoses with ketoconazole: emphasis on toxicity and clinical response in 52 patients: National Institute of Allergy and Infectious Diseases Collaborative Antifungal Study. Ann Intern Med 98:13-20 (1983)

34
Progressive Multifocal Leukoencephalopathy in AIDS

Lauren B. Krupp, Richard B. Lipton, Paul S. Shneidman

Progressive multifocal leukoencephalopathy (PML) is an uncommon demyelinating disease of the central nervous system caused by an opportunistic viral infection. PML produces progressive neurologic deterioration, usually terminating in death within three to six months. The disease was first described in 1958 (1). Although its association with lymphoproliferative disorders was emphasized, it was soon noted to occur with sarcoidosis, tuberculosis, cancer, chronic steroid therapy, and other immunosuppressive states (2)-(4). Electron microscopic examination of sections of infected brain tissue showed crystalline arrays of particles within oligodendrocytes, identical to papovavirus in size and morphology (5). Subsequently, viruses of the papovavirus group were isolated from brains of patients with PML (6), (7). One virus was SV40, which is indigenous to monkeys, and the other virus was named JC, after the initials of the first patient from whom this virus was recovered. (In retrospect this terminology was a poor choice, since it has frequently caused confusion with the unrelated Jakob-Creutzfeld agent). Subsequently, JC virus (JCV) has been isolated from numerous cases, while SV40 has been successfully grown from the brain of only two patients (8). The etiologic relationship between papovavirus and PML has been confirmed by immunohistochemical localization of viral antigen, in situ hybridization of JCV DNA, and numerous successful isolations of virus from the brain of affected patients (9),(10).

Recently, PML has been reported in patients with AIDS with

an incidence of 2% to 5% in clinical and pathologic series (11)-(15). As an increasing number of AIDS cases with PML have appeared, and since PML is often the initial manifestation of AIDS, it is timely to review the etiology, pathogenesis, and clinical characteristics of this disease.

CLINICAL FEATURES

Neurologic Presentation and Course

In patients with PML, an immunodeficient state is typically present for months to years prior to the development of the neurologic syndrome. The duration of the preceding immunocompromised state is unknown for patients with AIDS. Longitudinal studies of individuals at risk for AIDS from the time of development of human immunodeficiency virus (HIV) sero-positivity to the time of onset of PML might provide information on the duration of antecedent immunodeficiency in this setting. The clinical characteristics of 17 reported cases of PML and AIDS are summarized in Table 1 (15)-(25). PML was the initial opportunistic infection which led to the diagnosis of AIDS in 10 of 17 patients. For seven patients, the diagnosis of AIDS was established one to six months before PML developed. Conditions leading to the initial diagnosis of AIDS in patients who subsequently developed PML included: *Pneumocystis carinii* pneumonia, gastrointestinal cryptosporidiosis, miliary tuberculosis, esophageal candidiasis, and Kaposi's sarcoma (Table 1).

Early symptoms of PML include personality change, disturbance of memory and language, weakness, and sensory loss. Approximately 10 percent of patients present with coordination difficulties, poor balance, and other symptoms of cerebellar and brainstem disease. In a recent review of 230 pathologically confirmed cases (26), initial findings consisted of mental dysfunction (36%), visual field deficits (35%), and mono- or hemiparesis (33%). Seizures were uncommon as a presenting manifestation (6%). Neurologic dysfunction begins insidiously but relentlessly progresses to death within one year. Over 80% of patients are dead by eight months (26). Occasional patients, however, often with transient or mild immunodeficiency states, have had prolonged survival times (4).

In AIDS patients, clinical features are similar to those listed above. Of 17 reported cases (Table 1), the initial neurologic findings were: mono- or hemiparesis (eight patients), cognitive or memory loss (five patients), language disturbance (four patients), and visual field deficits (four patients). Three patients presented with symptoms referable to the posterior fossa. The average survival was four months (range: one to 13 months) (Table 2). It has been suggested that PML assumes a somewhat more rapid course in AIDS patients (8). The cases summarized in Tables 1 and 2 would support this observation.

Table 1. Progressive Multifocal Leukoencephalopathy (PML) in AIDS: Clinical Features

Reference	Risk Group	Preceding Infections or Neoplasia	PML was Presenting Opportunistic Infection	Neurologic Symptoms and Signs
16	homosexual	intestinal amebiasis (1 month before)	Yes	malaise numbness blurred vision monoparesis
17	IVDA	PCP(3 wks before)	No	confusion gait disturbance memory loss
18	homosexual	PCP (6 mo. before)	No	dysarthria monoparesis
18	homosexual	Kaposi's sarcoma	No	dementia hemiparesis
19	homosexual	none	Yes	field cut, dysphasia intellect loss
20	IVDA	cryptococcal meningitis	No	hemiparesis
21	Haitian	miliary tuberculosis muco-cutaneous *Herpes simplex* (5 mos before)	No	monoparesis
22	IVDA	none	Yes	ataxia malaise
23	homosexual	PCP (17 days before)	No	lethargy weakness memory loss
23	homosexual	none	Yes	dysarthria slow speech
24	homosexual	oral candidiasis (1 month before)	Yes	monoparesis

Table 1. Progressive Multifocal Leukoencephalopathy (PML) in AIDS: Clinical Features (Continued)

Reference	Risk Group	Preceding Infections or Neoplasia	PML was Presenting Opportunistic Infection	Neurologic Symptoms and Signs
25	homosexual	none	Yes	alexia without agraphia, homonymous hemianopsia
25	homosexual	cutaneous fungal infection	Yes	aphasia
15	IVDA	esophageal candidiasis (6 mos before) cryptosporidiosis (5 mos before)	No	hemiparesis aphasia
15	IVDA	none	Yes	ataxia facial numbness
15	IVDA	none	Yes	confusion field cut
15	IVDA	herpes zoster (5 mos before) oral candida (4 mos before)	Yes	monoparesis headache field cut

IVDA = Intravenous drug abuser
PCP = *Pneumocystis carinii* pneumonia

Radiographic Features

The CT scan plays a central role in the evaluation of AIDS patients with neurologic deficits. Though a characteristic CT scan may suggest PML, histologic confirmation is required for definitive diagnosis, as well as to exclude other treatable conditions (25)-(31). CT lesions most frequently appear as regions of decreased attenuation confined to the white matter which demonstrate no mass effect and are not enhanced after contrast

Table 2. Progressive Multifocal Leukoencephalopathy in AIDS: Diagnostic Methods, Treatment, Outcome

Reference	CT	DX Method	Treatment	Survival
16	one hypodense lesion	biopsy of cerebellum	vidarabine	4 months
17	atrophy	brain biopsy	acyclovir	9 weeks
18	one lucent lesion lesion	CT-guided needle biopsy	interferon	not stated
18	two focal lesions	autopsy	none	3 months
19	two focal lucent lesions	brain biopsy	not stated	not stated
20	one hypodense lesion	autopsy	none	4 months
21	normal	autopsy	none	1.5 months
22	normal	brain biopsy	steroids	13 months
23	one lucent lesion	brain biopsy	none	4 months
23	one lucent lesion	brain biopsy	none	3 months
24	one hypodense lesion	CT guided biopsy	cytosine arabinoside, adenine arabinoside, acyclovir, interferon	4 months
25	one hypodense lesion	autopsy	none	2 months
25	one hypodense lesion	open biopsy	steroids	2 months
15	two hypodense lesions	CT-guided biopsy	Adenine arabinoside	4 months
15	one hypodense lesion	open biopsy	none	1 month
15	one hypodense lesion	open biopsy	none	5 months
15	two hypodense lesions	CT-guided biopsy	none	4-1/2 months

injection. The location of the lesions bears no relationship to the vascular distribution or ventricular system. Early in the course of the illness, the CT may be normal or show only a small hypodense area. As the disease progresses, these areas enlarge, often extending to the subcortical gray-white junction and producing a scalloped appearance. Similar lesions on CT may occur in the cerebellum (16). Exceptions to this pattern do exist. Contrast enhancement along the peripheral border of lesions in non-AIDS patients has been reported (28). In a patient with PML (and systemic lupus erythematosus), repeated noncontrast and contrast scans were normal but a double dose delayed contrast scan revealed focal abnormalities (32). Early in the course of PML, the clinical signs on neurologic examination generally indicate more extensive disease than is visualized on CT scan, a "CT-clinical dissociation". The CT lesions progressively enlarge over time but often lag behind the clinical evolution (15).

In addition to CT, angiograms may occasionally be useful in evaluating these patients. A number of abnormal patterns have been described including: avascular zones (27); dilation of medullary veins, small arteries, or arterioles; or faint vascular blush (15). Rarely, a mild mass effect with stretching and separation of arterial branches occurs (28). More commonly, however, the angiogram is normal.

Because magnetic resonance imaging (MRI) is a highly sensitive method of identifying white matter disease, it should prove useful in the evaluation of these patients. Recently, it has been reported that MRI scans are able to detect PML lesions not apparent on CT (33).

Ancillary Diagnostic Tests

Electrophysiologic studies are another useful, although nonspecific, test for diagnosing PML (34). In patients with PML, the EEG may sometimes be abnormal before CT findings appear (35), or demonstrate more widespread cerebral dysfunction than the CT appearance would suggest. In supratentorial PML, the EEG may reveal focal abnormalities such as polymorphic slowing in the theta or delta frequencies or diffuse abnormalities such as disruption of the background activity (35). Focal polymorphic slowing probably reflects destructive lesions of the hemispheric white matter due to PML. The background slowing might be due to either PML, subacute encephalopathy of AIDS, or systemic disease. When PML involves the posterior fossa, the EEG is usually normal. However, evoked potentials may detect posterior fossa involvement. There is at least one report (35) of a patient whose CT revealed only a cerebellar lesion but whose clinical presentation suggested more extensive pathology. Somatosensory and brainstem auditory evoked potentials revealed abnormalities of the lower brainstem which were not apparent radiographically but which were subsequently confirmed at autopsy. EEG and evoked potentials, although nonspecific, are sensitive tests for identifying white matter dysfunction and may be useful in detecting early PML lesions.

Cerebrospinal (CSF) fluid examination is usually either normal or reveals only a slight protein elevation. Hypoglycorrhachia or CSF pleocytosis suggests a process other than PML, or in addition to PML.

Differential Diagnosis

The differential diagnosis of an AIDS patient with progressive cognitive or motor dysfunction and a focal lesion on CT includes toxoplasmosis, primary central nervous system (CNS) lymphoma, mycobacterial and/or fungal abscess, primary HIV infection of the central nervous system, stroke, and other disorders (36). Toxoplasmosis most commonly presents on CT as single or multiple ring enhancing lesions which are typically located at the cerebral gray-white junction or in the basal ganglia (37). There is generally little mass effect. The presence of contrast enchancement and the location in the gray matter helps to distinguish these lesions from PML. Rarely, toxoplasmosis may appear as an area of decreased density on CT which lacks contrast enhancement, thereby making the neuroradiographic differentiation more difficult. CNS lymphoma usually appears as a hyperdense lesion which enhances with contrast material and is easily distinguished from PML (18),(32). HIV infection is usually only associated with atrophy on CT. Strokes can be differentiated from PML in most cases by the rapid onset, the clinical course, and the vascular distribution of the CT lesion. The differential diagnosis of an immunosuppressed patient with progressive neurologic deterioration and leukoencephalopathy includes the effects of intrathecal or parenteral methotrexate therapy. Though occurring in a setting different from AIDS, methotrexate leukoencephalopathy can be confused with PML and is also associated with hypodense lesions of the cerebral white matter. Unlike PML lesions, however, the lesions in methotrexate leukoencephalopathy are typically symmetrical and periventricular in location. A syndrome similar to methotrexate induced leukoencephalopathy may occur months after radiotherapy to the brain.

Diagnosis

Stereotactic CT-guided biopsies generally provide rapid diagnosis. If insufficient tissue is obtained, a repeat stereotactic biopsy or an open biopsy should be considered. In cases of cerebellar involvement, open biopsy is the method of choice. Stereotactic biopsy may be complicated by small hemorrhages or focal seizures. However, serious complications rarely occur (38). Diagnostic points on biopsy are focal demyelination, bizzare appearing, enlarged astrocytes, and swollen oligodendrocytes with inclusions. Further confirmation involves demonstration of virus by electron microscopy, immunohistochemistry, in situ hybridization or culture (if available) (9),(39).

Treatment

Having established the diagnosis of PML, one is faced with

the problem of treatment. Currently, there is no proven therapy for PML. Most therapeutic attempts have been uncontrolled and empiric with variable results and no definite benefit (8). Favorable responses for biopsy proven cases of PML treated with cytarabine (cytosine arabinoside) have occasionally been reported (40). However, there are numerous cases in which cytarabine has had no benefit (15),(41). Other unsuccessful therapies attempted in AIDS patients include interferon, vidarabine, and acyclovir (Table 2). In conclusion, although definitive therapy is lacking, cytarabine represents the best option currently available but, because its benefit is unproven, we suggest that the drug be discontinued if bone marrow toxicity develops.

PATHOLOGY/PATHOGENESIS

Gross inspection of brain tissue from PML patients reveals foci of demyelination ranging from pinhead sized lesions to extensive areas of leukomalacia. The variation in size and the frequent finding of small foci adjacent to larger ones suggest that, as the disease advances, small lesions coalesce to form larger demyelinated areas (2),(3),(10). The cerebral hemispheres are generally more affected than the cerebellum or brainstem but in some cases this distribution is reversed. The microscopic features are distinctive and characteristic. The most striking finding is the presence of oligodendrocytes containing nuclei two to three times their normal size. With hematoxylin, these cells stain deeply, densely, and often have a glassy appearance. The swollen infected oligodendrocytes surround demyelinated zones and contain abundant viral particles. Most of the involved oligodendrocytes are found in small lesions which probably represent an early stage of disease. In chronic "burnt out" lesions, demyelination is complete and oligodendrocytes and viral particles are rarely found. The chronic lesions contain many macrophages and reactive astrocytes. These older lesions often contain another characteristic microscopic feature of PML - abnormal giant astrocytes with multilobulated, hyperchromatic, and pleomorphic nuclei which assume a bizzare and often malignant appearance.

The appearance of the abnormal astrocytes, coupled with the fact that JCV is known to produce tumors in other species, has led to speculation about JCV's oncogenic potential in man. Recently, both JCV DNA and viral capsid protein have been found in the abnormal astrocytes by in situ hybridization (42). This suggests that although these cells are profoundly altered by the virus, they are not malignant (42). Despite evidence of viral infection in PML, there is a notable lack of inflammatory changes in the cerebral tissue. This has been attributed to the deficient immune response of the infected host (3),(4).

Though the pathology of PML has been well studied and its viral etiology is clear, there are still certain questions regarding the pathogenesis of PML. For example, the mechanism of viral entry into the CNS remains unknown. It is also still unknown whether PML results from an acute infection, or from reactivation of a latent infection due to loss of normal immunosurveillance because of disease or immunosuppressive therapy. Despite these unresolved questions, investigators have clarified the sequence of events leading from infection to demyelination. Morphological studies (43) suggest that, following adsorption and penetration, the virus enters the cell nucleus and initiates viral assembly. As production of viral progeny proceeds, the cell's cytoplasm becomes increasingly vacuolated. The ribosomes disappear and mitochondria swell; eventually the nuclear membrane disintegrates, the cell undergoes cytolysis, and virions are released to infect nereby cells. The early stages of infection and viral replication occur at the periphery of demyelinated lesions. In these zones, there is a normal amount of myelin basic protein (MBP) and myelin associated glycoprotein (MAG). As one moves toward the center of the lesions, MAG begins to disappear. Since MAG is synthesized in the oligodendrocyte perikaryon, its loss reflects viral spread into oligodendroglial cytoplasm and processes (44). The relative distribution of MAP and MBP helps distinguish PML from other demyelinating conditions such as multiple sclerosis and acute measles encephalitis (45). As oligodendroglia continue to degenerate, myelin sheaths break down and viral spread is promoted. This sequence of viral spread occurs in areas of diminished MBP and MAG staining seen toward the center of the PML lesions (44). As lesions advance, macrophages and giant astrocytes accumulate while oligodendrocytes are lost. Gradually, with disease progression, scattered demyelinated areas enlarge and become confluent.

Biologic and Molecular Properties of JC Virus

Study of the molecular biology of JCV may help explain its tropism for oligodendroglia as well as provide a rational approach to novel treatment strategies. For example, a drug that selectively disrupts the function of viral specific proteins such as the viral T antigen might prove useful. Unlike herpes viruses, which encode for a variety of their own nucleotide biosynthetic enzymes and whose pathways can be inhibited by nucleotide analogues such as acyclovir, the papovaviruses depend exclusively on host enzymes for nucleotide synthesis (46).

JCV is extremely difficult to grow in tissue culture (47). Inferences about the molecular biology of JCV may be based on the similar but more extensively studied virus, SV40. JCV shares a 69% DNA sequence homology with SV40. JCV's genome is a convalently closed circular DNA of 5130 base pairs which codes for six proteins (48). The following findings established for SV40 will almost certainly apply to JCV. Two proteins are expressed early in lytic infection (prior to DNA replication); these are the large T antigen and small t antigen proteins. Four proteins are expressed late in the lytic phase (during and after replication) and consist of three capsid proteins and an agnoprotein. The promoter and transcriptional "start" sites (where the 5' end of mRNA begins) for early genes are found at one end of the regulatory noncoding region, and the promoter and start sites for the late genes are found at the opposite end (48). Therefore, the two sets of mRNAs are read in opposite directions of the molecule using different DNA strands as templates. The regulatory region also contains the origin of bidirectional DNA replication (48), (49). T antigen (a site specific DNA binding protein and ATPase) is absolutely required for replication. It is a multifunctional protein that can efficiently transform cells, both in vitro and in vivo, to a malignant phenotype (49),(50).

SV40 has a much broader host range and grows more readily than JCV. Nonetheless, JCV has been successfully grown in primary fetal glial cells and in primary human uroepithelial cells (47). It also efficiently transforms hamster brain cells. The reason for the difference in host range between the two viruses is probably multifactorial. However, one possible factor for which there is some experimental support is the difference in the respective promotor-enhancer sequences found within the noncoding regulatory regions (51).

The human population serves as the natural reservoir of JCV. Based on sero-epidemiologic data, JCV appears to be a ubiquitous virus (8). In the United States, the prevalence of serum antibody within the population ranges from 66% to 75%.

JCV has been recovered from the human kidney as well as brain although the virus does not produce clinical disease in the kidney. It presumably reaches both organs at the time of acute infection with an associated viremia.

CONCLUSION

In conclusion, PML occurs in 2-5% of AIDS patients. In 10 of 17 cases of PML and AIDS, PML was the initial symptomatic opportunistic infection. The disease is progressive and usually fatal within three to six months. At present, there is no proven therapy, however, progress in understanding the molecular biology of JCV may lead to new therapeutic approaches.

ACKNOWLEDGMENT

The authors thank Dr. Allen Aksamit for his thoughtful comments and review of the manuscript.

REFERENCES

1. Astrom, K.E., Mancall, E.L., Richardson, E.P., Jr., Progressive multifocal leukoencephalopathy. Brain 81:93-111 (1958)

2. Richardson, E.P., Progressive multifocal leukoencephalopathy. N Engl J Med 265:815-823 (1961)

3. Richardson, E.P., Progressive multifocal leukoencephalopathy. In: Handbook of Clinical Neurology (Vinken, P.J., Bruyn, G.W., eds) Elsevier Publishers, Amsterdam, Holland, Vol 9, p 489-499, (1970)

4. Walker, D.L., Progressive multifocal leukoencephalopathy: An opportunistic viral infection of the central nervous system. In: Handbook of Clinical Neurology (Vinken, P.J., Bruyn, G.W., eds.) Elsevier Publishers, Amsterdam, Holland, Vol 34, p 307-329, (1970)

5. Zurhein, G.M., Chou, S.M., Particles resembling papovaviruses in human cerebral demyelinating disease. Science 148:1477-1479 (1965)

6. Padgett, B.L., Walker, D.L., Zurhein, R.J., et al., Cultivation of papova-like virus from human brain with progressive multifocal leukoencephalopathy. Lancet 1:1257- 1260 (1971)

7. Weiner, L.P., Herndon, R.M., Narayan, O., et al., Isolation of virus related to SV40 from patients with progressive multifocal leukoencephalpathy. N Engl J Med 286:385-390 (1972)

8. Walker, D.L., Progressive multifocal leukoencephalopathy. In: Handbook of Clinical Neurology (Koetsier, J.C., eds) Elsevier Publishers, New York, Vol 47:503-529 (1985)

9. Padgett, B.L., Walker, D.L., Zurhein, R.J., et al., JC papovavirus in progressive multifocal leukoencephalopathy. J Infect Disease 133:686-690 (1976)

10. Johnson, R.T., Evidence for polyoma viruses in human diseases. In: Polyoma Viruses and Human Diseases, (Sever, J.L., Madden, D.L., eds.) Alan R. Liss, New York (1983)

11. Levy, A.M., Bredsen, D.E., Rosenblum, M.L., Neurological manifestations of the acquired immunodeficiency syndrome (AIDS): Experience at UCSF and review of the literature. J Neurosurg 62:475-495 (1985)

12. Niedt, G.W., Schinelle, R.A., Acquired immunodeficiency syndrome: Clinicopathologic study of 56 autopsies. Arch. Pathol Lab Med 109:727-734 (1985)

13. Amberson, J.B., DiCarlo, E.F., Metroka, C.E., et al., Diagnostic pathology in the acquired immunodeficiency syndrome. Arch Pathol Lab Med 109:345-351 (1985)

14. Moskowitz, L.B., Hensley, G.T., Chan, J.C., et al., The neuropathology of acquired immunodeficiency syndrome. Arch Pathol Lab Med 108:867-872 (1984)

15. Krupp, L.B., Lipton, R.B., Swerdlow, M.L., et al., Progressive multifocal leukoencephalopathy: Clinical and radiographic features. Ann Neurol 17:344-349 (1985)

16. Miller, J.R., Barret, R.B., Britton, C.B., et al. Progressive multifocal leukoencephalopathy in a male homosexual with T-cell immune deficiency. N Engl J Med 307:1436-1437 (1982)

17. Bedri, J., Weinstein, W., DeGregorio, P., et al., Progressive multifocal leukoencephalopathy in acquired immunodeficiency syndrome. N Engl J Med 309:492-493 (1983)

18. Snider, W.D., Simpson, D.M., Nielson, S., et al., Neurological complications of acquired immune deficiency syndrome: Analysis of 50 patients. Ann Neurol 14:403-418 (1983)

19. England, J.D., Hsu, C.Y., Garen, P.D., et al., Progressive multifocal leukoencephalopathy occurring with the acquired immune deficiency syndrome. South Med J 77:1041-1043 (1984)

20. Reichert, C.M., O'Leary, T.J., Levens, D.L., Autopsy pathology in the acquired immune deficiency syndrome. Am J Pathol 112:357-382 (1983)

21. Bernick, C., Gregorios, J.B., Progressive multifocal leukoencephalopathy in a patient with acquired immune deficiency syndrome. Arch Neurol 41:780-782 (1984)

22. Ho, J.L., Plldre, P.A., McEnry, D., et al., Acquired immunodeficiency with progressive multifocal leukoencephalopathy and monoclonal B-cell proliferation. Ann Intern Med 100: 693-696 (1984)

23. Blum, L.W., Chambers, R.A., Schwartzman, R.S., Progressive multifocal leukoencephalopathy in acquired immunodeficiency syndrome. Arch Neurol 42:137-139 (1985)

24. Speelman, J.D., ter Schegget, J., Bots, G., Progressive multifocal leukoencephalopathy in a case of acquired immunodeficiency syndrome. Clin Neurol Neurosurg 87:27-33 (1985)

25. Macher, A.B., Parisi, J.E., Aksamit, A.J., et al., AIDS case for diagnosis. Military Med (In press)

26. Brooks, B.R., Walker, D.L., Progressive multifocal leukoencephalopathy. Neurol Clin 2:299-313 (1984)

27. Carroll, B.A., Lane, B., Norman, D., et al., Diagnosis of progressive multifocal leukoencephalopathy by computed tomography. Radiology 122:137-141 (1977)

28. Heinz, E.B., Dreyer, B.P., Haenggell, C.A., et al., Computed tomography in white matter disease. Radiology 130:371-378 (1979)

29. Conomy, J.P., Weinstein, M.A., Agamanolis, D., et al., Computed tomography in progressive multifocal leukoencephalopathy. Am J Roentgenol 127:663-665 (1976)

30. Durham, D.S., Freyer, J.A., O'Neil, B.J., et al., Progressive multifocal leukoencephalopathy: CT and pathological features. Med J Aust 2:502-504 (1980)

31. Burstyn, M.E., Lee, B.C.P., Bauman, J., CT of the acquired immunodeficiency syndrome. AJNR 5:711-714 (1984)

32. Saxton, C.R., Farkis, R.A., Helderman, K., Progressive multifocal leukoencephalopathy in a renal transplant recipient - increased sensitivity of CT scanning by double dose contrast with delayed films. Am J Med 77:333-337 (1984)

33. Berger, J.R., Kasovitz, B., Post, J.D., et al., Progressive multifocal leukoencephalopathy in AIDS. Neurology 36:205 (1986)

34. Farrell, D.F., The EEG in progressive multifocal leukoencephalopathy. Electroenceph Clin Neurophysiol 26:357-360 (1972)

35. Lipton, R.B., Krupp, L.B., Horoupian, D.S., et al., Electrophysiologic findings in progressive multifocal leukoencephalopathy. Ann Neurol 18:135 (1985)

36. Britton, C.B., Miller, J.R., Neurologic complications in acquired immunodeficiency syndrome (AIDS). Neurol Clin 2:315-339 (1984)

37. Elkin, C.M., Leon, E., Grenell, S.L., et al., Intracranial lesions in the acquired immunodeficiency syndrome: radiological (computed tomographic) features. JAMA 253:393-396 (1985)

38. Apuzzo, M.L., Sabshin, J.K., Computed tomographic guidance stereotaxis in the management of intracranial lesions. Neurosurg 12:277-284 (1983)

39. Aksamit, A.J., Mourrain, P., Sever, J.L., et al., Progressive multifocal leukoencephalopathy: Investigation of three cases using in situ hybridization with JC virus biotinylated DNA probe. Ann Neurol 18:490-496 (1985)

40. Bauer, W., Turel, J.R., Johnson, K.P., Progressive multifocal leukoencephalopathy and cytarabine. JAMA 226:174-176 (1973)

41. Smith, C.R., Sima, A.A.F., Salit, I.E., et al., Progressive multifocal leukoencephalopathy: Failure of cytarabine therapy. Neurology 32:200-203 (1982)

42. Aksamit, A.J., Sever, J.L., Major, E.O., Progressive multifocal leukoencephalopathy: JC virus detection by in situ hybridization compared with immunohistochemistry. Neurology 36: 499-504 (1986)

43. Mazlo, J., Tariska, I., Morphological demonstration of the first phase of polyoma virus replication in oligodendroglial cells of human brain in progressive multifocal leukoencephalopathy (PML). Acta Neuropath (Berlin) 49:133-143 (1980)

44. Itoyama, Y., Webster, DeF., H., Sternberger, N.H., Distribution of papovavirus myelin-associated glycoprotein and myelin basic protein in progressive multifocal leukoencephalopathy lesions. Ann Neurol 11:396-407 (1982)

45. Gendelman, H.E., Pezeshkpour, G.H., Pressman, N.J., et al., A quantification of myelin associated glycoprotein and myelin basic protein loss in different demyelinating diseases. Ann Neurol 18:324-328 (1985)

46. Kornberg, A., 1982 Supplement to DNA Replication. W.H. Freeman & Co., San Francisco (1982)

47. Sever, J.L., Madden, D.L., Polyoma Viruses and Human Diseases, Alan R. Liss, New York (1983)

48. Frisque, R.J., Bream, G.L., Canella, M.T., Human polyoma virus JC virus genome. J Virol 51:458-469 (1984)

49. Tooze, J., DNA Tumor Viruses - Molecular Biology of Tumor Viruses, 2nd ed., Cold Spring Harbor Laboratory, Cold Spring Harbor, NY (1980)

50. DePamphilis, M.L., Wasserman, P.M., Organization and replication of papovavirus DNA. In: Organization and Replication of Viral DNA. (Kaplan, A.S., ed) CRC Press, p 37-114 (1982)

51. Kenney, S., Natarajan, V., Strike, D., et al., JC virus enhancer - promoter active in human brain cells. Science 226: 1337-1339 (1984)

35
Cryptosporidiosis in AIDS

Rosemary Soave

The coccidian protozoan, cryptosporidium, has been recently recognized as the cause of severe protracted diarrhea in immunocompromised humans, particularly those with the acquired immunodeficiency syndrome (AIDS), and self-limited, though significant, enteritis in the immunocompetent host. The organism however, is not a new pathogen. Cryptosporidium was first described in asymptomatic laboratory mice by Tyzzer in 1907 (1). It was considered a benign commensal of animals until 1955 when it was recognized as a cause of diarrhea in animals (2). The first human case of cryptosporidiosis was documented in 1976 (3) but by 1981 only six other cases had been reported (4)-(9) and the disease was considered rare. In 1981-82, 47 AIDS patients with cryptosporidiosis were reported to the Centers for Disease Control (CDC) and thus the pathogen was brought to the attention of the medical community (10). Since then, popularization of various techniques for detecting cryptosporidial oocysts in stool has resulted in the wider recognition of this organism's pathogenic potential, particularly in humans, and in a greater appreciation of its world wide distribution (ll)-(14a).

THE ORGANISM

Cryptosporidium was so named by Tyzzer to designate an organism in which spores are concealed in the oocyst. Based on its morphology, the genus Cryptosporidium has been assigned to the class Sporozoa in the order Eucoccidiida (15) . It is thus taxonomically related to other coccidia which infect humans including *Toxoplasma gondii*, *Isospora belli* and *Plasmodium species* and those which are primarily animal pathogens such as *Eimeria species* and *Sarcocystis species*. In its morphology and propensity to parasitize AIDS patients, cryptosporidium resembles the unclassified protozoan *Pneumocystis carinii*. Since 1907, approximately 18 species of cryptosporidium have been named according to the hosts in which they were found (16). However, cross transmission experiments indicate that the organism lacks host specificity, and in a manner similar to *T. gondii*, one species may parasitize a wide range of hosts (11),(12),(16)-(21). In a recent report, Upton and Current provided biologic and morphologic evidence that the species of cryptosporidium might be differentiated on the basis of size and they have suggested that the smaller *Cryptosporidium parvum* be considered a species distinct from the larger *Cryptosporidium muris* (22).

The life cycle of cryptosporidium was first described by Tyzzer in 1910 (23) and confirmed decades later in several electron microscopic investigations (24)-(27). The general pattern is similar to that of other coccidia, i.e., asexual multiplication followed by sexual development and discharge of oocysts in feces (Figure 1). However, it is important to note that cryptosporidium distinguishes itself from other coccidia by a number of unique biological characteristics, including its monoxenous (complete development occurs within a single host) life cycle, its ability to sporulate (mature) endogenously and its unique relationship to host target cells.

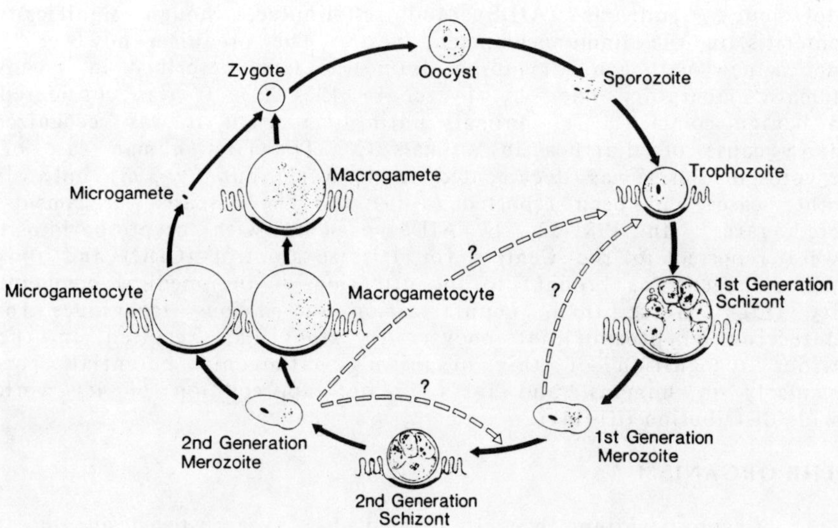

Figure 1. Proposed life cycle of cryptosporidium. (Reproduced with permission from reference 13).

The cryptosporidium oocyst is approximately 2-5 microns in diameter (Figure 2). When fully sporulated, it contains four sporozoites which are thin, flat, elliptical, motile and naked (not enveloped within a sporocyst) (Figure 3) (28). The sporozoites are released (excystation), presumably through the action of bile salts and digestive enzymes (29) (30), implant on epithelium and develop asexually (schizogony) to form merozoites and then sexually to form oocysts and thus complete the cycle. Due to its ability to sporulate endogenously, cryptosporidium may then reinitiate the cycle within the same host (31). Several features of the life cycle as represented in Figure 1 are controversial, including the presence of two generations of schizonts and the ability of first and second generation merozoites to reinfect intestinal epithelium rather than moving on to the sexual phase of the cycle. In addition, Current and Reese have recently proposed that two types of oocysts are formed: thin-walled which are immediately infective to the same host in which they developed and thick-walled which are excreted in feces (32). Despite the controversies, the unique features of cryptosporidium development provide a basis for the organism's high degree of infectivity and the persistence of infection and stool oocyst shedding in immunocompromised patients.

The cryptosporidium oocyst is quite hardy and able to withstand many laboratory disinfectants. Infectivity appears to be destroyed by ammonia, full-strength commercial bleach, formol saline and temperatures above 65°C and below O^{o}C (11),(14a), (33).

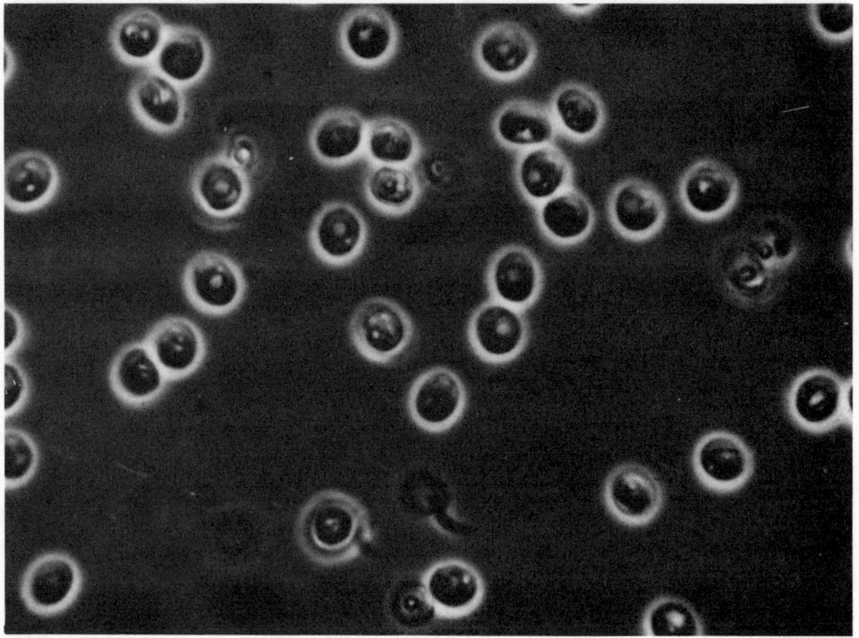

Figure 2. Cryptosporidium oocysts (Phase contrast.)

EPIDEMIOLOGY

Although much has been learned about the epidemiology of cryptosporidiosis in recent years, many questions remain unanswered (34). Transmission of cryptosporidium from animals (including pets) to humans has been well-documented (21),(35),(36) and animal handlers are known to be at high risk for acquiring the infection. Although initially thought to be the primary mode of transmission, it now appears that many humans do not acquire the pathogen from infected animals (35),(37),(38). Day care center outbreaks (39)-(42), nosocomial acquisition (43)-(45), and clustering of cases among close contacts of index cases (34),(46)-(48) suggest that person-to-person transmission is important. Reports of cryptosporidial infection in travelers (47),(49)-(52), and an out break in people exposed to a common water-supply (53) indicate that exposure to contaminated surfaces, food or water may be important in transmission of the parasite. Cryptosporidial infection has also been reported in homosexual men who do not have AIDS (54) but the role of sexual spread of the disease is uncertain.

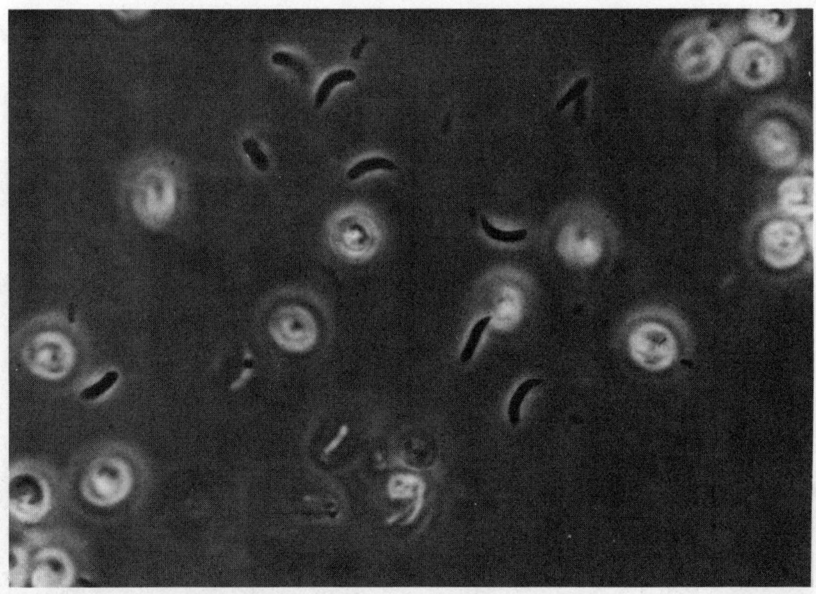

Figure 3. Cryptosporidium sporozoites (Phase contrast)

The actual prevalence of human cryptosporidiosis has not been determined. Although initially considered an opportunistic pathogen, it is now clear that cryptosporidium commonly infects immunocompetent hosts. Over the past four years there have been at least 25 published reports of epidemiologic surveys conducted in various parts of the world (14),(14a),(34),(50),(55)-(67). Data obtained from examination of stool specimens from approximately 20,000 persons, primarily in the developing world, indicate that cryptosporidium is, indeed, a common cause of infection worldwide, particularly in young children.

Cryptosporidiosis has been reported in approximately 3-4% of AIDS patients in the United States (CDC, unpublished). This is undoubtedly an underestimate since not all AIDS patients are examined for the parasite. In contrast, cryptosporidiosis appears to occur more commonly in AIDS patients in Haiti (68).

Cryptosporidiosis has been well documented in patients with congenital immunodeficiency (4),(5),(36),(69),(70) but it does not appear to occur commonly in organ transplant recipients and patients with neoplastic diseases. Asymptomatic carriage of the parasite has been described infrequently.

A serum antibody response has been documented in both humans and animals with cryptosporidial enteritis (71),(72). A recent study in which an enzyme-linked immunosorbent assay (ELISA) was used, showed that immunoglobulin G and M was present in the serum of immunocompetent as well as immunocompromised persons infected with cryptosporidium. In addition, a surprisingly large number of healthy individuals without previous knowledge of cryptosporidial infection were seropositive (73). Seroepidemiologic studies will be useful in describing the epidemiologic profile of cryptosporidial infection and in determining the true prevalence of the disease.

ENTERITIS IN AIDS

Diarrhea with profound wasting are major symptoms of the AIDS prodrome. Intestinal disease may be observed in 50-60% of patients with AIDS in the United States and close to 100% of AIDS patients in Africa and Haiti. While many infectious agents including cryptosporidium, *Isospora belli*, cytomegalovirus, *Herpes simplex* virus, *Mycobacterium avium-intracellulare*, *Salmonella sp.*, *Candida sp.*, as well as Kaposi's sarcoma may be associated with gastrointestinal disease in AIDS patients, often, the etiology is not determined (74)-(77). In the latter cases it is not known whether the patients are infected with other agents which are currently unrecognized or difficult to detect, e.g., viruses, or whether the enteric disease is a direct result of their immune dysfunction. The histopathologic changes present in patients with AIDS and enteritis are non-specific and cannot be correlated with the presence or absence of various pathogens (78). The immunopathogenesis of intestinal disease in immunocompromised patients is also poorly understood (79).

CLINICAL MANIFESTATIONS OF CRYPTOSPORIDIOSIS

Cryptosporidial infection in humans is characterized by watery diarrhea, cramping abdominal pain, weight loss and flatulence. Most patients report exacerbation of diarrhea and abdominal cramps with food ingestion. Nausea, vomiting, myalgias, and malaise may also be present. Physical examination frequently reveals signs of dehydration but is otherwise unremarkable. Fever and leukocytosis are uncommonly associated with cryptosporidiosis. Fecal examination reveals many cryptosporidial oocysts but no leukocytes or blood. Reversible lactase deficiency and fat malabsorption have been documented in several cases.

The severity and duration of human cryptosporidiosis appears to be determined primarily by immune competence. In patients with AIDS or other immunodeficiencies, symptoms usually begin insidiously and escalate as the immune defect becomes more severe (4),(5),(54),(80). Such patients may experience frequent (six to 25), voluminous (one to 25 liters), daily bowel movements, severe abdominal pain and profound weight loss. It is not unusual for AIDS patients with cryptosporidiosis to require hospitalization for parenteral hydration and alimentation. Clinical symptoms and oocyst shedding in stool commonly persist for months until the patient dies with other opportunistic infections and/or neoplasms.

Recently, a new constellation of signs and symptoms has been detected in AIDS patients with cryptosporidial enteritis (80)-(83). The symptom complex includes severe pain localized to the right upper quadrant, nausea and vomiting. Jaundice and hepatomegaly are usually absent. Laboratory studies reveal elevation, at times astronomical, of serum alkaline phosphatase, minimal elevation of serum transaminases and a normal bilirubin. Findings suggestive of sclerosing cholangitis including thickening of the gallbladder wall, dilated bile ducts, distal duct strictures and luminal irregularities may be demonstrated radiographically. Endoscopic retrograde cholangiopancreatography (ERCP) often reveals ampullary stenosis. Several of our patients who underwent either ERCP or cholecystectomy were found to have cryptosporidia in bile and attached to gallbladder epithelium (83). In addition, papillotomy or cholecystectomy resulted in a transient resolution of symptoms for most of the patients in whom these invasive procedures were performed. Concomitant infection with cytomegalovirus (CMV) has been described in several patients with cryptosporidial cholecystitis (82),(83). In addition, a few patients with the above described syndrome were found only to have CMV infection (83). Cryptosporidial cholecystitis and the role of CMV in biliary tract disease in AIDS patients awaits further definition.

Respiratory cryptosporidiosis, based on finding organisms in sputum or attached to bronchial epithelium in AIDS patients with pulmonary symptoms has also been described (70),(84)-(86). In these patients, however, it is not clear whether the organism gained access to the bronchial tree due to vomiting.

In the immunologically normal host, the symptoms of cryptosporidiosis are usually explosive in onset and last an average of 10-14 days (3),(7),(38),(40),(47),(48),(49),(49a),(87),(88). Clearance of the parasite from stool often lags behind clinical resolution of symptoms by two to three weeks thus creating obvious problems for infection control (49a). Although self-limited, symptoms may be severe and the duration of the illness may be prolonged such that therapeutic intervention, were it available, would be warranted.

PATHOLOGY AND PATHOGENESIS

Cryptosporidium has been found throughout the gastrointestinal tract (4)-(9),(54),(80),(89), in the gallbladder and bile ducts (80)-(83), on bronchial epithelium and in the sputum (70),(84)-(86) of infected (primarily AIDS) patients. Electron microscopic examination of infected tissue specimens from these patients has revealed a unique relationship between parasite and host target cell (Figure 4a) (24),(25). Characteristically, endogenous stages of cryptosporidium are found attached to the enterocyte surface, enveloped within a membrane believed to be derived from the host cell, but not within the cytoplasm (Figure 4b). Despite numerous parasitic forms there is usually a paucity of inflammatory cells and minimal cellular destruction. Histopathologic findings include villous atrophy, crypt elongation and minimal subjacent inflammatory infiltrates of the lamina propria resembling those seen in patients with giardiasis. Similar histopathologic findings have been reported for three immunocompetent patients with cryptosporidial enteritis (3),(87),(90). In the small number of reported cases of biliary cryptosporidiosis, organisms were seen in bile and adherent to gallbladder epithelium with edema, lymphocyte infiltration and destruction of the underlying mucosa (80)-(83). Biliary cryptosporidiosis has not been documented in the immunocompetent host.

In animals with cryptosporidiosis, the gastrointestinal tract is the most common site of involvement but bronchial, biliary, bursal and conjunctival infection has been reported as well. The histopathology is similar to that described for infected humans, with a few important differences (11)-(14a). Experimental infection of lambs (19), piglets (91), and gnotobiotic calves (92) has been associated with extensive lesions of the small intestine characterized by marked cellular infiltrates which extend into the lamina propria. In addition, recent studies of spontaneously infected guinea pigs revealed cryptosporidia deep within the cytoplasm of membranous epithelial (M) cells (93), the first description of intracytoplasmic organisms. This important finding provides a basis for antigenic sampling by the intestinal immune system and thus may shed light on the mechanisms by which cryptosporidial infection is self-limited in patients with intact immunity.

An association between cryptosporidium and other enteropathogens, primarily giardia (in immunocompetent patients) (51),(94) and CMV (in AIDS patients) (8),(74),(82),(83) has been reported

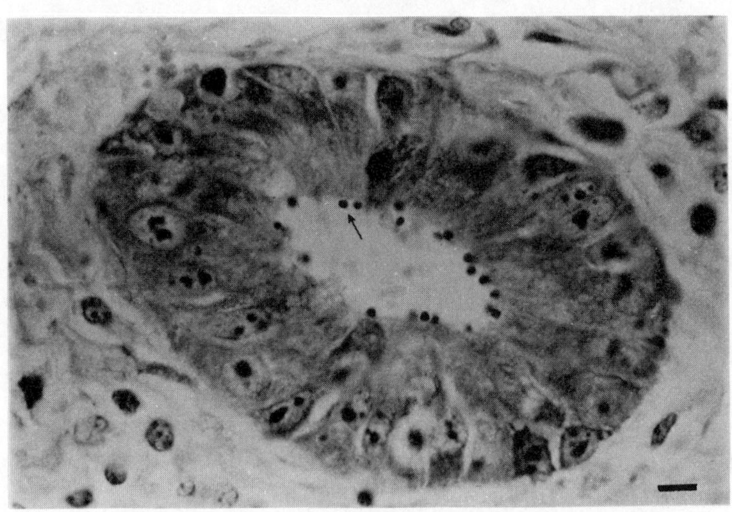

Figure 4a. Numerous cryptosporidial bodies on crypt epithelium of small intestine. Bar = 20*u*m. Giemsa stain.

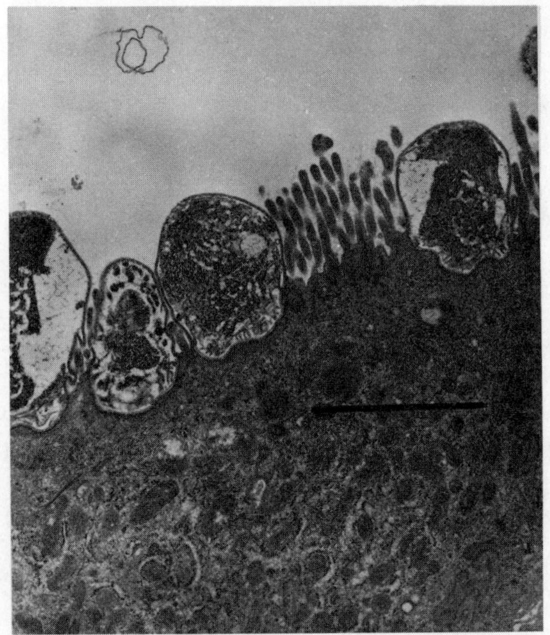

Figure 4b. Endogenous stages of cryptosporidium in the brush border of the small intestine of an AIDS patient. Bar = 5 *u*m.

by several investigators. The significance of concomitant infection is not known. That cryptosporidium is indeed an enteropathogen has been shown by Heine et al. in their study of gnotobiotic calves monoinfected with cryptosporidium (92).

The mechanisms by which cryptosporidium causes diarrhea are also not known. An enterotoxin mediated mechanism is suggested by the secretory nature of the diarrhea and the lack of inflammatory histopathologic changes. The malabsorptive changes are suggestive of giardiasis whereas destruction of the brush border is reminiscent of infection with rotavirus and enteropathogenic *Escherichia coli.*

DIAGNOSIS

Initially, the diagnosis of cryptosporidiosis was based on light and electron microscopic examination of intestinal tissue specimens obtained by biopsy. In 1978, Henricksen and Pohlenz showed that cryptosporidial oocysts are shed in feces and that they are acid fast positive (95). This latter property has been utilized to distinguish cryptosporidium (red staining) from the morphologically similar yeasts which do not retain carbol fuchsin (non-acid-fast) and hence stain green with counterstain. Since 1981, several techniques have been popularized for identifying oocysts in feces, including various modifications of the acid-fast stain (Ziehl-Neelsen, Kinyoun), the fluorescent auramine-rhodamine stain, the periodic acid Schiff (PAS) and carbolfuschin-negative stains (49a),(96)-(102). Recently a direct immunofluorescence method for detection of oocysts was reported (103). Although controlled studies comparing the sensitivity and specificity of stool examination with intestinal biopsies have not been conducted, most investigators feel that stool examination is more sensitive. Intestinal biopsies may be falsely negative due to autolysis of tissue specimens during processing, and the patchy distribution of cryptosporidia with few inflammatory changes to guide the endoscopist. The relative advantages of each of the various fecal stains have not been fully determined in controlled studies, but one study of 15 different methods suggests that the modified Ziehl-Neelsen staining of fecal-formalinether concentrates is most sensitive (97). It is generally agreed, however, that regardless of the staining method used, experienced observers have little difficulty in identifying cryptosporidia. The optimal number of negative stool specimens required to confirm the absence of cryptosporidial infection is also not known. During acute illness, both immunocompromised and immunocompetent patients shed large numbers of oocysts and the diagnosis is usually not subtle. Concentration techniques (including Sheather's sucrose flotation method and the formalinether method of Ritchie) may be used to optimize detection of fecal oocysts (104)-(106) but are not always necessary. Such techniques may have a role in detection of oocysts when they are rare, as with formed stool specimens, and for processing stool specimens from asymptomatic contacts and for examining environmental samples. Since these techniques expose laboratory workers to the risk of contamination from leakage, special caution is advised (21),(107).

THERAPY OF CRYPTOSPORIDIOSIS

There is currently no known effective therapy for human cryptosporidiosis. Inability to cultivate the organism in vitro and the absence of a symptomatic small animal model of the disease have severely hampered the identification of potentially active anticryptosporidial agents. Animal studies are few and have thus far failed to reveal useful treatment regimens (108).

Because of the severity of their disease, a vast array of antidiarrheal, antiparasitic and immunomodulating agents as well as special diets have been administered in an uncontrolled fashion to AIDS patients. Agents have been chosen on the basis of their activity against phylogenetically related parasites (*T. gondii, I. belli*), other intestinal protozoan pathogens (*G. lamblia, E. histolytica*) and other protozoa (*Plasmodium species*). Most of the attempts at therapeutic intervention have resulted in failure (10),(11),(13),(14a),(80),(109). Although most classes of nonspecific, antidiarrheal and antiperistaltic agents have been used, there is no information to support an advantage of any one over the others. Perhaps most promising and enduring have been reports of success in palliation of cryptosporidial diarrhea with spiramycin (46),(110),(111). The latter is a macrolide antibiotic widely used for bacterial infections and toxoplasmosis outside the United States. It is administered orally in a dose of two to three grams daily. Adverse side effects are rare and include gastrointestinal irritation (similar to other macrolide antibiotics) and the potential for hypersensitivity reactions. Its lack of toxicity and ease of administration have resulted in its widespread use for cryptosporidiosis. Since it is considered an investigational agent in the United States, it must be obtained directly from the Montreal-based manufacturer (Rhone-Poulenc Pharmaceuticals) and dispensed with permission of the U.S. Food and Drug Administration. Most of the AIDS patients treated with spiramycin achieve control of their diarrheal symptoms but not eradication of the parasite. There is currently an ongoing, multicenter, placebo-controlled trial of spiramycin designed to evaluate the clinical efficacy of this drug for treatment of chronic cryptosporidiosis in AIDS patients.

Recent studies have indicated that alpha-difluoromethylornithine (DFMO) is clinically useful against several protozoa including *Eimeria tenella*, African trypanosomes and *Pneumocystis carinii* (18),(112),(113). This agent is an irreversible inhibitor of ornithine decarboxylase a key enzyme in the biosynthesis of polyamines. In our experience, three of five AIDS patients treated with DFMO had significant palliation of their diarrhea, and a fourth had both a clinical and parasitologic response (114). Unfortunately, severe gastrointestinal and hematologic (bone marrow suppression) toxicity has limited use of this agent.

In addition to spiramycin and DFMO, other potentially promising anticryptosporidial agents currently undergoing evaluation include oral bovine transfer factor (115), and recombinant interleukin-2 (116). The veterinary coccidiostat, amprolium, has been minimally successful in treating animals with cryptosporidiosis but appears to be too toxic for human use (11).

Failure of therapeutic intervention for cryptosporidiosis in AIDS patients may reflect their profound immune defect rather than lack of drug efficacy. These patients with multiple, complex, concomitant problems are not an optimal population in which to conduct drug studies. Successful identification of efficacious anticryptosporidial agents hinges on development of techniques for in vitro study of the parasite (117), coupled with controlled clinical trials.

The supportive care needed for AIDS patients with chronic cryptosporidiosis differs from that given to other patients with enteritis only in magnitude and duration. The patients should be advised of possible lactose intolerance and instructed to avoid stimulants such as caffeine. Diet should be individualized and should optimize caloric intake in order to offset the accelerated wasting which AIDS patients with cryptosporidiosis experience. Maintenance of fluid and electrolyte balance and weight stabilization often requires parenteral hydration and alimentation.

Patients who develop cryptosporidiosis while on immunosuppressive agents, particularly corticosteroids, will resolve their illness with discontinuation of the drugs. The immunocompetent host with cryptosporidiosis usually has a self-limited illness. Often, however, these patients experience severe symptoms, protracted illness and/or prolonged stool oocyst shedding such that therapeutic intervention were it available, would be indicated.

ISOSPOROSIS IN AIDS

In the past isosporosis was synonymous with coccidiosis (118),(119), however, with the recent recognition of cryptosporidium's pathogenic potential in humans, this is no longer so. The coccidian protozoan parasite, *Isospora belli* is ubiquitously distributed in the animal kingdom but is a relatively rare cause of infection in humans. It is found more commonly in tropical and subtropical climates and, in fact, is endemic in certain parts of South America (e.g., Santiago, Chile), Africa and Southeast Asia (120). In the United States, *I. belli* has been implicated in various institutional outbreaks of diarrhea (120), and as a cause of enteritis in homosexual men with and without AIDS (120)-(126). The clinical manifestations of isosporosis include profuse watery diarrhea, steatorrhea, malabsorption, weight loss, and colicky abdominal pain (118)-(128). Diagnosis is made either by intestinal biopsy or by detection of the 10-20um by 20-30um, oval, acid fast positive isospora oocysts in stool (Figure 5) (123),(125), (126). As with cryptosporidial enteritis, the severity and duration of isosporosis varies with immune competence. Unlike cryptosporidiosis, isosporosis appears to respond to treatment with trimethoprim-sulfamethoxazole, pyrimethamine-sulfadiazine, metronidazole and other agents (119),(122),(124)-(128).

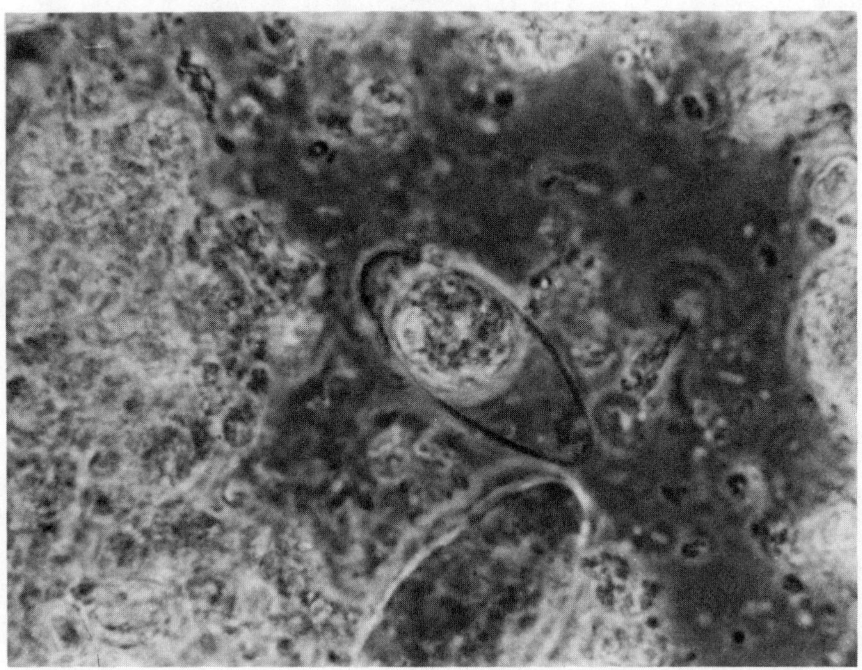

Figure 5. *Isospora belli* oocyst in fecal sample from an AIDS patient.

REFERENCES

1. Tyzzer, E.E., A sporozoan found in the peptic glands of the common mouse. Proc Soc Exp Biol Med 5:12-13 (1908).

2. Slavin, D., *Cryptosporidium meleagridis* (sp. nov.). J Comp Pathol 65:262-266 (1955)

3. Nime, F.A., Burek, J.D., Page, D.L., et al., Acute enterocolitis in a human being infected with the protozoan cryptosporidium. Gastroenterology 70:592-598 (1976).

4. Meisel, J.L., Perera, D.R., Meligro, C., et al., Overwhelming watery diarrhea associated with cryptosporidium in an immunosuppressed patient. Gastroenterology 70:1156-1160 (1976).

5. Lasser, K.H., Lewin, K.J., Ryning, F.W., Cryptosporidial enteritis in a patient with congenital hypogammaglobulinemia. Human Pathol 10:234-240 (1979).

6. Stemmermann, G.N., Hayashi, T., Glober, G.A., et al., Cryptosporidiosis. Report of fatal case complicated by disseminated toxoplasmosis. Am J Med 69:637-642 (1980)

7. Tzipori, S., Angus, K.W., Gray, E.W., et al., Vomiting and diarrhea associated with cryptosporidial infection. N Engl J Med 303:818 (1980)

8. Weinstein, L., Edelstein, S.M., Madara, J.L., et al., Intestinal cryptosporidiosis complicated by disseminated cytomegalovirus infection. Gastroenterology 81:584-591 (1981).

9. Weisburger, W.R., Hutcheon, D.F., Yardley, J.H., et al., Cryptosporidiosis in an immunosuppressed renal transplant recipient with IgA deficiency. Am J Clin Pathol 72:473-478 (1979)

10. CDC., Cryptosporidiosis: assessment of chemotherapy of males with acquired immune deficiency syndrome (AIDS). MMWR 31:589-592 (1982)

11. Tzipori, S., Cryptosporidiosis in animals and humans. Microbiol Rev 47:84-96 (1983)

12. Angus, K.W., Cryptosporidiosis in man, domestic animals and birds: a review. J Royal Soc Med 76:62-70 (1983)

13. Navin, T.R., Juranek, T.D., Cryptosporidiosis: clinical, epidemiologic and parasitologic review. Rev Infect Dis 6: 313-327 (1984)

14. Soave, R., Armstrong, D., Cryptosporidium and cryptosporidiosis. Rev Infect Dis 8:1012-1023 (1986)

14a. Fayer, R., Ungar, B.L.P., *Cryptosporidium spp.* and cryptosporidiosis. Microbiol Rev 50:458-483 (1986)

15. Leger L., *Caryospora simplex*, coccidie monosporee et la, classification des coccidies. Arch Protistenkd 22:71-78 (1911)

16. Levine, N.D., Taxonomy and review of the coccidian genus Cryptosporidium (Protozoa, Apicomplexa). J Protozool 31: 94-98 (1984)

17. Tzipori S., Angus K.W., Campbell I., et al., Cryptosporidium: evidence for a single-species genus. Infect Immun 30:884-886 (1980)

18. Moon, H.W., Schwartz, A., Welch, M.J., et al., Experimental fecal transmission of human cryptosporidia to pigs, and attempted treatment with an ornithine decarboxylase inhibitor. Vet Pathol 19:700-707 (1982)

19. Angus, K.W., Tzipori, S., Gray, E.W., Intestinal lesions in specific-pathogen-free lambs associated with a cryptosporidium from calves with diarrhea. Vet Pathol 19:67-78 (1982)

20. Reese, N.C., Current, W.L., Ernst, J.V., et al., Cryptosporidiosis of man and calf: a case report and results of experimental infections in mice and rats. Am J Trop Med Hyg 31: 226-229 (1982)

21. Current, W.L., Reese, N.C., Ernst, J.V., et al., Human cryptosporidiosis in immunocompetent and immunodeficient persons: studies of an outbreak and experimental transmission. N Engl J Med 103:256-259 (1983)

22. Upton, S.J., Current, W.L., The species of cryptosporidium (Apicomplexa: Cryptosporidiidae) infecting mammals. J Parasit 71:625-629 (1985)

23. Tyzzer, E.E., An extracellular coccidium, *Cryptosporidium muris* (gen. et sp. nov.), of the gastric glands of the common mouse. J Med Res 23:487-510 (1910)

24. Vetterling, J.M., Takeuchi, A., Madden, P.A., Ultrastructure of *Cryptosporidium wrairi* from the guinea pig. J Protozool 18:248-260 (1971)

25. Pohlenz, J., Benrick, W.J., Moon, H.W., et al., Bovine cryptosporidiosis: a transmission and scanning electron microscopic study of some stages in the life cycle and of the host-parasite relationship. Vet Pathol 15:417-427 (1978)

26. Isaki, M., *Cryptosporidium felis* sp. n. (Protozoa: Eimeriorina) from the domestic cat. Jpn J Parasitol 28:285-307 (1979)

27. Bird, R.G., Smith, M.D., Cryptosporidiosis in man: parasite life cycle and fine structural pathology. J Pathol 132:217-233 (1980)

28. Reduker, D.W., Speer, C.A., Blixt, J.A., Ultrastructure of *Cryptosporidium parvum* oocysts and excysting sporozoites as revealed by high resolution scanning electron microscopy. J Protozool 32:708-711 (1985).

29. Fayer, R., Leek, R.G., The effects of reducing conditions, medium, pH, temperature and time on in vitro excystation of cryptosporidium. J Protozool 31:567-569 (1984).

30. Reduker, D.W., Speer, C.A., Factors influencing excystation in cryptosporidium oocysts from cattle. J Parasitol 71:112-115 (1985)

31. Woodmansee, D.B., An in vitro study of sporulation in cryptosporidium species. J Parasit 72:348-349 (1986)

32. Current, W.L., Reese, N.C., A comparison of endogenous development of three isolates of cryptosporidium in suckling mice. J Protozool 33:98-108 (1986)

33. Anderson, B.C., Moist heat inactivation of *Cryptosporidium sp.* Am J Public Health 75:1433-1434 (1985)

34. Navin, T.R., Cryptosporidiosis in humans: Review of recent epidemiologic studies. Eur J Epidemiol 1:77-83 (1985)

35. Hart, C.A,, Baxby D, Blundell, N., Gastroenteritis due to cryptosporidium: a prospective survey in a children's hospital. J Infect 9:264-270 (1984)

36. Koch, L., Shankey, T.V., Weinstein, G.S., et al., Cryptosporidiosis in a patient with hemophilia, common variable hypogammaglobulinemia and the acquired immunodeficiency syndrome. Ann Intern Med 99:337 (1983)

37. Hunt, D.A., Shannon, R., Palmer, S.R. et al., Cryptosporidiosis in an urban community. Br Med J Clin Res 289:814-816 (1984)

38. Holten-Anderson, W., Gerstoft, J., Henriksen, S.A., et al., Prevalence of cryptosporidium among patients with acute enteric infection. J Infect 9:277-282 (1984)

39. CDC., Cryptosporidiosis among children attending day-care centers-Georgia, Pennsylvania, Michigan, California, New Mexico. MMWR 33:599-601 (1984)

40. Alpert, G., Bell, L.M., Kirkpatrick, C.E., et al., Outbreak of cryptosporidiosis in a day-care center. Pediatrics 77: 152-157 (1986)

41. Taylor, J.P., Perdue, J.N., Dingley, D., et al., Cryptosporidiosis outbreak in a day-care center. Am J Dis Child 139:1023-1025 (1986)

42. Combee, C.L., Collinge, M.L., Britt, E.M., Cryptosporidiosis in a hospital-associated day-care center. Pediatr Infect Dis 5:528-532 (1986)

43. Baxby, D., Hart, C.A., Taylor, C., Human cryptosporidiosis: a possible cause of hospital cross infection. Br Med J 287:1760-1761 (1983)

44. Koch, K.L., Phillips, D.J., Aber, R.C., et al., Cryptosporidiosis in hospital personnel. Evidence for person-to-person transmission. Ann Intern Med 102:593-596 (1985)

45. Dryjanski, J., Gold, J.W., Ritchie, M.T., et al., Cryptosporidiosis. Case report in a health team worker. Am J Med 80:751-752 (1986)

46. Collier, A.C., Miller, R.A., Meyers, J.D., Cryptosporidiosis after marrow transplantation: person-to-person transmission and treatment with spiramycin. Ann Intern Med 101:205-206 (1984)

47. Soave, R., Ma, P., Cryptosporidiosis: traveler's diarrhea in two families. Arch Intern Med 145:70-72 (1985)

48. Wolfson, J.S., Richter, J.M., Waldron, M.A., et al., Cryptosporidiosis in immunocompetent patients. N Engl J Med 312: 1278-1282 (1985)

49. Jokipii, L., Pohjola, S., Jokipii, A.M.M., Cryptosporidium: a frequent finding in patients with gastrointestinal symptoms. Lancet 2:358-361 (1983)

49a. Jokipii, L., Jokipii, A.M.M., Timing of symptoms and oocyst excretion in human cryptosporidiosis. N Engl J Med 315:1643-1647 (1986).

50. Tzipori, S., Smith, M., Birch, C., et al., Cryptosporidiosis in hospitalized patients with gastroenteritis. Am J Trop Med Hyg 32:931-934 (1983)

51. Jokipii, L., Pohjola, S., Valle, S.L., et al., Cryptosporidiosis associated with traveling and giardiasis. Gastroenterology 4:838-842 (1985)

52. Ma, P., Kaufman, D.L., Helmick, C.G., et al., Cryptosporidiosis in travelers returning from the Carribean. N Engl J Med 312:647-648 (1985)

53. D'Antonio, R.G., Winn, R.E., Taylor, J.P., et al., A waterborne outbreak of cryptosporidiosis in normal hosts. Ann Intern Med 103:886-888 (1985)

54. Soave, R., Danner, R.L., Honig, C.L., et al., Cryptosporidiosis in homosexual men. Ann Intern Med 100:504-511 (1984)

55. Mata, L., Bolanos, H., Pizarro, D., et al., Cryptosporidiosis in children from some highland Costa Rican rural and urban areas. Am J Trop Med Hyg 33:24-29 (1984)

56. Bogaerts, J., Lepage, P., Rouvroy, D., et al., *Cryptosporidium spp.* a frequent cause of diarrhea in central Africa. J Clin Microbiol 20:874-876 (1984)

57. De Mol, P., Mukashema, S., Bogaerts, J., et al., Cryptosporidium related to measles diarrhea in Rwanda. Lancet 2:42-43 (1984)

58. Weikel, C.S., Johnston, C.I., Auxilia Dora Sousa, M., et al., Cryptosporidiosis in northeastern Brazil: association with sporadic diarrhea. J Infect Dis 151:963-965 (1985)

59. Perez-Schael, I., Boher, Y., Mata, L., et al., Cryptosporidiosis in Venezuelan children with acute diarrhea. Am J Trop Med Hyg 34:721-722 (1985)

60. Issacs, D., Hunt, G.H., Phillips, A.D., et al., Cryptosporidiosis in immunocompetent children. J Clin Path 38:76-81 (1985)

61. Shahid, N.S., Rahman, A.S.M.H., Anderson, B.C., et al., Cryptosporidiosis in Bangladesh. Br Med J 290:114-115 (1985)

62. Mathan, M.M., Venkatesan, S., George, R., et al., Cryptosporidium and diarrhea in Southern Indian children. Lancet 2:1172-1175 (1985)

63. Addy, P.A.K., Aikins-Bekoe, P., Cryptosporidiosis in diarrheal children in Kumasi, Ghana. Lancet 1:735 (1986)

64. Hojlyng, N., Molbak, K., Jepsen, S., *Cryptosporidium spp.* a frequent cause of diarrhea in Liberian children. J Clin Microbiol 23:1109-1113 (1986)

65. Robinson, M., Hart, C.A., Baxby, D., et al., Cryptosporidium as a cause of gastroenteritis in Sudanese children. Ann Trop Pediatr 6:155-156 (1986)

66. Elsser, K.A., Moricz, M., Proctor, E.M., Cryptosporidium infections: a laboratory survey. Can Med Assoc J 135:211-213 (1986)

67. Van den Ende, G.M., Cryptosporidiosis among black children in a hospital in South Africa. J Infect 13:25-30 (1986)

68. Malebranche, R., Arnoux, E., Guerin, J.M., et al., Acquired immunodeficiency syndrome with severe gastrointestinal manifestations in Haiti. Lancet 2:873-877 (1983)

69. Sloper, K.S., Dourmashkin, R.R., Bird, R.B., et al., Chronic malabsorption due to cryptosporidiosis in a child with immunoglobulin deficiency. Gut 23:80-82 (1982)

70. Kocoshis, S.A., Cibull, M.L., Davis, T.E., et al., Intestinal and pulmonary cryptosporidiosis in an infant with severe combined immune deficiency. J Pediatr Gastroenterol Nutr 3:49 (1984)

71. Tzipori, S., Campbell, I., Prevalence of cryptosporidium antibodies in 10 animal species. J Clin Microbiol 14:455-456 (1981)

72. Campbell, P.M., Current, W.L., Demonstration of serum antibodies to *Cryptosporidium sp.* in normal and immunodeficient humans with confirmed infections. J Clin Microbiol 18: 165-169 (1983)

73. Ungar, B.L.P., Soave, R., Fayer, R., et al., Enzyme immunoassay detection of immunoglobulin M and G antibodies to cryptosporidium in immunocompetent and immunocompromised patients. J Infect Dis 153:570-578 (1986)

74. Kotler, D.P., Gaetz, H.P., Lange, M., et al., Enteropathy associated with the acquired immunodeficiency syndrome. Ann Intern Med 101:421-428 (1984)

75. Bodey, G.P., Fainstein, V., Infections of the gastrointestinal tract in the immunocompromised patient. Annu Rev Med 37:271-281 (1986)

76. Quinn, T.C., Bender, B.S., Bartlett, J.G., New developments in infectious diarrhea. Disease-a-Month 32:165-244 (1986)

77. Modigliani, R., Bories, C., LeCharpentier, Y., et al., Diarrhea and malabsorption in acquired immunodeficiency syndrome: a study of four cases with special emphasis on opportunistic protozoan infestations. Gut 26:179-187 (1985)

78. Dobbins, W.O., Weinstein, W.M., Electron microscopy of the intestine and rectum in acquired immunodeficiency syndrome. Gastroenterology 88:738-749 (1985)

79. Rodgers, V.D., Fassett, R., Kagnoff, M.F., Abnormalities in intestinal mucosal T cells in homosexual populations including those with the lymphadenopathy syndrome and acquired immunodeficiency syndrome. Gastroenterology 90:552-558 (1986)

80. Pitlik, S.D., Fainstein, V., Garza, D., et al., Human cryptosporidiosis: spectrum of disease. Report of six cases and review of the literature. Arch Intern Med 143:2269-2276 (1983)

81. Guarda, L.A., Stein, S.A., Cleary, K.A., et al., Human cryptosporidiosis in the acquired immune deficiency syndrome. Arch Pathol Lab Med 107:562-566 (1983)

82. Blumberg, R.S., Kelsey, P., Perrone, T., et al., Cytomegalovirus- and cryptosporidium-associated acalculous gangrenous cholecystitis. Am J Med 76:1118-1123 (1984)

83. Margulis, S.J., Honig, C.L., Soave, R., et al., Biliary tract obstruction in the acquired immunodeficiency syndrome. Ann Intern Med 105:207-209 (1986)

84. Forgacs, P., Tarshis, A., Ma, P., et al., Intestinal and bronchial cryptosporidiosis in an immunodeficient homosexual man. Ann Intern Med 99:793-794 (1983)

85. Miller, R.A., Wasserheit, J.N., Kirihara, J., et al., Detection of cryptosporidium oocysts in sputum during screening for mycobacterium. J Clin Microbiol 20:1192-1193 (1984)

86. Ma, P., Villanueva, T.G., Kaufman, D., et al., Respiratory cryptosporidiosis in the acquired immune deficiency syndrome. JAMA 252:1298-1301 (1984)

87. Babb, R.R., Differding, J.T., Trollope, M.L., Cryptosporidia enteritis in a healthy professional athlete. Am J Gastro 77:833-834 (1982)

88. Case Records of the Massachusetts General Hospital. Case 39-1985. N Engl J Med 313:805-815 (1985)

89. Lefkowitch, J.H., Krumholz, S., Feng-Chen, K-C., et al., Cryptosporidiosis of the human small intestine: A light and electron microscopic study. Hum Path 15:746-752 (1984)

90. Fletcher, A., Sims, T.A., Talbot, I.C., Cryptosporidial enteritis without general or selective immune deficiency. Br Med J 285:22-23 (1982)

91. Tzipori, S., McCartney, E., Lawson, G.H.K., et al., Experimental infection of piglets with Cryptosporidium. Res Vet Sci 31:358-368 (1981)

92. Heine, J., Pohlenz, J.F.L., Moon, H.W., et al., Enteric lesions and diarrhea in gnotobiotic calves monoinfected with *Cryptosporidium species*. J Infect Dis 150:768-775 (1984)

93. Marcial, M.A., Madara, J.L., Cryptosporidium: cellular localization, structural analysis of absorptive cell-parasite membrane - membrane interactions in guinea pigs and suggestion of protozoan transport by M cells. Gastroenterology 90: 583-594 (1986)

94. Wolfson, J.S., Hopkins, C.C., Weber, D.J., et al., An association between cryptosporidium and giardia in stool. N Engl J Med 310:788 (1984)

95. Henricksen, S.A., Pohlenz, J.F.L., Staining of cryptosporidia by a modified Ziehl-Neelsen technique. Act Vet Scand 22:594-596 (1981)

96. Ma, P., Soave, R., Three-step stool examination for cryptosporidiosis in 10 homosexual men with protracted watery diarrhea. J Infect Dis 147:824-828 (1983)

97. Garcia, L.S., Bruckner, D.A., Brewer, T.C., et al., Techniques for the recovery and identification of cryptosporidium oocysts from stool specimens. J Clin Microbiol 18:185-190 (1983)

98. Baxby, D., Blundell, N., Sensitive, rapid, simple methods for detecting cryptosporidium in faeces. Lancet 2:1149 (1983)

99. Horen, W.P., Detection of cryptosporidium in human fecal specimens. J Parasitol 69:622-624 (1983)

100. Bronsdon, M.A., Rapid dimethyl sulfoxide-modified acid-fast stain of cryptosporidium oocysts in stool specimens. J Clin Microbiol 19:952-953 (1984)

101. Casemore, D.P., Armstrong, M., Sands, R.L., Laboratory diagnosis of cryptosporidiosis. J Clin Pathol 38:1337-1341 (1985)

102. McNabb, S.J., Hensel, D.M., Welch, D.F., et al., Comparison of sedimentation and flotation techniques for identification of *Cryptosporidium sp.* oocysts in a large outbreak of

human diarrhea. J Clin Microbiol 22:587-589 (1985)

103. Sterling, C.R., Arrowood, M.J., Detection of *Cryptosporidium sp.* infections using a direct immunofluorescence assay. Pediatr Infect Dis 5(1Suppl):S139-142 (1986)

104. Sheather, A.L., The detection of intestinal protozoa and mange parasites by flotation technique. J Comp Pathol 36:268-275 (1953)

105. Levine, N.D., Protozoan Parasites of Domestic Animals and Man. Second Ed, Burgess, Minneapolis, p 227-230 (1973)

106. Ritchie, L.S., Pan, C., Hunter, G.W., A comparison of the zinc sulfate and the MGL (formalin-ether) techniques. J Parasit 38:16 (1983)

107. Blagburn, B.L., Current, W.L., Accidental infection of a researcher with human cryptosporidium. J Infect Dis 148:772-773 (1983)

108. Tzipori, S., Campbell, I., Angus, K.W., The therapeutic effect of 16 antimicrobial agents on cryptosporidium infection in mice. Aust J Exp Biol Med Sci 60:187-190 (1982)

109. Soave, R., Therapy and prevention of coccidiosis. In: Microbiology - 1984, American Society for Microbiology. (Schlessinger, D., ed), Wash D.C. p 232-236 (1984)

110. Portnoy, D., Whiteside, M.E., Buckley, E., III, et al., Treatment of intestinal cryptosporidiosis with spiramycin. Ann Intern Med 101:202-204 (1984)

111. CDC., Update: treatment of cryptosporidiosis in patients with acquired immunodeficiency syndrome (AIDS). MMWR 33:117-119 (1984)

112. McCann, P.P., Bacchi, C.J., Nathan, H.C., et al., Difluoromethylornithine and the rational development of polyamine antagonists for the cure of protozoan infection. Mechanisms of Drug Action. (Singer, T.R., Ondarza, R.N., eds). Academic Press, Inc., New York p 159 (1983)

113. Golden, J.A., Sjoerdsma, A., Santi, D.V., *Pneumocystis carinii* pneumonia treated with alpha-difluoromethylornithine. West J Med 141:613-623 (1984).

114. Soave, R., Sjoerdsma, A., Cawein, M.J., Treatment of cryptosporidiosis in AIDS patients with DFMO. International Conference on Acquired Immunodeficiency Syndrome (AIDS). Atlanta, Georgia (1985)

115. Louie, E., Borkowsky, W., Klesius, P.H., et al., Treatment of cryptosporidiosis with oral bovine transfer factor. International Conference on Acquired Immunodeficiency Syndrome (AIDS), Paris, France, (1986)

116. Kern, P., Toy, J., Dietrich, M., Preliminary clinical observations with recombinant interleukin-2 in patients with AIDS or LAS. Blut 50:1-6 (1985).

117. Current, W.L., Haynes, T.B., Complete development of cryptosporidium in cell culture. Science 224:603-605 (1984)

118. Brandborg, L.L., Goldberg, S.B., Breidebach, W.C., Human coccidiosis - a possible cause of malabsorption: the life cycle in small-bowel mucosal biopsies as a diagnostic feature. N Engl J Med 283:1306-1313 (1970)

119. Trier, J.S., Moxey, P.C., Schimmel, E.M., et al., Chronic intestinal coccidiosis in man: intestinal morphology and response to treatment. Gastroenterology 66:923-935 (1974)

120. Faust, E.C., Giraldo, L.E., Caicedo, G., et al., Human isosporosis in the Western Hemisphere. Am J Trop Med Hyg 10:343-349 (1961)

121. Pitchenik, A.E., Fischl, M.A., Dickinson, G.M., et al., Opportunistic infections and Kaposi's sarcoma among Haitians: evidence of a new acquired immunodeficiency state. Ann Intern Med 98:277-284 (1983)

122. Whiteside, M.E., Barkin, J.S., May, R.G., et al., Enteric coccidiosis among patients with the acquired immunodeficiency syndrome. Am J Trop Med Hyg 33:1065-1072 (1984)

123. Ng, E., Markell, E.K., Fleming, R.L., et al., Demonstration of *Isospora belli* by acid-fast stain in a patient with acquired immune deficiency syndrome. J Clin Microbiol 20:384-386 (1984)

124. Forthal, D.N., Guest, S.S., *Isospora belli* enteritis in three homosexual men. Am J Trop Med Hyg 33:1060-1064 (1984)

125. Ma, P., Kaufman, D., Montana, J., *Isospora belli* diarrheal infection in homosexual men. AIDS Res 1:327-338 (1984)

126. DeHovitz, J.A., Pape, J.W., Boncy, M., et al., Clinical manifestations and therapy of *Isospora belli* infection in patients with the acquired immunodeficiency syndrome. N Engl J Med 315:87-90 (1986)

127. Liebman, W.M., Thaler, M.M., DeLorimer, A., et al., Intractable diarrhea of infancy due to intestinal coccidiosis. Gastroenterology 78:579-584 (1980)

128. Westerman, E.L., Christensen, R.P., Chronic *Isospora belli* infection treated with co-trimoxazole. Ann Intern Med 91:413-414 (1979)

36
Tumors Associated with AIDS

Tauseef Ahmed

The epidemic of the acquired immunodeficiency syndrome (AIDS) has afforded basic scientists and clinicians a unique opportunity to examine the effects of viral induced immunosuppression. Immunosuppression, due to many causes, has been associated with the occurrence of malignancies, especially lymphoma (1),(2). As initially defined by the Centers for Disease Control (CDC), AIDS is characterized by the appearance of a serious opportunistic infection, Kaposi's sarcoma or a primary brain lymphoma in an otherwise well person (3). More recently, the CDC has expanded this definition to include patients with non-Hodgkin's lymphomas outside of the central nervous system who are seropositive for antibodies to human immunodeficiency virus (HIV) (4). Our own preliminary data would suggest that even this revised definition may underestimate the true incidence of AIDS-related lymphomas (5). Hodgkin's disease has also been described in patients at risk for AIDS (6), but convincing epidemiologic evidence for an increased risk of this lymphoma in AIDS patients is lacking at this time (5).

PRIMARY BRAIN LYMPHOMA IN AIDS

Primary brain lymphoma was one of the first malignancies to be associated with AIDS (7). At the Westchester County Medical Center (WCMC), we have had nine patients with primary brain lymphoma. All nine were intravenous drug abusers, seven were male and the median age was 31 years. Seven of these patients were also New York State prisoners, a group recognized to be at particularly high risk for AIDS because of the frequent history of past intravenous drug use (8). Eight of nine patients presented with altered mental status or obtundation and three had hemiparesis. In one patient, brain lymphoma was discovered incidentally at autopsy. In general, CT scanning disclosed single (two patients) or multiple (six patients) hypodense lesions. On brain biopsy, the diagnosis was often difficult to prove and in at least two patients the diagnosis could not be confirmed until post-mortem examination. Survival time after diagnosis was short, with no patients surviving beyond three months. In two patients whole brain radiation therapy was attempted but both died within one week of diagnosis. Three patients were treated with procarbazine and a nitrosourea followed by whole brain radiotherapy. However, all three treated in this manner expired two to three months after diagnosis. Four patients did not receive therapy specifically directed toward lymphoma. One patient was too unstable post biopsy to be moved from the intensive care unit for radiotherapy. Another had central nervous system toxoplasmosis diagnosed by brain biopsy which initially responded to pyrimethamine and a sulfonamide; the patient clinically deteriorated and a CT scan disclosed new lesions. At autopsy a primary brain lymphoma was noted in the cerebrum. The third patient died of interstitial pneumonia before therapy for lymphoma could be initiated. The fourth patient did not receive therapy because lymphoma was not suspected ante-mortem. Eight of the nine patients with primary brain lymphoma were autopsied and none had systemic evidence of lymphoma. Thus, in our experience, patients with primary brain lymphomas do extremely poorly despite early aggressive attempts to confirm the diagnosis and initiation of multimodal therapy. Gill et al. have described six patients with primary brain lymphoma and advocated radiotherapy to the whole brain (9). In their series two patients survived longer than six months following radiotherapy.

A major consideration in the differential diagnosis of patients with central nervous system mass lesions who are at risk for AIDS is cerebral toxoplasmosis. In a retrospective analysis, Small et al. (10) from our institution, reported on twelve patients with CNS lesions in the setting of AIDS. Seven had cerebral toxoplasmosis, all of whom were seropositive for antibodies to *Toxoplasma gondii*. Of the six patients with CNS lymphoma, five were tested for antibody to *T. gondii* and only two were found to be seropositive, including the one patient who had both toxoplasmosis and CNS lymphoma.

At present, we recommend that patients with CNS mass lesions in the setting of AIDS undergo serologic testing for serum antibody to *T. gondii*. Patients who are seropositive should be treated with pyrimethamine and a sulfonamide. If there is no clinical improvement within two weeks, or if the patient is seronegative for antibody, then a brain biopsy should be performed. If a primary lymphoma of the brain is diagnosed in the setting of AIDS, it may not be unreasonable to treat the patient symptomatically.

NON-HODGKIN'S LYMPHOMA OUTSIDE OF THE CENTRAL NERVOUS SYSTEM

Diffuse non-Hodgkin's lymphomas have been noted in patients at risk for AIDS by several observers (5),(11)-(13). Ziegler et al. described 90 homosexual men with lymphoma (12). The age distribution of these patients was identical of that of patients with AIDS. By histologic examination, 62% of the patients had high grade non-Hodgkin's lymphoma and 29% had intermediate grade lymphoma. Extra-nodal lymphoma was present in 98% of cases. Fifty-three percent of patients treated with combination chemotherapy, or radiotherapy, or both had complete responses, however, more than one-half of the complete responders relapsed. Patients had a markedly worse clinical course if they also had other manifestations of AIDS. Levine et al. described six homosexual men with B-cell lymphoma (13). They observed that these lymphomas were diffuse and intermediate to high grade histologically. They also noted a propensity to extranodal spread.

We have diagnosed non-Hodgkin's lymphomas not confined to the brain in 22 patients at risk for AIDS, the majority of which were New York State prisoners (5). In our experience, early stage (Stage I or II) non-Hodgkin's lymphoma is infrequent in patients at risk for AIDS. In the last five years, we have seen six patients with Stage I or Stage II diffuse non-Hodgkin's lymphomas. Two of these had tonsillar involvement. All six were treated with external beam radiotherapy and have had local control for 8+ to 72+ months. Two patients relapsed systemically and received salvage chemotherapy. They are alive five and 11 months following chemotherapy.

Sixteen patients at risk for AIDS presented with Stage III and IV non-Hodgkin's lymphoma. Six of these patients had Burkitt's lymphoma. The other ten patients had diffuse intermediate to high grade lymphoma. Fifteen patients with non-Hodgkin's lymphoma were treated with combination chemotherapy containing cyclophosphamide, doxorubicin, vincristine and prednisone. While these tumors were responsive, the median duration of survival was only five months. Patients frequently died of infectious complications or relapse of lymphoma. Two patients are still alive and free of disease more than 24 months after initial diagnosis. Given the poor survival seen in lymphoma patients who are in risk groups for AIDS, prospective clinical trials in patients with lymphoma should identify and separately analyze such patients.

In order to determine whether the frequent diagnosis of lymphoma among prisoners seen at WCMC represented a true increase in incidence, we analyzed data for the time period from January 1981 to December 1984 (5). During this interval the average daily inmate census for the sixteen New York State prisons referring patients to WCMC was 17,300. Using the U.S. population as a standard, the expected number of patients with lymphoma among these 17,300 prisoners was 2.28. Instead, eleven inmates were diagnosed during the four year period, a significantly greater number than would have been expected by chance alone ($p<0.001$) (Figure 1). If it is assumed that every prisoner who had lymphoma within the catchment area for WCMC was referred to this medical center during the study period, the annual crude incidence of lymphoma among New York State prisoners would be $15.9/10^5$. Figure 2 depicts the age breakdown of New York State prisoners. Among prisoners between the ages of 20 and 49 years the annual incidence of lymphoma would be $21.5/10^5$. However, only 32% of prisoners within the catchment area are referred to WCMC. The others are sent to four other hospitals. If this factor is taken into consideration, then the incidence of lymphoma among prisoners aged 20 - 49 years could be $67.2/10^5$. Previous studies (14) have shown that 41% of prisoners in New York abuse illicit drugs. Hence, if a history of drug abuse is factored into the incidence calculations, the annual incidence rate for lymphoma among New York State prisoners with a history of intravenous drug abuse could be as high as $165/10^5$. Within the National Cancer Institute SEER areas, the annual incidence of non-Hodgkin's lymphoma is $3.8/10^5$ in the population aged 20-49 years (15). The annual incidence of lymphoma is lower among non-whites and in males. Therefore, among prisoners the relative risk for lymphomas is 5.66 to 17.7 higher than the general population. Among prisoners with a history of intravenous drug abuse the relative risk may be 43 fold higher than the general population. The high incidence of non-Hodgkin's lymphoma in this population which is also at high risk for AIDS suggests an etiologic association. Among prisoners referred to WCMC, non-Hodgkin's lymphoma and Hodgkin's disease represent the most frequent cancer diagnosis. If these cases were all manifestations of AIDS, then lymphoma would be the second most frequent presentation of AIDS in the prisoner population (Figure 3).

It is interesting to note, however, that only two of our 22 patients with non-Hodgkin's lymphoma outside of the central nervous system would have been classified as having AIDS according to the original surveillance criteria of the Centers for Disease Control (4). Furthermore, of the five patients tested, only two demonstrated antibody against the HIV by an ELISA method. Whether the infrequent occurrence of antibody to this virus among prisoners with lymphoma is related to the small number of persons tested, or to an impairment of antibody formation to HIV in such patients, or whether there are other factors besides HIV infection to explain the elevated incidence of lymphomas in the intravenous drug abusing population is unknown. It is the author's feeling, however, that non-Hodgkin's lymphoma among prisoners who have a history of intravenous drug abuse should probably be treated as an AIDS related lymphoma until convincing data to the contrary become available. When tests for HIV antigen and/or retroviral cultures become generally available, the current surveillance definition of AIDS will probably undergo re-examination.

Lymphadenopathy is frequently noted in patients at risk for AIDS (16). Histologically, exuberant germinal center hyperplasia and follicle lysis are often noted (17). Occasionally, patients

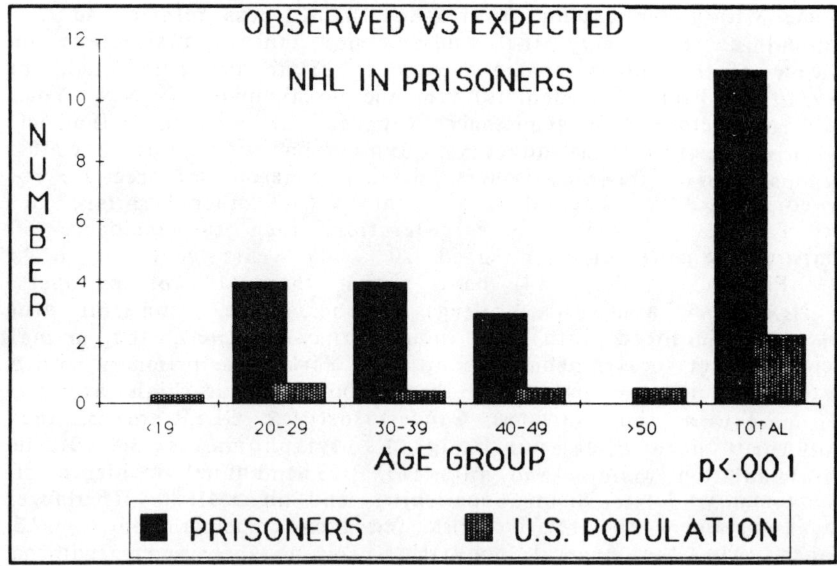

Figure 1. Observed versus expected number of prisoners with non-Hodgkin's lymphoma (NHL) diagnosed at Westchester County Medical Center between January 1981 and December 1984. Overall, 11 prisoners had NHL compared to an expected number of 2.28 ($p<0.001$)

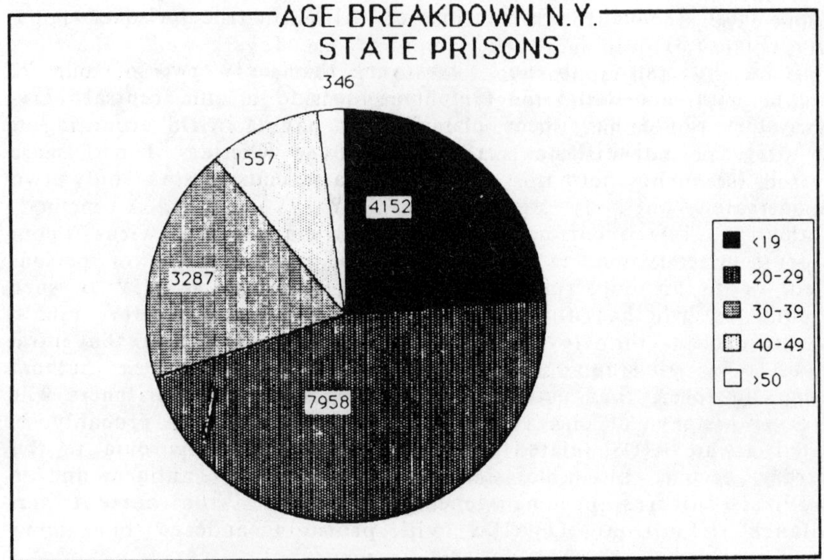

Figure 2. Age distribution of 17,300 New York State prisoners.

with lymph node hyperplasia in the setting of AIDS related complex (ARC) have been later diagnosed with lymphoma (6). However, in others without the histological appearance of lymphoma, there may still be evidence in tissue samples from lymph node biopsies of immunoglobulin gene rearrangement compatible with monoclonal B-lymphocytic lymphoma (18). Thus, the true incidence of lymphoma in patients at risk for AIDS may be higher than that observed in studies where only classic histopathologic techniques are used to confirm the presence of this tumor.

HODGKIN'S DISEASE

Hodgkin's disease has been reported in ARC patients with lymphadenopathy (6). Other observers have described patients at risk for AIDS with Hodgkin's disease (19). Ten patients with Hodgkin's disease who were intravenous drug abusers and/or prisoners were seen at WCMC since 1980. Of these, three patients had early stage disease ie. Stages I or II. They were treated with radiation therapy and all were alive and free of disease six to 21+ months later. Eight patients with Stages III to IV Hodgkin's disease were treated with combination chemotherapy including nitrogen mustard, vincristine, procarbazine, and prednisone (MOPP) or doxorubicin, bleomycin, vinblastine and dacarbazine (ABVD), or a variant there of. Of these patients, four are presently alive and appear to be free of disease at three to 48+ months after diagnosis. One patient who appeared to have been cured of Hodgkin's disease with chemotherapy demonstrated progressive generalized lymphadenopathy, but without evidence of recurrent tumor on multiple lymph node biopsies. In our anecdotal experience, Hodgkin's disease patients in risk groups for AIDS often exhibit more "B symptoms" i.e. fever, weight loss and night sweats, and appear to tolerate chemotherapy poorly compared to other patients with Hodgkin's lymphoma. In our study of prisoners with lymphoma, the number of who had Hodgkin's disease over the study period was too small to determine whether or not an increased frequency of this neoplasm was occurring in the prison population.

OTHER TUMORS

Before the AIDS epidemic, Kaposi's sarcoma was usually diagnosed in elderly patients of Jewish or Italian heritage (20). Classic Kaposi's sarcoma is usually an indolent disease. Among patients with AIDS related Kaposi's sarcoma, the disease may have a much more virulent course. A purplish red skin nodule is the most frequent initial presenting sign (Figure 4). The disease may disseminate systemically and involve lymph nodes, the gastrointestinal tract or other organs. Kaposi's sarcoma is responsive to a number of chemotherapeutic agents and biologic response modifiers (21),(22). For asymptomatic Kaposi's sarcoma, in the initial stages, only follow-up may be necessary. For symptomatic Kaposi's sarcoma in AIDS patients chemotherapeutic a-

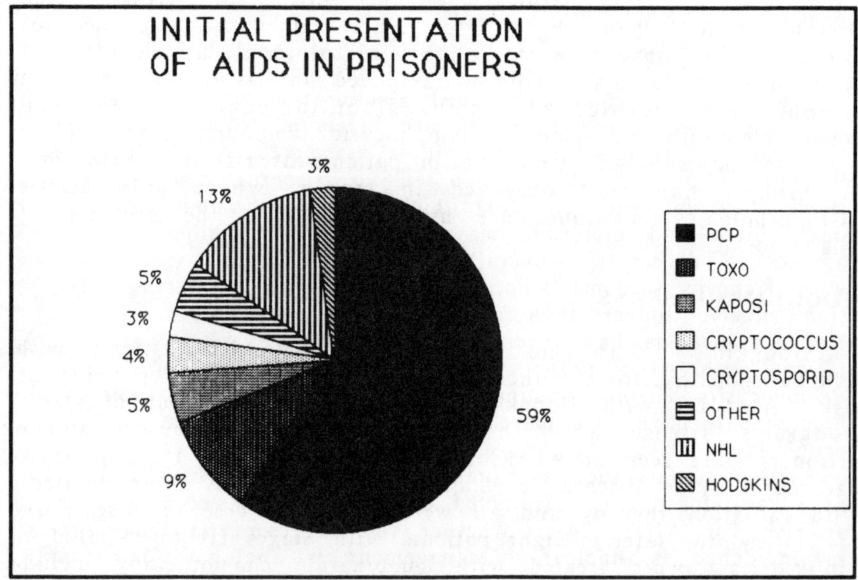

Figure 3. Initial presentation of AIDS in 85 consecutive prisoners seen at Westchester County Medical Center, assuming that all prisoners with lymphoma had AIDS. (PCP - *Pneumocystis carinii* pneumonia; Toxo = cerebral toxoplasmosis; Cryptosporid = cryptosporidiosis; NHL = non-Hodgkin's lymphoma)

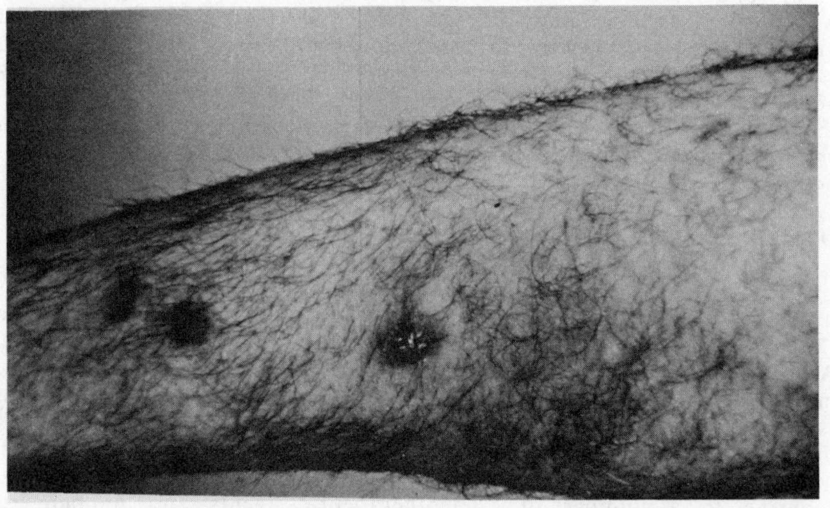

Figure 4. Lesions of Kaposi's sarcoma on the leg of an AIDS patient.

gents such as vincristine, vinblastine, or etoposide have all been associated with substantial tumor regression and improvement. Biological response modifiers such as interferon have also been tried successfully. Our own approach is to use vincristine 2 mg intravenously weekly until amelioration of cutaneous disease is noted. Patients with AIDS are often neutropenic and vincristine can be used safely since it is associated with minimal mycelosuppression. If there is extensive visceral disease, combinations of drugs such as doxorubicin, bleomycin and vinblastine or doxorubicin and etoposide may be used. Chemotherapy does not appear to effect the overall survival of these cases. Patients with Kaposi's sarcoma who do not develop an opportunistic infection survive longer than those who do. Difference in risk of Kaposi's sarcoma have been noted among the various patient populations with AIDS (23). Drug abusers have 33% more cases of *Pneumocystis carinii* pneumonia compared to homosexuals, while homosexuals have 31% more cases of Kaposi's sarcoma compared to drug addicts.

Other tumors such as squamous cell carcinoma of the head and neck or cloacogenic carcinoma are occasionally seen in patients at risk for AIDS (24). Whether this represents a true increase in incidence is unclear. Management is analogous to that for similar tumors in the general population.

CONCLUSION

Non-Hodgkin's lymphomas are a frequent manifestation of AIDS. These tumors may or may not be confined to the brain. Primary brain lymphomas are associated with an extremely poor prognosis. Hodgkin's disease is also seen in patients at risk for AIDS. Advanced (Stage IV) disease appears to be more frequent in these patients. Kaposi's sarcoma is principally found among homosexual men with AIDS and tends to disseminate widely. There is as yet no ideal standard therapy for patients with an AIDS- related tumor. This information will require much more experimental data. Simultaneous treatment of HIV may, however, turn out to be an essential component.

REFERENCES

1. Frizzera, G., Rosai, J., Dehner, L.P., et al., Lymphoreticular disorders in primary immunodeficiencies: New findings based on an up to date histologic classification of 35 cases. Cancer 46:692-699 (1980)

2. Gossett, T.C., Gale, R.P., Fleischman, H., et al., Immunoblastic sarcoma in donor cells after bone marrow transplantation. N Engl J Med 300:904-907 (1979)

3. CDC., Update on Kaposi's sarcoma and opportunistic infections in previously healthy persons - United States. MMWR 31:294-301 (1982)

4. CDC., Revision of the case definition of acquired immunodeficiency syndrome for national reporting. MMWR 34:373-375 (1985)

5. Ahmed, T., Wormser, G.P., Stahl, R.E., et al., Malignant lymphomas in prisoners and intravenous drug abusers: A clinical, pathologic and epidemiologic study. Cancer (In press)

6. Robert, N.J., Schneiderman, H., Hodgkin's disease and the acquired immunodeficiency syndrome. Ann Intern Med 101:142-143 (1984)

7. Snider, W.D., Simpson, D.M., Aronyk, K.E., et al., Primary lymphoma of the nervous system associated with the acquired immunodeficiency syndrome (Letter). N Engl J Med 308:45 (1983)

8. Gill, P.S., Levine, A.M., Meyer, P.R., et al., Primary central nervous system lymphoma in homosexual men. Clinical, immunologic, and pathologic features. Am J Med 78:742-749 (1985)

9. Wormser, G.P., Krupp, L.B., Hanrahan, J.P., et al., Acquired immunodeficiency syndrome in male prisoners: New insights into an emerging syndrome. Ann Intern Med 98:297-303 (1983)

10. Small, C.B., Ahmed, T., Stahl, R.E., et al., Comparison of cerebral toxoplasmosis with primary brain lymphoma in AIDS patients. Interscience Conference on Antimicrobial Agents Chemotherapy, Minneapolis (1985)

11. Ioachim, H.L., Cooper, M.C., Hellman, G.C., Lymphomas in men at high risk for acquired immunodeficiency syndrome (AIDS). Cancer 56:2831-2842 (1985)

12. Ziegler, J.L., Beckstead, J.A., Volberding, P.A., et al., Non-Hodgkin's lymphoma in 90 homosexual men. Relationship to generalized lymphadenopathy and the acquired immunodeficiency syndrome. N Engl J Med 311:565-570 (1984)

13. Levine, A.M., Meyer, P.R., Begandy, M.K., et al., Development of B-cell lymphoma in homosexual men: clinical and immunologic findings. Ann Intern Med 100:7-13 (1984)

14. Novick, L.F., Dello Penna, R., Schwartz, M.S., et al., Health status of New York City prison population. Med Care 15:205-216 (1977)

15. National Cancer Institute Surveillance, Epidemiology and End Results Program. Monograph 57, U.S. Department of Health and Human Services, p 72-73 (1980)

16. CDC., Persistent generalized lymphadenopathy among homosexual males. MMWR 31:249-251 (1982)

17. Burns, W., Wood, G., Dorfman, R., et al., The varied histopathology of lymphadenopathy in the homosexual male. Amer J Surg Path 9:287-297 (1985)

18. Pelicci, P.G., Knowles, D.M., II, Arlin, Z.A., et al., Multiple monoclonal expansion and C-myc oncogene rearrangements in AIDS related lymphoproliferative disorders: Implications for lymphomagenesis. J Exp Med (In press)

19. Schoeppel, S.L., Hoppe, R.T., Dorfman, R.F., et al., Hodgkin's disease in homosexual men with generalized lymphadenopathy. Ann Intern Med 102:68-70 (1985)

20. Oettle, A.G., Geographical and racial differences in the frequency of Kaposi's sarcoma as evidence for environmental or genetic causes. Acta Unio Int Contra Cancrum 18:330-363 (1962)

21. Rieber, E., Mittelman, A., Wormser, G.P., et al., Vincristine and Kaposi's sarcoma in the acquired immunodeficiency syndrome. Ann Intern Med 101:876 (1984)

22. Krown, S.E., Real, F.X., Cunningham-Rundles, S., et al., Preliminary observations on the effect of recombinant leukocyte A interferon in homosexual men with Kaposi's sarcoma. N Engl J Med 308:1071-1076 (1983)

23. Guinan, M.E., Thomas, P.A., Pinsky, P.F., et al., Heterosexual and homosexual patients with acquired immunodeficiency syndrome: A comparison of surveillance, interview, and laboratory data. Ann Intern Med 100:213-218 (1984)

24. Loazada, F., Silverman, S., Jr., Conant, M., New outbreak of oral tumors, malignancies and infectious diseases strikes young male homosexuals. Calif Dent Assoc J 10:39-42 (1982)

37
Kaposi's Sarcoma in AIDS

Kenneth B. Hymes

Kaposi's sarcoma (KS) has acquired new importance since the appearance of the acquired immune deficiency syndrome (AIDS). This tumor, which in the United States and Europe previously affected just a very small number of elderly patients and produced only moderate morbidity and mortality, has become a significant cause of illness and death among previously healthy young patients. Although some of the epidemiologic, virologic, and immunologic features of KS and AIDS are beginning to be understood, these diseases continue to pose new challenges as their natural histories evolve.

Prior to 1979, KS was known to occur in several different epidemiologic settings, each of which greatly influenced the clinical outcome of the disease. The "classical" form of KS has been characterized as an indolent tumor of elderly men of Ashkenazi Jewish or Mediterranian origin (1),(2). This tumor was occasionally associated with lymphoproliferative diseases or lymphedema and responded to radiation therapy or single agent chemotherapy (3). Median survival of patients with this form of KS was from 8-10 years, but when the median age of the patients (seventh decade) was taken into account, it was probable that the KS contributed little to mortality (4). In contrast to this experience from the United States and Europe, at least two distinct presentations were noted to exist in sub-Saharan Africa. Although elderly men in that region developed skin tumors with natural histories similar to those seen in the West, younger patients with histologically identical lesions developed a much more aggressive disease with spread of the tumor to lymph nodes and to other sites such as liver, spleen, lungs, and conjunctivae. This latter group of patients with lymphadenopathic KS had a much worse prognosis with a median survival of less than four to five years (5)-(7). In addition to classical KS and the African lymphadenopathic variety, a third form of KS has been described in patients receiving immunosuppressive therapy following renal transplantation (8),(9). Similar to the classical form, tumors in these patients were usually restricted to the lower extremities. More importantly, however, some patients had complete regression of the tumors upon the discontinuation of immunosuppressive treatment (10).

Since 1979 there has been a dramatic increase in the incidence of KS and a marked change in the clinical and epidemiologic pattern. Recent patients with KS are mostly homosexual men with histories of numerous sexual partners, multiple venereal diseases, and extensive recreational drug use (11),(12). The clinical course in such patients more closely resembles African lymphadenopathic KS than the classical form previously seen in North America. These distinguishing features of the epidemic form of KS permitted its recognition as a new entity associated with a syndrome of severe immunodeficiency, i.e., AIDS.

EPIDEMIOLOGY

Since the outbreak of the AIDS epidemic over 16,000 cases of this disorder have been reported in the United States (13),(14). The incidence of KS is approximately 30% among homosexual patients with AIDS while it is less than 5% among non-homosexual AIDS patients (15). This observation suggests that in addition to the immunosuppressive effect of human immunodeficiency virus (HIV), a cofactor is required for the appearance of KS. Among the cofactors which have been considered are other viruses (particularly herpes-viruses) which may be oncogenic in severely immunosuppressed patients, recreational drugs, or individual genetic susceptibility to KS.

Herpesvirus infections (both primary and reactivation) are clinically important problems in AIDS patients (16). Evidence of past infection with *Herpes simplex* virus (HSV) types I and II, Epstein-Barr virus (EBV), and cytomegalovirus (CMV) can be detected in most homosexual men with AIDS (17),(18). In other patient populations, HSV type II has been associated with an increased risk of epithelial malignancies (squamous carcinomas of the penis and the uterine cervix) (19), while EBV has been implicated in the pathogenesis of Burkitt's lymphoma in both homosexual and heterosexual patients (20),(21). CMV is ubiquitous is male homosexuals and often can be isolated from various sites including semen, urine, saliva, and blood as well as hepatic and pulmonary tissue (16). Infections with CMV may induce long lasting abnormalities in immune function including reversal of the ratio of T4 and T8 lymphocytes, similar (and perhaps additive) to the effect of HIV infection (22),(23). Although CMV DNA and RNA sequences have been identified in biopsies of KS tumors (24), and the virus has been isolated from an involved lymph node from a patient with African KS (25), CMV has not been isolated directly from the tumors of classical, African, or the AIDS-related form of KS (26). Additionally, early and late antigens of CMV have not been identified in biopsies of KS skin lesions or in tissue cultures derived from AIDS-related tumors (26). Although these data suggest an association of KS and CMV, it has not been established that CMV is etiologic. Since CMV infection is so prevalent in patients at risk for having either African or AIDS-related KS, the presence of viral nucleic acids in tissue samples may simply represent superinfection of the malignant endothelial cells with a common virus.

Inhaled amyl, butyl and isobutyl nitrites are common recreational drugs among male homosexuals (27). These drugs, which are popular as sexual stimulants, have in vitro immunosuppressive activity (28) and belong to the N-nitroso family of compounds which have mutagenic, teratogenic, and carcinogenic activity (27). Two epidemiologic studies of patients with KS and AIDS suggested an association of inhaled nitrites with the appearance of KS (12), (29). In the earliest of these (12), the use of nitrites correlated with sexual promiscuity and increased numbers of sexually transmitted infections, thus obscuring a direct relationhsip between nitrites and KS. Subsequent multivariate analysis of risk factors in a smaller group of patients (29) revealed a statistically significant correlation between sustained nitrite use and risk of KS, which was independent of number of sexual partners, other recreational drug use or episodes of non-B hepatitis. Since nitrites by themselves are not known to be immunotoxic or carcinogenic in intact animals, these observations lend support to the hypothesis that KS appears as a result of combined exposure to both immunosuppressive and carcinogenic agents. None of the studies implicating nitrites and AIDS-related KS, however, was designed to identify a specific mechanism for the effect of nitrites.

In classical KS an ethnic and sexual predisposition was noted in the earliest descriptions. That fact, plus the restricted epidemiologic pattern of KS in AIDS, suggests that there may be a genetic component to susceptibility to this disease. Although some patients with AIDS-related KS are of Ashkenazi Jewish or Mediterranian ancestry, there are large numbers of patients with this disease who are not from these ethnic groups; thus, the genetics of AIDS-related KS may involve markers which are less obvious, such as HLA related antigens. Early studies of these antigens showed an increased frequency of HLA DR5 in AIDS-associated KS patients compared with a healthy control population (30). As AIDS-related KS became more common, and these studies were extended to include more patients, the number of DR5 negative patients with KS began to increase lowering the overall frequency of this antigen in AIDS patients with KS towards the level found in control populations (31).

Of interest, however, is that the prevalence of DR5 is increased in populations with classical KS (31). It is possible that the predisposition to develop KS in the setting of immunosuppression is linked to the gene for DR5 or other genes of the major histocompatibility complex-II (MHC-II). This hypothesis has considerable theoretical appeal since products of MHC-II regulate lymphocyte recognition and activation during the immune response, modulate the intensity of immune responses to self and non-self antigens, and serve as markers for susceptibility to a variety of disorders of immune response, including type I diabetes mellitus, multiple sclerosis, and systemic lupus erythematosis (32). A gene which confers a high risk of developing KS may be closely linked to the gene directing production of the antigen serologically detected as DR5, while the same gene may be less frequently associated with genes directing a variety of other serologically defined HLA D antigens. Proof of this conjecture would require direct analysis of the MHC-II region of the genome by molecular biologic techniques, and until such information is known, the issue of genetic predisposition in AIDS-related KS will remain unsettled.

PATHOLOGY

KS in the setting of AIDS is histologically identical to the lesions found in the classical, African lymphadenopathic or transplantation-associated forms of the disease. Biopsies of the lesions show fasicles of spindled cells surrounding cleft-like spaces containing extravasated erythrocytes. Other areas within lesions show hemosiderin deposition, plasma cell and polymorphonuclear cell clusters and dilated lymphatic and capillary channels. Identical histologic findings are present regardless of whether the lesions are in skin, lymph nodes or other sites (33).

The origin of the malignant cell in KS remains a topic of some controversy. Factor VIII antigen has been identified in the spindled cells of KS lesions by immunoperoxidase staining (34), (35) suggesting that these cells arise from the vascular endothelium. Similar studies performed by other investigators (36), (37), however, were unable to identify this antigen by either immunoperoxidase or enzyme histochemical techniques on fresh frozen as well as paraffin embedded tissue. These latter data, therefore, implicate the lymphatic rather than the blood vessel endothelium as the origin of the malignant cell in KS.

CLINICAL MANIFESTATIONS OF KS IN AIDS

Cutaneous Lesions

The majority of AIDS patients with KS present with a limited number of pink, purple, or brown skin lesions. Although the lesions may appear at any location on the body, they most commonly present on the extremities (Figure 1). They are firm, nonblanching, and fixed to the underlying subcutaneous tissue. Lesions are usually nonpruritic, but occasionally patients report moderate pruritus prior to the appearance of a new tumor. Some rapidly growing lesions may present with an ecchymotic halo which fades as the tumor becomes more apparent (12).

The distribution of skin lesions in more advanced cases becomes quite typical with spread along skin cleavage lines creating a pattern resembling pityriasis rosea. The tumors also spread to acral areas involving the tip of the nose, ear pinna, posterior auricular region, fingers, toes and soles of feet. Periorbital lesions are fairly common and are often associated with extensive edema of the face, probably as a result of occlusion of vascular or lymphatic channels (38).

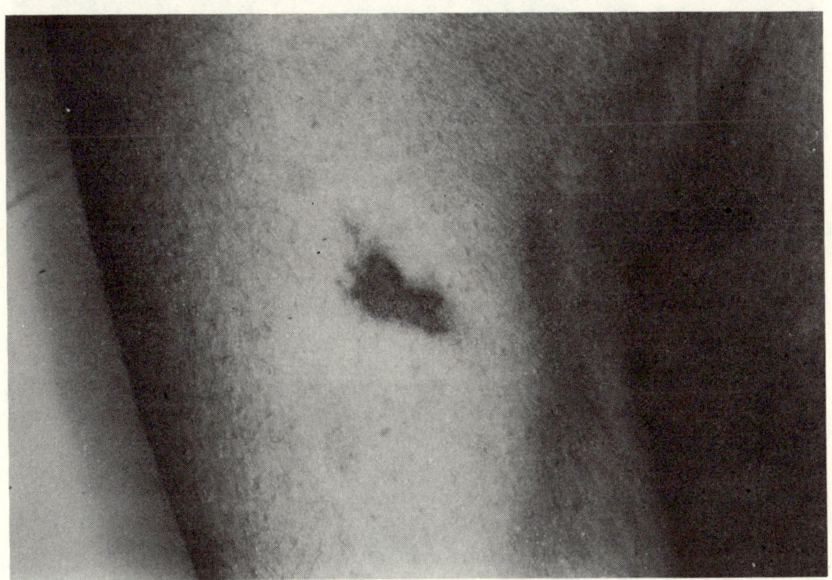

Figure 1. Lesion of Kaposi's sarcoma on the upper arm of a homosexual man with AIDS. (Photo courtesy of Dr. Gary P. Wormser)

Mucous membrane involvement is extremely common in KS. The oral mucosa including the hard and soft palate, buccal mucosa, and tongue may be the site of asymptomatic flat, smooth, violaceous lesions as well as exuberant polypoid growths which may interfere with swallowing, speech, and breathing (Figure 2). In at least one case, a random biopsy of a diffuse oral mucositis revealed KS suggesting that additional unexpected manifestations of this tumor may yet be discovered (39).

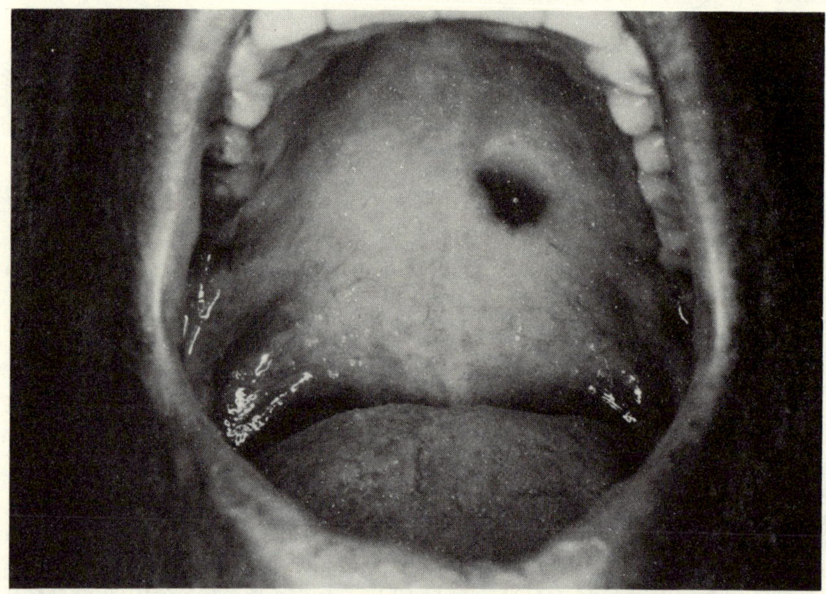

Figure 2. Lesion of Kaposi's sarcoma on the palate of an AIDS patient. (Photo courtesy of Dr. Theodore Lenox and Dr. Gary P. Wormser)

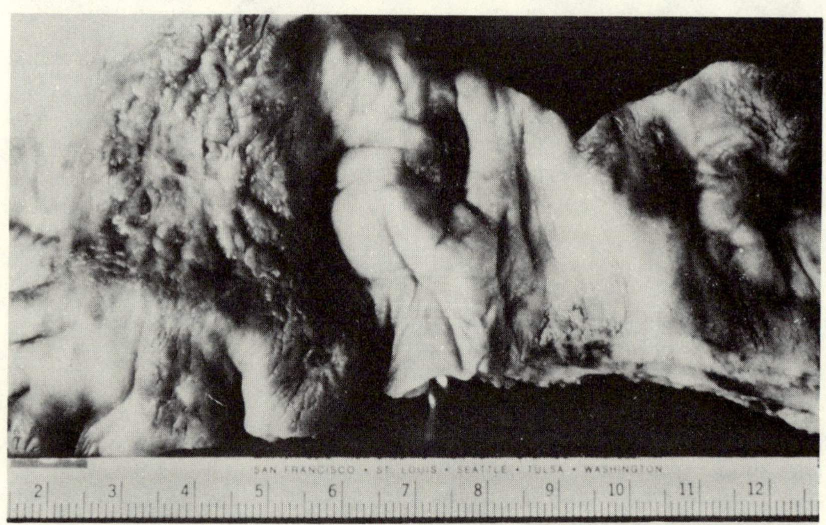

Figure 3. Kaposi's sarcoma involving the transverse colon in a patient with AIDS. (Photo courtesy of Dr. Gary P. Wormser)

Digestive System Lesions

In both autopsy (40),(41) and clinical (42) studies between 40-50% of all patients with KS have gastrointestinal involvement including lesions of the esophagus, stomach, colon, and small intestine in decreasing order of frequency (Figure 3). On endosocopy the tumors appear as cherry red, raised, nonulcerated, smooth masses covered by intact mucosa. Although lesions may be quite extensive, symptoms such as pain, hemorrhage, dysphagia, constipation or obstruction are uncommon.

Hepatic involvement is slightly less common, being found in 35% of cases in an autopsy series (40). As with gastrointestinal involvement it is usually asymptomatic although extention of the tumor from the hilar and portal regions may produce bile stasis and ascending cholangitis.

Pulmonary Lesions

Pulmonary involvement with KS is present in 30-40% of all cases (40),(43), however, unlike gastrointestinal disease, it is more often symptomatic. Patients may present with dyspnea, cough, hypoxemia, and hemoptysis (43),(44). Plain chest radiographs may show hilar adenopathy (either unilateral or bilateral), increased interstitial markings, pleural effusions, reticular-nodular infiltrates or well-defined tumor nodules (45). Since these radiographic findings are nonspecific, and since many patients with AIDS present with fevers and pulmonary infiltrates, the clinician is often faced with the problem of distinguishing between the diagnoses of progressive KS and opportunistic infections. Diagnostic studies such as bronchoscopy with bronchial lavage and transbronchial biopsy, thoracentesis with microbiologic and cytologic studies of pleural fluid, or Cope needle biopsy of pleura, are often useful in the diagnosis of infections due to *Pneumocystis carinii*, cytomegalovirus, or invasive fungi. These techniques, however, are less often successful in establishing the diagnosis of KS. Garay (44) has reported a 40% incidence of pulmonary involvement in patients with KS, however, in only 15% of cases could the diagnosis be established by bronchoscopy. Touboul (46) noted that the diagnosis of pulmonary KS may be suspected if bronchial lavage reveals evidence of intra-alveolar hemorrhage. However, the presence of KS was detected in only 10% of patients studied using this technique, suggesting that although the finding may be specific, it is no more sensitive than other diagnostic methods.

Open lung biopsy is also subject to a high false negative rate. Garay (44) described a group of nine patients with AIDS-related KS and abnormal chest radiographs, but with nondiagnostic fiberoptic bronchoscopic examinations. Open lung biopsies revealed KS in only five of the nine (56%), with four having the diagnosis made by mediastinoscopy or at autopsy. Because of difficulties in the diagnosis of pulmonary KS, physicians treating AIDS patients must rely on the clinical evidence of progressive tumor growth in the skin, lymph nodes, and other visceral sites and the absence of documented pulmonary infection in order to reach a decision to employ chemotherapy for the treatment of progressive pulmonary or pleural disease.

Pleural effusion secondary to progressive KS is a problem which deserves special mention. In 50% of patients with pulmonary KS, pleural fluid can be detected by physical examination, plain chest radiograph, or CT scans (43)-(45). With successful systemic treatment there is usually a dramatic reduction or complete disappearance of the fluid. It is the author's experience, however, that large pleural effusions do not respond well to local measures such as repeated thoracenteses or chest tube placement with, or without, instillation of sclerosing agents. These effusions respond best to systemic chemotherapy, and failure of the tumor to respond to treatment in this setting, carries a very poor prognosis. The majority of patients with AIDS who actually die of KS, usually do so in the setting of progressive pulmonary compromise due to recurrent pleural effusions.

Lymph Node and Splenic Involvement

Lymphadenopathy is commonly seen in patients with KS (13), (47), although the presence of enlarged lymph nodes does not insure that there will be histopathologic evidence of KS. Many co-morbid conditions seen in AIDS may also cause lymphadenopathy including infections with *Mycobacterium avium-intracellulare* (MAI), lymphomas or the lymphadenopathy seen as part of the HIV infection. Conversely, biopsy of enlarged lymph nodes may reveal foci of KS in the absence of evident cutaneous or mucous membrane tumors. These observations need to be considered when assessing the response of patients with KS to antineoplastic treatment. Failure of a lymph node mass to regress may reflect the presence of an opportunistic infection or another neoplasm, rather than failure of treatment to control the KS.

NATURAL HISTORY, PROGNOSIS, AND STAGING

In none of the earliest studies of either classical or African lymphadenopathic KS was there any attempt to stage patients systematically according to extent of disease, or to correlate a staging system with prognosis. Laubenstein et al. (48) described a staging system based upon a large experience with KS in AIDS patients seen at the New York University Medical Center. This system (Table 1) considers the anatomic extent of disease and the tumor associated symptoms (fever and weight loss), but discounts the presence or absence of concurrent or previous opportunistic infections as a variable in determining survival.

Current or previous opportunistic infections, however, significantly influence survival of patients with KS in AIDS as indicated by data subsequently presented by Laubenstein et al. (49) and Safai et al. (50). Patients with all stages of KS, but without opportunistic infections, had a survival rate of > 80% at 39 months (median survival not reached), while those with any stage of KS plus an opportunistic infection(s) had a median survival of only 16 months. If only patients without opportunistic infections are considered, survival correlated inversely with the anatomic extent of disease with stage I patients having a > 90% 36 month survival (median survival not reached), patients with stage IIIA and IVA disease having a > 60% 36 month survival (median not reached), and patients with stage IIIB and IVB disease having a median survival of 14 months. Patients with both KS (all stages) and opportunistic infections had a median survival almost exactly the same as patients with stage IIIB and IVB disease, suggesting either that the presence of fever and weight loss are good indicators of aggressive tumor growth and poor prognosis (as is the case for Hodgkin's disease and non-Hodgkin's lymphoma), or that these symptoms are related to an opportunistic infection which eluded diagnosis.

TABLE 1. A Staging System for Kaposi's Sarcoma in AIDS

Stage I	Cutaneous, locally indolent
Stage II	Cutaneous, locally aggressive with or without involvement of lymph nodes
Stage III	Generalized mucocutaneous or lymph node involvement
Stage IV	Visceral
A	No systemic signs or symptoms
B	Systemic signs: >10% weight loss or fever > 100°F orally lasting ≥ 2 weeks without identifiable source.

In an effort to define additional prognostic features in KS in AIDS patients, Safai et al. (50) and Taylor et al. (51) studied several immunologic parameters. Both groups found that reduction in the number of T4 lymphocytes correlated directly with poor prognosis, a finding which appeared to be independent of tumor stage or the presence or absence of constitutional symptoms. Those patients with absolute T4 counts of >300/*u*L and a T4/T8 ratio of >0.5 had an 85-95% one year survival, while those with <200 T4 cells/*u*L and a T4/T8 ratio of <0.2 had a 25% one year survival. Other laboratory findings correlating with a poor prognosis included reduced lymphocyte proliferation in response to concanavalin A or antigens, increased expression of the lymphocyte surface antigen OKT10, and elevated levels of serum IgA and immune complexes (51).

These data strongly suggest that simple clinical staging of patients is inadequate to predict prognosis both for purposes of clinical management and for planning clinical trials. A combination of extent of tumor, nature of opportunistic infections, and laboratory markers of immune dysfunction needs to be integrated in order to select and stratify patients accurately for clinical trials of antineoplastic or antiviral drugs, and to interpret the results of these trials.

TREATMENT

KS in AIDS responds to a variety of treatments, however, complete responses are rare, and a favorable impact of treatment upon overall survival has yet to be demonstrated. At least part of this failure is related to the high incidence of opportunistic infections which occur in these patients, whether or not they have treatment related myelosuppression (52). Infections such as *Pneumocystis carinii* pneumonia, *Toxoplasma gondii* encephalitis, or *Cryptococcus neoformans* meningitis may be responsible for acute mortality, while other infections such as cytomegalovirus colitis or retinitis, disseminated *Mycobacterium avium-intracellulare*, or cryptosporidial diarrhea may produce wasting syndromes which lower the performance status of the patients and leave them unable to tolerate even minimal toxicity from chemotherapy (49),(52).

Local Treatment

Although the very earliest clinical studies of classical KS suggested that some patients might have a prolonged remission following local surgical removal of a lesion, this therapeutic modality has only limited usefulness in the management of AIDS related KS (53). Excisional biopsy of suspicious lesions for diagnosis, or electrodessication for treatment of small localized extremity lesions is useful, but recurrence after careful, extensive surgical resection is the rule, reflecting the multifocal nature of this malignancy.

Radiotherapy (RT) has been employed for classical, African, lymphadenopathic, transplantation-related and AIDS-related forms of KS. Response rates varying from 33-100% for individual lesions irradiated have been reported, with the chief determinant of success being the size of dose administered (54)-(56). In the transplantation-related form, local doses of >800cGy administered by either kilovoltage or megavoltage techniques in a single fraction produce reliable responses in isolated facial and extremity lesions (54),(55). Higher doses, however, may be necessary for AIDS-related KS (e.g. 3000 cGy in 10 fractions), a subject currently under investigation.

The decision to employ RT for the treatment of KS should be

made with the understanding that it is a local palliative approach to a systemic disease. Suitable candidates for treatment with RT should have localized, slowly progressive lesions which are causing pain (as is commonly the case with extensive pedal lesions) or facial disfigurement.

Several unique complications of RT for KS have been noted. Oral and mucous membrane KS lesions may be a source of discomfort and require treatment even in the absence of extensive cutaneous or visceral disease. Attempts at local RT of these lesions, however, have been complicated by a severe necrotizing stomatitis of uncertain cause (56); thus the presence of symptomatic oral mucosal lesions is considered to be an indication for systemic chemotherapy, rather than local RT.

Irradiation of painful lesions of the feet is also followed by an exaggerated tissue reaction. In the majority of patients receiving RT for pedal lesions there is a period of severe pain, with or without necrosis and vesiculation of the KS lesions. This pain may last three to four weeks following completion of RT and is severe enough to require opiate analgesics; however, after resolution of this pain, good palliation of the lesions is achieved in most patients.

Finally, local RT to the pelvis for palliation of pain due to invasive rectal KS lesions may be complicated by severe proctitis and bacterial septicemia. It is felt that the marked radiosensitivity of the tumor leads to necrosis, with breakdown of the rectal mucosal barrier, and seeding of the bloodstream by bowel flora (56). Consequently, RT to lesions in this region should be used with extreme caution.

Chemotherapy

KS is known to respond to a variety of antineoplastic drugs. Triaziquone, actinomycin D, bleomycin, and ICRF-159 have single agent activity ranging form 50-75% in studies of the African lymphadenopathic form of KS (57)-(60). The combination of actinomycin D, vincristine and dacarbazine is capable of producing a response rate of 97% in patients with African KS with a high proportion of complete responses (61).

With the appearance of AIDS-related KS, studies were initiated based on the African experience. Initial treatment regimens employed vinblastine and bleomycin given together on an every three week schedule (11). Although there was a high response rate (60%), the duration of responses was very short (median approximately three months), prompting exploration of more aggressive investigational treatments (11). An early promising trial using etoposide at a dose of $100mg/M^2$ for three days every three weeks was started in 1981. This treatment produced a response rate of 76% (30% complete, 46% partial) in a group of 41 patients with tumor limited to the skin and without fevers or night sweats (49). In patients with evidence of visceral disease and/or constitutional symptoms, a more aggressive regimen of doxorubicin, bleomycin, and vinblastine (ABV) was employed (49). This combination produced a response rate of 84% (23% complete,

61% partial), although in both the ABV and the etoposide treated groups, the median duration of response was only eight months.

As indicated previously, the high incidence of opportunistic infections in patients with AIDS-related KS has a strong negative impact upon the results of chemotherapy trials. The results of etoposide and ABV trials indicate that the presence of an opportunistic infection either prior to, or during treatment, is associated with a poor prognosis regardless of tumor response. In an effort to reduce the contribution of treatment related toxicity to the development of infection, alternating weekly low dose bleomycin and vinblastine has been instituted for patients with early stage (skin and mucous membrane) lesions. Preliminary data on patients treated in this fashion (62) reveal a response rate of 62% (mostly partial responses) with a median duration of response of six months. Although these results compare favorably with more intensive treatment regimens, the incidence of opportunistic infections (50%) was no lower than that observed in patients receiving either etoposide or ABV treatment.

The observation that the alternating low dose bleomycin/vinblastine regimen produced results equivalent to those with ABV or etoposide therapy suggests that this multifocal tumor is susceptible to more chronic exposure to chemotherapeutic agents. In addition, the results of these trials underscore the importance of the associated immune deficiency in determining the ultimate fate of patients with AIDS. Successful treatment of KS may require treatment with both antineoplastic and immunorestorative therapy.

Biologic Response Modifiers

Attempts at restoration or stimulation of immune function in AIDS patients with KS are logical approaches to the management of this disease, especially in view of prior successes in transplantation-related KS following withdrawal of immunosuppressive therapy (63). Although the data are still preliminary, clinical trials with both natural and recombinant interferons, lymphokines, and pharmacologic immunomodulatory drugs are currently in progress.

Krown et al. (64) have reported response rates between 28-40% with recombinant interferon alpha$_2$ (rIFN-a$_2$) at a dose of 36-45x10^6 units/day intramuscularly for 28 days. Although a few durable complete responses have been reported from this study, the median duration of response was less than one year. There was a high incidence of adverse reactions to this treatment including fevers, malaise, and leukopenia, and despite attempts to ameliorate these toxicities by gradual dose escalation or administration of acetaminophen, drug dose had to be reduced in more than 30% of patients.

Although antitumor effects of rIFN-a$_2$ can be demonstrated, there is no evidence that this compound can consistently correct a reversal of the T4/T8 ratio, or that any improvement in immunologic parameters can be correlated with tumor response. This interferon preparation apparently exerts a direct anti-tumor effect rather than an immunostimulatory effect, and a second generation of studies combining rIFN-a_2 with vinblastine has been instituted in an attempt to enhance the clinical response (65). Preliminary results of this trial, however, have been disappointing with both the IFN and IFN plus vinblastine treatment arms showing response rates of only 18-20%. The failure of IFN to add to the efficacy of vinblastine may be the result of myelotoxicity from the IFN causing attenuation of the doses of vinblastine below an effective range. IFN may need to be combined with nonmyelosuppressive chemotheraputic agents such as vincristine or bleomycin in order to exploit its activity against KS.

Other biologic response modifiers in early clinical trials include both natural and recombinant beta and gamma interferons, lymphokines (particularly interleukin-2), imreg (an immunostimulatory substance derived from leukocytes), and a variety of pharmacologic interferon inducers. To date, none of these agents has demonstrated antitumor responses which approach those achievable with conventional chemotherapeutic agents, and none of these agents has been capable of producing a sustained improvement in laboratory or clinical measurements of immune function.

Future Prospects

Since the discovery of HIV as the etiologic agent responsible for AIDS, investigations have turned to the identification and clinical testing of agents which are capable of inactivating this virus. Most of these drugs function as inhibitors of reverse transcriptase (an enzyme unique to retroviruses), although some have other modes of action.

A number of drugs with antiviral activity including suramin (66),(67), 3' azido-3' deoxythymidine (azidothymidine, AZT)(68), ribavirin (69), and phosphonoformate (70) have entered early clinical trials. Although some of these agents are capable of eliminating HIV from peripheral blood, at least transiently, none has yet been shown to reduce the frequency of opportunistic infections or to induce resolution of AIDS associated malignancies. Perhaps these or other antiviral drugs will need to be combined with effective antineoplastic agents, immunostimulatory drugs, and possibly haplotype identical bone marrow or lymphoid cell transplantation in order to both eliminate the virus and reconstitute the damaged immune system, so that host defenses may effectively handle neoplasms such as KS.

CONCLUSION

Physicians experienced in the care of patients with AIDS and KS have become all too familiar with the relentless progression of these disorders. Although effective cytotoxic regimens for the treatment of KS have been identified, little impact has been made in improving survival. Contemporary shortcomings, however, should not be viewed with frustration or undue pessimism. In only five years medical and biological technologies have established AIDS as an entirely new disorder, elucidated many aspects of its pathophysiology, and identified HIV as its cause. These discoveries were made much more rapidly than those which led to the control of other viral diseases such as polio, small-pox, and measles. It is reasonable to expect that future clinical trials, based upon this foundation, will introduce pharmacologic, immunologic, and molecular biologic advances into the treatment and eventual eradication of KS and AIDS.

REFERENCES

1. Kaposi, M., Idiopathisches multiples pigmentsarkom der haut. Arch Derm Syph 4:265-273 (1872)

2. De Amicis, T., Studio clinico et anatomo-patologico su dodic nouve osservezioni di dermo polimelanosarcoma idiopatica. Napoli, Tipografica, A. Troni (1882)

3. Safai, B., Good, R.A., Kaposi's sarcoma: a review and recent developments. Clin Bull 10:62-69 (1980)

4. Reynolds, W.A., Winklemann, R.K., Soule, E.H., et al., Kaposi's sarcoma: a clinicopathologic study with particular reference to its relationship to the reticuloendothelial system. Medicine 44:419-443 (1965)

5. Kaminer, BV., Murray, J.P. Sarcoma idiopathicum multiple haemorrhagicum of Kaposi with special reference to its incidence in the South African Negro, and two case reports. S Afr J Clin Sci 4:1-25 (1950)

6. Taylor, J.F., Templeton, A.C., Vogel, C.L., et al., Kaposi's sarcoma in Uganda: a clinicopathological study. Int J Cancer 8:125-135 (1971)

7. Slavin, G., Cameron, H.M., Forbes, C., et al., Kaposi's sarcoma in East African children: a report of 51 cases. J Pathol 140:187-199 (1970)

8. Hardy, M.A., Goldfarb, P., Levine, S., De novo Kaposi's sarcoma in renal transplantation: case report and brief review. Cancer 38:144-148 (1976)

9. Penn, I., Kaposi's sarcoma in organ transplant recipients: a report of 20 cases. Transplantation 27:8-11 (1979)

10. Gague, R.W., Wilson-Jones, E., Kaposi's sarcoma and immunosuppressive therapy: a reappraisal. Clin Exp Dermatol 3:135-146 (1978)

11. Hymes, K.B., Cheung, T., Greene, J.B., et al., Kaposi's sarcoma in homosexual men: a report of eight cases. Lancet 2:589-600 (1981)

12. Friedman-Kien, A.E., Laubenstein, L.J., Rubenstein, P., et al., Disseminated Kaposi's sarcoma in homosexual men. Ann Intern Med 96 (Part 1):693-700 (1982)

13. CDC., Update: Acquired immunodeficiency syndrome - United States. MMWR 35:17-21 (1986)

14. CDC., Update: Acquired immunodeficiency syndrome (AIDS) - United States. MMWR 32:688-691 (1985)

15. Haverkos, H., Drotman, D.P., Morgan, M., Prevalence of Kaposi's sarcoma among patients with AIDS (letter). N Engl J Med 312:1518 (1985)

16. Quinnan, G.V., Masur, H., Rook, A.H., et al., Herpes infections in the acquired immune deficiency syndrome. JAMA 252: 72-77 (1984)

17. Drew, W.L., Mintz, L., Miner, R.C., et al., Prevalence of CMV infection in homosexual men. J Infect Dis 143:188-192 (1981)

18. Drew, W.L., Miner, R.C., Ziegler, J.L., et al., Cytomegalovirus and Kaposi's sarcoma in young homosexual men. Lancet 1:125-127 (1982)

19. Adam, E. Rawls, W.E., Melnick, J.L., The association of herpesvirus type-2 infection and cervical cancer. Prev Med 3:122-141 (1974)

20. Epstein, M.A., Achong, B.G., Barr, Y.M., Virus particles in cultured lymphoblasts from Burkitt's lymphoma. Lancet 1:702 (1983)

21. Ziegler, J.L., Drew, W.L., Miner, R.C., et al., Outbreak of Burkitt's-like lymphoma in homosexual men. Lancet 2:631-634 (1983)

22. Rinaldo, C.R., Stossel, T.P., Block, P.H., Leukocyte function during cytomegalovirus mononucleosis. Clin Immunol Immunpathol 12:331-334 (1979)

23. Carney, W.P., Rubin, R.H., Hoffman, W.P., Analysis of T lymphocyte subsets in infectious mononucleosis. J Immunol 126:2114-2116 (1981)

24. Giraldo, G., Beth, E., Henle, W., et al., Kaposi's sarcoma and its relationship to cytomegalovirus. III. CMV-DNA and CMV early antigens in Kaposi's sarcoma. Int J Cancer 26:23-29 (1980)

25. Fenoglio, C.M., Oster, M.W., Gerfo, P.L., et al., Kaposi's sarcoma following chemotherapy of testicular carcinoma in homosexual men: demonstration of CMV-RNA in sarcoma cells. Hum Pathol 13:955-959 (1982)

26. Civianto, F., Penneys, N.S., Haines, H., Kaposi's sarcoma: absence of cytomegalovirus. J Invest Derm 79:79-80 (1982)

27. Newell, G.R., Mossell, P.W.A., Spitz, M.R., et al, Volatile nitrites: use and adverse effects related to the current epidemic of the acquired immune deficiency syndrome. Am J Med 78:811-816 (1985)

28. Goeddert, J.J., Neuland, C.Y., Wallen, W.C., et al., Amyl nitrite may alter T-lymphocytes in homosexual men. Lancet 1: 412-416 (1982)

29. Haverkos, H., Pinsky, P.F., Drotman, D.P., et al., Disease manifestations among homosexual men with acquired immune deficiency syndrome (AIDS): a possible role of nitrites in Kaposi's sarcoma. Sex Trans Dis 12:203-208 (1985)

30. Rubenstein, O., Walker, N., Moller, N. et al., Immunogenetic aspects of epidemic Kaposi's sarcoma in homosexual men. In: AIDS: The Epidemic of Kaposi's Sarcoma and Opportunistic Infections. (Freidman-Kien, A., Laubenstein, L., eds.), Masson, New York, p 139-146 (1983)

31. Rubenstein, P., de Cordoba, S., Oestricher, R., et al., Immunogenetics and predisposition to Kaposi's sarcoma. In: Acquired Immune Deficiency Syndrome (Groopman, J., ed.) Alan J. Liss, New York, p 309-318 (1984)

32. Erclich, H., Stetler, D., Sheng-Dong, R., et al., Analysis by molecular cloning of human class II genes. Fed. Proc. 43:3025-3030 (1984)

33. Gottlieb, G., Ackerman, A.B., Kaposi's sarcoma. An extensively disseminated form in young homosexual men. Hum Pathol 13: 882-892 (1982)

34. Guarda, L.A., Silva, E.G., Ordornez, N.G., et al., Factor VIII in Kaposi's sarcoma. Am J Clin Pathol 76:197-200, (1981)

35. Nadji, M., Morales, A.R., Ziegles-Weisman, J., et al., Kaposi's sarcoma: immunohistologic evidence for an endothelial origin. Arch Pathol Lab Med 105:274-275 (1981)

36. Beckstead, J.H., Wood, G., Flectcher, V., Evidence for the origin of Kaposi's sarcoma from lymphatic endothelium. Am J Pathol 119:294-300, (1985)

37. Dorfman, R.F., Enzyme histochemistry and flourescence microscopy of Kaposi's sarcoma, malignant hemangioendothelioma, and post-mastectomy lymphangiosarcoma. S Afr Med J 36:989-990 (1962)

38. Friedman-Kien, A.E., Ostreicher, R., Overview of classical and epidemic Kaposi's sarcoma, in Friedman-Kien, A.E., Laubenstein, L.J. (eds.), AIDS, The Epidemic of Kaposi's Sarcoma and Opportunistic Infections, New York, Masson, p 23-24 (1984)

39. Laubenstein, L., personal communication (1985)

40. Niedt, G., Schinella, R.A., Acquired immunodeficiency syndrome: clinicopathologic study of 56 autopsies. Arch Pathol Lab Med 109:727-734 (1985)

41. Hui, A.N., Koss, M.N., Meyer, P.R., Necropsy findings in acquired immunodeficiency syndrome: a comparison of premortem diagnosis with postmortem findings. Hum Pathol 15:670-676 (1984)

42. Friedman, S.L., Wright, T.L., Altman, D.F., Gastrointestinal Kaposi's sarcoma in patients with the acquired immune deficiency syndrome - endoscopic and autopsy findings. Gastroenterology 89:102-108 (1985)

43. Murray, J.F., Felton, C.P., Garay, S.M., et al., Pulmonary complications of the acquired immune deficiency syndrome: report of a National Heart, Lung, and Blood Institute Workshop. N Engl J Med 310:1682-1688 (1984)

44. Garay, S.M., Fiberoptic bronchoscopic findings in patients with the acquired immune deficiency syndrome. Chest, (in press)

45. McCauley, D.I., Naidich, D.P., Leitman, B.S., et al., Radiographic patterns of opportunistic lung infections and Kaposi's sarcoma in homosexual men. Am J Roentgen 139: 661-666 (1982)

46. Touboul, J.L. Mayaud, C.M., Fouret, P., et al., Pulmonary lesions of Kaposi's sarcoma, intra-alveolar hemorrhage, and pleural effusion (letter). Ann Intern Med 103:808 (1985)

47. CDC., Persistent generalized lymphadenopathy among homosexual males. MMWR 31:249-252 (1982)

48. Kriegel, R.L., Laubenstein, L.J., Muggia, F.M., Kaposi's sarcoma: a new staging classification. Cancer Treat Rep 67:531-534 (1983)

49. Laubenstein, L.J., Kreigel, R.L., Odajnyk, C.M., et al., Treatment of epidemic Kaposi's sarcoma with VP-16-213 (etoposide) and a combination of doxorubicin, bleomycin, and vinblastine (ABV). J Clin Oncol 2:1115-1120 (1983)

50. Safai, B., Johnson, K.G., Myskowski, P.L., et al., The natural history of Kaposi's sarcoma in the acquired immune deficiency syndrome. Ann Intern Med 103:744-750 (1985)

51. Taylor, J., Afrasiabi, R., Fahey, J.L., et al., Prognostically significant classification of immune changes in AIDS with Kaposi's sarcoma. Blood 67:666-671 (1986)

52. Odajnyk, C., Muggia, F.M., Treatment of Kaposi's sarcoma: overview and analysis by clinical setting. J Clin Oncol 3:1277-1285 (1985)

53. McCarthy, W.D., Pack, G.T., Malignant blood vessel tumors: report of 56 cases of angiosarcoma and Kaposi's sarcoma. Surg Gynecol Obstet 91:465-482 (1950)

54. Harris, J.W., Reed, T.A., Kaposi's sarcoma in AIDS: the role of radiation therapy. Front Radiat Ther Onc 19:126-132 (Karger, Basel) (1985)

55. Cooper, J.S. Fried, P.R., Laubenstein, L.J. Initial observations of the effect of radiotherapy on epidemic Kaposi's sarcoma. JAMA 252:934-935 (1984)

56. Cooper, J.S. personal communication (1986)

57. Kyalwazi, S.K., Treatment of Kaposi's sarcoma. East Afr Med J 46:450-458 (1969)

58. Vogel, C.L., Templeton, C.J., Tempelton, A.C., et al., Treatment of Kaposi's sarcoma with actinomycin D and cyclophosphamide: results of a randomized clinical trial. Int J Cancer 8: 136-143 (1971)

59. Vogel, C.L., Clements, D., Wanuma, A.K., et al., Phase II clinical trials of BCNU (NSC-409962) and bleomycin (NSC-125066) in the treatment of Kaposi's sarcoma. Cancer Chemother Rep 57:325-333 (1973)

60. Olweny, C.L. Mababa, J.P., Sikyewunda, W., et al, Treatment of Kaposi's sarcoma with ICRF-159 (NSC-129943). Cancer Treat Rep 60:111-113 (1976)

61. Vogel, C.L., Primack, A., Dhru, D., et al., Treatment of Kaposi's sarcoma with a combination of actinomycin D and vincristine. Results of a randomized clinical trial. Cancer 31:1382-1391 (1973)

62. Wernz, J., Laubenstein, L., Hymes, K., et al., Chemotherapy and assessment of response in epidemic Kaposi's sarcoma with bleomycin and velban. Proc ASCO 5:4 (1986)

63. Harwood, A.R. Osoba, D., Hofstader, S., et al., Kaposi's sarcoma in recipients of renal transplants. Am J Med 67:759-765 (1979)

64. Krown, S.E., Real, F.X., Cunningham-Rundles, S., et al., Preliminary observations on the effect of recombinant leukocyte alpha interferon in homosexual men with Kaposi's sarcoma. N Engl J Med 308:1071-1076 (1983)

65. Krown, S.E., Real, F.X., Lester, T., et al., Interferon alpha 2a ± vinblastine in AIDS related Kaposi's sarcoma: a prospective randomized trial. Proc ASCO 5:6, (1986)

66. Mitsuya, H., Popovic, M., Yarchuon, R., et al., Suramin protection of T cells in vitro against the cytopathic effect of HTLV-III. Science 226:172-174 (1984)

67. Markham, P.D. Klecker, R.W., Redfield, R.R., et al., Effect of suramin on HTLV-III infection presenting as Kaposi's sarcoma or AIDS related complex: clinical pharmacology and suppression of viral replication in vivo. Lancet 1:874-878 (1985)

68. Mitsuya, H., Weinhold, K.J., Fenman, P.A., et al., 3' azido-3'deoxythymidine (BW A509V): an antiviral agent that inhibits the infectivity and cytopathic effect of human T lymphotropic virus type III/lymphadenopathy associated virus in vitro. Proc Natl Acad Sci (USA) 82:7096-7100 (1985)

69. McCormick, J.B., Getchell, J.P., Mitchell, W., et al., Ribavirin suppresses replication of lymphadenopathy associated virus in cultures of human adult T lymphocytes. Lancet 2: 1367-1369 (1984)

38
The Liver in AIDS

Edward Lebovics, Brad M. Dworkin

Patients with AIDS commonly have clinical and histologic hepatic abnormalities (1)-(9), yet human immunodeficiency virus (HIV) infection itself does not appear to have direct effects on the liver. This statement is supported by the lack of any predominant hepatic derangement that is characteristic of AIDS (1)-(3),(5),(7)-(9) and the occasional finding of normal hepatic histology in AIDS patients (1). However, thorough electron microscopic and immunopathologic studies of the liver in AIDS patients have not been reported to date. The recognized liver involvement in AIDS patients relates to: 1) coincident hepatotropic virus exposure; 2) complications, either infectious, malignant, or iatrogenic, of the immunodeficiency state; or 3) nonspecific changes associated with chronic debilitating illness.

HEPATITIS VIRUSES AND AIDS

Given the epidemiologic similarities of hepatitis B virus (HBV) and HIV infections, it is not surprising that markers of past HBV infection, namely hepatitis B surface antibody (anti-HBs) or hepatitis B core antibody (anti-HBc), are found in approximately 90% of AIDS patients (1)-(3),(5),(10)-(12). This prevalence rate is not substantially different from that of homosexuals, intravenous drug abusers or hemophiliacs without AIDS (11),(13). The prevalence of chronic HBV carriers, as determined by hepatitis B surface antigen (HBsAg) positivity, among AIDS patients with evidence of past HBV infection is about 10% (1)-(3),(5),(10), (11). This prevalence of antigenemia is similar to that of the general population including those epidemiologically at high risk for AIDS (13)-(20). However, it is less than that of certain immunosuppressed groups with impaired cell-mediated immunity, such as patients on renal dialysis, on corticosteroids or other immunosuppressive drugs, and patients with Down's syndrome or lepromatous leprosy (16),(21),(22). These findings are best explained by the fact that in most AIDS patients HBV infection and clearance occurred before the onset of immunodeficiency. In patients with established AIDS, de novo HBV infection would be expected to have a high chronicity rate, as adequate T cell function appears to be necessary for recovery from HBV infection (16),(23)-(26). However, this sequence must be rare and has not yet been reported.

Chronic HBV infection progresses from a stage of active viral replication to loss of viral replication. The former is associated with hepatitis B e antigen (HBeAg) positivity, HBV DNA or DNA polymerase in the serum, and in immunocompetent hosts, clinical and histologic evidence of hepatic inflammation (16), (23)-(25),(27),(28). Immunosuppressed hosts generally tolerate HBV replication without a significant inflammatory response (16),(29). In one report, two AIDS patients with evidence of active viral replication had minimal biochemical and histologic signs of inflammation, suggesting that AIDS reduces the inflammatory response to hepatitis B (10). While chronic hepatitis B with chronic active hepatitis and cirrhosis by histology has been reported in AIDS patients (1),(6), it appears to be unusual (2),(3),(5),(8). This is consistent with current thinking that HBV is not cytopathic and that hepatocyte damage is dependent primarily on the host's cell-mediated immunity (23),(24).

Non-AIDS homosexuals with chronic hepatitis B have been found to respond less well to anti-viral therapy (30), perhaps also due to a blunted immune response to HBV. Reactivation of chronic hepatitis B from the non-replicating to the replicating form has been found to occur commonly in non-AIDS homosexuals (31). This too may be a manifestation of immunosuppression in homosexuals, as reactivation has been described in association with immunosuppressive medications (32),(33). Whether these phenomena in non-AIDS homosexuals relate to incubating HIV infection remains to be elucidated. A study comparing chronic hepatitis B in non-AIDS homosexuals with and without antibody to HIV found that antibody positive patients had less severe histologic and biochemical evidence of inflammation despite higher levels of HBV DNA polymerase (34). This is consistent with an immunosuppressed pattern of reaction to HBV in non-AIDS homosexuals incubating HIV. Of interest, in a recent series, active HBV replication persisted longer and severe histologic damage occurred more frequently in homosexuals than in intravenous drug abusers with chronic hepatitis B; antibody to HIV was, however, absent in most patients in both groups (35).

Two studies seeking evidence for hepatitis delta virus infection in AIDS patients failed to detect serologic or immunopathologic signs of this agent (1),(10). This likely reflects the fact that the HBsAg positive patients (who alone are susceptible to delta infection) in these studies were homosexual men. Delta infection is felt to have entered the American population through intravenous drug abusers and is only more gradually spreading to male homosexuals (36),(37).

A history of non-B hepatitis and the presence of IgG anti-hepatitis A virus is more common in male homosexuals with AIDS than in homosexual controls (11). As with HBV, de novo infections with hepatitis A or hepatitis non-A, non-B hepatitis are uncommon in AIDS patients. Chronic non-A, non-B hepatitis accounts for the majority of chronic hepatitis in male homosexuals and intravenous drug abusers (38),(39). While its course in AIDS patients has not been specifically described, chronic active hepatitis was found to be less frequent in a series of AIDS patients predominantly comprised of intravenous drug abusers than in controls (5). Thus, the inflammatory response to any liver injury, not just HBV infection, may be depressed in AIDS. A notable exception to this hypothesis occurs in children. In a report of four children with AIDS or AIDS-related complex, hepatic histology showed piecemeal necrosis in all (40). The precise etiology for these histologic changes was unclear.

Fulminant hepatitis has not been reported in AIDS patients. In a review of 18 cases of fulminant hepatitis, including 13 of fulminant hepatitis B, no patient had antibody to HIV (41).

OTHER HEPATIC INFECTIONS AND AIDS

Hepatologic consultation is usually requested for AIDS patients to assist in the evaluation of unexplained fever, particularly when accompanied by hepatomegaly or abnormal liver biochemical tests. In our experience, the yield of liver biopsy in providing a diagnosis of an infectious disease is about 25% (1), (5), similar to the overall yield of liver biopsy in patients with fever of unknown origin (42). Others have reported higher yields (3),(4). While the presence of hepatomegaly or abnormal liver biochemical tests may increase the yield of liver biopsy in AIDS patients (1),(5), as in patients with fever of unknown origin (42), the presence or absence of these clinical findings is not sufficient to indicate or exclude significant hepatic pathology (1),(5).

The most commonly diagnosed hepatic infection in AIDS (exclusive of hepatitis B) is due to *Mycobacterium avium-intra-cellulare* (1),(9). Histologically, the organism can be found in granulomas, in clusters of foamy histiocytes, or within isolated Kupffer cells. The granulomas are typically small and poorly formed, without lymphocyte cuffing, multinucleated giant cells, caseation, or hyalinization (1),(9) (Figure 1). On acid-fast stain, granulomas are often teeming with numerous bacilli (Figure 2). This dramatic appearance is highly suggestive of AIDS. However, because the granulomatous response may be absent in AIDS patients, all liver biopsies should be acid-fast stained and

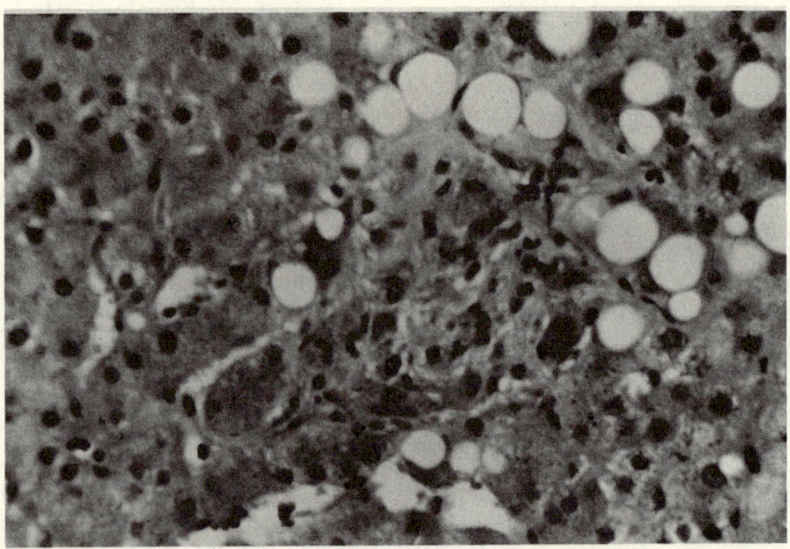

Figure 1. Liver biopsy specimen from a patient with AIDS showing a small, poorly formed granuloma accompanied by macrovesicular steatosis

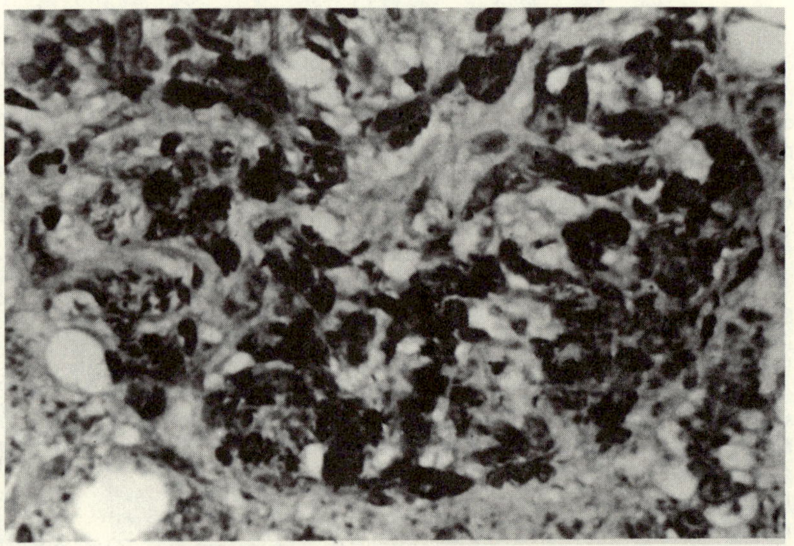

Figure 2. AFB stain of same specimen shown in Figure 1. The granuloma is teeming with acid-fast bacilli which appear clumped. Culture of the specimen was positive for *Mycobacterium avium-intracellulare*

carefully searched (1). Furthermore, biopsy specimens should be cultured for mycobacteria. Rarely, culture can be the sole means of diagnosis of *M. avium-intracellulare* infection (1).

Hepatic granulomas in AIDS patients have been reported secondary to *Mycobacterium tuberculosis* (3) and various fungal infections, including histoplasmosis (1),(5) and cryptococcosis (2)-(4). Toxoplasmosis and cytomegalovirus infection (CMV) are common infections in AIDS patients that can rarely evoke a granulomatous response in the liver (43)-(46). The histologic appearance of granulomas on hematoxylin-eosin stain is not helpful in identifying the causative organism, underscoring the need for special stains and culture of biopsy specimens. In patients with hepatic granulomas without histologic or culture evidence of an infectious agent, other causes of granulomatous disease must be considered (47),(48).

Other than the hepatitis viruses discussed above, viral infection of the liver in AIDS patients may be due to CMV (2),(5), (8),(9), *Herpes simplex* virus (HSV), and Epstein-Barr virus. These infections are typically associated with an acute hepatitis manifested by a hepatocellular pattern of abnormality in the liver biochemical tests (44)-(46),(49)-(52), but can occasionally present with marked cholestasis. Epstein-Barr virus may play a role in chronic hepatitis as well (40),(53). In AIDS patients, serologic diagnosis is hampered by the fact that antibody to these agents is present in nearly all homosexual patients (11), (51),(54). Cytomegalovirus and *H. simplex* virus hepatitis can be diagnosed histologically by the finding of characteristic inclusions in hepatocytes (44),(45),(49),(50). Immunopathologic staining, which is not widely available, can be used to confirm these diagnoses.

Biliary tract infections with unusual manifestations have been noted in AIDS patients. Acalculous cholecystitis has been reported in association with gallbladder infection by CMV or cryptosporidium (55)-(57). Infection of the bile ducts by these organisms may result in biliary obstruction with a cholangiographic appearance of focal stenoses and strictures reminiscent of primary sclerosing cholangitis (58),(59). A case of polymicrobial cholangitis with secondary sclerosing cholangitis due to *Klebsiella pneumoniae, Candida albicans* and cryptosporidium has been reported (60). Thus, in addition to intrahepatic disease, bile duct obstruction must be considered in AIDS patients with cholestasis.

HEPATIC NEOPLASMS IN AIDS

Kaposi's sarcoma (KS) has been seen only rarely in antemortem liver biopsy specimens (3). Autopsy liver specimens show KS more frequently (2),(6)-(9). As in non-AIDS patients with KS, when the liver is involved, the tumor is generally widely disseminated in multiple organs (61). KS appears to occur with greater frequency in AIDS patients who are homosexuals as compared to intravenous drug abusers (62),(63).

The liver may be involved by malignant lymphoma in AIDS patients (8). Typically, it is a monoclonal B-cell lymphoma with a morphologic pattern of B-cell follicular hyperplasia (64),(65). This may be related to Epstein-Barr virus-induced chromosomal translocations (66),(67). Notably, hepatic granulomas have been associated with Hodgkin's and non-Hodgkin's lymphomas (47),(48), (68),(69).

DRUG-INDUCED HEPATIC INJURY IN AIDS

During the course of their illness, AIDS patients are iatrogenically exposed to numerous medications that are potential hepatotoxins. In a recent review, 90% of hospitalized AIDS patients were ingesting at least one potentially hepatotoxic drug (5). A partial listing of drugs commonly used in AIDS patients and associated with hepatic abnormalities is shown in Table 1.

Adverse reactions to sulfonamides, such as sulfamethoxazole or sulfadiazine, appear to be more common in AIDS patients than in other patients (70),(71). Aminotransferase elevation is the liver biochemical abnormality most often observed with sulfonamide injury, but a mixed hepatocellular-cholestatic picture with a rise in alkaline phosphatase is also common (72). Of interest, granulomas may be found on histologic examination (73),(74); the presence of eosinophils and the absence of organisms on special stains suggests a drug-induced etiology (1).

Other commonly used, potentially hepatotoxic drugs include isoniazid, rifampin, and ketoconazole (75)-(77). These are primarily associated with a hepatocellular pattern of abnormality, although ketoconazole hepatic injury may present with cholestasis or a mixed pattern as well (75)-(77). Isoniazid has also been reported to cause hepatic granulomas (74). Of course, virtually any drug may be injurious to the liver. The concomitant protein-calorie malnutrition in AIDS patients may contribute by affecting both the plasma binding and hepatic metabolism of certain drugs, sometimes facilitating toxic effects (78), (79). The AIDS patient on multiple drugs who has fever and rising liver biochemical tests, in whom a specific infection cannot be identified or is not responding to appropriate therapy, represents a difficult clinical problem. Discontinuing non-essential or suspicious medications, when feasible, and observing for a brief period may uncover a drug-induced etiology.

NON-SPECIFIC HEPATIC HISTOPATHOLOGIC CHANGES

Despite the relatively low yield of percutaneous liver biopsy reported by most investigators in providing a specific clinical diagnosis, hepatic histology in AIDS is rarely completely normal (1)-(9). The most common histopathologic feature is macrovesicular steatosis (1). The steatosis is usually mild to moderate and scattered throughout the lobule. Occasionally it is distinctively periportal, typical of the pattern described in kwashiorkor (78). The most likely cause of steatosis in AIDS is marked malnutrition, recent weight loss, and chronic debilitating illness (80). Concomitant alcohol abuse may be a contributing factor in

Table 1. Commonly Used, Potentially Hepatotoxic Drugs In AIDS Patients

Acetaminophen
Cimetidine
Diphenylhydantoin
Isoniazid
Ketoconazole
Nafcillin
Oxacillin
Pentamidine Isethionate
Prochlorperazine
Rifampin
Sulfonamides
Trimethoprim - Sulfamethoxazole

some patients (1),(5). Parenteral nutritional support, particularly regimens including infusions with high concentrations of dextrose, can also contribute to the development of fatty liver (80)-(83).

Sinusoidal dilatation is occasionally present. In one autopsy series it was the most frequent abnormality (7). Its cause is unclear although it has been described in association with granulomas and tumors in the liver (84). Depletion of portal lymphocytes was found in all specimens in one series and attributed to general inhibition of the lymphoid system (6). Other abnormalities that occur include focal necrosis, Kupffer-cell hyperplasia, mild portal inflammation and/or fibrosis and mild hemosiderosis (1)-(9). These abnormalities are nonspecific, and could be either reactive to systemic disease or reflective of pre-existing liver injury.

INDICATIONS FOR LIVER BIOPSY

When early experience with AIDS indicated that the presence or absence of fever, hepatomegaly, or abnormal liver biochemical tests could not reliably predict whether liver biopsy would yield a meaningful diagnosis, it was suggested that all AIDS patients with any of these derangements undergo liver biopsy (1). While this approach would maximize the sensitivity of the procedure, it would expose a majority of patients to the risks of liver biopsy needlessly and in centers seeing a large number of AIDS patients, lead to an enormous volume of biopsies (85),(86).

A more conservative approach is based on the following reasoning. When opportunistic infections or malignancies can be diagnosed by liver biopsy, they are generally widespread through the body. Thus, less invasive procedures, including biopsies of bone marrow, skin, or gastrointestinal tract usually obviate the need for liver biopsy. Additionally, in the absence of fever or marked elevation of liver biochemical tests, the yield of liver biopsy rarely justifies its risks.

Therefore, we recommend that liver biopsy be performed in AIDS patients with unexplained fever or chronic significant abnormalities of liver biochemical tests in whom less invasive evaluations (i.e., biopsy of other possible sites, trial of medication withdrawal when feasible) fails to yield a diagnosis.

AIDS-PHOBIA AND THE HEPATITIS B VIRUS VACCINE

The release of a vaccine safe and effective in the prevention of HBV infection was a major medical breakthrough. Unfortunately, use of the vaccine has been limited due to fears that it may transmit HIV infection. Extensive data have revealed no rational basis for such concerns (87)-(91). The vaccine undergoes a threefold inactivation process using 8-molar urea, pepsin at pH2, and 1:4000 formalin. Representatives of all classes of viruses found in human blood, including HIV, are inactivated by this process (87). Several follow-up studies of vaccine recipients have failed to reveal anti-HIV seroconversion (88)-(90), other than that anticipated in high-risk groups (89). Furthermore, a decision-analysis study found that the risk of death from hepatitis B in groups with a 5% annual risk of hepatitis B infection exceeds any theoretical risk of AIDS that may deter vaccine use (91). Therefore, physicians should urge persons for whom the vaccine is recommended, to be vaccinated. Also, the recombinant DNA prepared hepatitis B vaccine is now available which should make the question of AIDS transmission irrelevant.

CONCLUSION

The crucial challenge facing AIDS investigators today is the development of both an effective therapy for those afflicted and a vaccine for those at risk of HIV infection. Meanwhile, this tragic experiment of nature has yielded important new information whose relevance extends beyond that of AIDS alone. Examples include the behavior of HBV in immunosuppressed hosts, the response of the liver to various metabolic and toxic phenomena and the yield of liver biopsy in systemic infections. Also, the observation that opportunistic infections may mimic other recognized disease states, for example, CMV or cryptosporidial infection of the bile ducts mimicking primary sclerosing cholangitis, may lead to new insights into poorly understood entities.

REFERENCES

1. Lebovics, E., Thung, S.N., Schaffner, F., et al., The liver in the acquired immunodeficiency syndrome: a clinical and histologic study. Hepatology 5:293-298 (1985)

2. Glasgow, B.J., Anders, K., Layfield, L.T., et al., Clinical and pathologic findings of the liver in the acquired immunodeficiency syndrome (AIDS). Am J Clin Pathol 83:583-588 (1985)

3. Devars du Mayne, J.F., Marche, C., Penalba, C., et al., Atteintes hepatiques au cours du syndrome d'immunodepression acquise: etude de 20 case. Presse Med 14:1177-1180 (1985)

4. Orenstein, M.S., Tairtian, A., Yonk, B., et al., Granulomatous involvement of the liver in patients with AIDS. Gut 26:1220-1225 (1985)

5. Dworkin, B.M., Stahl, R.E., Giardina, M.A., et al., The liver in AIDS: emphasis on patients with intravenous drug abuse. Am J Gastro (In press)

6. Nakunama, Y., Liew, C.T., Peters, R.L., et al., Pathologic features of the liver in acquired immune deficiency syndrome (AIDS). Liver 6:158-166 (1986)

7. Welch, K., Finkbeiner, W., Alpers, L.E., et al., Autopsy findings in the acquired immunodeficiency syndrome. JAMA 252:1152-1159 (1984)

8. Reichert, C.M., O'Leary, T.J., Levens, D.C., et al., Autopsy pathology in the acquired immune deficiency syndrome. Am J Path 112:357-382 (1983)

9. Guarda, L.A., Luna, M.A., Smith, J.L., et al., Acquired immunodeficiency syndrome: post-mortem findings. Am J Clin Pathol 81:549-557 (1984)

10. Rustgi, V.K., Hoofnagle, J.H., Gerin, J.C., et al., Hepatitis B virus infection in the acquired immunodeficiency syndrome. Ann Intern Med 101:795-797 (1984)

11. Rogers, M.F., Morens, D.M., Stewart, J.A., et al., National case-control study of Kaposi's sarcoma and *Pneumocystis carinii* pneumonia in homosexual men: Part 2, laboratory results. Ann Intern Med 99:151-158 (1983)

12. Ravenholt, R.T., Role of hepatitis B virus in the acquired immune deficiency syndrome. Lancet 2:885-886 (1983)

13. Keefe, E., Clinical approach to viral hepatitis in homosexual men. Med Clin NA 70:567-586 (1986)

14. Redeker, A.G., Viral hepatitis: clinical aspects. Am J Med Sci 270:9-16 (1975)

15. Nielson, J., Dietrickson, O., Elling, P., et al., Incidence and meaning of persistence of Australia antigen in patients with acute viral hepatitis: development of chronic hepatitis. N Engl J Med 285:1157-1160 (1971)

16. Wright, R., Type B hepatitis: progression to chronic hepatitis. Clin Gastro 9:97-115 (1980)

17. Shah, N., Ostrow, D., Altman, N., et al., Evolution of acute hepatitis B in homosexual men to chronic hepatitis B: prospective study of placebo recipients in a hepatitis B vaccine trial. Arch Intern Med 145:881-882 (1985)

18. White, C.G., Lesesne, H.R., Hemophilia, hepatitis and the acquired immunodeficiency syndrome. Ann Intern Med 98:403-404 (1983)

19. Cedarbaum, A.L., Blatt, P.M., Levine, P.H., Abnormal serum transaminase levels in patients with hemophilia A. Arch Intern Med 142:481-484 (1982)

20. Seeff, L.B., Hepatitis in the drug abuser. Med Clin NA 59:843-848 (1975)

21. Perillo, R.P., Aach, R.D., The clinical course and chronic sequelae of hepatitis B virus infection. Sem Liv Dis 1:15-25 (1981)

22. Anderson, M.G., Murray-Lyon, I.M., Natural history of the HBsAg carrier. Gut 26:848-860 (1985)

23. Thomas, H.C., Montano, L., Goodall, A., et al., Immunological mechanisms in chronic hepatitis B infection. Hepatology 2: 116S-120S (1982)

24. Mondelli, M., Eddeleston, A.L.W.F., Mechanisms of liver cell injury in acute and chronic hepatitis B. Sem Liv Dis 4:47-58 (1984)

25. Gerber, N.A., Thung, S.N., Biology of disease: molecular and cellular pathology of hepatitis B. Lab Invest 6:572-590 (1985)

26. Kukumu, S., Yata, K., Kashio, T., Immunoregulatory T-cell function in acute and chronic liver disease. Gastroenterology 79:613-619 (1980)

27. Realdi, G., Alberti, A., Ruzzi, M., et al., Seroconversion from HBe antigen to anti-HBe in chronic HBV infection Gastroenterology 79:195-199 (1980)

28. Hoofnagle, J., Dusheiko, G.M., Seeff, L.B., Seroconversion from hepatitis B e antigen to antibody in chronic type B hepatitis. Ann Intern Med 94:744-748 (1981)

29. Gudat, F., Bianchi, L., Sonnabend, W., et al., Pattern of surface and core expression in liver tissue reflects state of specific immune response in hepatitis B. Lab Invest 32:1-9 (1975)

30. Novick, D.M., Lok, A.S.F., Thomas, H.C., Diminished responsiveness of homosexual men to antiviral therapy for HBsAg-positive chronic liver disease. J Hepatol 1:29-35 (1984)

31. Perillo, R.P., Campbell, C.R., Sanders, G.E., et al., Spontaneous clearance and reactivation of hepatitis B virus infection among male homosexuals with chronic type B hepatitis. Ann Intern Med 100:43-46 (1984)

32. Weller, I.V.D., Bassendine, M.F., Murray, A.K., et al., Effects of prednisone/azathioprine in chronic hepatitis B infection. Gut 23:650-655 (1982)

33. Hoofnagle, J.H., Dusheiko, G.M., Schafer, D.F., et al., Reactivation of chronic hepatitis B infection by cancer chemotherapy. Ann Intern Med 96:447-449 (1982)

34. Perrillo, R.P., Regenstein, F.G., Roodman, S.T., Chronic hepatitis B in asymptomatic homosexual men with antibody to the human immunodeficiency virus. Ann Intern Med 105:382-383 (1986)

35. Moestrup, T., Hansson, B.G., Nordenfelt, E., et al., Long-term follow-up of chronic hepatitis B infection in intravenous drug abusers and homosexual men. Brit Med J 292:854-857 (1986)

36. Jacobson, I.M., Dienstag, J.L., The delta hepatitis agent: "viral hepatitis type D". Gastroenterology 86:1614-1617 (1984)

37. DeCock, K.M., Govindarajan, S., Chin, K.P., et al., Delta hepatitis in the Los Angeles area: a report of 126 cases. Ann Intern Med 105:108-114 (1986)

38. Cherubin, L.E., Rosenthal, W.S., Stenger, R.E., Chronic liver disease in asymptomatic narcotic addicts. Ann Intern Med 76:391-395 (1972)

39. Weller, I.V.D., Cohn, D., Sierralta, A., et al., Clinical, biochemical, serological, histological and ultrastructural features of liver disease in drug abusers. Gut 25:417-423 (1984)

40. Duffy, L.F., Daum, F., Kahn, E., et al., Hepatitis in children with acquired immune deficiency syndrome: histopathologic and immunocytologic features. Gastroenterology 90: 173-181 (1986)

41. Amoroso, A., Lettieri, G., Giorgio, A., et al., Lack of correlation between fulminant form of viral hepatitis and retrovirus infection associated with the acquired immune deficiency syndrome (AIDS) in drug addicts. Br Med J 292:376-377 (1986)

42. Mitchel, D.P., Hanes, T.E., Hoyumpa, A.M., et al., Fever of unknown origin. Assessment of the value of percutaneous liver biopsy. Arch Intern Med 137:1001-1004 (1977)

43. Martinez-Vazquez, J.M., Guardia, J., Pattiss, A., Granulomatous hepatitis in acquired toxoplasmosis in adults. Semaine des Hopitaux de Paris 51:963-965 (1975)

44. Ten Napel, H.H., Houthoff, H.J., The TH., Cytomegalovirus hepatitis in normal and immune compromised hosts. Liver 4:184-194 (1984)

45. Griffiths, P.D., Cytomegalovirus and the liver. Sem Liv Dis 4:307-313 (1984)

46. Clarke, J., Craig, R.M., Saffro, R., et al., Cytomegalovirus granulomatous hepatitis. Am J Med 66:264-269 (1979)

47. Simon, H.B., Wolff, S.M., Granulomatous hepatitis and prolonged fever of unknown origin: a study of 13 patients. Medicine 52:1-21 (1973)

48. Fauci, A.S., Wolff, S.M., Granulomatous hepatitis, In: Progress in Liver Diseases, (Popper, H., Schaffner, F., eds.) Grune & Stratton, New York, Vol. 5, p 609-621 (1976)

49. Henson, D.E., Grimley, P.M., Straus, A.S., Postnatal cytomegalovirus hepatitis: an autopsy and liver biopsy study. Hum Pathol 5:93-103 (1974)

50. Lee, J.C., Fortung, I.E., Adult *Herpes simplex* hepatitis. Hum Pathol 3:277-281 (1972)

51. Jacobson, I.M., Gang, D.L., Schapiro, R.H., Epstein-Barr viral hepatitis: an unusual case and review of the literature. Am J Gastro 79:628-632 (1984)

52. White, N.S., Juel-Jemen, B.E., Infectious mononucleosis hepatitis. Sem Liv Dis 4:301-306 (1984)

53. Schaffner, F., Epstein-Barr virus in chronic hepatitis. In: Trends in Hepatology. (Bianchi, L., Gerole, W., Popper, H., eds) MTP Press, Lancaster, England, p 209-216 (1985)

54. Fauci, A.S., Macher, A.M., Longo, D.L., et al., Acquired immunodeficiency syndrome: epidemiological, clinical immunologic and therapeutic considerations. Ann Intern Med 100:92-106 (1984)

55. Guarda, L., Stein, S.A., Cleary, K.A., et al., Human cryptosporidiosis in the acquired immunodeficiency syndrome. Arch Pathol Lab Med 107:562-566 (1983)

56. Kavin, N., Jonas, R.B., Chowdhury, L., et al., Acalculous cholecystitis and cytomegalovirus infection in the acquired immunodeficiency syndrome. Ann Intern Med 104:53-54 (1986)

57. Blumberg, R.S., Kelsey, P., Perrone, T., et al., Cytomegalovirus- and cryptosporidium-associated acalculous gangrenous cholecystitis. Am J Med 76:1118-1123 (1984)

58. Pitlik, S.D., Fainstein, V., Garza, D., et al., Human cryptosporidiosis: spectrum of disease. Report of six cases and review of the literature. Arch Intern Med 143:2269-2275 (1983)

59. Margulis, S.J., Honig, C.L., Soave, R., et al., Biliary tract obstruction in the acquired immunodeficiency syndrome. Ann Intern Med 105:207-210 (1986)

60. Cockerill, F.R., Hurley, D.V., Malagelada, J.R., et al., Polymicrobial cholangitis and Kaposi's sarcoma in blood product transfusion-related acquired immunodeficiency syndrome. Am J Med 80:1237-1241 (1986)

61. Anthony, C.U., Koneman, E.W., Visceral Kaposi's sarcoma. Arch Pathol 70:740-746 (1960)

62. Dworkin, B., Wormser, G.P., Rosenthal, W.S., et al., Gastrointestinal manifestations of the acquired immunodeficiency syndrome: a review of 22 cases. Am J Gastro 80:774-778 (1985)

63. Maayan, S., Wormser, G.P., Hewlett, D., et al., Acquired immunodeficiency syndrome in an economically disadvantaged population. Arch Intern Med 145:1607-1612 (1985)

64. Ziegler, J.L., Bekstead, J.A., Volberding, P.A., et al., Non-Hodgkin's lymphoma in 90 homosexual men. N Engl J Med 311:565-570 (1984)

65. Levine, A.M., Meyer, P.R., Begandy, M.K., et al., Development of B-cell lymphoma in homosexual men. Ann Intern Med 100:7-13 (1984)

66. Peterson, J.M., Tubbs, R.R., Savage, R.A., et al., Small non-cleaved B-cell Burkitt like lymphoma with chromosome t (8; 14) translocation and Epstein-Barr virus nuclear-associated antigen in a homosexual man with acquired immune deficiency syndrome. Am J Med 78:141-148 (1985)

67. Magrath, I., Erickson, J., Whang-Peng, J., et al., Synthesis of kappa light chains by cell lines containing an 8; 22 chromosomal translocation derived from a male homosexual with Burkitt's lymphoma. Science 222:1094-1098 (1983)

68. Aderka, D., Kraus, M., Avidor, I., et al., Hodgkin's and non-Hodgkin's lymphomas masquerading as "idiopathic" liver granulomas. Am J Gastro 79:642-644 (1984)

69. Braylan, C.R., Long, C.J., Jaffe, S.E., et al., Malignant lymphoma obscured by concomitant extensive epithelioid granulomas. Cancer 39:1146-1155 (1977)

70. Gordin, F.M., Simon, G.L., Wofsy, C.B., et al., Adverse reactions to trimethoprim-sulfamethoxazole in patients with the acquired immunodeficiency syndrome. Ann Intern Med 100:495-499 (1984)

71. Wharton, J.M., Coleman, D.L., Wofsy, C.B., et al., Trimethoprim-sulfamethoxazole or pentamidine for *Pneumocystis carnii* pneumonia in the acquired immunodeficiency syndrome: a prospective randomized trial. Ann Intern Med 105:37-44 (1986)

72. Dujovne, C.A., Chao, H.C., Zimmerman, H.J., Sulfonamide hepatic injury: review of the literature and report of a case due to sulfamethoxazole. N Engl J Med 277:785-788 (1967)

73. Expiritis, C.R., Kim, T.S., Levine, R.A., Granulomatous hepatitis associated with sulfadimethoxine hypersensitivity. JAMA 202:985-988 (1967)

74. McMaster, K.R., III, Hennigar, G.R., Drug-induced granulomatous hepatitis. Lab Invest 44:61-73 (1981)

75. Zimmerman, H.J., Hepatotoxicity, The Adverse Effects of Drugs and Other Chemicals on the Liver. Appleton-Century-Crofts, New York (1978)

76. Maddrey, W.C., Boitnott, J.K., Drug induced chronic liver disease. Gastroenterology 72:1348-1353 (1977)

77. Lewis, J.H., Zimmerman, H.J., Benson, G.D., et al., Hepatic injury associated with ketoconazole therapy: analysis of 33 cases. Gastroenterology 86:503-513 (1984)

78. McLaren, D.S., Bitar, J.G., Nasser, U.H., Protein-calorie malnutrition and the liver. In: Progress in Liver Diseases. (Popper, H., Schaffner, F., eds.) Grune & Stratton, New York, Vol. 4, p 527-536 (1972)

79. Hathcock, J.N., Metabolic interactions of nutrients and drugs. Fed Proc 44:123-129 (1985)

80. Alpers, D.H., Sabesin, S.M., Fatty liver: biochemical and clinical aspects. In: Diseases of the Liver. (Schiff, L., Schiff, E.R. eds.), J. B. Lippincott Co., Philadelphia, 5th ed., p 813-846 (1982)

81. Bower, R.H., Hepatic complications of parenteral nutrition. Sem Liv Dis 3:216-224 (1983)

82. Sheldon, G.F., Petersen, S.R., Sanders, R., Hepatic dysfunction during hyperalimentation. Arch Surg 113:504-508 (1978)

83. Buzby, G.P., Mullen, J.L., Stein, T.P., Manipulation of TPN caloric substrate and fatty infiltration of the liver. J Surg Res 31:46-54 (1981)

84. Bruguera, M., Aranguibel, F., Ros, E., et al., Incidence and clinical significance of sinusoidal dilatation in liver biopsy. Gastroenterology 75:474-478 (1978)

85. Perrault, J., McGill, D.B., Ott, B.F., et al., Liver biopsy: complications in 1000 inpatients and outpatients. Gastroenterology 74:103-106 (1978)

86. Sherlock, S., Dick, R., VanLeeuwen, D.J., Liver biopsy today. The Royal Free Hospital experience. J Hepatol 1:75-85 (1984)

87. Poiesz, B., Tomar, R., Lehr, B., et al., Hepatitis B vaccine: evidence confirming lack of AIDS transmission. MMWR 33:685-687 (1984)

88. Dienstag, J.L., Werner, B.G., McLane, M.F., et al., Absence of antibodies to HTLV-III in health workers after hepatitis B vaccination. JAMA 254:1064-1066 (1985)

89. Stevens, C.E., Taylor, P.E., Rubinstein, P., et al., Safety of hepatitis B vaccine. N Engl J Med 312:375-376 (1985)

90. Papavangelou, G., Kallinikos, G., Roumeliotou, A., et al., Risk of AIDS in recipients of hepatitis B vaccine. N Engl J Med 312:376-377 (1985)

91. Sacks, H.S., Rose, D.N., Chalmers, T.C., Should the risk of acquired immunodeficiency syndrome deter hepatitis B vaccination. JAMA 252:3375-3377 (1984)

39
Hematologic Findings in HIV Infection

Christina Walsh, Steve Savona

THROMBOCYTOPENIA IN GAY MEN

In 1982, Morris et al. reported a group of 11 homosexual men presenting with thrombocytopenia (1). Clinically these patients appeared to have idiopathic thrombocytopenia purpura (ITP), and they frequently responded to steroids or splenectomy. However, laboratory data revealed some unusual features. Several patients had very decreased T helper/suppressor cell ratios. Lymphopenia and polyclonal hypergammaglobulinemia were also seen. These findings immediately suggested that this cluster of cases with ITP might be related to the newly recognized syndrome of acquired immunodeficiency (AIDS). Over the last four years, several groups of such patients have been well studied, and the picture of ITP in gay men has become clearer. Characteristically, such patients are clinically well at the time of diagnosis of thrombocytopenia, aside from symptoms related to thrombocytopenia itself. However, as will be discussed below, emerging data have clearly identified thrombocytopenia as part of the expanding disease spectrum of human immunodeficiency virus (HIV) infection.

Natural History

As is the case for most HIV related illness, an understanding of the natural history of thrombocytopenia in these patients is still evolving. Three series have recently reported studies of cohorts of homosexual men with ITP (2)-(4) with a mean follow-up approaching two years. It is clear from these investigations that many of these patients, almost one-half in our NYU series, are mildly affected and do well without any specific treatment. Such patients can maintain platelet counts of 40,000 to 100,000/ mm^3 for years and do not suffer any complications. A few will spontaneously recover normal platelet counts and maintain them.

Nevertheless, recent reports have confirmed that this syndrome is part of the AIDS complex. In the NYU series 92% of patients tested had antibody to HIV (3). In the San Francisco series, antibody was detected in 100% of 25 patients tested by both ELISA and Western blot technique (2). Even more convincingly but unhappily, a small number of these patients have gone on to develop CDC-defined AIDS. In the NYU study, six out of 33 patients developed either pneumocystis pneumonia or Kaposi's sarcoma (KS) at periods ranging from one month to 37 months after diagnosis of thrombocytopenia. In the San Francisco study, three of 35 developed AIDS from 16 to 34 months after diagnosis. No predictive factors for this outcome have been noted; for example, development of AIDS was unrelated to severity of thrombocytopenia. As will be discussed more thoroughly below, development of AIDS also appeared to be independent of treatment modality or treatment outcome. Hence, at just under two years of mean follow-up, between eight and 18 percent of these patients have gone on to develop AIDS. Whether these numbers will continue to rise remains unclear. It is perhaps of interest to compare these observations on the probability of developing AIDS for thrombocytopenic homosexual men, with analogous data for other populations at high risk. Groopman et al. have followed 78 patients with generalized lymphadenopathy, 91% of whom were anti-HIV positive serologically (5). After approximately two years, six (8.0%) of 75 had developed AIDS. Goedert et al. have calculated the incidence of AIDS in cohorts of HIV antibody positive members of high risk groups followed for three years (6). Including patients who were antibody positive at time of study entry, as well as those who seroconverted during follow-up, 10.1% developed AIDS within three years.

Treatment

As with classic ITP, prednisone at a dose of approximately 1 mg/kg has been the initial therapy in the majority of patients. Most patients have been treated because of platelet counts less than 30,000/mm^3 or for bleeding or bruising manifestations. Although many patients derive a significant improvement in platelet count initially, few can be tapered off steroids successfully without a precipitous drop in count. In our series, only three of 17 patients retained platelet counts of >100,000/mm^3 after prednisone was tapered.

In both our patient series and the San Francisco series more than one-half of the patients initially treated with steroids required splenectomy. Splenectomy has been very successful, with 100% of our patients and 66% of San Francisco patients attaining normal platelet counts off all other therapy. In our experience, normal platelet counts have been maintained for a mean of 10 months. Of interest, in both series a few patients who failed steroids, but did not have splenectomy, developed normal platelet counts spontaneously and maintained them.

The very important question of whether steroid therapy or splenectomy increases the risk of AIDS development in these patients is unresolved. In the two largest series, the number of patients developing AIDS is still too small to permit conclusions, and there are no controlled studies. In the NYU series, two of the patients who developed AIDS had had no therapy for thrombocytopenia, while four others had had steroid therapy and splenectomy previously. The four latter patients were in remission off all therapy when AIDS was diagnosed. The time from splenectomy to AIDS diagnosis varied from one to 35 months. Six other splenectomized patients have been well with follow-up from 12 to 48 months.

No patients have been reported to develop conditions diagnostic of AIDS while on steroids for the treatment of thrombocytopenia. However, oral candidiasis has been seen commonly during steroid administration. While thrush has been suggested as a poor prognostic sign in ARC patients (7), there is no indication that it has the same significance in patients receiving corticosteroids.

Reports of use of other treatment modalities in these patients are anecdotal. Danazol has been used additively in a few patients at NYU without observed benefit (8). Based on prior experience of its favorable effect on classic ITP, it might still be expected to benefit some patients if more thoroughly tested (9). It should be noted, however, that Metroka observed poor outcomes in an anecdotal series of confirmed AIDS patients treated with danazol as a possible immune modulator (10). Vinca alkaloids have been used for patients presenting both with KS and severe thrombocytopenia. This group of patients may be intrinsically quite different from patients with thrombocytopenia alone. However, Mintzer et al. has reported that in a group of 18 evaluable patients with KS treated with weekly vincristine, three with platelet counts of 15,000, 30,000, and 68,000/mm^3 respectively, developed counts of >200,000/mm^3 during therapy (11). In two of these patients a normal platelet count was sustained for six and nine months respectively while on therapy.

Following several reports published in the early 1980's (12),(13), high dose intravenous gammaglobulin has become a therapeutic option for the treatment of ITP. Questions remain about the overall utility of this approach. Responses are usually transient, but some patients continue to respond to repeat booster infusions (14). This therapy has not been systematically studied in patients with HIV associated thrombocytopenia. Both success and failure have been described in brief reports concerning patients with AIDS associated thrombocytopenia treated this way (15)-(17). The mechanism of action of this therapy, as well as its effects on the immune system, are not totally understood. Fc receptor blockade has been considered one mechanism, but recent reports have suggested effects of intravenous gammaglobulin on T cell function in non-AIDS ITP patients. For example, some patients have shown increased T-cell numbers and increased T-cell response to phytohemagglutinin during remission following intravenous immunoglobulin therapy (18). How this would relate to immune defects in HIV positive patients is unclear. The high cost of a single course of treatment also remains a significant problem. In the setting of immune thrombocytopenia with severe or life threatening bleeding, a course of high dose gammaglobulin, possibly with platelet transfusion, should be considered (19). The role of this therapy in the treatment of stable patients with AIDS associated thrombocytopenia remains to be seen.

Overall, the clinical course of thrombocytopenia in these patients has been relatively benign. Therefore, we generally reserve treatment for patients with platelet counts <25,000/mm^3 or with bleeding complications. Steroids are used as initial therapy in most patients. If patients fail to respond or cannot be tapered to an acceptably low dose of prednisone within six to eight weeks, splenectomy is suggested. If patients must be maintained chronically on any dose of steroids, splenectomy should be considered. Although splenectomy has been a very successful treatment modality in our hands, the actual risk, if any, that steroids pose to these patients is not known.

Mechanism of Thrombocytopenia in Gay Men

Most patients with classic ITP have elevated levels of platelet associated IgG (20). Presumably this immunoglobulin promotes the destruction of platelets by the reticulo-endothelial system. Like classic ITP patients, homosexual patients with thrombocytopenia have been found to have elevated platelet bound IgG levels (2),(3). However, whether the mechanism of thrombocytopenia is precisely the same in the two groups of patients is controversial.

In studies at NYU, we have observed several differences between the two types of thrombocytopenic patients (21). When the serum of classic ITP patients is fractionated, the IgG fraction contains platelet binding activity. This IgG platelet binding activity could not be demonstrated in sera from homosexual men with ITP, even when the unfractionated serum had very high platelet binding activity. Similarly, when the platelets of classic ITP patients are properly treated, antiplatelet IgG can be eluted and shown to bind to fresh platelets. We could not elute antiplatelet IgG from nine of 10 homosexual patients studied; in the tenth case a very low titer of antiplatelet activity was seen.

Because of these results, we have suggested that the mechanism of thrombocytopenia may be different in homosexual men with ITP compared to classic ITP. Lack of evidence for antiplatelet IgG in the homosexual patients raises the possibility that the immunoglobulin on the platelet surface might be in the form of immune complexes. Although immune complex levels are often elevated in these patients (22), there has still been no direct demonstration of such complexes on platelets.

Using another methodology, a group in California has arrived at a different conclusion. With a very sensitive immunoblot technique, Stricker et al. demonstrated an immunoglobulin in the serum of 29 out of 30 homosexual patients that appeared to be directed to a platelet membrane antigen of 25,000 dalton size (23). This antibody was not detected in the serum of any of 30 patients with classic ITP or nonimmune thrombocytopenia. The investigators speculated that this antibody could be a cause of thrombocytopenia. The nature of the target platelet antigen remains unclear. It does not appear to be any of the previously well-studied platelet surface antigens. It is also distinct from the core protein of HIV. This antibody and antigen are undergoing further study. However, these investigators believe that homosexual men with ITP do have a serum antibody which binds to platelets.

Of interest, both our group and that of Stricker et al. (23) noted that homosexual "control" patients with normal platelet counts often had above normal levels of platelet associated IgG. Stricker et al. detected this antibody in 15 of 16 lymphadenopathy syndrome or AIDS patients with a mean platelet count of 192,000/mm^3. Therefore, clearly factors other than simply the presence of platelet associated antibody play a role in determining the extent of platelet destruction. In 1985 Bender et al. showed that 11 of 15 patients with AIDS had decreased reticuloendothelial system Fc receptor function (24). Some, but not all patients with ARC-type illnesses also had decreased receptor function. This interesting observation may be one important factor in determining whether or not thrombocytopenia will occur in HIV infected patients.

THROMBOCYTOPENIA IN INTRAVENOUS DRUG ABUSERS WITH HIV INFECTION

The association of HIV infection and thrombocytopenia has also been observed in hemophiliacs and in intravenous drug abusers (IVDA).

Before the AIDS epidemic, reports of thrombocytopenia in IVDA were principally confined to descriptions of acute episodes occurring in active users (25)-(29). In some instances, brown heroin was postulated as the etiological agent (25). In HIV infected addicts, thrombocytopenia is chronic and often not temporally related to illicit drug use. For example, among 69 IVDA studied by Savona et al. (30), at least 33 (48%) had claimed to have stopped intravenous drug use for an average of 21.2 (±4.7) months prior to the recognition of thrombocytopenia.

In this latter study of IVDA's, the mean platelet count (± SD) at time of presentation was 53,000/mm^3 (± 4000) (range 3000 - 140,000/mm^3). The ratio of female to male patients was 1:4, the reverse of that found in classical ITP. Aside from the common feature of illicit drug use, the patients were clinically heterogeneous. Eleven percent had chronic hepatitis, 30% had splenomegaly, 3% admitted to homosexual behavior, 4% had evidence of disseminated intravascular coagulation and 13% had

AIDS. Antibody to HIV was present in 87% of those tested.

Mechanism of Thrombocytopenia in IVDA

Studies on the pathogenesis of thrombocytopenia in IVDA show differences from the findings in gay men. Platelets from thrombocytopenic IVDA's have greatly elevated levels of bound IgG, IgM and complement when compared with contemporaneously tested platelets from patients with classical ITP or platelets from healthy controls. Circulating immune complexes were present (detected by polyethylene glycol precipitation), which bound to normal platelets (30). The structure of the immune complex has been studied by Yu, Lynette and Karpatkin (31), who found the presence of anti-$(FAB')_2$ antibody, suggesting that these immune complexes are comprised at least in part of anti-antibody complexes. However, 11 of 18 IVDA's with thrombocytopenia also had antiplatelet antibody in serum, which was shown to be present in the exclusion volume of a Sephadex G200 column as well as in the 7S gammaglobulin fraction (30). Thus, immunoreactivity for platelets in the serum of IVDA appears to be related to an immune complex as well as an auto-antibody.

Treatment

For symptomatic patients, steroids, or in a few cases, splenectomy have improved platelet counts analogous to the experience in gay men. There is no evidence that methadone usage during therapy impedes the therapeutic response.

HEMATOLOGIC CHANGES IN AIDS OTHER THAN THROMBOCYTOPENIA

Leukopenia and anemia are commonly observed in patients with AIDS or ARC and may be multifactorial in origin (32). Included among the causes are infections, such as disseminated *Mycobacterium avium-intracellulare* and *Pneumocystis carinii* pneumonia and neoplastic causes, such as metastatic lymphoma to bone marrow (33),(34). Treatment of *Pneumocystis carinii* pneumonia with trimethoprim-sulfamethoxazole may induce a temporally related drop in all blood counts of unknown cause, but apparently not due to interference with folic acid metabolism (35). Malnutrition may also contribute to bone marrow suppression, although hard data relating dietary deficiency to pancytopenia are lacking. AIDS patients generally do not have macrocytic or megaloblastic anemias. It is unclear if the anemia present in AIDS is an anemia of chronic disease. Sideroblastic abnormalities have not been generally noted in bone marrow aspirates of AIDS patients.

Immune hemolytic anemia was noted in four AIDS patients who had a positive direct 'IgG-type' Coombs test (36). One patient also had complement coating of the red blood cells. Heat eluates from these red cells did not show the presence of anti-red cell immunoglobulin, which suggested immune complex destruction. Only two of the four patients had a reticulocytosis.

Lymphopenia was noted early on in the description of AIDS, usually associated with an inversion of the T helper (T4) to T suppressor (T8) ratio. It appears that the HIV virus is selectively lymphotropic (and neurotropic) causing specific infection of T4 lymphocytes with their subsequent depletion and relative preservation of the number of T8 and B cells.

Granulocyte abnormalities have also been observed in AIDS. Murphy et al. (37) studied 20 AIDS patients and 59 pre-AIDS patients (lymphadenopathy syndrome) who were HIV positive. In this study, neutropenia was noted in 20% of AIDS patients and 22% of pre-AIDS patients, but it was not seen in asymptomatic HIV positive subjects. Seven of the 59 pre-AIDS patients progressed to AIDS and of these, four had prior neutropenia. One patient treated with steroids had an increase in neutrophil count, which fell when steroids were discontinued. Murphy et al. (38) described seven neutropenic or borderline neutropenic homosexual patients. All were HIV positive, six had lymphadenopathy and one had an opportunistic infection. In four of seven cases, neutrophil antibody activity was noted in a direct immunoflourescence test. An indirect test using these patients' sera was positive in one case. A distinction between antibody and immune complex activity was not established in this study.

Another mechanism of granulocytopenia may be bone marrow suppression. Leiderman et al. (39) have reported that AIDS patients have significantly decreased colony formation of their granulocyte-macrophage progenitor cells in vitro. AIDS marrow cells inhibited normal colony formation of granulocytes and macrophages in culture. Furthermore, eluates from bone marrow culture supernatant of AIDS patients also inhibited this process. Inhibition may be caused by a unique 84 Kd glycoprotein found in the supernatant of the AIDS bone marrow cultures. The 84Kd protein is not reactive with HIV antibodies, which suggests that it is not antigenic viral material. Depletion of interleukin-2 responsive lymphocytes may also contribute to bone marrow suppression, although T lymphocytes are not essential for hematopoietic colony formation. Interleukin-2 responsive T-cells may modulate erythroid colony growth in normal bone marrow (40).

Neutrophil function may also be impaired in AIDS and pre-AIDS. Ellis et al. (41) studied 14 patients with AIDS and three patients with pre-AIDS. Polymorphonuclear cells from both groups showed significantly less chemotactic responsiveness to *Escherichia coli* endotoxin in a modified Boyden chamber than normal cells exposed to endotoxin. Chemotaxis could be partially restored if patient cells were incubated in normal serum. Bacterial killing of *Staphylococcus aureus* was impaired in pre-AIDS and AIDS cells. No inhibition of granulocyte aggregration or degranulation was reported.

BONE MARROW FINDINGS IN AIDS

Bone marrow aspiration and biopsy are most often done in AIDS patients for one of two indications: cytopenias or fever. Despite the high incidence of anemia, neutropenia or thrombocytopenia in AIDS patients, an obvious cause for these abnormalities is rarely evident upon examining the marrow. Hypercellularity or normocellularity are more common than hypocellularity in biopsy specimens (32),(42). In contrast to biopsy samples, aspirates may appear less cellular, due in part to a high incidence of dry or very difficult taps. Spivak et al. (32) reported increased marrow reticulin in 10 of 12 patients studied, and felt this increased over time in the marrows of patients studied serially. Peripheral blood findings characteristic of myelofibrosis have not been reported, except in a single patient with accelerated myelofibrosis and HIV infection (43).

Plasmacytosis is repeatedly described in marrows of AIDS patients (32),(42), although actual percentages are infrequently given. Eosinophilia has also been seen (44), but the significance of this is unclear as many patients were receiving multiple drugs. Bone marrow necrosis has been described in several instances by one group (32).

Also frequently noted is prominent macrophage activity, as indicated by an apparent increase in the number of histiocytes or the presence of prominent erythrophagocytosis (32),(45). The latter finding is similar to the "hematophagic histiocytosis" reported by Risdall in immunosuppressed transplant patients with viral infection (46). However, in AIDS there has been no specific correlation with any viral culture results.

Another bone marrow finding that has received attention is the increased incidence of lymphoid aggregates. Castella et al. (42) reported one or more nonparatrabecular aggregates in five of 55 marrows, an observation which was confirmed by Osborne and Spivak (32),(47). Although marker studies have not been reported, these benign appearing aggregates have not been predictive of later lymphoma in the small number of patients studied to date.

Osborne et al. have suggested that there may be some confusion between lymphohistiocytic aggregates and granulomas in AIDS patients (47). Mycobacterial infection not infrequently involves the bone marrow in AIDS patients and as in other organs, may be associated with poorly formed granulomas, or none at all. Osborne reported one case in which a "lymphohistiocytic infiltrate", initially of concern as possibly malignant, appeared granulomatous on deeper sectioning.

CONCLUSION

The bone marrow is clearly an affected organ in AIDS. Anemia, neutropenia and thrombocytopenia are important clinical factors in these patients' illnesses, complicating and often limiting the administration of therapy for established diagnoses. Unfortunately, pathologic examination of bone marrow usually sheds little light on these clinical problems, except when a specific diagnosis such as lymphoma or infection can be made. No bone marrow findings have been found to be pathognomonic of AIDS. Abnormalities of lymphoid and plasma cell lines presumably reflect the disordered immune function of these patients, but the explanation for the cytopenias is little understood.

ACKNOWLEDGMENT

The authors wish to thank Mary Naber for her assistance in the preparation of this manuscript.

REFERENCES

1. Morris, L., Distenfeld, A., Amorosi, E., et al., Autoimmune thombocytopenic purpura in homosexual men. Ann Intern Med 96:714-717 (1982)

2. Abrams, D., Kiprov, D., Goedert, J., et al., Antibodies to T-lymphotropic virus type III and development of the acquired immunodeficiency syndrome in homosexual men presenting with immune thrombocytopenia. Ann Intern Med 104:47-50 (1986)

3. Walsh, C., Krigel, R., Lennette, E., et al., Thrombocytopenia in homosexual patients. Ann Intern Med 103:542-545 (1985)

4. Goldsweig, H., Grossman, R., William, D., Thrombocytopenia in homosexual men. Am J Hematology 21:243-247 (1986)

5. Groopman, J., Mayer, K., Sarngadharan, M., et al., Clinical and laboratory manifestations of human T cell leukemia virus type III among homosexual men. Proc ASCO 64:97a (1984)

6. Goedert, J., Biggar, R., Weiss, S., et al., Three year incidence of AIDS in five cohorts of HTLV-III infected risk group members. Science 231:992-996 (1986)

7. Klein, R., Harris, C., Small, C., et al., Oral candidiasis in high risk patients as the initial manifestation of AIDS. N Engl J Med 311:354-358 (1984)

8. Raphael, B., M.D., Personal communication (1985)

9. Ahn, Y., Harrington, W., Simon, S., Danazol for the treatment of ITP. N Engl J Med 308:1396-1399 (1983)

10. Metroka, C., Moore, A., Risks with danazol in AIDS. Ann Intern Med 101:564 (1984)

11. Mintzer, D., Real, F., Jovino, L., et al., Treatment of Kaposi's sarcoma and thrombocytopenia with vincristine in patients with AIDS. Ann Intern Med 102:200-202 (1985)

12. Imbach, P., Barandun, S., d'Apuzzo, V., et al., High dose intravenous gammaglobulin for idiopathic thrombocytopenic purpura in childhood. Lancet 1:1228-1231 (1981)

13. Fehr, J., Hotmann, V., Kappeler, C., Transient reversal of thrombocytopenia in idiopathic thrombocytopenic purpura by high dose intravenous gammaglobulin. N Engl J Med 306:1254-1258 (1982)

14. Bussel J., Aledort, L., Hilgartner, M., et al., Long term maintenance of adults with ITP using intravenous gammaglobulin. Blood:66N5S1:287a (1985)

15. Minzler, D.M., Real, F.X., Jovino, L., et al., Treatment of Kaposi's sarcoma and thrombocytopenia with vincristine in patients with the acquired immunodeficiency syndrome. Ann Intern Med 102:200-202 (1985)

16. Delfraissy, J.F., Tertian, G., Dreyfus, M., et al., Intravenous gammaglobulin, thrombocytopenia, and the acquired immunodeficiency syndrome. Ann Intern Med 103:478 (1985)

17. Ordi, J., Vilardell, M., Aligjotas, J., et al., Serum thrombocytopenia and high dose immunoglobulin treatment. Ann Intern Med 104:282 (1986)

18. Oral, A., Rabin, B., Jacob, H., et al., Modification of T cell function in idiopathic thrombocytopenic purpura with intravenous immunoglobulin. Blood 66N5S1:295a (1985)

19. Baumann, M.A., Menitour, J.E., Aster, R.H., et al., Single dose gammaglobulin followed by allogeneic platelet transfusion for urgent treatment of ITP. Blood 66N5S1:285a (1985)

20. Wintrobe, M., Lee, G., Boggs, D., et al., Clinical Hematology. Lea and Febiger, Philadelphia, p 1094 (1981)

21. Walsh, C., Nardi, M., Karpatkin, S., On the mechanism of thrombocytopenic purpura in sexually active homosexual men. N Engl J Med 311:635-639 (1984)

22. McDougal, J., Hubbard, M., Nicholson, J., et al., Immune complexes in the acquired immunodeficiency syndrome: Relationship to disease in manifestation, risk group, and immunologic defect. J Clin Immunol 5:130-135 (1985)

23. Stricker, R., Abrams, D., Corash, L., et al., Target platelet antigen in homosexual men with immune thrombocytopenia. N Engl J Med 313:1375-1380 (1985)

24. Bender, B., Frank, N., Lawley, J., et al., Defective R-E system Fc-Receptor function in patients with AIDS. J Infect Dis 152:409-412 (1985)

25. Adams, W., Rufo., R, Talarico, L., Thrombocytopenia and intravenous herion use. Ann Intern Med 89:207-211 (1978)

26. Kraut, R., Bahler, J., Heroin induced thrombocytopenic purpura. Oral Surg 46:637-640 (1978)

27. Taeltle, R., Browning, S., Thrombocytopenia associated with intravenous heroin abuse. West J Med 131:62-64 (1979)

28. Fishman, A., Thrombocytopenia and heroin. Ann Intern Med 94:280-281 (1981)

29. Ryan, D., Heroin and thrombocytopenia. Ann Intern Med 90:852-853 (1979)

30. Savona, S., Nardi, M., Lynnette, E., et al., Thrombocytopenic purpura in narcotic addicts. Ann Intern Med 102:737-741 (1985)

31. Yu, J., Lynnette, E., Karpatkin, S., Anti $(Fab^1)_2$ antibodies in thrombocytopenic patients at risk for acquired immunodeficiency syndrome. J Clin Invest 77:1756-1761 (1986)

32. Spivak, J., Bender, B., Quinn, T., Hematologic abnormalities in the acquired immune deficiency syndrome. Am J Med 77:224-228 (1984)

33. Groopman, J., Salahuddin, S., Sarnagadharan, M., et al., Clinical and laboratory manifestations of human T cell leukemia virus type III among homosexual men. Blood 64 N5 S1:97a (1984)

34. Moore, A., Lymphoma in 16 homosexual men with acquired immune deficiency syndrome. Blood 62 N5 S1:115a (1983)

35. Hollander, H., Leukopenia, trimethoprim-sulfamethoxazole and folinic acid. Ann Intern Med 102:138 (1985)

36. Schreiber, Z., Loh, S.H., Charles, M., et al., Autoimmune hemolytic anemia with the acquired immune deficiency syndrome. Blood N5 S1:117a (1983)

37. Murphy, M.F., Metcalfe, P., Carne, C., et al., Neutropenia and HTLV-III infection: Association with disease activity and progression to AIDS. Blood 66 N5 S1:115a (1985)

38. Murphy, M.F., Metcaffe, P., Waters, A.H., et al., Immune neutropenia in homosexual men. Lancet 2:217-218 (1985)

39. Leiderman, I.Z., Greenberg, M.L., Adelsberg, B.R., et al., Inhibition of granulopoeisis by 84 KD glycoprotein. Blood 66 N5 S1:130a (1985)

40. Eshow, Z., Grunberger, T., Roifman, C., et al., Interleukin 2 responsive T cells modulate human marrow hematopoeisis. Blood 66 N5 S1:150a (1985)

41. Ellis, M., Gupta, S., Vanderen, C., et al., Decreased polymorphonuclear chemotaxis secondary to serum inhibition and abnormal bacterial killing in preacquired immunodeficiency syndrome (pre-AIDS) and AIDS. Blood 66:110a (1985)

42. Castella, A., Croxson, T., Mildvan, D., et al., The bone marrow in AIDS. Am J Clin Path 84:425-432 (1985)

43. Darne, C., Solal-Celigny, P., Herrera, A., et al., Acute myelofibrosis and infection with the lymphadenopathy-associated virus/human T-lymphotropic virus type III. Ann Intern Med 104:130-131 (1986)

44. Hromas, R., Murray, J., Bone marrow in the acquired immunodeficiency syndrome. Ann Intern Med 101:877 (1984)

45. Abrams, D., Chinn, E., Lewis, B., et al., Hematologic manifestations in homosexual men with Kaposi's sarcoma. Am J Clin Path 81:13-18 (1984)

46. Risdall, R., McKenna, R., Nebit, M.E., et al., Virus associated hemophagocytic syndrome. Cancer 44:993-1202 (1979)

47. Osborne, B., Guarda, L., Butler, J., Bone marrow biopsies in patients with the acquired immunodeficiency syndrome. Hum Path 15:1048-1053 (1984)

40
Cutaneous Manifestations of AIDS Other Than Kaposi's Sarcoma

Clay J. Cockerell

By now, most physicians have had either direct or indirect contact with one or more patients having the acquired immune deficiency syndrome (AIDS). Because the skin is affected commonly in AIDS, it is of utmost importance that the dermatologist, as well as the dermatopathologist, be able to recognize certain skin conditions at their earliest possible stages. A very high index of suspicion for opportunistic infections with unusual cutaneous or histologic manifestations must be maintained. In addition, the non-infectious cutaneous manifestations that are sometimes associated with the syndrome must be considered. Life-saving antimicrobial therapy or, in the future, immunomodulatory therapy may be introduced based on such findings.

This chapter will review some of the clinical and histopathologic manifestations of AIDS as they occur in the skin. It should be remembered, however, that many new manifestations are being described in an ongoing fashion.

The cutaneous manifestations of AIDS other than Kaposi's sarcoma can be broadly divided into two groups. The first of these is infectious diseases that affect the skin (Table 1). The second of these are non-infectious cutaneous disorders that may lead one to suspect a diagnosis of AIDS (Table 2). These will be discussed in sequence.

CUTANEOUS INFECTIONS

Cytomegalovirus Infection

Cytomegalovirus (CMV) is a common pathogen in immunocompromised patients, including those with AIDS. Systemic manifestations of CMV infection are more common than cutaneous, but the skin may be involved. Petechiae and purpura related to thrombocytopenia induced by CMV are the most common cutaneous signs of this viral infection. Although vesicular or bullous eruptions are seen, these are rare manifestations. A generalized morbilliform skin eruption involving the trunk and extremities is more common (1). Occasionally, hyperpigmented indurated cutaneous plaques have been reported as heralding disseminated CMV infection (2). In one case, a generalized bullous toxic epidermal necrolysis-like eruption occurred in association with CMV hepatitis in a patient with AIDS (3). Bluish-red cutaneous papules and nodules have been reported in association with CMV infection in children with AIDS during the neonatal period; these lesions consisted of foci of extramedullary hematopoietic tissue (4).

An important cutaneous manifestation of CMV infection is that of persistent perianal ulcerations which resemble the perianal ulcerations seen with anogenital *Herpes simplex* infection (Figure 1) (5). Unlike herpetic ulcerations, ulcers due to CMV do not respond to topical treatments such as sitz baths and compresses. In our experience, all patients with ulcers due to CMV also had coexistent intractable proctitis and/or colitis with severe diarrhea that was caused by enteric CMV infection. Thus, the CMV induced ulcers most likely represent contiguous spread of infection to the skin from the gastrointestinal tract. Patients with CMV ulcerations are usually initially thought to have *Herpes simplex* infection. Light microscopic and electron microscopic examination of biopsy specimens and/or virus isolation are required to confirm the diagnosis and pathogenesis.

Microscopically, there is ulceration of the overlying epithelium, and in the dermis or lamina propria, depending on the site, there is a dense inflammatory cell infiltrate containing numerous lymphocytes, histiocytes, neutrophils, eosinophils and plasma cells. There is also abundant granulation tissue. On careful inspection, the characteristic CMV infected cells can be found usually in the deep portion of the biopsy rather than in the epithelium; however, the epithelium may be affected. Infected cells are typically either fibroblasts or endothelial cells which may enlarge to one and one-half to two times normal size. Only rarely is a keratinocyte infected. Inclusions may be found in either the cytoplasm, the nucleus, or both. The intranuclear inclusion is an elongated round or oval structure that stains slightly purplish with the hematoxylin-eosin stain. It is characteristically surrounded by a clear halo, sharply demarcating it from the nuclear membrane. The cytoplasmic inclusions are smaller basophilic structures found in clusters. There may be either many or relatively few cells that display these characteristic inclusions (Figure 2).

The presence of CMV induced perianal ulcers has been associated with a grave prognosis. Although experimental treatment with dihydroxypropoxylmethylguanine (DHPG) has showed some effect on this lesion, nevertheless, most patients died within two months

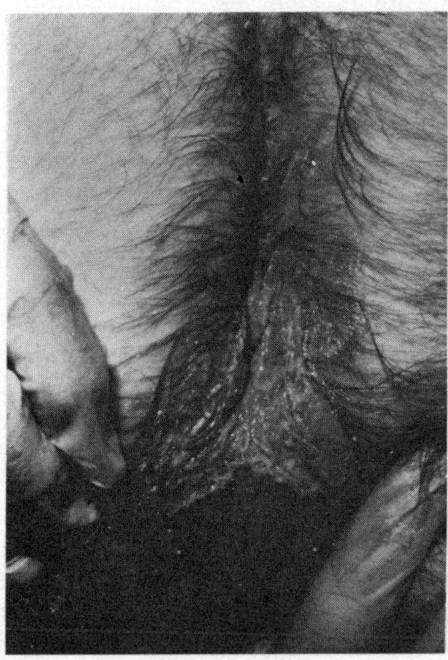

Figure 1. Perianal ulcerations caused by cytomegalovirus infection. These ulcerations are non-specific clinically and could be caused by a number of different organisms. When associated with persistent diarrhea in a patient with AIDS, a biopsy should be obtained to rule out cytomegalovirus infection.

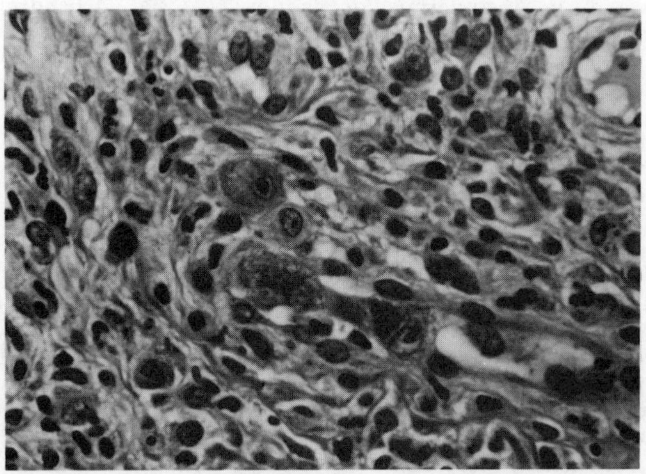

Figure 2. Fibroblasts infected with cytomegalovirus. Note the large rhomboidally-shaped intranuclear inclusion and small granular cytoplasmic inclusions. The cells are several times normal size

of diagnosis.

It should be remembered that occasionally skin ulcerations may be caused by more than one infectious agent. For example, it is not uncommon to find cells containing inclusions of CMV along with the characteristic multinucleated giant cells of *Herpes simplex* infection. In addition, one case has been reported where simultaneous infection occurred with acid fast bacilli, CMV and herpes virus (6). It is important to identify each individual infectious agent in order to give specific therapy.

Herpes Zoster and Herpes Simplex

Herpes zoster infection is thought to result from reactivation of a latent varicella-zoster virus infection in the dorsal root ganglion of patients with previous varicella infection. Zoster is usually manifested by painful clusters of vesicles in a localized neurodermatomal distribution. The vesicles often lie on a patch of erythema. In AIDS patients the initially localized zoster infection often becomes generalized with vesicles appearing at distant sites from the original dermatome involved. In some cases of disseminated zoster, lung and central nervous system involvement occurs. Often the patient will require hospitalization. The severe zoster infections seen in patients with AIDS or AIDS-related complex (ARC) tend to leave residual scars more often than is usually found in other patients; however, the incidence of post-herpetic neuralgia does not appear to be greater in AIDS patients despite the severity of the acute zoster infection.

Herpes zoster and *Herpes simplex* infections occur with greater frequency in patients with AIDS than in the normal population. It is known that herpes zoster infections also occur in other individuals with defects in cell-mediated immunity, such as in patients with Hodgkin's disease, chronic lymphocytic leukemia, and in iatrogenically immune-suppressed organ transplant recipients. Even otherwise "healthy" zoster patients have a diminished in vitro cell-mediated response to the varicella-zoster viral antigen during acute disease. The occurrence of herpes zoster infection in a patient from a high-risk group for developing AIDS may signal the possibility of the impending development of other AIDS related diseases (7).

Patients with AIDS, as well as those with other immunodeficiency disorders, are often plagued by severe recurrent *H. simplex* infections. These infections are often more extensive, last longer, and are less responsive to antiviral therapy with acyclovir than *H. simplex* infections occurring in healthy hosts (Figure 3).

When examining tissue histopathologically of patients suspected of having either varicella-zoster or *H. simplex* infection, rhomboidally-shaped eosinophilic intracytoplasmic inclusions should be looked for, as well as margination of the nucleoplasm against the nuclear membrane. Multinucleated epithelial giant cells are also characteristic (Figure 4). If an intact vesicle is seen, the multinucleated giant cells may be acantholytic and lie freely within the vesicle. The degree of inflammatory cell infiltrate varies with the stage of the infection. In fully developed ulcerations, there may be a dense inflammatory cell infiltrate consisting of lymphocytes, histiocytes, eosinophils, neutrophils and plasma cells. Early lesions may have only a sparse inflammatory cell infiltrate.

Although uncommon, *H. simplex* infection may also disseminate in AIDS patients with the entire skin surface becoming studded with individual lesions and clusters of erythematous papules and vesicles. Anogenital herpetic infections can be prolonged and painful, often with extensive ulcerations and erosions, which are susceptible to bacterial superinfection. Patients may require stool softeners and careful attention to maintenance of cleanliness in the infected area. Extensive herpetic infections are best treated with intravenous acyclovir; prophylaxis with oral acyclovir may be beneficial in reducing the number and frequency of recurrent attacks.

Molluscum Contagiosum

Molluscum contagiosum is an infection of the skin characterized by pearly, yellowish, waxy papular lesions often with a central umbilication, caused by a poxvirus which is spread by close contact. Mollusca contagiosa papules are commonly seen any place on the skin of children. In sexually active young adults, the pubic and inner thigh areas are frequently involved. In patients with AIDS, lesions of molluscum contagiosum are widely disseminated, being more numerous and often several times larger than those typically found in children. Occasionally, molluscum contagiosum may be confused with basal cell carcinomas or ordinary nevi. In order to make a definitive diagnosis, a biopsy is required. Histopathologically, characteristic purplish oval-shaped molluscum bodies are seen within the dilated infundibula of hair follicles. These follicles may coalesce to form the characteristic umbilicated papule. In general, molluscum papules are easily eradicated by simple curettage or cryosurgery with the topical application of liquid nitrogen; lesions found in AIDS patients, however, are frequently refractory to treatment and tend to recur and spread.

Verrucae vulgares and condylomata accuminata

Other viral skin infections, such as verrucae vulgares, are often seen in patients with AIDS. They tend to occur in the same areas as in healthy adults, but in greater numbers, and are often quite resistant to standard therapies. There are no data regarding which specific subtypes of human papilloma virus are involved. However, the warts may be of several different clinical varieties: extensive flat and filiform warts, often found in the bearded area of the face; exuberant cauliflower-like plaques of confluent condylomata accuminata in the anogenital region (Figure 5); or multiple and large hyperkeratotic verrucae vulgares, commonly seen on or around the fingers. Multiple plantar warts have

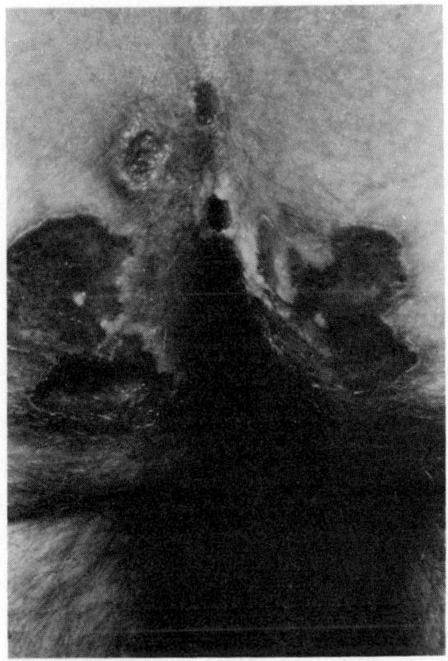

Figure 3. Perianal ulcerations caused by *Herpes simplex* virus infection. Deep, non-healing ulcerations caused by this agent are characteristically seen in patients with AIDS. These may appear identical to ulcerations caused by cytomegalovirus infection.

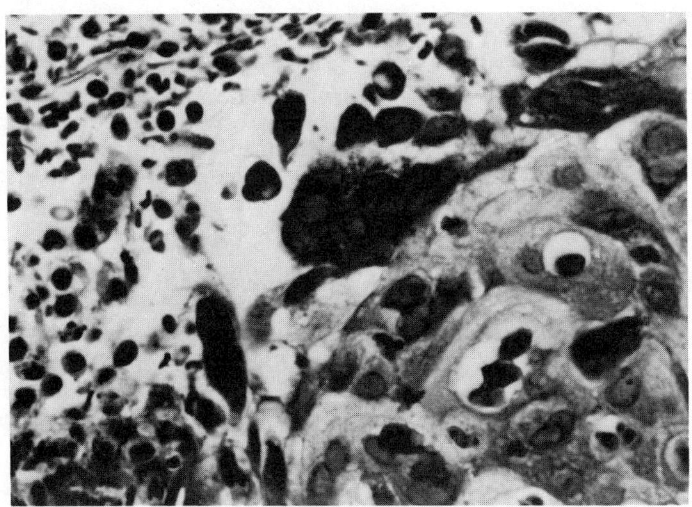

Figure 4. Multinucleated epithelial giant cell characteristic of herpes virus infection. These cells are pathognomonic of these infections

also been observed. If a biopsy is performed, the typical changes of verrucae vulgares or of condylomata accuminata are seen. Classically, digitated epidermal hyperplasia with dilated blood vessels and parakeratosis with hemorrhage at the tips of the papillae are found in common warts. There may also be koilocytosis and hypergranulosis in the epidermis. A gently papillated, slightly acanthotic epidermis with dilated blood vessels in the lamina propria are characteristic findings in condylomata accuminata. Occasionally, numerous atypical mitotic figures may be seen, raising the possibility of a form of squamous cell carcinoma in situ, Bowenoid papulosis. In light of the weakened immune system of these patients, if a diagnosis of Bowenoid papulosis is made, it would probably be wise to take more aggressive therapeutic measures, such as desiccation and curretage, to prevent the possible development of a more dangerous cutaneous neoplasm.

Hairy Leukoplakia

A unique oral mucosal lesion known as "hairy leukoplakia" has recently been described exclusively in AIDS patients or in those at risk for AIDS. Whitish, corrugated, verrucous plaques are seen on the lateral margins of the tongue and buccal mucosa (Figure 6) (8). Clinically, these lesions may resemble and may be misdiagnosed as candidiasis. Unlike thrush, when plaques of hairy leukoplakia are scraped with a tongue depressor or other blunt instrument, the whitish surface cannot be rubbed away. Histochemical and electron microscopic studies demonstrate the presence of human papilloma virus as well as Epstein-Barr virus particles in these lesions. It has been suggested that this unique mucosal lesion may be due to Epstein-Barr virus (9). Histologic examination of tissue is required for confirmation of the diagnosis. Microscopically, there is digitated epidermal hyperplasia with marked vacuolation of the mucosal epithelial cells. Tortuous dilated blood vessels are present within the digitations. Such a lesion may be confused with a mucosal verruca. Often, hyphae of *Candida albicans* may be superimposed on lesions of hairy leukoplakia. It is, therefore, important to do stains for fungi.

Folliculitis, Abscesses, Furuncles, and Impetigo

Because the B-cell arm of the immune system is defective in patients with AIDS, infections caused by common bacterial organisms, as well as those caused by more virulent bacteria, can cause serious, but not necessarily life-threatening diseases, in a given patient. Acneiform papules and pustules may be widely distributed over the trunk, extremities and face. Bacterial cultures of such lesions have been found to grow not only *Corynebacterium species* ("diphtheroids") but also *Staphylococcus aureus* and *Streptococcus pneumoniae*. In some cases, gram-negative organisms such as *Proteus species* were found. Like

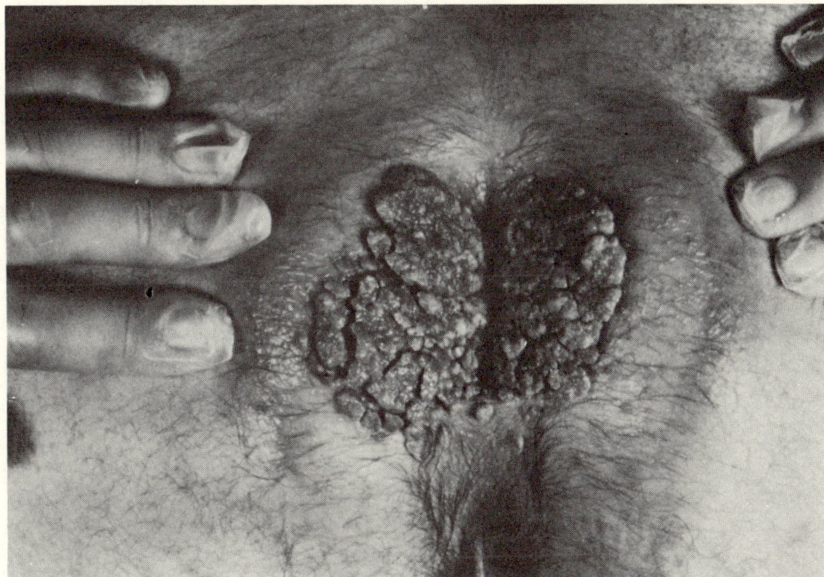

Figure 5. Condyloma accuminata. Infections from this common human papilloma virus may be very severe and result in anal obstruction.

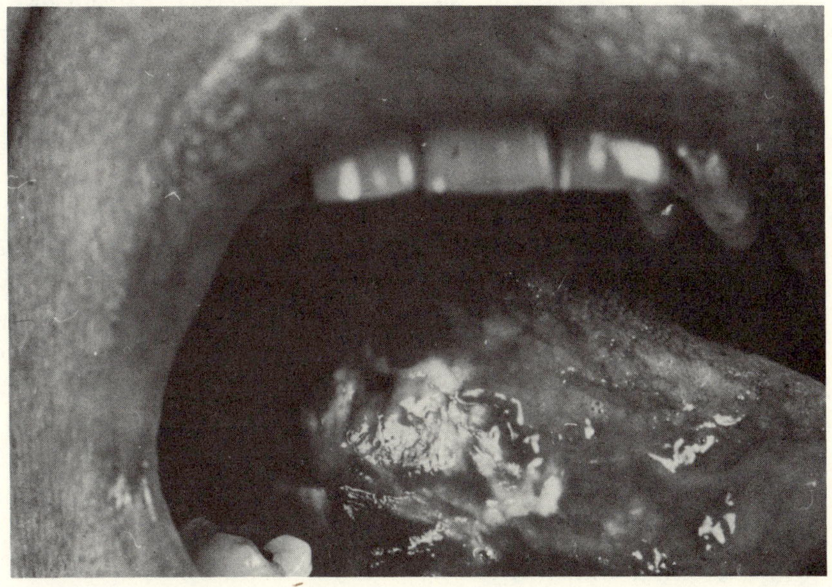

Figure 6. Hairy leukoplakia. A whitish verrucous plaque which does not rub away is characteristic of this condition.

many of the other infectious diseases encountered in the patient with AIDS, these bacterial infections are often refractory to usual therapeutic measures. Of interest is that in some cases a distinguishing feature of the histologic examination of pustules has been the presence of numerous eosinophils within the infundibula of hair follicles (10). The significance of this finding is not yet understood. In general, the usual findings include hair follicles filled with neutrophils and occasional lymphocytes and histiocytes. Often, there may be a dense acute inflammatory cell response present in the dermis surrounding the hair follicle.

Folliculitis may progress to form localized abscesses, furuncles and even carbuncles. Occasionally, cellulitis will supervene. Whereas an immunocompetent individual might be treated with oral antibiotics as an outpatient, the patient with AIDS often requires hospitalization and treatment with intravenous antimicrobial agents, since the risk of systemic spread of infection is much greater.

In determining the cause of an abscess, unusual opportunistic infectious organisms should be considered and cultures for bacteria, mycobacteria and fungi obtained. Clinically, one may not be able to distinguish an infection caused by staphylococcus from one caused by a mycobacterium. Delays in accurate diagnosis can be detrimental for the patient.

Another common skin infection childhood that is seen quite frequently among patients with AIDS is impetigo, which is caused by coagulase-positive staphylococci and/or by group A streptococci. While impetigo in children is seen most commonly on the face, in individuals at risk for AIDS and among patients with AIDS-related disease, impetigo is seen more often in the intertriginous, axillary and inguinal regions. Not infrequently, impetigo may be superimposed upon and may complicate a herpes infection of the skin. The infection usually begins as painful red macules which may develop into superficial vesicles that rupture, releasing serous or purulent fluid. A characteristic honey-colored surface crust forms and satellite and disseminated lesions develop. When biopsy material is obtained from such a lesion and examined histopathologically, a subcorneal vesicle containing scattered acantholytic keratinocytes with neutrophils, plasma cells and occasional bacteria is seen. When the lesions are fully crusted, a purulent scale-crust is present on the surface of an eroded epidermis. Usually, the infection responds readily to systemic antibiotics. However, in the patient with AIDS, therapeutic response may be delayed.

Mycobacterial Infections

Although extremely uncommon, AIDS patients with systemic mycobacterial infections may develop cutaneous lesions. Clinically, mycobacterial skin lesions appear as small papules and pustules that resemble folliculitis (11); however, cultures and specially stained biopsy specimens demonstrate mycobacteria. At our institution, four AIDS patients were found to have cutaneous

Table 1. Cutaneous and Mucosal Infections in AIDS
Abscesses
Candida infection (thrush)
Condylomata accuminata
Cryptococcosis
Cytomegalovirus infection
Dermatophyte infection
Folliculitis
Furuncles
Hairy leukoplakia
Herpes simplex infection
Histoplasmosis
Impetigo
Molluscum contagiosum
Mycobacterial infection
Plantar warts
Varicella-zoster infection
Verruca vulgaris

mycobacterial disease. All four were intravenous drug abusers. *Mycobacterium tuberculosis* was the cause in three cases and one had *Mycobacterium avium-intracellulare*. In the patients with *M. tuberculosis*, pustular lesions of the skin were secondary to reactivated pulmonary foci. Other cutaneous manifestations of tuberculosis, such as lupus vulgaris, are occasionally seen in patients with AIDS, albeit rarely.

Cutaneous mycobacterial lesions examined histopathologically, may show a granulomatous reaction with numerous multinucleated histiocytes surrounded by lymphocytes. This granulomatous dermatitis is present in the uppermost portion of the dermis and extends into the mid to lower reticular dermis associated with irregular psoriasiform hyperplasia and scale-crust. Alternatively, there may be a suppurative folliculitis in which neutrophils, histiocytes and eosinophils are present in the infundibula of hair follicles that rupture casing a granulomatous response in the dermis surrounding the follicles. In AIDS patients, stains for acid fast bacilli are usually positive, often showing innumerable organisms.

It should be reemphasized that individual tuberculous lesions appear virtually identical to those of simple folliculitis. Since the correct diagnosis can only be ascertained with certainty by culture or examination of tissue stained for acid fast bacilli, such studies should be performed on any patient with AIDS who has such lesions.

Superficial Fungal Infections

White patches on the buccal mucosa or tongue in a patient at risk for AIDS are suspicious for candidiasis (also known as moniliasis or thrush). The presence of thrush in a member of a risk group is a poor prognostic sign indicating a very high likelihood for the later development of AIDS (12). Clinically, oral candidiasis is characterized by whitish, curd-like exudates on the dorsal or lateral tongue, oro-pharynx, or buccal mucosa that can be easily scraped away with a cotton swab or tongue depressor. A reddish friable surface that may be associated with a burning sensation is found underneath the candidal exudate. Sometimes, only a beefy red, eroded surface of the tongue is seen and no exudate is evident. Microscopic examination of exudate shows numerous pseudohyphae and budding yeasts. Biopsy will reveal a dense infiltrate of lymphocytes, histiocytes and neutrophils is seen in the lamina propria with psoriasiform hyperplasia of the overlying epithelium. Spongiosis containing neutrophils with numerous yeast forms and pseudo-hyphae is found in the uppermost portion of the epithelium. *Candida species* can be easily demonstrated with periodic acid-Schiff (PAS) or Gomori methenamine silver stains. Oral candidiasis, with or without concomitant esophageal candidiasis, may be associated with dysphagia, which can lead to anorexia and consequent malnutrition. In addition to oral candidiasis, AIDS patients occasionally have cutaneous, perianal and vaginal candidal infections as well.

Treatment of thrush may be difficult since the condition often recurs following therapy. Oral administration of clotrimazole or nystatin may help to suppress candidal overgrowth. Ultimately, ketoconazole may be required.

In addition to *Candida species*, other fungi may cause severe cutaneous and/or systemic infections that fail to respond to available topical and systemic antifungal therapies. Widespread dermatophytosis, usually due to *Trichophyton rubrum*, involving palms, soles, nails, and intertriginous areas has been observed in individuals with, or at high risk, for AIDS. The histopathology of such infections is identical to that seen in patients who are non-immune compromised. A variably dense lympho-histiocytic infiltrate in the dermis is observed with psoriasiform epidermal hyperplasia, slight spongiosis, sometimes containing neutrophils, and parakeratosis containing neutrophils overlying the epidermis. With careful inspection, hyphae are often found between the parakeratotic and overlying orthokeratotic stratum corneum. Neither systemic griseofulvin nor topical antifungal medications have been found to be completely effective in eradicating such infections.

Systemic Fungal Infections

When highly pathogenic fungi, which often cause systemic disease in immuno-competent individuals, infect AIDS patients, the outcome may be fatal. The systemic fungal agents most commonly found among patients with AIDS are *Cryptococcus neoformans* and *Histoplasma capsulatum.*

Cryptococcosis is most often associated with meningitis and fungemia, but skin lesions may also occur. This fungus may cause single or multiple, red to purple, 5 mm to 1 cm, papules, nodules or indurated plaques of the integument that resemble the cutaneous lesions of bacterial cellulitis. Superficial erosion and crusting of cryptococcal skin lesions may be found. Another common presentation consists of widespread, skin-colored, dome-shaped, and sometimes slightly umbilicated papules that bear a striking resemblance to the papules of molluscum contagiosum (13). Occasionally, an AIDS patient may have cutaneous crytococcosis and molluscum contagiosum simultaneously, and individual lesions of each may be clinically indistinguishable. It is often necessary to examine histologically and culture biopsy samples of suspicious molluscum contagiosum papules to exclude the more serious diagnosis of cryptococcosis. Cutaneous involvement with cryptococcosis is distinctive histopathologically. In the papillary and reticular dermis are numerous clear staining areas that contain within them small hyperchromatic bodies which represent the viable component of the fungus. The clear staining material is the mucogelatinous capsule characteristic of *Cryptococcus neoformans.* There may be only a minimal inflammatory cell response to the fungus. The capsular material is best demonstrated with a mucicarmine stain which imparts a brilliant magenta to the capsule. Patients with cryptococcosis may vary from being totally asymptomatic to having one or more symptom complexes. Less severe illness includes subtle changes in personality and cognitive function or a poorly defined psychiatric illness. The most seriously ill have findings of overt meningitis or septicemia. Treatment of cryptococcosis requires systemic antifungal therapy with amphotericin B.

Cutaneous histoplasmosis is even rarer than cryptococcosis in patients with AIDS. Examination of the skin may reveal scattered acneiform papules, a widespread eruption of reddish macules and papules, or one to a few indurated, pinkish-red crusted plaques (14),(15). A specific diagnosis can only be made with certainty by fungal culture and/or histopathologic evaluation of biopsy specimens. Histopathologic examination may reveal an infiltrate of lymphocytes and histiocytes in the uppermost portion of the papillary dermis. Some of the histiocytes may have slightly vacuolated cytoplasm, and on careful inspection, small oval intracytoplasmic yeast cells can be seen. It is important to note that the fungus is quite difficult to visualize in hematoxylin and eosin stained sections, and special stains for fungi, as well as for acid fast bacilli, should be obtained. As in cryptococcosis, the inflammatory cell response may be relatively sparse. This may be a consequence of the invading organism itself or possibly the compromised state of the patient. It is important to alert the pathologist that the patient has, or is suspected of having AIDS, since the diagnosis of histoplasmosis can be subtle even with microscopic examination. As in the case with cryptococcosis, patients with cutaneous histoplasmosis may not be acutely ill or have any evidence of systemic involvement. AIDS patients with cutaneous histoplasmosis are usually not aware of prior pulmonary disease.

Any infectious disease in patients with AIDS may have an unusual appearance. The physician should maintain a high index of suspicion and should perform biopsies and viral, bacterial, mycobacterial and/or fungal cultures of any atypical skin lesion in order not to miss a potentially important infectious process.

NON-INFECTIOUS CUTANEOUS SIGNS

In addition to infectious diseases, a number of non-infectious cutaneous signs and symptoms have been described in patients with AIDS or ARC, such as non-specific severe pruritus or hives. It should be emphasized that AIDS should be included in the differential diagnosis when these complaints are elicited in members of high risk groups.

Table 2. Non-Infectious Non-Neoplastic Cutaneous Disorders in AIDS

Hives
Morbilliform drug eruption
Papular urticaria
Pruritus
Psoriasis
Seborrheic dermatitis-like eruption

Seborrheic Dermatitis-Like Eruption

One of the most commonly observed skin conditions associated with AIDS is an eruption that resembles serborrheic dermatitis, usually involving the scalp and face. This eruption appears as slightly indurated, diffuse, pinkish-red, scaly plaques (Figure 7). Occasionally, these may be large, thickened, and heavily crusted (16). This serborrheic dermatitis-like condition may occur on the upper anterior chest, back, groin, and on the extremities. The eruption tends to be somewhat refractory to the usual treatment modalities such as topical corticosteroids. In some patients, this eruption may be the first manifestation of AIDS. Histopathologically, the seborrheic dermatitis-like eruption seen in AIDS differs from that of ordinary seborrheic dermatitis in several respects. In AIDS patients there is usually a superficial perivascular lympho-histiocytic infiltrate with occasional plasma cells in the dermis (Figure 8,9). Slight psoriasiform hyperplasia of the epidermis is found. In contrast to non-AIDS-related seborrheic dermatitis, parakeratosis usually extends across the entire specimen rather than occurring only at the edges of the follicular ostia. A few neutrophils may also be present in the parakeratotic cornified layer. Of interest is that occasionally scattered necrotic keratinocytes are present within the epidermis (Figure 10). These cells, although not a constant finding in the seborrheic dermatitis-like eruption of AIDS, are highly suggestive of that entity.

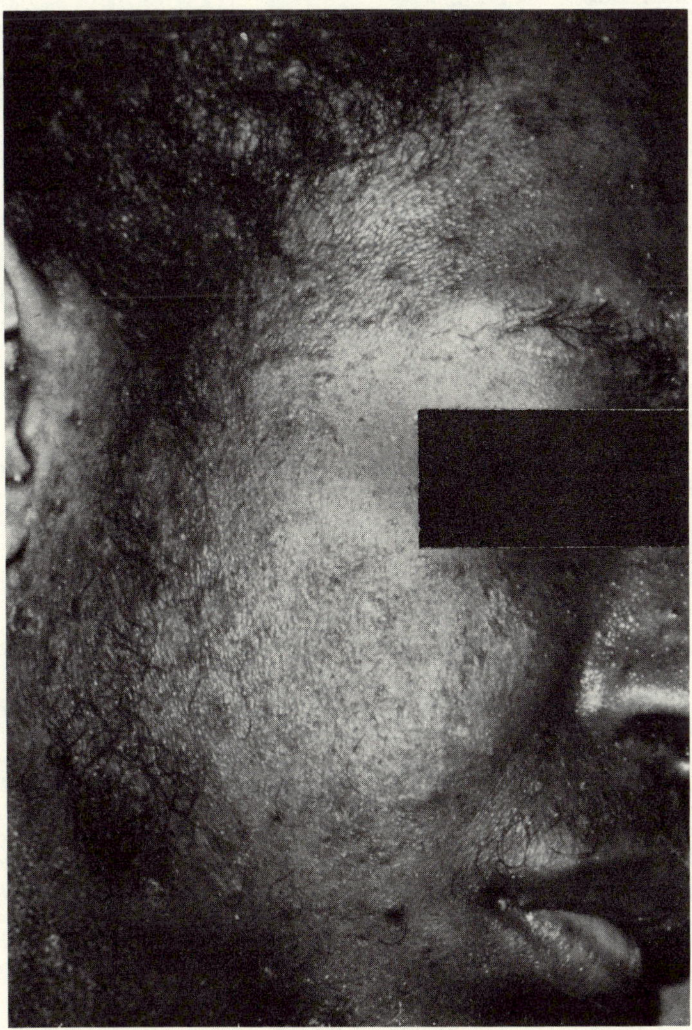

Figure 7. Seborrheic dermatitis-like eruption. An extensive eruption of scally pinkish plaques that is resistant to treatment is characteristic.

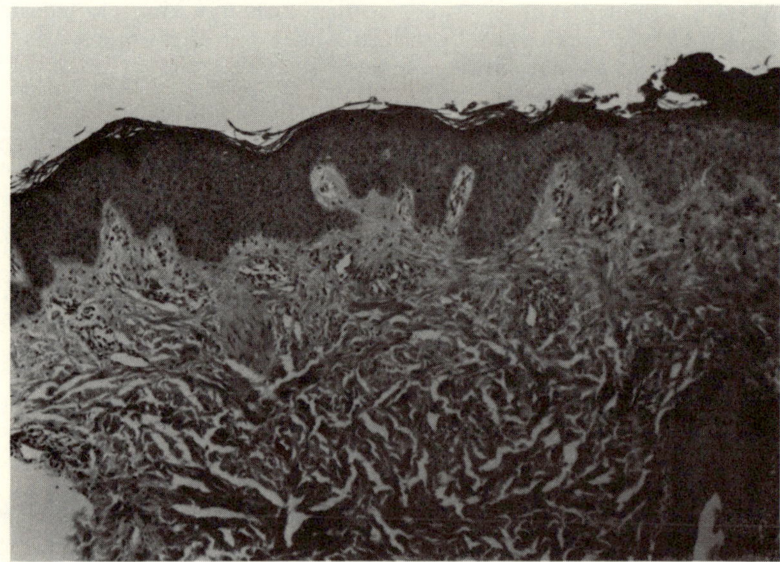

Figure 8. Seborrheic dermatitis-like eruption. The epidermis is hyperplastic and there is scale crust present over most of the specimen

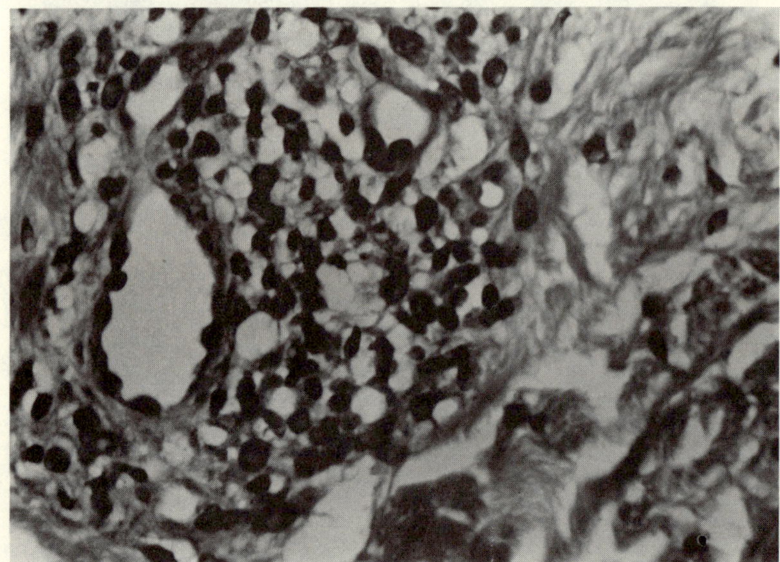

Figure 9. Seborrheic dermatitis-like eruption. An inflammatory cell infiltrate consisting of lymphocytes and plasma cells is highly characteristic of this condition

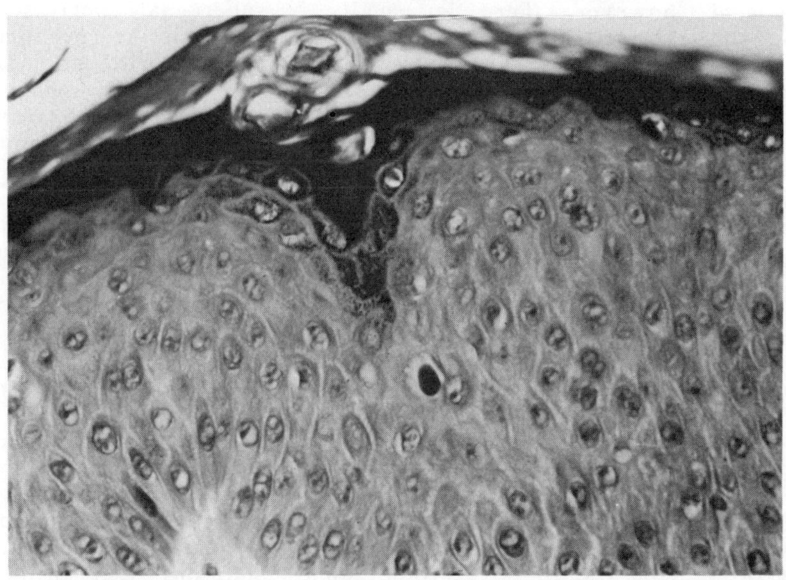

Figure 10. Seborrheic dermatitis-like eruption. Occasionally, necrotic keratinocytes, as pictured here, are seen scattered at random throughout the epidermis

When the eruption is especially florid, it may clinically resemble psoriasis; however, unlike psoriasis, the seborrheic dermatitis-like eruption does not involve extensor surfaces of the extremities, such as the elbows and knees, and has a superficial scale or crust rather than the thickened "micaceous" scale of typical psoriasis. Of course, patients with AIDS may also develop psoriasis, often of a severe and diffuse nature. In some individuals with a prior history of psoriasis, this condit- ion may be exacerbated and become widespread with the development of AIDS.

Morbilliform Drug Eruption

A widespread drug-related eruption consisting of pruritic, pinkish-red macules and papules, many often urticarial, frequently develops after administration of certain drugs in patients with AIDS. One agent which is especially likely to result in this complication is trimethoprim-sulfamethoxazole. Up to 60% of AIDS patients may develop a morbilliform drug eruption following administration of this medication (17). Although this drug eruption resembles the eruption which occurs from ampicillin in patients with infectious mononucleosis, no definite correlation with a viral infection has been established. Usually the clinical diagnosis of drug eruption is quite easily made, and for that reason, only rarely are such eruptions ever biopsied. When biopsied, however, there is usually a superficial, perivascular, slightly interstitial mixed-cell infiltrate consisting predominantly of lymphocytes, histiocytes and eosinophils with an occasional plasma cell. In some cases, there may be slight spongiosis of the epidermis, and sometimes the infiltrate in the dermis obscures the dermo-epidermal junction. On occasion, the eruption may be deep as well as superficial.

In some patients, the eruption will persist for several weeks, even months, after the drug has been discontinued. Both the high incidence and the tendency for persistence are distinguishing features in AIDS patients, compared to similar eruptions in normal populations. Treatment consists of antihistamines, cool compresses, emollients and topical steroids.

Papular Urticaria

One of the most peculiar and unusual, nonspecific cutaneous signs of AIDS is "papular urticaria," characterized by the onset of pruritic red to pink, urticarial, dome-shaped papules with a widespread distribution over the trunk and extremities. Individual lesions may resemble insect bites. The patients complain of severe pruritus, and like certain other conditions seen in AIDS patients, the symptoms, as well as the eruption are not readily responsive to conventional treatment modalities. The eruption may persist for several months, although the lesions may subside and recur intermittently. This cycle may continue relentlessly. Under the microscope, one sees a superficial and deep perivascular and interstitial mixed-cell infiltrate containing lymphocytes, histiocytes, eosinophils and occasional plasma cells. There may be slight spongiosis in the epidermis. There is often evidence of excoriation because of the intense pruritus. The histopathologic changes are, therefore, not specific, but they are most suggestive of insect bites.

CONCLUSION

In conclusion, AIDS is characterized by a number of unusual cutaneous manifestations that may, or may not, be related to underlying life-threatening conditions. It is essential that the dermatologist, as well as the dermatopathologist, be cognizant of both the clinical as well as the histopathological patterns of these conditions. Even though the prognosis of AIDS is grave, it remains an important part of the management of patients with this condition to recognize and treat both the infectious as well as the aggravating conditions.

ACKNOWLEDGMENT

Ellen C. Gendler, M.D., Clinical Instructor of Dermatology at New

York University Medical Center, assisted in the preparation of the sections on Herpes zoster and simplex, molluscum contagiosum, verrucae vulgares and condylomata accuminata, and impetigo.

Alvin E. Friedman-Kien, M.D., Professor of Dermatology at New York University Medical Center, also assisted in the preparation of this manuscript.

REFERENCES

1. Linn, C.S., Pinha, P.D., Krishnan, M.N., et al., Cytomegalic inclusion disease of the skin. Arch Derm 117:282-289 (1981)

2. Feldman, P.S., Walker, A.N., Baker, R., Cutaneous lesions heralding disseminated cytomegalovirus infection. J Am Acad Dermatol 7:545-550 (1982)

3. Muehler-Stamou, A., Sen, H.J., Emodi, G., Epidermolysis in a case of severe cytomegalovirus infection. Br Med J 3:609-612 (1974)

4. Medearis, D.N., Jr., Cytomegalic inclusion disease: An analysis of the clinical features based on the literature and six additional cases. Pediatrics 19:467-480 (1957)

5. Minars, N., Silverman, J.F., Escobar, N.R., et al., Fatal cytomegalic inclusion disease: associated skin manifestations in a renal transplant patient. Arch Dermatol 113:1569-1576 (1977)

6. Kwan, T.H., Kaufman, H.W., Acid fast bacilli with cytomegalovirus and herpes virus inclusions in the skin of an AIDS patient. Am J Clin Pathol 85:236-241 (1986)

7. Friedman-Kien, A.E., LaFleur, F.L., Gendler, E.C., et al., Herpes zoster: a possible early clinical sign for development of acquired immunodeficiency syndrome in high risk individuals. J Am Acad Dermatol 14:1023-1030 (1986)

8. Hollander, H., Schiodt, M., Greenspan, D., et al., Hairy leukoplakia and the acquired immunodeficiency syndrome. Ann Intern Med 104:892-895 (1986)

9. Greenspan, J.S., Greenspan, D., Lenette, E.T., et al., Replication of Epstein-Barr virus within the epithelial cells of oral "hairy" leukoplakia, an AIDS associated lesion. N Engl J Med 313:1564-1566 (1985)

10. Soeprono, F.F., Schinella, R.A., Eosinophilic pustular folliculitis and patients with acquired immunodeficiency syndrome. J Am Acad Dermatol 14:1020-1028 (1986)

11. Brown, F.S., Anderson, R.H., and Burnett, J.W., Cutaneous tuberculosis. J Am Acad Dermatol 6:101-106 (1982)

12. Klein, R.S., Harris, C.A., Small, C.B., et al., Oral candidiasis in high risk patients as the initial manifestation of the acquired immunodeficiency syndrome. N Engl J Med 311: 354-360 (1984)

13. Rico, N.J., Penneys, N.S., Cutaneous cryptococcosis resembling molluscum contagiosum in a patient with AIDS. Arch Derm 121:901-905 (1985)

14. Hazelhurst, J.A., Vismer, H.F., Histoplasmosis presenting with unusual skin lesions in acquired immunodeficiency syndrome (AIDS). Br J Dermatol 113:345-347 (1985)

15. Kalter, D.C., Tschen, J.A., Klima, M., Maculopapular rask in a patient with acquired immunodeficiency syndrome. Arch Dermatol 121:1455-1456 (1985)

16. Soeprono, F.F., Schinella, R.A., Cockerell, C.J., et al., Seborrheic-like dermatitis of acquired immunodeficiency syndrome. J Am Acad Dermatol 14:242-249 (1986)

17. Gordin, F.M., Simon, G.L., Wofsy, C.D., et al., Adverse reactions to trimethoprim-sulfamethoxazole in patients with the acquired immunodeficiency syndrome. Ann Intern Med 100:495-498 (1984)

41
HIV Disease in Childhood

Johanna Goldfarb, Asha Gupta

In 1983, a new syndrome was described in young children which had many similarities to the acquired immunodeficiency syndrome (AIDS) that had been recently described in adults (1),(2). These children had recurrent infections, failure-to-thrive, generalized lymphadenopathy, hepatosplenomegaly, parotid swelling and an interstitial pneumonitis. Acceptance of this apparently new entity in children as a pediatric AIDS was delayed in large part due to difficulty in distinguishing it from known congenital disorders in infancy. Over time, however, it was recognized that an epidemic of an immunodeficiency syndrome linked epidemiologically to adult cases of AIDS was occurring among children. Although the immunological spectrum of pediatric AIDS has similarities to that of adult AIDS, there is wide variation in the clinical illness and some unique features (3),(4). These unique characteristics also added to the initial confusion in linking pediatric cases to the AIDS epidemic. With the discovery of the causative agent, human immunodeficiency virus (HIV) (5),(6), the relationship of pediatric AIDS to adult AIDS has been confirmed.

CASE DEFINITION AND INCIDENCE

The Centers for Disease Control's (CDC) definition of pediatric AIDS requires the presence of either an opportunistic infection or a malignancy (such as Kaposi's sarcoma), at least moderately indicative of a cellular immunodeficiency state in a child less than 13 years of age. In addition, a primary or secondary immunodeficiency state from a congenital infection or other known cause besides HIV infection, must be excluded. The presence of a chronic lymphocytic interstitial pneumonitis (LIP) proven by lung biopsy was added to the definition of pediatric AIDS in June 1985. HIV infection (usually a positive HIV serology) should also be documented (7) (Table 1). From January 1982 to January 1985, 99 cases, or about 1% of total AIDS cases reported to the CDC were in children. The number increased to 231 or about 1.5% of the total cases by January 1986. This increase in reported cases was partly due to better recognition of the disease and partly due to the inclusion of LIP as a diagnostic criterion (7),(8).

Table 1. Provisional Case Definition for Acquired Immunodeficiency Syndrome (AIDS) Surveillance of Children (Ref 7)

For the limited purposes of epidemiologic surveillance, CDC defines a case of pediatric acquired immunodeficiency syndrome (AIDS) as a child who has had:

1. A reliably diagnosed disease at least moderately indicative of underlying cellular immunodeficiency; and

2. No known cause of underlying cellular immunodeficiency or any other reduced resistance reported to be associated with that disease.

The diseases accepted as sufficiently indicative of underlying cellular immunodeficiency are the same as those used in defining AIDS in adults. In the absence of these opportunistic diseases, a histologically confirmed diagnosis of chronic lymphoid interstitial pneumonitis will be considered indicative of AIDS unless test(s) for HIV are negative. Congenital infections, e.g., toxoplasmosis or *Herpes simplex* virus infection in the first month after birth or cytomegalovirus infection in the first six months after birth must be excluded.

Specific conditions that must be excluded in a child are:

1. Primary immunodeficiency diseases: severe combined immunodeficiency, DiGeorge syndrome, Wiskott-Aldrich syndrome, ataxia-telangiectasia, graft versus host disease, neutropenia, neutrophil function abnormality, agammaglobulinemia, or hypogammaglobulinemia with raised IgM.

2. Secondary immunodeficiency associated with immunosuppressive therapy, lymphoreticular malignancy, or starvation.

CDC statistics, however, clearly underestimate the number of symptomatic children with HIV infection. Many children with severe and even fatal disease associated with HIV infection are excluded by the CDC definition. In children, unlike adults, recurrent bacterial infections may occur in the absence of an opportunistic infection or malignancy and are not infrequently a cause of death. Also, in children, direct involvement of the central nervous system with HIV causes a distinctive syndrome which may occur without other CDC criteria for AIDS. As in adults, precisely defining this AIDS related complex of symptoms and signs (ARC) is difficult. Features of ARC in HIV positive children include: diffuse lymphadenopathy, hepatosplenomegaly, parotid swelling, autoimmune phenomena such as idiopathic thrombocytopenia purpura, a specific degenerative neurological syndrome and recurrent life threatening bacterial infections (9),(10).

TRANSMISSION

Of the 231 cases of pediatric AIDS accepted by the CDC as of January 1986, 75% were from the states of New York, New Jersey, California, and Florida. This geographical distribution parallels that of adult AIDS cases. Seventy-five percent of children had at least one parent who had AIDS or who was at increased risk for AIDS. Transfusion recipients (of blood or blood products) accounted for 20% of the total, a much higher proportion than the 1-2% seen in adult cases. As in adults, the risk factors are undetermined or unknown in about 5% of cases. This appears to be largely due to incomplete medical histories. The ratio of male to female cases is about equal in pediatric cases (8).

The epidemiology of AIDS in children suggests that in utero infection is the major route of transmission of HIV. Direct evidence for this includes demonstration of HIV viral antigen by immunological techniques in the tissue of a 20 day old premature baby delivered by cesarian section to a mother dying of AIDS (11) and actual isolation of the virus from the tissues of a 20 week fetus electively aborted of an HIV positive heroin addict (12). Indirect evidence includes the presence of AIDS and/or positive HIV serology in mothers of affected children and the observation that delivery by cesarean section and separation immediately after birth from an HIV infected mother was not protective of a child (13).

Onset of disease in congenitally infected children may occur early, often within the first three to four months of age. Most children are symptomatic by one year of age and by three years of age, approximately 80% are ill (10). Earlier dates of onset are found in cases presumed to be infected in the perinatal period compared to cases that are transfusion related, suggesting that the incubation period is shorter in perinatal infection. We have seen one baby (born to a woman with AIDS) who appeared to have severe HIV infection at birth, a case example of in utero transmission of virus (unpublished observation).

Theoretically, HIV transmission could occur during delivery. Indeed, other viruses, such as hepatitis B and *Herpes simplex*, are transmitted primarily during delivery. If this mode of transmission of HIV is proven, and if uninfected fetuses could be identified at term, elective cesarean sections might become a preventive measure. However, at present, it appears that transmission occurs predominantly in utero. Studies to elucidate this point are under way.

Transmission of virus through breastfeeding has been suggested by one reported case. A previously well woman without risk factors for AIDS received blood from an infected donor immediately after a cesarean section. Prepartum serologies from the mother were not available, but both she and her breastfed baby had positive serologies to HIV when tested more than a year later (14). Since some viruses can be transmitted during breastfeeding (eg., cytomegalovirus (CMV), rubella), this mode of transmission is possible and further study is warranted. The safety of breastfeeding during maternal HIV infection can not be assumed and probably is not advisable.

The majority of cases acquired by other than perinatal transmission are transfusion related cases, which account for about one-fifth of the total cases of pediatric AIDS. Many of these children received blood products as sick or premature newborns, but a significant number (about 5%) are hemophiliacs who have been on chronic clotting factor replacement therapy (15)-(19). As with adult cases, where blood transfusions have been traced a donor with risk factors for AIDS has been found and a positive HIV serology documented (15)-(19). The risk of developing AIDS after transfusion of infected blood products is unknown. Incubation periods may be shorter in childhood than in adult transfusion cases. Most of these young patients had received transfusions in the neonatal period, correlating with the period of greatest risk for multiple transfusions in the pediatric age group. Newborns are relatively immunoincompetent which might be important in explaining the somewhat shorter incubation period. However, there is undoubtedly great variability and at least one case of AIDS has occurred five years after a neonatal transfusion (20).

Transmission patterns of HIV in adolescents are similar to that of adults, with sexual contact accounting for about one-half of the cases, and parenteral exposure (blood product transfusion or intravenous drug abuse) the other major risk factor. How many older children will develop AIDS as a result of congenital infection is unknown. Cases in school age children have been seen which appear to be due to transmission in utero with a prolonged incubation period. These cases are unusual at present, and other routes of transmission, such as sexual abuse and exposure to contaminated needles, should be considered. Several studies have consistently demonstrated lack of seroconversion in household contacts of AIDS patients who had intimate but non-sexual exposures. In all age groups, therefore, including childhood, casual contact has not been associated with transmission of virus or disease (21)-(23).

CLINICAL PICTURE

Children with HIV disease are usually brought to medical attention because of an increased number of bacterial infections or because of an opportunistic infection. Rarely, neurological involvement, autoimmune phenomena or failure-to-thrive may be presenting signs. An individual child may have all or some of the clinical features discussed below.

The majority of children with HIV disease present in infancy, usually between four months and one year of age, with a few diagnosed later, up to five years of age and perhaps with time, even later. A significant number of children with congenital infection have been small for gestational age, but this appears to correlate with maternal drug abuse and may not be a direct effect of HIV (1)-(4). History of a parent with AIDS or risk factors for AIDS, or a history of transfusions in the several year period prior to onset of illness is helpful in considering the diagnosis in childhood.

Signs and Symptoms

Most children with HIV disease begin to grow poorly coincident with the development of other signs of disease. Some fail to gain weight normally while others lose weight and become wasted. Infants who were small for gestational age at birth frequently grow poorly from the start. We have seen one infant born with microcephaly, intracranial calcifications in the region of the basal ganglia, hepatosplenomegaly and autoimmune thrombocytopenia with no other apparent cause for these findings other than congenital HIV infection (unpublished observation). Most children with HIV disease, however, appear normal at birth.

With some exceptions, diffuse lymphadenopathy, often with hepatosplenomegaly, is present early on, frequently before the onset of other significant signs of disease. Bilateral parotid swelling has been described in some, perhaps 20%, but not all children with AIDS. Presumably this is due to lymphocytic infiltration of the glands. This clinical sign varies over time, often worsening during episodes of systemic infection and is one finding unique to children with AIDS.

Also distinctive to pediatric HIV disease is a chronic interstitial pneumonitis. Interstitial infiltrates on chest radiograph were reported in all of the original cases (1),(2) and in about one-half of the present CDC cases (8). Clinically, LIP may be asymptomatic but has been associated with hypoxemia with or without signs of respiratory distress. Among 11 pediatric patients we follow with HIV disease at the Westchester County Medical Center, four have had chronic interstitial infiltrates on chest x-ray (Figures 1, 2a, 2b).

Neurological disease in children with HIV disease, as in adults, can be due to direct involvement of HIV in the central nervous system (24). HIV apart from being tropic for the helper T lymphocyte, also appears to have an affinity for neural tissue. Shaw et al. were able to demonstrate the presence of the

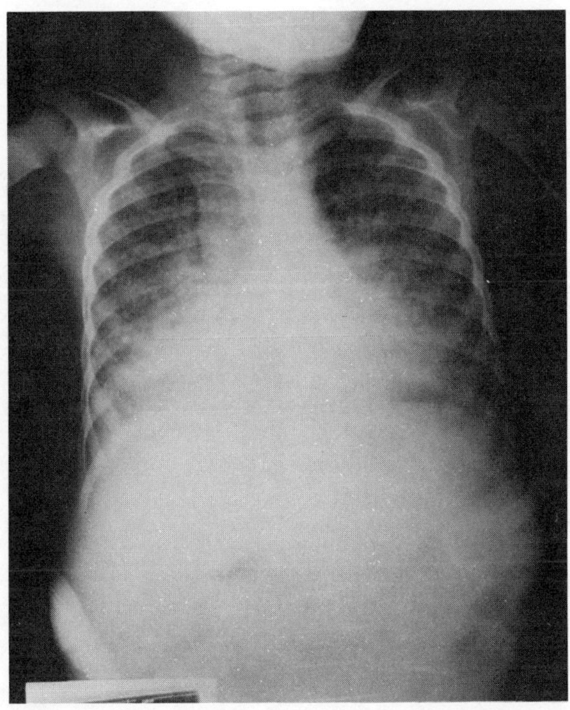

Figure 1. Chest roentgenogram of a five year-old child with AIDS and both lymphocytic interstitial pneumonitis and *Pneumocystis carinii* pneumonia.

viral genome in brain tissue of adults and children with AIDS and neurological disease (24). In adults, this involvement presents predominately as a progressive dementia. In children, there is a progressive encephalopathy beginning with mild spasticity and increased deep tendon reflexes. Loss of acquired major motor milestones with prominent pyramidal tract signs and lack of speech development follows thereafter. Eventually, the child may be left severely spastic with quadriplegia, without speech, but with an alert and aware affect. Routine studies of cerebrospinal fluid such as cell count and protein determination are usually unremarkable. Computerized tomography of the brain shows calcifications of the basal ganglia with varying degrees of cortical atrophy (25)-(27). This syndrome, which evolves over months in a child with previously normal development, is striking and distinctive for HIV disease.

Children, like adults with AIDS, have an increased incidence of autoimmune phenomena, such as thrombocytopenia and hemolytic anemia. Bone marrow examination may be useful in evaluating these conditions and in excluding infectious causes of pancytopenia in specific cases.

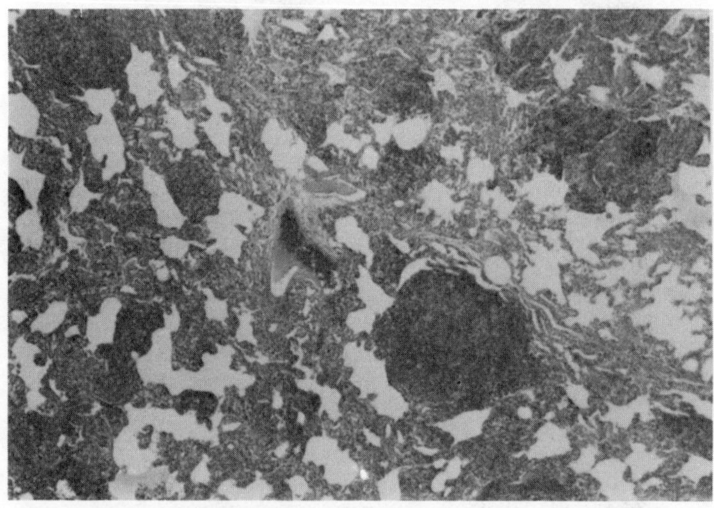

Figure 2a. Low power view of histologic section of lung in a child with lymphocytic interstitial pneumonitis (LIP)

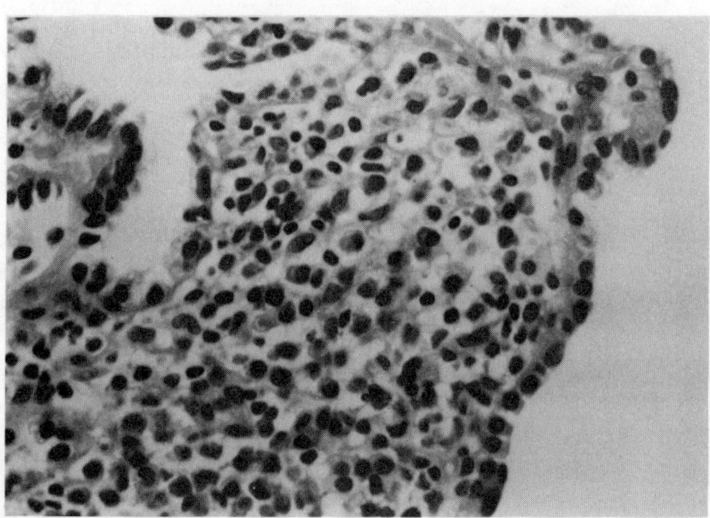

Figure 2b. Higher power view of same section of lung as in Figure 2a. There is marked infiltration of alveolar septae by mononuclear cells, mainly lymphocytes and plasma cells, focally forming nodular and/or sheet-like aggregates. Alveolar lining cells show bronchial metaplasia

An unexplained cardiomyopathy with enlarged cardiac silhouette on chest roentgenogram and poor muscle function on echocardiography has been present in three of our 11 patients with HIV disease. One has required digitalis and diuretic therapy for congestive failure. Known causes of cardiomyopathy such as CMV infection or toxoplasmosis are possible but not apparent in our cases.

Kaposi's sarcoma, common in adults with AIDS (especially in homosexual men), is rare in children with AIDS, but has occurred, as have other malignancies, such as non-Hodgkin's lymphoma.

Chronic diarrhea is also common and may be due to chronic bacterial or parasitic infections, such as salmonella enteritis and cryptosporidiosis, but may also be non-specific and without definite etiology. Diarrhea may add to the wasting and malnutrition seen in some children with HIV disease (28).

Recurrent bacterial infections and chronic oral candida infections are found in most children with HIV disease, and are discussed below.

INFECTIOUS DISEASE COMPLICATIONS

The spectrum of opportunistic infections seen in HIV disease in children is similar to that seen in adults and includes many previously exotic pathogens. As in adults, certain infections predominate. *Pneumocystis carinii* pneumonia (PCP) was present in 58% of CDC cases of pediatric AIDS reported as of January 1986, many of whom had disseminated infection with CMV simultaneously. Candida esophagitis occurred in 15% and cryptosporidiosis in 6% (8). Other opportunistic infections have included severe *Herpes simplex* stomatitis, progressive varicella-zoster infection, and disseminated *Mycobacterium avium-intracellulare* infection. Toxoplasmosis, so common in adults, is rare in pediatric cases.

Most striking, however, is the role of non-opportunistic pathogens in pediatric HIV disease. Bacterial infections, often recurrent and frequently life-threatening, are extremely common, accounting for significant morbidity and mortality. In one series of 46 children with either AIDS or ARC, 27 episodes of sepsis occurred in 21 patients, including five cases of meningitis (29). Other infections in that series included bacterial pneumonia, urinary tract infection, cellulitis, impetigo, perinephric abscess and enterocolitis. The pneumococcus appears to be the single most common bacterial pathogen. In our series of 11 patients, pneumococcal sepsis was documented in three patients, with one child dying of pneumococcal meningitis and sepsis. Another child has had three separate episodes of pneumococcal sepsis. Pneumococcal endocarditis occurred in a third child. Six of the 11 children have had recurrent otitis media, two with perforated tympanic membranes with isolation of *Streptococcus pneumoniae* from the purulent middle ear drainage. Episodes of lobar pneumonia have occurred in five patients. *Staphylococcus aureus* sepsis occurred in one patient and a second patient had *S. aureus* pneumonia.

The role of prophylactic antibiotics in these children remains to be determined, but may be important in preventing both minor and life-threatening infections. Certainly, the febrile child with AIDS who appears acutely ill and who is admitted to the hospital should be treated empirically with antibiotics to cover routine pediatric pathogens including *S. pneumoniae, Hemophilus influenzae, S. aureus*, and perhaps also *Salmonella species* when gastrointestinal complaints or signs are present. We have maintained younger children, those at greatest risk for bacteremia, and other children with episodes of recurrent otitis media or bacteremia, on chronic oral antibiotic therapy. While episodes of otitis media have occurred despite oral therapy, in our experience, bacteremia has been seen only in children not on prophylaxis.

We have used amoxicillin or penicillin most often for prophylaxis. Because of concerns about using trimethoprim/sulfamethoxazole (TMP/SMX) in patients with AIDS who have a higher than normal risk for adverse reactions to this drug (30), and also because it is intrinsically less safe when used chronically, we have avoided its long-term use. We reserve TMP/SMX for cases where PCP has occurred and where the patient tolerated the drug. Rarely a child who is allergic to the penicillins and cephalosporins has been kept on TMP/SMX chronically as bacterial prophylaxis. The use of intravenous gamma globulin has been advocated and may also decrease the number of bacterial infections (29). The use of either modality awaits confirmation of effectiveness in controlled studies.

Candidiasis

Oral candidiasis is probably the most commonly seen infection in children with HIV disease, almost universally present at some point. As in adults, the infection can be severe and may involve the esophagus. The infection is frequently resistant to conventional oral nystatin therapy, but usually responds to oral ketoconazole. Chronic administration of ketoconazole is frequently necessary and has been well tolerated in children, except in those with an underlying hepatitis.

Varicella-Zoster

Three of our children with HIV disease had varicella (chickenpox) prior to being diagnosed as having an immune deficiency. These children handled their infections without complications and healed spontaneously. One subsequently had a severe episode of shingles and was treated and responded to intravenous acyclovir. Varicella-zoster infection in the immuno-compromised child, however, is potentially life-threatening. There is a 7% mortality in the non-AIDS immunocompromised child. Lymphopenia is a risk factor for severe disease and death in such children (31). Children with HIV disease are also at risk for severe disease especially with primary infection. Varicella-zoster immune globulin should be given on exposure to chickenpox or shingles, and high dose acyclovir started if the disease develops. The new experimental chickenpox vaccines are live virus vaccines and are, therefore, contraindicated in children with HIV induced immunodeficiency. Unlike the situation in children on chemotherapy who have been successfully vaccinated, the immunodeficiency of HIV disease can not be reversed during the vaccine period. Also an immune response is unlikely to occur in children with HIV infection because of the associated severe B cell dysfunction.

Herpes Simplex

Primary *Herpes simplex* infection in childhood normally causes minimal local signs but may cause a severe stomatitis, which occasionally, especially in infancy, may require hospitalization for treatment of dehydration due to poor fluid intake. Children with HIV disease, like other immunodeficient children will frequently have a prolonged course with poor spontaneous healing. Intravenous acyclovir is very effective in such cases with prompt response to even low dose therapy. Recurrences after stopping therapy may necessitate retreatment, and oral prophylactic therapy may be useful.

Pneumocystis Carinii Pneumonia (PCP)

The prevalence of PCP in children with AIDS may be somewhat overestimated by the CDC figures because of the weighted case definition for those with proven opportunistic infection. However, clearly PCP is the most common opportunistic infection in children with AIDS from the United States, as it is in adults. The presence of fever and a peri-hilar interstitial pneumonia in a child with hypoxia is very suggestive of this diagnosis. LIP may be difficult to differentiate and may occur together with PCP. Lung biopsy is the most specific method to differentiate between these entities and is also necessary to diagnose other co-existing pathogens, especially CMV infection. Empiric therapy with TMP/SMX for interstitial pneumonias in these children is appropriate. Biopsy should probably be done, however, prior to initiating pentamidine treatment in children not responding to TMP/SMX. This will help to confirm the presence or absence of PCP and may also aid in diagnosing other treatable infections. PCP is a major cause of death in children, as in adults with AIDS, despite appropriate therapy.

IMMUNOLOGICAL MANIFESTATIONS

Abnormalities of both the cellular and the humoral components of the immune system have been seen in children with HIV disease. Lymphopenia, an almost uniform finding in adult AIDS, is not frequently present in children. When a decrease in the peripheral lymphocyte count is seen, usually late in the course of disease, it is due (as in adults) to a diminution of T cells bearing the helper/inducer phenotype OKT4 (1). This selective decrease of the helper set causes a relative increase in the proportion of the other major T cell subset, the suppressor/cytotoxic T cell identified by the monoclonal antibody OKT8. This causes a reduced or reversed T4/T8 ratio. In conjunction with other clinical features, such an inverted ratio is highly suggestive of HIV disease. It is, however, not diagnostic and may be seen in other viral diseases such as CMV and Epstein-Barr virus (EBV) infections (32). With viral infections, however, the reversal is usually caused by a relative increase in the OKT8 subset and may, therefore, be differentiated from the pattern seen in AIDS.

The loss of normal T cell function correlates clinically with the presence of unusual opportunistic, parasitic and viral infections. In adult patients a T cell defect is easily demonstrated at the bedside by the patient's inability to mount a delayed hypersensitivity skin test response to ubiquitously present antigens like candida and trichophyton (33). With young children, however, skin testing is of limited value as the absence of response may signify only lack of exposure to particular antigens (34). Therefore, in children, although the ability to mount a positive skin test to an antigen is indicative of intact T cell function, failure to do so cannot be accepted as proof of T cell dysfunction. In vitro tests of T cell function are more indicative of true abnormalities. Mitogens such as phytohemagglutinin, concanavalin A (con A) and pokeweed mitogen (PWM), require no prior exposure to stimulate lymphocyte blastogenesis and a good response is seen in the normal newborn (33). Children with AIDS have a reduced response, with the greatest reduction occurring to PWM, a T cell dependent B cell mitogen. This observation suggests a defect in helper cell function (1).

In vitro response to antigens such as candida, purified protein derivative (PPD), or streptokinase-streptodornase (SKSD) are also reduced in children with AIDS compared to age matched controls (1). However, like skin tests, the absence of such a response in a young child may indicate only lack of prior exposure and must be interpreted in light of other available clinical data (eg. absence of response to candida in a child with candida sepsis or absence of response to PPD in a child with tuberculosis).

The ability of lymphocytes to respond to alloantigens or the ability of an individual to reject a foreign graft is normally present in children at a very young age, and the inability to mount such a response represents a profound defect in T cell function. Mixed lymphocyte responses which are an in vitro correlate have been studied in a limited number of children with HIV disease and were found to be suboptimal (1).

A frequent and useful marker of pediatric HIV disease is the presence of hypergammaglobulinemia. This occurs despite the presence of a relative increase in the number of suppressor cells, suggesting suppressor cell dysfunction. The suppressor T cell may not be suppressing immunoglobulin producing B cells normally. Gupta et al. studied the suppressive action of T cells from children with HIV disease in vitro and found this activity to be abnormally low (35). A possible explanation for the lack of suppression is that the subset of helper T cells responsible for initiating suppressor cell function is diminished (36).

Abnormalities in the humoral immune system are also present in children with HIV disease (37). This correlates clinically with an increased number of infections due to pyogenic bacteria (29). As mentioned, hypergammaglobulinemia is very common in pediatric HIV disease with levels of IgG in the range of 3000-4000 mg/dL. Increases in levels of IgA and IgD are also seen. These high levels of immunoglobulins, however, are ineffective clinically. B cells in these patients are in a constant state of activation without any guidance from T cells. Although capable of secreting immunoglobulins spontaneously in vitro (37), they do not synthesize specific antibodies in response to antigenic challenge (35), (37).

Bernstein et al. (37) assessed specific antibody production in six children with HIV infection by immunizing them with bacteriophage phi x 174, a T cell dependent neoantigen, and also with pneumococcal vaccine (which stimulates B cells directly). Responses were abnormal in all patients: primary responses were blunted, secondary responses were markedly decreased, and the class switch (IgM-IgG) was absent in five of six. Other investigators have demonstrated a similar defect in response to the neoantigen keyhole limpet hemocyanin (KLH) in adult patients with AIDS (38). Thus, B cells in children with HIV disease are already activated, proliferating and secreting immunoglobulins, but are incapable of responding to signals that normally trigger resting B cells (38). Indication of B cell proliferation is also found in the increased incidence of B cell lymphomas in these patients.

The degree of polyclonal activation of cells, along with clinical evidence of lymphoproliferation, suggests direct viral infection and transformation of B cells as seen in EBV infection. Montagnier et al. demonstrated that EBV-transformed B cell lines are readily infected with HIV (39). EBV can be isolated from throat washings of 90% of adult AIDS patients (40) and EBV DNA has been found in lung biopsy specimens from children with LIP (41). Therefore, the polyclonal proliferation of B cells may be due to concurrent infection with EBV and HIV.

DIFFERENTIAL DIAGNOSIS

Two groups of conditions must be differentiated from pediatric HIV disease. These are: 1) primary immunodeficiency disorders, and 2) immunodeficiency states secondary to congenital infections other than HIV. Nezeloff's syndrome is an ill-defined syndrome of defective T cell immunity with normal levels of serum antibodies, which may be confused with HIV disease in a particular child. The characteristics of HIV disease that set it apart from primary immunodeficiencies are: A) the presence of risk factors in the child or parent, B) distinctive clinical features which may include: parotid swelling, LIP, degenerative neurological syndrome, and C) the immunological findings, specifically the extremely high gamma globulin levels seen in HIV disease and the lack of findings associated with primary immunodeficiency states, such as impaired maturation of the T cell system, or abnormal erythrocyte adenosine deaminase and purine nucleoside phosphorylase levels. In addition, while thymulin levels are decreased as in other congenital thymic deficiencies, thymosin alpha 1 levels, which are diminished in all other thymic congenital disorders, are markedly elevated in AIDS (42) (also see page 314).

In the young infant, differentiation from other immunosuppressive congenital infections, such as CMV or rubella, can be made by serologic or culture techniques. Introduction of HIV antibody testing has made the diagnosis much easier. In the newborn or infant under seven months of age, however, the presence of antibody can represent transplacentally transferred antibody and not true infection. Techniques that may help resolve whether antibody represents infection or passive transfer include:

1. Demonstration of HIV antibody of the IgM class in the baby.

2. Demonstration by the Western blot method that the baby and mother possess different antibodies to the virus. (The virus may change so quickly that mother and child could have different antibody patterns in true infection.)

3. Persistence of antibody beyond seven or eight months of age, when maternal antibody should no longer be present.

4. Successful culture of the virus from the baby.

So far, only the last two methods may be considered reliable.

PATHOLOGY

Major abnormalities have been described in autopsy studies of pediatric HIV disease patients in the lung, thymus, lymph nodes, and brain. A nonspecific hepatitis has also been reported (43)-(47).

Lung findings frequently include those of PCP, CMV infection or LIP (43). Lymphocytic interstitial pneumonitis is characterized by a diffuse lymphocytic infiltration of the alveolar septa and bronchiolar areas. Plasma cells and immunoblasts may also be present with nodular areas containing germinal centers. Clinically, LIP is associated with moderate, persistent elevation of serum lactate dehydrogenase (48). The etiology of LIP is unknown but infection with EBV is suggested by a study which found EBV DNA in lung biopsy material from children with LIP (41). The use of steroids in this disease, although described as beneficial (41), remains controversial, especially since opportunistic pathogens may coexist with LIP. A desquamative interstitial pneumonitis (DIP), described in some specimens, correlated with poor prognosis, while LIP can be compatible with long (months) survival (44).

Lymphadenopathy is common in pediatric AIDS as it is in adult cases. On pathologic examination the following patterns have been described: follicular hyperplasia with normal paracortical cellularity, follicular hyperplasia with depletion of the paracortex and atrophy of the follicles with depletion of paracortex (43). Lymph node biopsy is sometimes useful in diagnosing opportunistic infection and appropriate cultures and staining for fungi and acid fast bacteria is essential, as typical host response to infection may be lacking.

The presence of a normally placed thymus is helpful in distinguishing this syndrome from other immunodeficiencies. In pediatric HIV disease there is a normally placed gland with severe depletion of lymphocytes and Hassall's corpuscles. Thymocyte depletion and patchy fibrosis is present and the normal demarcation of the junction of cortex and medulla is lost (45),(46).

The neuropathology of children with HIV associated encephalopathy includes cortical atrophy, microglial nodules, and intranuclear inclusions similar to those seen in subacute encephalitis (24).

Non-specific abnormalities have also been described on liver biopsy in children with clinical hepatitis (47).

SOCIAL CONSIDERATIONS

The social implications of pediatric HIV disease are monumental. Issues of schooling for sick children, as well as for those who are well, but HIV antibody positive, are most visible in the public eye. The care of chronically ill children, many of whom are in foster care, is an important concern (7) (Table 2). With present information documenting no transmission of virus by even close family type contact, the alarming fear surrounding this illness is vastly disproportionate to the actual risk (49). However, until effective preventive measures are developed, concerns about public health issues will continue (50).

CONCLUSION

Some states presently require informed consent before HIV serologies can be performed. Issues of confidentiality and the rights of the individual versus those of society are severely tested by this illness. As the present generation of children grows older, the prognosis of a child with positive serology for HIV will be learned. Whether these children will survive, whether some will be carriers of the virus to future sexual contacts, or to their progeny, are serious questions to be answered over time.

Table 2. Recommendations for Education and Foster Care of Children Infected with HIV (Ref 7)

1. Decisions regarding the type of educational and care setting for HIV-infected children should be based on the behavior, neurologic development, and physical condition of the child and the expected type of interaction with others in that setting. These decisions are best made using the team approach including the child's physician, public health personnel, the child's parent or guardian, and personnel associated with the proposed care or educational setting. In each case, risks and benefits to both the infected child and to others in the setting should be weighed.

2. For most infected school-aged children, the benefits of an unrestricted setting would outweigh the risks of their acquiring potentially harmful infections in the setting and the apparent nonexistent risk of transmission of HIV. These children should be allowed to attend school and after-school day-care and to be placed in a foster home in an unrestricted setting.

3. For the infected preschool-aged child and for some neurologically handicapped children who lack control of their body secretions or who display behavior, such as biting, and those children who have uncoverable, oozing lesions, a more restricted environment is advisable until more is known about transmission in these settings. Children infected with HIV should be cared for and educated in settings that minimize exposure of other children to blood or body fluids.

4. Care involving exposure to the infected child's body fluids and excrement, such as feeding and diaper changing, should be performed by persons who are aware of the child's HIV infection and the modes of possible transmission. In any setting involving an HIV-infected person, good handwashing after exposure to blood and body fluids and before caring for another child should be observed, and gloves should be worn if open lesions are present on the caretaker's hands. Any open lesions on the infected person should also be covered.

5. Because other infections in addition to HIV can be present in blood or body fluids, all school and day-care facilities, regardless of whether children with HIV infection are attending, should adopt routine procedures for handling blood or body fluids. Soiled surfaces should be promptly cleaned with disinfectants, such as household bleach (diluted 1 part bleach to 10 parts water). Disposable towels or tissues should be used whenever possible, and mops should be rinsed in the disinfectant. Those who are cleaning should avoid exposure of open skin lesions or mucous membranes to the blood or body fluids.

Table 2: Continued

6. The hygienic practices of children with HIV infection may improve as the child matures. Alternatively, the hygienic practices may deteriorate if the child's conditions worsens. Evalution to assess the need for a restricted environment should be performed regularly.

7. Physicians caring for children born to mothers with AIDS or at increased risk of acquiring HIV infection should consider testing the children for evidence of HIV infection for medical reasons. For example, vaccination of infected children with live virus vaccines, such as the measles-mumps-rubella vaccine (MMR), may be hazardous. These children also need to be followed closely for problems with growth and development and given prompt and aggressive therapy for infections and exposure to potentially lethal infections, such as varicella. In the event that an antiviral agent or other therapy for HIV infection becomes available, these children should be considered for such therapy. Knowledge that a child is infected will allow parents and other caretakers to take precautions when exposed to the blood and body fluids of the child.

8. Adoption and foster-care agencies should consider adding HIV screening to their routine medical evaluations of children at increased risk of infection before placement in the foster or adoptive home, since these parents must make decisions regarding the medical care of the child and must consider the possible social and psychological effects on their families.

9. Mandatory screening as a condition for school entry is not warranted based on available data.

10. Persons involved in the care and education of HIV infected children should respect the child's right to privacy, including maintaining confidential records. The number of personnel who are aware of the child's condition should be kept at a minimum needed to assure proper care of the child and to detect situations where the potential for transmission may increase (e.g., bleeding injury).

11. All educational and public health departments, regardless of whether HIV-infected children are involved, are strongly encouraged to inform parents, children, and educators regarding HIV and its transmission. Such education would greatly assist efforts to provide the best care and education for infected children while minimizing the risk of transmission to others.

REFERENCES

1. Rubinstein, A., Sicklick, M., Gupta, A., et al., Acquired immunodeficiency with reversed T4/T8 ratios in infants born to promiscuous and drug-addicted mothers. JAMA 249:2350-2356 (1983)

2. Oleske, J., Minnefor, A., Cooper, R., et al., Immune deficiency syndrome in children. JAMA 249:2345-2349 (1983)

3. Scott, G.B., Buck, B.E., Leterman, J.G., et al., Acquired immunodeficiency syndrome in infants. N Engl J Med 310:76-81 (1984)

4. Amman, A.J., The acquired immunodeficiency syndrome in infants and children. Ann Intern Med 103:734-737 (1985)

5. Broder, S., Gallo, R.C., A pathogenic retrovirus (HTLV-III) linked to AIDS. N Engl J Med 311:1292-1297 (1984)

6. Laurence J., Brun-Vezinet, F., Schutzer, S.E., et al., Lymphadenopahty-associated viral antibody in AIDS. N Engl J Med 311:1269-1273 (1984)

7. CDC., Education and foster care of children infected with human T-lymphotropic virus type III/lymphadenopathy-associated virus. MMWR 34:517-521 (1985)

8. CDC., Update: Acquired immunodeficiency syndrome - United States. MMWR 35:17-20 (1986)

9. Parks, W.P., Scott, G.B., Pediatric AIDS: a disease spectrum causally associated with HTLV-III infection. Cancer Res 45(s):4659-4661 (1985)

10. Rogers, M.F., AIDS in children: a review of the clinical, epidemiologic and public health aspects. Ped Infect Dis 4:230-236 (1985)

11. Lapointe, N., Michaud, J., Pekovic, D., et al., Transplacental transmission of HTLV-III virus. N Engl J Med 312:1325 (1985)

12. Jovaisas, E., Koch, M.A., Schafer, A., et al., LAV/HTLV-III in 20 week fetus. Lancet 2:1129 (1985)

13. Vilmer, E., Fischer, A., Griscelli, C., et al., Possible transmission of a human lymphotropic retrovirus (LAV) from mother to infant with AIDS. Lancet 2:229-230 (1984)

14. Ziegler, J.B., Johnson, R.O., Cooper, D.A., et al., Postnatal transmission of AIDS-associated retrovirus from mother to infant. Lancet 1:896-897 (1985)

15. Wykoff, R.F., Pearl, E.R., Saulsbury, F.T., Immunologic dysfunction in infants infected through transfusion with HTLV-III. N Engl J Med 312:294-296 (1985)

16. Church, J.A., Isaacs, H., Transfusion-associated acquired immune deficiency syndrome in infants. J Ped 105:731-737 (1984)

17. Curran, J.W., Lawrence, D.N., Jaffe, H., et al., Acquired immunodeficiency syndrome associated with transfusions. N Engl J Med 310:69-75 (1984)

18. Evatt, B.L., Ramsey, R.B., Lawrence, D.N., et al., The acquired immunodeficiency syndrome in patients with hemophilia. Ann Intern Med 100:499-504 (1984)

19. Feorino, P.M., Jaffe, H.W., Palmer, E., et al., Transfusion-associated acquired immunodeficiency syndrome. N Engl J Med 312:1293-1296 (1985)

20. Maloney, M.J., Cox, F., Wray, B.B., et al., AIDS in a child 5-1/2 years after a transfusion. N Engl J Med 312:1256 (1985)

21. Kaplan, J.E., Oleske, J.M., Getchell, J.P., et al., Evidence against transmission of human T-lymphotropic virus/lymphadenopathy-associated virus (HTLV-III/LAV) in families of children with the acquired immunodeficiency syndrome. Ped Infect Dis 4:468-471 (1985)

22. Lewin, E.B., Zack, R., Ayodele, A., Communicability of AIDS in a foster care setting. International Conference on Acquired Immunodeficiency Syndrome (AIDS), Atlanta, April 1985

23. Friedland, G.H., Saltzman, B.R., Rogers, M.F., et al., Lack of household transmission of HTLV-III infection. N Engl J Med 314:344-348 (1986)

24. Shaw, G.M., Harper, M.E., Hahn, B.H., et al., HTLV-III infection in brains of children and adults with AIDS encephalopathy. Science 227:177-180 (1985)

25. Suri, M., Asaiker, S., Gupta, A., et al., Neurological disease in infants with AIDS. Ped Res 19:395A #1708 (1985)

26. Epstein, L.G., Sharer, L.R., Joshi, V.V., et al., Progressive encephalopathy in children with acquired immunodeficiency syndrome. Child Neurology Society, October 1984

27. Belman, A.L., Ultmann, M.H., Horoupian, D., et al., Neurologic complications in infants and children with AIDS. Ann Neurol 18:560-566 (1985)

28. Benkov, K.J., Stawski, C., Sirlin, S.M., et al., Atypical presentation of childhood acquired immunodeficiency syndrome mimicking Crohn's disease: nutrition considerations and management. Am J Gastro 80:260-264 (1985)

29. Bernstein, W., Krieger, B.Z., Novick, B., et al., Bacterial infection in the acquired immunodeficiency syndrome of children. Ped Infect Dis 4:472-475 (1985)

30. Wormser, G.P., Krupp, L.B., Hanrahan, J.P., et al., Acquired immunodeficiency syndrome in male prisoners. New insights into an emerging syndrome. Ann Intern Med 98:297-303 (1983)

31. Feldman, S., Hughes, W.T., Daniel, C.B., Varicella in children with cancer: seventy-seven cases. Pediatrics 56:388-397 (1975)

32. De Waele, M., Thielemans, C., Van Camp, B.K.G., et al., Characterization of immunoregulatory T-cells in EBV induced infectious mononuclosis by monoclonal antibodies. N Engl J Med 304:460-462 (1981)

33. Fauci, A.S., Immunologic abnormalities in the acquired immunodeficiency syndrome (AIDS). Clin Res 32:491 (1984)

34. Ammer, J., Hong, R., Disorders of the T-cell system. In: Immunologic Disorders in Infants and Children. (Stiehm, E.R., Fulginiti, V.A. eds), W.B. Saunders Co., Philadelphia (1983)

35. Gupta, A., Novick, B., Rubinstein, A., Restoration of suppressor T-cell functions in children with AIDS following intravenous gammaglobulin. Amer J Dis Child 140:143-146 (1986)

36. Reinherz, E.L., Morimoto, C., Fitzgerald, K., et al., Heterogeneity of human T4 inducer T-cells defined by a monoclonal antibody that delineates two functional subpopulations. J Immunol 128:463-468 (1982)

37. Bernstein, L.J., Ochs, H.D., Wedgewood, R.J., et al., Defective humoral immunity in pediatric acquired immunodeficiency syndrome. J Ped 107:352-357 (1985)

38. Lane, H.C., Masur, H., Edgar, L.C., et al., Abnormalities of B lymphocyte activation and immunoregulation in patients with the acquired immunodeficiency syndrome. N Engl J Med 309:453-458 (1983)

39. Montagnier, L., Gouest, J., Chamaret, J., et al., Adaption of lymphadenopathy-associated virus (LAV) to replication in EBV-transformed B lymphoblastoid cell lines. Science 225:63-66 (1984)

40. Quinnan, G.V., Masur, H., Rook, A.H., et al., Herpes virus infections in the acquired immunodeficiency syndrome. *JAMA* 252: 72-77 (1984)

41. Andiman, W.A., Eastman, R., Martin, K., et al., Opportunistic lymphoproliferations associated with Epstein-Barr viral DNA in infants and children with AIDS. *Lancet* 2: 1390-1393 (1985)

42. Rubinstein, A., Bernstein, L., Novick, B., et al., Thymulin and thymosin alpha 1 -- diagnostic criteria for AIDS in children. *Pediatr Res* 18:264A (1984)

43. Joshi, V.V., Oleske, J.M., Minnefor, A.B., et al., Pathology of suspected acquired immunodeficiency syndrome in children: a study of eight cases. *Pediatr Pathol* 2:71-87 (1984)

44. Joshi, V.V., Oleske, J.M., Minnefor, A.B., et al., Pathologic pulmonary findings in children with the acquired immunodeficiency syndrome: a study of ten cases. *Hum Pathol* 16:241-246 (1985)

45. Davis, A.E., The histopathological changes in the thymus gland in the acquired immune deficiency syndrome. *Ann NY Acad Sci* 437:493-502 (1984)

46. Joshi, V.V., Oleske, J.M., Pathologic appraisal of the thymus gland in acquired immunodeficiency syndrome in children. *Arch Pathol Lab Med* 109:142-146 (1985)

47. Duffy, L.F., Daum, F., Kahn, E., et al., Hepatitis in children with acquired immune deficiency syndrome. *Gastroenterology* 90:173-181 (1986)

48. Silverman, B.A., Rubinstein, A., Serum lactate dehydrogenase levels in adults and children with acquired immunodeficiency syndrome (AIDS) and AIDS related complex: possible indicator of B-cell lymphoproliferation and disease activity. Effect of intravenous gammaglobulin on enzyme levels. *Am J Med* 78:728-736 (1985)

49. Sande, M.A., Transmission of AIDS: the case against casual contagion. *N Engl J Med* 314:380-382 (1986)

50. Osborn, J.E., The AIDS epidemic: multidisciplinary trouble. *N Engl J Med* 314:779-782 (1986)

Part V
Pathology of HIV Infection

42
General Pathology of AIDS

Rosalyn E. Stahl

The acquired immunodeficiency syndrome (AIDS) is associated with a variety of morphologic lesions which are neither specific nor diagnostic of AIDS or human immunodeficiency virus (HIV) infection, but which are characteristic of the disease. The pathologic features include lymphadenopathy and thymic abnormalities, manifestations of infection by HIV or opportunistic pathogens, and neoplasms, mainly Kaposi's sarcoma (KS) and lymphomas.

This chapter reviews the general pathology of AIDS based on our experience with 27 consecutive autopsies performed on prisoners with AIDS at Westchester County Medical Center and on published autopsy studies of other patient populations with AIDS, excluding children (1)-(8). Since 26 (96%) of the 27 prisoners were intravenous drug abusers (and all but two of the 27 were heterosexual), this series may be considered representative of autopsy findings in heterosexual intravenous drug abusers. Ultrastructural changes or pathologic findings caused directly by HIV infection will not be discussed here.

AUTOPSY FINDINGS

At autopsy in AIDS patients, the characteristic features are the multiplicity of serious diseases present simultaneously, the overwhelming number of organisms in infection, and the lack of a normal inflammatory response in infected tissue.

Table 1 lists the predominant autopsy findings in 27 prisoners with AIDS. Over one-third of these patients had two or more of the diseases listed simultaneously. Compared to autopsy studies of AIDS patients who were predominantly male homosexuals (1)-(3),(5)-(8) (Table 2), prisoner-intravenous drug abusers with AIDS have a much lower incidence of KS, a lower incidence of cytomegalovirus infections and a higher incidence of lymphomas and cirrhosis.

Table 1. Autopsy Findings in 27 Prisoners with AIDS*

Bronchopneumonia	12	(44%)
Pneumocystis carinii pneumonia	12	(44%)
Cytomegalovirus infection	10	(37%)
Cirrhosis	9	(33%)
Toxoplasmosis	4	(15%)
Brain lymphoma	3	(11%)
Candidiasis	3	(11%)
Histoplasmosis	2	(7%)
Cryptococcosis	2	(7%)
Mycobacteriosis	2	(7%)
Kaposi's sarcoma	1	(4%)

* Autopsies were performed by the Medical Examiner's Office of Westchester County. Although gross pathologic examinations were complete, except for lungs and adrenals, microscopic sections from other organs were not obtained for every case.

INFECTIONS

Pneumocystis Carinii Pneumonia

The most common opportunistic infection found in prisoner intravenous drug abusers at autopsy was *Pneumocystis carinii* pneumonia (PCP). It is also the most common presenting manifestation of AIDS (1),(9). In our experience and those of others (5) many patients have persistent PCP at necropsy despite having received antimicrobial therapy directed against the pathogen during life.

Lungs infected with PCP are heavy and consolidated and cut with increased resistance. Histologically, several different patterns can occur. Invariably, there is an eosinophilic, intra-alveolar, foamy exudate on routine hematoxylin-eosin (H&E) stain, and methenamine silver stain reveals multiple cup-shaped, oval or round structures, 4-7 microns in diameter, representing the cyst wall of the organisms. Sometimes, a central dot can be detected within these structures representing a focal thickening of the

Table 2. Opportunistic Infections and Neoplasms on Post-mortem Examination of AIDS Patients

	Reference and First Author								
	1 Niedt	2 Reichert	3 Welch	4 Moskowitz	5 Hui	6 Mobley	7 Guarda	8 Macher	Stahl**
No.of Patients Studied	56	10	36	54	12	12	13	15	27
Patient Population*	47 Homo 4 IVDA 1 Haitian 2 Other	8 Homo or bisex 1 Haitian 1 IVDA	32 Homo 2 Children 1 Haitian 1 No known risk	25 Haitian 19 Homo 5 IVDA 2 Hemophiliac 3 No known risk	12 Homo	10 Homo 2 IVDA	13 Homo	NM	26 IVDA 1 homo
Opportunistic Infections									
Pneumocystis carinii pneumonia	18(32%)	1(10%)	13(36%)	16 (30%)	8(67%)	5(42%)	3(23%)	3(20%)	12(44%)
Cytomegalovirus	43(77%)	9(90%)	25(69%)	10(19%)	10(83%)	10(83%)	12(92%)	14(93%)	10(37%)
Toxoplasmosis	5(9%)	1(10%)	0	12(22%)	0	3(25%)	1(8%)	NM	4(15%)
Mycobacteriosis	9(16%)	6(60%)	5(14%)	1(2%)	3(25%)	5(42%)	1(8%)	NM	2(7%)
Candidiasis***	33(59%)	7(70%)	3(8%)	0	2(17%)	1(8%)	1(8%)	NM	3(11%)
Cryptococcosis	7(13%)	3(30%)	3(8%)	0	0	2(17%)	1(8%)	NM	2(7%)
Histoplasmosis	0	0	1(3%)	0	0	0	1(8%)	NM	2(7%)
Aspergillosis	5(9%)	0	0	0	1(8%)	0	1(8%)	NM	0
Cryptosporidiosis	1(2%)	0	1(3%)	0	0	1(8%)	4(31%)	NM	0
Neoplasms									
Kaposi's sarcoma	29(52%)	3(30%)	18(50%)	6(11%)	2(17%)	4(33%)	13(100%)	NM	1(4%)
Lymphoma	5(9%)	2(20%)	4(11%)	0	2(17%)	0	1(8%)	NM	3(11%)

NM = Not mentioned.
* Heirarchically ordered; patients with multiple risk factors are tabulated only in the group listed first.
** Unpublished data.
*** Candidiasis includes non-disseminated forms as well as visceral involvement.
Homo = Homosexual men
IVDA = Intravenous drug abusers

cyst wall (10) (Figures 1a, 1b). In some patients, the alveolar septae are thin and perfectly normal, manifesting no inflammatory response to the infection. Other patients have an interstitial pneumonitis with infiltration of alveolar septae by mononuclear cells and proliferating fibroblasts. This pattern can be seen in varying degrees ranging from mild to severe, and may be associated with marked interstitial fibrosis (Figures 2a, 2b, 2c).

Bronchopneumonia

A very common autopsy finding (44% of cases) in the prisoner intravenous drug abusing population was bronchopneumonia which was often necrotizing, implying that AIDS patients, despite their immunodeficiency, can still mount a florid neutrophilic reaction to what probably represents a bacterial infection. (Tissue Gram stains of microscopic sections of pneumonia are usually negative, however, since most patients have been treated with multiple antibiotics before death.)

Cytomegalovirus Infection

Disseminated cytomegalovirus (CMV) infection is the most common necropsy finding in patients with AIDS (1)-(3),(5)-(8), other than intravenous drug abusers and Haitians (4) (Table 2). For example, in autopsy series of homosexual men, disseminated CMV infection has been found in 77-93%. In contrast, only 37% of prisoner intravenous drug abusers with AIDS had evidence of CMV infection at autopsy. The lower prevalence of CMV infections in prisoner intravenous drug abusers may reflect less frequent or intensive exposure to this virus among this group compared to homosexual men. The most common sites of involvement by CMV are the lungs and adrenal glands. Another frequent focus of CMV infection in AIDS patients is the gastrointestinal tract.

CMV lesions can have a range of histologic manifestations. Numerous enlarged cells with characteristic intranuclear and intracytoplasmic inclusions are found in all cases (Figure 3). In the lungs, CMV can cause a focal or diffuse interstitial pneumonitis sometimes with areas of frank necrosis. Characteristic inclusions are typically present in alveolar lining cells but other cells such as endothelial cells can also be infected. In the adrenal glands, CMV causes necrotizing hemorrhagic lesions, which, although variable in size from patient to patient, typically involve the medulla; in some cases, however, the entire adrenal glands are infarcted and hemorrhagic.

Toxoplasmosis

Toxoplasma encephalitis is the most common cause of death in Haitian AIDS patients, accounting for 40% of deaths in one autopsy study (4) (Table 2). Brain toxoplasmosis was present in 15% (4/27) of our prisoner intravenous drug abusers with AIDS. The prevalence in other populations at postmortem has varied from

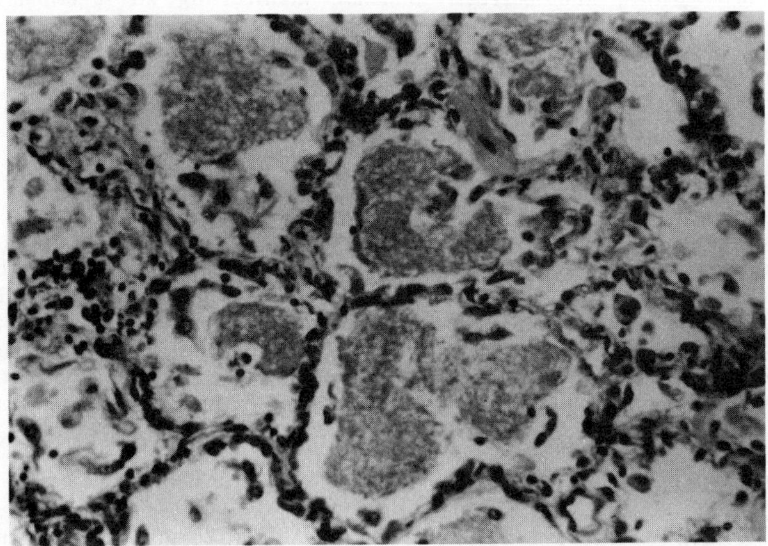

Figure 1a. *Pneumocystis carinii* pneumonia. Histological section of lungs infected with *Pneumocystis carinii* with a characteristic eosinophilic foamy exudate.

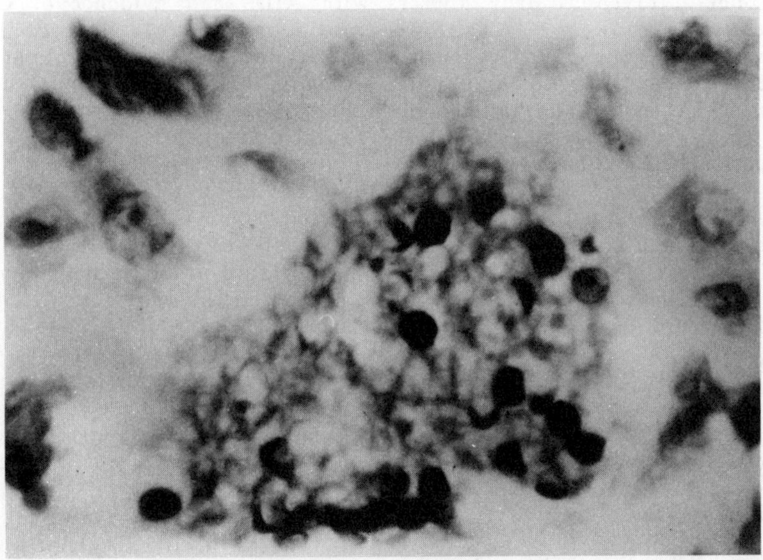

Figure 1b. *Pneumocystis carinii* pneumonia. High power methenamine silver stain of foamy exudate revealing characteristic "cup" or "football shaped" cyst walls of the pneumocystis organisms. Note the central dot present in some of the cysts.

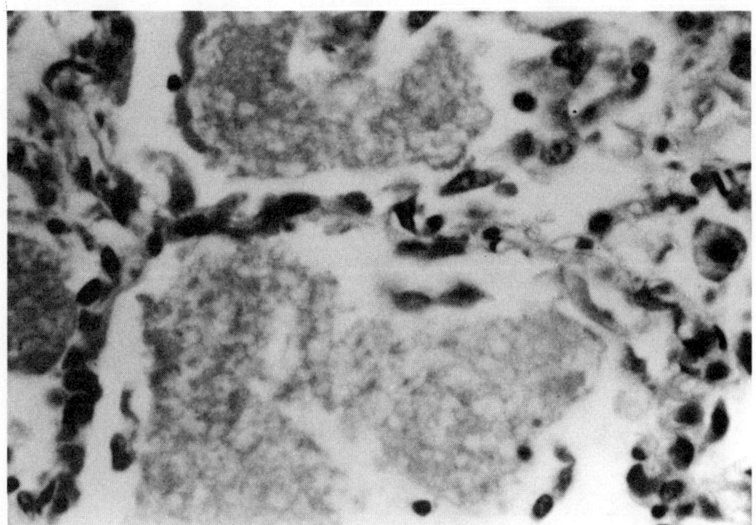

Figure 2a. *Pneumocystis carinii* pneumonia. Histologic sections of three different patterns of lung tissue reaction to *Pneumocystis carinii* are shown in Figures 2a, b, c. Note the eosinophilic foamy intra-alveolar exudate present in all three figures. In Figure 2a, the alveoli are of normal thickness with practically no inflammatory cells.

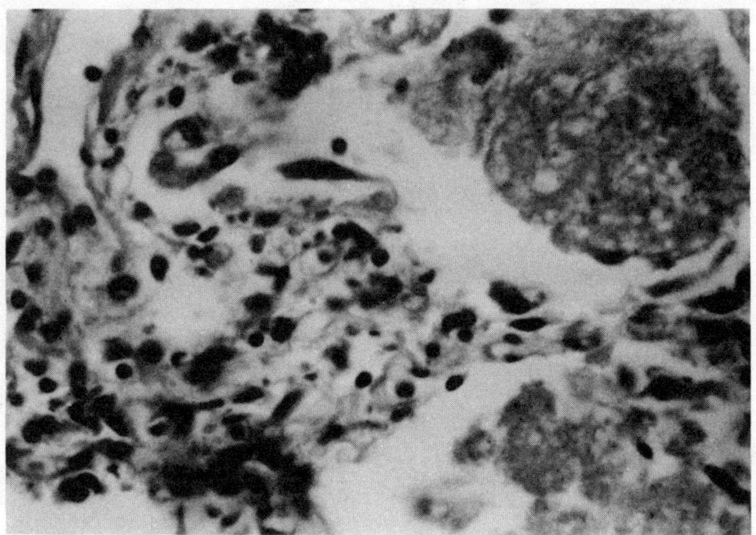

Figure 2b. *Pneumocystis carinii* pneumonia with interstitial pneumonitis. The alveolar septae are mildly thickened by an infiltrate of mononuclear cells and small numbers of proliferating fibroblasts.

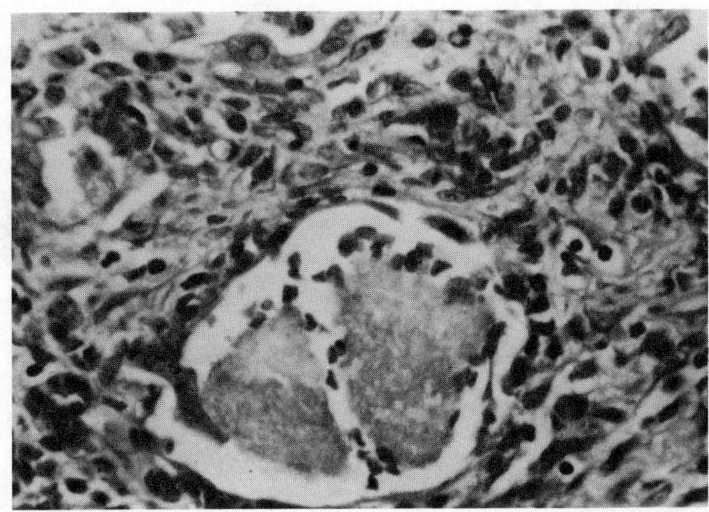

Figure 2c. *Pneumocystis carinii* pneumonia associated with severe interstitial fibrosis. In this example, the alveoli are markedly thickened by many proliferating fibroblasts, dense fibrosis and a small number of mononuclear cells.

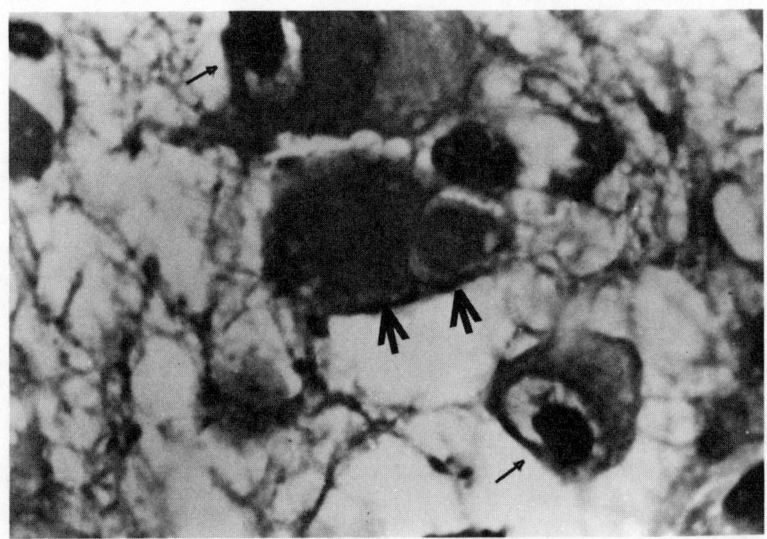

Figure 3. Histologic section of brain with cytomegalovirus infection. Note the enlarged cells with classic intra-nuclear (thin arrows) and intracytoplasmic inclusions (thick arrows).

8% to 25% (Table 2). In two of our patients, toxoplasma organisms were also found in myocardium associated with myocarditis (Figures 4 and 5a). In one of these patients, the myocardium was also invaded by candida organisms (Figure 5b).

Histologic diagnosis of toxoplasmosis requires visualization of the characteristic 2 by 6 micron tachyzoites or the larger cyst forms on H&E stained sections or Giemsa stained smears. Theoretically, free tachyzoites must be visualized to make a diagnosis of active infection. However, in the proper clinical setting and in an area of necrosis, the presence of a toxoplasma cyst is usually sufficient to support a diagnosis of active toxoplasmosis. In an immunocompetent host, the tachyzoites remain encysted after primary infection and do not cause cellular damage. However, under conditions of severe immunodeficiency, such as exists in AIDS, the tachyzoites multiply asexually within human host cells, which eventually rupture, releasing free tachyzoites to infect additional cells. The destruction of parasitized cells results in foci of necrosis. The pathologist should be aware, however, that nuclear debris in an area of necrosis due to other causes can often be confused with free tachyzoites.

Histologically, toxoplasmosis of the brain in AIDS patients can also be misdiagnosed as primary brain lymphoma. Toxoplasmosis can elicit a very atypical mononuclear inflammatory reaction with areas of perivascular infiltration by mononuclear cells and large areas of necrosis. All these features are also characteristic of lymphomas. Unless the organism can clearly be recognized, differentiating toxoplasmosis from lymphoma histologically, as well as clinically, can be extremely difficult and sometimes impossible. Immunoperoxidase stains, using antibody against toxoplasma, has been helpful in detecting the organism (11).

Candidiasis

Candida albicans is the most common opportunistic fungal pathogen reported in AIDS. Oral candidiasis also frequently occurs in patients at risk for the development of AIDS and its presence is indicative of a high likelihood of progression to full-blown AIDS (12). Candida esophagitis is one of the CDC surveillance criteria for the diagnosis of AIDS.

Although candidiasis is often a serious disseminated disease in debilitated or immunosuppressed non-AIDS patients, in patients with AIDS widespread visceral dissemination is infrequent. Only three (11%) of our 27 patients with AIDS had invasive candidiasis at death, although higher percentages of patients, up to 50%, have had evidence of visceral candidiasis at necropsy in other studies (2).

Histologically, in infected tissues, one sees 3 to 4 micron budding yeast cells (blastospores) and pseudohyphae invading tissue often with underlying necrosis (Figures 5a, 5b). The organisms can be seen, albeit with some difficulty, on a routine H&E stain, but they are much more apparent on periodic acid Schiff (PAS) or silver stains.

Cryptococcosis

Cryptococcosis is a fungal disease caused by *Cryptococcus neoformans.* AIDS patients with cryptococcal infection usually develop disseminated cryptococcosis involving, in decreasing order of frequency, central nervous system, lungs, lymph nodes, adrenal glands, liver, spleen, pancreas, and bone marrow. Two (11%) of our 27 prisoner intravenous drug abusers had cryptococcosis, one involving mainly the lung and the other involving virtually every organ with literally sheets of organisms on histologic sections. Also, in the latter case there was absolutely no inflammatory response (Figures 6a, 6b). This patient had in addition disseminated Kaposi's sarcoma and *Pneumocystis carinii* pneumonia.

Histologically, cryptococci appear as pale, narrow-pore, encapsulated budding yeasts, which like all yeasts, stain strongly with PAS and methenamine silver. They are, however, uniquely mucin positive, i.e., the yeast capsule will stain a bright magenta on mucicarmine stain. This is a very helpful diagnostic feature. The yeast capsule also imparts a unique mucoid gross appearance to cryptococcal tissue lesions. As has been described by Bottone et al. (13) and Bottone and Wormser (14), the cryptococcal organism in AIDS patients seems to have a thinner capsule than is usually seen in immunocompetent individuals (Figure 7). This characteristic affects their histologic appearance, and it is encumbent upon the pathologist to perform mucicarmine stains when budding yeasts are seen in a patient at risk for AIDS.

Histoplasmosis

Histoplasmosis is a fungal infection that is acquired by inhalation of *Histoplasma capsulatum* microconidia (spores) from contaminated soil. Dissemination from the lung or gastrointestinal tract (in patients whose initial lesions are in the mouth or pharynx) through the bloodstream may result in lesions at distant sites including lymph nodes, liver, meninges, adrenal glands and bone marrow. Although disseminated histoplasmosis can occur among healthy, immunocompetent people, an increased incidence of disseminated histoplasmosis has been reported among patients at high risk for AIDS (15)-(17). These patients usually live or have lived in endemic geographic locations, the latter implying that reactivation of a latent infection can be important in pathogenesis. Two of our 27 prisoner intravenous drug abusers with AIDS had disseminated histoplasmosis at autopsy. Both presented with fever of unknown origin and at postmortem, virtually every organ, including skin and mucus membranes, was teaming with organisms (Figures 8a-e). In contrast to the experience with non-AIDS patients with disseminated histoplasmosis, there was a total lack of inflammatory response to the organism despite their huge numbers. The organisms are oval, 2 to 4 micron budding yeast

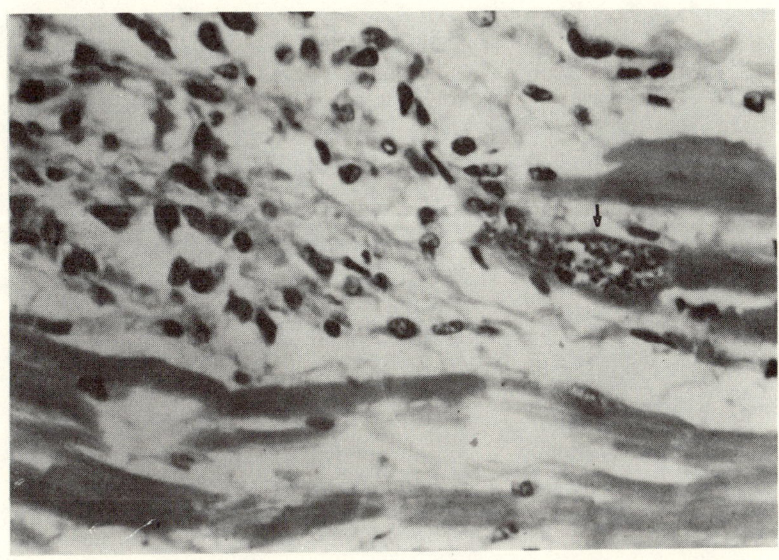

Figure 4. Toxoplasmosis in heart; note toxoplasma cyst in myocardial fiber (arrow) associated with inflammatory cell infiltrate in myocardium (myocarditis).

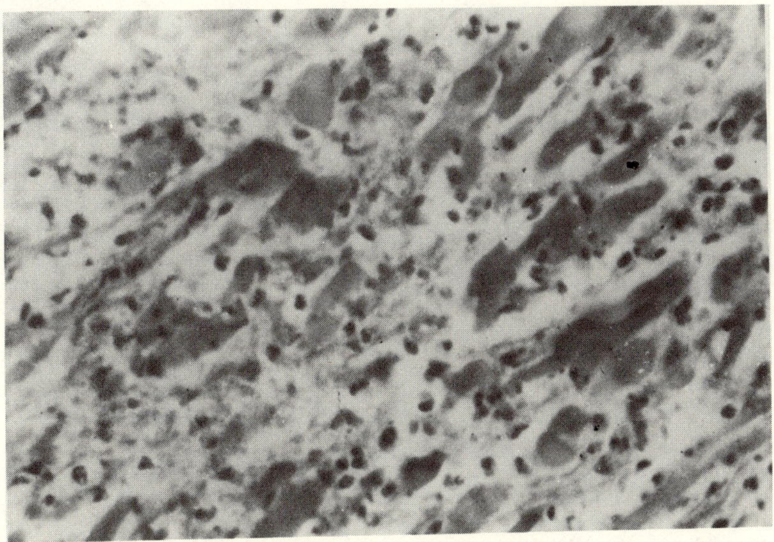

Figure 5a. Additional section of myocardium from the same patient as in Figure 4 showing severe necrotizing myocarditis.

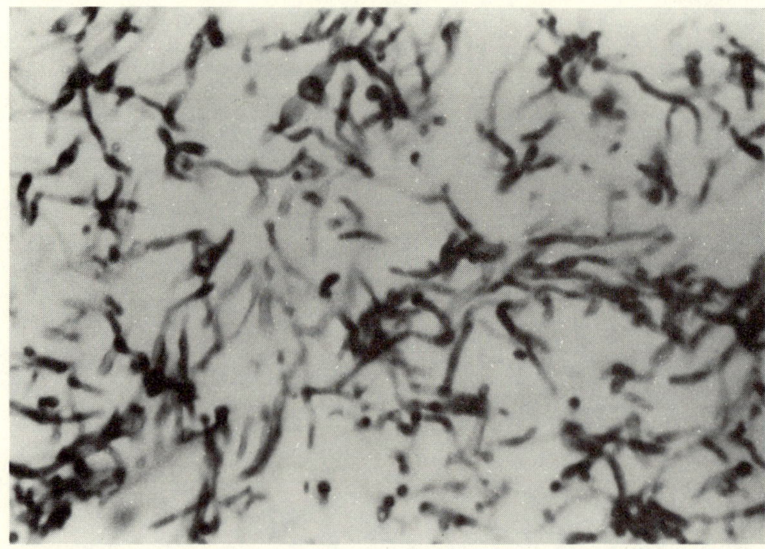

Figure 5b. Methenamine silver stain of same area as in Figure 5a revealing sheets of pseudohyphae and budding yeasts characteristic of candida.

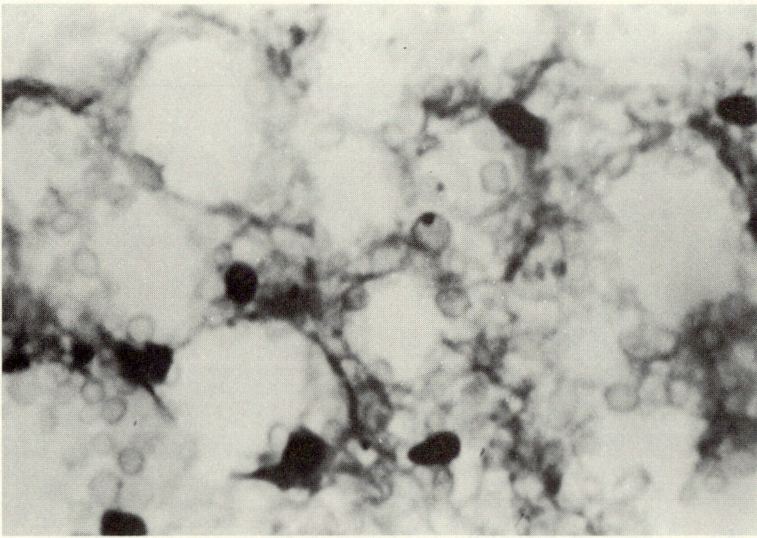

Figure 6a. Microscopic section of peripancreatic fat stained with H&E in an AIDS patient with disseminated cryptococcosis. Note the lack of inflammation and the huge number of organisms visible even on routine H&E stain.

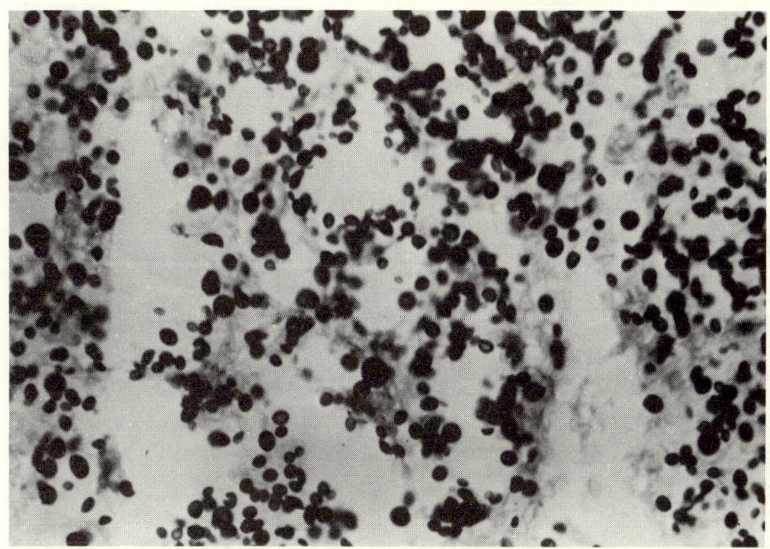

Figure 6b. Methenamine silver stain of same section as in Figure 6a demonstrating swarms of cryptococcal organisms.

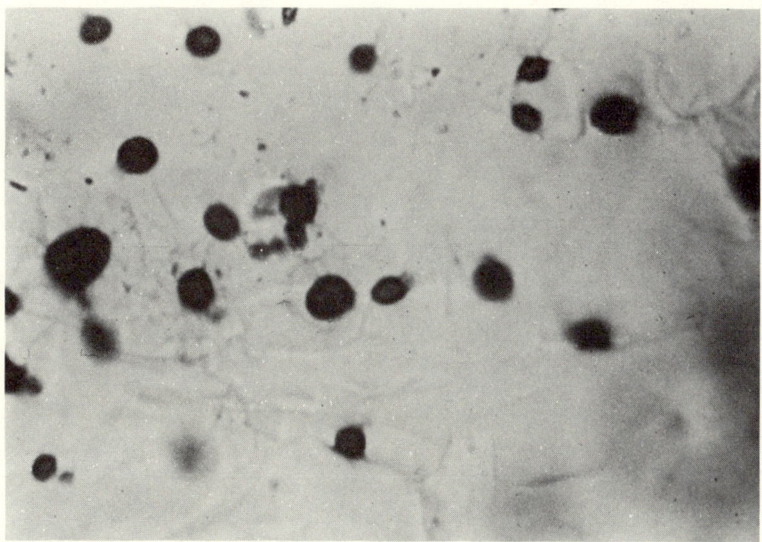

Figure 7. Mucicarmine stain of cerebrospinal fluid submitted during the life of same patient as in Figure 6 demonstrating mucin positive cryptococcal organisms. Note thickness of capsule which is much thinner than usually found in the non-AIDS patient with cryptococcal meningitis.

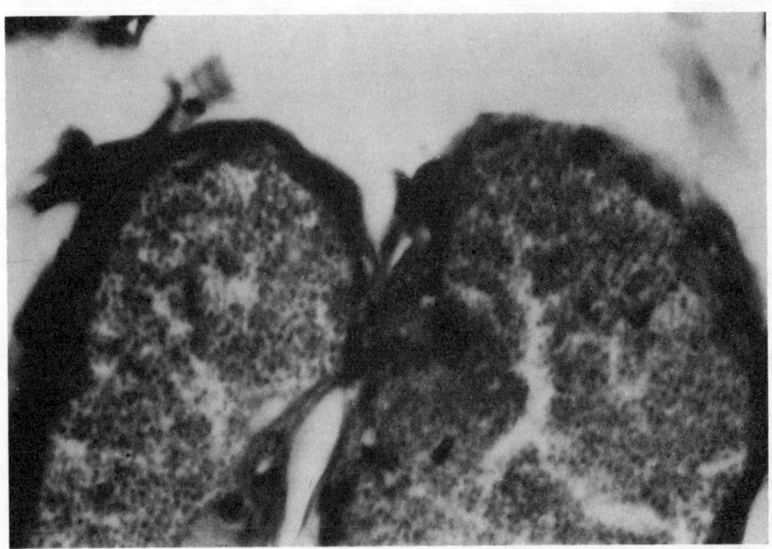

Figure 8a. Histologic section of tongue in a patient with disseminated histoplasmosis. Papillae of lamina propria are filled with sheets of organisms visible even on this H&E stain.

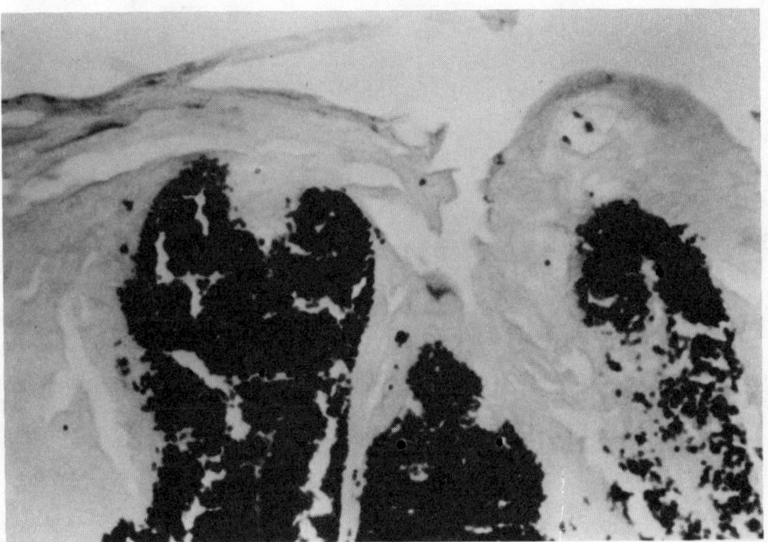

Figure 8b. Histoplasmosis. Methenamine silver stain of section in Figure 8a. Note intensity of stain due to the multitude of histoplasma organisms.

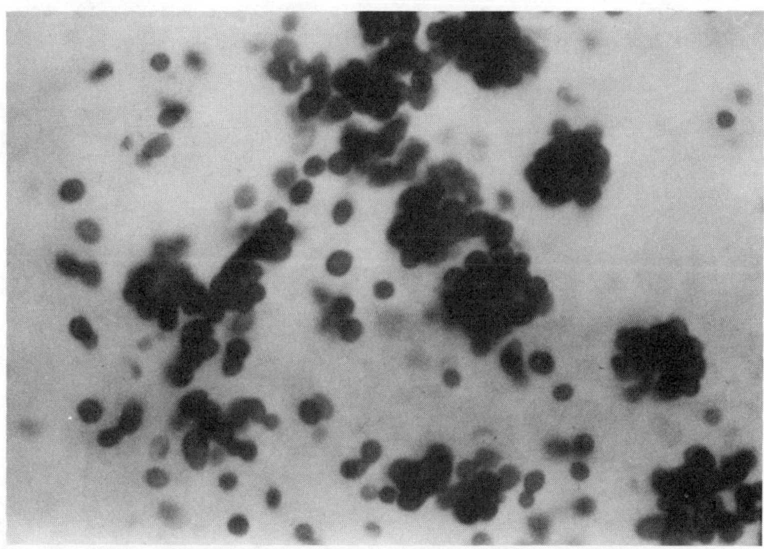

Figure 8c. Histoplasmosis. Higher power view of methenamine silver stain of section of spleen from same patient demonstrating budding yeasts of histoplasma.

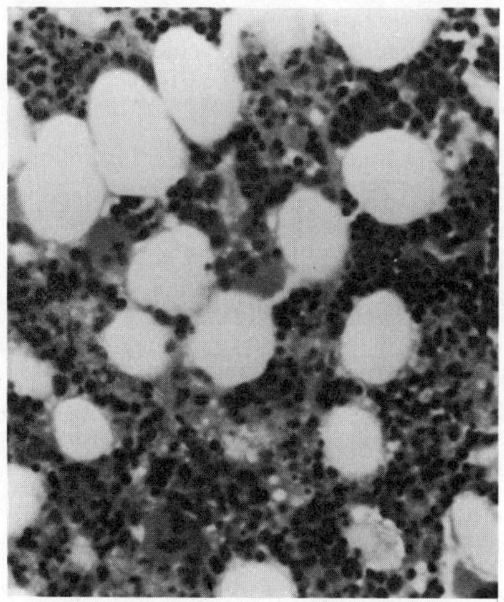

Figure 8d. Histoplasmosis. Section of bone marrow biopsy on same patient stained with H&E. Note relatively unremarkable histology.

cells, which are present both intra- and extracellularly and are extremely difficult, if not impossible in some cases, to see on routine H&E stains. A silver or PAS stain is required.

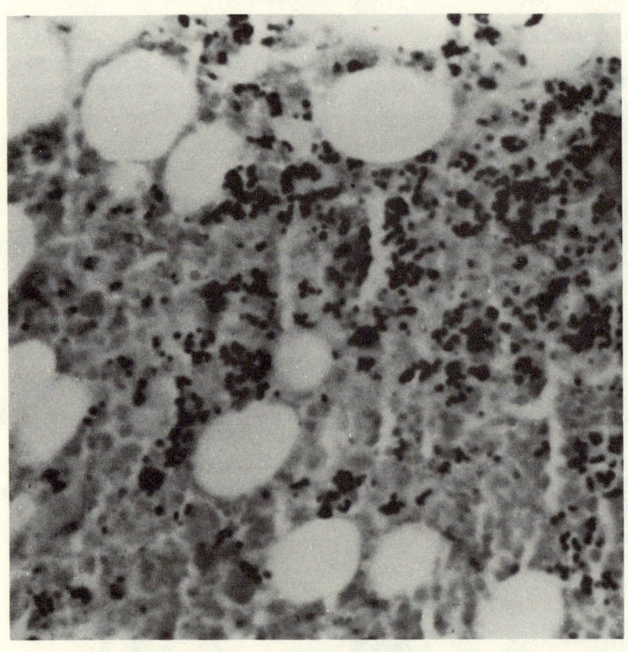

Figure 8e. Histoplasmosis. This figure shows a methenamine silver stain of same section as in Figure 8d revealing budding yeasts of histoplasma.

In lung specimens, histoplasma organisms can be confused with *Pneumocystis carinii*. The important distinction is that histoplasma is a budding yeast and pneumocystis organisms do not bud. The central dot present in pneumocystis organisms (vide supra) is also a distinguishing feature. In addition, pneumocystis organisms are intra-alveolar, whereas histoplasma organisms can be present both intra-alveolarly and within alveolar septae. Of course, a patient can have dual infection with both *Pneumocystis carinii* and histoplasma and precise diagnosis requires very careful examination.

Aspergillosis

Aspergillus is a ubiquitous mold and aspergillosis is an extremely common and frequent cause of death among non-AIDS immunocompromised patients, particularly granulocytopenic oncology patients. It is noteworthy, therefore, that aspergillosis is rare among AIDS patients. It has been reported as a terminal infection in one homosexual patient with AIDS (18), and has been present in up to 9% of reported autopsied AIDS patients (1),(5), (7) (Table 2).

Mycobacteriosis

Mycobacterium avium-intracellulare is a ubiquitous environmental saprophyte that before the AIDS epidemic, was rarely a cause of disseminated disease. However, *Mycobacterium avium-intracellulare* is a common pathogen in patients with AIDS and is usually disseminated.

In contrast to the caseating granulomas and giant cell reactions with epithelioid histiocytes that have been classically observed in mycobacterial infections, histologic sections of infected AIDS tissues show either perfectly normal histology on routine H&E stains or collections and/or sheets of foamy histiocytes with otherwise minimal inflammation and poorly formed or absent granulomas. Occasionally sheets of histiocytes can replace normal tissue architecture, and these lesions have occasionally been misdiagnosed as tumors. Involvement of the small bowel may mimic Whipple's disease (19),(20). Because of the lack of inflammatory or granulomatous response, even overwhelming infections may go undetected unless special acid fast stains (Ziehl-Neelsen, Fite, Kinyoun) are performed. (Although mycobacteria are also methenamine silver and PAS positive, acid fast stains are more specific and stain the organisms more intensely.) Also, in contrast to classic tuberculosis in which only a few, difficult to detect, acid-fast organisms are present, acid fast stains in tissues from infected AIDS patients usually reveal swarms of organisms generally in histiocytes (Figures 9a, 9b) but also in parenchymal cells (e.g. hepatocytes).

Mycobacterium tuberculosis, also a common infection in AIDS patients, cannot be differentiated histologically from *Mycobacterium avium-intracellulare*. A culture is required to distinguish these two organisms. Furthermore, specimens can be positive by culture but acid fast stain negative. Therefore, a portion of all biopsies performed to rule out tuberculosis should be sent for culture. Two (7%) of our 27 prisoner intravenous drug abusers had disseminated mycobacteriosis at postmortem while the incidence of disseminated mycobacterial infection in other autopsy studies has ranged from 2% to 60% (1)-(7) (Table 2). These prevalence rates, however, may indeed be underestimations since acid fast stains are too tedious to perform routinely on autopsy slides and, as mentioned above, mycobacterial infections can often be undetectable on routine H&E stains.

NEOPLASMS

Kaposi's Sarcoma

Kaposi's sarcoma (KS) is a common manifestation of AIDS among homosexuals but is rare in the other high risk groups (Table 2).

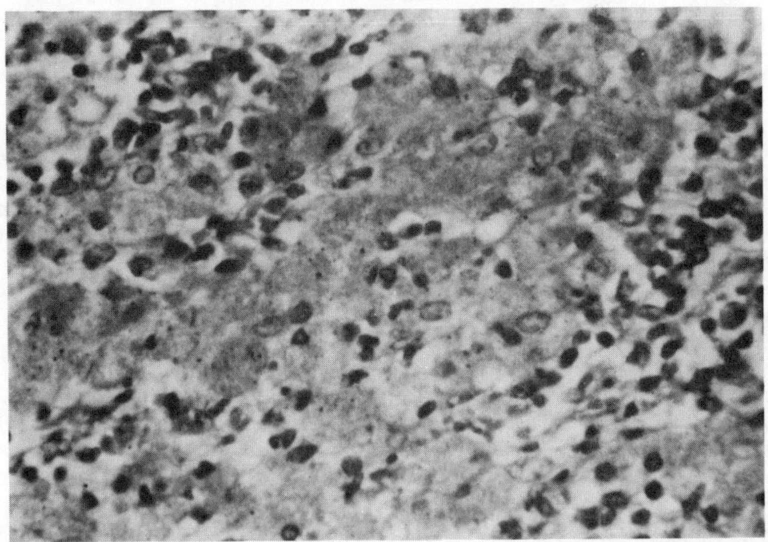

Figure 9a. High power microsection of lymph node showing infiltration by collections of histiocytes which on H&E stain have a bluish-gray hue.

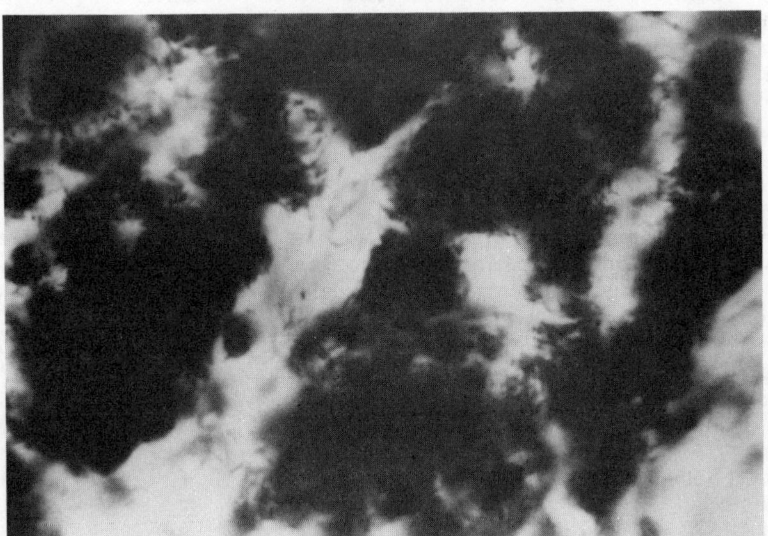

Figure 9b. Acid fast stains of same lymph node as in Figure 9a revealing millions of acid fast organisms within histiocytes and several in the intervening tissue.

The reason for this is unclear since the exact etiology of KS is unknown at the present time. In our series of prisoner intravenous drug abusers only 1 (4%) had KS. In this patient the neoplasm involved skin at multiple sites, lymph nodes, pharynx, gastrointestinal tract, lung, kidney, mesentery and liver. The prevalence of KS in autopsy studies of homosexual men has been as high as 100% (7) and other sites of this neoplasm have included spleen, gallbladder, bone marrow, conjunctiva, testes, epididymis, heart, pericardium, periadrenal fat, oral mucosa and larynx (1).

Prior to the AIDS epidemic, KS in this country and in Europe was generally an indolent disease of elderly Jewish and Italian men, with lesions often confined to the skin of the lower extremities. In AIDS patients, KS also usually presents in the skin, but often at multiple sites over the body. It may then spread to lymph nodes (lymphadenopathic disease) and/or to viscera. Some patients, however, present with lymph node involvement before the development of noticeable skin lesions.

Skin lesions in AIDS patients may be seen at different stages of development, namely patches, plaques or nodules. Patches, which represent the earliest stage, are irregularly shaped macules, usually violaceous in color, although they may appear hyperpigmented in some patients, especially black patients. It is at this stage that the histopathologic changes are very subtle and the diagnosis very difficult to render. These early lesions histologically resemble granulation tissue - the blood vessels in the dermis are dilated and increased in number and may have large endothelial cells which protrude into the lumen. The vessels in KS, as opposed to granulation tissue, however, have bizarre, irregular arborizing lumenae (Figures 10a, 10b) (21). Frequently, one sees small groups of extravasated erythrocytes, deposits of hemosiderin and a perivascular and diffuse inflammatory cell infiltrate, varying in severity, composed of lymphoid cells, plasma cells and some histiocytes.

Plaques are slightly elevated, irregularly shaped, violaceous or hyperpigmented lesions. Histologically, one sees variously sized endothelial lined spaces with strange arborizing shapes throughout the dermis with increased numbers of spindle shaped cells and a patchy mononuclear infiltrate containing plasma cells (Figures 11a, 11b) (22).

Nodular KS is histologically characterized by a well circumscribed tumor in the dermis composed of interweaving fascicles of spindle cells with many extravasated erythrocytes in the interstices between spindle cells. Nuclei vary in size and staining qualities and can be atypical. Occasional mitotic figures may also be present (Figures 12a and b). Lymph node and visceral lesions are usually identical in histologic appearance to nodular skin lesions.

Lymphomas

AIDS patients have an increased incidence of non-Hodgkin's (23)-(28) and Hodgkin's lymphomas (29). Lymphomas in AIDS pa-

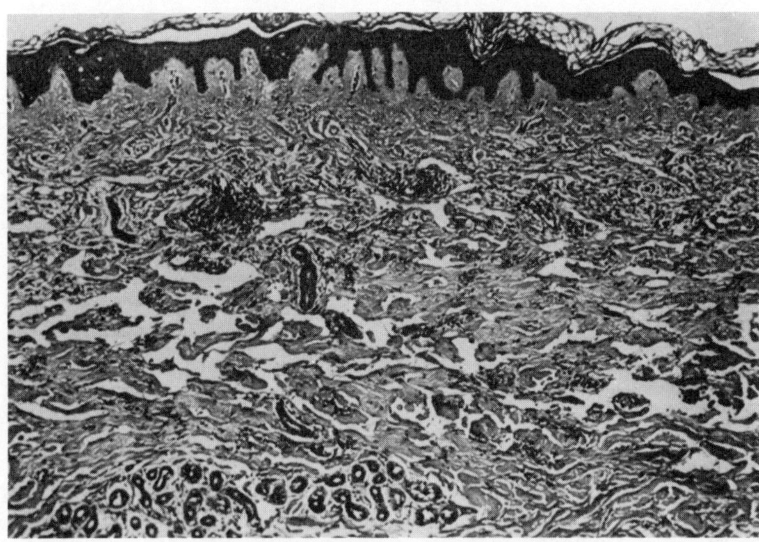

Figure 10a. Section of skin of a patient with early or patch stage of Kaposi's sarcoma. Note abnormal vasculature in dermis more clearly demonstrated in Figure 10b. Reproduced with permission from reference 21.

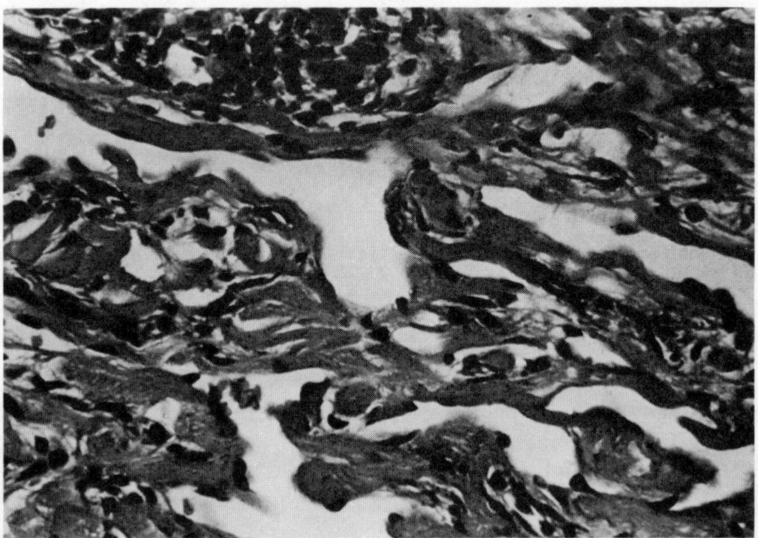

Figure 10b. Kaposi's sarcoma. Higher power view of same section as in Figure 10a. Vessels have peculiar and unique arborizing shapes. Note that the endothelial cells are not necessarily prominent or atypical in Kaposi's sarcoma. There is also a mild interstitial mononuclear infiltrate. Reproduced with permission from reference 21.

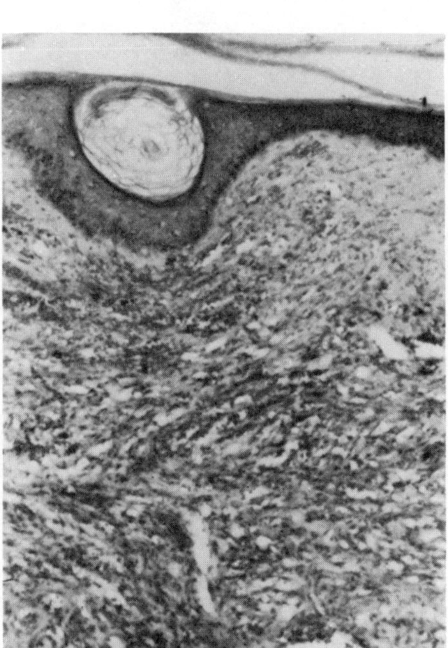

Figure 11a. Plaque stage of Kaposi's sarcoma. See legend of Figure 11b for more detailed description.

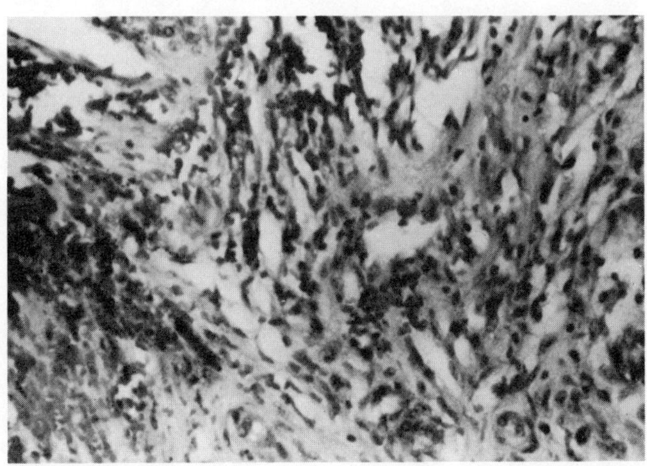

Figure 11b. Plaque stage of Kaposi's sarcoma, higher power view of section seen in Figure 11a. There are irregularly shaped, variously sized endothelial lined spaces throughout the dermis with increased numbers of spindle shaped cells and a patchy mononuclear infiltrate.

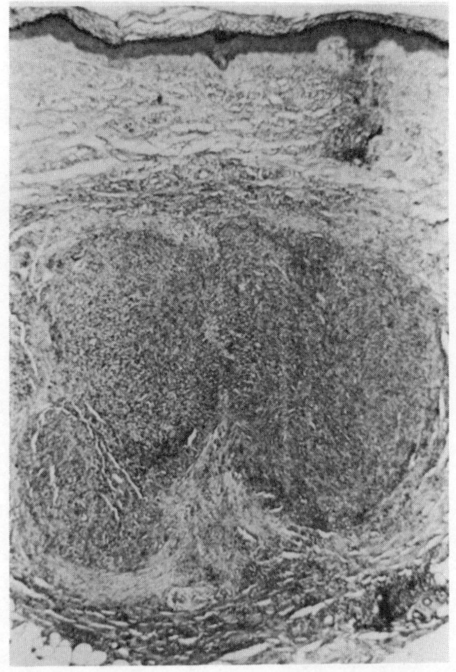

Figure 12a. Nodular Kaposi's sarcoma. Note fairly well circumscribed tumor in mid and reticular dermis.

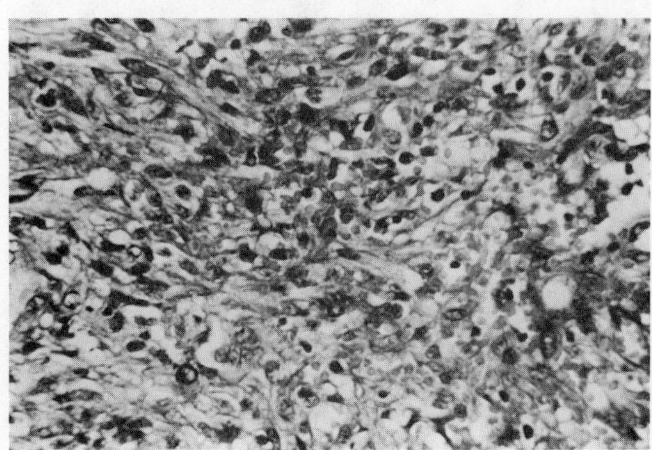

Figure 12b. Nodular Kaposi's sarcoma, higher power view of tumor in Figure 12a. Fascicles of atypical spindle cells with extravasated erythrocytes are shown.

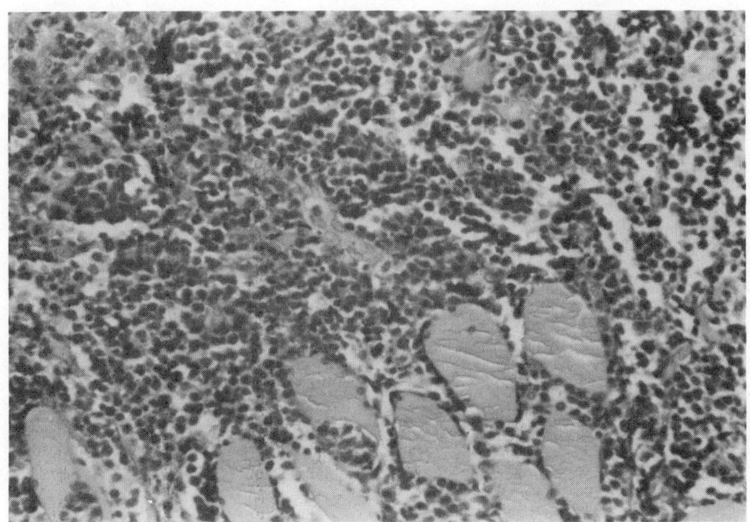

Figure 13a. Small, non-cleaved malignant lymphoma (Burkitt's lymphoma) presenting as a submandibular mass in a 26 year-old male. Note lymphoma cells invading striated muscle fibers.

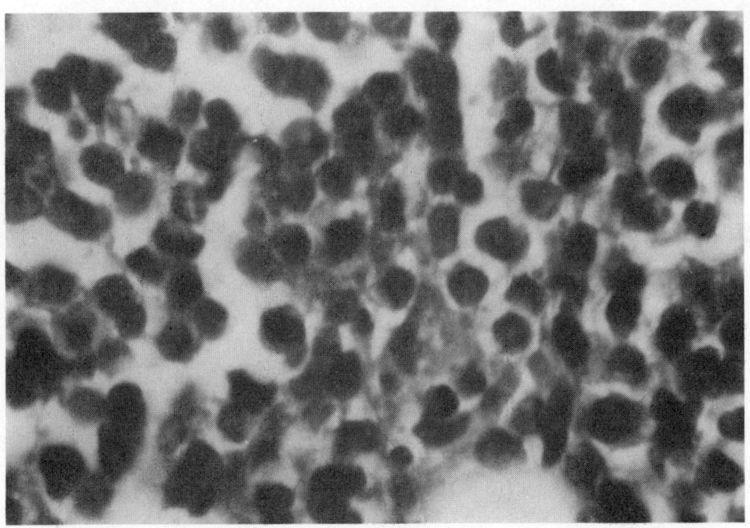

Figure 13b. Small, non-cleaved malignant lymphoma (Burkitt's lymphoma). Higher power view of section seen in Figure 13a showing a uniform population of small, non-cleaved cells.

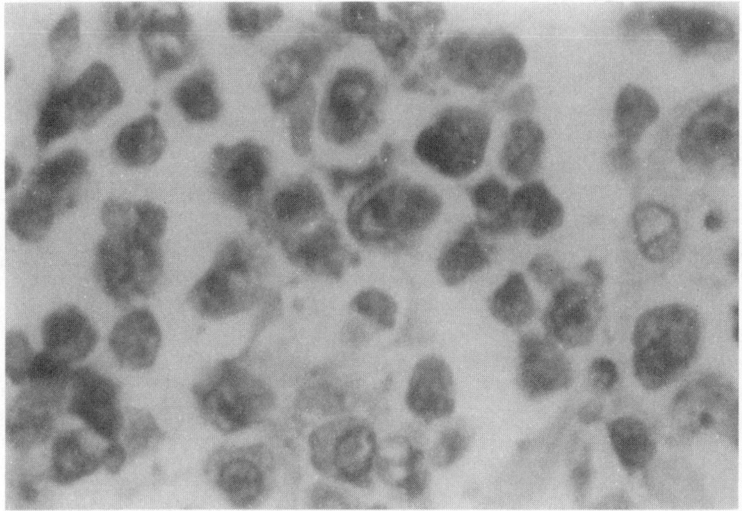

Figure 14. Large cell, immunoblastic sarcoma presenting as skin nodule. Note the large atypical plasmacytoid cells with prominent nucleoli.

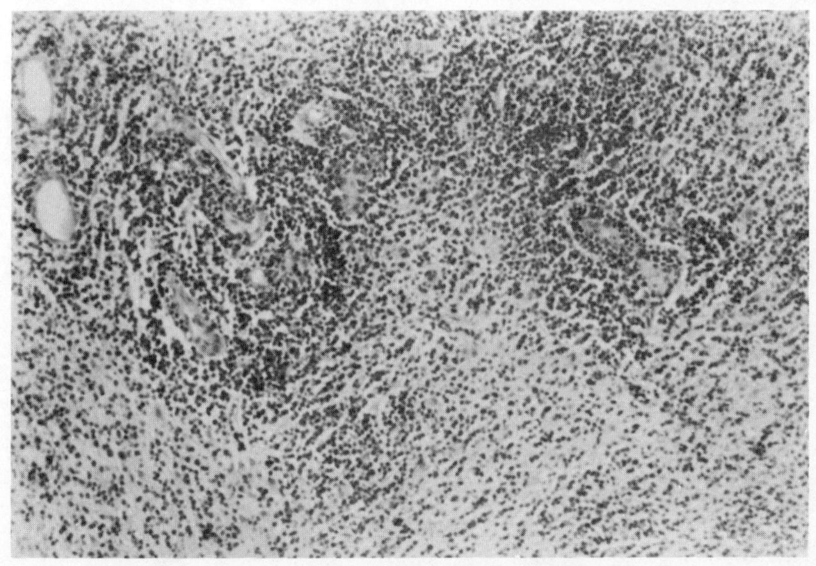

Figure 15a. Diffuse, small cleaved cell lymphoma in brain. Note large areas of necrosis with complete replacement of normal brain architecture by tumor cells.

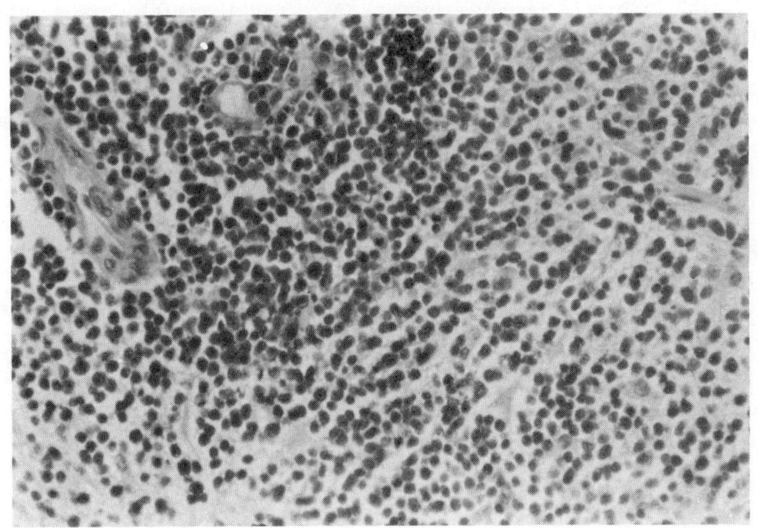

Figure 15b. Brain lymphoma. Higher power view of section seen in Figure 15a demonstrating perivascular infiltrate of tumor cells.

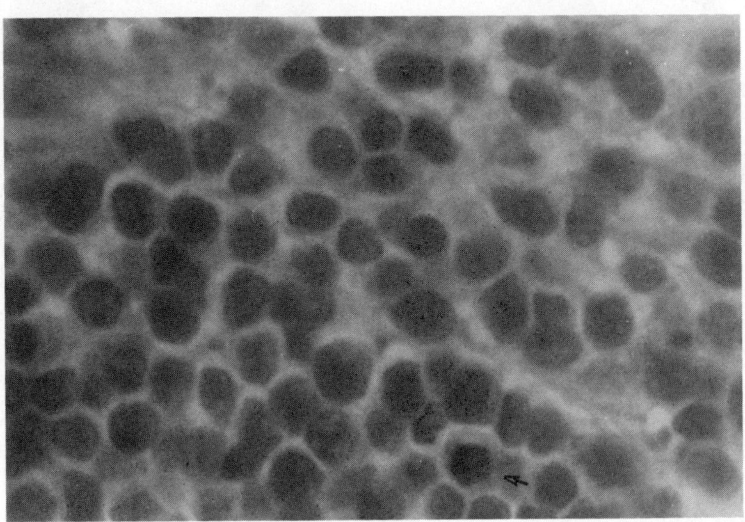

Figure 15c. Brain lymphoma. High power view of tumor cells seen in Figure 15b. Note mitotic figure in lower portion of picture (arrow).

tients, in contrast to the general population, are often primary within the central nervous system, are usually high grade undifferentiated types, have a younger age distribution and have a terrible prognosis with very poor responses to conventional therapy. They are also usually classifiable as B-cell lymphomas.

The histology of these lymphomas is somewhat variable from patient to patient. Table 3 summarizes the different types of non-Hodgkin's lymphomas found in five studies comprising a total of 157 homosexual men. Ninety-eight (63%) were categorized as high grade, 47 (30%) as intermediate grade and only 10 (6%) as low grade malignant lymphomas.

In the majority of patients, the lymphomas were present in extranodal sites including gastrointestinal tract, lungs, skin, bone, liver, salivary gland, and orbit. A large number of patients had involvement limited to the brain. Selected examples of the histology of lymphomas seen in patients in risk groups for AIDS treated at Westchester County Medical Center are demonstrated in Figures 13 - 16.

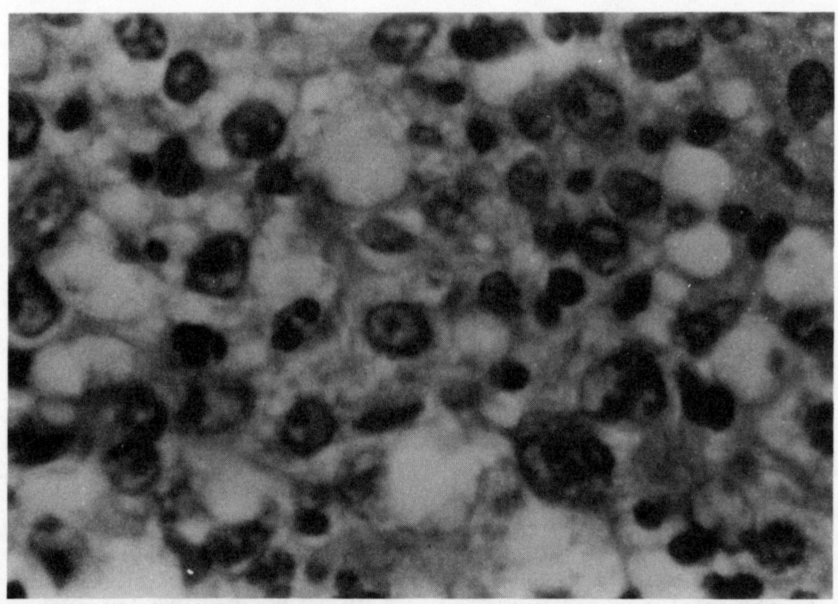

Figure 16. Diffuse, large cell lymphoma in brain. Note markedly atypical, pleomorphic cells with prominent nucleoli. A small number of inflammatory cells are also present probably because of the large amount of necrosis that was present in this tumor.

Table 3. Types of Non-Hodgkin's Lymphomas in Different Studies of Homosexual Men

Reference	23	24	25	27	28
No. of Subjects	90	6	6	27	28
Histologic Subtype					
High-grade malignant lymphoma					
Small, noncleaved cell	32(36%)	2(33%)	0	10(37%)	3(11%)
Large cell, immunoblastic	22(24%)	3(50%)	5(83%)	11(41%)	7(25%)
Lymphoblastic	2(2%)	0	0	0	1(4%)
Total	56(62%)	5(83%)	5(83%)	21(78%)	11(39%)
Intermediate-grade malignant lymphoma					
Diffuse, large cell	17(19%)	0	0	0	14(50%)
Diffuse, small cleaved cell	8(9%)	0	0	4(15%)	2(7%)
Diffuse, mixed	1(1%)	0	0	0	1(4%)
Total	26(29%)	0	0	4(15%)	17(61%)
Low-grade malignant lymphoma					
Small lymphocytic, plasmacytoid	3(3%)	1(17%)	1(17%)	2(7%)	0
Follicular, small cleaved cell	3(3%)	0	0	0	0
Total	6(7%)	1(17%)	1(17%)	2(7%)	0
Miscellaneous					
Unclassified	2(2%)	0	0	0	0

CONCLUSION

AIDS patients can have a multitude of severe life-threatening diseases simultaneously with unusual clinical and histopathologic manifestations. Biopsy and culture of even the most subtle lesions in these patients is extremely important. Performing routine acid fast and methenamine silver stains in addition to H&E stains on all histologic material from an AIDS or suspected AIDS patient is mandatory, no matter what the histology of the lesion. Furthermore, the pathologist should be alerted to the possibility of finding several different pathologic conditions within one biopsy specimen.

REFERENCES

1. Niedt, G.W., Schinella, R.A., Acquired immunodeficiency syndrome. Clinicopathologic study of 56 autopsies. Arch Path Lab Med 109:727-734 (1985)

2. Reichert, C.M., O'Leary, T.J., Levens, D.L., et al., Autopsy pathology in the acquired immune deficiency syndrome. Am J Path 112:357-382 (1983)

3. Welch, K., Finkbeiner, W., Alpers, C.E., et al., Autopsy findings in the acquired immune deficiency syndrome. JAMA 252:1152-1159 (1984)

4. Moskowitz, L., Hensley, G.T., Chan, J.C., et al., Immediate causes of death in acquired immunodeficiency syndrome. Arch Path Lab Med 109:735-738 (1985)

5. Hui, A.N., Koss, M.N., Meyer, P.R., Necropsy findings in acquired immunodeficiency syndrome: a comparison of premortem diagnosis with postmortem diagnosis with postmortem findings. Hum Path 15:670-676 (1984)

6. Mobley, K., Rotterdam, H.Z., Lerner, C.W., et al., Autopsy findings in the acquired immune deficiency syndrome. Path Ann Part 1:45-65 (1985)

7. Guarda, L.A., Luna, M.A., Smith, J.L., et al., Acquired immune deficiency syndrome: postmortem findings. Am J Clin Path 81:549-557 (1985)

8. Macher, A.M., Reichert, C.M., Straus, S.E., et al., Death of the AIDS patient: role of cytomegalovirus. N Engl J Med 23: 1454 (1983)

9. CDC., Update on acquired immunodeficiency syndrome (AIDS) - United States. MMWR 31:507-514 (1982)

10. Watts, J.C., Chandler, F.W., *Pneumocystis carinii* pneumonitis. The nature and diagnostic significance of methenamine silver-positive "intracystic bodies". Am J Surg Path 9:744-751 (1985)

11. Conley, F.K., Jenkins, K.A., Remington, J.S., *Toxoplasma gondii* infection of the central nervous system: use of the peroxidase method to demonstrate toxoplasma in formalin fixed, paraffin-embedded tissue sections. Hum Path 12:690-698 (1981)

12. Klein, R.S., Harris, C.A., Small, C.B., et al., Oral candidiasis in high risk patients as the initial manifestation of the acquired immune deficiency syndrome. N Engl J Med 311: 354-358 (1984)

13. Bottone, E.J., Toma, M., Johansson, B.E., et al., Poorly encapsulated *Cryptococcus neoformans* from patients with AIDS: I. preliminary observations. AIDS Research 2:211-218 (1986)

14. Bottone, E.J., Wormser, G.P., Poorly encapsulated *Cryptococcus neoformans* from patients with AIDS. II. Correlation of capsule size observed directly in cerebrospinal fluid with that after animal passage. AIDS Research 2:219-225 (1986)

15. Pasternak, J., Bolivar, R., Histoplasmosis in acquired immunodeficiency syndrome (AIDS): diagnosis by bone marrow examination. Arch Intern Med 143:2024 (1983)

16. Kaur, J., Myer, A.M., Homosexuality, steroid therapy, and histoplasmosis. Ann Intern Med 99:567 (1983)

17. Small, C.B., Hewlett, D., Duncanson, F.P., et al., The acquired immunodeficiency syndrome and disseminated histoplasmosis in a non-endemic area. International Conference on Acquired Immunodeficiency Syndrome (AIDS) Atlanta, GA (1985)

18. Jones, P.G., Cohen, R.L., Batts, D.H., et al., Disseminated histoplasmosis, invasive pulmonary aspergillosis and other opportunistic infections in a homosexual patient with acquired immunodeficiency syndrome. Sex Transm Dis 10:202-204 (1983)

19. Strom, R.L., Gruninger, R.P., AIDS with *Mycobacterium avium-intracellulare* lesions resembling those of Whipple's disease. N Engl J Med 309:1323-1324 (1983)

20. Roth, R.I., Owen, R.L., Keren, D.F., AIDS with *Mycobacterium avium-intracellulare* lesions resembling those of Whipple's disease. N Engl J Med 309:1324-1325 (1983)

21. Krigel, R.L., Friedman-Kien, A.E., Kaposi's sarcoma in AIDS. In: AIDS--Etiology, Diagnosis, Treatment and Prevention (De Vita, V.T., Hellman, S., Rosenberg, S.A., eds) J.B. Lippincott, Co., Philadelphia, PA, p 185-211 (1985)

22. Gottlieb, G.J., Ragaz, A., Vogel, J.V., et al., A preliminary communication on extensively disseminated Kaposi's sarcoma in young homosexual men. Am J Dermatopath 3:111-114 (1981)

23. Ziegler, J.L., Beckstead, J.A., Volberding, P.A., et al., Non-Hodgkin's lymphoma in 90 homosexual men. N Engl J Med 311:565-570 (1984)

24. Levine, A.M., Meyer, P.R., Begandy, M.K., et al., Development of B-cell lymphoma in homosexual men. Ann Intern Med 100:7-13 (1984)

25. Gill, P.S., Levine, A.M., Meyer, P.R., et al., Primary central nervous system lymphoma in homosexual men. Am J Med 78:742-748 (1985)

26. Ahmed, T., Wormser, G.P., Stahl, R.E., et al., Malignant lymphomas in prisoners and intravenous drug abusers: evidence for an etiologic relationship with the acquired immunodeficiency syndrome. Cancer (In press)

27. Levine, A.M., Parkash, S.G., Meyer, P.R., et al., Retrovirus and malignant lymphoma in homosexual men. JAMA 254:1921-1925 (1985)

28. DiCarlo, E.P., Amberson, J.B., Metroka, C.E., et al., Malignant lymphomas and the acquired immunodeficiency syndrome. Evaluation of 30 cases using a working formulation. Arch Pathol Lab Med 110:1012-1016 (1986)

29. Schoeppel, S.L., Hoppe, R.T., Dorfman, R.F., et al., Hodgkin's disease in homosexual men with generalized lymphadenopathy. Ann Intern Med 102:68-70 (1985)

43

Pathology and Immunohistology of Lymph Nodes in HIV Infection

Gary S. Wood

INTRODUCTION

Human immunodeficiency virus (HIV) retroviral infection can be asymptomatic, result in the persistent generalized lymphadenopathy syndrome (PGL) (1) (or other manifestations of the acquired immunodeficiency syndrome complex (ARC)), or result in the acquired immunodeficiency syndrome (AIDS) (2). Patients with either PGL or AIDS may exhibit generalized lymph node enlargement, a decreased peripheral blood helper/cytotoxic-suppressor T-cell ratio and nonspecific constitutional symptoms such as fever, malaise and weight loss. AIDS is further characterized by the presence of opportunistic infections and/or neoplasms such as Kaposi's sarcoma or lymphoma. These variable clinical features are reflected by the broad spectrum of histopathologic and immunohistologic alterations that have been observed in lymph nodes obtained from these patients.

LYMPH NODE ANATOMY

In order to appreciate the histopathologic alterations that occur in PGL and AIDS, it is useful to review briefly lymph node anatomy and histology (3),(4). The lymph node is surrounded by a connective tissue capsule. Afferent lymphatics empty into a subcapsular sinus which connects to paratrabecular sinuses that follow connective tissue trabeculae into the substance of the lymph node and eventually converge at the hilum as efferent lymphatics. The outer lymph node parenchyma, the cortex, contains primary lymphoid follicles or nodules composed of B cells set within a unified meshwork of follicular dendritic cells (FDC). FDC are involved in antigen trapping and accessory cell functions. In response to antigenic stimulation, the primary follicle becomes a reactive secondary follicle containing a germinal center composed of mitotically active small and large cleaved and noncleaved cells. This germinal center is surrounded by a mantle or cuff or small mature B lymphocytes. In contrast to the follicles which comprise the B cell domain, the adjacent paracortex comprises the T cell domain. Admixed with T cells are "interdigitating cells" which have accessory cell function. Adjacent to the paracortex are the medullary cords which lie between the paratrabecular sinuses as they course to the hilum. The medullary cords are rich in plasma cells.

HISTOPATHOLOGY

The morphologic alterations of lymph nodes associated with HIV infection fall into two basic categories: reactive and neoplastic (5)-(10). The reactive changes generally consist of either florid follicular hyperplasia or lymphocyte depletion. The neoplastic changes involve Kaposi's sarcoma or lymphoma.

REACTIVE LYMPHADENOPATHY

The most common type of reactive pattern is florid follicular hyperplasia. It is characteristic of the vast majority of patients with PGL. There is a marked increase in the number and size of secondary B cell follicles, often with partial or total effacement of the mantle zone. In at least one-half of such cases, some follicles exhibit a characteristic change referred to as "follicle lysis" (9),(11). This consists of disruption of the normally unified germinal center by aggregates of small mature lymphocytes and extravasated erythrocytes (Figures 1 and 2). The paracortex is generally also hyperplastic with prominent vasculature and scattered immunoblasts. Another feature seen in approximately one-half of cases is collections of "monocytoid" cells, often admixed with neutrophils, within lymph node sinuses (Figure 3). The histologic triad found in the lymphadenitis associated with toxoplasmosis (follicular hyperplasia, clusters of epithelioid histiocytes and sinusal monocytoid cells) has also been noted in occasional cases, some confirmed by positive serology for *Toxoplasma gondii* (9). Although cytologically similar to monocytes, monocytoid cells have been shown to be of B cell lineage (12). Additional findings that have been observed in a minority of cases include focal dermatopathic change, paracortical histiocytosis and plasmacytosis. Dermatopathic change involves expansion of the paracortex by HLA-DR$^+$ dendritic histiocytes including CD1$^+$ Langerhans cells (13).

Polykaryocytes, resembling the Warthin-Finkeldey giant cells of measles, have been noted in several cases within the germinal center or paracortex (9),(10). These cells have been documented in a variety of reactive and neoplastic lymphoid disorders and

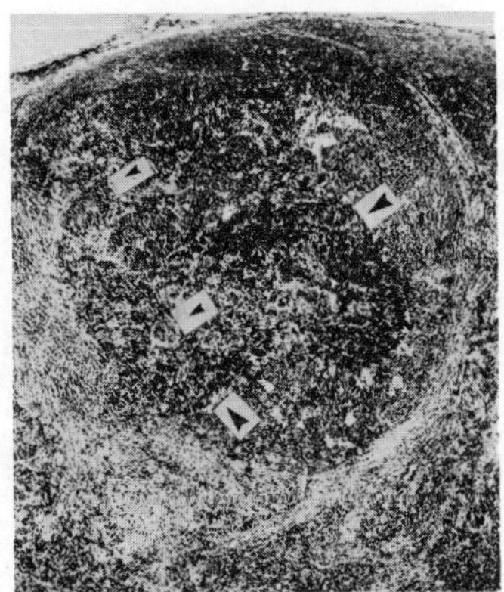

Figure 1. The histopathology of follicle lysis (see Figure 2 also).

Paraffin section of a subcapsular B cell follicle in a lymph node biopsy from a homosexual man with PGL. The mantle zone is poorly developed. Within the germinal center are dark aggregates of small, mature lymphocytes admixed with extravasated erythrocytes (large arrowheads). Germinal center cells in some areas are organized into cohesive cell clusters (small arrow-heads). Hematoxylin and eosin stain.
(Reprinted from Ref. 11 with permission.)

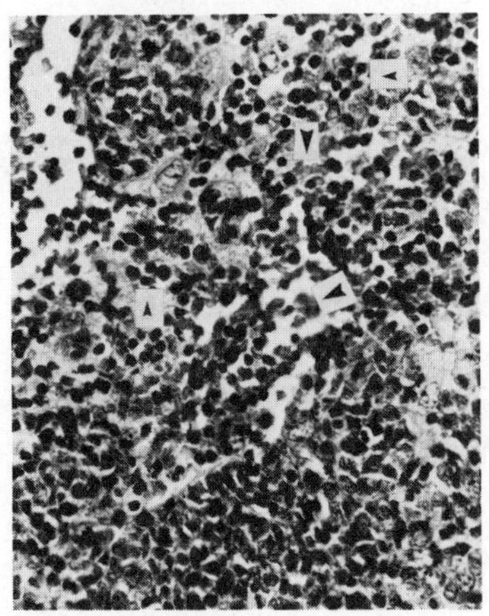

Figure 2. Higher magnification of a serial section of the germinal center shown in Figure 1 demonstrates numerous dark, small mature lymphocytes (small arrowheads) admixed with small grey erythrocytes (large arrowheads). In the background are larger residual germinal center cells. Hematoxylin and eosin stain. (Reprinted from Ref. 11 with permission.)

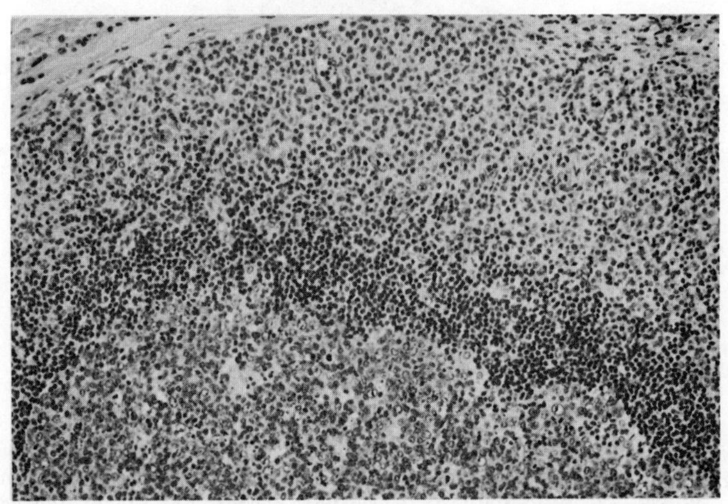

Figure 3. Monocytoid cells.

Sinusal distension by monocytoid cells and rare neutrophils (above) in a lymph node showing reactive follicular hyperplasia (below). Hematoxylin and eosin stain.
(Reprinted for Ref. 9 with permission.)

are not specific for HIV infection (9),(14). However, it is well known that viruses can induce polykaryocytosis in vitro (15). This includes giant cell formation by T cells infected with HIV retrovirus (16),(17). Splenic and thymic multinucleated cells obtained from AIDS patients have been shown to be helper T cells infected by HIV (18).

The second major reactive pattern observed in lymph nodes from patients with HIV infection has been termed "lymphocyte depletion" (Figure 4). These lymph nodes exhibit a "washed-out" appearance with few or absent reactive follicles and an overall depletion of small lymphocytes. Scattered "burned-out" or regressively transformed germinal centers (4) are often present, characterized by concentric layers of follicular dendritic cells, blood vessels and a few lymphocytes forming a small, compact follicle. Other features that are variably seen in these cases include histiocytosis, plasmacytosis, increased paracortical immunoblasts, paracortical fibrosis with increased vascularity, dermatopathic change and sinusal monocytoid cells. Although sinus histiocytosis with hemophagocytosis can be seen in association with any of the reactive patterns, it is most common in nodes exhibiting the lymphocyte depletion pattern (10).

A third, uncommon "paracortical hyperplasia" reactive pattern has also been reported in lymph nodes from HIV-infected patients, and has been postulated to represent a transition between the former two (10). Regression of B cell follicles parallels that seen in the lymphocyte depletion pattern; however, there is diffuse paracortical hyperplasia associated with immunoblasts, plasma cells and a prominent vasculature.

NEOPLASTIC LYMPHADENOPATHY

Kaposi's sarcoma in patients with AIDS may present in either the skin or lymph nodes (9). The histologic appearance of the tumor is similar in both sites and consists of characteristic bundles of spindle cells containing cleft-like spaces and extravasated erythrocytes. Eosinophilic hyaline globules can often be observed within macrophages or tumor cells. Kaposi's sarcoma can totally efface the normal lymphoid architecture or, in early involvement, can be present as only a tiny focus within the lymph node capsule or sinuses. This is also characteristic of early lymph node involvement in African children, where Kaposi's sarcoma is often clinically aggressive (9). Cytomegalovirus (CMV) infection of tumor cells has been documented in Kaposi's sarcoma in AIDS, leading to speculation that it may be CMV-induced (19). Uninvolved areas of lymph nodes partially effaced by Kaposi's sarcoma can exhibit either follicular hyperplasia or lymphocyte depletion. They often contain regressively transformed germinal centers bearing some similarity to the lymph node lesion described initially as "hypervascular follicular hyperplasia" (20) and more recently as resembling Castleman's disease (21).

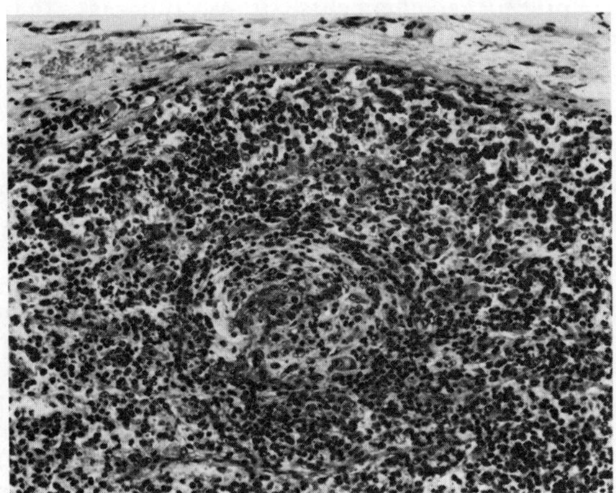

Figure 4. Lymphocyte depletion reactive pattern.

There is lymphocyte depletion in the paracortex with a small, regressively transformed germinal center. Hematoxylin and eosin stain. (Reprinted from Ref. 9 with permission.)

Most of the lymphomas described in association with HIV infection have been of B cell lineage (22). They often exhibit follicular center cell differentiation including small noncleaved, small cleaved and large cell types. They are histologically similar to their counterparts unassociated with HIV infection; however, they are clinically more aggressive. Other types of lymphoma, including Hodgkin's disease, have also been observed (9),(22),(23). The CD4 antigen, or a spatially related structure, is an essential component of the cell surface receptor necessary for HIV infection (24),(25). Because HIV can infect $CD4^+$ B lymphoblastoid cell lines transformed by Epstein-Barr virus (EBV) (25), it is theoretically possible that HIV infection of B cells in vivo might trigger the development of B cell lymphoma in AIDS (26). However, studies of one such B cell lymphoma documented infection of tumor cells by EBV but not HIV (26). The c-myc oncogene was also rearranged. These results suggest that at least some B cell lymphomas in patients with AIDS might arise from clonal expansion of an EBV-transformed B cell exhibiting deregulation of oncogene expression in the mileau of a depressed host response secondary to HIV infection of T cells (26). In this context, HIV-infected patients have been shown to exhibit abnormally high numbers of EBV-infected circulating B cells capable of spontaneous outgrowth in vitro (27). Evidence for aneuploid cell lines (28) and abnormal immunoglobulin light chain ratios (29) have been obtained from studies of lymph nodes from PGL patients and may represent early manifestations of HIV associated lymphoma.

CLINICAL RELEVANCE OF LYMPH NODE HISTOPATHOLOGY

From the preceding comments, it is apparent that HIV-associated lymphadenopathy has a large differential diagnosis. A significant proportion of cases will be caused by infectious diseases or neoplasms with some potential for treatment, e.g. mycobacterial infections, toxoplasmosis, lymphomas or Kaposi's sarcoma. It is also apparent that any of these disorders may occur in a patient with prior biopsies showing only reactive changes. Therefore, close follow-up of these patients, with biopsy of lymph nodes when clinically indicated, is an important part of overall patient care.

The histopathology of lymph nodes showing only reactive features may also be clinically relevant. PGL patients characteristically exhibit follicular hyperplasia (5)-(10), although occasionally paracortical hyperplasia (6),(8)-(10) and rarely lymphocyte depletion (7)-(9) have been reported. Lymph nodes in AIDS may also exhibit follicular hyperplasia (5),(9),(10), paracortical hyperplasia (5),(9),(10) or lymphocyte depletion (5),(9). End-stage AIDS is typically associated with the latter pattern (5),(9). These findings suggest that patients with the lymphocyte depletion pattern of preterminal AIDS may have evolved from prior follicular hyperplasia (10). This transition has been documented histologically in monkeys with an AIDS-like disease (30); however, similar serial biopsy studies in humans are lacking. Although it is uncertain what percentage of PGL patients will go on to develop AIDS, this transition has been reported in some cases (8),(31)-(33), particularly those with constitutional symptoms, oral candidiasis, depressed antigen-stimulated lymphocyte proliferation or impaired gamma interferon generation (33), or the histopathologic features of paracortical hyperplasia or lymphocyte depletion (6),(8),(10). Furthermore, AIDS has resulted from HIV exposure up to seven years prior to diagnosis and longer incubation periods may be possible (2). This implies that long-term monitoring of PGL patients will be required before the risk of subsequent AIDS is clarified. In a small percentage of PGL patients, lymphadenopathy has regressed without subsequent AIDS within a limited follow-up period; however, tests of immune function have not normalized (31).

IMMUNOHISTOLOGY

The immunohistologic features of lymph nodes in PGL and AIDS have been delineated by staining frozen sections with monoclonal antibodies directed against a variety of lymphoid antigens. Representative antibodies and their relevant reactivities are summarized in Table 1. Most studies have focused upon follicle lysis, T cell subsets or non-T cells.

FOLLICLE LYSIS

As noted above, follicle lysis is a characteristic alteration of B cell follicles originally described in lymph node biopsies from homosexual men (9),(11),(34),(35). Although similar changes have been noted in other clinical settings (36), follicle lysis has been reported principally in association with HIV infection. It consists of disruption of germinal centers by aggregates of small mature lymphocytes variably associated with erythrocyte extravasation (Figures 1 and 2).

Immunohistologic studies of follicle lysis have documented disruption of the normal, unified follicular meshwork of R4/23$^+$ T05$^+$ FDC (Figure 5) by aggregates of small lymphocytes predominantly of either polytypic mantle B cell phenotype (T015$^+$/Leu 8$^+$/mu$^+$/delta$^+$/kappa$^+$ or lambda$^+$) (11),(36),(37), or mature T cell phenotype (mixed CD4$^+$ and CD8$^+$) (11),(34),(35). Unlike the minor population of T cells present in normal germinal centers, these T cells have been Leu 8$^+$ (11),(35). This is the principal phenotype of T cells in the mantle and paracortex (38). These observations suggest migration of T cells into the germinal center or abnormal expression of Leu 8 by germinal center T cells in follicle lysis. Immunohistologic studies employing antibodies reactive with HIV antigens, have documented reactivity localized to the FDC network (39),(40). These results correlate with ultrastructural observations of typical retroviral particles between (41),(42), and occasionally within (43), the cell processes of FDC in PGL. Interestingly, other lymph node cells, including CD4$^+$ T cells, were unreactive with these antibodies (39),(40). This may be explained by the fact that less than 0.01% of mono-

Table 1. Monoclonal Antibodies Employed in Immunohistologic Studies of Lymph Nodes in PGL and AIDS.

Antigen Specificity	Relevant Reactivity
Leu 2 (CD8)	T_C, T_S
Leu 3 (CD4)	T_H, histiocytes
Leu 4 (CD3)	T cells
9.3	T_H, T_C
Leu 8	Blood: Majority of T_H, $T_{C/S}$, B cells and some NK/K, monocytes and granulocytes. Lymph Node: Majority of T_H, $T_{C/S}$, mantle B. Virtually no cells in germinal centers.
T015	B cells
Immunoglobulin	B cells
T05	FDC
R4/23	FDC
Leu 6 (CD1)	Langerhans cells and precursors (seen in dermatopathic nodes)
Leu 7	NK/K cells
Leu M3	Histiocytes
T10	Plasma Cells
HLA-DR	B cells, histiocytes, activated T cells
TAC	Interleukin-2 receptor
Ki-67	Nuclei of proliferating cells

T_C - cytotoxic T cells; T_S - suppressor T cells;
T_H - helper T cells; NK/K - natural killer and killer cells;
FDC - follicular dendritic cells.

nuclear cells from the blood or lymph nodes of HIV-infected patients contain retrovirus detectable by an in situ RNA hybridization technique (44). In tissue sections, these cells appear to lie within germinal centers (45).

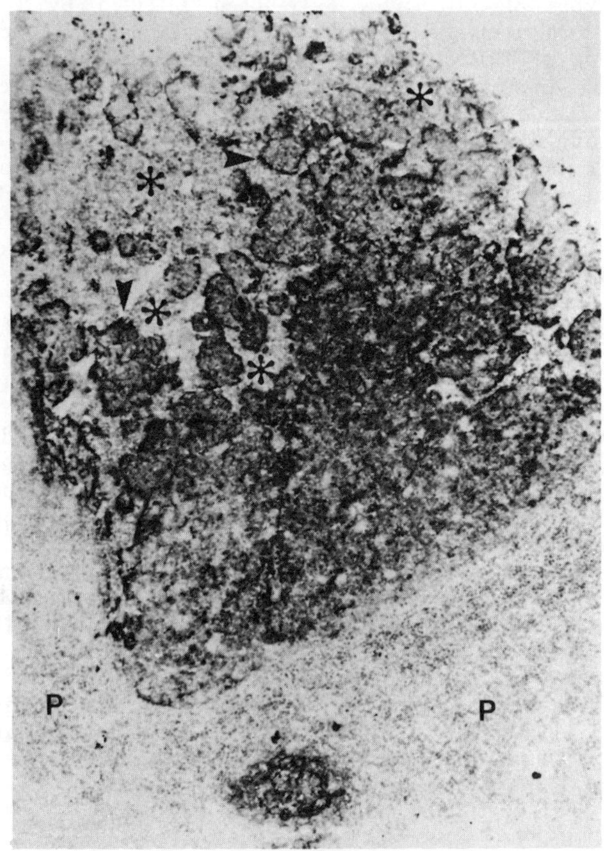

Figure 5. R4/23$^+$ follicular dendritic cells (FDC) in follicle lysis.

Frozen sections of a B cell follicle in a lymph node biopsy from a homosexual man with PGL. The darkly stained R4/23$^+$ FDC are severely disrupted into multiple discrete aggregates (arrowheads). These aggregates contain the germinal center cells apparent as cohesive cell clusters in paraffin sections such as in Figures 1 and 2. The unstained cells between R4/23$^+$ areas (*) expressed the mantle B cell phenotype. The lower portion of the figure is composed predominantly of unstained paracortical T cells (P). Immunoperoxidase stain, original magnification x 80. (Reprinted from Ref. 11 with permission.)

Although initially described in T cells, the CD4 antigen is expressed by most types of histiocytic dendritic cells and macrophages, including FDC which express it weakly (46). Because the CD4 antigen is essential to penetration and infection of cells by HIV (24),(25), it is possible that FDC as well as $CD4^+$ T cells are targets for retroviral infection in PGL and AIDS. Indeed, certain types of histiocytes have been infected by HIV in vitro (24). Alternatively, HIV antigens may simply be concentrated on the surface of FDC in the form of immune complexes (39). However, such immune complex concentration of other relevant viral antigens, including CMV and hepatitis B, has not been detectable in PGL using similar techniques (39).

Follicular dendritic cells, which have polyclonal immune complexes on their surfaces, provide accessory cell function essential to the homeostasis of the normal germinal center microenvironment (4). It is possible that HIV accumulation within germinal centers might both physically and functionally disrupt the FDC network, resulting in deregulation of B cell proliferation with consequent florid follicular hyperplasia, mantle zone attenuation and hypergammaglobulinemia (39). Clonal B cell proliferations, manifest clinically as lymphoma, might evolve as a direct consequence of this, or perhaps as a result of concurrent EBV infection. EBV infection can produce B cell activation with follicular hyperplasia, hypergammaglobulinemia and an inverted $CD4^+/CD8^+$ T cell ratio (47). Such preactivation of B cells in vivo has been offered as an explanation for the decreased responsiveness of B cells from PGL and AIDS patients to T cell-dependent and T cell-independent mitogens in vitro (47). In this context, EBV has been documented both within an increased number of circulating B cells (27) and within some B cell lymphomas in AIDS (26). It has been noted previously that HIV infection of humans may be somewhat analogous to infection of cats with another lymphotropic retrovirus, the feline leukemia virus (39). This virus, which causes feline leukemia and immunodeficiency, has been localized within the hyperplastic B cell follicles of lymph nodes in infected cats (39).

T CELL SUBSETS

Patients with PGL or AIDS exhibit quantitative and qualitative abnormalities of peripheral blood T cells including decreased total T cells, a decreased helper/cytotoxic-suppressor (T_H/T_{CS} or $CD4^+/CD8^+$) ratio, reduced response to mitogens, diminished helper activity in vitro, increased suppressor activity in vitro, and defective reactivity in the allogeneic and autologous mixed lymphocyte reactions (38). Several immunohistologic studies have documented a reduced T_H/T_{CS} ratio within lymph nodes in AIDS (38),(48),(49) and PGL (37),(49)-(54) analogous to that noted initially in the peripheral blood (1),(2),(37),(38). Within individual lymph nodes, the most severe reduction was in the paracortical T cell domain, while in general the T_H/T_{CS} ratio was relatively preserved (>1.0) within the follicular B cell domain. Although results vary, several studies of lymph nodes have documented less reduction of this ratio in PGL relative to AIDS (37),(53),(54). This may correlate with a more intact immune system protective against the opportunistic infections and neoplasms that distinguish PGL from AIDS (37).

In order to dissect T cell subset alterations in HIV infection further, immunohistologic studies of lymph nodes have also employed novel monoclonal antibodies such as 9.3 and anti-Leu 8 (Table 2) (37),(38). 9.3 allows the dissection of $CD8^+$ T_{CS} into $CD8^+$ 9.3^+ T_C and $CD8^+$ 9.3^- T_S (55). Anti-Leu8 allows the dissection of $CD4^+$ T_H into functionally distinct subsets (56). These studies indicated that the reversal of the paracortical T_H/T_{CS} ratio in AIDS and PGL was due to an increase in T_S with a concomitant decrease in T_H. These changes were also reflected in a reduction of the normal paracortical T_C/T_S ratio (3.0). Except for decreased paracortical T_C in AIDS, normal numbers of lymph node T_C were observed in PGL and AIDS. Alterations of T_H, T_C and T_S in AIDS lymph nodes are detailed in Figure 6.

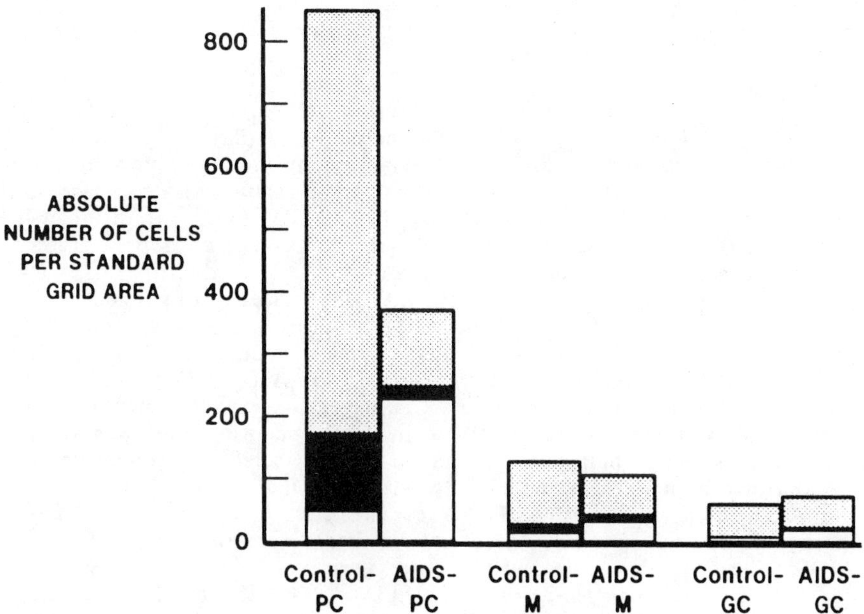

Figure 6. Alterations of T cell subsets in AIDS vs. controls.

The histogram is based on the mean values for T_H (gray), T_C (black), and T_S (white). Within the paracortex (PC) in AIDS, there was a marked reduction in total T cells, T_H, and T_C, while T_S were increased ($P \leq .01$). No statistically significant quantitative alterations were noted within the mantle (M); however, with the germinal center (GC), T_S were increased ($P \leq .01$). (Reprinted from Ref. 38 with permission.)

Table 2. In Vitro Functions of Phenotypically Defined T Cell Subsets.

Phenotype	Function
$CD8^+9.3^+$	T_C
$CD8^+9.3^-$	T_S
$CD4^+Leu8^+$	Inducer of T_C and T_S
$CD4^+Leu8^-$	Inducer of T_C and B

T_C = Cytotoxic T cells
T_S = Suppressor T cells

In AIDS, there was also a marked reduction in paracortical $CD4^+Leu8^+$ T_H (38) which are important in cell-mediated immunity as inducers of T_C and T_S, and which exert feedback inhibition of immunoglobulin production through a T_S intermediary (56). These features might help to explain the deficient cell-mediated immunity and hypergammaglobulinemia noted in HIV infection (38). While other studies have shown a decrease of peripheral blood $CD4^+$ $Leu8^+$ T_H in PGL (57), alterations in paracortical T cell subsets in PGL did not reflect those present in the peripheral blood where a more severe reduction in $CD4^+$ T_H and an increase in $CD8^+9.3^+$ T_C were observed (37). Furthermore, the $CD4^+$ $Leu8^+$ T_H population was relatively preserved in the paracortex of PGL lymph nodes, again suggesting a more intact immune system relative to AIDS (37). In vitro studies indicate that the Leu 8 antigen, as well as the CD4 antigen, may somehow be involved in HIV reception and penetration (24). This may help to account for the selective reduction of T_H that are both $CD4^+$ and $Leu8^+$ in AIDS and PGL (37),(38).

Although $CD8^+9.3^-$ T_S are increased in both T cell (paracortex) and B cell (germinal center) domains in PGL and AIDS, the T_H/T_S ratio within the germinal center is generally preserved (greater than 1.0) (37),(38). Furthermore, virtually all germinal center $CD4^+$ T_H belong to the Leu 8^- subset (37),(38). Normal levels of $CD4^+Leu8^-$ T_H have been documented in the peripheral blood of PGL patients (57). These $CD4^+Leu8^-$ T_H provide the major help for B cell differentiation in vitro (56). Their preservation in blood and lymph nodes may help to explain the follicular hyperplasia, hypergammaglobulinemia and plasmacytosis noted in PGL and AIDS (37),(38).

TAC, the interleukin-2 receptor, can be expressed by activated T cells as well as some non-T cells. AIDS patients have impaired production of interleukin-2 (58) and other lymphokines

(59) in their peripheral blood. There were decreased TAC^+ cells within the germinal center in PGL with a trend towards a similar decrease in the mantle and paracortex. This correlates with decreased TAC expression by circulating lymphocytes in AIDS and PGL (60),(61). A trend towards increased $HLA\text{-}DR^+$ cells within the paracortex has been noted in PGL (37). This might be due to activation of paracortical T cells or hyperplasia of paracortical histiocytes. Within this and other series, there was also an increase in circulating $HLA\text{-}DR^+$ T cells (37),(57).

NON-T CELLS

While much attention has focused upon T cell abnormalities in PGL and AIDS, additional findings indicate abnormalities among non-T cells as well (62). Despite the superficial appearance of intact humoral immunity as indicated by hypergammaglobulinemia (5)-(7),(47),(57),(63)-(66), there is evidence of primary B cell abnormalities including decreased circulating (7),(63),(66) or lymph node (48),(50) B cells in some cases, an increased incidence of B cell lymphoma (22), monoclonal gammopathy (62), abnormal kappa/lambda immunoglobulin light chain ratios suggestive of monoclonal B cell proliferations (29), increased spontaneous immunoglobulin production in vitro (47),(57), and defective responsiveness to B cell mitogens (47),(49),(57),(63)-(66). Abnormalities among histiocytes have been suggested by increased or decreased circulating macrophage precursors (63), (64), increased serum lysozyme levels (64), decreased cutaneous Langerhans cells (67) and defective antigen presentation by circulating mononuclear cells (68). Although natural killer/killer (NK/K) cell activity was normal in some studies (64),(65), decreased NK activity has also been noted (31),(66), (69). These findings have prompted immunohistologic evaluation of non-T cells in lymph nodes from PGL and AIDS.

B LINEAGE CELLS

Some studies have documented a decreased absolute number of blood (7) or total lymph node (48),(50) B cells in PGL and AIDS. Immunohistologic studies have not revealed an absolute decrease in paracortical B cells in AIDS (62) or in paracortical, mantle or germinal center B cells in PGL (37). There was, however, a relative increase in paracortical B cells in AIDS secondary to the absolute decrease in T cells (62). A trend towards increased lymph node $T10^+$ plasma cells was also noted in both AIDS (paracortex) (62) and PGL (paracortex, mantle and germinal center) (37). This is consistent with prior morphologic studies noting plasmacytosis in some cases (6),(8)-(10),(70). Ki-67 defines a nuclear antigen expressed by proliferating cells (71). Increased $Ki\text{-}67^+$ cells were noted within the mantle zones of PGL lymph nodes (37). This may be related to altered B cell follicle homeostasis in HIV infection with consequent abnormal control of B cell proliferation.

In the context of these findings, it is evident that the depletion of B cell follicles seen in some lymph nodes in PGL and AIDS cannot be due to random depletion of lymph node B cells. Rather, it is likely related to specific events within the germinal center such as the follicle lysis discussed earlier.

HISTIOCYTES (MACROPHAGES AND DENDRITIC CELLS)

Leu $M3^+$ histiocytes were increased within the paracortex of AIDS lymph nodes (62). A similar trend was noted within the paracortex of PGL lymph nodes but not within the mantle or germinal center (37). This correlates with reports of elevated serum lysozyme in AIDS (64) and morphologic observations of paracortical and sinus histiocytosis (5)-(10),(50),(62). This hyperplasia may be secondary to the functional histiocyte deficiency noted in AIDS (70),(72). Circulating monocytes were increased in some cases (63) but decreased in several others (63),(64), possible reflecting recruitment of circulating histiocyte precursors into lymphoid tissue. In this way, a more primitive form of cell-mediated immunity, phagocytosis, might partially compensate for the immune deficits caused by progressive HIV-mediated T cell depletion (62).

A trend towards increased $CD1^+$ paracortical cells has been noted in both PGL (37) and AIDS (62). This increase generally correlated with the presence of dermatopathic change, a process wherein there is an increase in HLA-DR^+ cells, including $CD1^+$ Langerhans cells and Langerhans cell precursors, within the paracortex (13). These cells probably originated in the skin with subsequent transit to lymph nodes via afferent lymphatics (13),(62). This mechanism would be consistent with the decreased number of $CD1^+$ Langerhans cells noted in the skin of HIV infected patients (67). Langerhans cells, like other histiocytes, are variably $CD4^+$ and, like T_H and FDC, might be potential targets for HIV infection (62).

The effects of HIV infection upon $R4/23^+$ $T05^+$ FDC have been discussed earlier in the context of follicle lysis.

NK/K CELLS

$Leu7^+$ NK/K cells were increased within the paracortex but not the mantle or germinal center compartments of AIDS lymph nodes (62). This parallels the observation of increased $Leu7^+$ cells in the blood of AIDS patients (69). Because some NK/K cells express a $Leu7^-11^+$ phenotype, these studies may represent an underestimate of nodal NK/K cells (62).

SUMMARY

A broad spectrum of histopathologic and immunohistologic findings within lymph nodes has been associated with HIV infection. The histopathologic alterations fall into two major categories--reactive and neoplastic. The reactive changes consist predominantly of florid follicular hyperplasia or lymphocyte depletion. The neoplastic changes consist of Kaposi's sarcoma or lymphoma. Lymph node evaluation by serial biopsy is sometimes clinically important because individual patients may exhibit different findings over time.

Immunohistologic studies, interpreted in the context of in vitro studies of HIV infection, suggest certain pathogenetic mechanisms for the findings associated with PGL and AIDS. There appear to be at least two principal targets of HIV in lymph nodes -- T_H and FDC. Infection results in gradual depletion of $CD4^+$ $Leu8^+T_H$ associated with a reduced T_H/ T_{CS} ratio and impaired cell-mediated immunity. In this milieu of diminished host response, patients exhibit an increased incidence of opportunistic infections, Kaposi's sarcoma and B cell lymphoma. Transformation of tumor cells by CMV or EBV, respectively, may also be involved in the pathogenesis of these latter two neoplasms. Although peripheral blood T cell subset alterations are often similar in PGL and AIDS, the absence of opportunistic infections and neoplasms in PGL may be related to the relative preservation of $CD4^+Leu8^+T_H$ within the lymph node paracortex in PGL. Localization of HIV in or on FDC may play a role in the follicle lysis associated with PGL and AIDS. This architectural disruption of germinal centers might result in a disruption of FDC function with deregulation of B cell proliferation predisposing to B cell lymphoma. In some cases, FDC might be destroyed eventually. This would be expected to result in regression of B cell follicles, such as seen in lymph nodes exhibiting the lymphocyte depletion reactive pattern characteristic of preterminal AIDS, because FDC are an important component of the follicular microenvironment.

REFERENCES

1. CDC., Persistent, generalized lymphadenopathy among homosexual males. MMWR 31:249-251 (1982)

2. CDC., Update on acquired immunodeficiency syndromes (AIDS) - United States. MMWR 35:17-21 (1986)

3. Beckstead, J.H., The evaluation of human lymph nodes using plastic sections and enzyme histochemistry. Am J Clin Pathol 80:131-139 (1983)

4. Stein, H., Gerdes, J., Mason, D.Y., The normal and malignant germinal center. Clin Hematol 11:531-559 (1982)

5. Ioachim, H., Lerner, C.W., Tapper, M.L., Lymphadenopathies in homosexual men. Relationships with the acquired immune deficiency syndrome. JAMA 250:1306-1309 (1983)

6. Brynes, R.K., Chan, W.C., Spira, T.J., et al., Value of lymph node biopsy in unexplained lymphadenopathy in homosexual men. JAMA 250:1313-1317 (1983)

7. Guarda, L.A., Butler, J.J., Mansell, P., et al., Lymphadenopathy in homosexual men. Morbid anatomy with clinical and immunologic correlations. Am J Clin Pathol 79:559-568 (1983)

8. Fernandez, R., Mouradian, J., Metroka, C., et al., The prognostic value of histopathology in persistent generalized lymphadenopathy in homosexual men. N Engl J Med 309:185-186 (1983)

9. Burns, B.F., Wood, G.S., Dorfman, R.F., The varied histopathology of lymphadenopathy in the homosexual male. Am J Surg Pathol 9:287-297 (1985)

10. Ewing, E.P., Jr, Chandler, F.W., Spira, T.J., et al., Primary lymph node pathology in AIDS and AIDS-related lymphadenopathy. Arch Pathol Lab Med 109:977-981 (1985)

11. Wood, G.S., Garcia, C.F., Dorfman, R.F., et al., The immunohistology of follicle lysis in lymph node biopsies from homosexual men. Blood 66:1092-1097 (1985)

12. Sohn, C.C., Sheibani, K., Winberg, C.D., et al., Monocytoid B lymphocytes: Their relation to the patterns of the acquired immunodeficiency syndrome (AIDS) and AIDS-related lymphadenopathy. Hum Pathol 16:979-985 (1985)

13. Weiss, L.M., Beckstead, J.H., Warnke, R.A., et al., Leu-6-expressing cells in lymph nodes: Dendritic cells phenotypically similar to interdigitating cells. Hum Pathol 17:179-184 (1986)

14. Kjeldsberg, C.R., Kim, H., Polykaryocytes resembling Warthin-Finkeldey giant cells in reactive and neoplastic disorders. Hum Pathol 12:267-272 (1981)

15. Roizman, B., Polykaryocytosis induced by viruses. Proc Natl Acad Sci 48:228-234 (1962)

16. Barre-Sinoussi, F., Chermann, J.C., Rey, F., et al., Isolation of a T-lymphotropic retrovirus from a patient at risk for acquired immune deficiency syndrome (AIDS). Science 220:868-871 (1983)

17. Popovic, M., Sarngadharan, M.G., Read, E., et al., Detection, isolation, and continuous production of cytopathic retroviruses (HTLV-III) from patients with AIDS and pre-AIDS. Science 224:497-500 (1984)

18. Pekovic, D.D., Chausseau, J.P., Lapointe, N., et al., Involvement of HTLV-III in immunopathogenic reactions in thymus and spleen of patients with AIDS. International Conference on Acquired Immunodeficiency Syndrome (AIDS), Atlanta, (1985)

19. Fenoglio, C.M., Oster, M.W., Lo Gerfo, P., et al., Kaposi's sarcoma following chemotherapy for testicular cancer in a homosexual man: Demonstration of cytomegalovirus RNA in sarcoma cells. Hum Pathol 13:955-959 (1982)

20. Lubin, J., Rywlin, A.M., Lymphoma-like lymph node changes in Kaposi's sarcoma. Arch Pathol 92:338-341 (1971)

21. Harris, N.L., Hypervascular follicular hyperplasia and Kaposi's sarcoma in patients at risk for AIDS. (letter) N Engl J Med 310:462-463 (1984)

22. Ziegler, J.L., Beckstead, J.H., Volberding, P.A., et al., Non-Hodgkin's lymphoma in 90 homosexual men. Relation to generalized lymphadenopathy and the acquired immunodeficiency syndrome. N Engl J Med 311:565-570 (1984)

23. Schoeppel, S.L., Hoppe, R.T., Dorfman, R.F., et al., Hodgkin's disease in homosexual men with generalized lymphadenopathy. Ann Intern Med 102:68-70 (1985)

24. Dalgleish, A.G., Beverley, P.C.L., Clapham, P.R., et al., The CD4 (T4) antigen is an essential component of the receptor for the AIDS retrovirus. Nature 312:763-767 (1984)

25. Klatzmann, D., Barre-Sinoussi, F., Nugeyre, M.T., et al., Selective tropism of lymphadenopathy-associated virus (LAV) for helper-inducer T lymphocytes. Science 225:59-63 (1984)

26. Groopman, J.E., Sullivan, J.L., Mulder, C., et al., Pathogenesis of B cell lymphoma in a patient with AIDS. Blood 67:612-615 (1986)

27. Birx, D.L., Redfield, R.R., Tosato, G., Defective regulation of Epstein-Barr virus infection in patients with acquired immunodeficiency syndrome (AIDS) or AIDS-related disorders. N Engl J Med 314:874-879 (1986)

28. Srigley, J.R., Barlogie, B., Butler, J.J., et al., Lymphadenopathy and malignant lymphoma in homosexual males; acridine orange deoxyribonucleic acid-ribonucleic acid flow cytometric observations. Lab Invest 50:65A (1984)

29. Levy, N., Nelson, J., Meyer, P., et al., Reactive lymphoid hyperplasia with single class (monoclonal) surface immunoglobulin. Am J Clin Pathol 80:300-308 (1983)

30. King, N.W., Hunt, R.D., Letvin, N.L., Histopathologic changes in macaques with an acquired immunodeficiency syndrome (AIDS). Am J Pathol 113:382-388 (1983)

31. Gold, J.W.M., Weikel, G.S., Godbold, J., et al., Unexplained persistent lymphadenopathy in homosexual men and the acquired immune deficiency syndrome. Medicine 64:203-213 (1985)

32. Mathur-Wagh, U., Enlow, R.W., Spigland, I., et al., Longitudinal study of persistent generalized lymphadenopathy in homosexual men: Relation to acquired immunodeficiency syndrome. Lancet 1:1033-1098 (1984)

33. Murray, H.W., Hillman, J.K., Rubin, B.Y., et al., Patients at risk for AIDS-related opportunistic infections. Clinical manifestations and impaired gamma interferon production. N Engl J Med 313:1504-1510 (1985)

34. Janossy, G., Pinching, A.J., Bofill, M., et al., An immunohistological approach to persistent lymphadenopathy and its relevance to acquired immune deficiency syndrome. Clin Exp Immunol 59:257-266 (1985)

35. Biberfeld, P., Porwit-Ksiazek, A., Bottiger, B., et al., Immunohistopathology of lymph nodes in HTLV-III infected homosexuals with persistent adenopathy or AIDS. Cancer Res (Suppl) 45:4665s-4670s (1985)

36. Guettier, C., Gatter, K.C., Heryet, A., et al., Dendritic reticulum cells in reactive lymph nodes and tonsils: An immunohistological study. Histopathol 10:15-24 (1986)

37. Garcia, C.F., Lifson, J.D., Engleman, E.G., et al., The immunohistology of the persistent generalized lymphadenopathy syndrome (PGL). Am J Clin Pathol (In press)

38. Wood, G.S., Burns, B.F., Dorfman, R.D., et al., In situ quantitation of lymph node helper, suppressor, and cytotoxic T cell subsets in AIDS. Blood 67:596-603 (1986)

39. Tenner-Racz, K., Bofill, M., Schulz-Meyer, A., et al., HTLV-III/LAV viral antigens in lymph nodes of homosexual men with persistent generalized lymphadenopathy and AIDS. Am J Pathol 123:9-15 (1986)

40. Parravicini, C.L., Vago, L., Costanzi, G.C., et al., Follicle lysis in lymph nodes from homosexual men (letter). Blood 68:595-596 (1986)

41 Armstrong, J.C., Horne, R., Follicular dendritic cells and virus-like particles in AIDS-related lymphadenopathy. Lancet 2:370-372 (1984)

42. Tenner-Racz, K., Racz, P., Dietrich, M., et al., Altered follicular dendritic cells and virus-like particles in AIDS and AIDS-related lymphadenopathy. Lancet 1:105-106 (1985)

43. Armstrong, J.A., Dawkins, R.L., Horne, R., Retroviral infection of accessory cells and the immunological paradox in AIDS. Immuno Today 6:121-122 (1985)

44. Harper, M.E., Marselle, L.M., Gallo, R.C., et al., Detection of lymphocytes expressing human T-lymphotropic virus type III in lymph nodes and peripheral blood from infected individuals by in situ hybridization. Proc Natl Acad Sci 83:772-776 (1986)

45. Harper, M.E., Marselle, L.M., Gallo, R.C., et al., Detection of rare HTLV-III-infected cells in primary tissue from AIDS patients by in situ hybridization. International Conference on Acquired Immunodeficiency Syndrome (AIDS), Atlanta (1985)

46. Wood, G.S., Turner, R.R., Shiurba, R.A., et al., Human dendritic cells and macrophages: In situ immunophenotypic definition of subsets that exhibit specific morphologic and microenvironmental characteristics. Am J Pathol 119:73-82 (1985)

47. Lane, H.C., Masur, H., Edgar, L.C., et al., Abnormalities of B-cell activation and immunoregulation in patients with the acquired immunodeficiency syndrome. N Engl J Med 309:453-458 (1983)

48. Zeigler, T., Tubbs, R., Alanis, A., et al., Lymph node immunohistology in homosexual males with acquired immunodeficiency. Lab Invest 48:97A (1983)

49. Modlin, R.L., Meyer, P.R., Hofman, F.M., et al., T-lymphocyte subsets in lymph nodes from homosexual men. JAMA 250:1302-1305 (1983)

50. Said, J.W., Shintaku, I.P., Teitelbaum, A., et al., Distribution of T-cell phenotypic subsets and surface immunoglobulin-bearing lymphocytes in lymph nodes from male homosexuals with persistent generalized adenopathy: An immunohistochemical and ultrastructural study. Hum Pathol 15:785-790 (1984)

51. Meyer, P.R., Modlin, R.L., Powers, D., et al., Altered distribution of T lymphocyte subpopulations in lymph nodes from patients with acquired immunodeficiency-like syndrome and hemophilia. J Ped 103:407-410 (1983)

52. Mangkornkanok-Mark, M., Mark, A.S., Dong, J., Immunoperoxidase evaluation of lymph nodes from acquired immune deficiency patients. Clin Exp Immunol 5:581-586 (1984)

53. Raphael, M., Pouletty, P., Cavaille-Coll, M., et al., Lymphadenophathy in patients at risk for acquired immunodeficiency syndrome. Arch Pathol Lab Med 109:128-132 (1985)

54. Chan, W.C., Byrnes, R., Spira, T.J., et al., Lymphocyte subsets in lymph nodes of homosexual men with generalized unexplained lymphadenopathy. Arch Pathol Lab Med 109:133-137 (1985)

55. Damle, N.K., Engleman, E.G., Immunoregulatory T cell circuits in man. Alloantigen-primed inducer T cells activate alloantigen-specific suppressor T cells in the absence of the initial antigenic stimulus. J Exp Med 158:159-173 (1983)

56. Kansas, G.S., Wood, G.S., Fishwild, D.M., et al., Functional analysis of human T lymphocyte subsets distinguished with anti-Leu-8. J Immunol 134:2995-3002 (1985)

57. Nicholson, J.K.A., McDougal, J.S., Spira, T.J., et al., Immuno-regulatory subsets of the T helper and T suppressor cell populations in homosexual men with chronic unexplained lymphadenopathy. J Clin Invest 73:191-201 (1984)

58. Fauci, A.S., Macher, A.M., Longo, D.L., et al., Acquired immuno-deficiency syndrome: epidemiologic, clinical, immunologic and therapeutic considerations. Ann Intern Med 100:92-106 (1984)

59. Murray, H.W., Rubin, B.Y., Masur, H., et al., Impaired production of lymphokines and immune (gamma) interferon in the acquired immunodeficiency syndrome. N Engl J Med 310:883-889 (1984)

60. Tsang, K.Y., Fudenberg, H.H., Galbraith, S.M.P., In vitro augmentation of interleukin-2 production and lymphocytes with the TAC antigen marker in patients with AIDS. N Engl J Med 310:987 (1984)

61. Prince, H.E., Kermani-Arab, V., Fahey, J.L., Depressed interleukin-2 receptor expression in acquired immune deficiency and lymphadenopathy syndromes. J Immunol 133:1313-1317 (1984)

62. Wood, G.S., Burns, B.F., Dorfman, R.F., et al., The immunohistology of non-T cells in the acquired immunodeficiency syndrome. Am J Pathol 120:371-379 (1985)

63. Masur, H., Michelis, M.L., Greene, J.B., et al., An outbreak of community-acquired *Pneumocystis carinii* pneumonia: Initial manifestation of cellular immune dysfunction. N Engl J Med 305:1431-1438 (1981)

64. Reuben, J.M., Hersh, E.M., Mansell, P.W., et al., Immunological characterization of homosexual males. Cancer Res 44: 897-904 (1983)

65. Schroff, R.W., Gottlieb, M.S., Prince, H.E., et al., Immunological studies of homosexual men with immunodeficiency and Kaposi's sarcoma. Clin Immunol Immunopathol 27:300-314 (1983)

66. Siegal, F.P., Lopez, C., Hammer, G.S., et al., Severe acquired immunodeficiency in male homosexuals, manifested by chronic perianal ulcerative *Herpes simplex* lesions. N Engl J Med 305:1439-1444 (1981)

67. Belsito, D.V., Thorbecker, G.J., Reduced Ia-positive Langerhans' cells in AIDS (corres). N Engl J Med 311:858 (1984)

68. Kirkpatrick, C.H., Davis, K.C., Horsburgh, C.R., Reduced Ia-positive Langerhans' cells in AIDS (corres). N Engl J Med 311:857-858 (1984)

69. Lifson, J.D., Benike, C.J., Mark, D.F., et al., Human recombinant interleukin-2 partly reconstitutes deficient in vitro immune responses of lymphocytes from patients with AIDS. Lancet 1:698-702 (1984)

70. Fligiel, S., Naeim, F., Immunopathologic findings in male homosexual patients with acquired immunodeficiency syndrome (Abstr). Lab Invest 48:25A (1983)

71. Gerdes, J., Lemke, H., Baisch, H., et al., Cell cycle analysis of a cell proliferation associated human nuclear antigen defined by the monoclonal antibody Ki-67. J Immunol 133:1710-1715 (1984)

72. Pinching, A.J., The acquired immune deficiency syndrome. Clin Exp Immunol 56:1-13 (1984)

44 Ultrastructural Changes in HIV Infection

Gurdip S. Sidhu, Wafaa El-Sadr

Early in 1981, in the course of electron microscopic examination of a lymph node from a patient with disseminated *Mycobacterium avium-intracellulare* infection, one of us (GSS) noticed the presence of a large number of cytoplasmic tubuloreticular structures (TRS), similar to those first described in systemic lupus erythematosus (1)-(4), in paracortical lymphocytes and blood vascular endothelial cells (Figure 1). These structures were also known to be associated with a variety of viral infections (1),(3),(5)-(9).

The purpose of the examination had been to look for evidence of digestion of mycobacteria by macrophages. This search had been prompted by the absence of a granulomatous reaction to the infection (10) in a patient who was anergic and had no detectable helper-T cells in peripheral blood. No microorganisms were present in the sample examined, but a large number of strange cytoplasmic structures with ring-shaped and tubular profiles were observed in lymphocytes (Figure 2). They had a thick electron-dense layer which seemed to be penetrated at places by cytoplasm containing ribosomes. Spaces were present on both the inner and outer surfaces of the dense layer, and these spaces were bound by ribosome-coated membranes. The structures resembled no known microorganism; in fact, they appeared to be comprised of two lamellae of endoplasmic reticulum, one invaginated within the other, with a layer of dense material laid between them. A brief examination of the literature revealed the presence of such structures in a case of adult T-cell leukemia from Japan (11). The authors had described them as "test-tube and ring-shaped

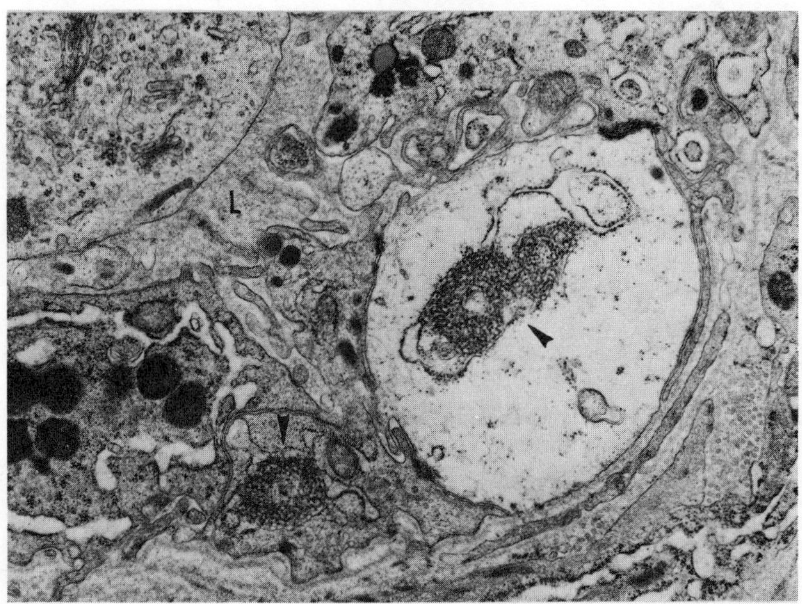

Figure 1. Lymph node - AIDS. Blood vessel showing TRS (arrowheads) in two endothelial cells, one of which has rarefied cytoplasm. Lumen (L)

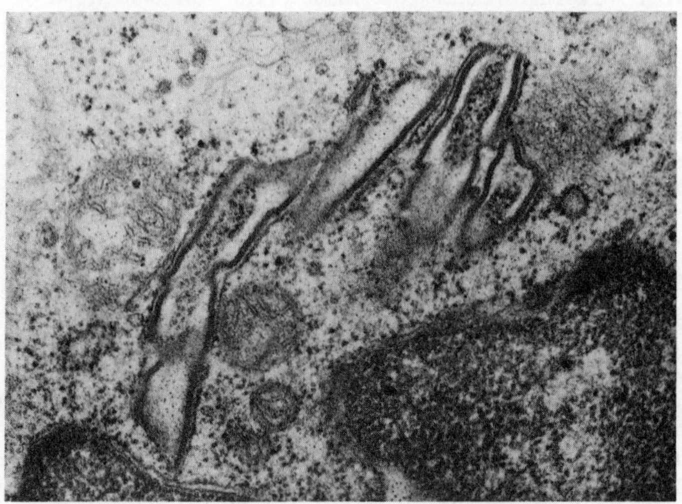

Figure 2. Lymph node - AIDS. Lymphocyte with CCC cut along their long axis, resulting in a test tube-shaped configuration.

forms", so this term was adopted in our initial reports on the ultrastructure of AIDS (12)-(17). The name of these structures has now been changed to the more pathogenesis-oriented term cylindrical confronting cisternae (CCC); but it must be kept in mind that the presence of the dense amorphous layer implies more than just the apposition or confrontation of two cisternae. Processing for paraffin embedding dissolves away the apposing membranes of the cisternae but leaves intact the dense material (12)-(15), helping differentiate this type of formation from the more ubiquitous ones seen as apposing remnants of nuclear membrane in dividing cells and occasionally post-mitotically (Figures 3, 4) (18)-(20).

By early 1982, we had seen six cases of what was then referred to as the "gay-related immune deficiency" (GRID) syndrome. The immunological findings revealed a profound depression of helper-T cell function (21)-(24), and the ultrastructural findings suggested the presence of an underlying viral infection. The fact that the immune depression was permanent, indeed worsened with time, suggested an assault by an agent that continued to be present in the patients. A self-replicating cause such as a microorganism was the most plausible choice, and since this putative organism had resisted all efforts to be isolated by that time, a bacterium was unlikely but a virus was a distinct possibility. The syndrome lacked resemblance to any known viral infection, so other, as yet unknown or little known, viruses had to be sought for.

Human T-cell leukemia virus (now known as human T-lymphotropic virus I or HTLV-I) had recently been discovered by Gallo and coworkers (25). It was recovered from the same type of patients with adult T-cell leukemia in which CCC, and incidentally also TRS, had been described (11). In addition, it had a helper-T cell tropism. The possibility that this or a related unknown retrovirus might be the cause of AIDS seemed quite likely on purely circumstantial grounds. Accordingly, sera from our six patients were screened by Dr. Gallo for antibodies against HTLV-I. One was found to have anti-HTLV-I antibodies, and subsequently the virus was successfully grown from his peripheral blood lymphocytes (26),(27). The remaining sera and six more sent later were negative for these antibodies. One out of 12 cases was not a particularly promising result. Of course, it was also difficult to explain how a virus that causes neoplasia as its major manifestation, would cause another disease in which the characteristic feature was cell destruction. This dilemma was finally solved by Barre-Sinoussi's (28) and Gallo's (29) subsequent discovery of lymphadenopathy-associated virus (LAV) and human T-cell lymphotropic virus III (HTLV-III), respectively. This retrovirus is new referred to as human immunodeficiency virus (HIV) (30)-(33).

THE SCOPE OF THE STUDY

This chapter summarizes the ultrastructural findings in AIDS based on the author's experience with 214 cases. One hundred

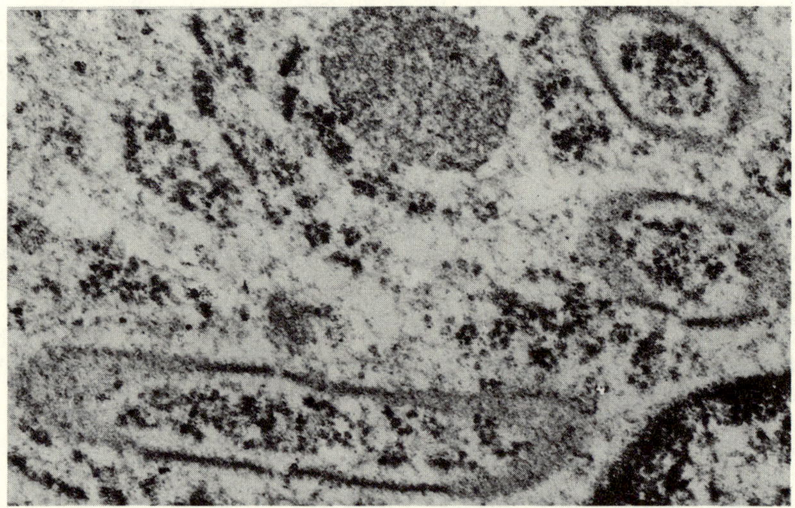

Figure 3. Lymph node - AIDS. Deparaffinized tissue. The dense material of the CCC in this lymphocyte appears unaffected by the lipid solvents used in paraffin embedding, whereas the membranous component of the structures has been dissolved away.

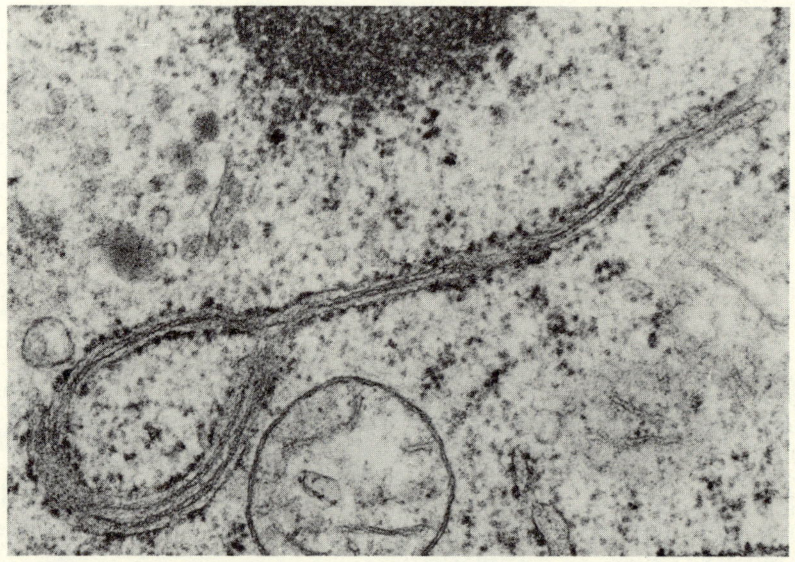

Figure 4. Lymph node - ARC. Paired cisternae of nuclear membrane in a dividing lymphocyte. Note the absence of electron-dense material between the adjoining membranes of the cisternae.

sixty-five of the patients studied either presented with AIDS as defined by the CDC criteria or developed it during the course of the study. The other 49 had AIDS related complex (ARC). Eighty of the AIDS cases and 19 of the ARC cases were homosexual or bisexual males. Of these, nine and two respectively were also intravenous drug users. In total, 78 AIDS cases and 28 ARC cases were heterosexual intravenous drug users. One case developed AIDS secondary to a blood transfusion. In six AIDS and two ARC cases, the patients denied any risk factors. Only one of the patients was female; she was a drug addict and had AIDS. A total of 515 specimens were examined. The breakdown of these by organ system or body site is shown in Table 1.

Table 1. Number and Distribution of Specimens Examined

Total Specimens - 515

Blood	170	Lung	6
Transbronchial biopsy	99	Stomach	5
Marrow	54	Kidney	3
Lymph Node	50	Duodenum	2
Skin	44	Mouth	2
Liver	41	Pericardium	2
Endobronchial biopsy	13	Smintest*	2
Brain	11	Esophagus	1
Colon	9	Rectum	1

* Smintest = small intestine

THE ULTRASTRUCTURAL CHANGES

The major ultrastructural changes of diagnostic importance are TRS, CCC, and HIV virions. Other changes seen in HIV infection are present in a variety of organs in varying degree and are of interest in explaining several manifestations of the disease, but are usually not in-and-of themselves of diagnostic importance. These include derangements of iron metabolism in erythroid precursors, megakaryocytic maturation abnormalities, changes suggesting immunological capping in peripheral blood lymphocytes, lipid engorgement of Ito cells (hepatic perisinusoidal fibroblasts or lipocytes), hepatocytic cytoplasmic changes, and renal glomerular changes (15). Finally, of purely morphological interest are the ultrastructural features of the wide variety of opportunistic organisms flourishing in AIDS patients, including protozoa such as *Pneumocystis carinii* and *Toxoplasma gondii*, cytomegalovirus and other herpesviruses, the JC virus of progressive multifocal leukoencephalopathy, fungi such as cryptococci, and mycobacteria.

Tubuloreticular Structures and Cylindrical Confronting Cisternae

TRS are comprised of anastomosing tubules of 24 nm outer diameter present within cisternae of endoplasmic reticulum. They were originally thought to be paramyxovirus particles, but this contention was untenable on morphological grounds. Paramyxoviruses have a smaller outer diameter of about 18 nm and occur free in the cytosol, not in the endoplasmic reticulum as do TRS. It has also been demonstrated that TRS are composed of an acidic glycoprotein and lack any nucleic acid (4). Whether the protein is of viral or host origin is not known. Any component of the endoplasmic reticulum, including granular endoplasmic reticulum, agranular endoplasmic reticulum, the perinuclear cistern, and the Golgi complex may be involved (15). Tubuloreticular structures may even occur within the space of the inner lamella of CCC (Figure 5), or within annulate lamellae (15).

TRS can be induced in tissue culture with interferon administration or with substances that induce interferon production and in human volunteers with interferon administration (3),(6),(34)-(38). They can be induced by both alpha-interferon and beta-interferon (29),(39),(40), but not by gamma interferon (35). In cultured human endothelial cells, only beta-interferon produces TRS (36). Their presence in large numbers in systemic lupus erythematosus and in AIDS may be related to the very high levels of an acid-labile alpha-interferon present in the sera of patients with both these diseases (2),(3),(41)-(46). TRS are also found in other collagen-vascular diseases of unknown cause (1),(3),(5),(9),(47),(48). In none of the latter entities has a viral etiology been definitely excluded.

TRS are seen most frequently in lymphocytes, monocytes and endothelial cells, including the neoplastic endothelial cells of Kaposi's sarcoma. Less often, they are seen in macrophages (including Kupffer cells), pericytes, fibroblasts, interdigitating cells and dendritic reticulum cells of lymph nodes, Schwann cells, squamous epithelial cells of skin appendages and mucosae (Figure 6), and type 1 pneumocytes. In any one cell type, they occur with approximately equal frequency throughout the body, regardless of the presence or absence of a pathological lesion. One exception is macrophages. TRS are quite frequent in marrow macrophages and Kupffer cells, less common in lymph nodal macrophages, and rare in alveolar macrophages.

Table 2 compares the prevalence of TRS in AIDS and ARC patients. It is evident that when only the presence or absence of the structures is considered, there is no significant difference between the two stages of HIV disease.

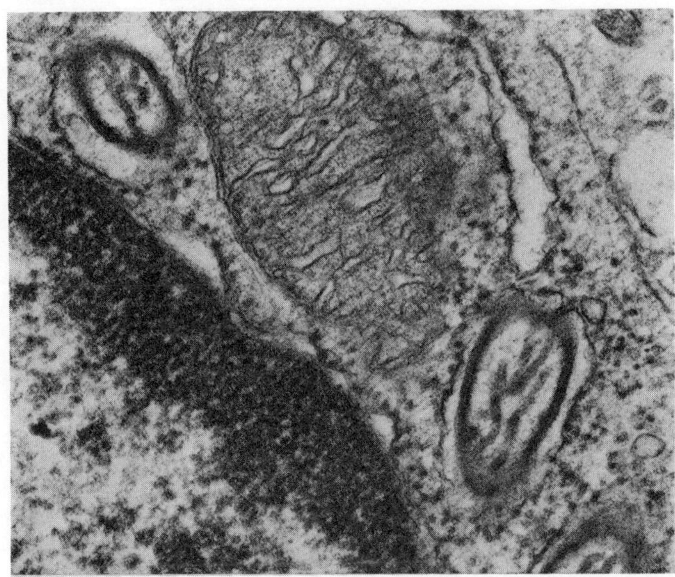

Figure 5. Lymph node - AIDS. Lymphocyte with TRS tubules present within the inner cisternae of CCC.

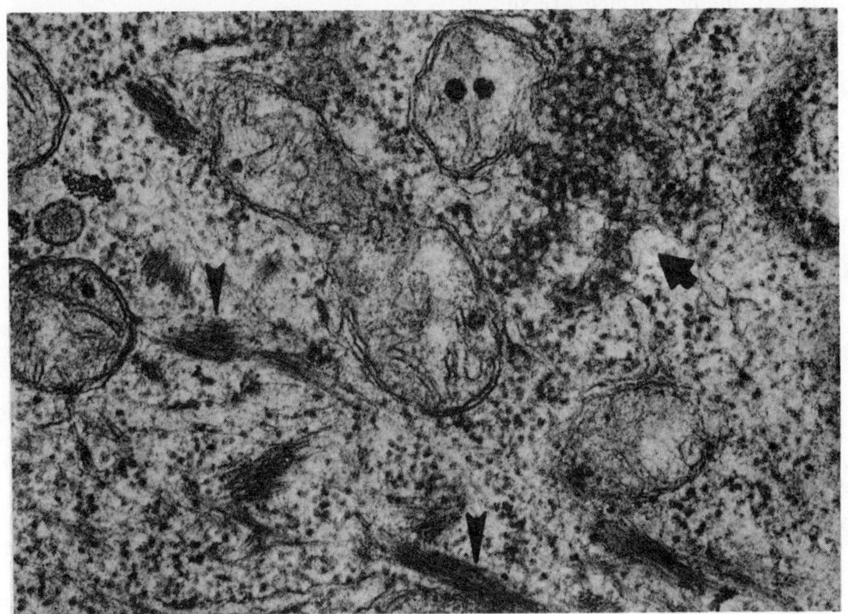

Figure 6. Tongue biopsy - ARC. TRS (arrow) within a squamous cell of the surface epithelium. The many tonofibrils (arrowheads) present in the cytoplasm attest to the squamous nature of the cell.

Table 2. Prevalence of TRS and CCC in AIDS and ARC

		%
AIDS cases with TRS	153	92.7[a]
AIDS cases with CCC	83	50.3[b]
ARC cases with TRS	48	98.0[a]
ARC cases with CCC	9	18.4[b]

a p>0.05 for the comparison between AIDS and ARC cases.
b p<0.05 for the comparison between AIDS and ARC cases.

Table 3 shows the distribution and frequency of TRS in the various tissues sampled. Only those sites with 10 or more observations performed are shown.

Table 3. TRS and CCC by Site

	AIDS CASES				ARC CASES			
Site	Total Tests	Cases (No.)	TRS+ Cases	CCC+ Cases	Total Tests	Cases (No.)	TRS+ Cases	CCC+ Cases
Blood	128	98	89(91%)	41(42%)	41	35	31(89%)	6(17%)
Transbr Bx	91	78	78(100%)	3(4%)	8	8	7(88%)	0
Marrow	50	45	35(78%)	34(76%)	4	4	2(50%)	1(25%)
Skin	42	34	28(82%)	3(9%)	2	2	0	0
Lymph Node	35	30	23(77%)	17(57%)	15	14	12(86%)	3(21%)
Liver	39	36	34(94%)	9(25%)	2	2	2(100%)	0
Endobr Bx	12	12	11(92%)	9(75%)	1	1	1(100%)	0
Brain	11	11	10(91%)	5(45%)				

Transbr Bx = transbronchial biopsy specimen
Endobr Bx = endobronchial biopsy specimen

It is evident from the data that TRS are ubiquitously distributed. One reason which may account for this wide distribution is their presence in endothelial cells of blood vessels, including marrow and liver sinusoids. Accordingly, the highest frequency of TRS is in the most vascular sites, such as lung parenchyma and renal glomeruli (not shown in table).

Forty-eight of the 49 cases with ARC had TRS. The duration for which these structures had been present ranged from three to 41 months, with a mean duration of 18.9 months. It is obvious then that TRS may be detectable well before the onset of AIDS. However, this conclusion is valid only to the extent that one assumes that ARC cases will ultimately develop AIDS. This assumption can only be tested with time.

Table 4. Discovery of TRS and/or CCC Prior to AIDS Diagnosis

	No. of Cases	Average Period (mo)	Range (mo)
Cases with EM prior to AIDS dx	42(25%)*	9.6	1-47
TRS found prior to AIDS dx	38(90%)	7.8	1-47
CCC found prior to AIDS dx	21(50%)	6.5	1-32
Total AIDS Cases	165		

* Four of these cases did not have TRS at any time
EM = electronmicroscopic studies
dx = diagnosis

In Table 4, the frequency of TRS was examined for the 42 AIDS cases (25% of the total AIDS cases) in which material was available before the onset of AIDS. In four, these structures were not found at any time during the entire course of their illness. In the remaining 38, they were detected one to 47 months (average 7.8 months) before the development of AIDS. In the vast majority of cases, TRS were first discovered at the very first ultrastructural examination.

In Table 5, the distinction between AIDS and ARC based on the presence of TRS is analyzed further. The abundance of TRS in each specimen was graded from 1 to 3. A grade of 1 implied that only rare TRS were found; in grade 2, they were not rare, but required a fair amount of searching before a small to moderate number of them were detected; in grade 3, they were abundant and found in numerous cells with ease. As shown in the table, the difference, based on the chi-square test, between AIDS and ARC in the number of cases with grade 3 specimens, is highly significant. The data imply that the abundance of TRS is directly proportional to the progression or increasing severity of HIV disease.

Table 5. Abundance of TRS and CCC in AIDS and ARC

	TRS (amount)			CCC (amount)		
	3	2	1	3	2	1
AIDS (no.)	135[a]	10	11	51[b]	13[b]	20
(%)	82	6	7	31	8	12
ARC (no.)	26[a]	12	10	1[b]	3[b]	5
(%)	53	24	20	2	6	10

a p<0.001 for the comparison between AIDS and ARC.
b (CCC 3 and 2 combined) p<0.001 for the comparison between AIDS and ARC.

CCC are formed by a test tube-like stacking of two or more cisternae of endoplasmic reticulum, one within the other. When these structures are cut perpendicular to their long axis, they have a ring-shaped appearance. When cut in the long axis, they have a test tube-shaped form (Figure 7). Interposed between the cisternae comprising the CCC is a layer of amorphous dense material, which is resistant to lipid solvents (15),(49). It has been shown that this material has a periodicity (transverse striation) and is composed of at least two proteins, but lacks any nucleic acid (49). Whether the proteins are of viral or host origin is not known.

The spectrum of diseases in which CCC occur is small. Besides HTLV-I-associated adult T-cell lymphoma-leukemia (11), they also develop in the hepatocytes of chimpanzees injected with the sera of patients with non-A, non-B hepatitis (49)-(56). In fact, they were first described in this latter setting. They are absent in human patients with this disease and are not seen in lymphocytes of infected chimpanzees. Recent reports suggest that the non-A, non-B hepatitis virus may also be a retrovirus (57). Other diseases not known to be retroviral in etiology in which CCC have been reported include multiple sclerosis (58) and systemic lupus erythematosus (59), albeit in rare instances, and hepatitis B-infected chimpanzees injected with delta hepatitis virus-containing human sera (60). Thus, CCC may be a marker of retroviral infection, but also occur to a lesser extent in diseases in which the etiology may or may not be retroviral.

CCC have been induced in tissue culture cells exposed to concentrations of alpha-interferon greater than those required to

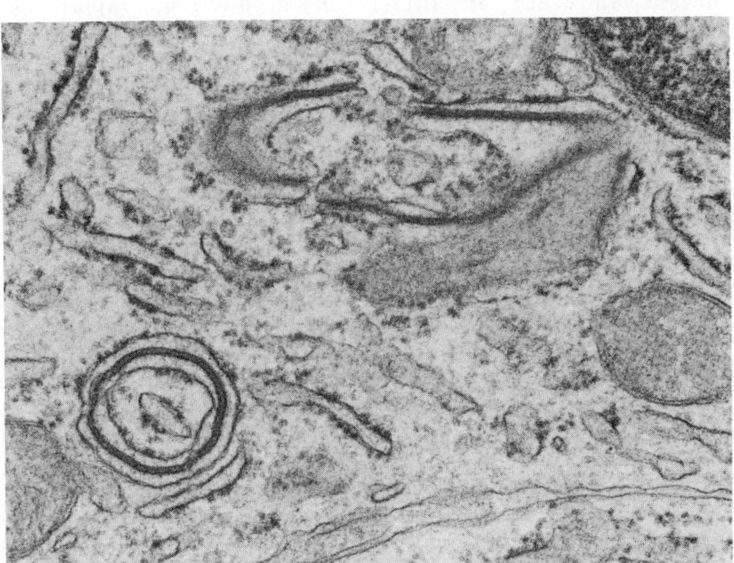

Figure 7. Lymph node - AIDS. Interdigitating cell with ring and test tube-shaped sections of CCC.

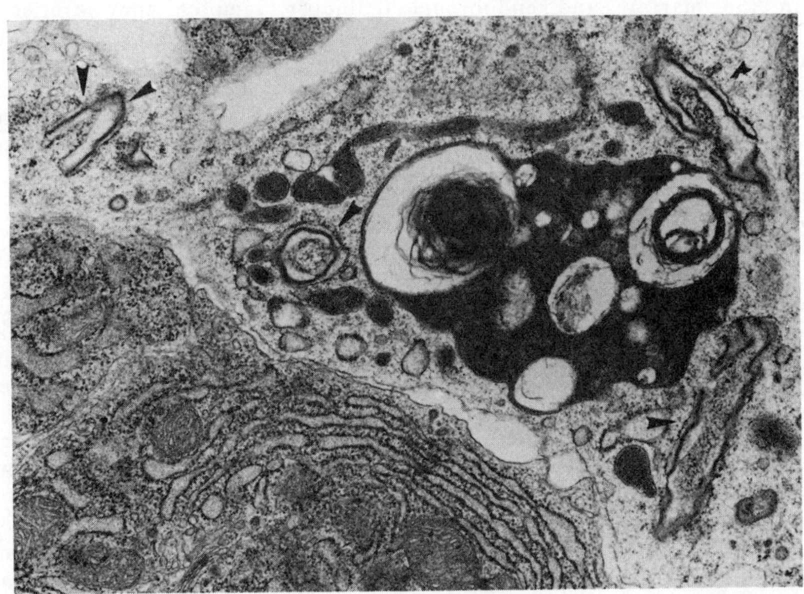

Figure 8. Bone marrow - AIDS. Macrophage with phagocytosed material and four CCC (arrowheads).

produce TRS (39). It may well be that retroviruses are among the most potent inducers of interferon production, explaining the presence of CCC in the diseases they cause.

The case frequency of CCC in AIDS patients is significantly greater than that in ARC patients (Table 2). Furthermore, as shown in Table 5, an abundance of CCC is far more likely in AIDS patients than in ARC patients. It is evident that not only the number of CCC present in a patient's cells, but also their mere presence is a more ominous sign than the presence of TRS. Even though nine of the 49 ARC patients had CCC and five had them for 17, 22, 22, 27 and 35 months respectively, in only one case were the CCC abundant. Among the AIDS patients, five of the 21 patients with CCC present in the pre-AIDS period (Table 4) had them for durations of 10 or more months prior to developing AIDS. These durations were 10, 10, 13, 15, and 32 months respectively. Obviously, the presence of CCC is compatible in individual cases with a long delay in the development of AIDS, though apparently of shorter duration than in those who only have TRS.

CCC are not as ubiquitous in different tissues as TRS, primarily because CCC are present in a lesser number of cell types. CCC are most frequently found in lymphocytes, marrow macrophages (Figure 8) and sinusoidal endothelial cells (Figure 9), and bronchial ciliated and intermediate epithelial cells (Figure 10). They are seen infrequently in macrophages and endothelial cells in other sites (Figure 11), plasma cells (Figure 12), interdigitating cells and dendritic cells of lymph nodes, and oligodendroglial and microglial cells of brain. In all tissues other than the marrow and endobronchial biopsy samples, they are seen in a much smaller number of cells than are TRS. In decreasing order, the tissues in which CCC are most likely to be found are bone marrow, endobronchial biopsy samples (because of the presence of CCC in the lining epithelial cells), lymph nodes, brain and blood (Table 3). The number of involved cases is also lower than with TRS, both in AIDS and in ARC, though the difference is greater for ARC patients (Table 2). This agrees with the contention that they are a sign of more advanced disease.

CCC sometimes occur in the same cells (generally lymphocytes) as TRS (Figure 13), and occasionally, the two structures are combined, the TRS occurring within the inner cisternae of a CCC (Figure 5). In some instances, three cisternae are involved in CCC formation, producing a double layer of dense material (Figure 14). On rare occasions, particularly in monocytes and sometimes macrophages, the outer cisterna of a CCC is wrapped around a mitochondrion (15). Though the shape of CCC is unique, they are not always cylindrical and may sometimes be formed of just two flat cisternae attached to each other (Figure 12). This reemphasizes the point that the feature of paramount importance in CCC is the dense amorphous material and not the shape, even though they are usually cylindrical.

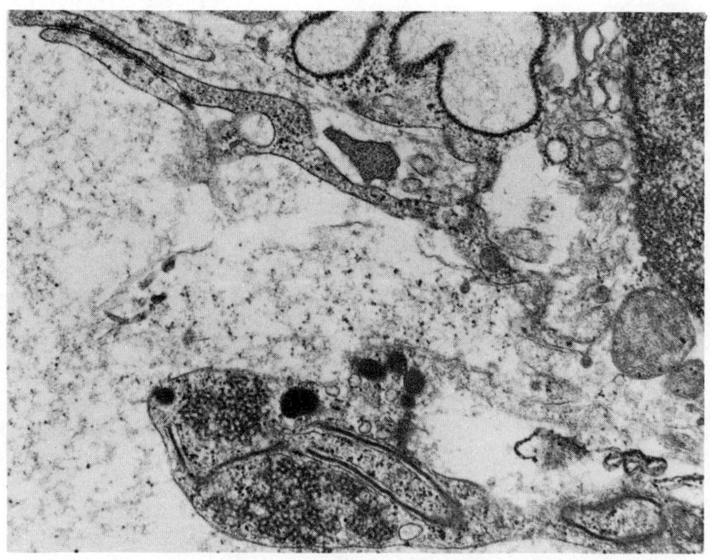

Figure 9. Bone marrow - AIDS. CCC and TRS are seen together in a sinusoidal endothelial cell.

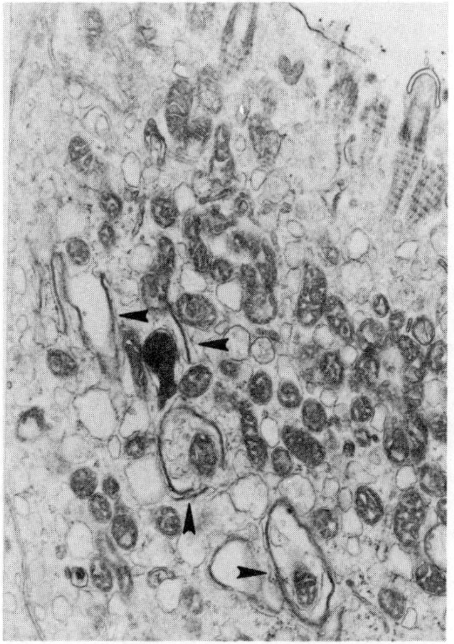

Figure 10. Endobronchial biopsy - AIDS. Multiple CCC (arrowheads) are seen in the cytoplasm of a ciliated epithelial cell. Darkly stained structures in cytoplasm are mitochondria.

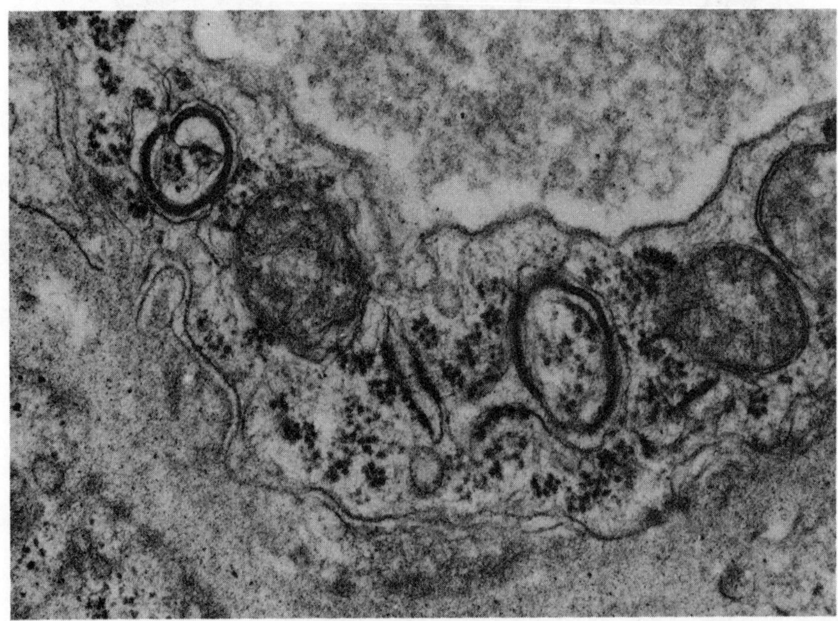

Figure 11. Brain biopsy - AIDS. Two CCC are seen in a capillary endothelial cell of a case with progressive multifocal leukoencephalopathy.

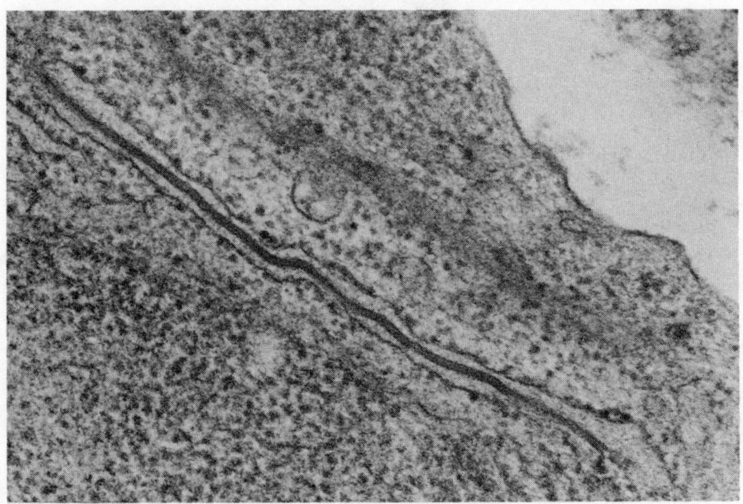

Figure 12. Bone marrow - AIDS. A CCC in a plasma cell. This shows an uncommon variant configuration in which the structure is straight instead of curved.

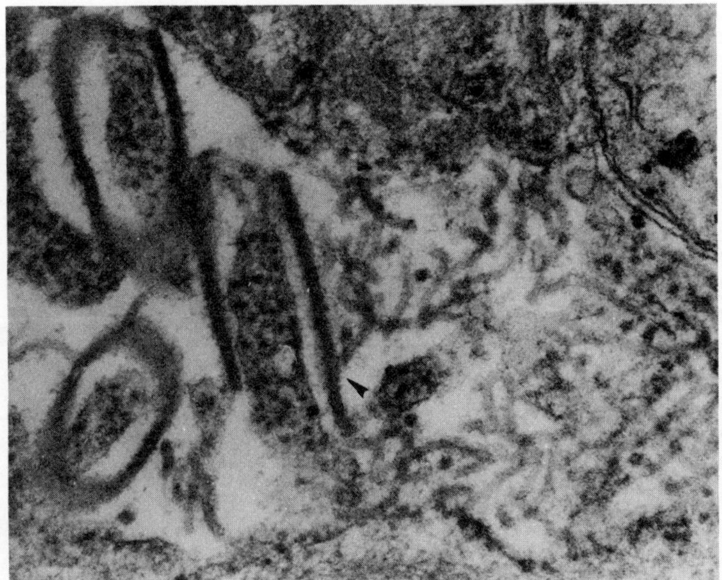

Figure 13. Lymph node - ARC. Lymphocyte showing intimate association of TRS and CCC. A TRS tubule appears to be arising from the surface of a CCC (arrowhead).

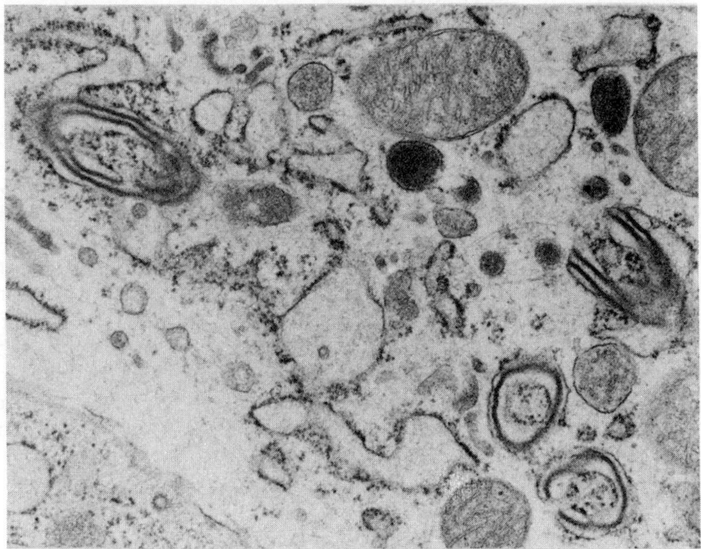

Figure 14. Bone marrow - AIDS. Macrophage with four CCC, two of which have a double layer of dense material indicating that they are comprised of three confronting cisternae each instead of the more usual two.

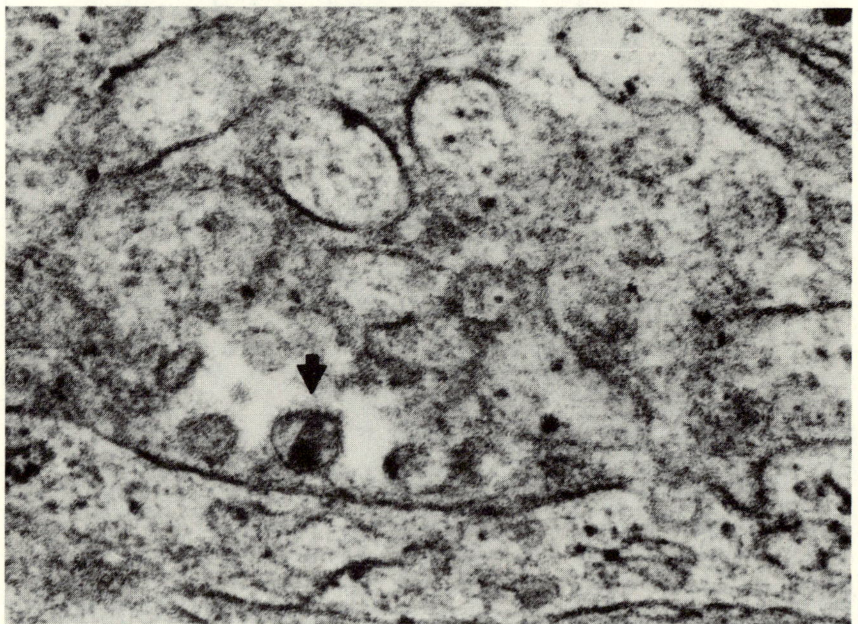

Figure 15. Lymph node - ARC. Germinal center area showing proliferated processes of dendritic reticular cells with a viral particle (arrow), morphologically consistent with HIV, in the intercellular space. Note the conical core with the eccentric nucleoid in the wider end.

Other Ultrastructural Features

HIV virions are present within the enlarged germinal centers of lymph nodes seen in ARC and the earlier stages of AIDS before the centers are totally effaced. In germinal centers, a complex arborization of dendritic cell processes much beyond anything seen in other types of follicular hyperplasia is a consistent feature. The virions are found in the intercellular space between these processes, (61)-(63). They are quite difficult to find, but when present have a morphological appearance typical of lentiviruses (64). This includes an eccentrically-located nucleoid in a conical core shell with the larger end containing the nucleoid (Figure 15). The viral envelope surrounds the core shell and has an outer diameter of 115 to 120 nm.

LITERATURE REVIEW

The presence of TRS (40),(54),(65)-(70) and CCC (54),(65), (66),(68),(69) in AIDS has been amply confirmed by other workers. It has also been shown that both TRS and CCC may be present in ARC (40),(65)-(67),(69). Although initially several of the studies showed that TRS in lymphocytes were confined to T cells (66) or T suppressor/cytotoxic cells (40), it is evident from their presence in plasma cells (15),(65) and natural killer (NK) cells (15),(68) that all types of lymphocytes may be involved, though the T cell is the most intensely affected. The latter is consistent with our observation that paracortical lymphocytes more frequently have TRS than follicular lymphocytes.

Several studies have attempted to quantitate the changes (40),(66),(67),(69). In peripheral blood lymphocytes in AIDS, TRS were present in 3-12% (mean 5%) of lymphocytes (66) or 1.5-10% of total mononuclear cells (40). The highest percentage of TRS-positive cells was seen in those patients with a T4:T8 ratio of <0.2 (40). In one study in which 59 patients with ARC were studied, though only 44% of the patients had TRS in their peripheral blood, they were present in 2-10% of lymphocytes in the positive specimens (69). In addition, their number was inversely proportional to the T4:T8 ratio, suggesting that TRS-bearing cells increase in number with worsening disease. In lymph nodes from AIDS patients (only two cases), they were present in an average of 21% of lymphocytes, and in lymph nodes from ARC patients (nine cases) they were present in 4% (1-9% range) of lymphocytes (67).

In one study, CCC were observed in peripheral blood lymphocytes of 20% of 59 ARC patients, generally being found only in those with the lowest T4:T8 ratios (≤ 0.3) (69). CCC were not found in specimens lacking TRS. AIDS developed in six of the 59 cases. TRS, and sometimes CCC, were present in four of these cases for as long as 16 months before the diagnosis of AIDS. In one ARC patient, Kostianovsky et al. (66) found CCC in 10% of peripheral blood lymphocytes. In the study by Onerstein et al. (67), no CCC were seen in specimens of 11 lymph nodes from ARC patients while they were present in 4% of lymphocytes from one lymph node from an AIDS patient. Their conclusion that CCC are not a feature of lymph nodes from ARC patients is not supported by our findings, probably because we studied a larger number of cases. However, CCC in lymph nodes from ARC patients are generally rare, though there are exceptions. Ewing et al. (65) observed the presence of CCC in lymph nodes of four of 31 patients with ARC. All four went on to develop and die of AIDS. It is apparent that, although CCC are much less common in ARC than in AIDS, they can, nevertheless, be abundant in an occasional patient. The suggestion from one group that CCC may be more common in ARC than in AIDS patients (66) is refuted by almost all other studies. Our data and those of others suggest that CCC are a sign of more advanced disease.

So far, virions morphologically compatible with HIV have been seen only in the enlarged germinal centers of lymph nodes. In ARC, and in the early stages of AIDS, the germinal centers of lymph node follicles are markedly enlarged, and frequently show changes of regressive transformation (71). The processes of dendritic reticular cells are markedly expanded, producing a labyrinthine pattern more complex than that seen in any other type of follicular hyperplasia. There may even be evidence of fragmentation of the dentritic cell networks (71). HIV-like virus particles are seen in the intercellular spaces between the dendritic cell processes (61)-(63), and in one report were seen budding from the plasma membrane of a cell process, although the cell to which the process belonged could not be identified (63). It has been proposed that the normal antigen-trapping function of dendritic reticular cells helps concentrate the HIV virions in follicular centers, and the possibility is left open that these cells may even harbor the virus. This localization may explain the markedly enlarged follicular germinal centers, polyclonal B cell proliferation, and the loss of function due to the ultimate degeneration of the dendritic cells (which may be the reason for the absence of follicles and dendritic cells in the later stages of AIDS and for the impairment of the B-cell system) (63),(71), (72).

CONCLUSION

TRS and CCC are interferon-related cytoplasmic structures that can be of major value in the diagnosis of ARC and AIDS. TRS are present almost universally in both ARC and AIDS. They are ubiquitous in their distribution in different tissues, so that examination of blood buffy coat or biopsy of any tissue with blood vessels, whether a lesion is present or not, will reveal their presence. The percentage of TRS-positive cells is directly proportional to the progression of HIV disease, whether judged by clinical or immunological parameters.

CCC are less frequent than TRS, and in any one particular case, they are also less abundant than TRS, though occasional exceptions do occur. Cells with CCC are more likely to be found in blood buffy coat, and in marrow, endobronchial and lymph node biopsies, than in other sites. Their presence signifies more advanced disease than the presence of TRS alone. As with TRS, the percentage of CCC-positive cells increases with increasing severity of disease. Though they may be seen rarely in other diseases, their high frequency in retroviral diseases makes them a reliable though somewhat insensitive marker for these entities.

When both TRS and CCC are abundant, they may occur within the same cell, and occasionally may even occur as a combined structure, highlighting their common pathogenesis, if not nature.

HIV virions can be found, though with some difficulty, among the spaces of the expanded labyrinthine network of dendritic reticular cell processes in lymph nodes of ARC patients. Preliminary evidence of budding from cell surfaces suggests that they may even infect these antigen concentrating and presenting cells. The virions are more difficult to find in AIDS because the follicular architecture tends to be obliterated, possibly due to degeneration of the dendritic cells. The presence of virions in the follicular centers may explain the stimulation and later impairment of the B-lymphocyte system.

ACKNOWLEDGMENTS

The authors wish to express their gratitude to Nicholas D. Cassai and Eulee M. Forrester for the enormous amount of expert technical work and its excellence on their part that made this study possible.

REFERENCES

1. Gyorkey, F., Sinkovics, J.G., Min, K.W., et al., A morphologic study on the occurrence and distribution of structures resembling viral nucleocapsids in collagen diseases. Am J Med 53:148-158 (1972)

2. Klippel, J.H., Grimley, P.M., Decker, J.L., Lymphocyte inclusions in newborns of mothers with systemic lupus erythematosus. N Engl J Med 290:96-97 (1974)

3. Preble, A.T., Friedman, R.M., Interferon-induced alterations in cells: Relevance to viral and nonviral diseases. Lab Invest 49:4-18 (1983)

4. Schaff, Z., Barry, D.W., Grimley, P.M., Cytochemistry of tubuloreticular structures in lymphocytes from patients with systemic lupus erythematosus and in cultured human lymphoid cells. Comparison to a paramyxovirus. Lab Invest 29:577-586 (1978)

5. Beringer, J.R., Tubular aggregates in endoplasmic reticulum in *Herpes simplex* encephalitis. N Engl J Med 285:943-945 (1971)

6. Grimley, P.M., Davis, G.L., Kang, Y-H., et al., Tubuloreticular inclusions in peripheral blood mononuclear cells related to systemic therapy with alpha-interferon. Lab Invest 52: 638-649 (1985)

7. Hammar, S.P., Winterbauer, R.H., Bockus, D., et al., Endothelial cell damage and tubuloreticular structures in interstitial lung disease associated with collagen vascular disease and viral pneumonia. Am Rev Respir Dis 127:77-84 (1983)

8. Hanissian, A.S., Hashimoto, K., Paramyxovirus-like inclusions in rubella syndrome. J Ped 81:231-237 (1972)

9. Uzman, B.G., Saito, H., Kasac, M., Tubular arrays in the endoplasmic reticulum in human tumor cells. Lab Invest 24:492-498 (1971)

10. Greene, J.B., Sidhu, G.S., Lewin, S., et al., *Mycobacterium avium-intracellulare*: a cause of disseminated life-threatening infection in homosexuals and drug abusers. Ann Intern Med 97:539-546 (1982)

11. Shamoto, M., Murukami, S., Zenke, T., Adult T-cell leukemia in Japan: an ultrastructural study. Cancer 47:1804-1811 (1981)

12. Sidhu, G.S., Stahl, R.E., El-Sadr, W., et al., Ultrastructural markers of AIDS. Lancet 1:990-991 (1983)

13. Sidhu, G.S., Ultrastructure of AIDS lymph nodes. N Engl J Med 309:1188-1189 (1983)

14. Sidhu, G.S., Stahl, R.E., El-Sadr, W., et al., Ultrastructural features of acquired immune deficiency syndrome. Lab Invest 50:54A (1984) (abstract)

15. Sidhu, G.S., Stahl, R.E., El-Sadr, W., et al., The acquired immunodeficiency syndrome: An ultrastructural study. Hum Pathol 16:377-386 (1985)

16. Sidhu, G.S., Weisman, J., Case for the panel. Cytoplasmic structures in endothelial cells of the choroid. Ultrastruct Pathol 8:378-379 (1985)

17. El-Sadr, W., Stahl, R., Sidhu, G., et al., The acquired immune deficiency syndrome: Laboratory findings, clinical features, and leading hypotheses. Diagnostic Immunol 2:73-85 (1984)

18. Ghadially, F.N., Ultrastructural Pathology of the Cell and Matrix. Butterworths, Sevenoaks 372, 376-377 (1981)

19. Paintrand, M.R., Pignoi, I., Navelbine: an ultrastructrual study of its effects. J Electron Microscopy 32:115-124 (1983)

20. Sato, S., Murphy, G.F., Harrisi, T.J., The genesis of paired cisternae during the mitotic cycle. Am J Pathol 107:150-160 (1982)

21. Goedert, J.J., Neuland, C.Y., Wallen, W.C., et al., Amyl nitrite may alter T lymphocytes in homosexual men. Lancet 1:412-416 (1982)

22. Marmor, M., Friedmen-Kien, A.E., Laubenstein, L., et al., Risk factors for Kaposi's sarcoma in homosexual men. Lancet 1:1083-1087 (1982)

23. Hurtenbach, U., Shearer, G.M., Germ cell-induced immune suppression in mice. Effects of inoculation of syngeneic spermatozoa on cell mediated immune response. J Exp Med 155:719-729 (1982)

24. Shearer, G.M., Allogeneic leukocytes as a possible factor in induction of AIDS in homosexual men. N Engl J Med 308:223-224 (1983)

25. Poiesz, B.J., Ruscetti, F.W., Gazdar, A.F., et al., Detection and isolation of type C retrovirus particles from fresh and cultured lymphocytes of a patient with cutaneous T-cell lymphoma. Proc Natl Acad Sci, USA 77:7415-7419 (1980)

26. Gallo, R.C., Sarin, P.S., Gelmann, E.P., et al., Isolation of human T-cell leukemia virus in acquired immune deficiency syndrome (AIDS). Science 220:865-867 (1983)

27. Gelmann, E.P., Popovic, M., Blayney, D., et al., Proviral DNA of a retrovirus, human T-cell leukemia virus, in two patients with AIDS. Science 220:862-865 (1983)

28. Barre-Sinnoussi, F., Chermann, J.C., Rey, F., et al., Isolation of a T-lymphotropic retrovirus from a patient at risk for acquired immune deficiency syndrome (AIDS). Science 220:868-876 (1983)

29. Gallo, R.C., Salahuddin, S.Z., Papovic, M., et al., Frequent detection and isolation of cytopathic retroviruses (HTLV-III) from patients with AIDS and at risk for AIDS. Science 224:500-503 (1984)

30. Popovic, M., Sarngadharan, M.G., Reed, E., et al., Detection, isolation, and continuous production of cytopathic human T lymphotropic retrovirus (HTLV-III) from patients with AIDS and pre-AIDS. Science 224:497-500 (1984)

31. Safai, B., Sarngadharan, M.G., Groopman, J.E., et al., Seroepidemiological studies of HTLV-III in AIDS. Lancet 1:1438-1440 (1984)

32. Sarngadharan, M.G., Popovic, M., Bruch, L., et al., Antibodies reactive with a human T-lymphotropic retrovirus (HTLV-III) in the sera of patients with acquired immune deficiency syndrome. Science 224:506-508 (1983)

33. Schupbach, J., Popovic, M., Gilden, M., et al., Serological analysis of a subgroup of human T-lymphotropic retroviruses (HTLV-III) associated with AIDS. Science 224:503-505 (1984)

34. Grimley, P.M., Rutherford, M.N., Kang, Y-H., et al., Formation of tubuloreticular inclusions in human lymphoma cells compared to the induction of 2'-5' A synthetase by interferon in dose effect and kinetic studies. Cancer Res 144:3480-3488 (1984)

35. Grimley, P.M., Kang, Y-H., Silverman, R.H., et al., Blood lymphocyte inclusions associated with alpha-interferon. Lab Invest 48:30A-31A (1983)

36. Luu, J., Bockus, D., Remington, F., et al., Selective induction of tubuloreticular structures in cultured human endothelial cells by recombinant beta-interferon. Lab Invest 54: 39A (1986)

37. Rich, S.A., Human lupus inclusions and interferon. Science 213:772-775 (1981)

38. Rich, S.A., Owens, T.R., Bartholomew, L.E., et al., Immune interferon does not stimulate formation of alpha and beta interferon induced human lupus inclusions. Lancet 1:127-128 (1983)

39. Bockus, D., Remington, F., Luu, J., et al., Induction of cylindrical confronting cisternae (CCC) in Daudi lymphoblastoid cells by recombinant alpha-interferon. Lab Invest 54:7A (1986)

40. Grimley, P.M., Kang, Y-H, Frederick, W., et al., Interferon-related leukocyte inclusions in acquired immune deficiency syndrome: localization in T cells. Am J Clin Pathol 81:147-155 (1984)

41. Buimovici-Klein, E., Lange, M., Klein, R.J., Is presence of interferon predictive for AIDS? Lancet 2:344 (1983)

42. DeStefano, E., Friedman, R.M., Friedman-Kien, A.E., et al., Acid-labile leukocyte interferon in homosexual men with Kaposi's sarcoma and lymphadenopathy. J Infect Dis 146:451-455 (1982)

43. Preble, O.T., Vilcek, J., Friedman-Kien, A.E., et al., Acid-labile leukocyte interferon in homosexual men with Kaposi's sarcoma and lymphadenopathy. In: The Acquired Immune Deficiency Syndrome and Infections of Homosexual Men, (Ma, P., Armstrong, D., eds) Yorke Medical Books, New York, p 381-386 (1984)

44. Hooks, J.J., Jordan, G.W., Cupps, T., et al., Multiple interferons in the circulation of patients with systemic lupus erythematosus and vasculitis. Arthritis Rheum 25:396-400 (1982)

45. Preble, O.T., Black, R.J., Friedman, R.M., et al., Systemic lupus erythematosus: presence in human serum of an unusual acid-labile leukocyte interferon. Science 216:429-431 (1982)

46. Ytterberg, S.R., Schnitzer, T.J., Serum interferon levels in patients with systemic lupus erythematosus. Arthritis Rheum 25:401-406 (1982)

47. Helder, A.W., Feltkamp-Vroom, T.M., Tubuloreticular structures and antinuclear antibodies in autoimmune and non-autoimmune diseases. J Pathol 119:49-56 (1976)

48. Schaff, Z., Lapis, K., Grimley, P.M., Undulating membraneous structures associated with the endoplasmic reticulum in tumor cells. Int J Cancer 18:697-702 (1976)

49. Schaff, Z., Gerety, R.J., Grimley, P.M., et al., Ultrastructural and cytochemical study of hepatocytes and lymphocytes during experimental non-A, non-B infections in chimpanzees. J Exp Pathol 2:25-36 (1985)

50. Gerety, R.J., Tabor, E., Schaff, Z., et al., Non-A, non-B hepatitis agents. Proceedings of the 1984 International Symposium on Viral Hepatitis, San Francisco, Orlando, FL (1984)

51. Jackson, D., Tabor, E., Gerety, R.J., Acute non-A, non-B hepatitis: Specific ultrastructural alterations in the endoplasmic reticulum of infected hepatocytes. Lancet 1:1249-1250 (1979)

52. Pfeifer, U., Thomssen, R., Legler, K., et al., Experimental non-A, non-B hepatitis: Four types of cytoplasmic alterations in hepatocytes of infected chimpanzees. Virchows Arch (Cell Pathol) 33:233-243 (1980)

53. Schaff, Z., Tabor, E., Jackson, D.R., et al., Ultrastructural alterations in serial liver biopsy specimens from chimpanzees experimentally infected with a human non-A, non-B hepatitis agent. Virchows Arch (Cell Pathol) 45:301-312 (1984)

54. Schaff, Z., Tabor, E., Jackson, D.R., et al., AIDS-associated ultrastructural changes. Lancet 1:1336 (1983)

55. Shimizu, Y.K., Feinstone, S.M., Purcell, R.H., et al., Non-A, non-B hepatitis: Ultrastructural evidence for two agents in experimentally infected chimpanzees. Science 205:197-200 (1979)

56. Kunze, K.D., Kemmer, C., Porst, H., et al., Non-A, non-B hepatitis: ultrastructural findings in human liver biopsies. Exp Pathol 21:36-45 (1982)

57. Seto, B., Coleman, Jr., W.G., Iwarson, S., et al., Detection of reverse transcriptase activity in association with the non-A, non-B hepatitis agent(s). Lancet 2:941-943 (1984)

58. Prineas, J.W., Wright, R.G., Macrophages, lymphocytes, and plasma cells in the perivascular compartment in chronic multiple sclerosis. Lab Invest 38:409-421 (1978)

59. Hammer, S.P., Bockus, D., Remington, F., et al., More on ultrastructure of AIDS lymph nodes. N Engl J Med 310:924-925 (1984)

60. Govindarajan, S., Fields, H.A., Humphrey, C.D., et al., Pathologic and ultrastructural changes of acute and chronic delta hepatitis in an experimentally infected chimpanzee. Am J Pathol 122:315-322 (1986)

61. Armstrong, J.A., Horne, R., Follicular dendritic cells and virus-like particles in AIDS-related lymphadenopathy. Lancet 2:370-372 (1984)

62. Min, K.W., Localization of retroviruses in lymph nodes of AIDS-related lymphadenopathy. Lab Invest 54:44A (1986)

63. Tenner-Racz, K., Racz, P., Dietrich, M., et al., Altered follicular dendritic cells and virus-like particles in AIDS and AIDS-related lymphadenopathy. Lancet 1:105-106 (1985)

64. Munn, R.J., Marx, P.A., Yamamoto, J.K., et al., Ultrastructural comparison of the retroviruses associated with human and simian acquired immunodeficiency syndromes. Lab Invest 53:194-199 (1985)

65. Ewing, E.P. Jr., Spira, T.J., Chandler, F.W., et al., Ultrastructural markers in AIDS. Lancet 2:285 (1983)

66. Kostianovsky, M., Kang, Y-H, Grimley, P.M., Ultrastructural and immunoelectron microscopic studies of cells with abnormal cytoplasmic inclusions in patients with AIDS. AIDS Research 1:181-196 (1984)

67. Onerheim, R.A., Wang, N-S., Gilmore, N., et al., Ultrastructural markers of lymph nodes in patients with acquired immune deficiency syndrome and in homosexual males with unexplained persistent lymphadenopathy. A quantitative study. Am J Clin Pathol 82:280-288 (1984)

68. Orenstein, J.M., Ultrastructural markers in AIDS. Lancet 2: 284-285 (1983)

69. Orenstein, J.M., Simon, G.L., Kessler, C.M., et al., Ultrastructural markers in circulating lymphocytes of subjects at risk for AIDS. Am J Clin Pathol 84:603-609 (1985)

70. Rozman, C., Feliu, E., Ultrastructural markers in AIDS. Lancet 2:285 (1983)

71. Wood, G.S., Burns, B.F., Dorfman, R.F., et al., The immunohistology of non-T cells in the acquired immunodeficiency syndrome. Am J Pathol 120:371-379 (1985)

72. Zolla-Pazner, S., Sidhu, G., The possible pathogenic role of the hyperactive B-lymphocytes in AIDS. In: AIDS: The Epidemic of Kaposi's Sarcoma and Opportunistic Infections. (Friedman-Kien, A.E., Laubenstein, L.J., eds), Masson Publishing USA, New York, p 161-168 (1984)

45
Pathology of AIDS in Children

Vijay V. Joshi, James M. Oleske

Since 1979, a disease complex resembling the acquired immune deficiency syndrome (AIDS) has been noted in children from the Newark metropolitan area (1)-(6). This chapter will describe the pathologic changes found in children with AIDS on the basis of study of biopsy and/or autopsy material from 25 children treated at The Children's Hospital of New Jersey. The significance of these pathologic changes with respect to pathogenesis and diagnosis of AIDS will also be briefly discussed. Lesions in different organs related to opportunistic infections and B cell lymphoid proliferation will be described under those two sections separately.

LYMPHORETICULAR SYSTEM

Thymus

The thymus is usually in its normal location, with a normal configuration and vascularity (2),(3),(7). However, at postmortem, a marked reduction in size and weight has been noted. On microscopic examination the following features are characteristic: a) dysinvolution defined as involution which mimics the thymic dysplasia seen in severe combined immunodeficiency syndrome characterized by a marked reduction in, or virtual absence of, lymphocytes and Hassall's corpuscles (HC) with loss of corticomedullary differentiation (7) (Figure 1); b) precocious involution defined as involution which antedates changes normally associated with age and stress and which are characterized by the presence of readily demonstrable microcystic HC (7),(8) (Figure 2); c) thymitis, characterized by medullary lymphoid follicles (Figure 3), lymphomononuclear/plasmacytic infiltrate or the presence of multinucleated giant cells in the medulla. Foci of hyalinization are frequently present in association with these lesions.

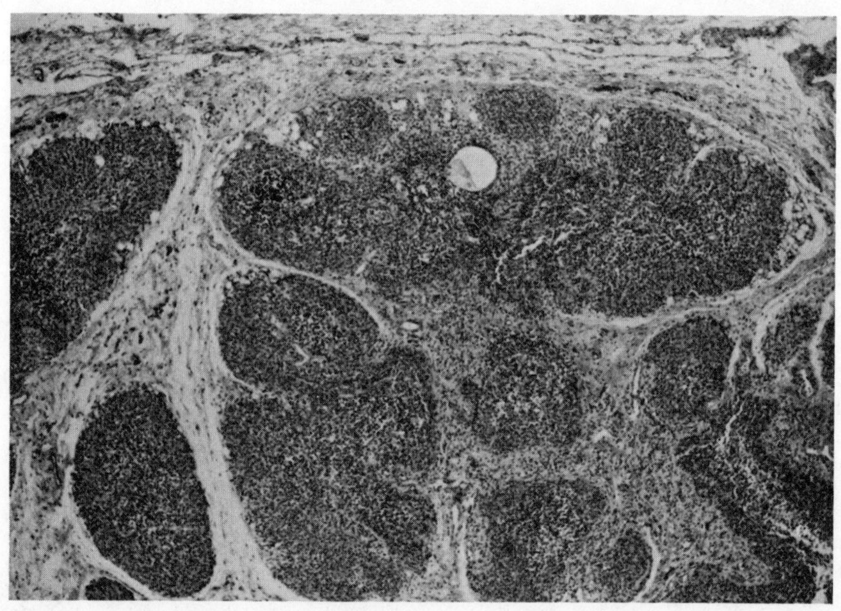

Figure 1. Thymus showing marked reduction in number of Hassall's corpuscles in lobules, loss of corticomedullary differentiation, and lymphocytic depletion in lobules. Small clusters of lymphocytes are seen in a few lobules (hematoxylin-eosin) (Reproduced with permission from ref. 3).

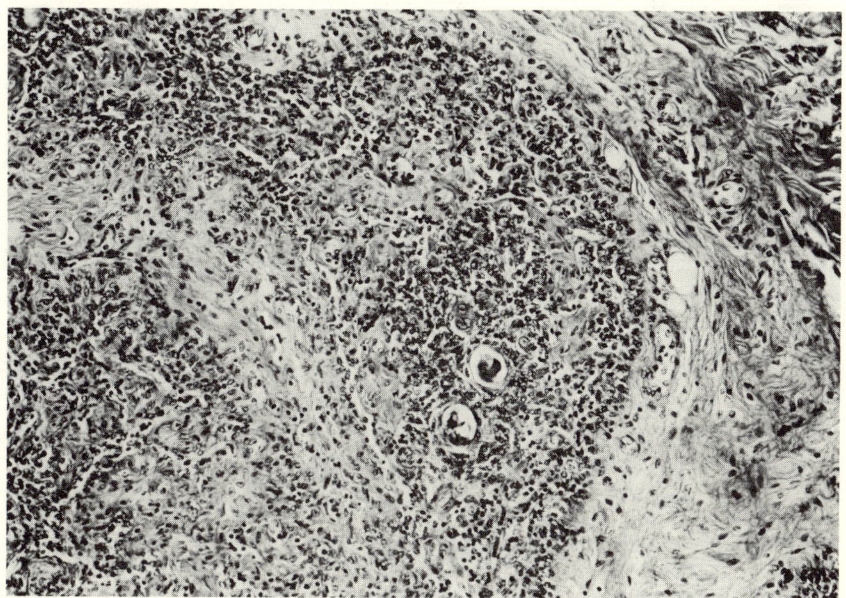

Figure 2. Thymic lobule showing marked lymphocytic depletion of cortex and medulla and microcystic Hassall's corpuscles in the medulla. (Hematoxylin and eosin) (Reproduced with permission from ref. 7).

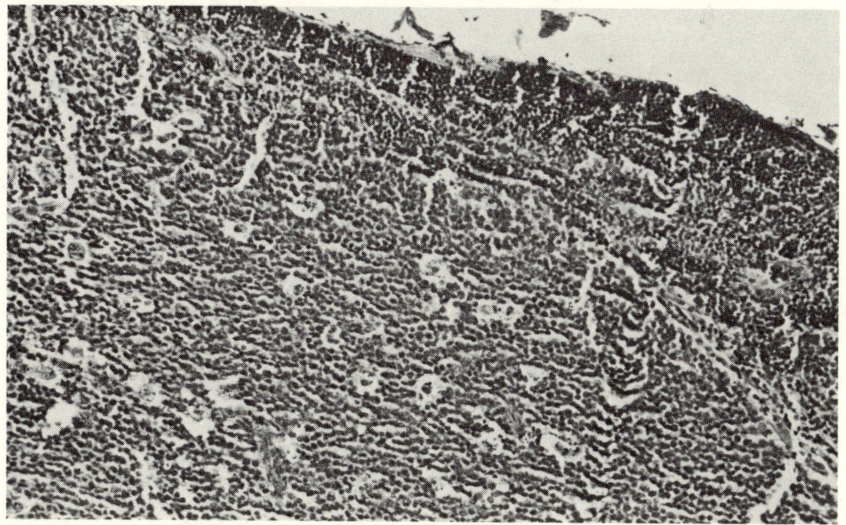

Figure 3. Thymic lobule showing a lymphoid follicle in the medulla. Note compression of the overlying cortex. (Hematoxylin-eosin)

Lymph Nodes

Three different patterns of lymph node pathology (2) have been observed. The first is follicular hyperplasia, often of a florid type with normocellular paracortical zones and proliferation of plasma cells, plasmacytoid lymphocytes, immunoblasts, lymphocytes and capillaries in the interfollicular zones. Multinucleated giant cells, resembling Warthin-Finkeldey giant cells which are seen in prodromal stages of measles and in reactive lymphoid proliferations (9), have been noted in the lymphoid follicles in some cases. A few scattered pale staining histiocytes and rare neutrophils are present in the interfollicular zones, but appreciable focal collections of these cells of the type described in the lymph nodes in adults with AIDS by Ioachim et al. (10) are not seen. The second is follicular hyperplasia with lymphocytic depletion of the paracortical zones. The third pattern is characterized by atrophy of follicles with absence of germinal centers and lymphocytic depletion of paracortical zones. Multinucleated giant cells are seen in these atrophic follicles in some cases.

Immunohistochemical studies done on frozen sections of lymph nodes and on cell suspensions from lymph nodes of adults with AIDS or AIDS related complex (ARC) have shown that the number of T suppressor cells is increased while the number of T helper cells is decreased (11),(12). Using the methodology described by Koziner et al. (13),(14), fluorescence activated flow cytometric analysis of cell suspensions prepared from lymph nodes from some of our patients have shown similar results (15).

Other Lymphoreticular Tissues

The bone marrow is generally slightly hypercellular and an increased number of plasma cells may be seen. In some cases, however, hypocellularity with increase in reticulin is present. Spleens were available for examination only in autopsy cases. In most of these cases, there was severe lymphocytic depletion, particularly of the periarteriolar lymphoid sheath. Lymphocytic depletion of appendix and Peyer's patches of small intestine was also seen in most of the autopsy cases.

CENTRAL NERVOUS SYSTEM

AIDS Encephalopathy

A clinicopathologic syndrome labelled as AIDS encephalopathy (16) is characterized pathologically by cortical atrophy, inflammatory cell infiltrates in basal ganglia, pons and white matter, vascular inflammation, vascular calcifications and typically multinucleated giant cells both in the parenchyma and in perivascular locations (Figure 4). Human immunodeficiency virus (HIV) can be demonstrated in these giant cells by electron microscopy (Figure 5) and by hybridization techniques (17),(18). Perivascular inflammatory infiltrates and multinucleated giant cells have been

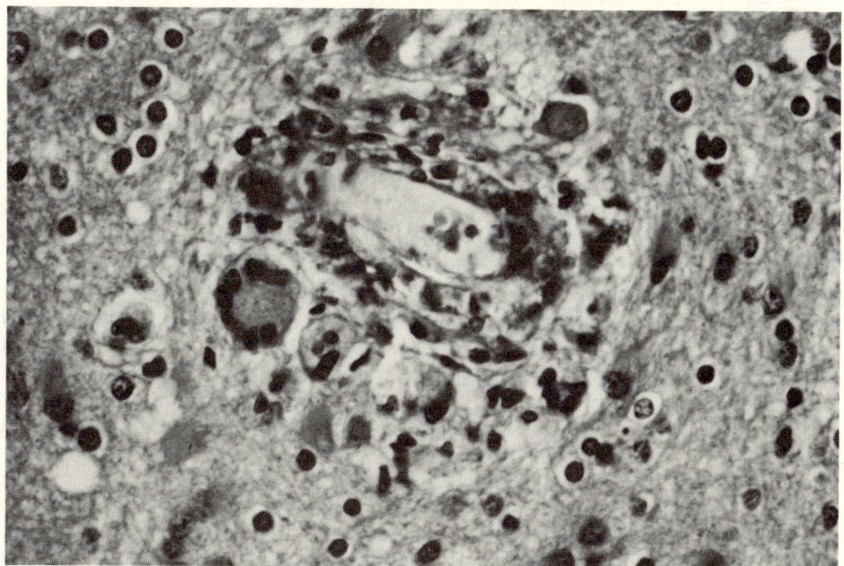

Figure 4. Cerebral cortex showing vasculitis and a perivascular multinucleated giant cell with peripherally arranged nuclei (hematoxylin-eosin)

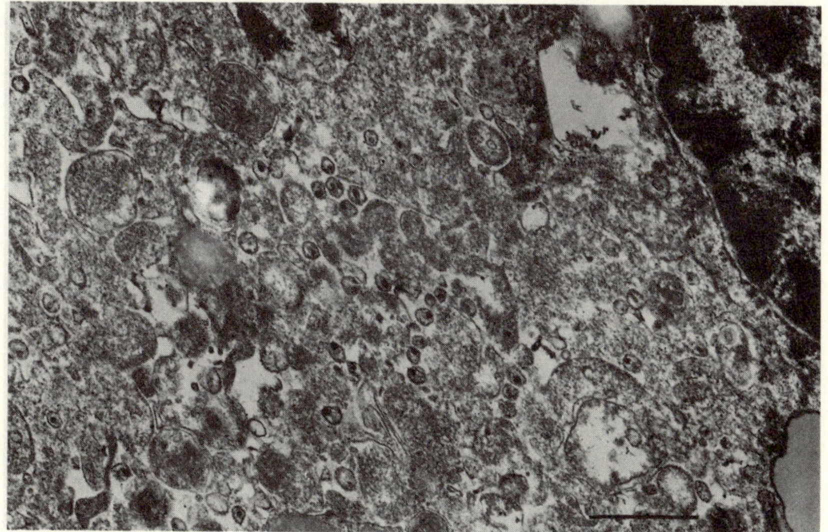

Figure 5. Electron micrograph of a giant cell in the hippocampal area of brain of the type shown in Figure 4. Note the HIV viral particles in the cytoplasm. Note the eccentric and cylindrical nucleoids. (Formalin fixed tissue, uranyl acetate and lead citrate, bar represents 500 nm) (Reproduced with permission from ref. 17)

observed in the spinal cord in a few cases. Vacuolar myelopathy seen in adults with AIDS (19) has not been observed in children with AIDS, with the exception of one recent case.

RESPIRATORY SYSTEM

Other than opportunistic infections (described below), four different types of lesions have been noted in the lungs of children with AIDS (2),(4). Diffuse alveolar damage characterized by varying degrees of edema, hyaline membranes, cuboidal metaplasia of alveolar epithelium and interstitial fibrosis has been seen, but usually in autopsy cases (Figure 6). Pulmonary lymphoid hyperplasia (PLH) (2) is a lesion which is characterized by nodular aggregates of lymphoid cells with or without germinal centers. These lymphoid aggregates consist of immature and mature lymphocytes, plasma cells, plasmacytoid lymphocytes and immunoblasts and are primarily peribronchiolar in location, but parenchymal nodules may also be seen. Lymphoid interstitial pneumonitis (LIP) is a process which is characterized by diffuse alveolar septal infiltrates by the same type of cells described in PLH above, with or without nodular aggregates, and germinal centers (Figure 7). In some cases overlap between PLH and LIP occurs suggesting that PLH and LIP may represent a continuum and for practical purposes that both could be designated under the single heading of PLH/LIP complex (20). Desquamative interstitial pneumonitis (DIP) (4) has also been observed and is characterized by large intra-alveolar collections of mononuclear cells, minimal to mild lymphoid infiltrate of alveolar septa and cuboidal metaplasia of alveolar epithelial cells (Figure 8).

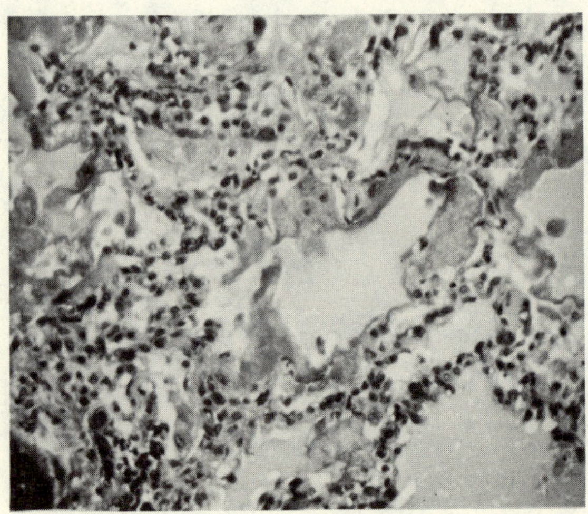

Figure 6. Portions of lung showing diffuse alveolar damage characterized by hyaline membrane formation, edema and a few macrophages in the alveolar lumina. (Hematoxylin and eosin)

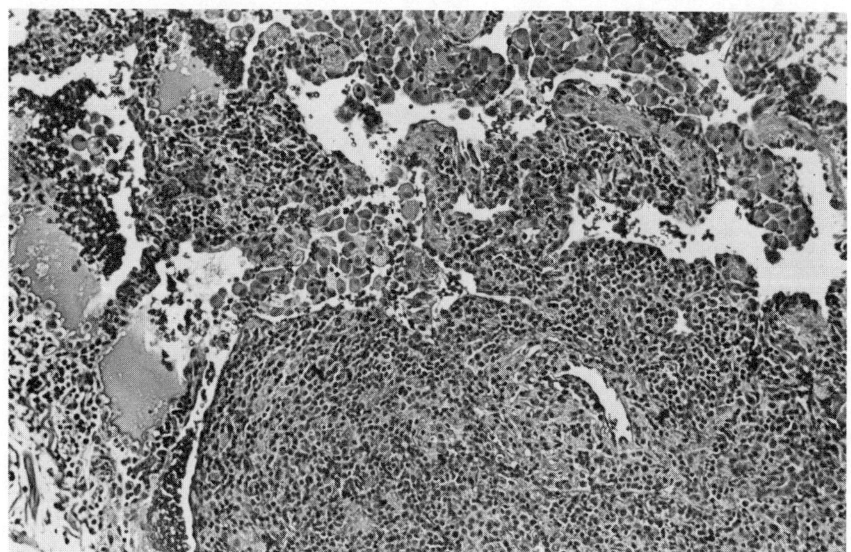

Figure 7. Lung showing a parenchymal nodular lymphoid aggregate with infiltration of the alveolar septa by lymphoid cells. Note clusters of macrophages in some of the alveoli. (Hematoxylin-eosin)

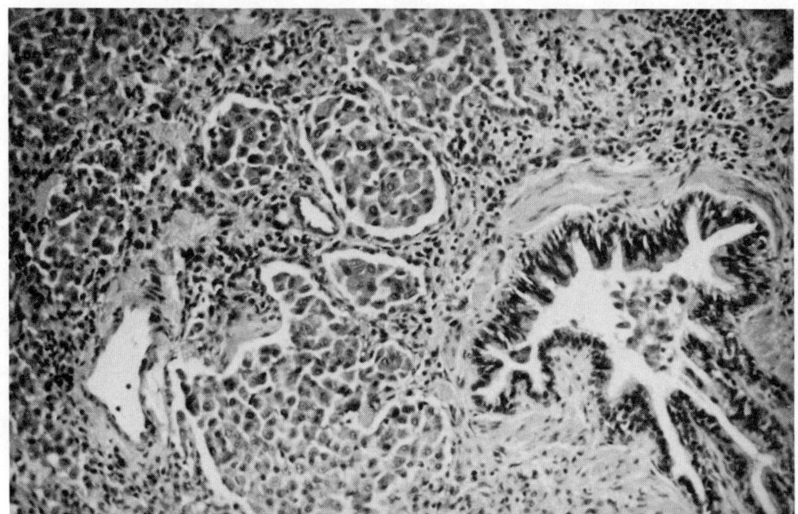

Figure 8. Portion of lung showing clusters of large mononuclear cells in the alveoli. Cuboidal metaplasia of alveolar lining cells and a mild focal lymphocytic infiltrate of the alveolar septa are also seen. (Hematoxylin and eosin) (Reproduced with permission from ref. 4)

DIGESTIVE SYSTEM

Gastrointestinal Tract

Variable degrees of villous atrophy of small intestinal mucosa have been noted in biopsy and autopsy specimens. Necrotizing segmental jejunitis with perforation requiring surgical resection was seen in one patient (21). As mentioned above, lymphocytic depletion of the appendix and Peyer's patches of the small intestine was seen in most of the autopsy cases.

Liver

Prominent lymphoid nodular aggregates composed of lymphocytes, plasma cells, plasmacytoid lymphocytes and rare immunoblasts can be seen in the portal triads (2). Lesions resembling chronic active hepatitis have been described by Duffy et al. (22) but were not present in our series. Also, variable degrees of fatty change and cholestasis with portal fibrosis were observed in some cases. In one, early cirrhosis was present. An additional patient had *Serratia marcescens* cholecystitis (21).

UROGENITAL SYSTEM

Kidneys

Kidneys are generally unremarkable in children with AIDS, however, focal segmental glomerulosclerosis presenting as nephrotic syndrome was seen in one case.

Testes

Delayed maturation was present in all autopsy cases of adolescents with AIDS.

CARDIOVASCULAR SYSTEM

Heart

In three of the fatal cases in our series we observed cardiomegaly with a slight to moderate increase in cardiac weight and biventricular dilatation. Microscopic findings included myocardial hypertrophy, swelling of myocytes with vacuolation, and minimal to mild interstitial fibrosis and edema. In two of these three patients congestive heart failure was present clinically.

Blood Vessels

In five fatal cases we observed calcification involving the adventitia and media of medium sized or small arteries particularly in the brain but also in the spleen, kidneys, lungs, skeletal muscle, heart and thymus. In one case, an aneurysm of the right coronary artery with thrombosis and myocardial infarction was seen. In the brain, vasculitis was also present as described above.

ENDOCRINE AND MUSCULOSKELETAL SYSTEMS

No specific or significant lesions, except for involvement by opportunistic infections or B cell lymphoid proliferation, have been seen at autopsy.

OPPORTUNISTIC INFECTIONS (OI)

A variety of OI's have been noted in 15 children with AIDS seen at our Medical Center (23): parasitic infections included *Pneumocystis carinii* pneumonia in seven of the 15 children, four diagnosed by lung biopsy and three on the basis of autopsy specimens. In lung biopsy specimens of two of the cases, the number of organisms was very small and the inflammatory reaction sparse or absent. A careful examination of the sections stained with Gomori's methanamine silver stain is, therefore, essential in every lung biopsy. Toxoplasmosis of brain was present in one case.

Fungal infections included candida esophagitis which was documented by biopsy and culture in two patients and aspergillus pulmonary granulomata which were demonstrated at autopsy in one patient. Oral thrush was present in all 15 patients at some time during their clinical course.

Among the bacterial infections, *Mycobacterium avium-intracellulare infection* (MAI) involving liver, spleen, lymph nodes and gastrointestinal tract was present in two patients. In one case the diagnosis was made on a jejunal biopsy. The morphologic features of the biopsy resembled those of Whipple's disease (24) but the stain for acid-fast bacilli was markedly positive (Figure 9). At autopsy of the same case the mesenteric nodes were partially replaced by a nodular mass composed of fusiform to spindle shaped cells arranged in sheets and bundles resembling a mesenchymal tumor-like lesion. Special stains for acid fast organisms demonstrated intracellular organisms. This represents the "histoid" variety of reaction to *Mycobacterium avium-intracellulare* (25). In addition, repeated infections (more than three times) with the following common pathogenic bacteria were noted clinically in seven of the 15 patients: *Streptococcus pneumoniae, Hemophilus influenzae, Staphylococcus aureus* and *Salmonella species* (23).

Herpes infections were the most common viral infections observed. Disseminated cytomegalovirus (CMV) infection was seen in four patients at autopsy, two cases involved the lymphoreticular system, gastrointestinal tract, lungs, kidneys, brain and adrenal glands. In one of these cases, infection of the posterior pituitary was characterized by focal necrosis. In the other two cases, CMV infection was confined to the lungs and occurred in association with *P. carinii* pneumonia. Chronic mucocutaneous *Herpes simplex* infection was seen in four patients.

EXTRANODAL AND NODAL B-CELL LYMPHOID PROLIFERATION

As described above, LIP, follicular hyperplasia of lymph nodes, nodular lymphoid aggregates in the portal traids of the liver, and lymphoid hyperplasia of Peyer's patches and submucosa of colon were present in some of our cases (2). These lymphoid aggregates consisted of polymorphic polyclonal B cells (lymphocytes, plasma cells, plasmacytoid lymphocytes and immunoblasts) (Figure 10), as indicated by histologic features, immunoperoxidase stains for light chains of immunoglobulins done on paraffin sections (20) and by fluorescence activated cytometric analysis of cell suspensions (15) (according to the methodology described by Koziner et al. (13),(14)).

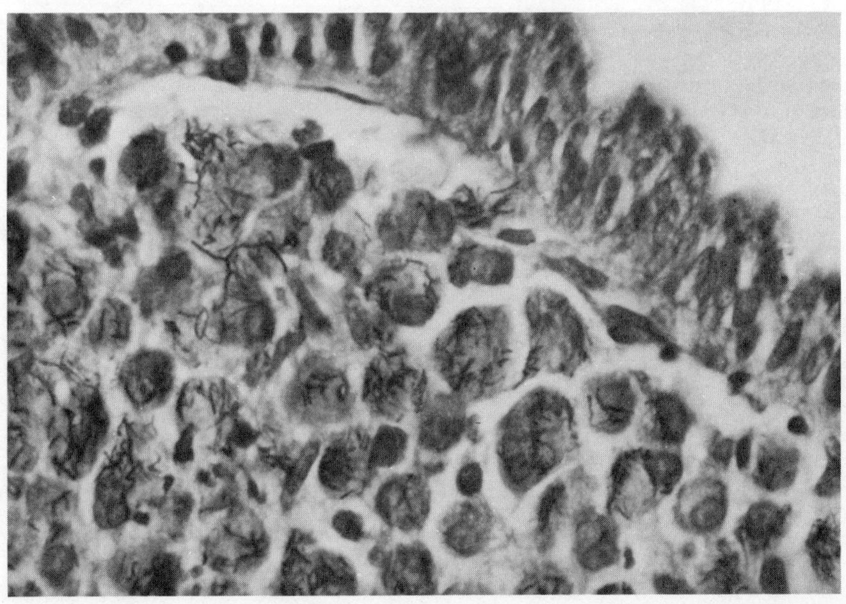

Figure 9. Jejunum showing lamina propria containing macrophages with intracytoplasmic acid-fast bacilli (Kinyoun's acid fast stain)

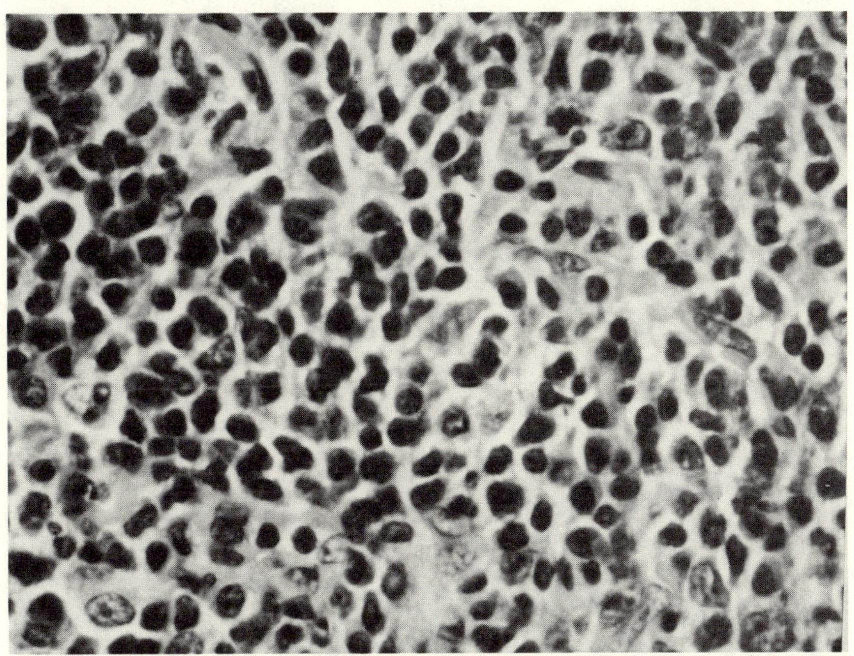

Figure 10. Lymphoid infiltrate in lung showing admixture of lymphocytes, plasma cells, plasmacytoid lymphocytes and occasional immunoblasts. (Hematoxylin-eosin)

It has been suggested that these lesions might represent B cell lymphoid hyperplasia involving extranodal and nodal sites (2). In two recent autopsy cases we noted grossly demonstrable nodular aggregates of B cells in lungs (Figure 11) and spleen with microscopic infiltrates of polymorphic B cells in liver, kidneys, adrenals, skeletal muscle, lymph nodes and soft tissue of the cervical region. The lymphoid cells in these lesions did not show cellular atypia, prominent mitotic activity or foci of necrosis. In the spleen and kidneys lymphoid cells had infiltrated the walls of blood vessels with micronodular subendothelial projections (Figure 12). Besides the presence of B cells, the lymphoid infiltrates in the lungs also contained pale epithelioid type of cells and multinucleated giant cells with granuloma-like collections of these cells in some areas (4).

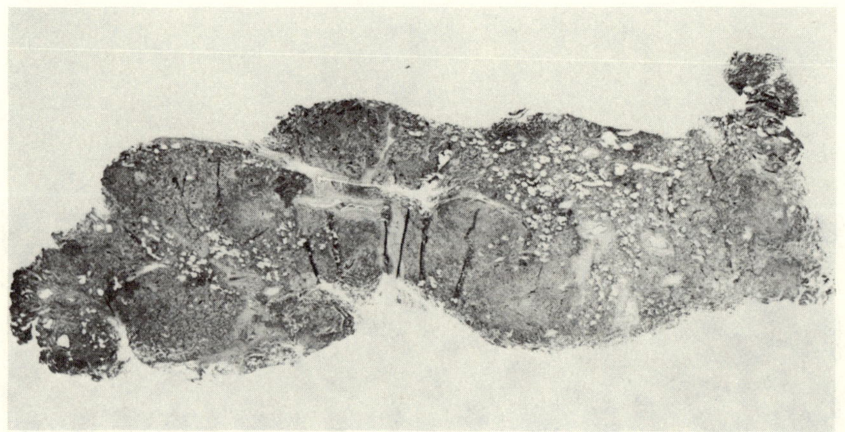

Figure 11. Lung showing large nodular aggregates of lymphoid cells. (Hematoxylin-eosin)

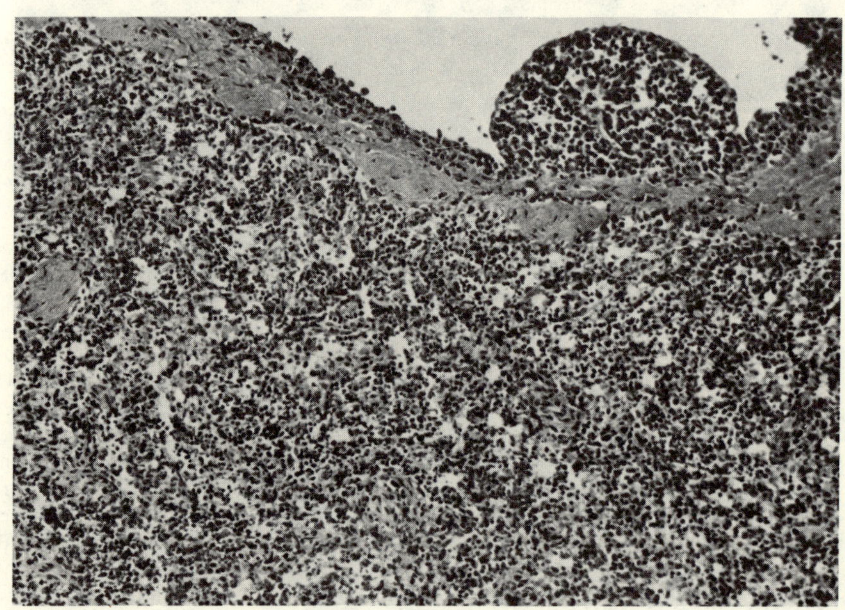

Figure 12. Spleen showing a diffuse lymphoid infiltrate with subendothelial infiltration of a trabecular vein and formation of a micronodule projecting into the lumen. (Hematoxylin-eosin)

OPPORTUNISTIC MALIGNANCIES

We have not observed Kaposi's sarcoma in our series, but a few children with AIDS have been reported to have this tumor (26),(27). Malignant lymphoma (small cell, non-cleaved Burkitt-like) of the central nervous system was seen in one case.

PATHOGENESIS OF PATHOLOGIC LESIONS IN CHILDREN WITH AIDS

HIV is now accepted as the etiologic agent of AIDS (28). Evidence in some of the children with AIDS in our series which supports such a conclusion is as follows: isolation of HIV from peripheral blood lymphocytes (28), demonstration of HIV DNA and RNA by Southern blot and in situ hybridization techniques in brain (18), presence of HIV antibody in serum, successful transmission of infection from children to chimpanzees by inoculation of brain and other tissues (29), and ultrastructural demonstration of HIV in giant cells of brain (17).

Pathogenesis

The pathologic lesions in different organ systems in children with AIDS can be divided into two broad groups: a) primary pathologic lesions due to direct infection of different cells and tissues by HIV; and b) associated lesions resulting from secondary immunologic effects of HIV infection (opportunistic infections), lymphoid proliferation, chronic debilitating disease, iatrogenic injury, or uncertain pathogenesis.

Primary Pathologic Lesions

Destruction of T4 helper cells by HIV infection reflects morphologically in the depletion of T cell areas of lymphoreticular tissues and more specifically in a reduced number of T4 helper cells in lymph nodes (11),(12),(15).

Pathologic lesions of the thymus viz. precocious involution, dysinvolution and thymitis may represent different and/or progressive expressions of thymic epithelial injury (3),(7). Thus, thymitis may be the earliest manifestation as seen in thymic biopsies taken during the active early stages, whereas precocious involution and dysinvolution may be the late manifestations seen in preterminal or terminal stages of the syndrome. In one of our autopsy cases, although the predominant features were those of precocious involution, a few small medullary lymphoid follicles with hyalinized germinal centers indicative of "burnt out" thymitis were also present. In another case, dysinvolution was seen in a thymic biopsy, while at autopsy the thymus showed normal histologic features suggesting that in this case reconstitution of the thymus might have occurred. It is possible that the type of thymic injury may also be related to the timing of injury. Dysinvolution (i.e. involution mimicing dysplasia) may thus be the result of thymic injury during the embryonic development of the thymus when there is transplacental HIV infection. Evidence that the thymus may be directly involved in the HIV infection is inconclusive but includes the demonstration of HIV by an immunofluorescence technique in the thymus of a newborn infant born to a mother with AIDS (30), and the isolation of HIV from a thymic biopsy specimen in a child with AIDS (31).

Direct HIV involvement of the brain has been described above. Therefore, it is reasonable to conclude that the pathologic lesions related to AIDS encephalopathy are due to HIV infection of brain and its sequelae.

Associated Pathologic Lesions

Lesions Resulting from Secondary Immunologic Effects of HIV Infection

The lesions seen in different organ systems due to OI described above fall into this category. The thymic lesions described above contribute to defective cell mediated immunity and lymphocytic depletion of thymus dependent areas of lymph nodes and spleen. It is to be noted that the brain and lymphoreticular system can be the site of both primary and associated pathologic lesions, since OI such as toxoplasmosis or CMV infection can also affect the brain or lymphoreticular system.

Lesions Related to Lymphoproliferative Disorders

It is suggested that the lesions described in the section on extranodal and nodal B cell lymphoid proliferation and other lesions such as LIP constitute a polyclonal polymorphic B cell lymphoproliferative disorder (LD). This LD has a spectrum extending from follicular hyperplasia of lymph nodes or localized lymphoid infiltration of organs, to systemic lymphoid proliferation, as seen in two recent autopsy cases in our series in whom nodular or diffuse B cell lymphoid infiltrates were present in various organs and tissues. Although there were foci of vascular invasion, the different lesions seen in our series were composed of polyclonal B cells and lacked cellular atypia, prominent mitotic activity or foci of necrosis. Therefore, we believe that LD seen in our patients had not progressed to malignancy. However, a case of malignant lymphoma of the brain has been described by Andiman et al. (26) and thus, it appears that the LD in children with AIDS has a broader spectrum. The lymphoid proliferation may be etiologically related to Epstein Barr virus (EBV) infection, since the EBV genome has been demonstrated in lung biopsy and CNS lymphoma tissue in children with AIDS (26),(32). In our patients with AIDS, the incidence of EBV infection, based on serum antibody titers, was about 33%. It is of interest to note that similar EBV related LD occurs in patients with congenital immune deficiency syndromes (33),(34) and in renal transplant recipients (35). It is possible that there is synergism between HIV and EBV in the pathogenesis of LD since latent EBV infection may be activated in children with AIDS, HIV can be adapted by in vitro passage to infect EBV infected B cell lines, which can then serve as reservoirs of HIV (36), and EBV genome has been demonstrated in lung tissue of children with LIP (26) while lymphadenopathy-associated virus (LAV) has been isolated from cells obtained by bronchoalveolar lavage in an adult with LIP and AIDS (37).

Lesions Related to Chronic Debilitating Disease

Besides the specific effects of HIV infection on the thymus and T4 cells, the lymphocytic depletion and atrophy of different lymphoreticular tissues is also related to the effects of failure to thrive and inanition. Villous atrophy of small intestine and fatty change of liver are also probably related to the same factors.

Iatrogenic Lesions

These lesions include the diffuse alveolar damage seen in the lungs at autopsy associated with respiratory supportive therapy, and the fatty change with portal fibrosis of liver and villous atrophy of small intestine associated with hyperalimentation (38).

Lesions of Uncertain Pathogenesis

The lesions seen in the heart may constitute an AIDS cardiomyopathy, the pathogenesis of which is not clear. Alternatively, some of lesions may be secondary to pulmonary disease of different types seen in these children, although a significant degree of pulmonary fibrosis has not been noted in our series. Nutritional deficiencies associated with inanition and vascular factors (see below) may also be involved in the pathogenesis of the cardiac abnormalities (39).

The presence of vascular calcification in the brain and other organs is unexplained. Vascular calcification with or without vasculitis can occur in certain viral infections such as rubella (40),(41). It is possible that HIV may induce similar vascular lesions (17). It is not certain whether these lesions interfere with regional perfusion. It is possible that lesions such as mild interstitial fibrosis of myocardium or cerebral gliosis and atrophy may be partly related to the vascular lesions.

Although DIP was originally described as a clinicopathologic entity (42), it has become apparent that pathologic features resembling DIP may be seen in the lung parenchyma around space-occupying lesions such as eosinophilic granuloma, hamartoma or infections such as tuberculosis (43). We have noted in our cases DIP-like collections of mononuclear cells in the alveoli within or around nodular or diffuse lesions of LIP (Figure 7). It, therefore, appears that in some cases DIP is not a specific pulmonary lesion in children with AIDS but may be a reflection of the response of pulmonary parenchyma around other specific pulmonary pathologic lesions (20).

Multinucleated Giant Cells in Tissues of Children with AIDS

Giant cells resembling Warthin-Finkeldey giant cells have been detected in hyperplastic and atrophic lymph nodes, in lungs with LIP, in brains with AIDS encephalopathy and in thymuses and spleens (2),(4),(7),(17). HIV has been demonstrated in the giant cells in the brain by electron microscopy (17). It is of interest to note that multinucleated giant cells have been described as a cytopathogenic effect during in vitro culture of HIV (44). Although such giant cells can occur in the tissues in other viral infections or in reactive lymphoid hyperplasia (9), their presence can be helpful in the diagnosis of AIDS.

SIGNIFICANCE OF PATHOLOGY OF AIDS IN CHILDREN

Pathologic information derived from study of children with AIDS has contributed much to our understanding of this syndrome. For example, the thymic findings played an extremely important role in helping to distinguish AIDS from congenital immunodeficiencies. Furthermore, the discovery of LIP has added an important additional diagnostic criterion for this syndrome. Clearly more study is needed in this important area.

ACKNOWLEDGMENTS

The authors thank Dr. L. R. Sharer for providing the electron micrograph of HIV in the brain. We are grateful to Ms. Joyce Jackson and Ms. Beinvenida M. Janeck for typing the manuscript.

REFERENCES

1. Oleske, J.M., Minnefor, A.B., Cooper, R., et al., Immune deficiency syndrome in children. JAMA 249:2345-2349 (1983)

2. Joshi, V.V., Oleske, J.M., Minnefor, A.B., et al., Pathology of suspected acquired immune deficiency syndrome in children. Pediatr Pathol 2:71-87 (1984)

3. Joshi, V.V., Oleske, J.M., Pathologic appraisal of the thymus gland in acquired immune deficiency syndrome in children. Arch Pathol Lab Med 109:142-146 (1985)

4. Joshi, V.V., Oleske, J.M., Minnefor, A.B., et al., Pathologic pulmonary findings in children with acquired immune deficiency syndrome. Human Pathol 16:241-246 (1985)

5. CDC., Revision of case definition of AIDS for national reporting -- United States. MMWR 34:373-375 (1985)

6. Amman, A.J., The acquired immune deficiency syndrome in infants and children. Ann Intern Med 103:734-737 (1985)

7. Joshi, V.V., Oleske, J.M., Saad, S., et al., Thymus biopsy in children with acquired immune deficiency syndrome. Arch Path Lab Med 110:837-842 (1986)

8. Seemayer, T.A., Bolande, R.P., Thymic involution mimicking thymic dysplasia: A consequence of transfusion-induced graft vs. host disease in a premature infant. Arch Path Lab Med 104:141-144 (1980)

9. Delsol, G., Pradere, M., Voigt, J.J., et al., Warthin-Finkelday-like cells in benign and malignant lymphoid proliferations. Histopathol 6:451-465 (1982)

10. Ioachim, H.L., Lerner, C.W., Tapper, M.L., The lymphoid lesions associated with the acquired immune deficiency syndrome. Am J Surg Pathol 7:543-553 (1983)

11. Chan, W.C., Brynes, R.K., Spira, J.J., et al., Lymphocyte subsets in lymph nodes of homosexual men with generalized unexplained lymphadenopathy: Correlation with morphology, blood changes, and prognosis. Arch Pathol Lab Med 109:133-137 (1985)

12. Said, J.W., Shintaku, I.P., Teitelbaum, A., et al., Distribution of T-cell phenotypic subsets and surface immunoglobulin-bearing lymphocytes in lymph nodes from male homosexuals with persistent generalized adenopathy. Human Pathol 15:785-790 (1984)

13. Koziner, B., Gebhard, D., Denny, T.N., et al., Analysis of T cell differentiation antigen in acute lymphatic leukemia using monoclonal antibodies. Blood 63:752-757 (1982)

14. Koziner, B., Gebhard, D., Denny, T.N., et al., Characterization of B cell type chronic lymphocytic leukemia cells by surface markers and a monoclonal antibody. Am J Med 73:802-807 (1982)

15. Oleske, J.M., Joshi, V.V., Denny, T., Unpublished data.

16. Epstein, L.G., Sharer, L.R., Joshi, V.V., et al., Progressive encephalopathy in children with acquired immune deficiency syndrome: Clinical and neuropathological findings. Ann Neurol 7:488-496 (1984)

17. Sharer, L.R., Epstein, L.G., Cho, E.S., et al., Pathologic features of AIDS encephalopathy in children. Human Pathol 17:271-284 (1986)

18. Shaw, G.M., Harper, M.E., Hahn, B.H., et al., HTLV-III infection in brains of children and adults with AIDS encephalopathy. Science 227:177-182 (1985)

19. Petito, C.K., Navia, B.A., Cho, E.S., et al., Vacuolar myelopathy pathologically resembling subacute combined degeneration in patients with AIDS. N Engl J Med 312:874-879 (1985)

20. Joshi, V.V., Oleske, J.M., Pulmonary lesions in children with AIDS: A reappraisal based on data in additional cases and follow-up of previously reported cases. Human Pathol 17:641-642 (1986)

21. McLaughlin, L., Joshi, V.V., Nord, K.S., et al., The spectrum of gastrointestinal involvement in children with AIDS. J Ped Gastroenterol Nutr (In press)

22. Duffy, L.F., Daum, F., Kahn, E., et al., Hepatitis in children with AIDS. Gastroenterology 90:173-181 (1986)

23. Joshi, V.V., Oleske, J.M., Saad, S., et al., Pathology of opportunistic infections in children with AIDS (Submitted for publication)

24. Stram, R.L., Gruninger, R.P., AIDS with *Mycobacterium avium-intracellulare* lesions resembling those of Whipple's disease. N Engl J Med 309:1323-1324 (1983)

25. Wood, C., Nickoloff, B.J., Todes-Taylor, N.R., Pseudotumor resulting from atypical mycobacterial infection: A "histoid" variety of *Mycobacterium avium-intracellulare* complex lesion. Am J Clin Pathol 83:524-527 (1984)

26. Andiman, W.A., Eastman, R., Nartin, K., et al., Opportunistic lymphoproliferation associated with Epstein-Barr viral DNA in infants and children with AIDS. Lancet 2:1390-1393 (1985)

27. Buck, B.E., Scott, G.B., Valdes-Dapena, M., et al., Kaposi's sarcoma in two infants with AIDS. J Pediatr 103:911-913 (1983)

28. Gallo, R.C., Salahuddin, S.Z., Popovic, M., et al., Frequent detection and isolation of cytopathogenic retrovirus (HTLV-III) from patients with AIDS and at risk for AIDS. Science 224:500-503 (1984)

29. Gajdusek, D.C., Gibbs, C.J., Rodger-Johnson, P., et al., Infection of chimpanzees by human T-lymphotropic retrovirus in brain and other tissues from AIDS patients. Lancet 1:55-56 (1985)

30. Lapointe, N., Michaud, J., Pekovic, D., et al., Transplancental transmission of HTLV-III virus. N Engl J Med 312:1325-1326 (1985)

31. Oleske, J.M., Unpublished data.

32. Fackler, J.C., Nagel, J.E., Adler, W.H., et al., Epstein-Barr virus infection in a child with acquired immune deficiency syndrome. Am J Dis Child 139:1000-1004 (1985)

33. Frizzera, G., Rosai, J., Dehner, L.P., et al., Lymphoreticular disorders in primary immunodeficiencies. Cancer 46:692-699 (1980)

34. Purtilo, D.T., Immune deficiency, Epstein-Barr virus and lymphoproliferative disorders: In: Immune Deficiency and Cancer: Epstein-Barr Virus and Lymphoproliferative Malignancies (Purtilo, D.T., ed), Plenum Medical Books, New York, p 1-10 (1984)

35. Frizzera, G., Hanto, D.W., Gajl-Peczalska, K.J., et al., Polymorphic diffuse B cell hyperplasias and lymphomas in renal transplant recipients. Cancer Res 41:4262-4269 (1981)

36. Casareale, D., Sinangil, F., Sonnabend, J., et al., Establishment of retrovirus, Epstein-Barr virus positive B lymphoblastoid cell lines derived from individuals at risk for acquired immune deficiency syndrome (AIDS). AIDS Res 1:253-270 (1985)

37. Ziza, J.M., Brun-Vezinet, F., Venet, A., et al., Lymphadenopathy associated with virus isolated from bronchoalveolar lavage fluid in AIDS related complex with lymphoid interstitial pneumonitis. N Engl J Med 313:183 (1985)

38. Cohen, C., Olesen, M.M., Pediatric total parenteral nutrition. Arch Pathol Lab Med 105:152-156 (1981)

39. Alexander, C.S., Nutritional heart disease. Cardiovascular Clin 4:222-244 (1972)

40. Townsend, J.J., Stroop, W.G., Baringer, J.R., et al., Neuropathology of progressive rubella panencephalitis after childhood rubella. Neurology 32:185-190 (1982)

41. Esterly, J.R., Oppenheimer, E.H., Intrauterine rubella infection. Persp Pediatr Pathol 1:313-338 (1973)

42. Liebow, A.A., Steer, A., Billingsley, J.G., Desquamative interstitial pneumonia. Am J Med 39:369-404 (1965)

43. Bedrossian, C.W.M., Kuhn, C., Luna, M.A., et al., Desquamative interstitial pneumonia-like reaction accompanying pulmonary lesions. Chest 62:166-169 (1977)

44. Popovic, M., Sarngadharan, M.G., Read, E., et al., Detection, isolation, and continuous production of cytopathic retrovirus (HTLV-III) from patients with AIDS and pre-AIDS. Science 224:497-500 (1984)

46
Neuropathology of AIDS

Marius P. Valsamis

The recognition of the acquired immune deficiency syndrome (AIDS) as a nosologic and infectious entity has resulted in an unprecedented intensive search to elucidate the pathogenetic, epidemiologic, clinical and therapeutic features of the disease. At the present time, our knowledge of the neuropathologic aspects of the disease, although increasing, is incomplete (1)-(5). The purpose of this chapter is to provide a survey of the lesions encountered and to discuss certain patterns of disease which we feel deserve greater emphasis.

A striking feature of the brain involvement in AIDS is the multiplicity and variety of infections encountered. Nervous system lesions are caused by opportunistic infections and neoplasms arising as a result of a compromised immune system, and by spread of the primary agent, human immunodeficiency virus (HIV), to the brain. A question which may be important is why particular infectious agents have affected the brain while others have not. It may very well be that the absence or rarity of certain central nervous system (CNS) infections in AIDS, despite the ubiquity of the causative agents in the environment, may be as significant in the understanding of the immune process as those which are found. AIDS has provided an unusual opportunity to dissect the immune process in such a way that important, possibly fundamental advances in our understanding of host defenses may be disclosed.

GENERAL CONCERNS OF THE NEUROPATHOLOGIST

The multiplicity of lesions found in brains of AIDS patients poses a challenge for the diagnostic neuropathologist. One cannot simply select a single lesion for microscopic analysis with the assumption that all other lesions which have a similar gross appearance are identical. Instead, the multiple areas of necrosis, the areas of pallor, or the areas of overt cavitary softening, may very well represent separate pathologic processes with distinctly different etiologies. On occasion, the same lesion may harbor two or more infectious agents. It is, therefore, incumbent upon the pathologist to sample every lesion and to take great care in examining each lesion, to achieve a complete and proper diagnostic evaluation.

In AIDS, the alterations in the immune state sometimes result in patterns of reaction and infiltration which differ from those encountered in the same disease process in the non-immunocompromised host. Toxoplasma and cryptococcal infections are associated with such differences and will be discussed below. The inflammatory response in AIDS is altered depending upon the stage of the disease. In early cases of AIDS, lymphocytes may be numerous, but as the disease progresses and lymphopenia appears, the cellular exudates are altered and the rising percentage of reactive macrophages in the cellular responses may cause diagnostic problems. It is our experience that in advanced cases the pathologist may be hard pressed to discriminate, for example, between toxoplasma infection and primary lymphoma.

Lesions may be poorly demarcated with a tendency for the process to spread into adjacent tissues. Furthermore, it is only recently that direct involvement of the nervous system by HIV has been recognized (6)-(8). The morphologic changes associated with this involvement have not yet been definitively evaluated.

INFECTIONS

Bacterial Infections

Considering the severity of the immunosuppression in AIDS, bacterial infections appear to involve the CNS less frequently than might be anticipated. One might expect to find an increased incidence of the classic meningitides: due to *Hemophilus influenzae*, pneumococcal or meningococcal. Instead, a constellation of unusual infections which form a part of the opportunistic infectious spectrum which characterizes AIDS is most commonly found. The most commonly reported bacterial infections are due to atypical mycobacteria, particularly *Mycobacterium avium-intracellulare* (9). Tuberculosis has also been reported (9), (10). Because of their decreased "acid-fastness", non-tuberculous mycobacteria may be more easily demonstrated with the special variants of the acid-fast procedure previously developed to demonstrate the lepra bacillus, such as the Fite stain. Caseous necrosis may be present. In late cases of AIDS, the chronic granulomatous inflammatory response is modified in that there is a smaller proportion of lymphocytes and multinucleated giant cells.

Nocardia infections have also been described in AIDS patients but appear to be very rare (9).

Fungal Infections

Among the fungi, *Cryptococcus neoformans* is a frequent cause of meningitis and disseminated disease in AIDS (5),(9). The pathologic presentation is no different from that seen in other immunosuppressed patients. Encapsulated, narrow-pore, budding yeasts within the cerebrospinal fluid may be detected utilizing standard India ink preparations. Organisms have been cultured from brain, cerebrospinal fluid, bone marrow, lymph nodes, liver, lungs, blood and urine. Hematoxylin and eosin preparations reveal pale cell walls of yeast from 4 to 7 microns in diameter. Silver impregnation stains are commonly used to demonstrate the organism. Positive mucicarmine stains are helpful in distinguishing cryptococcal yeast forms from those of *Blastomyces dermatitidis* or *Histoplasma capsulatum*. Cryptococcal organisms are surrounded by a characteristic carminophylic mucoid capsule. One should be aware that the thickness of the capsule itself is modified relative to the immune state. Bottone et al. (11) have demonstrated that the capsule thickness is reduced parallel to the reduction of the immune response.

Other fungi, such as aspergillus and mucor have also been reported (2),(5),(9). These organisms present as typical vasculitides and the features of infection are not different from those encountered in non-AIDS cases. Candidiasis may also present as a vasculitis with coagulative necrosis and parenchymal involvement.

Protozoa

Protozoal infections of the CNS in AIDS are relatively few in number. Reported cases have been limited to toxoplasmosis (2),(5),(9),(12) and amebiasis (13). Toxoplasma has been the most frequently encountered protozoan invader of the brain. It has presented both as an encephalitis and as a mass lesion (9). The pattern of toxoplasma infection in the nervous system in AIDS is frequently modified due to alterations in the immune system. In 1969, Frenkel (14) described, in an experimental model, variations in the pathologic features of infections of toxoplasma and toxoplasma-like organisms in hamsters with and without immune suppression. In untreated animals, pseudocysts were the most striking morphologic feature and only a relatively small number of extracellular organisms were found in areas of necrosis. With immunosuppression, however, the number of pseudocysts was vastly reduced. Large numbers of individual organisms were found scattered in broad areas of coagulative necrosis. The latter picture resembles the pattern seen in AIDS; i.e. individual organisms are found scattered through areas of coagulative necrosis (Figure 1). Occasional pseudocysts may also be encountered. When pseudocysts are not evident, the diagnosis requires a sharp eye and a bit of luck as well as an awareness of the possibility of toxoplasmosis on the part of the diagnostician as the organisms may be mistaken for nuclear fragments. Definitive diagnosis requires visualization of the characteristic tachyzoites and/or cysts in hematoxylin and eosin- or Giemsa-stained specimens. A peroxidase-antiperoxidase method has proven useful (15). In fresh tissue, the tachyzoites may be crescentic, but in fixed tissue sections, they are rounded and thus may be confused with nuclear dust (9).

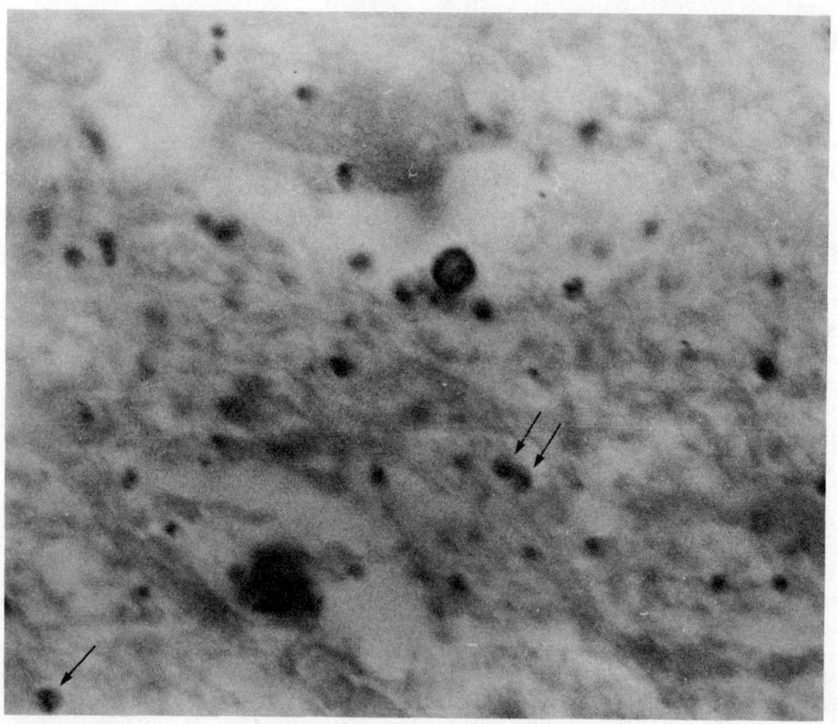

Figure 1. An area of necrosis with many toxoplasma organisms scattered in the debris; three are indicated by arrows (hematoxylin and eosin stain)

In the acute phase of toxoplasma infection, organisms multiply asexually within engorged host cells. Destruction of these cells results in foci of necrotic lesions which may be detected both grossly and microscopically. Encysted forms are seen most often at the periphery of such lesions; free organisms are most easily found at the interface between viable and necrotic tissue. An arteritis with a characteristic concentric fibrosis involving the vessel media and adventitia is also prominent. This arteritis may provide a clue to the presence of toxoplasma in the absence of detectable organisms, but the organism must be demonstrated to make a definitive diagnosis. It should also be pointed out that as a result of the immune depression, lymphocytes are reduced in the reactive response but there may be a concomitant increase in reactive, cytologically atypical macrophages, thus mimicing the microscopic appearance of lymphoma. Appropriate stains utilizing monoclonal antibodies to the protozoan may be useful in making the distinction (15).

Katz et al. (13) have encountered a case of amebiasis (thought to be acanthomeba) of the central nervous system in an AIDS patient. A significant feature was that the distribution of organisms did not follow the pattern seen when the presumed route of infection is intranasal. Instead, the distribution of organisms suggested vascular dissemination. In other respects the lesions did not differ from those in non-AIDS cases.

Viral Infections

The most common viral infections of the nervous system in AIDS have been those of cytomegalovirus, polyomavirus and *Herpes simplex*. Epstein-Barr virus has been demonstrated in the genome of Burkitt lymphomas of the CNS (9). Recently, evidence for direct brain involvement by HIV has been presented.

Viral diseases in AIDS have no unusual histologic appearance with the exception of cytomegalovirus infection which has been found to involve a greater variety of structures and to be associated with a greater degree of necrosis than described previously. Sites of CMV infection have included optic nerve, retina, and dorsal root ganglia (presenting as a Guillain-Barre syndrome) (16), as well as the more traditional parenchymal lesions (9),(16),(17).

Chorioretinitis due to cytomegalovirus has been a frequent occurrence in some series (9),(17),(18). An interesting feature has been the coexistence of toxoplasma infection within lesions containing the characteristic cytomegalic inclusion bodies. The coexistence of toxoplasma and viral infections has also been reported in immunosuppressed non-AIDS patients. Cheever et al. (19) and Vietzke et al. (20) reported cases in whom the combined infection caused mass lesions or an encephalitis. Subsequently, Gelderman et al. (21) performed an in vitro study in which tissue cultures were infected with cytomegalovirus and then secondarily infected with toxoplasma organisms. Different patterns of infection were noted which led the investigators to theorize that coexistence of certain viruses with toxoplasma infection might lead to enhancement of the growth of the toxoplasma organism. Multiple infectious agent interactions in AIDS have yet to be explored, but such interactions may very well prove to be of more than passing interest.

Evidence of progressive multifocal leukoencephalopathy (PML) including demyelinating lesions, inclusion bodies and demonstration of the etiologic viral agent (JC virus) has been found in AIDS (9),(16),(22). JC virus, when injected into hamsters (23), has produced gliomas. PML with subsequent multiple gliomas has been reported in a human case (24); in the future, should a patient survive long enough, other cases of gliogenous neoplasm in the CNS following JC virus infection may be seen.

HIV INFECTION OF THE NERVOUS SYSTEM

Recently, attention has been given to the existence and prevalence of direct infection of the nervous system by HIV (4),(6), (25),(26). Clinically, many patients have shown personality changes or signs of encephalitis and/or progressive dementia. Symptoms have sometimes appeared years before the patient's demise or before signs of immunodeficiency. Histologic descriptions have appeared noting the presence of multinucleated cells (26),(27). The authors did not discriminate between two different types of giant cells recognized by pathologists. We have examined several cases in which the virus has been demonstrated and have noted the following:

1. Multinucleated cells in which the nuclei have a peripheral distribution (Langhan's type) are often seen (Figure 2). In addition, multinucleated cells in which the nuclei are centrally aggregated (Warthin-Finkeldey type) can be found, especially in areas of necrosis, or scattered throughout the interstitium. These cells are frequently present in close proximity to blood vessels, in areas where, under routine hematoxylin-eosin staining, no abnormalities could be noted in the surrounding tissue (Figure 3).

2. Microglial nodules are found in gray matter (Figure 4).

3. Scattered throughout areas of gray matter and less frequently in white matter are elongated activated microglial cells ("rod cells") (Figure 5).

These findings are in agreement with those previously reported (4),(26), save for the distinction between Langhans and Warthin-Finkeldey cells. The two types of multinucleated cells are probably a response to different stimuli and may have separate significance. The Langhan's type of giant cell is most likely a reaction to phagocytosis of lipid material. Such cells have classically been described in cases of tuberculosis within granulomas. Similar cells have been found in the brains of patients with multiple sclerosis at sites where there has been

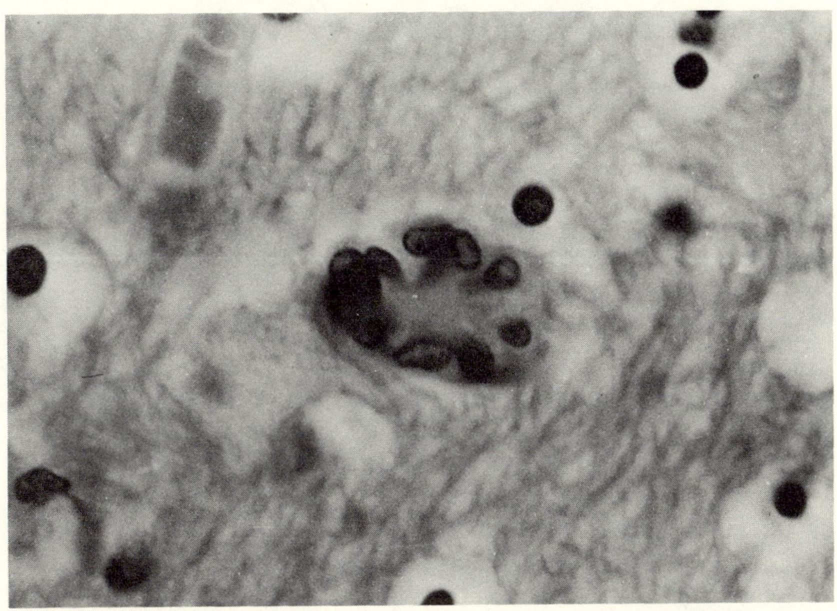

Figure 2. A multinucleated cell of the Langhans type (hematoxylin and eosin stain)

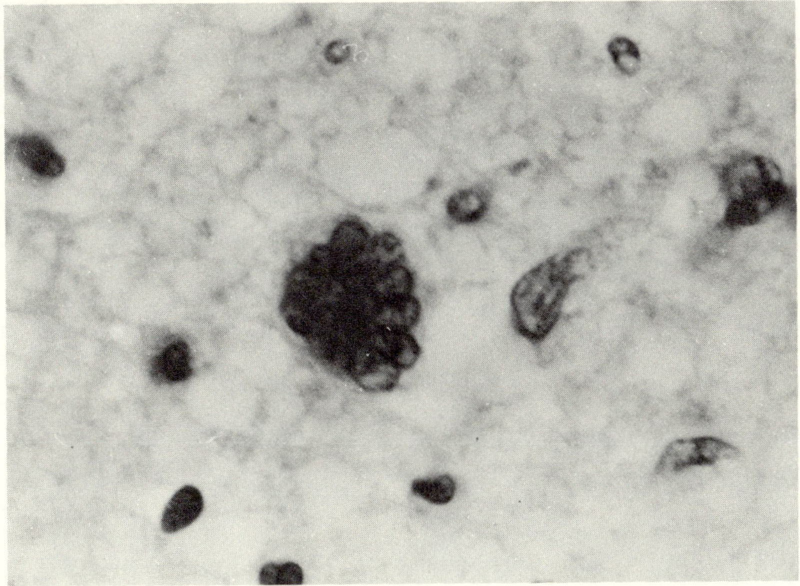

Figure 3. A multinucleated cell of the Warthin-Finkeldey type (hematoxylin and eosin stain)

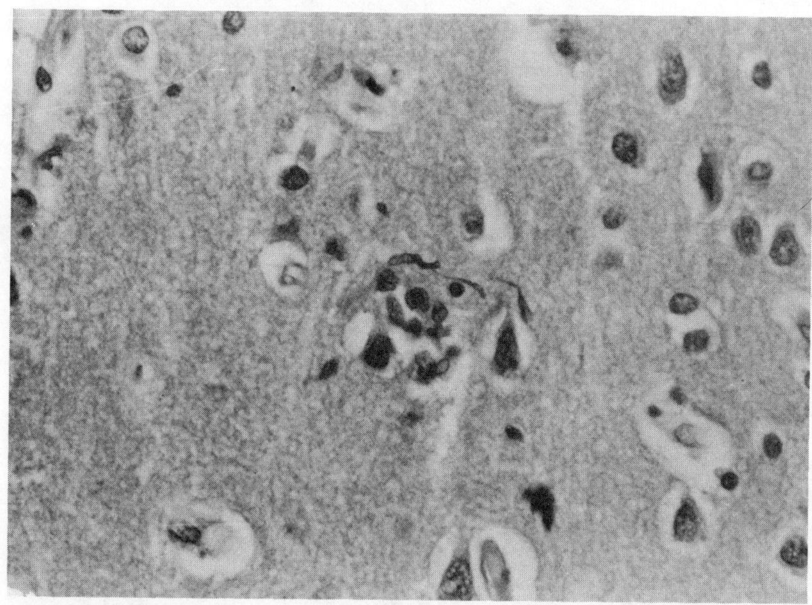

Figure 4. A microglial nodule flanked by two neurones (hematoxylin and eosin stain)

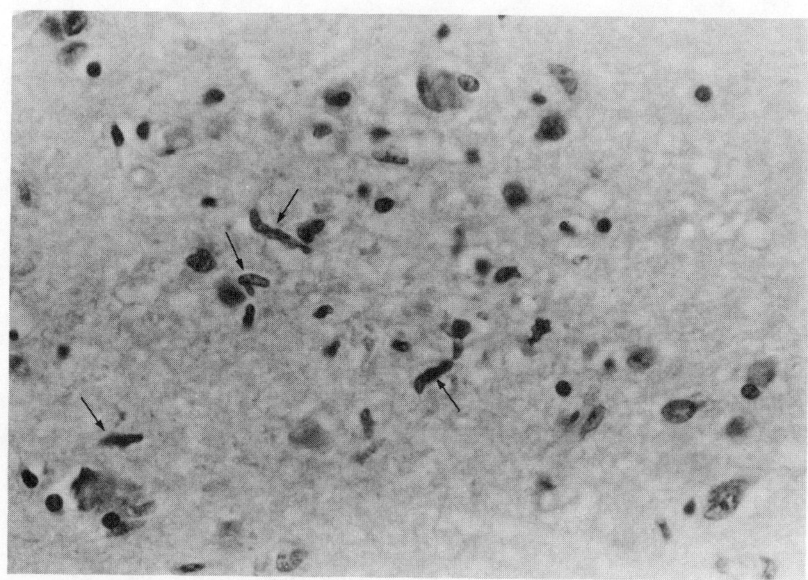

Figure 5. Activated microglia or "rod cells" (arrows) scattered in cortex (hematoxylin and eosin stain)

breakdown of lipid material (28). This type of cell may very well phagocytize viral particles. Therefore, studies which have reported the presence of viral antigen and other debris within the cytoplasm of such cells (27) do not constitute evidence for primary involvement with HIV.

The Warthin-Finkeldey type of cell has been reported in both benign and malignant lymphoid proliferations (29). In the past, such cells have been regarded as specific for virus infections (29). They have also been considered as derived from endothelial cells (30). The Warthin-Finkeldey type of cell may very well represent a virally induced multinucleated cell.

We would suggest that in a routine examination of the brain, the diagnosis of presumptive HIV infection be based on the following:

1. The presence of a progressive dementia in a patient with AIDS.

2. The presence of rod cells in significant numbers scattered throughout the cortex and white matter along with glial nodules in cortex and white matter.

3. The presence of Warthin-Finkeldey cells; both in areas of necrosis and within normal tissue.

The validity of such diagnostic criteria could be tested in a series of autopsy cases in which clinical data are available and the tissues examined for viral antigen.

Recently, Yankner et al. (31) have reported a granulomatous angiitis associated with isolation of HIV from the nervous system. The causative agent is not known. There is some evidence that HIV is present in endothelial cells (25) and in macrophages (6), but the pathogenesis of granulomatous angiitis in AIDS has yet to be fully elucidated.

NEOPLASMS

Immune deficiency states have been associated with an increased incidence of several neoplasms (32). In AIDS, Kaposi's sarcoma and primary intracranial lymphomas have been most prominent. However, we are unaware of any case of Kaposi's sarcoma primary in the CNS. Central nervous system lymphomas have frequently been the cause of presenting symptoms in AIDS (9),(33),(34). These have been of the non-Hodgkin's type and are unusual in that they are frequently primary within the central nervous system, whereas spontaneous non-Hodgkin's lymphomas are rarely encountered in this location. The lymphomas encountered in AIDS are usually non-differentiated lymphomas of the relatively rare Burkitt's-like type. The malignant lymphocytes most often have small non-cleaved nuclei, multiple small nucleoli and scanty cytoplasm. In those cases where immunohistology has been performed, the lymphomas were determined to be of B cell lineage with the expression of either kappa or lambda light chains and a heavy chain, most commonly IgM. Both large cell immunoblastic and small non-cleaved lymphomas have been seen, and in one series of 11 cases (34), all were multicentric.

The clinical and radiographic appearance of lymphomas is non-specific. Histologic confirmation is necessary to discriminate between neoplasm and infectious lesions. As mentioned above, the reduced number of lymphocytes in chronic inflammatory exudates with a concomitant increase in atypical macrophages may cause difficulty in differentiating between lymphomas and infections. The prognosis has been extremely poor, with an average survival of less than two months after diagnosis (34).

An insight into the possible pathogenesis of these lymphomas was obtained in a series of experiments performed by Krueger (35), who reviewed the clinical literature extensively and determined that there was strong evidence for immunosuppression preceding the appearance of lymphoma. He then proceeded to study an animal model in which persistent antigenic stimulation was coupled with chronic immunosuppression. T-cell lymphomas were produced in a more than tenfold greater frequency than the baseline incidence. The analogy of this experimental model with AIDS is striking.

SUMMARY

The plethora of neuropathologic findings in AIDS places a significant responsibility on the diagnostic neuropathologist. The multiplicity of organisms and the coexistence of multiple pathologic processes within individual lesions make a thorough, all-inclusive examination necessary to achieve diagnostic completeness. Morphologic criteria for the presence of HIV infection are now being defined and may very well not be as specific as one would like. It would be valuable to have established reliable criteria which could be applied using the light microscope and routine stains. If absolute proof of HIV encephalitis is dependent upon techniques of molecular biology, definitive diagnosis might be expensive and labor-intensive. A study correlating prospective psychological and clinical evaluation with morphologic and molecular biologic studies on brains, would represent an excellent opportunity to gain further insights into the neurobiology of AIDS. Certainly, easily applied, inexpensively determined criteria for detection of early encephalitic changes due to the HIV would be of great value to the practicing clinician, and indirectly, to those afflicted with the disease.

ACKNOWLEDGMENT

The author would like to express his thanks to Dr. David Katz, Dr. Abe Macher, Dr. Carol Petito, Dr. Cheryl Reichert, for fruitful discussions and opportunities to review material.

REFERENCES

1. Joshi, V.V., Oleske, J.M., Minnefor, A.B., et al., Pathology of suspected acquired immune deficiency syndrome in children: A study of eight cases. Ped Path 2:71-87 (1984)

2. Levy, R.M., Bredesen, D.E., Rosenblum, M.L., Neurological manifestations of the acquired immunodeficiency syndrome (AIDS): Experience at UCSF and review of the literature. J Neurosurg 62:475-495 (1985)

3. Moskowitz, L.B., Hensley, G.T., Chan, J.C., et al., The neuropathology of acquired immune deficiency syndrome. Arch Pathol Lab Med 108:867-872 (1984)

4. Petito, C.K., Cho, E.S., Leman, W., et al., Neuropathology of acquired immunodeficiency syndrome (AIDS): An autopsy review. J Neuropath Exptl Neurol 45: 635-646 (1986)

5. Snider, W.D., Simpson, D.M., Neilsen, S., et al., Neurological complications of acquired immune deficiency syndrome: Analysis of 50 patients. Ann Neurol 14:403-417 (1983)

6. Koenig, S., Gendelman, H.E., Orenstein, J.M., et al., Detection of AIDS virus in macrophages in brain tissue from AIDS patients with encephalopathy. Science 233:1089-1093 (1986)

7. Nielsen, S.L., Petito, C.K., Urmacher, C.D., et al., Subacute encephalitis in acquired immune deficiency syndrome: A postmortem study. Am J Clin Pathol 82:678-682 (1984)

8. Navia, B.A., Cho, E.S., Petito, C.K., et al., The AIDS dementia complex: II. Neuropath Ann Neurol 19:525-535 (1986)

9. Reichert, C.M., O'Leary, T.J., Levens, D.L., et al., Autopsy pathology in the acquired immune deficiency syndrome. Am J Path 112:357-382 (1983)

10. Mata-Gonzalez, P.R., Vazquez, H.C., Joachim, G.F., et al., Tuberculous brain abscess. J Neurosurg 52:419-422 (1980)

11. Bottone, E.J., Wormser, G.P., Poorly encapsulated *Cryptococcus neoformans* from patients with AIDS II: Correlation of capsule size observed directly in cerebrospinal fluid with that after animal passage. AIDS Res 2:219-225 (1986)

12. Anders, K., Steinsapir, K.D., Iverson, D.J., et al., Neuropathologic findings in the acquired immunodeficiency syndrome (AIDS). Clinic Neuropath 5:1-20 (1986)

13. Katz, D., Pathologic Anatomy Branch National Cancer Institute, National Institute Health, Bethesda, MD., Personal communication. (1986)

14. Frenkel, J.K., Pathogenesis of toxoplasmosis and of infections with organisms resembling toxoplasma. Ann NY Acad Sci 64:215-251 (1956)

15. Conley, F.K., Jenkins, K.A., Remington, J.S., *Toxoplasma gondii* infection of the central nervous system; Use of the peroxidase-antiperoxidase method to demonstrate toxoplasma in formalin-fixed, paraffin-embedded tissue sections. Hum Pathol 12:690-698 (1981)

16. Tucker, T., Dix, R.D., Katzen, C., et al., Cytomegalovirus and *Herpes simplex* virus ascending myelitis in a patient with acquired immune deficiency syndrome. Ann Neurol 18: 740-749 (1985)

17. Friedman, A.H., Freeman, W.R., Orellana, J., et al., Cytomegalovirus retinitis and immunodeficiency in homosexual males. Lancet 1:959 (1982)

18. Pepose, J.S., Hilborne, L.H., Cancilla, P.Q., et al., Concurrent *Herpes simplex* and cytomegalovirus retinitis and encephalitis in the acquired immune deficiency syndrome (AIDS). Ophthal 91:1669-1677 (1984)

19. Cheever, A., Valsamis, M.P., Rabson, A., Necrotizing toxoplasmic encephalitis and herpetic pneumonia complicating treated Hodgkin's disease. N Engl J Med 272:26-29 (1965)

20. Vietzke, W.M., Gelderman, A.H., Grimley, P.M., et al., Toxoplasmosis complicating malignancy. Cancer 215:816-827 (1968)

21. Gelderman, A.H., Grimley, P.M., Lunde, M.N., et al., *Toxoplasma gondii* and cytomegalovirus: Mixed infection by a parasite and a virus. Science 160:1130-1132 (1968)

22. Gia Russo, M.H., Koeppeu, A.H., Atypical progressive multifocal leukoencephalopathy and primary cerebral malignant lymphoma. J Neurol Sci 35:391-398 (1978)

23. Walker, E.L., Padgent, B.L., Zurhein, G.M., et al., Human papovavirus (J.C.): Induction of brain tumors in hamsters. Science 181:674-676 (1973)

24. Castaigne, P., Rondot, P., Escourolle, R., et al., Leukoencephalopathie multifocale progressive et "gliomes" multiples: Revuew Neurologue (Paris) 130:379-392 (1974)

25. Gabuzda, D.H., Ho, D., de la Monte, S.M., et al., Immunohistochemical identification of HTLV-III antigen in brains of patients with AIDS. Ann Neurol 1986 20:289-295 (1986)

26. Shaw, G.M., Harper, M.E., Hahn, B.H., et al., HTLV-III infection in brains of children and adults with AIDS encephalopathy. Science 227:177-182 (1985)

27. Sharer, L.R., Cho, E., Epstein, L.G., Multinucleated giant cells and HTLV-III in AIDS encephalopathy. Hum Path 16:760 (1985)

28. Bise, K., Mehraeim, P., Hubner, G., et al., Multinucleated giant cells unlike those of histiocytic or glial origin: A unique cell formation in acute demyelination. Abstract #836 X International Congress of Neuropathology, Stockholm (1986)

29. Delson, G., Pradere, M., Voigt, J.J., et al., Warthin-Finkeldey-like cells in benign and malignant lymphoid proliferation. Histopathology 6:451-465 (1982)

30. Lennert, K., Lymphknoten diagnostik in Schnitt and Ausstrich. Bandteil A. Cytologie und Lymphadenitis, Springer Verlag, Berlin, 134-136 (1961)

31. Yankner, B.A., Skolnik, P.R., Showkimas, T.M., et al., Cerebral granulomatous angiitis associated with isolation of HTLV-III from the central nervous system. Ann Neurol 20: 362-364 (1986)

32. Waldmann, T.A., Struber, W., Blaese, R.M., Immunodeficiency disease and malignancy. Ann Intern Med 77:605-628 (1972)

33. Snider, W.D., Simpson, D.M., Aronyk, K.E., et al., Primary lymphoma of the central nervous system associated with acquired immune deficiency syndrome. N Engl J Med 308:45 (1983)

34. So, Y.T., Beckstead, J.H., David, R.L., Primary central nervous system lymphoma in acquired immune deficiency syndrome: A clinical and pathological study. (In press)

35. Krueger, G.R.F., Chronic immunosuppression and lymphomagenesis in man and mice. National Cancer Institute, Monograph 35:183-190 (1972)

Part VI
Infection Control Considerations

47
Infection Control Considerations in HIV Infection

Eugene McCray, William J. Martone

Acquired immunodeficiency syndrome (AIDS) was first recognized in 1981 (1)-(3). The epidemiology of AIDS suggested that it was caused by a transmissible infectious agent (4),(5), and in 1983 the etiologic agent that caused AIDS (human immunodeficiency virus [HIV]) was discovered (6)-(9). Serologic tests were developed to detect antibody to HIV, thereby providing an indicator of past or present infection with the virus (9)-(16). Serologic evidence of exposure to HIV is seen in most AIDS patients (10),(12),(13),(17)-(20) and in up to 70% of asymptomatic persons in certain populations at increased risk for AIDS (10),(13),(17)-(22). The prevalence of antibody to HIV is, however, less than 0.1% in individuals who are not in identified risk groups for infection with HIV (e.g., blood donors) (12),(21)-(23).

Early in the AIDS epidemic, there was concern that health-care personnel taking care of AIDS patients might face an increased risk of acquiring AIDS or infection with HIV. In contrast to hepatitis B, however, data indicate that this risk is small (<1%) and is related to parenteral exposure to blood (24)-(29).

In this chapter we will briefly review the epidemiology of HIV infection with specific reference to common infectious diseases affecting these patients and will outline infection control strategies to prevent transmission of HIV and opportunistic infections that may be associated with HIV infection in the health-care setting.

EPIDEMIOLOGY OF HIV INFECTION

The natural history of infection with HIV has not yet been clearly defined. However, preliminary data show that up to 60% of persons infected with HIV, as measured by the presence of antibody to HIV, may have virus isolated from their blood (30)-(32). Viremia has been shown to persist for up to 52 months (32),(33). These persons may serve as a reservoir of infection for others. After infection with the virus, a person may have an acute, mild self-limited illness (34)-(37) or may remain asymptomatic for months or years. A variable percentage of those infected with HIV will develop AIDS-related conditions (ARC) (23%-26%) or AIDS (7%-15%) (19),(32),(33),(38).

Between 1981 and June 9, 1986, 21,517 cases of AIDS were reported in the United States. Centers for Disease Control (CDC) projects that over 30,000 cases of AIDS will be reported in the United States by the end of 1986. The risk factors for AIDS are well-defined, and the percentage of AIDS cases with the various risk factors have remained relatively constant since the beginning of the epidemic.

Some AIDS patients reported to CDC have indicated the health care profession as their occupation. These health-care workers with AIDS are epidemiologically similar to other reported patients with AIDS, that is, 95% belong to groups recognized to be at increased risk for AIDS. In those health-care workers with no identified risk factors for AIDS, no specific occupational exposure could be identified as the source of HIV infection (39). Results from several studies suggest that health-care workers caring for, or working with specimens from, patients infected with HIV are at extremely low risk for acquiring HIV (26),(28), (29),(39). Whatever low risk exists, appears to be related to parenteral exposure to blood from a patient infected with HIV.

TRANSMISSION OF HIV

Transmission of HIV occurs in the following ways: 1) through sexual contact, 2) through parenteral exposure to blood or its components, and 3) perinatally from infected mother to child before, at, or shortly after the time of birth. Although the virus has been isolated from a number of body fluids other than blood and semen (e.g., saliva, tears, breast milk, and cerebrospinal fluid) (40)-(43), there are no instances in which exposure to these body fluids has been conclusively shown to result in transmission of the virus. In the one case in which parenteral exposure to pleural fluid was implicated in transmission of HIV, the fluid was described as "bloody" (43a). Transmission of HIV does not occur through ordinary social or occupational contact with persons infected with the virus or through air, water, or food. Studies of people living in the same household with persons infected with HIV show that transmission does not occur except through direct sexual contact with infected persons (44), (45).

No unusual or extreme precautions are necessary to prevent

transmission of the virus in the health-care environment. Published recommendations have stressed that patients infected with HIV should be placed on blood and body fluid precautions (27), (46)-(49). In addition, emphasis was given to precautions targeted at preventing needlesticks and other injuries caused by the use of sharp instruments by health-care workers caring for patients. However, such injuries continue to occur even during the care of patients who are known to be infected with HIV (28). Commonly reported preventable injuries resulting in parenteral exposures to blood of AIDS patients have been defined in the CDC Prospective Surveillance System for health-care workers with parenteral or mucous-membrane exposures to blood or other body fluids from patients infected with HIV (Table 1).

Table 1. Health-Care Workers with Preventable Exposures to Body Fluids of Patients with AIDS or AIDS-Related Illnesses by Circumstance of Exposure.

August 15, 1983 - March 31, 1986

Circumstance of the Exposure	Percent of Health-Care Workers (n = 992)
Recapping a used needle	16%
Injury from improperly disposed needle or sharp object	13%
Contamination of an open wound	10%
Using needle cutting device	1%
Total	40%

OPPORTUNISTIC INFECTIONS IN PATIENTS WITH AIDS

Patients infected with HIV who are immunocompromised may develop a number of infections or conditions, some of which will require specific precautions. Most of the microorganisms that may infect AIDS patients (Table 2) take advantage of the T-lymphocyte defect in the immune system of these patients (50). For others, immunoglobulin defects appear to be responsible for invasive or persistent diseases (e.g., *Hemophilus influenzae; Streptococcus pneumoniae*) or the defect responsible is unknown (e.g., *Staphylococcus aureus*). Many of the infectious diseases associated with AIDS require specific isolation precautions (Table 2) (51).

MANAGEMENT OF PATIENTS INFECTED WITH HIV

Patients infected with HIV include persons who test positive for antibody to HIV, and persons with AIDS, ARC, or other manifestations of infection with HIV. The basic techniques and precautions for managing patients infected with HIV are appropriate for routine care of all patients. Because all infected patients cannot be identified by history, physical examination, or readily available laboratory tests, the same infection control precautions should be applied to all patients receiving medical care.

PREVENTING HIV EXPOSURE AMONG PATIENTS AND STAFF

Patient-Care Precautions

Handwashing is the single most important means of preventing spread of infection. Personnel should always wash their hands after taking care of patients, even when gloves are used. In addition, personnel should wash their hands after touching excretions (feces, urine, or materials soiled with them) and secretions (from wounds, skin infections, etc.) and before touching any patient again. Hands should also be washed before performing invasive procedures, touching wounds, or touching immunocompromised patients.

Private Versus Multiple-Bed Rooms

A private room is not necessary for patients infected with HIV unless the patient's hygiene is poor, or the presence of other infections makes a private room necessary, e.g., *Mycobacterium tuberculosis*. Care should be exercised in placing other HIV-infected patients, or patients immunosuppressed because of other factors, in the same room because of the potential risk of cross infection with opportunistic pathogens.

It will frequently be necessary to care for HIV-infected patients in intensive care units (ICU), operating rooms, and other special care facilities. Health-care facilities must not deny HIV-infected patients the potential benefits of such facilities, if medically indicated. If ICU care is required, a bed in an open ICU may be used as long as the patient has no other transmissible infections that necessitate a private room and the additional requirements of blood and body fluid precautions can be observed. Otherwise, an isolation room is desirable.

Blood and Body Fluid Precautions

As is true in the case of all patients, when the possibility of exposure to blood or other body fluids exists, routinely recommended precautions should be followed. The anticipated exposure may require gloves alone, as in handling items soiled with blood or equipment contaminated with blood or other body

Table 2. Microorganisms Causing Opportunistic Infections in Patients with Acquired Immunodeficiency Syndrome and Recommended Isolation Procedures

Microorganisms	Syndrome	Precautions
Bacteria		
Mycobacteria Nontuberculous (atypical)	Pulmonary or Disseminated	None
	Wound	Drainage/Secretion
Mycobacterium tuberculosis	Extrapulmonary, draining lesion	Drainage/Secretion
	Extrapulmonary, meningitis	None
	Pulmonary	Tuberculosis
Nocardia asteroides	Draining lesions	None
	Other	None
Salmonella species	Gastroenteritis	Enteric
	Bacteremia	Enteric*
Listeria monocytogenes	Infection at any site	None
Legionella species	Pneumonia	None
Streptococcus pneumoniae	Pneumonia	None
Hemophilus influenzae	Adults	None
	Infant/Children	Respiratory
Staphylococcus aureus	Skin, wound, or burn infection	
	Major	Contact
	Minor or limited	Drainage/Secretion
	Pneumonia or draining lung abscess	Contact
Shigella species	Gastroenteritis	Enteric
	Bacteremia	Enteric*
Viruses		
Cytomegalovirus	Infection at any site	Pregnant personnel may need special counselling

Table 2. (Continued)

Microorganisms	Syndrome	Precautions
Herpes simplex	Encephalitis	None
	Mucocutaneous, disseminated or primary, severe (skin, oral, and genital)	Contact
	Mucocutaneous, recurrent (skin, oral, and genital)	Drainage/Secretion
Herpes-zoster (varicella-zoster)	Localized in immunocompromised patient, or disseminated	Strict
Epstein-Barr	Infectious mononucleosis	None
Adenoviruses	Respiratory infection in infants and young children	Contact
Parasites		
Pneumocystis carinii	Pneumonia	None
Toxoplasma gondii	Encephalitis, brain abscess	None
Cryptosporidium species	Gastroenteritis	Enteric
Fungi		
Candida species	Infection at any site, including mucocutaneous (thrush, moniliasis)	None
Cryptococcus neoformans	Infection at any site	None
Histoplasma capsulatum	Infection at any site	None
Aspergillus species	Infection at any site	None

* unless stool culture negative.

fluids, or may also require gowns, masks, and eye coverings when performing procedures involving more extensive contact with blood or potentially infective body fluids, as in some dental or endoscopic procedures or postmortem examinations. Hands should be washed thoroughly and immediately if they accidentally become contaminated with blood.

Mouth-to-Mouth Resuscitation

Pulmonary resuscitation equipment, e.g., mouth pieces and resuscitation bags, should be immediately available for use in areas where the need for resuscitation is predictable.

Masks and Protective Eyewear

Masks are not necessary for the routine care of HIV infected patients unless other infectious diseases are present which would indicate their use. As is true in the case of all patients, the use of protective eyewear, such as goggles with masks, is recommended in situations in which splattering with blood, body secretions, or body fluids is possible. This is particularly recommended in the performance of procedures such as endotracheal intubation, bronchoscopy and endoscopy, and during many common dental procedures. Precautions during other procedures should be determined on an individual basis.

Pregnant Health-Care Workers

Pregnant health-care workers are not known to be at greater risk of contracting HIV infections than health-care workers who are not pregnant; however, if a health-care worker develops HIV infection during pregnancy, the infant is at increased risk of infection resulting from perinatal transmission (52). Because of the risk of parenteral transmission, pregnant health-care workers should be educated about precautions for preventing HIV transmission (27),(52). Many patients with AIDS are infected with and excrete cytomegalovirus (CMV). Infection with CMV during pregnancy may result in transmission to the fetus. When hygiene precautions (appropriate handwashing) are satisfactory, the risk of acquiring CMV infections through patient contact is low (53),(54). Therefore, a practical approach to reducing the risk of infection with CMV is to stress careful handwashing after all patient contacts and avoid direct contact with materials that are potentially infective. Other measures, such as serologic screening of pregnant personnel, with reassignment of those susceptible, are controversial (55). All pregnant patient-care personnel should at least be counseled about precautions for preventing acquisition of CMV (56),(57).

Immunosuppressed Health-Care Workers

Health-care workers with defective immune systems are not known to be at greater risk of acquiring HIV infection than health care workers with normal immune systems. However, they may have an increased risk of acquiring or experiencing serious complications of other infectious diseases. Of particular concern is the risk of severe infection following exposure to patients infected with HIV who may be infected with microorganisms that are easily transmitted if appropriate precautions are not adhered to (e.g., *M. tuberculosis*). Health-care workers with defective immune systems should be counseled about the potential risk associated with taking care of patients with transmissible infections and should follow existing recommendations for infection control to minimize their risk of exposure to other infectious agents (27),(56).

PATIENT CARE AND LABORATORY PRACTICES

Disposal of Needles, Syringes, and Other Sharp Objects

As with other blood-borne diseases, the potential for transmission is greatest when needles and other sharp instruments are used in patient care. Therefore, needles and syringes should be disposable, when feasible, and should be disposed of in rigid, puncture-resistant containers. Needles should not be recapped, removed from disposable syringes, or purposely bent or broken, because needlestick injuries are most likely to occur during these activities. Needle-stick injuries have been reported when personnel used needle cutting devices (Table 1). Currently, no data are available from controlled studies examining the effect, if any, of needle cutting devices on the incidence of needlestick injuries. Parenteral injections and blood drawing should be carried out by trained personnel.

Handling of Blood and Other Specimens

All blood and other specimens should be considered potentially infectious and should be handled with special precautions to prevent percutaneous and mucous membrane exposures. Blood and other specimens from patients with known or suspected infection with HIV should be labeled prominently with a warning such as "Blood/Body Fluid Precautions" (46),(49). The label should accompany the specimen through all phases of processing until appropriate disposal. The label should not indicate the patient's diagnosis. If the outside of any specimen container is visibly contaminated with blood, it should be cleaned with a hospital disinfectant or a freshly prepared (once daily) 1:10 dilution of 5.25 percent sodium hypochlorite (household bleach) with water. All blood specimens should be placed in a second container, such as an impervious bag, for transfer. Soiled linens and other laundry should be bagged, appropriately labeled or color coded, and processed according to the hospital's policy regarding linens from patients in isolation. Nondisposable articles contaminated with blood or body fluids should be bagged and labeled before being sent for decontamination and reprocessing.

Sterilization and Disinfection Procedures

An important infection control issue is whether routine sterilization and disinfection procedures are adequate for HIV. This issue has been addressed, in part, in a number of laboratory studies. In general, two laboratory assay methods for assessing inactivation of HIV by chemical and physical agents have been reported (Table 3) (58)-(64). The first method does not directly measure the effect of these agents on viral infectivity, but rather measures inactivation of the viral enzyme reverse transcriptase (RT). The second, and preferred, method compares the infectivity of treated and untreated virus preparations for T-cell culture systems. Infection of cell cultures inoculated with treated and untreated viral preparations is determined by: 1) assays of supernatant RT activity, 2) ELISA capture assay for HIV, 3) cellular immunofluorescence for viral antigens, 4) cellular cytopathic effect and/or 5) combinations of the above. The results of an assay may be reported in dichotomous fashion, either as an inactivation failure or success with failure defined as any cell culture showing viral replication, or as the log reduction in the ID_{50} at various levels of exposure.

Assays for virus inactivation by chemical germicides are technically difficult. Inconsistent results may be obtained if certain conditions are not controlled for or specified. These might include the strain of the virus; the initial concentration of virus; the physical condition of viral preparation (e.g., liquid suspension or dried preparation); the relative humidity and/or the status of hydration of dried preparations; the presence in suspending media of substances which might inactivate the germicide or protect virus particles from germicide-virus interaction (e.g., protein); the inactivation of the germicide by the diluent; the effect of residual germicide on the test cell system; temperature; time; and the sensitivity of the assay for determining if cell culture infection has occurred.

In spite of these limitations, a growing body of evidence strongly suggests that HIV does not possess unusual resistance properties. Several liquid chemical germicides commonly used in laboratories and health-care facilities kill HIV at concentrations much lower than are used in practice (58),(59),(62),(63). For example, Martin and colleagues (58) have found that after 2-10 minutes of exposure, at 21-25°C, the ID_{50} of HIV suspensions was reduced to less than measurable by 0.3% hydrogen peroxide, 0.1% household bleach, 50% ethanol, 35% isopropanol, and 0.5% of a phenolic disinfectant.

Sterilization and disinfection procedures currently recommended for use in health care and dental facilities are adequate to sterilize or disinfect instruments, devices, or other items contaminated with blood or other body fluids from individuals infected with HIV (27),(65)-(67). For the disinfection or sterilization of instruments or medical devices, chemical germicides that are registered with and approved by the U.S. Environmental Protection Agency (EPA) as sterilants and/or hospital disinfect-

Table 3. Published Methods Used to Assess Inactivation of HIV by Physical and Chemical Agents

Ref. No.	Assay	Method for Detecting Growth of Virus in Cell Cultures	Reporting of Assay Results	Physical and/or Chemical Agents Tested
59	RT* inactivation	NA**	NA	Sodium hypochlorite B-propionolactone, glutaraldehyde, sodium hydroxide, ethanol, formalin.
60	RT inactivation Cell infectivity	NA Supernatant RT	NA +/-***	Heat (liquid media), gamma-radiation, uv light
58	Cell infectivity	ELISA	Reduction in in ID_{50}	pH, heat (liquid media), hydrogen peroxide, ethanol, isopropanol, paraformaldehyde, a phenolic, sodium hypochlorite, nonidet-p40, tween-80
61	Cell infectivity	Supernatant RT	+/-	Heat (liquid media), drying
62	Cell infectivity	Supernatant RT Cellular immunofluorescence (IF)	+/- Reduction in IF	Sodium chlorite/ lactic acid solution
63	Cell infectivity	Supernatant RT Cellular cytopathic effect	Reduction in ID_{50}	Quaternary ammonium chlorides, nonidet-P40, drying, heat (liquid media), sodium hypochlorite, alcohol, alcohol-acetone fixation
64	Cell infectivity	ELISA	Reduction in ID_{50}	Heat (liquid media and lyophilized)

*RT = Reverse transcriptase
**NA = Not applicable
***+/- = Detection of virus indicates a failure at the given dilution

ants which have tuberculocidal activity can be used.

General procedures to be followed to ensure adequate disinfection/sterilization are discussed in the CDC Guidelines for Handwashing and Environmental Control, 1985 (66). Several important considerations are worth reemphasizing. Instruments or other nondisposable items that enter normally sterile tissue or the vascular system (or those which act as conduits for blood), should be sterilized before reuse. After use and before sterilization, surgical instruments should be decontaminated rather than just rinsed with water. Decontamination can be done by machine or by hand by trained personnel wearing appropriate attire (68) and by using appropriate chemical germicides. Instruments or other nondisposable items that touch intact mucous membranes should receive high-level disinfection (65),(66). Finally, an important principle to follow whenever chemical germicides are used for disinfection or sterilization is that the item should be thoroughly cleaned before exposure to the germicide and that the manufacturer's instructions for the use of the germicide be closely followed.

Housekeeping and Laundry

Housekeeping procedures commonly used in hospitals are adequate for cleaning rooms of all patients with HIV infection.

Laundry and dishwashing cycles commonly used in hospitals are adequate to decontaminate linens, dishes, glassware, and utensils. When cleaning environmental surfaces, housekeeping procedures commonly used in hospitals and laboratories are adequate; surfaces exposed to blood and body fluids should be cleaned with a detergent followed by decontamination using an EPA-approved hospital disinfectant (27). Individuals cleaning up such spills should wear disposable gloves. (Information on specific label claims of commercial germicides can be obtained by writing to the Disinfectants Branch, Office of Pesticides, Environmental Protection Agency, 401 M Street, S.W., Washington, D.C. 20460). In addition to hospital disinfectants, a freshly prepared solution of sodium hypochlorite (household bleach) is an inexpensive and very effective germicide (58),(59). Concentrations ranging from 5,000 ppm (a 1:10 dilution of household bleach) to 500 ppm (a 1:100 dilution of household bleach) sodium hypochlorite are effective, depending on the amount of organic material (e.g., blood, mucus, etc) present on the surface to be cleaned and disinfected.

Disposal of Solid Waste

Sharp items should be considered as potentially infectious and should be handled and disposed of with extraordinary care to prevent accidental injuries. Other potentially infective waste should be contained and transported in clearly identified impervious plastic bags. If the outside of the bag is contaminated with blood or other body fluids, a second outer bag should be used. Recommended practices for disposal of infective waste are adequate for disposal of waste contaminated by HIV (66). Personnel involved in the handling and disposal of solid waste should be informed of the potential health and safety hazards and trained in the appropriate handling and disposal methods. Infective waste, in general, should be incinerated, or should be decontaminated by autoclaving before disposal. Blood and other body fluids may be carefully poured down a utility sink drain or toilet connected to a sanitary sewer.

Hemodialysis and Peritoneal Dialysis

Patients infected with HIV may occasionally require hemodialysis or peritoneal dialysis. Currently recommended procedures for disinfection, sterilization, and sanitation in dialysis facilities are adequate to prevent transmission of HIV (69)-(71). These recommendations emphasize applying blood precautions and barrier techniques, aseptic techniques, and use of good environmental control procedures, especially adequate disinfection and sterilization procedures.

When peritoneal dialysis is used in the management of patients infected with HIV, peritoneal dialysis bags and other disposable items can be disposed of in the same fashion as other solid waste (66). Bags containing peritoneal dialysis fluid should be handled with care but extraordinary precautions are not needed. Disposable gloves should be worn when handling bags containing peritoneal dialysis fluid. In the home environment, the peritoneal dialysis fluid can be carefully poured down a toilet. The empty bag should be wrapped securely in an impervious plastic bag or double bagged and discarded in the conventional trash system.

Dental and Oral Surgical Procedures

Dental and oral surgery personnel may be exposed to a variety of microorganisms in the blood and saliva of patients (68). These include *Mycobacterium tuberculosis*, hepatitis B virus, cytomegalovirus, *Herpes simplex* virus, HIV, staphylococci, streptococci, and several other bacteria and viruses that may be present in the upper respiratory tract or blood. Because all infected patients cannot be identified by history, physical examination, or readily available laboratory tests, the same infection control precautions should be applied to all patients receiving dental or oral surgical procedures. The U.S. Public Health Service (PHS) has recommended a common set of infection control strategies which are designed to prevent transmission of hepatitis B, HIV, and other bloodborne infectious diseases in dental practices (67). These recommendations are similar to those for other health-care workers and stress handwashing, use of protective attire and barrier technique, appropriate use, care, and disposal of sharp instruments and needles, disinfection and sterilization of instruments, and decontamination of environmental surfaces, laboratory supplies and materials.

Precautions for Infectious Diseases Occurring with High Frequency in HIV Infected Patients

Table 2 lists the microorganisms that may infect AIDS patients and the isolation precautions recommended for preventing transmission of the microorganism in the health-care setting. Most of these microorganisms are not transmitted in health-care settings if appropriate precautions are applied. The specifics of each isolation category are outlined in the "CDC Guideline for Isolation Precautions in Hospitals" (51). For some of the diseases or conditions listed in Table 2, more stringent isolation precautions may be needed for infants and young children than for adults, since the risk of spread and the consequence of infection may be greater in infants and young children (i.e., *Hemophilus influenzae*).

Postmortem Care

The procedures followed before, during, and after postmortem examination of a person infected with HIV are similar to those for persons infected with hepatitis B virus (48). All persons involved in performing an autopsy should wear gloves, masks, protective eyewear, gowns, waterproof aprons, and shoe coverings. Instruments and surfaces contaminated during the postmortem examination should be handled as potentially infective items.

As part of the immediate postmortem care, it has been recommended that the body of patients known to have died with HIV or other blood-borne diseases (hepatitis B, Creutzfeldt-Jakob, etc.) should be labelled "blood/body fluid precautions" and that such identification should remain with the body, whether or not an autopsy is carried out, for delivery to the morticians (48),(49). In many instances, the HIV antibody status of the deceased patient will not be known. Thus, all deceased patients receiving postmortem care should be considered infectious, and appropriate precautions should be taken to prevent parenteral or mucous membrane exposure of personnel to blood or other body fluids.

MANAGEMENT OF HEALTH-CARE WORKERS INFECTED WITH HIV

There is no evidence that health-care workers infected with HIV have transmitted infection to patients during routine patient care or during operative, obstetric, or dental procedures. A risk of transmission from infected health-care workers to patients would theoretically exist in situations where there is both: 1) a high degree of trauma to the patient that provides a portal of entry for the virus (e.g., during surgery), and 2) access of blood or serous fluid from the infected health-care worker to the open tissue of the patient, as could occur if the worker sustains a needlestick or scapel injury during an invasive procedure. Thus, special emphasis should be placed on recommended precautions to prevent transmission of bloodborne agents between all patients and all health-care workers (27),(49),(72). All health-care workers should be educated regarding the epidemiology, modes of transmission, and prevention of HIV infection and the need for routine use of appropriate barrier precautions when handling instruments contaminated with blood or other body fluids. All health care workers should wear gloves when touching mucous membranes or nonintact skin of all patients. Health-care workers infected with HIV need not be restricted from work unless they have evidence of other infections or illnesses for which any such worker should be restricted. However, all health-care workers who have exudative lesions or weeping dermatitis should refrain from direct patient care and from handling patient care equipment until the condition resolves. Persons with AIDS or other manifestations of infection with HIV may develop neuropsychiatric illnesses that may compromise their ability to provide patient care adequately and safely (73)-(76). Thus, all health-care workers with evidence of any illness that may compromise their ability to provide patient care adequately and safely should be evaluated medically to determine whether they are physically and mentally competent to perform invasive procedures (27),(72).

Management of Health-Care Workers and Patients Following an Accidental Parenteral Exposure

Routine serologic testing of health-care workers and patients for antibody to HIV is not recommended to prevent transmission (27),(49),(72). The risk of transmitting HIV from an infected health-care worker to patients or from infected patients to health-care workers is extremely low and can further be minimized when routinely recommended infection control precautions are followed.

The management of parenteral or mucous membrane exposure of health care workers should follow the recommendations of the Public Health Service (27).

If a health-care worker has a parenteral (e.g., needlestick, cut, or bite) or mucous membrane (e.g., splash to the eye or mouth) exposure to blood or other body fluids, the source patient should be assessed clinically and epidemiologically to determine the likelihood of HIV infection. If the assessment suggests that an infection may exist, the patient should be informed of the incident and requested to consent to serological testing for evidence of HIV infection. If the source patient is seronegative and has no other evidence of HIV infection, no further follow-up of the health-care worker is necessary. If the source patient cannot be identified, decisions regarding appropriate follow-up should be individualized based on the type of exposure and the likelihood that the source patient was infected. If the source patient has AIDS or other evidence of HIV infection, declines testing, or has a positive test, the health-care worker should be evaluated clinically and serologically for evidence of HIV infection as soon as possible after the exposure, and, if seronegative, retested after six weeks and on a periodic basis thereafter (e.g., three, six and 12 months following exposure) to determine if transmission has occurred. During this follow-up period, especially the first 6-12 weeks, when most infected persons are expected to seroconvert, exposed health-care workers should receive counseling about the risk of infection and follow Public Health Service recommendations for preventing transmission of AIDS (76)-(78), including the following:

a. Refrain from donating blood.
b. Avoid exchange of saliva and/or deep kissing.
c. Avoid sexual intercourse or use condoms during sexual intercourse.

Similarly, if a patient has a parenteral or mucous membrane exposure to blood or other body fluids of a health care worker, the patient should be informed of the incident and the management of such exposures followed as described above.

OTHER INFECTION CONTROL CONSIDERATIONS

Patient Confidentiality

Hospitals and other health-care institutions should be careful to balance the need to ensure appropriate precautions to prevent the spread of disease with the need to ensure patient confidentiality. Patients with AIDS and others known to be infected with HIV will need laboratory tests, and some may need surgery or other specialized invasive procedures. In addition, some will need to be transported to other hospital departments for proper management. The hospital should emphasize its procedures to ensure that staff who care for these patients in other departments know what precautions should be taken.

Due to the publicity that AIDS and HIV have received, however, special care must be taken to preserve the dignity and confidentiality of the AIDS or HIV-infected patient. The modes of transmission of HIV are similar to hepatitis B, but the risk of transmission is substantially lower in the hospital setting; therefore, application of the general category of "blood/body fluid precautions" as recommended in the CDC Guideline for Isolation Precautions in Hospitals (51) is sufficient, if used uniformly throughout the hospital. The precautions, but not the diagnosis, should be clearly identified.

Additionally, local and state regulations regarding confidentiality and reporting of HIV test results and patient care information should be observed.

Blood and Blood Products

The risk of acquiring infection with HIV from transfusion of blood and blood products has been significantly reduced as the consequence of several interventions. In March 1983, the Public Health Service published recommendations for preventing AIDS (76). Members of high risk groups were advised not to donate blood. Additionally, it was recommended that a safer clotting factor product be developed for persons with hemophilia. HIV was shown to be sensitive in vitro to heat (79). Heat-treated factor VIII concentrates are now commercially available and are recommended by the National Hemophilia Foundation to treat patients with hemophilia A (74).

Finally, in March 1985, specific serologic tests for antibody to HIV were licensed and became commercially available for screening of blood and plasma. Testing is now being done in blood banks and plasma centers throughout the United States. All units positive for antibody to HIV by an ELISA test are not transfused or manufactured into other products capable of transmitting infectious agents.

Immune globulin products manufactured before April 1985, were derived from plasma of human donors who were not screened for antibody to HIV. Tests conducted by Public Health Service agencies (Food and Drug Administration and Centers for Disease Control) have shown that as many as two-thirds of hepatitis B immune globulin (HBIG) lots, as well as some lots of immune globulin (IG) and intravenous immune globulin (IVIG) produced between 1982 and 1985, may have been positive for antibody to HIV (80). However, epidemiologic and laboratory studies have shown that immune globulin preparations are safe and that current indications for their clinical use should not be changed (80)-(83).

Hepatitis B virus (HBV) vaccine was licensed in 1981 and became available for general use in July 1982. Since HBV vaccine is made from human plasma and the source of the plasma has been homosexual men at risk for HIV infection, there has been concern regarding the risk of acquiring HIV following receipt of the vaccine. In March 1983, the PHS reported that HBV vaccine was safe and carried no etiologic or epidemiologic risk of AIDS (84). The manufacturing process for HBV vaccine includes several procedures that inactivate representative viruses of all known types, and epidemiologic data from vaccine studies have identified no AIDS cases outside recognized risk groups for AIDS that could be attributed to the vaccine (84),(85).

Use of Vaccines in Persons Infected with HIV

The indications and contraindications for use of vaccines in persons infected with HIV are not known. Of concern is the risk of disseminated illness or significant adverse reactions following administration of live-virus (e.g., mumps, measles, rubella, poliovirus) vaccine. Several factors need to be considered before any patient is vaccinated. These include the susceptibility of the patient, the risk of exposure to the disease, the risk from the disease, and the benefits and risks from the immunizing agent. The Immunization Practices Advisory Committee (ACIP) has generally recommended against the use of live or live attenuated vaccine in immunocompromised patients (86). Recommendations regarding the use of vaccines in children infected with HIV have recently been published (87).

CONCLUSION

Infection control strategies currently recommended for use in health-care institutions are adequate to prevent transmission of HIV. Health-care personnel should be educated about the epidemiology of HIV and the precautions recommended to prevent transmission. Health-care institutions should develop education programs directed towards all levels of personnel and this program should be reviewed regularly for accuracy and presented periodically to update the staff about HIV infection.

REFERENCES

1. CDC., Pneumocystis pneumonia - Los Angeles, MMWR 30:250-252 (1981).

2. CDC., Kaposi's sarcoma and pneumocystis pneumonia among homosexual men. New York City and California. MMWR 30:305-308 (1981).

3. Gottlieb, M.S., Schroff, R., Schanker, H.M., et al., *Pneumocystis carinii* pneumonia and mucosal candidiasis in previously healthy homosexual men: evidence of a new acquired cellular immunodeficiency. N Engl J Med 305:1425-1431 (1981)

4. Francis, D.R., Curran, J.W., Essex, M., Epidemic acquired immune deficiency syndrome (AIDS). Epidemiologic evidence for a transmissible agent. J Nat Cancer Inst 71:1-4 (1983).

5. Jaffe, H.W., Choi, K., Thomas, P.A., et al., National case-control study of Kaposi's sarcoma and *Pneumocystis carinii* pneumonia in homosexual men: Part 1, epidemiologic results. Ann Intern Med 99:145-151 (1983).

6. Barre-Sinoussi, F., Chermann, J.C., Rey, F., et al., Isolation of a T-lymphotropic retrovirus from a patient at risk for acquired immune deficiency syndrome (AIDS). Science 220:868-871 (1983).

7. Popovic, M., Sarngadharan, M.G., Read, E., et al., Detection, isolation, and continuous production of cytopathic retroviruses (HTLV-III) from patients with AIDS and pre-AIDS. Science 224:497-500 (1984).

8. Gallo, R.C., Salahuddin, S.Z., Popovic, M., et al., Frequent detection and isolation of cytopathic retroviruses (HTLV-III) from patients with AIDS and at risk for AIDS. Science 224:500-502 (1984).

9. Sarngadharan, M.G., Popovic, M., Bruch, L., et al., Antibodies reactive with human T-lymphotropic retroviruses (HTLV-III) in the serum of patients with AIDS. Science 224:506-508 (1984).

10. Brun-Vezinet, F., Barre-Sinoussi, F., Saimot, A.G., et al., Detection of IgG antibodies to lymphadenopathy-associated virus in patients with AIDS or lymphadenopathy syndrome. Lancet 1:1253-1256 (1984).

11. Laurence, J., Brun-Vezinet, F., Schutzer, S.E., et al., Lymphadenopathy associated viral antibody in AIDS. N Engl J Med 311:1269-1273 (1984).

12. Safai, B., Sarngadharan, M.G., Groopman, J.E., et al., Sero-epidemiological studies of human T-lymphotropic retrovirus type III in acquired immunodeficiency syndrome. Lancet 1:1438-1440 (1984).

13. CDC., Antibodies to a retrovirus etiologically associated with acquired immunodeficiency syndrome (AIDS) in populations with increased incidence of the syndrome. MMWR 33:377-379 (1984).

14. Saxinger, C., Gallo, R.C., Application of the indirect enzyme-linked immunosorbent assay microtest to the detection and surveillance of human T cell leukemia-lymphoma virus. Lab Invest 49:371-377 (1983)

15. Tsang, V.C.W., Peralta, J.M., Simons, A.R., The enzyme-linked immunoelectrotransfer blot techniques (EITB) for studying the specificity of antigens and antibodies separated by gel electrophoresis. Methods Enzymol 92:377-391 (1983)

16. Kalyanaraman, V.S., Cabradilla, C.D., Getchell, J.R., et al., Antibodies to the core protein of lymphadenopathy associated virus (LAV) in patients with AIDS. Science 225:321 (1984).

17. Barre-Sinoussi, F., Mathur-Wagh, U., Rey, F., et al., Isolation of lymphadenopathy-associated virus (LAV) and detection of LAV antibodies from U.S. patients with AIDS. JAMA 253:1737-1739 (1985)

18. Ramsey, R.B., Palmer, E.L., McDougal, J.S., et al., Antibody to lymphadenopathy-associated virus in hemophiliacs with and without AIDS. Lancet 2:397-398 (1984)

19. Goedert, J.J., Sarngadharan, M.G., Biggar, R.J., et al., Determinants of retrovirus (HTLV-III) antibody and immunodeficiency conditions in homosexual men. Lancet 2:711-716 (1984)

20. Gazzard, B.G., Farthing, C., Shanson, D.C., et al., Clinical findings and serological evidence of HTLV-III infection in homosexual contacts of patients with AIDS and persistent generalized lymphadenopathy in London. Lancet 2:480-482 (1984)

21. Schupbach, J., Haller, O., Vogt, M., et al., Antibodies to HTLV-III in Swiss patients with AIDS or pre-AIDS and in groups at risk for AIDS. N Engl J Med 312:265-270 (1985)

22. Cheingsong-Popov, R., Weiss, R.A., Dalgleish, A., et al., Prevalence of antibody to human T-lymphotropic virus type III in AIDS and AIDS-risk patients in Great Britain. Lancet 2:477-480 (1984)

23. Results of human T-lymphotropic virus type III test kits reported from blood collection centers - United States, April 22 - May 19, 1985. MMWR 34:375-376 (1985)

24. Hirsch, M.S., Wormser, G.P., Schooley, R.T., et al., Risk of nosocomial infection with human T-cell lymphotropic virus III (HTLV-III). N Engl J Med 312:1-4 (1985)

25. Weiss, S.H., Saxinger, W.C., Rechtman, D., et al., HTLV-III infection among health care workers: association with needle-stick injuries. JAMA 284:2089-2093 (1985)

26. CDC., Update: Evaluation of HTLV-III/LAV infection in health-care personnel-United States. MMWR 34:575-578 (1985)

27. CDC., Recommendations for preventing transmission of infection with human T-lymphotropic virus type III/lymphadenopathy-associated virus in the workplace. MMWR 34:681-695 (1985)

28. McCray E., The CDC Cooperative Needlestick Study Group. Occupational risk of acquired immunodeficiency syndrome (AIDS) for health-care workers. N Engl J Med 314:1127-1132 (1986)

29. Henderson, D.K., Saah, A.J., Zak, B.J., et al., Risk of nosocomial infection with human T-cell lymphotropic virus type-III/lymphadenopathy-associated virus in a large cohort of intensively exposed health-care workers. Ann Intern Med 104:644-647 (1986)

30. Kaplan, J.E., Spira, T.J., Feorino, P.M., et al., HTLV-III/LAV viremia in homosexual men with generalized lymphadenopathy. N Engl J Med 312:1572-1573 (1985)

31. Ward, J., Grindon, A., Feorino, P., et al., Laboratory and epidemiologic evaluation of an enzyme immunoassay test for antibody to human T-lymphotropic virus type-III. JAMA (In press)

32. Francis, D.P., Jaffe, H.W., Fultz, P.N., et al., The natural history of infection with the lymphadenopathy-associated virus/human T-lymphotropic virus type III. Ann Intern Med 103:719-722 (1985)

33. Feorino, P.M., Jaffee, H.W., Palmer, E., et al., Transfusion-associated acquired immunodeficiency syndrome: evidence of persistent infection in blood donors. N Engl J Med 312:1293-1296 (1985)

34. Editorial. Needlestick transmission of HTLV-III from a patient infected in Africa. Lancet 2:1376-1377 (1984)

35. Cooper, D.A., Gold, J., Maclean P., et al., Acute AIDS retrovirus infection. Lancet 1:537-540 (1985)

36. Ho, D.D., Sarngadharan, M.G., Resnick, L., et al., Primary human T-lymphotropic virus type III infection. Ann Intern Med 103:880-883 (1985)

37. Tucker, J., Ludlam, C.A., Craig, A., et al., HTLV-III infection associated with glandular-fever-like illness in a hemophiliac (letter). Lancet 1:585 (1985)

38. Jaffee, H.W., Darrow, W.W., Echenberg, D.R., et al., The acquired immunodeficiency syndrome in a cohort of homosexual men: A 6-year follow-up study. Ann Intern Med 103:210-204 (1985)

39. Lifson, A.R., Castro., K.G., Narkunas, J.P., et al., "No identified risk" cases of acquired immunodeficiency syndrome (abstract). Epidemic Intelligence Service Conference, U.S. Department of Health and Human Services, Public Health Service, Centers for Disease Control, Atlanta, GA April 14-18, (1986)

40. Groopman, J.E., Salahuddin, S.Z., Sarngadharan, M.G., et al., HTLV-III in saliva of people with AIDS-related complex and healthy homosexual men at risk for AIDS. Science 226:447-449 (1984)

41. Fujikawa, L.S., Palestine, A.G., Nussenblatt, R.B., et al., Isolation of human T-lymphotropic virus type III from the tears of a patient with acquired immunodeficiency syndrome. Lancet 2:529-530 (1985)

42. Thiry, L., Sprecher-Goldberger, S., Johckheer, T., et al., Isolation of AIDS virus from cell-free breast milk of three healthy virus carriers. Lancet 2:891-892 (1985)

43. Levy, J.A., Shimabukuro, J., Hollander, H., et al., Isolation of AIDS associated retrovirus from cerebrospinal fluid and brain of patients with neurological symptoms. Lancet 2:586-588 (1985)

43a. Oksenhendler, E., Harzic, M., Le Roux, J-M., et al., HIV infection with seroconversion after a superficial needlestick injury to the finger. N Engl J Med 315:582 (1986)

44. Friedland, G.H., Saltzman, B.R., Rogers, M.F., et al., Lack of transmission of HTLV-III/LAV infection to household contacts of patients with AIDS or AIDS-related complex with oral candidiasis. N Engl J Med 314:344-349 (1986)

45. Jason, J.M., McDougal, J.S., Dixon, G., et al., HTLV-III/LAV antibody and immune status of household contacts and sexual partners of persons with hemophilia. JAMA 255:212-215 (1986)

46. CDC., Acquired immune deficiency syndrome (AIDS): precautions for clinical and laboratory staffs. MMWR 32:577-580 (1982)

47. Conte, J.E., Hadley, W.K., Sande, M., and the University of California, San Francisco Task Force on the Acquired Immunodeficiency Syndrome. Special Report: Infection control guidelines for patients with the acquired immunodeficiency syndrome (AIDS). N Engl J Med 309:740-744 (1983)

48. CDC., Acquired immunodeficiency syndrome (AIDS): precautions for health-care workers and allied professionals. MMWR 32: 101-103 (1983)

49. American Hospital Association. Management of HTLV-III/LAV infection in the hospital. Recommendations of the Advisory Committee on Infections within Hospitals. 1-23 (1986)

50. Armstrong D, Hold, J.W.M., Dayjanski, J., et al., Treatment of infections in patients with the acquired immunodeficiency syndrome. Ann Intern Med 103:738-743 (1985)

51. Garner, J.S., Simmons, B.P., Guideline for isolation precautions in hospitals. Infect Control 4:245-325 (1983)

52. CDC., Recommendations for assisting in the prevention of perinatal transmission of human T-lymphotropic virus type III/lymphadenopathy-associated virus and acquired immunodeficiency syndrome. MMWR 34:721-732 (1985)

53. Ahlfors, K., Ivanson, S-A., Johnson, T., et al., Risk of cytomegalovirus infection in nurses and congenital infections in their offsprings. Acta Paediatr Scand 70:819-823 (1981)

54. Dworsky, M.E., Welch, K., Cassady, G., et al., Occupational risk for primary cytomegalovirus infection among pediatric health care workers. N Engl J Med 309:150-153 (1983)

55. Plotkins, S.A., Cytomegalovirus in hospitals. Pediatr Infect Dis 5:177-178 (1986)

56. Williams, W.W., Guidelines for infection control in hospital personnel. Infect Control 4:245-325 (1983)

57. Onorato, I.M., Morens, D.M., Martone, W.J., et al., Epidemiology of cytomegalovirus infections: Recommendations for prevention and control. Rev Infect Dis 7:474-497 (1985)

58. Martin, L.S., McDougal, J.S., Loskoski, S.L., Disinfection and inactivation of the human T-lymphotropic virus type III/ lymphadenopathy-associated virus. J Infect Dis 152:400-403 (1985)

59. Spire, B., Barre-Sinoussi, F., Montagnier, L., et al., Inactivation of lymphadenopathy associated virus by chemical disinfectants. Lancet 2:899-901 (1984)

60. Spire, B., Dormont, D., Barre-Sinoussi, F., et al., Inactivation of lymphadenopathy-associated virus by heat, gamma rays and ultra-violet light. Lancet 1:188-189 (1985)

61. Barre-Sinoussi, F., Nugeyre, M.T., Chermann, J.C., Resistance of AIDS virus at room temperature (letter). Lancet 2:721-722 (1985)

62. Sarin, P.S., Scheer, D.I., Kross, R.D., Inactivation of human T-cell lymphotropic retrovirus (HTLV-III) by LD (letter). N Engl J Med 313:1416 (1985)

63. Resnik, L., Veren, K., Salahuddin, S.Z., et al., Stability and inactivation of HTLV-III/LAV under clinical and laboratory environments. JAMA 255:1887-1891 (1986)

64. McDougal, J.S., Martin, L.S., Cort, S.P., et al., Thermal inactivation of the acquired immunodeficiency syndrome virus, human T-lymphotropic virus-III/lymphadenopathy-associated virus, with special reference to antihemophilic factor. J Clin Invest 76:875-877 (1985)

65. Favero, M.S., Sterilization, disinfection, and antisepsis in hospitals. In: Manual of Clinical Microbiology, Fourth Ed. (Lennette, E.H., Balows, A., Hausler, W.J., Shadomy, H.J., eds) American Society for Microbiology, p 127-137, (1985)

66. Garner, J.S. Favero, M.S. Guideline for handwashing and hospital environmental control, 1985. Publication No. 99-1117, Centers for Disease Control, Atlanta, GA (1985)

67. CDC., Recommended infection-control practices for dentistry. MMWR 35:237-242 (1986)

68. Kneedler, J.A., Dodge, G.H., Perioperative Patient Care, Blackwell Scientific Publications, Boston, p. 210-211, (1983)

69. Favero, M.S., Dialysis-associated diseases and their control. In: Hospital Infections, Second Ed. (Bennett, J.V., Brachman, P.S., eds). Little, Brown, and Co., Boston, p. 267-284 (1985)

70. CDC., Recommendations for providing dialysis treatment to patients infected with human T-lymphotropic virus type-III/ lymphadenopathy associated virus. MMWR 35:376-378, 383 (1986)

71. Favero, M.S., Recommended precautions for patients undergoing hemodialysis who have AIDS or non-A, non-B hepatitis. Infect Control 6:301-305 (1985)

72. CDC., Recommendations for preventing transmission of infection with HTLV-III/LAV during invasive procedures. MMWR 35:221-223 (1986)

73. Snider, W.D., Simpson, D.M., Nielson, S., et al., Neurological complications of acquired immune deficiency syndrome: analysis of 50 patients. Ann Neurol 14:1403-1418 (1983)

74. Petito, C.K., Navia, B.A., Cho, E.S., et al., Vacuolar myelopathy pathologically resembling subacute combined degeneration in patients with the acquired immunodeficiency syndrome. N Engl J Med 312:874-879 (1985)

75. Holland, J.C., Tross, S., The psychosocial and neuropsychiatric sequelae of the acquired immunodeficiency syndrome and related disorders. Ann Intern Med 103:760-764 (1985)

76. CDC., Prevention of acquired immune deficiency syndrome (AIDS): report of inter-agency recommendations. MMWR 32:101-103 (1985)

77. CDC., Provisional public health services inter-agency recommendations for screening donated blood and plasma for antibody to the virus causing acquired immunodeficiency syndrome. MMWR 34:1-5 (1985)

78. CDC., Additional recommendations to reduce sexual and drug abuse-related transmission of HTLV-III/LAV. MMWR 35:152-155 (1986)

79. CDC., Update: acquired immunodeficiency syndrome (AIDS) in persons with hemophilia. MMWR 33:589-591 (1984)

80. CDC., Safety of therapeutic immune globulin preparations with respect to transmission of human T-lymphotropic virus type III/lymphadenopathy-associated virus infection. MMWR 35: 231-233 (1986)

81. Tedder, R.S., Uttley, A., Cheingsong-Popov, R., Safety of immunoglobulin preparations containing anti-HTLV-III (letter) Lancet 1:815 (1985)

82. Steele, D.R., HTLV-III antibodies in human immune-globulin (letter). JAMA 255:609 (1986)

83. Wells, M.A., Wittek, A.E., Epstein, J.S., et al., Inactivation and partition of human T-cell lymphotropic virus type III during ethanol fractionation of plasma. Transfusion 26:210-213 (1986)

84. CDC., The safety of hepatitis B virus vaccine. MMWR 32:134-136 (1983)

85. CDC., Hepatitis B virus vaccine safety: report of inter-agency groups. MMWR 31:465-467 (1982)

86. CDC., Adult immunizations. Recommendations of the Immunization Practices Advisory Committee (ACIP). MMWR 33:1-68 (1984)

87. CDC., Immunization of children infected with human T-lymphotropic virus type III/lymphadenopathy-associated virus. MMWR 35:595-606 (1986)

48
Practical Clinical Perspectives in Infection Control of HIV

Carol Joline

At present, there is no known cure for the acquired immunodeficiency syndrome (AIDS), no vaccine available for prevention, and no proven method for eliminating the infectivity of the human immunodeficiency virus (HIV) carrier. For these reasons, great emphasis must be placed on preventing transmission of HIV.

In addition to the members of the known risk groups for this disease (1), health care workers and those in related services may be at special risk (2)-(4). The major modes of transmission for HIV are through sexual contact with an infected person and from contaminated blood, predominantly among intravenous drug abusers who share needles and syringes. There is no evidence of transmission through casual contact (food, dishes, toilets, sneezing) (5),(5a). While HIV has been isolated from blood, semen, saliva, tears, breast milk, urine, lymph nodes, brain tissue, cerebrospinal fluid and bone marrow, blood and semen are the only body fluids to date, which have been epidemiologically linked to transmission (5),(6).

Since many unknowns still exist about HIV infection, it seems prudent to consider all body fluids, tissues, secretions and excretions from all patients as potentially infectious, particularly if they contain blood and/or lymphocytes, and to avoid any parenteral or mucous membrane exposure to them. Potentially infective individuals are those persons with documented AIDS, AIDS related complex (ARC), asymptomatic carriers of HIV or HIV antibody, and those in the risk groups for AIDS, whose antibody status is uncertain.

Guidelines have been developed by the Centers for Disease Control (1),(5),(7)-(12) to minimize the risk of exposure to blood and body fluids, and to reduce the transmission of HIV to health care workers and others.

GENERAL GUIDELINES

Hospitalized patients with HIV infection and those suspected of being infected should be placed on Blood/Body Fluid Precautions (13). In addition, appropriate precautions should be added for any concurrent infections the patient may have. In applying the precautions, one must consider the following: the condition of the patient, the level of care required, the type of contact to be made at each visit, and the patient's ability to understand and comply with good hygiene. Unfortunately, media publicity has generated misconceptions about AIDS and its mode of spread, generating the belief that AIDS is highly contagious. Emotions must not be allowed to supercede logic when caring for these patients. We must isolate the disease, not the patient. Some, or all of the precautions shown in Table 1 may be necessary, and will be discussed. In addition, recommendations will be made for the handling of specimens, infective wastes, and performing special patient care activities.

Table 1. Precautions to Prevent Transmission of HIV in the Hospital

1. Needles and other sharps: avoid accidental injury; dispose of properly.
2. Handwashing: before and after each patient contact.
3. Gloves: for touching infective material.
4. Gowns: if soiling with blood and body fluids is anticipated.
5. Masks: for prolonged contact with coughing patient and for suctioning.
6. Protective eyewear: if mucous membrane exposure is anticipated.
7. Private room: if patient's hygiene is poor.

Sharps Disposal

The Centers for Disease Control (5) has stated that the highest risk for transmission of HIV in the workplace would involve parenteral exposure to a needle or other sharp instrument contaminated with the blood of an infected patient. Although it has been shown (2),(14) that accidental needle-stick exposure appears to provide little additional risk of HIV transmission, needles, scalpel blades, trocars, and other sharps should be handled with extreme care to prevent such exposures (1),(5),(15)-(17). Needles should not be recapped, clipped, bent, broken, or removed from disposable syringes. Syringes with needles attached should be dropped into rigid puncture-resistant containers conveniently located (if possible, in the patient's room). Vacutainer needles may be safely removed by twisting into the special opening provided for that purpose on the tops of sharps disposal containers that have this feature. Devices for destroying needles by clipping should not be used. It has been shown that a significant amount of potentially infectious material is released in aerosols and splatter by these devices during cutting (18),(19). This material has the potential for being inhaled and reaching deep lung tissue, as well as for contaminating environmental surfaces.

Handwashing

Handwashing is the single most important means of preventing transmission of infection (18),(20),(21). A minimum 10 second wash of all lathered surfaces followed by a rinse under running water is recommended. Hands must be washed before and after each patient contact, and after coming into contact with infective materials, regardless of whether gloves are worn. Since antimicrobial handwashing agents are reported to be more effective against resident skin microorganisms, it is reasonable to recommend their use in the care of patients on isolation as well as for immunocompromised patients.

Gloves

Gloves should be worn when there is any chance that hands may come in contact with blood, body fluids, secretions or excretions, or items or areas soiled with them (1). Gloves should be worn by persons performing phlebotomies, endoscopies, invasive procedures, dental procedures and autopsies.

Gowns

Gowns should be worn when it is anticipated that clothing may become soiled with blood or body fluids, including secretions and excretions. Gowns should be worn for performing the special procedures listed above. Gowns need not be worn for casual contact such as delivering a food tray.

Masks

Masks are not usually necessary. Masks should be worn, however, for prolonged contact with a coughing patient, for suctioning a patient, and by those performing endoscopies, autopsies, surgical procedures, vaginal deliveries, and dental procedures.

Protective Eyewear

Protective eyewear, such as goggles, is recommended for any situation or procedure in which splashing or aerosolization of blood or any body fluid is possible (5),(10),(11). Protective eyewear should be worn for surgical procedures in the operating room, delivery room (including vaginal deliveries), for dental procedures, endoscopies, bronchoscopies, autopsies, endotracheal intubation, handling peritoneal dialysis fluid (if risk of splash) and for suctioning patients.

Isolation Garb

All isolation garb should be removed and discarded in a container in the patient's room, after which hands should be washed.

Private Room

A private room is indicated for those patients whose hygiene is poor (13). Many patients may be too ill or confused to comply with good hygienic requirements such as handwashing after touching infective material. Such patients may inadvertently contaminate the environment with infective material or share certain personal articles with other patients.

Specimens

If the outside of a specimen container is visibly soiled with blood or other body fluids it should be wiped with a disinfectant solution such as a 1:10 solution of 5.25% sodium hypochlorite (household bleach) and water. The specimen container should be placed in a ziplock bag and sealed to prevent leakage. The outside of the bag must remain clean for transport personnel to handle. The laboratory slip should be attached to the outside of the bag. Bag and lab slip should be labeled "Blood/Body Fluid Precautions".

Infectious Waste

The handling of potentially infectious waste from isolation patients has previously been addressed (13), and is adequate for processing waste contaminated by HIV (5). This waste would include excretions, exudates, secretions, suctionings, disposable medical supplies, pathological waste, renal dialysis waste, and surgical and laboratory waste. Disposable items which have come in contact with blood, body fluids, secretions or excretions should be placed in sturdy bags and tied securely. Double-bagging is not necessary unless the outside of the bag becomes contaminated. Bags should be color-coded or labeled to designate infectious waste. This waste should be incinerated, and/or processed according to local and state regulations. If an incinerator is not available, solid waste may be autoclaved before disposal. Bulk blood and other body fluids may be poured down a drain connected to a sanitary sewer.

Laundry

Soiled laundry should be bagged and tagged appropriately to identify it as isolation linen. Ideally, an inner water-soluble bag should be used to eliminate pre-wash handling of linen by laundry personnel. Laundry should be placed in the bag in a way that will prevent the outside of the bag from becoming soiled.

Laundry cycles and temperatures used in hospitals are adequate for decontamination of linen contaminated with blood and other body fluids containing HIV (5). Both a hot-water and a low-temperature wash may be used: for hot-water washing: 71°C (160°F) with detergent for 25 minutes (18); for low-temperature (below 70°C) washing: follow instructions for the specified chemical used for the low-temperature wash cycle.

Housekeeping

Guidelines for concurrent and terminal cleaning of isolation rooms have been published (13). Any U.S. Environmental Protection Agency (EPA) registered disinfectant-detergent designed for hospital use may be used for cleaning environmental surfaces (18). Blood and body fluid spills should be wiped up with a freshly prepared 1:10 solution of sodium hypochlorite as described above. A one minute contact time with the bleach solution is generally considered sufficient to kill the virus (23). All cleaning equipment, including mopheads and buckets should be cleaned and disinfected before being used elsewhere. Large equipment such as wheelchairs and stretchers should be cleaned with a disinfectant-detergent and hot water, and then wiped with a bleach solution. Mattresses and pillows should be covered with impervious plastic which is easily cleaned. Housekeeping personnel should wear gloves and protective garb while cleaning.

Sterilization and Disinfection

Current recommendations for sterilization and disinfection of patient care items used in hospitals and dental facilities (18), (24), are adequate for use with items from individuals infected with HIV (5). Surgical instruments should be washed and decontaminated before being processed for future use. Ideally, steam-autoclavable instruments should be placed directly into a washer-sterilizer (for decontamination), with minimal handling.

Work-room personnel should use appropriate barrier precautions to prevent accidental exposure.

Endoscopes, cystoscopes, and other instruments that cannot withstand exposure to steam under pressure should be washed, decontaminated and gas sterilized with ethylene oxide. (Procedures of this type should be scheduled at the end of the work day to allow for gas sterilization of the instruments over night). If gas sterilization is not practical or tolerated by the scopes, the instruments should receive high-level disinfection. Chemical germicides approved by the Environmental Protection Agency as sterilants can be used for this purpose, although the choice of agent may be dependent on the composition and tolerance of the equipment.

Dishes

Disposable dishes and utensils are generally no longer recommended, but may be used as a convenience (13),(25). If used, they should be discarded with the infectious waste. Hot water and detergent in dishwashing cycles used in hospitals are adequate for inactivation of HIV (5).

PREVENTION OF TRANSMISSION FOR SPECIFIC GROUPS

Laboratory Workers

Precautions for laboratory workers working with clinical specimens from HIV infected patients should be the same as those followed for patients with hepatitis B infection (1). Workers should avoid parenteral, skin and mucous membrane exposure with blood and body fluids. Protective garb (gloves, gowns, masks, goggles) should be worn if indicated, as described under the general guidelines. Hands should be washed after removing protective garb. Biological safety cabinets (class I or II) are recommended for procedures which may result in aerosolization of blood and other potentially infectious materials.

Phlebotomists

Persons performing phlebotomies should use extreme care when handling needles and syringes. (See sharps disposal). Vacutainer needles may be safely removed from the holder and discarded without touching the hands: twist into the opening on the top of sharps containers which have been designed specifically for this purpose.

Dental Care Personnel

Infection control guidelines specific for dentistry have been published (11),(26)-(28).

Dental care personnel are continuously exposed to blood and saliva through direct contact as well as from droplets and aerosols. While a thorough medical history taken from each patient may identify some who are at risk for HIV infection, many may be missed. Therefore, it is prudent to take appropriate barrier precautions with all patients. The recommended practices for infection control in dentistry from the Centers of Disease Control are interpreted as follows:

1. Gloves should be worn by all dental care personnel when touching blood, saliva, and mucous membranes, and any items or surfaces contaminated with them. Gloves should be examined frequently for signs of perforation during the procedure. If perforations should occur, gloves should be removed immediately and hands washed thoroughly before regloving.

2. Masks and protective eyewear, such as goggles or chin-length plastic face shields, should be worn when splashing with potentially infective materials is anticipated.

3. Reusable or disposable gowns or laboratory coats should be worn whenever splashing with potentially infective material is anticipated. Gowns should be changed and/or discarded when visibly soiled with blood and between patients.

4. Surfaces that are difficult to disinfect such as light handles and x-ray unit heads should be covered with sturdy aluminum foil or plastic wrap. The covering should be changed between each patient.

5. Every effort should be made to minimize splashing and aerolization of potentially infective materials. Use of high-speed evacuation and rubber dams is recommended. High-speed evacuation used during tooth preparation (drilling of a tooth for a filling or crown) removes any aerosol spray of water and debris, including the patient's saliva, as fast as it is produced. (This is a marked improvement over the old-fashioned saliva ejector.) The use of a rubber dam (a thin sheet of rubber with a hole to fit over the tooth), isolates the tooth being worked on from the rest of the oral cavity. This prevents patients from aspirating foreign material, as well as maintains a clear field (29).

6. Hands must be washed before and after each patient contact even though gloves have been worn. Dental care personnel with exudative lesions or dermatitis on the hands should avoid direct patient contact until the condition clears.

7. Needles and sharps should be handled and disposed of as described in the general guidelines.

8. All instruments should be cleaned and sterilized or undergo high-level disinfection after each use. Disposable items and instruments that are steam autoclavable should be used whenever possible. Sterilizers should undergo weekly spore tests to verify proper functioning.

9. All environmental surfaces contaminated with blood or saliva should be cleaned at the end of the procedure, and decontaminated with a 1:10 bleach solution.

10. Impression materials and other laboratory items should be cleaned and disinfected before being handled. Items returned from the dental laboratory should receive similar treatment before being placed in the patient's mouth.

11. Autoclavable handpieces are recommended. However, when non-sterilizable handpieces and ultrasonic scalers are used, they should be thoroughly flushed, scrubbed with detergent and water, and wiped with a registered sterilant solution. A cloth saturated with the solution should remain in contact with the instrument for the length of time recommended by the manufacturer of the solution.

12. Check valves should be installed to prevent aspiration of infective materials into the handpiece and water line. Water-cooled handpieces should be flushed for 30 seconds after each patient use, and at the beginning of each day.

13. Wastes should be disposed of as described under general guidelines.

Persons Performing Invasive Procedures

Surgeons, obstetricians, emergency room personnel and others who perform invasive procedures should observe the precautions outlined to prevent transmission of bloodborne infections such as HIV (10):

1. Persons performing invasive procedures and their assistants should be made aware of the modes of transmission and prevention of HIV infections, and instructed in the use of barrier precautions.

2. Gloves should be worn for contact with blood, mucous membranes, open wounds, body fluids, instruments and articles contaminated with them. Gloves should be changed immediately if a cut or perforation occurs.

3. Masks, protective eyewear (such as goggles), and gowns should be worn in situations where splashing or aerosolization of potentially infective material may occur. Shoe covers may be indicated in certain situations.

4. Barrier precautions as described above should be used by persons performing or assisting in vaginal deliveries and cesarean sections. Precautions should be taken while handling the placenta and newborn infant.

5. Extreme care should be taken to avoid accidental cuts and puncture wounds, as described under sharps disposal.

6. Persons with exudative lesions on the hands should not perform or assist in invasive procedures until the condition clears.

7. All surgical cases should be considered potentially contaminated, as one must be prepared for unknown carriers as well as identified HIV infected patients (30). Guidelines for operating room sanitation are detailed in the April 1984 issue of the Association of Operating Room Nurses Journal.

8. Instruments and other articles which have come in contact with blood or other body fluids must be cleaned and terminally disinfected before being processed for re-use. Decontamination room personnel should wear protective barrier garb.

9. Infectious waste and contaminated linen should be handled as previously described.

Ophthalmologists and Optometrists

Although HIV has been isolated from the tears of an AIDS patient (9), there is no evidence that the virus can be transmitted through contact with tears. Guidelines have been developed for individuals performing eye examinations and fitting trial contact lenses, and are summarized below. Careful attention should be paid to handwashing after patient contact. Gloves should be worn if there are cuts on the hands. Instruments that come in direct contact with the eye should be decontaminated with either 3% hydrogen peroxide, a 1:10 solution of 5.25% sodium hypochlorite and water, or 70% alcohol, depending on the material in the instrument. Re-usable trial lenses should be disinfected by using the hydrogen peroxide solution or heat, depending on the type of lens. Chemical disinfectants used in standard contact lens solution have not yet been tested for activity against HIV.

Emergency Service Personnel

Emergency service personnel should avoid parenteral and mucous membrane exposure to blood, saliva, and all potentially infective body fluids. Because of the hypothetical risk of transmission of HIV through saliva during mouth-to-mouth resuscitation, disposable airway equipment, resuscitation bags, and mechanical ventilation equipment are recommended (5). Gloves should be worn when contact with blood or any body fluid is anticipated.

Disposable cardio-pulmonary resuscitation (CPR) equipment and gloves should be available in all ambulances, first aid transport units, and fire and police vehicles.

Persons Performing Cardiopulmonary Resuscitation

Resuscitation bags and disposable CPR devices should be available for use in all areas where AIDS patients and suspected AIDS patients may be seen and treated.

Recommendations for decontaminating manikins used for CPR instruction have been published (31). CPR recertification should include training with resuscitation bags and other disposable mouth-to-mouth devices. Mouth-to-mouth contact with the manikin during the two person exercise should be simulated. (The correct timing for chest decompression and lung inflations, as well as the exchange position by the two resuscitators can be learned without actual mouth contact with the manikin.)

Endoscopists

Persons performing endoscopies should wear masks, gowns, caps, and protective eyewear. Booties may also be worn. When possible, patients should be scheduled at the end of the work day to allow time for the endoscopes to be gas sterilized over night. If gas sterilization is not feasible, high-level disinfection, as described above, should be used. Linen and disposable items should be handled as contaminated. Environmental surfaces should be cleaned with the 1:10 bleach solution.

Dialysis Personnel

Precautions for patients undergoing hemodialysis or peritoneal dialysis who have AIDS or any evidence of HIV infection have been published (32). Guidelines for prevention of transmission of hepatitis B, using the established Blood/Body Fluid Precautions should be followed. Methods already in place for disinfection of the internal circuits of dialysis machines are adequate for inactivating HIV. Special attention should be paid to the cleaning of frequently touched environmental surfaces and the external areas of the machine (33). Disposable hemodialyzers and other supplies are recommended for use with AIDS patients. However, nondisposable supplies may be used if sterilized between patients. If hospital policy permits reuse of disposable dialyzers, the dialyzers should be cleaned and disinfected for reuse only on the same patient. The precautions described under general guidelines pertaining to strict attention to handwashing, use of barrier garb, and proper disposal of sharps and contaminated waste should be followed.

Radiology Department

Precautions described under general guidelines should be used. Protective garb should be worn as indicated for the specific task to be performed. Soiled laundry and disposable items should be handled as contaminated. For special procedures (barium enema, arteriogram) use disposable items whenever possible. Decontaminate and re-sterilize non-disposable items before use on another patient.

Pregnant Health Care Workers

There has been no documentation that pregnant health care workers are at increased risk for developing infection when caring for AIDS patients (34),(35) and no restrictions in work activities are recommended.

Visitors

Generally, visitors need not wear barrier garb. However, if the AIDS patient has a concomitant infection which requires additional isolation, the visitor must wear the appropriate garb. It is best that small children not visit patients on isolation or precautions. Visitors should not visit if they have infections to which the AIDS patient may be susceptible (eg. varicella).

Food Service Workers

There has been no evidence that bloodborne and sexually

transmitted diseases are transmitted during the preparation or serving of food (5). Food handlers should observe proper hygiene including handwashing practices and sanitary food preparation. If an accidental injury occurs causing a blood spill onto food, the contaminated food should be discarded. Food handlers who are HIV antibody positive need not be restricted from work unless they have other illnesses which warrant it.

Personal Service Workers

Persons whose work involves close personal contact with clients such as hairdressers, barbers, manicurists, tatoo artists, acupuncturists and those involved in ear piercing should be thoroughly instructed in the modes of transmission of HIV (5). Instruments and equipment which may potentially come into contact with blood or serum, such as scissors, razors, cuticle instruments, etc., should be disinfected and sterilized between clients. Disposable equipment should be used whenever possible. Persons with exudative lesions should avoid direct contact with clients until the condition clears.

Other Workers Sharing the Work Environment

There is no known risk of transmission of HIV from an infected worker to others in settings such as offices, schools, factories, and construction sites (5). Workers with HIV infection should not be restricted from work on this basis alone. They should not be restricted from using telephones, toilets, drinking fountains and office equipment. Equipment contaminated with blood or body fluids from any worker should be wiped with a disinfectant solution such as sodium hypochlorite and water.

Hospital Employees with AIDS

Employees with AIDS or any form of HIV infection should be counseled in precautions to take in order to eliminate the risk of infecting others. Gloves should be worn for all invasive procedures and for mucous membrane contact. Employees with exudative lesions on the hands or other overt symptoms may be necessarily removed from direct patient contact.

Schools

Recommendations for the prevention of transmission of HIV infections in schools have been published, and are summarized as follows (12):

1. Decisions regarding the admission of children with HIV infection to the classroom should be made on an individual basis. A multidisciplinary approach should examine the child's behavior, physical condition, and the expected type of interaction with others.

2. Preschool-aged children, and those who lack control over their bodily functions, or who exhibit unsociable behavior, (bit-

ing) should be educated in an environment that restricts exposure of other children to blood and body fluids.

3. Educators and caregivers should be aware of the modes of transmission of HIV, and instructed in good handwashing techniques, and methods for cleaning surfaces soiled with blood or body fluids.

4. The child should be observed on a continuing basis to assess the improvement or deterioration of his hygienic practices.

5. While confidentiality must be maintained, key personnel should be aware of the child's disease in order to monitor his/her progress and to determine whether his/her condition or any incident which may occur (e.g. bleeding) should require that activities be restricted.

Postmortem Care

During postmortem care, the same precautions should be used in handling the body as pertained when the patient was alive (13). All mortuary tags should state that the patient expired while on Blood/Body Fluid Precautions, along with the diagnosis. This identification should remain with the body, whether or not an autopsy is performed, for delivery to morticians. The Pathology Department should be notified of the disease and the cause of death. Although this information appears on the patient's chart, it may be overlooked.

Autopsy Precautions

Barrier garb for persons performing autopsies should include double gloves, masks, protective eye wear, gowns, waterproof aprons, and waterproof shoe coverings (8). Methods that avoid aerosolization of infectious materials should be used. For example, bones should be cut with a hand saw rather than an electric device. Care should be taken to avoid parenteral and mucous membrane exposure to patient's blood and body fluids. Autopsy tables, equipment, and instruments should be decontaminated at the conclusion of the autopsy. A 1:10 sodium hypochlorite and water solution should be used. Contaminated surfaces should be flooded with the bleach solution for at least one minute to kill the virus (23). Disposable barrier garb should be discarded as infectious waste.

REFERENCES

1. CDC., Acquired immune deficiency syndrome (AIDS): precautions for clinical and laboratory staffs. MMWR 31:577-580 (1982)

2. Hirsch, M.S., Wormser, G.P., Schooley, R.T., et al., Risk of nosocomial infection with human T-cell lymphotropic virus III (HTLV-III). N Engl J Med 312:1-4 (1985)

3. Shanson, D., The risks of transmission of the HTLV-III and hepatitis-B virus in the hospital. Infect Control 7:128-132 (1986)

4. Garibaldi, R.A., Transmission of hepatitis B and AIDS. Infect Control 7:132-134 (1986)

5. CDC., Recommendations for preventing transmission of infection with HTLV-III/LAV in the workplace. MMWR 34: 682-695 (1985)

5a. Conte, J.E., Infection with human immunodeficiency virus in the hospital. Ann Intern Med 105:730-736 (1986)

6. Marwick, D., AIDS-associated virus yields data to intensifying scientific study. JAMA 254:2865-2870 (1985)

7. CDC., Prevention of acquired immune deficiency syndrome (AIDS): report of inter-agency recommendations. MMWR 32:101-103 (1983)

8. CDC., Acquired immunodeficiency syndrome (AIDS): precautions for health-care workers and allied professionals. MMWR 32:450-451 (1983)

9. CDC., Recommendations for preventing possible transmission of human T-lymphotropic virus type III/lymphadenopathy-associated virus from tears. MMWR 34:533-534 (1985)

10. CDC., Recommendations for preventing transmission of infection with HTLV-III/LAV during invasive procedures. MMWR 35:221- 223 (1986)

11. CDC., Recommended infection-control practices for dentistry. MMWR 35:237-242 (1986)

12. CDC., Education and foster care of children infected with HTLV-III/LAV. MMWR 34:518-521 (1986)

13. Garner, J.S., Simmons, B.P., CDC guideline for isolation precautions in hospitals. Infect Control 4:245-325 (1983)

14. Wormser, G.P., Joline, C., Duncanson, F., et al., Needle-stick injuries during the care of patients with AIDS. N Engl J Med 310:1461-1462 (1984)

15. Salome, P., Uncapped needle receptacles reduce puncture injuries. Hospitals 57:63 (1983)

16. Reed, J.S., Anderson, A.C., Hodges, G.R., Needlestick and puncture wounds: definition of the problem. Am J Infect Control 8:101-106 (1980)

17. Jacobson, J.T., Burke, J.P., Conti, M.T., Injuries of hospital employees from needles and sharp objects. Infect Control 4:100-102 (1983)

18. Garner, J.S., Favero, M.S., CDC guideline for handwashing and hospital environmental control, 1985, Infect Control 7:231-243 (1986)

19. Binley, R.J., Fleming, D.O., Swift, D.L., Release of residual material during needle cutting. Am J Infect Control 12: 282-288 (1984)

20. Larson, E., Handwashing and skin, physiologic and bacteriologic aspects. Infect Control 6:14-23 (1985)

21 Larson, E., Current handwashing issues. Infect Control 5: 15-17 (1984)

22. Soule, B.M. (ed), The APIC Curriculum for Infection Control Practice, Kendall/Hund. Dubuque (1983)

23. Resnick, L., Veren, K., Salahuddin, S.Z., et al., Stability and inactivation of HTLV-III/LAV under clinical and laboratory environments. JAMA 225:1887-1891 (1986)

24. Favero, M.S., Sterilization, disinfection, and antisepsis in the hospital. In: Manual of Clinical Microbiology (Linnette, E.H., Balows, A., Hausler, W.J., Jr., Shadomy, H.J., eds) 4th ed, American Society for Microbiology, Washington, DC, p 129-137, (1985)

25. Jackson, M.M., From ritual to reason - with a rational approach for the future: an epidemiologic perspective. Am J Infect Control 12:213-220 (1984)

26. Colley, R.L., Lubow, R.M., AIDS, an occupational hazard? J Am Dent Assoc 107:28-31 (1983)

27. Crawford, J.J., State-of-the-art: practical infection control in dentistry. J Am Dent Assoc 110:629-633 (1985)

28. Council on Dental Therapeutics and Council on Prosthetic Services and Dental Laboratory Relations. Guidelines for infection control in the dental office and the commercial dental laboratory. J Am Dent Assoc 110:969-972 (1985)

29. Rechtschaffer, B., personal communication (1986)

30. AORN Recommended Practices Subcommittee, Recommended practices, O.R. sanitation. AORN J 39:838-844 (1984)

31. Recommendations for decontaminating manikins used in CPR training, 1983 update. Infect Control 5:399-401 (1984)

32. CDC., Recommendations for providing dialysis treatment to patients infected with human T-lymphotropic virus type III/lymphadenopathy-associated virus. MMWR 35:376-384 (1986)

33. Favero, M.S., Recommended precautions for patients undergoing hemodialysis who have AIDS or non-A, non-B hepatitis. Infect Control 6:301-305 (1985)

34. Williams, W.W., CDC guideline for infection control in hospital personnel. Infect Control 4:326-349 (1983)

35. Valente, W.M., Infection control and the pregnant health care worker. Am J Infect Control 14:200-227 (1986)

Part VII
Treatment and Prevention of HIV Infection

49

Current Status of the Immunotherapy of AIDS and the AIDS-Related Complex

John W. Hadden

The immunologic perturbations which are associated with the acquired immunodeficiency syndrome (AIDS) and the AIDS-related complex (ARC) have been well described in numerous reports (1),(2). Central to the immune destruction would appear to be infection of helper T lymphocytes with a lymphotrophic retrovirus, human immunodeficiency virus (HIV). In addition to hematopoietic cells, the central nervous system is now recognized as a target for this retrovirus. In addition to T cells themselves, thymic epithelial cells which secrete thymic hormones are also destroyed (3), apparently by autoimmune and/or infectious mechanisms, resulting in thymic hormone deficiency (4). Circulating anti-T-cell antibodies and otherwise uncharacterized immunosuppressive substances are also found in the circulation which are envisioned to impair function of surviving T lymphocytes. Thus, the T cell system and resultant cellular immune responses are progressively compromised and replenishment is prevented. Defects of natural killer cell (NK), monocyte, and B lymphocyte function also occur which may be secondary to T cell dysregulation and destruction or to direct viral infection with the lymphotrophic virus or with other viruses associated with these disorders. Some of the more consistent defects of immunity observed in AIDS and ARC are summarized in Table 1.

In considering the immunotherapeutic approaches to AIDS and ARC it is important to understand the immune defects and the nature of host-virus interaction. It has been estimated that at least 500,000-1,000,000 people in the United States

TABLE 1. Immunologic Findings in AIDS and ARC

	ARC	AIDS
Total Lymphocytes		
T lymphocytes (T3, T11)	N/D	D
B lymphocytes	N	N
T helper cells	N/D	VD
T suppressor cells	I	D
Th/Ts ratio	D	VD
Mitogen Responses		
Phytohemagglutinin (PHA)	D	VD
Concanavalin A (Con A)	D	VD
Pokeweed mitogen (PKWD)	D	VD
Mixed Leukocyte Culture Responses (MLR)	D	VD
IL-2 production	D	VD
Cytotoxic lymphocyte generation	D	VD
Immunoglobulin levels (Ig)	I	I
In vitro Ig production	I	I
Autoantibodies	N/I	I

N = No Change I = Increased D = Decreased VD = Very Decreased

have been exposed to this virus and have developed serum antibodies. Only a fraction of this population has developed signs and symptoms of ARC (estimated to be 10-20%). In turn, only a small proportion of ARC patients have converted to AIDS (10-20%). Thus, less than 5% of the individuals exposed have developed the most serious consequences of infection.

We do not know to what extent positive serology in asymptomatic individuals reflects protective immunity. Nothing is known about cellular immune responses to this virus. Since cellular immune responses are critical to defense against most viruses, this information is essential for assessing the degree and nature of protective immunity. The frequency of latency with this virus is considered to be high so that under circumstances of immunosuppression (steroids, cancer, chemotherapy, etc.) or of immune senesence with aging, viral activation and disease progression may also be high. Conversely, the knowledge that more than 95% of individuals can keep the virus quiescent, offers some hope that immunotherapy may yield a degree of immune compensation sufficient to keep the virus under control and allow a symptom-free life.

Control of spread of the lymphotrophic retrovirus is essential to prevention. Avoidance of exposure to infected blood products and bodily fluids, like serum and semen, capable of transmitting the virus is of utmost importance. The prospects for a vaccine are real (5). However, because of the immunosuppressive effect of inactivated virus (6) and the genetic variability of viral proteins (7), development of an effective vaccine will probably require several years. Application of DNA recombinant technology, in conjunction with coupled immunoadjuvants like muramyl peptides (8), offers the prospect of eliciting both antibody and cellular immune responses by vaccination with better correlation of immune response to resistance. The extent to which such vaccines are capable of producing a cellular immune response may define their possible usefulness in immunotherapeutic strategies in patients already infected but incapable of eradicating the virus.

In order to achieve immune reconstitution those immunosuppressive influences which contribute to conversion of the asymptomatic patient with positive serology to ARC, and ARC to AIDS, must be controlled to the greatest extent possible. Infection with other immunosuppressive viruses like Epstein-Barr virus (EBV), hepatitis B, cytomegalovirus (CMV), and *Herpes simplex* viruses, if not already present, should be avoided. Rectal delivery of semen may be deleterious since not only is it a vector for various viruses, but semen by this route is also immunosuppressive (9). Correction of malnutrition and avoidance of immunosuppressive recreational drugs may also contribute to immune stabilization or improvement. Collectively, these efforts have not reversed AIDS or ARC so that more active therapies have had to be considered. These efforts have been reviewed previously (1), (10)-(14).

The prospects of therapeutic immunorestoration in AIDS and ARC depend on viral containment and/or eradication. In addition to bolstering natural antiviral mechanisms, the use of exogenous antiviral agents like alpha interferon, suramin, HPA23, ribavirin, ansamycin, 3-azido-3'-deoxy thymidine, or trisodium phosphonoformate will probably be essential, particularly in AIDS (14)-(16). It is clear from past experience with this and other viruses that antiviral therapy, in the absence of effective immunity, is associated with inhibition of viral replication during therapy, but with recurrence of virus replication upon discontinuation of therapy. Only immune reconstitution plus antiviral therapy can be expected to be effective in curing ARC and AIDS. Whether immune restorative therapy alone will contain ARC remains to be determined; however, immunorestorative therapy alone for AIDS has generally been a fruitless effort, as was predicted several years ago (1). It is the purpose of this chapter to assess the current status of the immunotherapy of AIDS and to discuss the prospects for improving this approach using synergistic combination strategies. The therapeutic approaches employed in AIDS and ARC are summarized in Table 2.

ADOPTIVE IMMUNOTHERAPY

Bone marrow transplantation has been attempted in AIDS using

TABLE 2. Immunotherapeutic Approaches to ARC and AIDS

Adoptive Therapy	Biological Therapy
Bone marrow transplantation	Alpha interferon
Lymphocyte infusion	Gamma interferon
Gamma globulin therapy	Thymic hormones
	Thymosin Fr V & alpha 1
	Thymostimulin (TP-1)
Drug Therapy	Thymopentin
	Thymulin
Levamisole	Thymic humoral factor (THF)
Isoprinosine	Interleukin II
Imuthiol (DTC)	Imreg (DLE)
Azimexone	

twin or matched-related donors in at least 10 patients (17-19). In several patients transient immunologic improvement was observed, but each investigator concluded that the effort was without success. Three AIDS patients have been recently treated with suramin plus bone marrow transplantation (19). In one, an increase in T helper cells ($300/mm^3$ - $600/mm^3$) occurred with development of delayed type hypersensitivity (DTH) dermal responses to recall antigens. Only transient effects were seen in two other patients who received lymphocyte transfusions (20),(21). Transplantation of thymic epithelial cell fragments in 11 AIDS patients yielded some evidence of immunological reconstitution in five patients who developed increased OKT8 but not OKT4 cells (2); no other details were reported.

GAMMA GLOBULIN THERAPY

AIDS patients show defects in new responses to B-cell antigens but have hyperglobulinemia and intact memory responses for B cell antigens. Thus, adult AIDS patients do not generally have difficulty with infections to which antibody responses form the major defense (e.g pneumococci, streptococci, staphylococci). For this reason, the use of gamma globulin therapy has been centered on the pediatric population of AIDS sufferers who have a high incidence of infections with these pathogens. Rubinstein (22),(23) has reported beneficial effects of intravenous gamma globulin in 30/32 pediatric patients with AIDS or ARC. Further studies are needed to confirm the usefulness of this therapy.

BIOLOGICAL THERAPY

Interferons

Alpha, beta and gamma interferons (IFN) all have immunomodulating properties as well as antiviral and growth inhibitory effects (24). The immunomodulating effects are generally positive at low doses. IFN's enhance killing by natural killer cells, macrophages, and cytotoxic T cells. At low doses of IFN, T and B cell responses may be augmented in vitro and in vivo, but at higher doses, which promote killer cell responses, antiproliferative effects of IFN impair T and B cell responses. At very high doses all immunologic responses are generally suppressed. The principle use of interferon in ARC and AIDS has been to treat Kaposi's sarcoma. In several trials from New York City, San Francisco, Los Angeles, and Houston complete and partial response rates in Kaposi's sarcoma have averaged from 30-50% (25)-(30). No studies have reported a consistently positive effect of IFN's on lymphocyte-mediated immune response parameters. In one preliminary report gamma IFN increased monocyte-mediated killing and natural killer cell activity at doses near 0.1 mg/m^2 (19). It has been noted that interferon-induced anti-tumor responses generally occur in patients with better preserved immune responses (31). A low frequency of opportunistic infections is often noted during interferon therapy (26),(27),(30); however, whether the regression of Kaposi's sarcoma or the decreased frequency of opportunistic infections translates into prolonged survival remains to be determined. The superiority of IFN therapy to multidrug chemotherapy is underscored not only by the response rate but by the absence of potent immunosuppression induced by the latter. Alpha interferon treatment has been associated with depressed retrovirus recovery in patients with AIDS (19) so that its use as an antiviral agent in conjunction with immunorestorative therapies seems logical. Based on the clinical responses, licensing approval of the use of interferon for Kaposi's sarcoma in AIDS would appear warranted, since in the absence of such licensing, it will be difficult, if not impossible, to utilize combined protocols.

THYMIC HORMONES

Thymosin Fraction V

Thymosin fraction V is a partially purified protein extracted from bovine thymus containing 35 or more distinct peptides apparently including other thymic hormones like thymosin alpha 1, thymopoietin, and thymulin. This preparation induces prothymocyte differentiation and modulates a variety of T cell functions in vitro and in vivo. It has been used experimentally with some success in primary immunodeficiencies and cancer (32). Several reports describe the effects of thymosin administration to 20 seropositive patients with ARC (32)-(35). An initial study with intramuscular doses of 30, 60, and 120 mg/day indicated that only 60 mg/day produced favorable effects. In six evaluable patients with ARC treated daily with 60 mg for 10 weeks, then twice weekly for four weeks, no changes were observed in levels of OKT4 and T8 cells, in the T4/T8 ratios, or in the NK cell activity. Significant increases in mixed leukocyte culture responses (MLR) were observed at six (but not two) weeks of therapy and in cell mediated lysis (CML) and PHA-induced IL-2 production at two and six weeks. No major toxicity was observed, although local reactions to herterologous bovine proteins led to discontinuation of therapy in three patients. While clinical responses were not reported, none of the patients showing immunologic response converted to AIDS, while six of the remaining patients did progress to AIDS. A controlled trial is under consideration (A. Goldstein, personal communication).

Thymosin alpha 1

Thymosin alpha 1 is a pure peptide component of thymosin fraction V produced by recombinant DNA technology. It induces T cell differentiation and modulates T cell functions both in vitro and in vivo (33),(34). Ten patients with ARC have been treated with 0.6 mg daily for 10 weeks then twice daily for four weeks. No change was observed in OKT4 and T8 cell numbers or ratio, NK cell activity, CML, MLR or IL-2 production. No toxicity, clinical effects, seroconversion, or conversion to AIDS was observed during the study period.

Thymopentin

Thymopentin is the 32-36 amino acid sequence of the 49 amino acid peptide thymopoietin, another putative thymic hormone. Both thymopentin and thymopoietin induce prothymocyte differentiation and modulate a variety of T cell functions. Thymopentin has been reported to have activity in DiGeorge syndrome and rheumatoid arthritis. One group of investigators (36) used intravenous thymopentin (1 mg/kg as a 30 minute infusion every other day for varying times) in one ARC and two AIDS patients. No significant beneficial effects on lymphocyte or leukocyte number were observed. All three patients responded with increased PHA responses and Newcastle disease virus-induced interferon production. In another study (37), 11 ARC and five AIDS patients were given subcutaneous injection or intravenous infusion of varying doses of thymopentin (15-50 mg) thrice weekly for a month. The five patients with AIDS showed an apparent drug-related depression of OKT4 cells, T4/T8 ratio, and PHA response. Five ARC patients treated with subcutaneous thymopentin showed no significant immunologic response. Six ARC patients treated with intravenous thymopentin showed small, but in some cases, significant increases in total lymphocyte count, OKT3 and OKT8 lymphocyte levels, and significant increases in PHA mitogen responses. Conversion of DTH skin test responses to positive occurred in five of six patients. Four patients showed clinical improvement with weight gain lasting eight months, while the other two patients progressed to AIDS at three and seven months. Both reports cite no toxicity but conclude that thymopentin is not useful in AIDS, although ARC patients may benefit from thymopentin administered by infusion.

Thymulin

Thymulin is a zinc binding oligopeptide isolated from thymus which induces prothymocyte differentiation and modulates T cell functions. It has shown clinical activity in human patients with DiGeorge syndrome and rheumatoid arthritis (38). It has been employed in four patients with AIDS with no effect but has not yet been tried in ARC patients (JF Bach, personal communication).

Thymic Humoral Factor (THF)

Thymic humoral factor (THF) is a partially characterized small peptide extracted from bovine thymus (39). It modulates a number of T cell functions and has been reported to modify infection in immunodepressed hosts. Notably THF has been reported to increase lymphocyte counts, an effect not generally observed with other thymic hormone preparations. THF given to one AIDS patient (40) apparently induced weight gain, increased lymphocyte counts (T3, T4, and T8 levels) without increase in PHA or Con A response. Despite immunologic improvement, the patient died while still on therapy. THF was administered by injection for two 12 day periods with a one week interim to seven male homosexuals with immune defects (ARC equivalent) and compared to seven placebo-treated controls (39),(41),(42). Immune studies were performed at days 0, 15, and 35. Either no change or a decrease was observed in circulating total lymphocytes and T cell subpopulations in the placebo treated controls. In contrast, significant increases in total lymphocytes, T lymphocytes and their subpopulations, occurred in five of seven THF-treated patients, and mitogen responses improved in two. No clinical changes were described in this apparently asymptomatic group of patients.

Thymostimulin (TP-1)

Thymostimulin, like thymosin fraction V, represents a collection of bovine thymic peptides. The effects of TP-1 on T cell responses in vitro and in vivo are similar to those reported for thymosin (43). One study with seven ARC patients by Byrom, Dixey, Farthing, and Gazzard in London (N. Byrom, personal communication and report at Rome AIDS meeting, 1983) used TP-1 by injection twice a week for one month. No toxicity was observed and lymphocyte counts normalized in five of seven patients who had abnormal counts to begin with. No changes in mitogen responses or clinical signs were reported. Dr. M. Fischl in Miami (personal communication) has observed encouraging results in another open study of 15 patients with ARC.

On the basis of these initial reports, an FDA-approved, multicenter controlled trial of TP-1 in approximately 180 ARC patients has been initiated in New York City, Chicago, and Los Angeles. Another controlled trial has been instituted in London. The major endpoint of these studies will be clinical (symptoms, conversion of ARC to AIDS); however, immune parameters will be monitored.

Summary of Thymic Hormone Studies

What is notable from these studies are the encouraging results in ARC but not AIDS patients. Thymosin, thymopentin, TP-1 and THF (but not thymosin alpha 1) all have been reported to have positive effects in ARC patients. Irrespective of the type of thymic hormone preparation, 23 of 27 reported patients have improved by laboratory criteria, but only a few have been described to be clinically improved, and a modification of the rate of conversion to AIDS has not been clearly established. Toxicity has been limited to local reactions to heterologous proteins. Also notable in these studies are those immune parameters which have not responded to therapy. Except for THF, no real effects of thymic hormones on T lymphocyte numbers have been observed. Depressed functional responses (IL-2 and IFN production, mitogen responses, etc.) have generally been improved. These data indicate that the effects of these thymic hormones are in the direction of improving the function of existing T cells; reconstitution of T cell number remains to be clearly established.

INTERLEUKIN 2

Interleukin 2 (IL-2) is a T cell secretory product which promotes clonal proliferation of T lymphocytes and perhaps B lymphocytes. It also enhances killing by natural killer cells and lymphokine-activated killer cells (LAK cells). Recent observations indicate that several stages of T cell ontogeny are positively regulated by IL-2 (44). Several groups (45)-(48) have shown effects of IL-2 treatment in vitro to restore various deficits observed in AIDS and ARC including mitogen responses, natural killer cell activity, and cytolytic T cell generation. Although it might be postulated that IL-2 would favor lymphotrophic retrovirus replication, the converse effect has apparently been observed in vivo (19).

Lotze and coworkers (49),(50) employed escalating doses of purified Jurkat IL-2 in five AIDS patients using intravenous bolus injection or infusion over 24 hours on a weekly basis for one month without significant change in lymphocyte count (except for an acute decrease), function, or surface markers, in NK and LAK activity, in skin test responses, or in clinical status. Similar negative findings were observed by Lane et al. (51) in 12 AIDS patients and Mertelsman et al. (52) in seven AIDS patients using escalating doses of human buffy coat IL-2 and by Kern et al. (53) in three AIDS and six ARC patients with escalating doses of recombinant IL-2. Isolated findings from these studies included several observations of decreased immunoglobulin levels (51),(52), increased neopterin levels (53), minor changes in Kaposi's sarcoma lesions (53), and partial restoration of platelet count in one patient (52). Toxicities observed in these trials included fever, chills, malaise, headache and nausea in many patients. In contrast to these negative reports, Fauci and Lane (19) have described marked immunomodulation in more than 50 AIDS patients treated with continuous infusion of cloned IL-2 (2 x 10^6 units/days). Observed were increases in blood lymphocyte counts (1500 cells/mm^3 -> 4000 cells/mm^3) and enhanced spontaneous lymphocyte proliferation. In some cases this was associated with minor tumor regression and clearance of HIV viremia. The place of IL-2 in the treatment of AIDS remains to be determined.

DIALYZED LEUKOCYTE EXTRACTS (IMREG 1; TRANSFER FACTOR)

Imreg represents a partially purified low molecular weight constituent of lymphocytes (54), (55). No claims are made for a relationship of this material to transfer factor. Imreg has been reported to increase cutaneous delayed type hypersensitivity reaction in vivo and to enhance in vitro antigen-induced lymphokine production (but not proliferative responses) by human buffy coat cells. The enhancement of lymphokine production includes macrophage and leukocyte migration inhibitory factors (MIF and LIF), IL-2, and gamma IFN. On the basis of these findings an initial trial of imreg 1 in 33 patients with AIDS and ARC was carried out.

Preliminary data from this trial (55, and Gottlieb abstract and presentation at International Symposium On "Current Problems in Testing and Evaluation of Experimental and Clinical Effects of Immunomodulators", Prague, May 13, 1985) indicated that addition of Imreg 1 in vitro increases mitogen-induced IL-2 and gamma IFN production and given with antigen in vivo, restored delayed type hypersensitivity responses in some subjects. Monitoring of 33 Imreg 1-treated patients showed improvement of mitogen-induced proliferative responses and IL-2 production in 64% (21/33), peaking at 7-14 days after administration, and declining by day 21-30. No toxicity was observed. Other details were omitted from the report.

Another dialyzed leukocyte extract with similar properties has been termed transfer factor. Dwyer (2) treated three AIDS patients with nonspecific transfer factor and was unable to see effects on T cell number or on DTH responses.

DRUG THERAPY

Sulfur-containing thymomimetic drugs (levamisole; diethyldithiocarbamate [DTC]; imuthiol).

These drugs stimulate various aspects of the immune system (56). The central feature of their immunopharmacologies appears to be the induction in vivo of a thymic hormone-like factor from liver, called hepatosin. Thus, many of their actions can be explained by thymic hormone-like effects on T lymphocytes. One study of levamisole in five AIDS patients noted considerable toxicity (skin rash, flu-like syndrome) without a consistent beneficial effect and concluded that the risks outweighed any benefit observed (57). DTC is notably less toxic and has been employed in several studies of ARC patients. Pompidou and coworkers (58), (59) have studied the effects of oral DTC, 5 mg/kg administered weekly, in five ARC patients and noted an increase in OKT4 cells in three (129/mm^3 to 420/mm^3) after six months of therapy; clinical improvement was also noted in three patients with increased DTH skin tests and decreased lymphadenopathy. Lang et al. (60) employed 10 mg/kg DTC weekly for six months in six ARC patients and observed increased E rosette forming cells (2/2), OKT3 levels (3/6), OKT4 levels (3/6) and increased DTH skin test responses (3/6). Slow clinical improvement and no toxicity was noted in all six patients. Recently Pompidou et al. (61) have described the ability of DTC to inhibit manifestations of HIV infection (i.e., reverse transcriptase, p15, and p24 expression) in peripheral blood lymphocytes and H9 cells in culture. A randomized, double-blind, cross-over clinical trial with 20 ARC patients is currently in progress in Houston.

Thymomimetic Purines

Isoprinosine

Isoprinosine (inosine pranobax - inosiplex) is a molecular complex of inosine and the p-acetamidobenzoic acid salt of N, N-dimethylamino-2-propanol in a 1:3 molar ratio. Isoprinosine has been shown to induce prothymocyte differentiation in both mouse and human precursor cells and to augment various functions of mature T lymphocytes; the effects of isoprinosine in vitro and in vivo to augment T lymphocyte responses has been characterized as a thymomimetic action (56). In addition, NK cell activity (58), (62), (63) and macrophage functions (64) are also enhanced by isoprinosine. Isoprinosine has been shown to restore depressed immune responses in both animals (65)-(70) and man (71)-(75). The efficacy of isoprinosine treatment has been demonstrated in controlled trials in *Herpes simplex* virus infections (66),(76)-(78), influenza (79) and rhinovirus infection (80), viral hepatitis (81), as well as in subacute sclerosing panencephalitis (SSPE) (82).

The immunopharmacologic effects of isoprinosine have been studied in vitro on cells of patients with AIDS and ARC. Incubation of peripheral blood lymphocytes from patients with AIDS and ARC with isoprinosine resulted in significant increases, and in some cases, normalization of mitogen-induced lymphocyte proliferative responses, with the greatest increases seen in cells from ARC patients (83)-(87). It has also been reported that incubation of isoprinosine with lymphocytes from ARC patients resulted in a significant increase in both the percentage and absolute number of T helper lymphocytes (58).

Tsang et al. (83) demonstrated that isoprinosine increases IL-1 production by monocytes from both normal subjects and AIDS patients and that lymphocytes from AIDS patients absorbed more IL-1 and produced significantly greater quantities of IL-2 following incubation with isoprinosine (83), (87). The depressed production of IL-2 by lymphocytes from AIDS patients was nearly normalized in the presence of isoprinosine. Isoprinosine also increased the expression of TAC antigen, the putative IL-2 receptor on the Leu 2+ subset (suppressor/cytotoxic) of T-lymphocytes, to normal or near normal levels.

Isoprinosine has also been demonstrated to have a direct inhibitory effect on the expression of HIV (58),(61). Peripheral blood lymphocytes infected with HIV exhibited a 48% decrease in reverse transcriptase activity when virus and cells were coincubated with isoprinosine at a concentration of 200 *u*g/ml; no reproducible inhibitory effects were obtained by preincubation of cells or virus with the drug four hours before virus infection. Pompidou et al. (61) concluded that isoprinosine is active against HIV during the first steps of viral infection of T helper cells, either at the stage of viral transduction through the cell membrane, or at the point of integration into the nucleus of the viral DNA transcript.

A pilot clinical study involving both AIDS and ARC patients indicated that while isoprinosine at 4 g/day for 28 days enhanced mitogen-induced lymphocyte proliferative responses in ARC patients, this effect was not seen in patients with frank AIDS (88), (89). Mansell et al. (90), however, have cautioned that a treatment and observation period of only 28 days may not be sufficient in patients with AIDS.

Based on these findings, a double-blind, placebo-controlled clinical study was undertaken to evaluate the effect of isoprinosine in a group of immunodeficient male homosexuals (91)-(94). Patients were treated with isoprinosine (3 g/day) or placebo for 28 days, and were followed clinically and immunologically for one year. Isoprinosine had a significant enhancing effect on several immune parameters, including NK cell activity, total lymphocytes and T helper lymphocytes. By day seven of treatment, NK cell activity had increased 60% relative to the initial baseline value. Total T-cells showed an increase at day 28, and T helper cells were increased at day 90. All three of these immunologic parameters remained elevated at day 180, five months after termination of drug treatment, and NK cell activity remained significantly elevated at 11 months after completion of the treatment period (Figure 1).

In addition, the 20 patients in the 3g/day isoprinosine treatment group showed significant and progressive declines in previously elevated levels of serum immunoglobulin levels, antigen-antibody complexes, and cytoplasmic and secreted immunoglobulin of circulating B lymphocytes. Also significant were the normalization of HLA DR levels, Leu 7+ and 11+ (NK)

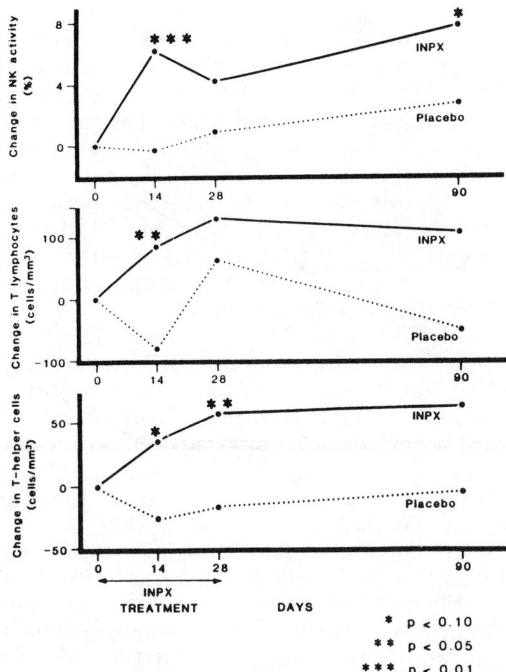

Figure 1. Change in NK cell activity, total lymphocytes and T helper cells following treatment with isoprinosine (INPX) or placebo (provided by A. Glasky from (95). *p<.10, **p<.05, ***p<.01.

cells, and the T cell subsets of T helper/inducer and T suppressor/cytotoxic. The internal consistency of the isoprinosine-induced correction of altered immune parameters manifest in these ARC patients is impressive and unmatched in any other controlled study in this disease.

Clinical status of the treated patients was similarly beneficially affected by isoprinosine. Cumulative clinical scores indicated that isoprinosine-treated patients experienced a substantially better clinical response than placebo-treated patients (Figure 2). Also observed was a lower and delayed conversion to AIDS in the 3 g/d isoprinosine-treated group.

Interim data from two multicenter trials following similar protocols confirm these findings (95). Preliminary analysis of a total of 157 immunodepressed patients at risk of developing AIDS indicate that isoprinosine has a significant immunoenhancing effect manifested by substantial and sustained increases in NK cell activity, total T lymphocytes and T helper lymphocytes. Like the Wallace and Bekesi study (91), the isoprinosine treated group experienced a delay in progression to AIDS (Figure 3). By day 210, six placebo-treated patients had progressed to AIDS, as compared to only three isoprinosine-treated patients.

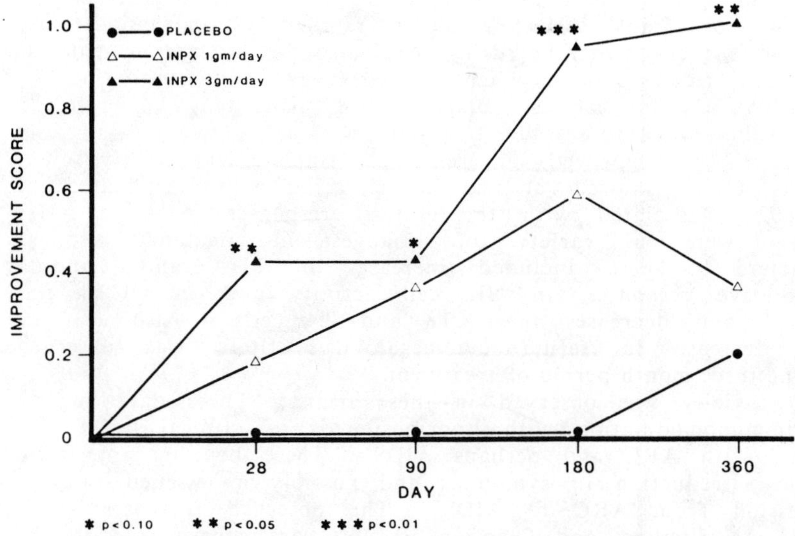

Figure 2. Effect of two doses of isoprinosine (INPX) on cumulative clinical improvement scores. Clinical improvement was scored as: improved = 2, slightly improved = 1, unchanged = 0, slightly worse = -1, worse = -2. *p<.1, **p<.05, ***p<.01 (significantly different from placebo: two sided Mann-Whitney u test) (from Wallace and Bekesi (91) with permission).

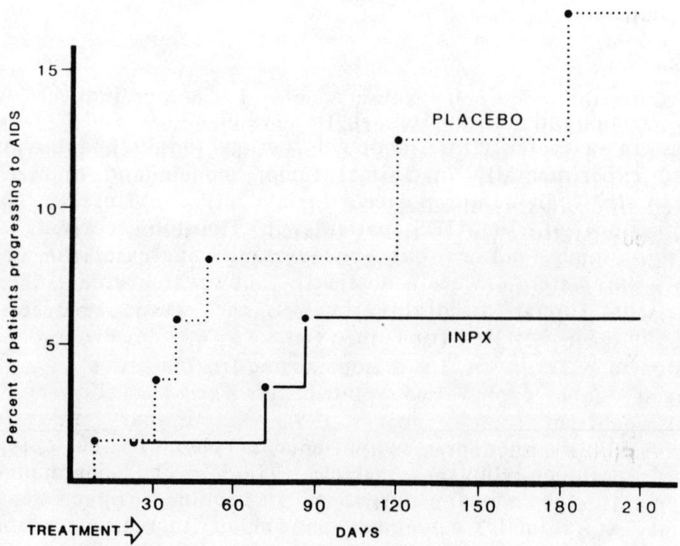

Figure 3. Kaplan-Meier life table estimate of the proportion of patients developing AIDS in the isoprinosine (INPX) and placebo treated groups (Provided by A. Glasky).

Interim results from an ongoing study of isoprinosine in the treatment of frank AIDS, conducted under a compassionate-use protocol, suggest that the drug may also be useful in patients with more serious disease when administered for longer periods of time (95). Out of a total of 48 patients who received isoprinosine at a dose of 3 g/day for at least 60 days, 40 patients (84%) improved or remained stable, while only eight patients (16%) showed clinical deterioration when evaluated at day 60. Associated with the clinical responses in these AIDS patients were a variety of changes in immune response parameters. These included increases in PHA and Candida proliferative responses, in NK cell activity and in OKT4 cell numbers, and decreases in OKT8 and T4 cells. Also a three $\log_{10}$ decrease in serum cytomegalovirus titers was observed over the three month period of treatment.

No toxicity was observed in these trials. These data suggest that immunomodulation with isoprinosine is of clinical benefit in patients with ARC and perhaps AIDS. These benefits appear to include a reduction in symptoms and possibly a lessened rate of progression from ARC to AIDS. The observed increases in T lymphocyte numbers and function in ARC are consistent with the proposed thymomimetic drug action of isoprinosine (56). Based upon these findings, isoprinosine would appear to be the only immunotherapeutic agent ready to be considered for licensing in the treatment of ARC; however, post licensing monitoring would seem warranted to evaluate whether longer term treatment maintains or improves the effects of isoprinosine on immune response parameters and clinical signs and symptoms.

Other Compounds

Azimexon

This compound stimulates both lymphocyte and macrophage activities in a potentiator mode of action (96),(97) and has been employed experimentally in animal tumor models and human cancer patients. In an unreported trial (P. Mansell, personal communication) of 70 AIDS patients in Houston receiving 200mg/m^2 daily, some minor but encouraging increases in selected immune parameters were observed; however, toxic hemolytic complications forced discontinuation of the study. A less toxic analog (ciamexon) is slated for future trials.

Glucan

Soluble glucan has been employed experimentally as a stimulant of the reticuloendothelial system (98). The macrophage is thought to be the primary target of its action. Experimental use of glucan in animals has been shown to increase resistance to bacterial, viral, fungal, parasitic and tumor challenges. Soluble intravenous glucan (up to 100 gm/m^2 twice weekly) has been administered to 13 ARC patients and six AIDS patients (P. Mansell personal communication). Significant increases in T helper number, IL-1 production, and weight gain were observed. Toxicity included fever, headache, hypertension and diaphoresis in the majority of patients and palmar plantar hyperkeratosis in five patients. Further studies with lower doses in combination with other agents are under discussion.

PROSPECTS FOR THE FUTURE: COMBINED THERAPY

The rational for use of combined immunotherapy is based upon a number of observations demonstrating synergism between two or more immunotherapeutic agents. The following are three strategies employing combinations of immunotherapeutic agents which may be applicable in AIDS.

T Cell Reconstitution

The thymic hormones have received considerable attention as therapeutic agents for treating immunodeficiency secondary to thymus dysfunction. The clinical results to date with thymic hormones in various diseases including ARC, although encouraging, have not been dramatic. Abundant evidence supports the notion that thymic hormones induce the differentiation of pre-T cells and modulate the function of mature T cells; however, efforts to show that any of the thymic hormones induce intrathymic maturation of T cells have been unsuccessful. In previously published experiments (99), we showed that T cell growth factor (IL-2) is a potent inducer of cell surface receptor changes of immature thymocytes which correlate with the normal maturation sequence. Our recent experiments (44) further indicate that IL-2 induces prothymocyte differentiation. It also induces immature thymocyte differentiation in vitro to the point of mitogen responsiveness. These experiments cast IL-2 in a new role as an inducer of differentiation, in addition to the generally accepted role as co-mitogen in T lymphocyte proliferation, or activation of lymphocyte activated killer (LAK) cells and NK cells.

The therapeutic implications of these observations are that the combination of thymic hormones and IL-2 together or in sequence may be required to reconstitute the T-cell system. One may predict that thymic hormones and IL-2 will be synergistic in vivo in yielding T cell reconstitution. Similarly, the thymomimetic drugs like isoprinosine and imuthiol (DTC) are more active in vivo in inducing T cell markers in nude mouse spleens than either thymosin or IL-2 (unpublished data); and they may also be synergistic with IL-2 in inducing T cell function as well as maturation. Based upon these considerations, these seem ideal combinations to apply to patients with AIDS in an attempt to reconstitute T cell function.

Augmentation of Antiviral Resistance

It has been shown that the antiviral action of interferon can be potentiated by immunostimulants (100),(101). From an immunopharmacologic standpoint, interferon is an ambivalent agent with potentially immunosuppressive activity, particularly at high doses. The rationale for combining interferon with isoprinosine is based on observations that their immunopharmacologies are complementary. Experiments have demonstrated that isoprinosine, while inactive alone, significantly potentiates the effects of interferon in protecting animals against a lethal challenge with encephalomyocarditis virus. Similar but less dramatic results in this model were obtained with interferon in combination with *Corynebacterium parvum*, cyclomunine or staphylococcal lysate, thus further confirming the principle that potentiation is possible. Thus, the combination of isoprinosine and interferon may be considered for future clinical trials in HIV infected patients to attempt to reconstitute nonspecific viral resistance.

Interleukin 2 is an effector in nonspecific resistance mechanisms involving NK cells and perhaps LAK cells as well. Combining IL-2 with interferon, particularly in an intermittent protocol, may also offer synergistic augmentation of viral resistance.

Augmentation of Macrophage Mediated Resistance

Better treatment of opportunistic infections represents one approach to the management of AIDS. Persistence of these infections is principally the result of deficiency of T cell-mediated immunity; however, the primary mechanism for the destruction of the involved pathogens is the macrophage. Resistance to facultative intracellular pathogens requires macrophage activation. This activation process is induced by lymphokines produced by the T cell, operationally termed macrophage activating factors, of which there are several, including gamma interferon. Their use alone, or in combination with antimicrobial chemotherapy, where available, should yield enhanced resistance to such pathogens both prophylactically and therapeutically. Since the microbicidal activity of the macrophage can be nonspecifically enhanced, i.e., enhanced for a broad spectrum of intracellular bacteria and parasites, it seems feasible that a general and prolonged enhancement of resistance might be achieved, allowing patients to be free of such infections for relatively long periods.

Alternatively, the same purpose might be achieved by use of one or more of several chemically defined agents which can directly activate macrophages for microbicidal activity. One example is muramyl dipeptide which is a direct activator of macrophages for both microbicidal and tumoricidal activity (102). This substance is the smallest active component of the mycobacterial cell wall having adjuvant effects and protective effects against pathogen challenge. It is water soluble, orally active, and nontoxic in initial phase I human clinical trials. In addition to its considerable potential as a single agent, muramyl dipeptide has been demonstrated to have a potentiative action on lymphokine-induced macrophage activation in vitro and in vivo. Therefore, combination of this agent with lymphokines may prove synergistic in augmenting resistance of AIDS patients to pathogen challenge.

CONCLUSION

In conclusion, AIDS offers a unique opportunity for clinical immunologists to employ what is known about immunopharmacology in the design of treatment for these patients. Strategies to utilize biologicals and drugs to restore T cell-mediated immune response and to enhance both microbicidal and antiviral resistance should ameliorate AIDS and ARC. Cure of these diseases will predictably require effective antiviral therapy used in conjunction with immunotherapeutic agents and strategies.

REFERENCES

1. Hadden, J., Perspectives on the immunotherapy of AIDS. Ann NY Acad Sci 437:76-89 (1984)

2. Dwyer, J.M., McNamara, J.G. Sigal, L.H., et al., Immunological abnormalities in patients with the acquired immune deficiency syndrome (AIDS): A review. Clin Immunol Rev 3:25-129 (1984)

3. Savino, W., Dardenne, M., Marche, C., et al., Thymic epithelium in AIDS: An immunoholistic study. Am J Pathol 122:98-103 (1986)

4. Dardenne, M., Bach, J-F., Low serum thymic hormone levels in patients with acquired immunodeficiency syndrome. N Engl J Med 309:48-49 (1983)

5. Frances, D.P., Petricciani, J.C., The prospects for and pathways toward a vaccine for AIDS. N Engl J Med 313: 1586-1590 (1985)

6. Pahwa, S. Pahwa, R., Saxinger, C., et al., Influence of the human T-lymphotrophic virus/lymphadenpathy-associated virus on functions of human lymphocytes: Evidence for immunosuppressive effects and polyclonal B-cell activation by banded viral preparations. Proc Natl Acad Sci 82:8198-8202 (1985)

7. Musina, M.A., Smith D.H., Cabradilla, E.D., et al., Nucleic acid structure and expression of the human AIDS/lymphadenopathy retrovirus. Nature 313:450-458 (1985)

8. Audibert, F., Jolivet, M., Amar, O., Role of adjuvants and carriers in synthetic vaccines. In: Immunopharmacology (Miescher, P.A., Bolis, L., Ghione, M., eds.) Raven Press, NY, Vol. 23:91-100 (1985)

9. Witkin, S.S., Richards, J.M., Bongiovanni, A.M., et al., Inhibition of lymphocyte proliferation by sera from rectally inseminated male rabbits. Ann NY Acad Sci 437:504-507 (1984)

10. Lane, H.C., Fauci, A.S., Immunologic reconstitution of the acquired immunodeficiency syndrome. Ann Intern Med 103:714-718 (1985)

11. Masur, H., Immunotherapy and therapy of complications of AIDS, Topics in Clin Nursing 6:53-60 (1984)

12. Klatzman, D., Montagnier, L., Approaches to AIDS therapy. Nature 319:10-11 (1986)

13. Lane, H.C., Masur, H., Gelman, E.P. et al., Therapeutic approaches to patients with AIDS. Cancer Res (Suppl.) 45:4674s-4676s (1985).

14. Gupta, S., Gottlieb M.S., Treatment of the acquired immunodeficiency syndrome. J Clin Immunol (In press)

15. Bolognesi, D.P., Fischinger, P.J., Prospects for treatment of human retrovirus-associated diseases. Cancer Res (Suppl.) 45:4700s-4705s (1985)

16. Hersh, M.S., Kaplan, J.C., Prospects of therapy for infections with human T-lymphotropic virus type III. Ann Intern Med 103:750-755 (1985)

17. Hassett, J.M., Zaroulis, C.G., Greenberg, M.L., et al., Bone marrow transplantation in AIDS. N Engl J Med 309:655-660 (1985)

18. Mitsuyasu, R., Volberding, P., Groopman, J., et al., Bone marrow transplantation for patients with AIDS and Kaposi's sarcoma. Blood 62 (suppl.) 226a (1983)

19. Fauci, A., Lane, H.C., Therapeutic approaches to the underlying immune defect in patients with AIDS. International Conference on Acquired Immunodeficiency Syndrome (AIDS), Paris, France (1986)

20. Lane, H.C., Masur, H., Longo, D.L., et al., Partial immune reconstitution in a patient with the acquired immunodeficiency syndrome. N Engl J Med 311:1099-1103 (1984)

21. Davis, K.C., Hayward, A., Ozturk, G., et al., Lymphocyte transfusion in a case of acquired immunodeficiency syndrome. Lancet 1:599-600 (1983)

22. Rubenstein, A., Sicklick, M., Bernstein, L., et al., Treatment of AIDS with intravenous gammaglobulin. Pediatr Res 18:264a (Abstract #1010) (1984)

23. Silverman, B., Rubenstein, A., Possible vertical transmission of acquired immunodeficiency in intravenous drug users. Pediatr Res 18:265a (Abstract #1017) (1984)

24. Stewart, W.E., The Interferon System, Springer-Verlag, Vienna (1981)

25. Volberding, P., Valero, R., Rothman, J., et al., Alpha interferon therapy of Kaposi's sarcoma in AIDS. Ann NY Acad Sci 437:439-446 (1986).

26. Krown, S.E., Real, F.X., Krim, M., et al., Interferons and other biological response modifiers in the treatment of Kaposi's sarcoma. Front Radiat Ther Onc 19:138-149 (1985)

27. Rios, A., Mansell, P., Newell, G. R., et al., Treatment of acquired immunodeficiency syndrome-related Kaposi's sarcoma with lymphoblastoid interferon. J Clin Oncol 3:506-512 (1985)

28. Frederick, W.R., Epstein, J.S., Gelman, E.P., et al., Viral infections and cell-mediated immunity in immunodeficient homosexual men with Kaposi's sarcoma treated with human lymphoblastoid interferon. J Infect Dis 152:162-170 (1985)

29. Groopman, J.E., Gottlieb, M.S., Goodman, J., et al., Recombinant alpha-2 interferon therapy for Kaposi's sarcoma associated with the acquired immunodeficiency syndrome. Ann Intern Med 100:671-676 (1984)

30. Volberding, P.A., Mitsuyasu, R., Recombinant interferon alpha in the treatment of acquired immune deficiency syndrome-related Kaposi's sarcoma. Sem Onc 12:2-6 (1985)

31. Vadhan-Raj, S., Wong, G., Gnecco, C., et al., Immunological variables as predictors of prognosis in patients with Kaposi's sarcoma and the acquired immunodeficiency syndrome. Cancer Res 46:417-425 (1986)

32. Goldstein, A.L., Naylor, P.H., Schulof, R.S., et al., Thymosin in the staging and treatment of HTLV-III positive homosexuals and hemophiliacs with AIDS-related immune dysfunction. Proceedings on AIDS-associated Syndromes, Plenum Press, NY (In press)

33. Naylor, P.H., Schulof, R.S., Sztein, M.B., et al., Thymosin in the early diagnosis and treatment of high risk homosexuals and hemophiliacs with AIDS-like immune dysfunction. Ann NY Acad Sci 437:88-99 (1986)

34. Schulof, R.S., Simon, G.L., Sztein, M.B., et al., Phase I/II trial of thymosin fraction 5 and thymosin alpha one in HTLV-III seropositive subjects. J Biol Resp Mod (In press)

35. Schulof, R., Simon, G., Sztein, M., et al., In vivo effects of thymosin fraction 5 in male homosexuals and hemophilics at risk for AIDS. Proceedings of ASCO (abstract) 4:1 (1985).

36. Mascart-Lemone, F., Huygen, K., Clumeck, N., et al., Stimulation of cellular function by thymopentin (TP-5) in three AIDS patients. Lancet 2:735-736 (1983).

37. Clumeck, N., Cran, S., Van de Perre, P., et al., Thymopentin treatment in AIDS and pre-AIDS patients. Surv Immunol Res 4:suppl 1:58-62 (1985)

38. Dardenne, M., Bach, J.F., Recent data on the structure, localization, and function of the serum thymic factor (thymulin). In: Immunomodulation: New Frontiers and Advances (Fudenberg, H., Whitten, H.D., Ambrogi, F., eds.), Plenum Press, New York, p 35-42 (1984)

39. Trainin, N., Burstein, Y., Buchner, V., et al., Immunity and Immunodeficiency (Szentivanyi, A., Friedman, H., eds), Plenum Press, NY (In press)

40. Berner, Y., Pecht, M., Bentwich, Z., et al., Attempted treatment of acquired immunodeficiency syndrome (AIDS). Isr Med Sci 20:1195-1196 (1984)

41. Ze'ev, H.T., Bentwich, A., Burstein, R., et al., Anti-viral properties of thymic humoral factor and other thymic hormones. Clin Immunol Newsletter 6(5):68-71 (1985)

42. Hendzel, Z.T., Berner, Y., Burstein R., et al., Immunomodulation of the "immunodeficiency of homosexuals" using THF - a thymic hormone (abstract). 14th Conference on Clinical Immunology, Toronto, July (1986)

43. Falchetti, R., Bergesi, G., Eshkol, A., et al., Pharmacological and biological properties of a calf thymus extract (TP-1). Drugs Exp Clin Res 3:39-47 (1977)

44. Hadden, J.W., Specter, S., Galy, A., et al., Thymic hormones, interleukins, endotoxin, and thymomimetic drugs in T lymphocyte ontogeny. In: Advances in Immunopharmacology III, Pergamon Press, Oxford (In press)

45. Rook, A.H., Masur, H., Lane, H.C., et al., Interleukin 2 enhances the depressed natural killer cell and cytomegalovirus-specific cytotoxic activities of lymphocytes from patients with the acquired immunodeficiency syndrome. J Clin Invest 72:398-403 (1983)

46. Gupta, S., Gillis S., Thornton, M., et al., Autologous mixed lymphocyte reaction in man. XIV Deficiency of the autologous mixed lymphocyte reaction in acquired immune deficiency syndrome (AIDS) and AIDS-related complex (ARC). In vitro effect of purified interleukin 1 and interleukin 2. Clin Exp Immunol 58:395-401 (1984).

47. Sharma, B., Gupta. S., Antigen-specific primary cytotoxic T lymphocyte (CTL) responses in acquired immune deficiency syndrome (AIDS) and AIDS-related complex (ARC). Clin Exp Immunol 62:296-303 (1985).

48. Rubin, B.Y., Mertelsmann, R., Roberts, R.B., Production of and in vitro response to interleukin 2 in the acquired immunodeficiency syndrome. J Clin Invest 76:1959-1964 (1985)

49. Lotze, M.T., Robb, R.J., Sharrow, S., et al., Systemic administration of interleukin-2 in humans. J Biol Res Mod 3:475-482 (1984)

50. Lotze, M., Frana, L., Sharrow, S., et al., In vivo administration of purified human interleukin 2. I. Half-life and immunologic effects of the jurkat cell line-derived interleukin 2. J Immunol 134(1):157-166 (1985)

51. Lane, H.C., Siegal, J., Rook, A., et al., Use of interleukin-2 in patients with acquired immunodeficiency syndrome. J Biol Resp Mod 3:512-516 (1984)

52. Mertelsmann, R., Welte, K., Sternberg C., et al., Treatment of immunodeficiency with interleukin-2: Initial exploration. J Biol Resp Mod 4:483-490 (1984)

53. Kern, P., Toy, J., Dietrich, M., Preliminary clinical observations with recombinant interleukin-2 in patients with AIDS or LAS. Blut 50:1-6 (1985)

54. Gottlieb, A.A., Farmer, J., Matzura, C., et al., Modulation of human T cell production of migration inhibitory lymphokines by cytokines derived from human leukocyte dialysates. J Immunol 132(1):256-260 (1984)

55. Gottlieb, A.A., Advances in the treatment of the immune defect in AIDS/ARC (abstract). Proceeding of ASCO, Los Angeles, March (1986)

56. Hadden, J.W., Thymomimetic drugs. In: Immunopharmacology (Miescher, P.A., Bolis, L., Ghione, M., eds.), Serono Symposia Publications, Raven Press, NY. Vol 23, p 183-192, (1985)

57. Surapaneni, N., Raghunathan, R., Beall, G., et al., Levamisole, immunostimulation, and the acquired immunodeficiency syndrome. Ann Intern Med 101:137-142 (1984)

58. Pompidou, A., Delsauz, M.C., Talvi, L., et al., Isoprinosine and imuthiol, two potentially active compounds in patients with AIDS-related complex symptoms. Cancer Research (suppl). 45:4671s-4673s (1985)

59. Pompidou, A., Lang, J-M., Talvi, L., et al., Influence of immunomodulators on T lymphocyte differentiation in ARC patients and resistance to LAV/HTLV-III infection. In: Comparative Immunology, Microbiology and Infectious Diseases (In press)

60. Lang, J-M., Oberling, F., Aleksijevic, A., et al., Immunomodulation with diethyldithiocarbamate in patients with AIDS-related complex. Lancet 2:1066 (1985)

61. Pompidou, A., Zagury, D., Gallo, R., et al., In vitro inhibition of LAV/HTLV-III infected lymphocytes by dithiocarb and inosine pranobax. Lancet 2:1423 (1985)

62. Balestrino, C., Montesoro, E., Nocera, A., et al., Augmentation of human peripheral blood natural killer activity by methisoprinol. J Biol Resp Mod 2:577-585 (1983)

63. Tsang, K.Y., Fudenberg, H.H., Pan, J.F., et al., An in vitro study on the effects of isoprinosine on the immune responses in cancer patients. Int J Immunopharm 5:481-490 (1983)

64. Hadden, J. W., Englard, A., Sadlik, J.R., et al., The comparative effects of isoprinosine, levamisole, muramyl dipeptide and SM1213 on lymphocyte and macrophage proliferation and activation in vitro. Int J Immunopharm 1:17-27 (1979)

65. Tsang, K.Y., Fudenberg, H.H., Gnagy, M.J., Restoration of immune responses of aging hamsters by treatment with isoprinosine. J Clin Invest 71:1750-1755 (1983)

66. Fischback, M., Talal, N., Restoration of interleukin-2 production and immune function in autoimmune mice. Clin Exp Immunol 61:242-247 (1985)

67. Cerutti, I., Chany, C., Schlumberger, J., Isoprinosine increases the antitumor action of interferon. Cancer Treat Rep 62:1971-1974 (1978)

68. Tsang, K.Y., Fudenberg, H.H., Isoprinosine as an immunopotentiator in an animal model of human osteosarcoma. Int J Immunopharm 3:383-389 (1982)

69. Binderup, L., Effects of isoprinosine on animal models of depressed T-cell function. Int J Immunopharm 7:93-101 (1985)

70. Ohnishi, H., Kosuzume, H., Inaba, H., et al., Mechanism of host defense suppression induced by viral infection: Mode of action of inosiplex as an antiviral agent. Infect Immun 38:243-250 (1982)

71. Bradshaw, L., Sumner, H., In vitro studies of cell-mediated immunity in patients treated with inosiplex for herpes virus infection. Ann NY Acad Sci 284:190-196 (1977)

72. Corey, L., Chiang, W., Reeves, W., et al., Effect of isoprinosine on the cellular immune response in initial genital herpes virus infection. Clin Res 27:41 (1979)

73. Fenton, J., Double-blind study of the effect of isoprinosine upon immunity tests in patients with pelvic radiation. Bull Cancer 68:200 (1981)

74. Fridman, H., Calle, R., Morin, A., Double-blind study of isoprinosine influence on immune parameters in solid tumor-bearing patients treated by radiotherapy. Int J Immunopharm 2:194 (1980)

75. Gui, D., Borgogone, A., Pittiruti, M., et al., Immunostimulation of the anergic surgical patient with methisoprinol. Clin Eur 21:3-8 (1982)

76. Sato, O., Lassus, A., Treatment of recurrent genital herpes with isoprinosine. Eur J Sex Trans Dis 1:101-105 (1983)

77. Bouffaut, P., Saurat, J., Isoprinosine as a therapeutic agent in recurrent mucocutaneous infections due to herpes virus. Int J Immunopharm 2:193 (1980)

78. Galli, M., Lazzarin, A., Moroni, M., et al., Inosiplex in recurrent *Herpes simplex* infections. Lancet 2:331-332 (1982)

79. Khakoo, R., Watson, G., Waldman R., et al., Effect of inosiplex (isoprinosine) on induced human influenza: An infection. J Antimicrob Chemother 7:389-397 (1981)

80. Waldman, R., Ganguly, R., Therapeutic efficacy of inosiplex in rhinovirus infection. Ann NY Acad Sci 84:153-160 (1978)

81. Scasso, A., Paladini, A., Della Santa, M., Methisoprinol in the treatment of acute B viral hepatitis: Controlled clinical study. Curr Ther Res 34:423-435 (1983)

82. Jones, C., Dyken, P., Huttenlocher, P., et al., Inosiplex therapy in subacute sclerosing panencephalitis. Lancet 2:1034-1037 (1982)

83. Tsang, P., Lew, F., O'Brien, G., et al., Immunopotentiation of impaired lymphocyte functions in vitro by isoprinosine in prodromal subjects and AIDS patients. Int J Immunopharm 7:511-514 (1985)

84. Tsang, P., Tangnavard, K., Solomon, S., et al., Modulation of T and B-lymphocyte functions by isoprinosine in homosexual subjects with prodromata and in patients with acquired immune deficiency syndrome (AIDS). J Clin Immun 4:469-478 (1984)

85. Tsang, K.Y., Donnely, R.P., Galbraith, G., et al., Isoprinosine effects on interleukin-1 production in acquired immune deficiency syndrome (AIDS). Int J Immunopharm (In press)

86. Tsang, K.Y., Boutin, B., Pathak, S., et al., Effect of isoprinosine on the sialylation of interleukin-2. Int J Immunopharm (In press)

87. Tsang, K.Y., Fudenberg, H.H., Galbraith, G., Partial restoration of impaired interleukin-2 production and tac antigen (putative interleukin-2 receptor) expressions in AIDS patients by isoprinosine treatment in vitro. J Clin Invest 75:1538-1544 (1985)

88. Manvar, D., Ahuja, K., Reddy, M., et al., Immunomodulation with isoprinosine in AIDS. J Allerg Immunol 71:133-138 (1983)

89. Grieco, M., Reddy, M., Manvar, D., et al., In vitro immunomodulation by isoprinosine in patients with acquired immunodeficiency syndrome (AIDS) and related complexes. Ann Intern Med 101:206-207 (1984)

90. Mansell, P., Reuben, J., Odem, M., et al., The use of isoprinosine in an attempt to improve function in AIDS and AIDS related complex. Proc Am Soc Clin Oncol (abstract) 4:1 (1985)

91. Wallace, J.I., Bekesi, J.G., A double-blind clinical trial of the effects of inosine pranobex in immunodepressed patients with prolonged generalized lymphadenopathy. Clin Immunol Immunopath 39:179-186 (1986)

92. Tsang, P., Warner, N., Bekesi, J.G., Impaired B and T-lymphocyte subsets and function restored by isoprinosine in prodromal homosexuals and AIDS patients. Cancer Detect Prev 8:580 (1985)

93. Tsang, P.H., Wallace, J.I., Robox, J.P., et al., Potentiation of impaired lymphocyte functions by isoprinosine in AIDS patients and prodromal subjects in vitro and in vivo data (abstract). Proc Am Soc Clin Oncol 4:4 (1985)

94. Bekesi, G., Wallace, J., Tsang, P., et al., Normalization of immunoregulatory T helper and T suppressor sublineage and cell mediated immunity by isoprinosine in pre-clinical homosexual males: an in vivo study. Cancer Detect Prev (In press)

95. Glasky, A.J., Gordon, J.G., Isoprinosine (inosine pranobex) in the treatment of AIDS and other acquired immunodeficiencies of clinical importance. Cancer Detect Prev (In press) (1986)

96. Bicker, U., In: Progress in Cancer Research and Therapy: Augmenting Agents in Cancer Therapy (Hersh, E., Chirigos, M. A., Mastrangelo, M.J., eds.) Raven Press, NY. Vol 16:523-538, (1981)

97. Hadden, J.W., Effects of BM 12, 531 (Azimexon) in in vitro lymphocyte and macrophage proliferation. Recent Results. Cancer Res 75: 171-173 (1980)

98. DiLuzio, N.R., Immunopharmacology of glucan: A broad spectrum enhancer of host defense mechanisms. Trends in Pharmacol Sci 4:344 (1983)

99. Chen, S.S., Tung, J.S., Gillis, S., et al., Changes in surface antigens of immature thymocytes under the influence of T cell growth factor and thymic factors. Proc Natl Acad Sci 80:5980-5984 (1983)

100. Cerutti, I., Chany, C., Schlumberger, J.F., Isoprinosine increases the antitumor action of interferon. Int J Immunopharm 1:58-63 (1979)

101. Chany, C., Cerutti, I., Enhancement of antiviral protection against encephalomyocarditis virus by a combination of isoprinosine and interferon. Arch Virol 55:225-231 (1977)

102. Lederer, E., Chedid, L., Immunomodulation by synthetic muramyl peptides and trchalose diesters. In: Immunological Approaches to Center Therapeutics (Michich, E., ed.). Wiley Interscience, New York, p 108-135 (1982)

50
An Overview of Antiviral Therapy of HIV Infection

Markus W. Vogt, Robert T. Schooley

Despite much progress in treating many bacterial and fungal infections, only a few clinically useful antiviral drugs are available today. Attempts to reduce the incidence and severity of viral diseases have focused on development of effective vaccines. Vaccines were responsible for the eradication of smallpox and, in several countries, for the control of polio, measles, rubella and mumps. Recent advances in molecular biological techniques suggest that new genetically engineered vaccines or subunit vaccines will further enhance efforts in prophylaxis of viral infections.

While vaccines have been successfully used for over 150 years, antiviral chemotherapy has a much shorter history. Viruses are obligate intracellular organisms. In contrast to bacteria, fewer specific replicative and metabolic functions are utilized by viruses. Thus, there are fewer potential targets for the action of candidate antiviral drugs Because viral replication occurs exclusively in a cellular environment, proposed antiviral drugs must also exhibit acceptable toxicity for mammalian cells, a consideration which has eliminated numerous agents from further testing. Furthermore, many viruses survive as integrated genomic proviral sequences, and are, therefore, not affected by agents which are dependent on replication for activity.

Recent insights into viral replicative mechanisms have led, however, to the development and licensure of several effective antiviral agents. Currently three antiviral drugs are licensed for systemic use in the United States - amantadine, vidarabine, and acyclovir.

Two years after the first patients with acquired immunodeficiency syndrome (AIDS) were described, the etiologic agent was established as a human retrovirus. The discovery of HTLV-III (human T-cell lymphotropic virus III) (1) or LAV (lymphadenopathy associated retrovirus) (2) has provided an enormous challenge to develop a potent vaccine and antiviral drugs against this newest member of the lentivirus family (3). The International Committee on Taxonomy of Viruses recently proposed the unifying name HIV (human immunodeficiency virus) (4). AIDS has by now reached epidemic proportions not only in the USA but in Central African countries and Europe. Although progress has been made toward the development of an effective vaccine, the 25,000+ residents of the United States with AIDS and the more than a million infected, but currently healthy, persons cannot expect to benefit from this approach. An effective vaccine will be most important for high risk individuals who are not yet infected. Antiviral agents are thus necessary to prevent viral morbidity in individuals who have already been infected (5).

The biology and clinical behavior of the AIDS-virus is by now at least partly understood. An ideal antiviral agent to treat persons infected with HIV should have demonstrable activity against HIV in vitro and should fulfill several additional criteria (Table 1):

1. Since HIV has been isolated from the brain and cerebrospinal fluid of infected individuals (6)-(9), agents with little or no ability to penetrate the blood brain barrier would not be ideal.

2. Because the virus is integrated as latent proviral DNA in the genome (10) of host helper T-lymphocytes and monocytes (7), (11) (Figure 1), it would be anticipated that viral replication would only be temporarily reduced during treatment in most patients. Results from the first clinical trials have confirmed this expectation. This outcome was anticipated since no currently available drug affects latent integrated viral DNA. Such infected cells may act as lifelong reservoirs, potentially treatable only with chronic suppressive therapy. This means that an ideal antiviral drug must show minimal long-term toxicity in chronic treatment regimens and exhibit great virus specificity (5).

3. Considering the number of individuals currently infected with HIV on a worldwide basis, drugs with the following additional properties should be favored: inexpensive, adequately absorbed when given orally, long half-life, stable at room temperature.

Another important issue is the timing of therapy. Patients who are still immunologically competent might profit more significantly from antiviral therapy, and thus early recognition of asymptomatic infection is important. However, apparently not all

Table 1. Important Attributes of Antiviral Compounds with Activity Against HIV

Name of Drug	CSF Entry	Oral Regimen	Longterm Toxicity	Stability (4°C)*	Low Price
Ideal Drug	+	+	-	+	+
Azidothymidine	+	+	?	+	?
Phosphonoformate	+	-	?	+	?
Ribavirin	+	+	?	+	?
Suramin	-	-	+	+	+
HPA-23	?	-	?	+	?
Recombinant Interferon-alpha	-	-	?	-	-

CSF = Cerebrospinal Fluid
* Drug stored in crystalline powder form.

patients with HIV infection go on to develop demonstrable clinical or immunologic sequelae of infection. Thus, methods for identification of individuals at greatest risk for subsequent illness would help determine which subsets of healthy, but HIV infected, individuals would be most likely to benefit from antiviral treatment. Additional treatment with immunomodulators might also be necessary in selected cases.

HIV REPLICATION AND POSSIBLE DRUG ACTION

The replicative cycle of HIV is initiated by binding of HIV to cellular T4 receptors (Figure 1) (12),(13). Recent studies indicate that the viral envelope glycoprotein (gp120) binds to only a portion of the T4 molecule (14). At least one compound (AL 721) has been developed that might inhibit penetration without interfering with cellular function (15).

After penetration into the cell, the virus is uncoated and the HIV enzyme, reverse transcriptase (RT), makes a circular double stranded proviral DNA molecule coded by the viral RNA genome. A variety of different drugs such as suramin, azidothymidine, phosphonoformate, ansamycin and HPA-23 are capable of interrupting this specific step (Table 2).

New viral messenger RNA molecules (mRNA) are expressed by transcription of proviral DNA, and mRNA is then translated into different viral capsid proteins, envelope glycoproteins and enzymes (5),(16). Ribavirin may act at this stage of replication. The amount of protein synthesis seems to be regulated by a positive feedback regulation. The existence of transregulatory genes (tat, art) makes HIV more complex than other retroviruses which contain only gag, env and pol (17)-(19). In contrast to other unique HIV genes (3'-orf, sor) the genes tat and art are always necessary for efficient viral replication. The products of both genes accelerate overall viral gene expression; thus, compounds which inhibit these genes or their products might have a profound effect on viral replication.

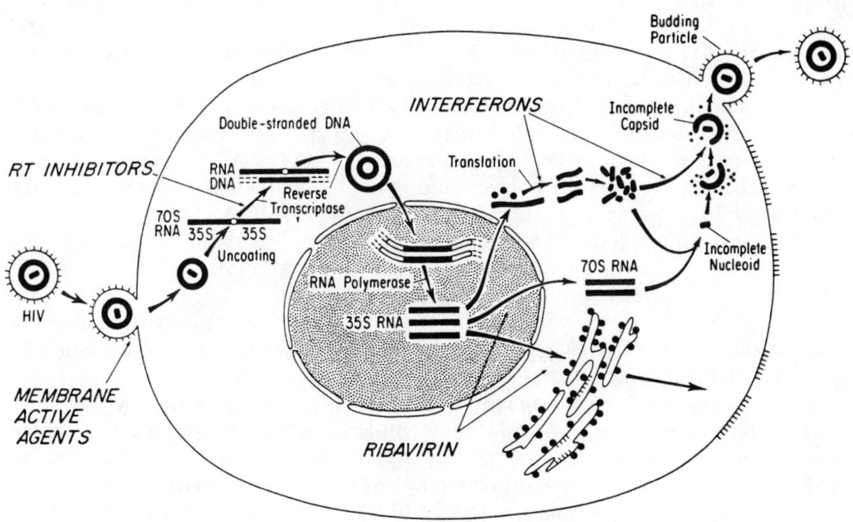

Figure 1. Replicative cycle of HIV.

Assembly followed by release of the viral particle are the last steps of viral replication. Interferons inhibit one or both of these steps in other retroviral systems but the precise mechanism of action against HIV is still unclear (20). Budding virus may be vulnerable to virus specific antibodies and sensitized lymphocytes which might prevent virus spread from cell to cell.

Azidothymidine (AZT)

Azidothymidine is a thymidine analogue (3'-azido-3'-deoxythymidine) which was formerly known as compound S or BW A509U. Azidothymidine has potent in vitro activity against two murine retroviruses, Friend leukemia virus and Harvey sarcoma virus (21), and can inhibit in vitro feline leukemia virus replication (22). Further in vitro studies have revealed a marked antiviral effect on HIV replication (23),(24) at concentrations that were non toxic for T-cells in tissue culture.

Cellular kinases phosphorylate AZT over several steps to AZT triphosphate which is inhibitory to viral reverse transcriptase, but not to cellular DNA polymerases (23),(24). AZT seems to act as an inhibitor of DNA chain elongation. Antiviral effect was demonstrated in vitro at concentrations between 0.05-10*u*M (24).

The terminal half-life in humans after infusion is about one hour; peak plasma concentrations of approximately 5*u*M can be achieved with intravenous (2.5 mg/kg AZT over one hour) and oral (5 mg/kg AZT) regimens. After oral dosage the bioavailability is about 60%. Virustatic concentrations of drug in vitro can be achieved in the cerebrospinal fluid.

During a six week phase I trial, 11 patients with AIDS and eight patients with AIDS related complex (ARC) were treated with different intravenous and oral regimens of AZT (25). The treatment was generally well tolerated. Patients receiving the highest dose regimen showed evidence of partial immune reconstitution and a possible virustatic effect (25). Fifteen of 19 patients had increases in numbers of circulating T4-lymphocytes and six patients who were previously anergic, showed positive skin test responses to at least one of four antigens. In two patients chronic fungal nailbed infections healed without specific antifungal treatment. Furthermore, patients gained an average of 2.2 kg of weight. This promising phase I study prompted a multicenter double-blind, placebo controlled trial. Between February 1986 and June 1986, 282 patients with AIDS who had had a recent episode of a *Pneumocystis carinii* pneumonia, or with ARC as manifested by oral thrush, fever, herpes zoster or significant weight loss were enrolled in the trial (26). The trial was halted in September when an evaluation by an independent Data Safety Monitoring Board found a significantly increased survival in patients receiving AZT. One of the 145 patients receiving AZT died compared to 16 of 137 patients receiving placebo. Although the data analysis is not yet complete, the drug seems to have increased the number of T4 cells. In addition, a subgroup of patients with neurologic disease showed improvement. The available data further suggest that HIV replication is not significantly reduced although the culture techniques used might not discriminate subtle reductions in viremia (26).

The most common side effect was megaloblastic anemia and 40 of the 145 AZT recipients required blood transfusions compared to 11 patients from the placebo group. Another relatively frequent side effect was mild headache. The effectiveness of AZT was thus only established in a particular subgroup of individuals with HIV infection. Possible long-term toxic effects of AZT, and the questions of long-term efficacy remain to be elucidated in future studies. The approval process for AZT is underway at the Food and Drug Administration, and the drug will probably be licensed in early 1987. Until AZT is commercially available Burroughs Wellcome supplies the drug free of charge to patients with a recent episode of *Pneumocystis carinii* pneumonia.

Other Nucleoside Derivatives

Recent in vitro studies showed that purine (adenosine, guanosine, inosine) and pyrimidine (cytidine and thymidine) analogues inhibit HIV replication substantially. The active antiviral portion of the compound is coupled to the ribose moiety in a 2', 3'-dideoxy configuration. To date, the exact mechanism of action is unclear, but an inhibitory effect on reverse transcriptase is most likely (27).

Phosphonoformate

Trisodium phosphonoformate hexahydrate (foscarnet, PFA) was first synthesized in 1924 (Tables 2,3). It has been used in Sweden in topical form for mucocutaneous *Herpes simplex* virus infections since 1980 (28).

Phosphonoformate is structurally similar to pyrophosphate and inhibits viral DNA polymerases of herpes viruses (*Herpes simplex* virus, cytomegalovirus (CMV), Epstein-Barr virus) as well as the RNA polymerase of influenza virus at concentrations that do not inhibit cellular DNA polymerases (28)-(30).

To date, intravenous phosphonoformate has been utilized in uncontrolled trials in several immunocompromised patients with severe CMV infections (31),(32). Although there were suggestions that several of the patients benefited from the drug, properly controlled, large scale studies will be required before the utility of the drug in this setting is fully understood.

Phosphonoformate was also found to inhibit the reverse transcriptase of several retroviruses, including visna virus, Moloney murine leukemia virus, and avian myeloblastosis virus (33)-(35). Our group has shown that the RT-activity of HIV is inhibited by 50% at concentrations of 0.1*u*M and that RT-activity is completely inhibited at 5*u*M (36). In lymphoid cell cultures, a concentration of 132*u*M partially inhibited HIV replication with complete inhibition at 680*u*M. These concentrations are equivalent to the serum levels achieved in patients treated for severe CMV infections. At this concentration, we observed no marked negative effect on cell growth in vitro (36). An increase of the number of cells of the helper surface phenotype was observed in one in vitro study in which phosphonoformate was added to infected cells from patients with ARC or AIDS (37). Preliminary results from a phase I study in Europe suggest that PFA can cross the blood brain barrier and that it may be virostatic in vivo (38). Common side effects were phlebitis at sites of intravenous administration. Clinical trials are now underway in the United States.

Ribavirin

Ribavirin is a synthetic nucleoside derivative of the antibiotic pyrazomycin with a broad spectrum of activity in vitro against both DNA and RNA viruses (Tables 2,3) (39),(40). Ribavirin acts as an analogue of the nucleoside, guanosine. After intracellular phosphorylation, this compound interferes with the guanylation step for 5' capping of viral messenger RNA (39),(40). The antiviral affect can be inhibited by adding guanosine to infected cultures (39),(40).

In addition to inhibiting certain animal retroviruses, such as the Gross murine leukemia virus and the Rauscher murine leukemia virus, ribavirin temporarily inhibits replication of HIV in vitro at concentrations between 10-100*u*g/ml (39)-(41). In vitro experiments are, however, severely limited by the drug's cytotoxic effect on leukocytes at concentrations over 10*u*g/ml (unpublished observation). The drug can be administered to patients orally or intravenously. Ribavirin is excreted largely unmetabolized by renal mechanisms and the terminal half-life is approximately 24 hours. The drug is selectively concentrated in red blood cells ($t_{1/2}$ ~ 40 days) (39),(40). Preliminary studies suggest that the drug penetrates the blood brain barrier at least to some extent. (C. Crumpacker, personal communication). In early human trials the usual total daily dose was 1000 mg, given for five days. However, in trials in patients with advanced cancer much higher doses (up to 12 g/day) have been given (39). Because ribavirin shows a broad spectrum of antiviral activity in vitro, several clinical trials have been carried out for viral infections other than HIV. Unfortunately, the quality of design of many of these studies makes them difficult to interpret. Three double-blind trials with oral ribavirin have shown favorable results against measles (40).

Other trials have been conducted in patients with acute and chronic hepatitis, herpes genitalis, and herpes zoster. Results have been variable (39). Aerosolized ribavirin is beneficial in infants with respiratory syncytial viral infections. Symptoms in patients with upper respiratory influenza infections have also been reduced by aerosolized ribavirin (42),(43).

The drug has efficacy for Lassa fever, an often fatal arenavirus infection and is recommended for postexposure prophylaxis (45).

Although the drug shows considerable cytotoxicity in vitro, clinical studies have revealed relatively few side effects (39),

(40). Hemolytic anemia is the most serious reversible adverse reaction (44). At higher doses, CNS toxicity has also been encountered.

In a small phase I study, patients with AIDS and ARC were treated with varying oral doses of ribavirin. In this study the drug decreased the rate of isolation of HIV from peripheral blood. In addition, virostatic drug levels were achieved in the cerebrospinal fluid (45). Patients showed signs of immunologic improvement such as a rise of T4 cells and a return of proliferative responses to Con A. A larger placebo controlled multicenter study is currently underway.

Suramin

Suramin is the hexasodium salt derivative of naphthalene trisulfonic acid (46) (Tables 2,3). It was first produced in 1916 by the Bayer Company as an antiparasitic drug and is still widely used in Africa to treat trypanosomiasis and onchoncerciasis. The drug inhibits a variety of different enzymes of many organisms. Its inhibitory action on the reverse transcriptase of three murine retroviruses and avian myeloblastosis virus was first reported in 1979 by DeClercq (46). Suramin inhibits the reverse transcriptase of HIV and inhibits the replication of this virus in vitro at concentrations of greater than 50 *u*g/ml (47).

Suramin is usually given by a slow intravenous infusion over at least 20 minutes. Intramuscular injections are painful. Because of rare idiosyncratic anaphylactoid reactions (0.1-0.5%), patients should first receive a test dose of 200 mg (5),(48). The drug is strongly bound to plasma proteins and is slowly excreted through the kidneys with a half-life of 40 days (48). Suramin is extremely polar and does not penetrate the blood-brain-barrier. It is, therefore, not used in patients with trypanosomiasis of the central nervous system (48).

Early clinical trials with HIV infected individuals were designed to evaluate safety, pharmacokinetics, and possible efficacy of suramin over a limited time. Six patients with AIDS (Kaposi's sarcoma) and four with ARC were treated at the National Institute of Health for five weeks each receiving 1 gram of suramin each week (48). There was no apparent clinical or immunological improvement and virus replication was inhibited only temporarily during treatment. Side effects such as fever, skin rash, burning skin sensations, proteinuria and elevated liver enzymes were frequent but usually self-limited (48).

Therefore, several studies addressing the risk and benefit of the long-term use of suramin were initiated in 1985. In one study 12 patients with AIDS were treated with weekly maintenance doses of 500 mg after six weekly induction doses of 1 gram. HIV viremia was suppressed in three and significantly reduced in two of 11 evaluable patients. In the remaining six patients, however, suramin was not associated with HIV suppression although drug levels were adequate (49). There was only one patient with clinical improvement and no immunologic improvement was observed in the study population (49). In this and other studies, toxic side effects were very frequent and often severe. Side effects included malaise and fatigue (11/12); transient skin rash (10/12); fever (9/12); clinical adrenal insufficiency (2/12); moderate proteinuria (10/12); hepatic enzyme elevations (9/12); anemia (non hemolytic) (8/12); neutropenia (4/12); and thrombocytopenia (2/12) (49). In other studies severe side effects such as hepatic failure and agranulocytosis were also observed. Further clinical trials are, therefore, unlikely in the United States.

Other polyanionic compounds which are chemically related to suramin such as Evans blue, direct yellow 50 and congo red also appear to inhibit replication of HIV in vitro (50).

Antimoniotungstate (HPA-23)

HPA-23 is a condensed polyanion of ammonium 5-tungsto-2-antimoniate with a molecular weight of 6800 (51),(52). Several reports have shown a broad spectrum of activity against RNA and DNA viruses. Mice were partially protected from tumors or leukemias induced by Friend leukemia virus, a variant of a murine sarcoma virus, and the Moloney murine sarcoma virus (51). HPA-23 is a potent inhibitor of isolated preparations of HIV reverse transcriptase at concentrations of 30ug/ml (52). Despite the marked inhibition of HIV-RT only a weak reduction of viral replication was found in infected H9 cells by other investigators (50). The reason for this difference is unclear.

The drug has a short half-life ($t_{1/2}$ < 20 minutes) after intravenous bolus injection, and, therefore, infusions over three hours (generally 200 mg per day over 15 days) are preferred (53). Over 50 patients have received HPA-23 in France in uncontrolled trials. The drug suppressed virus growth in some patients at least during therapy, but the patients showed no clear clinical improvement (54). The same results seem to be occurring in ongoing trials in the United States (54).

Interferons

Interferon was discovered in 1957 by Isaacs and Lindenmann. Interferons are proteins induced by viral infection of mammalian cells which interfere with viral replication. Research in the following years indicated that different interferon types are produced by different cells during viral infections or in response to other stimuli, such as exposure to RNA polymers, bacteria or chemical substances (55).

Three major interferon types exist:

1. Interferon alpha (HuIFN-alpha) (virus induced leukocyte)
2. Interferon beta (HuIFN-beta) (virus induced fibroblast)
3. Interferon gamma (HuIFN-gamma) (immune)

Interferon-alpha and interferon-beta have a molecular weight of approximately 20,000 and contain 166 amino acids. Gamma interferon is an oligomer with a molecular weight of approximately 58,000 (20).

Table 2. In Vitro Activity of Antiviral Agents Against HIV

Name of Drug	Mode of Action	Inhibitory Concentration	References
Azidothymidine	RT*-Inhibition	0.05-10 *u*M	24, 25, 61
Phosphonoformate	RT-Inhibition	100-680 *u*M	36
Ribavirin	Inhibition of proviral DNA transcription?	10-100 *u*g/ml	39, 41
Suramin	RT-Inhibition	50-100 *u*g/ml	47, 48
Antimoniotungstate (HPA-23)	RT-Inhibition	?	50, 52
Interferon alpha	Inhibition of assembly and release?	4-256 U/ml	20, 57 56

*RT = Reverse Transcriptase

Interferon-alpha and interferon-beta inhibit replication of diverse types of viruses and have, therefore, been evaluated in several clinical studies (see below). Interferon-alpha and interferon-beta have a common cellular receptor, while interferon-gamma has a separate receptor and exhibits immunomodulatory functions as well as antiviral activity (20),(56).

After binding to cellular receptors, interferons induce the production of other proteins with antiviral activity. The predominant mechanisms of action differ from virus to virus and include inhibition of transcription, translation, assembly or release (2),(55),(56). In murine retrovirus infections, interferon mainly acts in the late stage of viral morphogenesis, e.g., assembly and release of mature viral particles.

We have studied the effects of recombinant interferon-alpha (Hoffmann-LaRoche) on the replication of HIV in vitro. Virus replication was completely inhibited at concentrations between

256 and 1024 U/ml and the drug showed a partial effect at concentrations of 4-64 U/ml (57). Pharmacokinetic data in humans show that after intramuscular injection of 36 x 10^6U IFN-alpha, serum interferon peak levels were approximately 200-400 U/ml; the serum $t_{1/2}$ is 1.5 to 4.5 hours and levels of approximately 10-20 U/ml remain after 24 hours (58). CSF penetration of interferons, however, is poor (20).

Several therapeutic or prophylactic clinical studies have shown beneficial effects of topical or parenteral interferon alpha preparations against a broad variety of viruses (rhinoviruses, *Herpes simplex*, cytomegalovirus, Epstein-Barr virus, hepatitis B virus, papillomaviruses) (20).

Table 3. Selected Properties of Compounds Active Against HIV in Clinical Studies

Name of Drug	Route of Administration	CSF-Penetration	Side Effects	Reference
Azidothymidine	Oral Intravenous	Yes	headache, leukopenia	25,26
Phosphonoformate	Intravenous	Some	rise in serum creatinine	32,38
Ribavirin	Oral, Intravenous	Yes	anemia	39,44,45
Suramin	Intravenous	No	fever, renal dysfunction	48,49
HPA-23	Intravenous	?	thrombocytopenia, liver dysfunction	5,53
Interferon-alpha	Intramuscular	Poor	fever, bone marrow suppression, neurologic symptoms	20

CSF = Cerebrospinal fluid

In preliminary trials, recombinant interferon-beta had less effect on HIV replication than interferon-alpha. Interferon-gamma was even less active than interferon-beta (K. Harthshorn, M.S. Hirsch, unpublished observations). The conclusions from a recent double-blind placebo controlled trial using different doses of interferon-alpha are expected in late 1986.

Other Compounds with Anti-HIV Activity

AL 721 is a lipid compound which extracts cholesterol from cellular membranes in vitro and in vivo (15). Treatment of infected H9 cells diminished infectivity of HIV. Preliminary reports from early human pharmacokinetic trials showed no apparent side effects at daily doses of 10-15 g (15). Clinical trials are underway in this country.

Ansamycin (rifabutine) is a rifamycin S derivative and inhibits reverse transcriptase of HIV. In vitro studies suggest that HIV replication is partly inhibited at concentrations of 0.2-0.5ug/ml (59). Ansamycin is presently being used as an investigational drug in AIDS patients with *Mycobacterium avium-intracellulare* infections.

Drug Combinations

We evaluated several combinations of drugs individually active against HIV. Synergistic effects could be seen with PFA and rIFN-alpha (60), PFA and ribavirin (M. Vogt, K. Harthshorn, unpublished data) and azidothymidine and rIFN-alpha (61). Multi-center clinical trials comparing AZT given alone or in combination with interferon are currently being planned. Not all drug combinations, however, act synergistically. Preliminary data suggest that antagonism is also possible (M. Vogt, unpublished data).

FUTURE DIRECTIONS

Over the past 24 months the number of agents with demonstrable activity against HIV in vitro has been growing at a relatively rapid pace. Although the activity of several of these agents against HIV was discovered as a result of previous experience with these agents in other viral systems, recent insights into the replicative mechanisms of HIV have provided the groundwork for a much more directed search for new antiviral compounds. As this understanding is broadened, it is likely that an increasing array of agents with anti-HIV activity in vitro will become available for clinical testing. New strategies for inhibiting HIV replication such as the development of agents which interfere with tat will possibly emerge from these basic studies. Furthermore, with an increased understanding of the mechanism of action of these agents, trials with rational combinations of agents with activity against different points in the replication process may be undertaken.

Greater knowledge is needed of those factors that regulate the state of HIV replication, and of the aspects of viral replication responsible for cytotoxicity. Understanding the mechanism responsible for the apparent relative sparing of HIV infected monocytes from cytopathic effects may provide new clues for anti-viral intervention. If the retroviral variant (HTLV-IV) recently isolated from West African prostitutes proves to be less pathogenic than HIV, as it appears to be, this may also provide new clues for the development of antiviral agents and/or vaccines (62).

Identification of patients early in the course of infection and at greatest risk for clinical progression should help in the selection of the most suitable candidates for antiviral intervention. In certain patients it may be necessary to combine immunomodulators to provide optimal benefit to the patient.

Although HIV is a newly described agent, progress in the understanding of the pathogenesis of AIDS, and of the molecular biology of the virus have contributed to the relatively rapid proliferation of candidate antiviral drugs for clinical testing. Recent coordinated efforts by the National Institutes of Allergy and Infectious Disease and the National Institutes of Health to develop new antiviral compounds, and to test these agents in well-designed clinical trials will hasten the time when questions regarding clinical benefits of drug therapy may be answered. These efforts can be sustained only if the current level of commitment by both governmental and industrial sources is maintained. With the current level of interest on the part of a large number of laboratories, there is every reason to hope that effective antiviral compounds will reach clinical application in the very near future.

ACKNOWLEDGMENT

Supported by NIH grants 37461 and the Mashud A. Mezerhane B fund; Markus Vogt is supported by the Swiss National Science Foundation.

REFERENCES

1. Gallo, R.C., Salahuddin, S.Z., Popovic, M., et al., Frequent detection and isolation of cytopathic retroviruses (HTLV-III) from patients with AIDS and at risk for AIDS. Science 224:500-503 (1984)

2. Barre-Sinoussi, F., Chermann, J.C., Rey, F., et al., Isolation of a T-lymphotropic retrovirus from a patient at risk for acquired immune deficiency syndrome. Science 220:868-871 (1983)

3. Gonda, M., Wong-Staal, F., Gallo, R.C., et al., Sequence homology and morphologic similarity of HTLV-III and visna virus, a pathogenic lentivirus. Science 227:173-177 (1985)

4. Coffin, J., Haase, A., Levy, J.A., et al., Human immunodeficiency viruses. Science 232:697 (1986)

5. Vogt, M., Hirsch, M.S., Prospects for the prevention and therapy of HTLV-III infections. Rev Infect Dis 8:991-1000 (1986)

6. Ho, D.D., Rota, T.R., Schooley, R.T., et al., Isolation of HTLV-III from cerebrospinal fluid and neural tissues of patients with neurologic syndromes related to the acquired immunodeficiency syndrome. N Engl J Med 313:1493-1497 (1985)

7. Koenig, S., Gendelman, H.E., Orenstein, J.M., et al., Detection of AIDS virus in macrophages in brain tissue from AIDS patients with encephalopathy. Science 233:1089-1093 (1986)

8. Shaw, G.M., Harper, M.E., Hahn, B.H., et al., HTLV-III infection in brains of children and adults with AIDS encephalopathy. Science 227:177-182 (1985)

9. Resnick, L., DiMarzo-Veronese, F., Schuepbach, J., et al., Intra-blood-brain-barrier synthesis of HTLV-III specific IgG in patients with neurologic symptoms associated with AIDS or AIDS related complex. N Engl J Med 313:1498-1504 (1985)

10. Shaw, G.M., Hahn, B.H., Arya, S.K., et al., Molecular characterization of human T-cell leukemia (lymphotropic) virus type III in the acquired immune deficiency syndrome. Science 226:1165-1171 (1984)

11. Ho, D.D., Rota, T.R., Hirsch, M.S., Infection of monocyte/macrophages by human T-lymphotropic virus type III. J Clin Invest 77:1712-1715 (1986)

12. Dalgleish, A.G., Beverly, P.C.L., Clapham, P.R., et al., The CD4 (T4) antigen is an essential component of the receptor of the AIDS retrovirus. Nature 312:763-767 (1984)

13. Klatzmann, D., Champagne, E., Chamaret, S., T-lymphocyte T4 molecule behaves as the receptor for human retrovirus LAV. Nature 312:767-768 (1984)

14. McDougal, J.S., Kennedy, M.S., Sligh, J.M., et al., Binding of HTLV-III/LAV to T4+ T cells by a complex of the 110K viral protein and the T4 molecule. Science 231:382-385 (1986)

15. Sarin, P.S., Gallo, R.C., Scheer, D.I., et al., Effect of a novel compound (AL 712) on HTLV-III infectivity in vitro. N Engl J Med 313:1289-1290 (1985)

16. Hirsch, M.S., Kaplan, J.C., Prospects of therapy for infections with human T-lymphotropic virus type III. Ann Intern Med 103:750-755 (1985)

17. Rosen, C.A., Sodroski, J.G., Goh, W.C., et al., Post-transcriptional regulation accounts for the transactivation of the human T-lymphotropic virus type III. Nature 319:555-559 (1986)

18. Sodroski, J., Goh, W.C., Rosen, C., et al., A second post - transcriptional trans-activator gene required for HTLV-III replication. Nature 321:412-417 (1986)

19. Chen, I.S.Y., Regulation of AIDS virus expression. Cell 47:1-2 (1986)

20. Hartshorn, K.L., Hirsch, M.S., Interferons, In: Antimicrobial Agents Annual I (Peterson, P.K., Verhoef, J., eds) Elsevier Science Publishers, Amsterdam, p 344-357 (1986)

21. Furman, P.A., St. Clair, M., Weinhold, K., et al., Selective inhibition of HTLV-III by BW A509U. Interscience Conference Antimicrobial Agents Chemotherapy, Minneapolis, Minn (1985)

22. Hardy, W.D., Zuckerman, E.E., Nusinoff-Lehrmann, S., et al., Antiviral effects of BW A509U against a naturally occurring feline acquired immune deficiency syndrome (FAIDS)-inducing retrovirus. Interscience Conference Antimicrobial Agents Chemotherapy, Minneapolis, Minn. (1985)

23. Furman, P.A., Fyfe, J.A., St. Clair, M., et al., Phosphorylation of 3'-azido-3'-deoxythymidine and selective interaction of the 5'-triphosphate with human immunodeficiency virus reverse transcriptase. Proc Natl Acad Sci USA 83:8333-8337 (1986)

24. Mitsuya, H., Weinhold, K.J., Furman, P.A., et al., 3'-Azido-3'-deoxythymidine (BW A509U): An antiviral agent that inhibits the infectivity and cytopathic effect of human T-lymphotropic virus type III/lymphadenopathy-associated virus in vitro. Proc Natl Acad Sci USA 82:7096-7100 (1985)

25. Yarchoan, R., Klecker, R.W., Weinhold, K.J., et al., Administration of 3'-azido-3'-deoxythymidine, an inhibitor of HTLV-III replication, to patients with AIDS and AIDS-related-complex. Lancet 1:575-580 (1986)

26. Barnes, D.M., Promising results halt trial of anti-AIDS drug. Science 234:15-16 (1986)

27. Mitsuya, H., Broder, S., Inhibition of the in vitro infectivity and cytopathic effect of human T-lymphotropic virus type III/lymphadenopathy-associated virus (HTLV-III/LAV) by 2'-3'-dideoxynucleosides. Proc Natl Acad Sci USA 83:1911-1915 (1986)

28. Oberg, B., Antiviral effects of phosphonoformate (PFA, foscarnet sodium). Pharmac Ther 19:387-415 (1983)

29. Larsson, A., Oberg, B., Selective inhibition of herpesvirus DNA synthesis by foscarnet. Antiviral Research 1:55-62 (1981)

30. Margalith, M., Manor, D., Usieli, V., et al., Phosphonoformate inhibits synthesis of Epstein-Barr virus (EBV) capsid antigen and transformation of human cord blood lymphocytes by EBV. Virology 102:226-230 (1980)

31. Apperley, J.F., Marcus, R.E., Goldman, J.M., et al., Foscarnet for cytomegalovirus pneumonitis. Lancet 1:1151 (1985)

32. Klintmalm, G., Lonnqvist, B., Oberg, B., et al., Intravenous foscarnet for the treatment of severe cytomegalovirus infection in allograft recipients. Scand J Infect Dis 17:157-163 (1985)

33. Sundquist, B., Larner, E., Phosphonoformate inhibition of visna virus replication. J Virol 30:847-851 (1979)

34. Margalith, M., Falk, H., Panet, A., Differential inhibition of DNA polymerase and RNase H activities of the reverse transcriptase by phosphonoformate. Molec Cell Biochem 43:97-103 (1982)

35. Eriksson, B., Stening, G., Oberg, B., Inhibition of reverse transcriptase activity of avian myeloblastosis virus by pyrophosphate analogues. Antiviral Res 2:81-95 (1982)

36. Sandstrom, E.G., Kaplan, J.C., Byington, R.E., Inhibition of human T-cell lymphotropic virus type III in vitro by phosphonoformate. Lancet 1:1480-1482 (1985)

37. Beldekas, J.C., Levy, E.M., Black, P., In vitro effect of foscarnet on expansion of T-cells from people with LAS and AIDS. Lancet 2:1128-1129 (1985)

38. Farthing, C.F., Dalgleish, A.G., Clark, A.L., et al., Pilot study on the treatment of AIDS and ARC patients with intravenous foscarnet (Abstract). International Conference on Acquired Immunodeficiency Syndrome (AIDS), Paris (1986)

39. Chang, T.W., Heel, R.C., Ribavirin and inosiplex: a review of their present status in viral diseases. Drugs 22:111-128 (1981)

40. Gilbert, B.E., Knight, V., Biochemistry and clinical applications of ribavirin. Antimicrob Agents Chemother 30:201-205 (1986)

41. McCormick, J.B., Getchell, J.P., Mitchell, S.W., et al., Ribavirin suppresses replication of lymphadenopathy associated virus in cultures of human adult T lymphocytes. Lancet 2: 1367-1369 (1984)

42. Hall, C.B., McBride, J.T., Walsh, E.E., et al., Aerosolized ribavirin treatment of infants with respiratory syncytial viral infection. N Engl J Med 308:1443-1447 (1983)

43. Knight, V., McClung, H.W., Wilson, S.Z., et al., Ribavirin small-particle aerosol treatment of influenza. Lancet 2:945-949 (1981)

44. McCormick, J.B., King, I.J., Webb, P.A., Lassa fever. Effective therapy with ribavirin. N Engl J Med 314:20-26 (1986)

45. Crumpacker, C., Bubley, G., Hussey, S., et al., Evaluation of oral ribavirin therapy on immunologic and viral parameters in AIDS and ARC. International Conference on Acquired Immunodeficiency Syndrome (AIDS), Paris (1986)

46. DeClercq, E., Suramin: A potent inhibitor of the reverse transcriptase of RNA tumor viruses. Cancer Letters 8:9-22 (1979)

47. Mitsuya, H., Popovic, M., Yarchoan, R., et al., Suramin protection of T-cells in vitro against infectivity and cytopathic effect of HTLV-III. Science 226:172-174 (1984)

48. Broder, S., Yarchoan, R., Collins, J.M., et al., Effects of suramin on HTLV-III/LAV infection presenting as Kaposi's sarcoma or AIDS related complex: Clinical pharmacology and suppression of virus replication in vivo. Lancet 2:627-630 (1985)

49. Levine, A.M., Gill, P.S., Cohen, J., et al., Suramin antiviral therapy in the acquired immunodeficiency syndrome. Ann Intern Med 105:32-37 (1986)

50. Balzarini, J., Mitsuya, H., DeClercq, E., et al., Comparative inhibitory effects of suramin and other selected compounds on the infectivity and replication of human T-cell lymphotropic virus (HTLV-III)/lymphadenopathy associated virus (LAV). Int J Cancer 37:451-457 (1986)

51. Jasmin, C., Chermann, J.C., Herve, G., et al., In vivo inhibition of murine leukemia and sarcoma viruses by the heteropolyanion 5-tungsto-2-antimoniate. J Natl Cancer Inst 53: 469-474 (1974)

52. Dormont, D., Spire, B., Barre-Sinoussi, F., Inhibition of RNA-dependent DNA polymerases of AIDS and SAIDS retroviruses by HPA-23 (Ammonium-21-tungsto-9-antimoniate). Ann Inst Pasteur/Virol 136E:75-83 (1985)

53. Rozenbaum, W., Dormont, D., Spire, B., et al., Antimoniotungstate (HPA 23) treatment of three patients with AIDS and one with prodrome. Lancet 1:450-451 (1985)

54. Norman, C., AIDS therapy: New push for clinical trials. Science 230:1355-1357 (1985)

55. Baron, S., Grossberg, S.E., Klimpel, G.R., et al., Immune and interferon systems. In: "Antiviral agents and viral diseases of man", (Galasso, G.J., et al., eds), 2nd edition, Raven Press, New York, p 123-178 (1984)

56. Sen, G.C., Mechanisms of interferon action. Prog Nucleic Acid Res Mol Biol 27:105-156 (1982)

57. Ho, D.D., Hartshorn, K.L., Rota, T.R., et al., Recombinant human interferon alpha suppresses HTLV-III replication in vitro. Lancet 1:602-604 (1985)

58. Wills, R.J., Dennis, S., Spiegel, H.E., et al., Interferon kinetics and adverse reactions after intravenous, intramuscular, and subcutaneous injection. Clin Pharmacol Ther 35: 722-727 (1984)

59. Anand, R., Moore, J., Feorino, P., Rifabutine inhibits HTLV-III. Lancet 1:97-98 (1986)

60. Hartshorn, K.L., Sandstrom, E.G., Neumeyer, D., et al., Synergistic inhibition of human T-cell lymphotropic virus type III replication in vitro by phosphonoformate and recombinant alpha-A interferon. Antimicrob Agents Chemother 30:189-191 (1986)

61. Hartshorn, K.L., Vogt, M.W., Chou, T-C., et al., Synergistic inhibition of human immunodeficiency virus in vitro by azidothymidine and recombinant interferon alpha-A. Antimicrob Agents Chemother (In press)

62. Kanki, P.J., Barin, F., M'Boup, S., et al., New human T-lymphotropic retrovirus related to simian T-lymphotropic virus type III (STLV-III agm). Science 232:238-243 (1986)

51
Use of Vaccination in Prevention of HIV Infection

Gordon R. Dreesman, Jorg W. Eichberg, Tran C. Chanh, Patrick Kanda, Ronald C. Kennedy

Acquired immune deficiency syndrome or AIDS was first recognized as a new disease associated with the gay population in 1981 (1)-(3). Approximately 2-1/2 years later a family of closely related viruses known as human T-lymphotropic virus type III (HTLV-III) (4),(5), lymphadenopathy-associated virus (LAV) (6) and AIDS-associated retrovirus (ARV) (7) was isolated, and shown to be the etiologic agent. In a short time period, these viruses were cloned (8) and the nucleotide sequences of the RNA genomes determined (9)-(12). This family of viruses recently has been collectively referred to as human immunodeficiency virus (HIV).

Two observations have clearly established that this new infection poses a major problem of worldwide public health significance. First, more than 20,000 people have been diagnosed with AIDS in the United States (13). Furthermore, the cumulative mortality rate of AIDS two or more years after diagnosis has been estimated to be approximately 85% (14). Second, and of much greater concern, serosurveys indicate that between one and two million people have circulating antibody to the virus in the United States alone (13). The most important route of spread for the virus is sexual contact, both heterosexual and male homosexual, both in Africa (15) and the United States (16). DeGruttola and coworkers (17) present a strong argument that the potential magnitude of the epidemic is unknown, and thus current predictions may seriously underestimate the scope of this disease. In fact, results of the first three months of testing of new military recruits show a confirmed HIV antibody positivity rate of 1.4 per thousand (Col. W. Bancroft, personal communication).

The above considerations indicate the paramount importance of developing control measures. It has been suggested that changes in sexual behavior may be the only way to retard spread of HIV at present (17). In the absence of effective antiviral drugs, research in vaccine development becomes an especially high priority to protect the general population not yet exposed to HIV.

SPECIAL CONCERNS IN DEVELOPMENT OF AN HIV VACCINE

The first essential step in the development of a safe effective vaccine for a given disease is to find a relevant animal model. This model was established for HIV infection when it was shown that lymphadenopathy syndrome and seroconversion to anti-HIV took place in chimpanzees that had been inoculated with plasma derived from human AIDS and lymphadenopathy patients (18). The susceptibility of chimpanzees to HIV infection was soon confirmed by other investigators (19)-(22).

The process of generating a safe effective HIV vaccine for protection of humans presents several major challenges. Two critical questions have not as yet been answered with certainty. The first question deals with transfer of the virus. Present epidemiologic observations show that the virus is most efficiently spread from an infected individual to a susceptible host by exchange of contaminated blood or blood products. However, it has not been conclusively established whether the primary infection takes place by transmission of cell-free plasma or by cell-to-cell transmission (23). In the absence of an unequivocal answer to this question, it is reasonable to assume that a potential vaccine should be able to induce both a strong humoral and cellular immunity to HIV. The second major question arises from the considerable genomic diversity of HIV (24),(25); basically, is it possible for any vaccine to induce a solid protective immunity to HIV? Of greatest concern is that the most divergent part of the genomes are found clustered within the major envelope gene product of HIV. In this regard, HIV loosely resembles the ungulate lenti retroviruses, particularly visna virus and equine infectious anemia virus, which can mutate within a host, escape immune surveillance and continue a progressive infection (24)-(26).

Several laboratories have reported that sera obtained from AIDS patients or patients with AIDS related complex (ARC), contain specific viral neutralizing activity in vitro (27)-(31). Even in the presence of high titered antibody activity to envelope glycoprotein, neutralizing titers are generally low. Presumably, infection occurred in these patients before development of neutralizing antibody. Consequently, the protective capabilities of preexisting neutralizing antibody, antedating viral exposure, is unknown. To date, the structure and precise location of HIV associated viral neutralizing epitopes have not yet been identified. However, we have recently shown that antibody induced in rabbits in response to synthetic peptides 735-752 (gp41) and peptide 503-532 (gp120) do have the capacity to neutralize HIV infectivity in vitro (32). Obviously, the antigenic determinants which induce protective antibodies will have to be defined before an effective vaccine against HIV can be developed.

A number of special challenges have to be considered in the development of a vaccine to protect against HIV infections. The major antigenic determinants associated with the induction of neutralizing antibodies to a number of retroviruses appear to reside within the surface envelope glycoproteins (33)-(38). The env gene product of HIV is synthesized as a polyprotein precursor and is subsequently glycosylated within infected cells. This glycosylated polyprotein of HIV with a molecular weight of 160 Kd (gp160) (for HTLV-III) is processed into an amino terminus subunit, gp120, and a carboxyl transmembrane subunit, gp41 (24). The env gene product for LAV is referred to as gp150 and the amino terminus subunit as gp110. For the remainder of this chapter, we will refer to the gp160/gp150 and the gp120/ gp110 envelope glycoproteins as gp160 and gp120, respectively. The envelop glycoproteins of HIV have been demonstrated to be the most immunogenic component (39)-(41). The gp120 subunit of HIV is also required for infection of susceptible cells and mediates attachment of the virus to the CD4 receptor of the T4 positive lymphocytes (42).

A second major surface glycoprotein associated with the retrovirus envelope is a hydrophobic transmembrane glycoprotein, which in most retroviruses anchors the envelope glycoprotein to the virus particle (36). In HIV, the transmembrane glycoprotein has been identified as the carboxyl terminus of the gp160 precursor glycoprotein with a molecular weight of 41 Kd (12),(43). The transmembrane protein is of interest as a possible vaccine candidate since Fischinger and coworkers (33) have reported that the transmembrane protein of Friend murine leukemia virus induces neutralizing antibodies. Although HIV exhibits a wide degree of genomic diversity (24),(25), the gp41 subunit is an attractive vaccine candidate since its amino acid sequence is relatively constant among the different isolates (44). In keeping with this observation, Thiel and coworkers (45) have demonstrated that the most conserved epitopes of the retrovirus group are associated with the transmembrane protein.

Of added potential importance to vaccine development, both the retrovirus envelope glycoprotein and transmembrane protein are found on the surface of infected cells (46), and as such, represent a target for immune surveillance (47). Furthermore, we have recently identified HIV epitopes associated with gp120 and gp41 on the surface of chronically infected A3.01 and HUT-78 cells (48),(49).

Both envelope glycoproteins, gp120 and gp41, are heavily glycosylated; for example, gp120 contains 32 potential glycosylation sites (9),(12). The polypeptide backbone of gp120 has an approximate molecular weight of 88 Kd (39)-(43). Presently, the role of the carbohydrate moieties in inducing immunity, in maintaining critical secondary structures or possibly blocking potential neutralizing epitopes on the polypeptide backbone is unknown. However, our laboratories have recently shown that antibody prepared to non-glycosylated synthetic peptide analogues of gp41 and gp120 respectively, each neutralize HIV infectivity in vitro (32).

VACCINE CANDIDATES

A number of HIV vaccine candidates will be discussed in this review (Table 1). Each method of vaccine preparation has been successful for one or more viral diseases (50).

Table 1. Vaccine Candidates for Induction of Protective HIV Immunity

Vaccine Candidates
Inactivated Virus (Native)
Virus Subunit Vaccines
Envelope glycoprotein (gp120, gp41, or gp120-gp41 complex)
Live Attenuated Virus
Natural variants
Engineered variants
Recombinant Live Virus Vaccine
Genetically Engineered Recombinant Protein
Synthetic Peptides
Anti-Idiotype Internal Image Antibodies

Inactivated Virus and Subunit Vaccines

The vaccine which would be easiest to produce against HIV would be a native inactivated virus. However, a number of potential difficulties and dangers mitigate against the production of an inactivated HIV vaccine. Typically, a relatively large antigenic mass is required and, therefore, a huge quantity of virus would have to be produced, with the potential risk of contamination with live viruses and/or foreign proteins. In addition, a purification procedure is usually employed in the preparation of inactivated viral vaccines, which is of concern since it has been noted that the major gp120 subunit is extremely labile (39). Furthermore, presently all HIV stocks are grown in continuous malignant lymphoblastic cell lines (24), while most approved virus vaccine stocks are propagated in human diploid cells (50). Most importantly, an inactivated whole virus vaccine would contain viral nucleic acid whose potential activity in the human host is unknown. Alternatively, a purified subunit vaccine without nucleic acid could be considered. Purified retrovirus glycoproteins linked to transmembrane protein have been shown to induce protective immunity both in mice (51) and in cats (52). It is anticipated, however, that the cost of producing a subunit vaccine for HIV would be prohibitive.

Live Attenuated Virus Vaccine

A family of viruses closely related to HIV has been isolated from healthy,wild-caught African green monkeys (53) and from captive, ill rhesus macaque monkeys (54). These viruses have been designated the simian T-lymphotropic viruses (STLV-III). Recent studies by Kanki and coworkers (55) have also described a new human T-lymphotropic virus isolated from apparently healthy people in West Africa. The virus is referred to as HTLV-IV. Sera obtained from individuals infected with HTLV-IV strongly reacted with both HTLV-IV and STLV-III and weakly cross-reacted with HIV (HTLV-III) antigens. Thus, nonpathogenic virus isolates are available for study and can be considered as future vaccine candidates. Certainly the virology, immunobiology and genetic stability of these agents require further evaluation. In addition, nonmalignant cell culture systems for virus propagation should be developed and examined.

Because of the difficulties mentioned above with use of conventional vaccine approaches, along with such practical issues, as safety and economy, greater impetus has been given to a number of molecular engineering approaches. These include recombinant live virus vaccines, genetically engineered recombinant proteins and synthetic peptides. The present state-of-development for each of these approaches is summarized.

Recombinant Live Virus Vaccines

A number of viral proteins have been produced by inserting defined viral gene sequences into recombinant vaccinia virus (56),(57), *Herpes simplex* virus (58) or adenovirus (59). Two groups of investigators have reported the expression of HIV (HTLV-III) env gene products by a recombinant vaccinia virus (60),(61). In the first study, the complete gp160 was inserted into vaccinia vectors and the env gene product was synthesized, glycosylated, processed and transported (60). Both the gp120 and gp41 subunits were identified. However, a single inoculation of this construct into mice induced only a gp120 antibody response. It is unclear why an anti-gp41 response was not induced. Since a neutralizing epitope is associated with gp41, it might be advantageous to produce a specific response directed against directed against gp41. In the second study, gp150 of LAV was inserted into vaccinia virus, and both gp120 (gp110 for LAV) and gp41 were produced (61). Mice produced an antibody response to both gp120 and gp41, and in addition, seven of eight vaccinated macaques developed a specific anti-HIV gp160 response. Together these data indicate the feasibility of using vaccinia virus recombinants to induce an immune response to HIV. However, as emphasized by Hu and coworkers (61), the use of live vaccinia virus in individuals who are in high risk groups and have already been infected with the virus would be contraindicated because of the potential suppression of their immune system.

Recombinant Protein Vaccines

A number of research groups have begun investigation of vaccines produced by molecular engineering techniques. As outlined above, most, if not all, of these studies involve the production of recombinant proteins containing sequences derived from the precursor gp160 subunit. A precedent for this approach has been the successful use of a recombinant protein as a vaccine against hepatitis B virus (62),(63).

Chang and coworkers (64) have developed 20 recombinant clones expressed in *Escherichia coli*. Each specified a fusion protein containing HIV (HTLV-III) encoded peptides that reacted immunologically with antibodies in sera from AIDS patients. These polypeptides were derived from the gag, pol and env-lor coding regions. Results of this study indicate that antibody is produced to a number of distinct viral epitopes. A protein encoded by the portion of env-lor region, referred to as ORF clone 120, reacts with sera obtained from most, if not all, AIDS patients. This may represent a logical vaccine candidate. Crowl and coworkers (65) inserted a large segment of the env gene into *Escherichia coli*. A protein with a molecular weight of 68 Kd was produced along with a number of smaller polypeptides. The 68 Kd protein contains amino acid residues 44-640 of gp160 which encompasses regions from both gp120 and gp41. This protein has vaccine potential in that it contains hydrophilic regions which are relatively well conserved among different isolates of HIV.

Synthetic Peptide Vaccines

If the major gp160 epitopes which induce protective antibodies are linear, it would be advantageous to utilize a synthetic peptide approach for production of a vaccine Our laboratories have recently pursued this avenue. These studies have examined potential neutralizing epitopes associated with the HIV envelope glycoprotein utilizing synthetic peptide methodology. We used a computer program that utilizes the parameters of hydrophilic values developed by Hopp and Woods (66) to predict possible antigenic determinants present on the envelope glycoprotein gp120 of three virus isolates (67). The rationale behind this selection was that peak hydrophilic areas have been shown to coincide with known antigenic determinants (66). Putative antigenic determinants on the precursor envelope glycoprotein were identified as hydrophilic areas containing potential beta turn regions.

Based on computer analysis, a highly hydrophilic area containing predicted beta turns was associated with residues 735-752 from gp41 of HIV (67). This region also possessed a relatively invariant stretch of amino acids when comparing the predicted amino acid sequences of HIV isolates. Synthetic peptide 735-752 coupled to keyhole limpet hemocyanin was used to immunize rabbits. The resulting rabbit anti-peptide antisera reacted with lysates of HIV infected cells and more specifically recognized the precursor envelope glycoprotein (gp160) of HIV (68). Some, but not all, human sera positive for antibody to HIV also reacted with this peptide. These findings indicate that synthetic peptides can be utilized to induce an immune response directed against a native envelope glycoprotein epitope of HIV.

Antisera produced in rabbits against the 735-752 peptide, along with a peptide corresponding to the carboxyl terminal peptide sequences of gp120, including some residues from the amino terminus of gp41 (amino acid sequences 503-532), have been shown to neutralize HIV infectivity in vitro (32). These data suggest that at least two epitopes associated with gp120 and gp41 subunits can induce neutralizing activity. Based on our observations that a gp41 synthetic peptide induced neutralizing activity against HIV (32), we have begun immunizing chimpanzees with peptide 735-752 conjugated to keyhole limpet hemocyanin. The chimpanzees have responded with a vigorous response to gp160 as determined by radioimmunoprecipitation and to HIV infected cell lysates by ELISA. These animals will soon be challenged with an infectious HIV inoculum. If the animals are indeed protected in this early study, we will be able to ascertain the feasibility of developing an effective peptide vaccine against HIV.

Synthetic peptides are usually weak immunogens and, therefore, must be incorporated with carrier proteins and/or adjuvants. However, this difficulty has recently been circumvented. DiMarchi (69) induced protection in cattle against a challenge of infectious foot-and-mouth disease virus (FMDV) by inoculation of two distinct synthetic peptides free of any carrier protein. These two peptide sequences of FMDV VP1 were linked together by cysteine residues at, or near, each terminus for the purpose of polymerization. These two peptides were separated by a Pro-Pro-Ser amino acid sequence to increase the likelihood of interaction between the two sites through a presumed induction of a secondary structural turn. The resultant 40-residue peptide, absorbed to aluminum hydroxide-saponin adjuvant, induced full protective immunity. A similar approach has been successful in inducing an immune response to hepatitis B surface antigen (HBsAg) in mice (70).

A defined structure, termed an immunostimulatory complex (ISCOM), has been recently described (71). Briefly, surface glycoproteins derived from enveloped viruses are solubilized with detergent and then complexed with glycoside to form ISCOMs. In these micelle-like structures the hydrophilic antigenic portion of the envelope glycoprotein is present on the exterior of the particles (71). Osterhaus and coworkers (72) reported that ISCOMs containing feline retrovirus subunits elicited a solid protective immune response in cats. These observations suggest that presentation of recombinant polypeptides or synthetic peptides incorporated in micelles (70) or ISCOM structures (71),(72) may provide a valuable approach in the development of a safe effective vaccine against HIV.

Anti-Idiotype Internal Image Vaccine

Another possible approach to vaccine development which has recently gained popularity is the use of anti-idiotype antibodies (anti-Id) for inducing protective viral immunity (73),(74). Anti-Id alone are capable of mimicking antigen since anti-Id and antigen bind to the V region and the combining site of an antibody, the idiotope and the paratope sites, respectively. If the idiotope and paratope are the same site on the antibody, then anti-Id and antigen should have a similar conformation. It is the idiotope on the anti-Id (Ab-2) that is the basis of the vaccine potential of anti-Id antibodies (75).

We have shown that if anti-Id is given prior to immunization of mice with HBsAg, an enhanced humoral and cellular anti-HBs response occurs (76),(77). More recently it has also been demonstrated that anti-Id alone may serve as an alternate vaccine for hepatitis B virus (HBV). Chimpanzees immunized with anti-Id were protected from experimental infection with HBV (78). Because chimpanzees are the relevant animal model for human HBV (as well as for HIV) infections, it follows that anti-Id may represent a viable alternative as a vaccine candidate in humans.

DEVELOPMENT OF PEDIGREED AND STANDARDIZED INOCULA

For the proper evaluation of AIDS related vaccines, immunoglobulins and inactivating agents, it will be necessary to have standardized HIV inocula for efficacy testing. These standardized inocula should be uniformly infectious, but not so virulent that they would overwhelm the system and mask any protective effect. Such standardized inocula have been invaluable in assessing HBV related vaccines and inactivation procedures. The goal would be to establish one or more infectious inocula for which infectivity titers are established both in vitro and in vivo. The standardized inocula would be centrally stored and made available to investigators throughout the world. Additional experience gained through continued use of this stock would permit a constant upgrading of their validity. The cumulative experience with the HBV standardized inocula has validated this approach and has enhanced the utilization of chimpanzees in efficacy studies; therefore, the number of animals required for each experiment has decreased. It is probable that the development of standardized HIV inocula will be a collaborative effort among several government organizations.

CONCLUSION

Recent epidemiologic observations clearly show that AIDS is a lethal sexually transmitted disease. The high mortality and rapid spread of HIV to as many as two or more million people in the United States alone clearly indicate that control measures are of paramount importance. Vaccine development research is an extremely high priority to protect the population who have not yet been exposed to the virus. Concern over the potential lethality of the etiologic viral agent makes development of a conventional vaccine (inactivated virions, purified virion subunits, or a live attenuated virus) less attractive than some newer vaccine approaches. These innovative methods include the use of recombinant live viruses, genetically engineered recombinant proteins, synthetic peptides and internal image anti-idiotype antibodies. The first order of business in the development of an effective HIV vaccine will be to define the viral epitopes which elicit neutralizing antibodies. Later, the candidate vaccine preparations will have to be tested for induction of protection in a susceptible non-human host, the chimpanzee.

The great urgency of the work clearly warrants testing each of the above strategies simultaneously. Ideally, parallel studies by a number of research groups will shorten the time period required to develop an effective first-generation vaccine. It would be highly advantageous to develop a pedigreed and standardized HIV challenge inocula. This would facilitate a fair comparison of the various vaccine candidates, and enable a reasonable decision as to which should be developed further. Hopefully, these studies will bear fruit soon so that an effective and economical vaccine will be available in the near future.

ACKNOWLEDGMENTS

This work was supported by grants R01-HL-32505, R01-AI-23472, U01-AI-23619 and R23-AI-22307 from the National Institutes of Health.

REFERENCES

1. Gottlieb, M.S., Schroff, R., Schanker, H.M., et al., *Pneumocystis carinii* pneumonia and mucosal candidiasis in previously healthy homosexual men: evidence of a new acquired cellular immunodeficiency. N Engl J Med 305:1425-1431 (1981)

2. Masur, H., Michelis, M.A., Greene, J.B., et al., An outbreak of community-acquired *Pneumocystis carinii* pneumonia. Initial manifestations of cellular dysfunction. N Engl J Med 305:1431-1438 (1981)

3. Siegal, F.P., Lopez, C., Hammer, G.S., et al., Severe acquired immunodeficiency in male homosexuals manifested by chronic perianal ulcerative *Herpes simplex* lesions. N Engl J Med 305:1439-1444 (1981)

4. Gallo, R.C., Salahuddin, S.Z., Popovic, M., et al., Frequent detection and isolation of cytopathic retroviruses (HTLV-III) from patients with AIDS and at a risk for AIDS. Science 224: 500-503 (1984)

5. Popovic, M., Sarngadharan, M.G., Read, E., et al., Detection, isolation, and continuous production of cytopathic retroviruses (HTLV-III) from patients with AIDS and pre-AIDS. Science 224:497-500 (1984)

6. Barre-Sinoussi, F., Cherman, C., Axler-Blin, C., et al., Isolation of a T-lymphotropic retrovirus from a patient at risk of acquired immune deficiency syndrome (AIDS). Science 220:868-871 (1983)

7. Levy, J.A., Hoffman, A.D., Kramer, S.M., et al., Isolation of lymphocytopathic retrovirus from San Francisco patients with AIDS. Science 225:840-842 (1984)

8. Shaw, G.M., Hahn, B.H., Arya, S.K., et al., Molecular characterization of human T-cell leukemia (lymphotropic) virus type III in the acquired immune deficiency syndrome. Science 226: 1165-1171 (1984)

9. Ratner, L., Haseltine, W., Patarca, R., et al., Complete nucleotide sequence of the AIDS virus, HTLV-III. Nature 313: 277-284 (1985)

10. Wain-Hobson, S., Sonigo, P., Danos, O., et al., Nucleotide sequence of AIDS virus, LAV. Cell 40:9-17 (1985)

11. Sanchez-Pescador, R., Power, M.D., Barr, P.J., et al., Nucleotide sequence and expression of an AIDS-associated retrovirus (ARV2). Science 227:484-492 (1985)

12. Muesing, M.A., Smith, D.H., Cabradilla, C.D., et al., Nucleic acid structure and expression of the human AIDS/lymphadenopathy retrovirus. Nature 313:450-458 (1985)

13. CDC., Additional recommendations to reduce sexual and drug abuse - related transmission of HTLV-III/LAV MMWR 35:152-155 (1986)

14. Fischinger, P.J., Bolognesi, D.P., In: AIDS: Etiology, Diagnosis, Treatment and Prevention (DeVita, V.T., Jr., Hellman, S., Rosenberg, S.A., eds.), J.B. Lippincott Co., New York, p 55-87 (1985)

15. Van de Perre, P., Clumeck, N., Carael, M., et al., Female prostitutes: a risk group for infection with human T-cell lymphotropic virus type III. Lancet 2:524-527 (1985)

16. Redfield, R.R., Markham, P.D., Salahuddin, S.Z., et al., Heterosexually acquired HTLV-III/LAV disease (AIDS related complex and AIDS): epidemiologic evidence for female-to-male transmission. JAMA 254:2094-2096 (1985)

17. DeGruttola, V., Mayer, K., Bennett, W., AIDS: has the problem been adquately assessed? Rev Infect Dis 8:295-305 (1986)

18. Alter, H.J., Eichberg, J.W., Masur, H., et al., Transmission of HTLV-III infection from human plasma to chimpanzees: an animal model for AIDS. Science 226:549-552 (1985)

19. Francis, D.P., Feorino, P.M., Broderson, J.R., et al., Infection of chimpanzees with lymphadenopathy-associated virus. Lancet 2:1276-1277 (1984)

20. Gajdusek, D.C., Amyx, H.C., Gibbs, C.J., et al., Infection of chimpanzees by human T-lymphotropic retroviruses in brain and other tissues from AIDS patients. Lancet 1:55-56 (1985)

21. Eichberg, J.W., Alter, H.J., Dreesman, G.R., Longitudinal study of HTLV-III infected chimpanzees by lymphocytic subpopulation analysis. J Med Primatol 14:317-326 (1985)

22. Fultz, P.N., McClure, H.M., Swenson, R.B., et al., Persistent infection of chimpanzees with human T-lymphotropic virus type III/lymphadenopathy-associated virus: a potential model for acquired immunodeficiency syndrome. J Virol 58:116-124 (1986)

23. Zagury, D., Fouchard, M., Vol, J.C., et al., Detection of infectious HTLV-III/LAV virus in cell-free plasma from AIDS patients. Lancet 2:505-506 (1985)

24. Wong-Staal, F., Gallo, R.C., Human T-lymphotropic retrovirus. Nature 317:395-403 (1985)

25. Rabson, A.B, Benn, S., Willey, R.L., et al., In: Vaccines 86, New Approaches to Immunization (Brown, F., Channock, R.M., Lerner, R.A., eds.) Cold Spring Harbor Laboratory, Cold Spring Harbor, p 351-358 (1986)

26. Gonda, M.A., Braun, M.J., Clements, J.E., et al., Human T-cell lymphotropic virus type III shares sequence homology with a family of pathogenic lentiviruses. Proc Natl Acad Sci USA 83:4007-4001 (1986)

27. Robert-Guroff, M., Brown, M., Gallo, R.C., HTLV-III neutralizing antibodies in patients with AIDS and AIDS-related complex. Nature 316:72-74 (1985)

28. Weiss, R.A, Clapham, P.R., Cheingsong-Popov, R., et al., Neutralization of human T-lymphotropic virus type III by sera of AIDS and AIDS-risk patients. Nature 316:69-72 (1985)

29. McDougal, J.S., Cort, S.P., Kennedy, M.S., et al., Immunoassay for the detection and quantitation of infectious human retrovirus, lymphadenopathy-associated virus (LAV). J Immunol Meth 76:171-183 (1985)

30. Ho, D.D., Rota, T.R., Hirsch, M.S., Antibody to lymphadenopathy-associated virus in AIDS. N Engl J Med 312:649-650 (1985)

31. Clavel, F., Klatzmann, D., Montagnier, L., Deficient LAV neutralizing capacity of sera from patients with AIDS or related syndromes. Lancet 1:879-880 (1985)

32. Chanh, T.C., Dreesman, G.R., Kanda, P., et al., Induction of anti-HTLV-III/LAV neutralizing antibodies by a synthetic peptide. (In press)

33. Fischinger, P.J., Schafer, W., Bolognesi, D.P., Neutralization of homologous and heterologous oncornaviruses by antisera against the p15(e) and gp 71 polypeptides of Friend murine leukemia virus. Virology 71:169-184 (1976)

34. Hunsmann, G., Pedersen, N.C., Theilen, G.H., Active immunization with feline leukemia virus envelope glycoprotein suppresses growth of virus-induced feline sarcoma. Med Microbiol Immunol 171:233-241 (1983)

35. De Noronha, F., Essex, M., Bolognesi, D.P., Influence of antisera to oncornavirus glycoprotein (gp71) on infection of cats with feline leukemia virus. Virology 85:617-621 (1978)

36. Schafer, W., Bolognesi, D.P., Mammalian C-type oncornaviruses: relationships between viral structural and cell-surface antigens and their possible significance in immuno-

logical defense mechanisms. Contemp Top Immunobiol 6:127-167 (1977)

37. Schwartz, H., Ihle, J.N., Wecker, E., et al., Properties of mouse leukemia viruses, XVII. Factors required for successful treatment of spontaneous AKR leukemia by antibodies against gp71. Virology 111:568-578 (1981)

38. Earl, P.L., Moss, B., Chesebro, B., In: Vaccines 86, New Approaches to Immunization (Brown, F., Channock, R.M., Lerner, R.A., eds.) Cold Spring Harbor Lab, Cold Spring Harbor, p 299-302 (1986)

39. Allan, J.S., Colligan, J.E., Barin, F., et al., Major glycoprotein antigens that induce antibodies in AIDS patients are encoded by HTLV-III. Science 228:1091-1094 (1985)

40. Barin, F., McLane, M.F., Allan, J.S., et al., Virus envelope protein of human T-cell leukemia virus type III (HTLV-III) represents the major target antigen for antibodies in AIDS patients. Science 228:1094-1096 (1985)

41. Montagnier, L., Clavel, F., Krust, B., et al., Identification and antigenicity of the major envelope glycoprotein of lymphadenopathy-associated virus. Virology 144:283-289 (1985)

42. McDougal, J.S., Kennedy, M.S., Sligh, J.M., et al., Binding of HTLV-III/LAV to T4$^+$ T-cells by a complex of the 110K viral protein and the T4 molecule. Science 231:382-385 (1986)

43. Robey, W.G., Safai, B., Oroszlaw, S., et al., Characterization of envelope and core structural gene products of HTLV-III with sera from AIDS patients. Science 228:593-595 (1985)

44. Starcich, B.R., Hahn, B.H., Shaw, G.M., et al., Identification and characterization of conserved and variable regions in the envelope gene of HTLV-III/LAV, the retrovirus of AIDS. Cell 45:637-648 (1986)

45. Thiel, H.J., Broughton, E.M., Matthews, T.J., et al., Interspecies reactivity of type C and D retrovirus p15E and p15C proteins. Virology 111:270-274 (1981)

46. Schwarz, H., Hunsmann, G., Moennig, V., et al., Properties of mouse leukemia viruses, XII. Immunoelectron microscopic studies on viral structural antigens on the cell surface. Virology 69:169-178 (1976)

47. Hunsmann, G., Claviez, M., Moennig, V., et al., Properties of mouse leukemia viruses, X. Occurrence of viral structural antigens on the cell surface as revealed by a cytotoxicity test. Virology 69:157-168 (1976)

48. Kennedy, R.C., Kanda, P., Chanh, T.C., et al., Use of resin bound sythetic peptide for identifying a native antigenic determinant associated with the HTLV-III/LAV envelope. (Submitted)

49. Chanh, T.C., Kennedy, R.C., Kanda, P., et al., Human Immunodeficiency virus glycoprotein gp120 detected by a monoclonal antibody to a synthetic peptide. Europ J Immunol (In Press)

50. Hillelman, M.R., Newer directions in vaccine development and utlization. J Infect Dis 151:407-419 (1985)

51. Hunsmann, G., Schneider, J., Schulz, A., Immunoprevention of Friend virus-induced erythroleukemia by vaccination with viral envelope glycoprotein complexes. Virology 113:602-612 (1981)

52. Hunsmann, G., Pedersen, N.C., Theilen, G.H., et al., Active immunization with feline leukemia virus envelope glycoprotein suppresses growth of virus-induced feline sarcoma. Med Microbiol Immunol 171:233-241 (1983)

53. Kanki, P.J., McLane, M.F., King, N.W., et al., Serologic identification and characterization of a macaque T-lymphotropic retrovirus closely related to HTLV-III. Science 228: 1199-1201 (1985)

54. Daniel, M.D., Letvin, N.L., King, N.W., et al., Isolation of T-cell tropic HTLV-III-like retrovirus from macaques. Science 228:1201-1204 (1985)

55. Kanki, P.J., Barin, F., M'Boup, S., et al., New human T-lymphotropic virus type III (STLV-III$_{AGM}$). Science 232:238-243 (1986)

56. Smith, G.L, Mackett, M., Moss, B., Infectious vaccinia virus recombinants that express hepatitis B virus surface antigen. Nature 302:490-495 (1983)

57. Paoletti, E., Lipinskas, B.R., Samsanoff, C., et al., Construction of live vaccines using genetically engineered poxviruses: Biological activity of vaccinia virus recombinants expressing the hepatitis B virus surface antigen and the *Herpes simplex* virus glycoprotein D. Proc Natl Acad Sci, USA 81:193-197 (1984)

58. Shih, M.F., Arsenakis, M., Tiollais, P., et al., Expression of hepatitis B virus S gene by *Herpes simplex* virus type 1 vectors carrying alpha and beta-regulated gene chimeras. Proc Natl Acad Sci USA 81:5867-5870 (1984)

59. Davis, A.R., Kostek, B., Mason, B.B., et al., In: Vaccines 86, New Approaches to Immunization (Brown, F., Channock, R.M., and Lerner, R.A., eds.) Cold Spring Harbor Laboratory, Cold Spring Harbor, p 283-287 (1986)

60. Chakrabarti, S., Robert-Guroff, M., Wong-Staal, F., et al., Expression of the HTLV-III envelope gene by a recombinant vaccinia virus. Nature 320:535-537 (1986)

61. Hu, S.L., Kosowski, S.G., Dalrymple, J.M., Expression of AIDS virus envelope gene in recombinant vaccinia viruses. Nature 320:537-540 (1986)

62. Valenzuela, P., Coit, D., Kuo, C.H., Synthesis and assembly in yeast of hepatitis B surface antigen particles containing the polyalbumin receptor. Bio/Technology 3:317-320 (1985)

63. Patzer, E.J., Gregory, T.J., Nakamura, G.R., et al., Recombinant hepatitis B surface antigen vaccine from a continuous cell line. In: Vaccines 85. Molecular and Chemical Basis of Resistance to Parasitic, Bacterial and Viral Diseases. (Lerner, R.A., Chanock, R.M., Brown, F., eds.) Cold Spring Harbor Laboratory, Cold Spring Harbor, p 261-264 (1985)

64. Chang, N.T., Chanda, P.K., Barone, A.D., et al., Expression in *Escherichia coli* of open reading frame gene segments of HTLV-III. Science 228:93-96 (1985)

65. Crowl, R., Ganguly, K., Gordon, M., et al., HTLV-III env gene products synthesized in *E. coli* are recognized by antibodies present in the sera of AIDS patients. Cell 41:979-986 (1986)

66. Hopp, T.P., Woods, K.R., Prediction of protein determinants from amino acid sequences. Proc Natl Acad Sci USA 78:3824-3828 (1981)

67. Pauletti, D., Simmonds, R., Dreesman, et al., Application of a modified computer algorithm in determining potential antigenic determinants associated with the AIDS virus glycoprotein. Anal Biochem 151:540-546 (1985)

68. Kennedy, R.C., Henkel, R.D., Pauletti, D., et al., Antiserum to a synthetic peptide recognizes the HTLV-III envelope glycoprotein. Science 231:1556-1559 (1986)

69. DiMarchi, R., Brooke, G., Gale, C., et al., Protection of cattle against foot-and-mouth disease by a synthetic peptide. Science 232:639-641 (1986)

70. Sanchez, Y., Ionescu-Matiu, I., Sparrow, J.T., et al., Immunogenicity of conjugates and micelles of synthetic hepatitis B surface antigen peptides. Intervirol 88:209-213 (1982)

71. Morein, B., Sundquist, B., Hoglund, S., et al., Iscom, a novel structure for antigenic presentation of membrane proteins from enveloped viruses. Nature 308:457-460 (1984)

72. Osterhaus, A., Weijer, K., Uytdehaag, F., et al., Induction of protective immune response in cats by vaccination with feline leukemia virus ISCOM. J Immunol 135:591-596 (1985)

73. Dreesman, G.R., Kennedy, R.C., Anti-idiotypic antibodies: implications of internal image-based vaccines for infectious diseases. J Infect Dis 151:761-765 (1985)

74. Koprowski, H., Unconventional vaccines: immunization with anti-idiotype antibody against viral disease. Cancer Res (Suppl) 45:4895-4905 (1983)

75. Kennedy, R.C., Dreesman, G.R., In: International Reviews of Immunology (Kohler, H., Bona, C., eds.), Harwood Academic Ltd, New York, p 67-78, (1985)

76. Kennedy, R.C., Adler-Storthz, K., Henkel, R.D., et al., Immune response to hepatitis B surface antigen: enhancement by prior injection of anti-idiotype antibodies. Science 221: 853-855 (1983)

77. Kennedy, R.C., Dreesman, G.R., Enhancement of the immune response to hepatitis B surface antigen: in vivo administration of anti-idiotype induces anti-HBs which expresses a similar idiotype. J Exp Med 159:655-665 (1984)

78. Kennedy, R.C., Eichberg, J.W., Lanford, R.E., et al., Anti-idiotype vaccine for type B viral hepatitis in chimpanzees. Science 232:220-223 (1986)

52
Behavioral Change in Response to AIDS

Don C. Des Jarlais, Susan Tross, Samuel R. Friedman

Until either effective treatment and/or an effective vaccine is developed for AIDS, behavioral changes to reduce the risk of exposure to human immunodeficiency virus (HIV) will have to be the primary method of controlling the spread of AIDS, and a critical strategy for controlling the epidemic. In this chapter studies of behavioral change among homosexual men and intravenous (IV) drug users, the two largest groups at increased risk for AIDS in the United States, are reviewed.

BEHAVIORS RESPONSIBLE FOR SPREAD OF HIV AMONG HOMOSEXUAL MEN AND INTRAVENOUS DRUG ABUSERS

The dominant modes of transmission of HIV in homosexual men and IV drug abusers are sexual intercourse, particularly unprotected anal intercourse for the former, and the sharing of equipment ("works") for injecting illicit drugs for the latter. Both of these modes of transmission pose severe difficulties for public health prevention campaigns. For the gay man living in the era of gay liberation, unrestricted sexual experience has often served as an important expression of positive gay identity and community--beyond the obvious fulfillment of sexual and intimacy needs. For IV drug users, sharing of needles was often associated with the strongest positive social relationships within the group. Thus, both modes of transmission have played a central role in the lives of the risk group members, and this must be considered in any behavioral interventions to reduce transmission of HIV. There are few if any precedents in public health prevention campaigns that require such change in individual behavior, social relationships and sense of group identity.

From a behavior theory perspective, these behaviors can be described as "overlearned". They are behaviors that prior to the AIDS epidemic, were very frequently practiced, and were very frequently positively reinforced. The behavior patterns were generalized to the extent that they, independent of reinforcement for any specific instance, have become resistant to change even when the individual is strongly motivated to change.

Behaviors related to HIV transmission are also interpersonal; they involve patterned interactions between individuals. Change in these behaviors entails changes in the social relationships between members of the risk groups. Thus, a sociological perspective, including the concepts of self, social norms and subcultures, is useful in describing these changes. Widespread and sustained change in these behaviors will require changes in the social organization of the gay (1)-(4) and IV drug use (5)-(7) subcultures in the United States.

Reducing multiple partner sex and anal intercourse among homosexual men, and the sharing of "works" among IV drug users, are not simple social changes within the two subcultures. Multiple partner sexuality emerged as an expression of gay power, pride and identity during the gay rights movement in the 1970's in the United States. Changing to monogamous relationships will require new definitions of what it means to be "gay" within contemporary America.

The sharing of "works" for injecting drugs was similarly central to the IV drug use subculture prior to AIDS. Sharing served multiple purposes: it symbolized the joining of the group at initiation into IV drug use and the positive social relationships between "running buddies" (IV drug users who pool efforts to obtain money and drugs). Sharing works also served practical functions; legal restrictions on syringes and needles lead to higher prices for sterile equipment, and the possibility of arrest for possessing narcotics paraphernalia deters many IV drug users from carrying their own sets with them (8).

When change involves behaviors that are fundamental to a subculture, the change process is quite complex (9). Such change may produce increased solidarity within the subculture, but also typically involves factionalization into groups and conflict between the groups. Some groups will be advocating the new ways, while others defend the previous ways. Within subcultures that are considered to be socially deviant, this conflict may be exacerbated by the general alienation from conventional society, and alliances between some of the factions and power groups within conventional society. When the conflict involves changes in behavior and values that are fundamental to the subculture, "resolution" of the conflict through a consensus is quite rare. Resolution usually occurs over generations, and the form of the resolution is typically determined by which faction gains control over recruitment of new members into the subculture.

GAY MEN

Epidemiology and Special Obstacles to Change

Throughout the six years of CDC surveillance, gay or bisexual men have continued to account for approximately 72% of all AIDS cases (although 8% of the gay/bisexual cases also involve drug injection) (10). The threat of AIDS, naturally, extends far beyond persons with AIDS themselves -- to the vastly larger asymptomatic gay male population who may be assumed to have been exposed to HIV, and to the others who are currently at risk for exposure. In a 1984 retrospective study of 6,875 members of a San Francisco hepatitis B study cohort, recruited as early as 1978, HIV seroprevalence was estimated to be 28 times more frequent than the AIDS diagnosis proper. Absolute seroprevalence in this cohort was 68% (11). Seroprevalence in urban gay men has otherwise been estimated at anywhere between 17% and 67%, with the variance accounted for by geographic and sampling differences (12)-(16). The earliest generation of case-control studies highlighted the number of sexual partners as the primary risk factor for developing AIDS (17)-(21). The earliest Public Health Service sexual behavior precautions for AIDS cautioned risk group members against relations with multiple sexual partners (22). However, since the discovery of HIV as the etiological agent of AIDS (23),(24), increased emphasis has been given to type of sexual behavior, along with number of partners, in AIDS epidemiology. In particular, receptive anal intercourse without protection by condom, has been implicated as the sexual behavior carrying the highest risk for AIDS (25),(26). Indeed, as long as the necessary and sufficient conditions for HIV infection remain undetermined, AIDS prevention initiatives must adopt the broadest appropriate definition of the conditions of risk.

Because of the grave medical consequences of AIDS, and in the absence of either vaccine or effective medical treatment, behavioral change has become the primary approach to prevention. For the gay male risk group, these behavior changes have generally involved restriction of sexual activities to those which do not exchange bodily fluids (i.e., semen, blood, urine, feces) and limitation of numbers of sexual partners with whom "safe" sexual practices may be negotiated. Recent risk reduction guidelines have been formulated and disseminated by self-help AIDS organizations in the gay community. The recommendations in Table 1, authored by the New York Physicians For Human Rights (27) and distributed by the Gay Men's Health Crisis in 1984 in New York City, although not all valid, exemplify these considerations.

In addition to the general obstacles to changing highly valued individual behavior and subcultural organization, there is one additional obstacle to reduction of HIV transmission among gay men that deserves special comment. This is the considerable uncertainty regarding what constitutes "safe sex" and/or "safer sex". Within the scientific community, there has been continuing debate on what changes in gay sexual activities are needed to provide what level of protection against HIV infection. Additional confusion has centered around the finding of HIV in saliva (28), leading to questions regarding the safety of oral sex and kissing, even though there is no epidemiologic evidence of salivary transmission.

TABLE 1. Sexually Transmitted Disease and AIDS Risk Reduction Guidelines Suggested by the Gay Men's Health Crisis of New York City in 1984

CHOOSE FAMILIAR PARTNERS
LEARN ABOUT THEIR HEALTH AND LIFE STYLE

USE GOOD HYGIENE DURING SEXUAL RELATIONS

USE SEXUAL METHODS THAT DO NOT INVOLVE EXCHANGE OF BODY FLUIDS (i.e., Semen, Urine, Feces):

CARESSING
MUTUAL MASTURBATION
ANAL INTERCOURSE WITH CONDOMS

USE A LUBRICANT DURING ANAL INTERCOURSE AND AVOID FISTING TO PREVENT ANAL WOUNDS

URINATE AFTER HAVING SEX

REDUCE SUBSTANCE AND ALCOHOL USE TO PROTECT IMMUNE FUNCTION AND JUDGEMENT

MAINTAIN GOOD HEALTH (i.e., Rest, Diet, Exercise)

Humans are generally not good at decisions involving low probability events, particularly when the events in question are associated with strongly negative consequences (29). They tend either to round the low probability to zero, and behaviorally ignore the possible event, or to exaggerate the likelihood of the event and feel compelled to do all possible to prevent its occurrence. The difficulties in defining just what constitutes "safe sex" make it hard for gay men to know the extent to which they are actually protecting themselves against HIV exposure, thus diminishing cognitive reinforcement for the new behavior.

Individual Behavior Change Among Gay Men

Despite the difficulties in changing sexual behavior, there is consistent evidence that the majority of gay men in the United States have altered their behavior in response to AIDS epidemic.

Major research programs are currently in progress in three

cities, San Francisco (30),(31), New York (32),(33) and Chicago (34),(35), to characterize the behavioral and emotional impact of AIDS on gay men. As described below, risk reduction is being observed by investigators in all three locations. Although all research programs are examining a wide variety of psychological/ behavioral aspects of AIDS in gay men, only preliminary results are available at this time from these programs and only descriptive findings of AIDS-related sexual behavior change will be presented.

In November 1983, McKusick and his colleagues (30),(36) initiated a longitudinal panel study of 655 gay men in San Francisco. Four subsamples were developed: a bathhouse sample, a bar sample, a non-bathhouse/non-bar sample, and a couple relationship sample. AIDS-related behavioral change is measured both in terms of the persistence of "higher risk behavior" (i.e., "rimming", "fisting", anal intercourse without condoms, "water sports", and "swallowing semen") and the converse, "health conscious behavior" (i.e., anal intercourse with condoms, coitus interruptus, and mutual masturbation). Relations with primary partners are considered separately from secondary partners. Behavioral change is defined as the difference in frequency of a given behavior for the time frame of the past month as compared to the time frame of the year prior to study. In the three non-bathhouse subsamples, a considerable decrement was observed in number of sexual contacts in public locations; the bathhouse sample failed to show any change. Behavior change varied with type of partner. That is, little change in high risk behavior was detected within monogamous relationships; the authors argue that, for these subjects, monogamy itself may have been perceived as sufficient health protection. A considerable decrease in high risk behavior (especially oral-genital contact) was reported for relations with secondary partners and casual partners. Whereas the absolute number of monogamous subjects actually slightly decreased between the time periods, there was an increase in the proportion of non-monogamous relationships shifting into monogamy (30). Comparable data for a later assessment (i.e., May 1984) were available for 454 subjects. Considerable decrements were reported for several risk parameters including: number of partners; frequency of high risk sexual behavior; and frequency of general sexual activity. At the same time, the affirmative adoption of "safe" sexual precautions appeared more difficult than the exercise of restraint in "high risk behavior"; no change was observed on the health conscious behaviors (30).

Pluckett and his colleagues (31) obtained consistent findings for a random probability panel study of 500 gay men surveyed by telephone in San Francisco between August 1984 (Wave 1) and April 1985 (Wave 2). Efforts for partner and behavior restriction alike increased considerably during this interval. The proportion of respondents restricting themselves to monogamy, celibacy, or high risk behavior with a primary partner only, increased from 49% to 81%. The proportion of respondents with more than one sexual partner during the 30 days prior to survey decreased from 49% to 35%. The proportion of respondents who had had anal intercourse without a condom with a secondary partner during these (respective) time periods decreased from 18% to 12%. The proportion of respondents having oral intercourse ending in ejaculation with swallowing semen during the same periods dropped from 15% to 7%. "Objective" corroboration of these self-report data may be found in a 73% decline in the rate of rectal gonorrhea for San Francisco men from 1980 to 1984 (11).

Between May and October of 1985, Martin (32) initiated a community-based study of the health behavioral, social psychological and mental health impact of AIDS in 750 healthy gay men in the metropolitan New York area. Data are being collected in two waves -- at entry into the study and one year later. Retrospective reports on the year prior to when the subject first learned of the subject of AIDS, are used as a pre-AIDS era baseline for the quantification of change.

Change in sexual behavior has been computed for the interval between this baseline and entry on study. There was marked evidence of AIDS risk reduction on multiple indices of sexual-behavior, including number of partners, frequency of specific sexual behaviors and visits to "extra-domestic" locations for sex. Annual number of extra-domestic sexual partners decreased by 82%, while number of domestic sexual partners decreased by 56%. The ratio of domestic sexual episodes to domestic partners doubled from 5:1 to 11:1. There was a 67% drop in annual frequency of visits to extra-domestic locations for sex. There were marked decrements in the frequency of a wide variety of sexual behaviors, including passive (72%) and active (67%) anal intercourse, anal intake of semen (75%), oral intercourse (60%), swallowing of semen (80%), and others. At the same time, there was an 80% rise in the frequency of condom use during anal intercourse. There was no change in the frequency of sexual abstinence.

Siegel and her colleagues (33) observed similar trends in a control sample of 54 gay men, without AIDS-related symptoms, in a hospital based study of AIDS and ARC patients at the Memorial Sloan-Kettering Cancer Center. Eighty-five percent of the sample initiated at least one of the following AIDS reduction measures: (1) decreased number of partners (83%); (2) decreased number of anonymous partners (74%); (3) decreased drug use during sex (38%); (4) increased own condom use (30%); and (5) increased requests for partner condom use (28%).

Corroboration of these self-report data may be inferred from a 59% drop in the rectal and pharyngeal gonorrhea rates for men enrolled in the sexually transmitted disease clinics of the New York City Department of Health from 1980 to 1983 (37).

In 1983, Joseph and her colleagues (34),(35) initiated a study of gay men in Chicago, as part of the Multi-Center AIDS Cohort Study of the National Institute on Allergy and Infectious Diseases. Three subgroups were recruited: (1) asymptomatic men attending a local gay men's screening clinic; (2) participants in an ongoing hepatitis B vaccine research program at the same clinic; and (3) men with AIDS spectrum symptoms. Behavioral and emotional outcomes, and their possible psychological and social determinants, are being assessed along with medical and immunological status at six month intervals for a two and one-half year period. One report described a significant drop in the frequency of all risk behaviors measured for the period between 1982 and 1983 among the first 700 men in the study (35). This was especially true for so-called "high risk" behaviors, i.e., anal intercourse and rimming, for which decrements of at least 60% were observed. Fifteen percent of the sample became abstinent. Another report described an 81% rate of adherence to at least one risk reduction measure among 300 men (34).

These authors emphasize the critical issue of the psychological cost of risk reduction. Seventy-five percent of their sample experienced daily stress as a result of their risk reduction efforts; 67-81% doubted the efficacy of these efforts. Furthermore, levels of both stress and doubt were found to be predictors of self-reported general psychological distress.

The role of emotional distress in the life of the gay man in the AIDS era is formidable. Even among gay men without AIDS spectrum symptoms in New York City, mean levels of psychological symptoms generally lie between one and two standard deviations above norms for a healthy male reference population (38). This distress is greater among AIDS patients and even greater among AIDS related complex (ARC) patients. Distress levels for the latter lie between two and three standard deviations above these norms. Similar results have been documented for a sample of gay men in San Francisco (39). Such findings clearly represent clinically, as well as statistically, meaningful levels of distress in these populations, which may easily be expected to impact on any aspect of behavioral adaption, including AIDS risk reduction.

As yet, there are limited data available to identify specific motivational and/or sociodemographic determinants of AIDS risk reduction behavior. McKusick and his colleagues (30) reported an association between history of having seen a gravely ill AIDS patient and a (relatively) low number of sexual partners during the month prior to study. In contrast, a higher number of partners was associated with positive values about uninhibited sexual activity as: (1) an expression of gay identity and (2) a major mode of tension relief. Siegel and her colleagues (33) observed a correlation between severity of perceived threat of AIDS and number of risk reduction measures undertaken. Ostrow et al. (35) identified the following attitudinal factors as primary reasons for persistence of high risk behaviors: (1) perception of safety of one's partners; (2) conviction of inability to adhere to risk reduction; (3) belief in a multiple HIV exposure model of transmission; and (4) reluctance to initiate risk reduction in the face of medical uncertainty about AIDS.

Changes in the Gay Subculture

A number of studies of AIDS-related changes in the gay subculture in the United States have been conducted (40)-(42). One component of the change in the gay subculture is the emergence of gay organizations that are carrying on specific AIDS-related activities. These activities include political lobbying, education/prevention efforts and provision of services to persons with AIDS or to those who are concerned that they may develop AIDS (the "worried well"). The Gay Men's Health Crisis in New York City, the Shanti Project in San Francisco, and the AIDS Project in Los Angeles are among the better known of these organizations. A national lobbying group has been formed, the AIDS Action Council, which includes 110 member organizations. The great majority of these, between 75% and 90%, were organized by gay men. (Others were organized by social workers, health care advocates, clergy and families of persons with AIDS) (43).

The recent off-Broadway play "The Normal Heart" by Larry Kramer recounts the early days of the Gay Men's Health Crisis from the perspective of one of the founders. It illustrates some of the intra- and interpersonal conflicts that are to be expected when fundamental behavior patterns within a subculture undergo rapid change.

An aspect of gay subculture that is clearly in need of greater study is initiation into the subculture, both in terms of "coming out" and initial gay experiences. How has the need for "safer sex" and the greatly increased potential for discrimination against gay men affected willingness to identify with the gay subculture? Has concern about AIDS influenced the emotional tone of the homo-erotic experiences of adolescent males that have always been common in American society? If so, has this led to any changes in the frequency of behaviors associated with HIV transmission? It is important to study these questions, for they will provide insight into the long-term adaption to the risk reduction reviewed in the section above.

BEHAVIORAL CHANGE AMONG IV DRUG USERS

Intravenous drug users have constituted the second largest group of persons to have developed AIDS throughout the epidemic in the United States. Drug injection has been the primary risk factor in 17% of all AIDS cases, and an additional 8% of cases have occurred in homosexual/bisexual men who also inject drugs (44).

The IV drug use AIDS cases have been heavily concentrated in the metropolitan New York City area; over 70% of such cases to date have been from the states of New York, New Jersey and Connecticut (44). Seroprevalence studies of HIV among IV drug users reflect this concentration, but also show the potential for substantial numbers of IV drug use cases to develop in other areas. The studies in New York (45) and in northern New Jersey show seroprevalence rates of 50% or greater, while studies in San Francisco and Chicago show rates of approximately 10% (46), and studies in Washington, D.C. and New Orleans show 7% and 2% respectively (47).

For IV drug users, there are several special obstacles to AIDS risk reduction, above and beyond those generally associated with changing overlearned behavior, that need to be mentioned (48). The alienation between IV drug users and conventional society is considerably greater than that between the gay subculture and conventional society, particularly since the successes of the gay rights movement. The social organization of the IV drug use subculture is dominated by the drug distribution networks. This type of social structure is not conducive to organized efforts to promote health interest among IV drug users. Drug users and drug dealers frequently find themselves in intense economic competition over scarce resources (the drugs, and, to a lesser extent, the equipment to inject). Since the entire drug distribution business is illegal, the competition is not restrained by adherence to laws. Disputes are not settled by taking people to court, but rather by threats and violence.

Another specific obstacle to risk reduction among IV drug users is the onset of withdrawal symptoms. While not life-threatening, withdrawal creates intense physical discomfort and considerable anxiety. In this situation, IV drug users will tend to use whatever works are available, even if they have previously been used by another person (8).

Individual Behavior Change Among IV Drug Users

Compared to research on gay men, there have been relatively few studies of AIDS-related behavioral change in IV drug users. The studies that have been conducted have been primarily in the New York City area, where the largest number of cases have occurred. There is a great public health and scientific need to conduct behavioral change studies in areas of low incidence to determine appropriate intervention strategies for such areas.

Knowledge of AIDS and modes of transmission can be considered a prerequisite for successful risk reduction. Intravenous drug users in New York City seem to have considerable knowledge about AIDS. In 1984, all of a sample of 59 methadone maintenance patients whom we interviewed had heard of AIDS; 55 (93%) of them knew that IV drug use is a mode of transmission of the disease. The majority (61%) of these subjects also were able to name at least one AIDS symptom correctly, with the most frequently named symptoms being weight loss (36%) and fatigue (31%) (49). In the summer of 1985, Selwyn et al. (50) studied IV drug users in jail (n = 115) as well as methadone maintenance clients (n = 146) and found similar knowledge; 97% of both groups said that sharing needles could transmit AIDS.

The common stereotype that IV drug users are "self destructive" and not concerned about their health make it seem doubtful that knowledge would lead to behavioral change in this group. Contrary to this notion, the majority of IV drug users in both our and the Selwyn studies (50) reported risk reduction. In our 1984 interviews, 59% of those interviewed reported some form of risk reduction to avoid AIDS and 54% reported changes in injection-related behavior. The most common changes were increased use of clean needles and/or the cleaning of needles (reported by 31%) and a reduction in needle sharing (reported by 29%). Fifty-one per cent of the group also reported that friends had changed their behaviors to avoid AIDS. The Selwyn group found that over 60% of their subjects reported risk reduction. Reduction in needle sharing was the most common change in this study, with 42% of the methadone patients and 23% of the IV drug users interviewed in jail reporting that they had stopped sharing needles, and 24% and 38% of the two groups respectively reporting that they had reduced needle sharing (without stopping completely).

Individual users may also be changing their route of administration of drugs in order to avoid exposure to HIV. We have received reports from individual IV drug users that they have switched from injecting cocaine to smoking free base cocaine (in the form of "crack") in order to reduce their risk of AIDS. Drug abuse treatment statistics in New Jersey also show that, among heroin users, there has been a decrease in the percentage who inject the drug and an increase in the percentage who are using it intranasally ("sniffing") over the last two years. The New Jersey treatment statistics also show that approximately one-half of the IV drug users entering treatment in the last year give fear of AIDS as one reason for entering treatment (51).

Concern about AIDS and risk reduction to avoid exposure to the virus have developed among IV drug users in the New York metropolitan area, where HIV seroprevalence is approximately 50%, and there are literally thousands of IV drug users who have already developed AIDS using the CDC surveillance definition. An important question for control of the epidemic among IV drug users in other areas is whether risk reduction will occur prior to extensive spread of the virus. Preliminary data from San Francisco, where seroprevalence is estimated to be approximately 10% (46),(52) are encouraging on this point.

Biernacki and Feldman (53) have been conducting ethnographic research on IV drug users not in treatment in San Francisco. They report that AIDS is already a topic of "grave concern" among IV drug users there, and that the drug users want to learn how to protect themselves against exposure, including how to sterilize needles and syringes. Prior to any widespread prevention campaigns, a "substantial minority" had already reduced the number of persons with whom they would share needles.

Changes in the IV Drug Use Subculture

Studies of AIDS-related changes in the IV drug use subculture have focused on the marketing of sterile needles and syringes. They show evidence of a large-scale change in the demand for sterile "works". In the spring of 1985, we conducted interviews with persons selling needles and syringes in the drug dealing areas of New York City (54). Eighteen of 22 needle sellers reported that sales had increased over the previous year. When asked why this had occurred, six reported increased demand in general terms, five said it was easier to get new needles, and four specifically mentioned AIDS. It is interesting to note that not only has demand for sterile works increased but also the supply. The major source of supply in New York City is diversion from legitimate medical sources, and it appears that there may have been a decrease in the security of medical supplies.

The persons selling needles and syringes were also asked if they had ever sold used needles as new; 10/21 (48%) reported that they had repackaged used equipment and then sold it as new. This phenomenon had not been observed in the city prior to AIDS. The demand for sterile "works" is now sufficiently strong that it will support a market in counterfeit sterile "works".

More recently, we have observed additional AIDS-related changes in the marketing of needles and syringes for illicit drug injection. Some needle sellers are now including an extra needle with the sale of a "set" of a needle and syringe. If the first needle gets clogged, it can immediately be replaced with the extra needle, greatly reducing the chances that the immediate need to inject would lead to renting a used needle or using the needle of a friend. Finally, drug dealers have been including a new set of "works" as a marketing device with $25 and $50 bags of heroin (55).

With respect to self-help groups specifically focused on AIDS, IV drug users have been much slower to organize than have gay men. This is not surprising given the different social structures within the subcultures, the economic differences between the two groups, and the differences in their pre-existing relationships with conventional society.

In New York City, organization to respond to AIDS among IV drug users began in the Fall of 1985. The initiative was taken by a handful of ex-drug users employed in public and private drug agencies and programs. Additional members were recruited from others in similar positions, from other drug treatment personnel with no history of IV drug use, from current program clients, and from drug injectors who were not in treatment. The organization was named ADAPT (Association for Drug Abuse Prevention and Treatment, Inc.).

ADAPT has produced educational literature, including several posters aimed at conveying the message that sharing "works" can be fatal, and informational sheets written in a language familiar to drug users. The organization has also participated in several conferences on AIDS among IV drug users. Members of ADAPT are also currently conducting face-to-face AIDS education in the drug dealing areas of New York City. Additional planned activities include a hotline, services for drug users with AIDS, educational programs, and referral procedures to help IV drug users enter drug treatment programs.

Whether ADAPT will be as successful in promoting behavioral change and in providing AIDS-related services to IV drug users as organizations like the Gay Men's Health Crisis remains to be seen. One possible limit on organizational effectiveness is conflict between ex-IV drug users, particularly those employed in treatment programs, and current IV drug users who do not wish to be in treatment. Clearly these groups have important differences, including a different evaluation of stopping drug injection as a means of avoiding exposure to HIV. These two groups may also be treated differently by representatives of conventional society. Despite these potential organizational problems, the current and planned activities of ADAPT are an indication of the power of AIDS to change the subculture of IV drug use in the United States.

CONCLUSION

Research on risk reduction in gay men and IV drug users shows that substantial numbers of both groups are modifying their behavior to reduce the risk of developing AIDS, but also that a substantial residue of transmission-related behavior remains. Whether the degree of risk reduction achieved to date will be sufficient to control the epidemic (in the absence of an effective vaccine) cannot be determined yet, but will depend upon a number of factors. First among these is the seroprevalence among the risk group within a geographic area. The risk of infection for an individual from any one specific act, i.e., unprotected anal intercourse or sharing of a needle, depends upon the likelihood that the partner is carrying the virus. Since HIV appears to lead to lifelong infection, with the great majority of infected persons also being infectious, effective risk reduction becomes more difficult with time. As the number of infected persons within the risk groups cumulates over time, greater reductions in the number of partners for transmission-related behavior are needed, even to maintain a constant probability of transmission for a given act. The problem of cumulating infective persons appears particularly relevant for gay men, since, with the exception of the New York City area, seroprevalence among gays is generally higher than among IV drug users. Preliminary data from ongoing research in San Francisco (56), Baltimore (57), and New York (26) indicate that risk reduction among gay men in those cities has reduced the rate of seroconversion to between 5% and 10% per year among seronegatives. This is one-quarter to one-half of what might be expected in the absence of risk reduction, but can only be considered a slowing of the epidemic.

In our opinion, the chance that risk reduction efforts will lead to total monogamy within the gay subculture is extremely low. Even within heterosexual sexuality, where there is strong institutional support for monogamy, serial monogamy rather than exclusive monogamy appears to be the rule. Risk reduction through limiting the number of sexual partners may certainly reduce the rate of HIV transmission among gay men but does not appear likely to stop the spread.

Prevention of AIDS among gay men will thus probably have to rely on substitution of "safe sex" activities for other activities that are more likely to result in viral transmission. As noted above, uncertainties regarding what sexual activities can be considered "safe" have been an obstacle to risk reduction among gay men. Current research suggests that anal intercourse is by far the most likely act to lead to viral transmission (26),(56),(57). While no one can guarantee safety for other forms of sexual activity, it is certainly possible that eliminating anal intercourse transmission might be sufficient to control the epidemic among gay men. The extent to which condoms provide protection during anal intercourse is not yet known. There is also the possibility that if present condoms are not very effective, better ones can be developed. Having effective protection for anal intercourse would greatly reduce the magnitude of the behavioral changes needed for control of AIDS among gay men.

Among IV drug users, there are still many areas in the country with low seroprevalence rates. Thus, reduction in needle sharing may greatly reduce HIV transmission in those areas. Whether reduction in sharing needles would merely slow the epidemic or would lead to actual control within geographic areas, cannot be predicted at this point.

In New York, preliminary data from our follow-up studies of IV drug users indicate a seroconversion rate of approximately 7% per year among seronegatives. This is equivalent to that observed among gay men, and should be considered as a major reduction due to changes in transmission-related behavior. It also must be considered only a slowing of the epidemic within the risk group.

The substitution of other forms of intensive drug use for injection also might considerably change the course of the epidemic. In New York City, there are some indications of a change from injecting cocaine to smoking free-base cocaine (in the form called "crack"). Heroin can also be smoked, with an effect that rivals injecting in its intensity. This, however, requires a high purity in the drug preparation, 40% pure or better. Street heroin preparations in the US are generally around 5% pure. A street form of heroin called "black tar" has been reported in New York and elsewhere with high enough purity for smoking (58), and there also is the possibility that illicit chemists may develop "designer drug" narcotic analogs that can be marketed with enough purity for smoking.

For both risk groups, long-term prevention of AIDS in the absence of a vaccine will require changes in the ways in which new members are initiated into the subcultures. It is at this early stage that safe sexual practices and methods of avoiding blood transfer while using drugs, will have to be inculcated. Unfortunately, it is in this area of the initiation into the subcultures where we most need risk reduction research, but have the least.

ACKNOWLEDGEMENTS

We would like to acknowledge the assistance of Jo Sotheran, Drs. Jimmie Holland and Dan Hirsch in the preparation of this chapter. Support was provided by grants 2-R01-DA-03574 from the National Institute on Drug Abuse and 2-R01-MH-39326 from the National Institute on Mental Health.

REFERENCES

1. Bell, A.P., Weinberg, M.S., Homosexualities: A Study of Diversity Among Men and Women. Simon and Schuster, New York (1978)

2. Humphreys, R.A.L., The tearoom trade: Impersonal Sex in Public Places. Aldine, Chicago (1970)

3. Humphreys, R.A.L., Out of the Closets: The Sociology of Homosexual Liberation. Prentice-Hall, Englewood Cliffs (1972)

4. Weinberg, M.S., Williams, C.J., Male Homosexuals: Their Problems and Adaptations. Penguin, New York (1975)

5. Agar, M.H., Ripping and Running: A Formal Ethnography of Urban Heroin Addicts. Seminar Press, New York (1973)

6. Hanson, B., Beschner, G., Walters, J.M., et al., Life with Heroin: Voices from the Inner City. Lexington Books, Lexington (1985)

7. Johnson, B.D., Goldstein, P., Preble, E., et al., Taking Care of Business: The Economics of Crime by Heroin Abusers. Lexington Books, Lexington (1985)

8. Des Jarlais, D.C., Friedman, S.R., Strug, D., AIDS among intravenous drug users: A sociocultural perspective. In: The Social Dimensions of AIDS: Methods and Theory. (Feldman, D., Johnson, T. eds). Praeger, New York (1986)

9. Garner, R.A., Social Change. Rand McNally, Chicago (1977)

10. Centers for Disease Control, AIDS Surveillance (1986)

11. Curran, J.W., Morgan, W.M., Hardy, A.M., et al., The epidemiology of AIDS: current status and future prospects. Science 229:1352-1357 (1985)

12. CDC., Update: acquired immunodeficiency syndrome in the San Francsico cohort study 1978-1985. MMWR 34:573-575 (1985)

13. Safai, B., Sarngadharan, M.G., Groopman, J.E., et al., Sero-epidemiological studies of human T-lymphotropic retrovirus type III in acquired immune deficiency syndrome. Lancet 1: 1438-1440 (1984)

14. Schupach, J., Haller, O., Vogt, M., et al., Antibodies to HTLV-III in Swiss patients with AIDS and pre-AIDS and in groups at risk for AIDS. N Engl J Med 312:265-270 (1985)

15. Cheingsong-Popov, R., Weiss, R.A., Dalgleish, A., et al., Prevalence of antibody to human T-lymphotropic virus type III in AIDS and AIDS-risk patients in Britain. Lancet 2:477 (1984)

16. Francis, D.P., Jaffee, H.W., Fultz, P.N., et al., The natural history of infection with the lymphadenopathy-associated virus/human T-lymphotropic virus type III. Ann Intern Med 103:719-722 (1985)

17. Jaffe, H.W., Choi, K., Thomas, P.A., et al., National case-control study of Kaposi's sarcoma and *Pneumocystis carinii* pneumonia in homosexual men: Part 1 epidemiological results. Ann Intern Med 99:145-151 (1983)

18. Marmor, M., Friedman-Kien, A.E., Zolla-Pazner, S., et al., Kaposi's sarcoma in homosexual men. Ann Intern Med 100:809 (1984)

19. Goedert, J.J., Sarngadharan, M.G., Biggar, R.J., et al., Determinants of retrovirus (HTLV-III) antibody and immunodeficiency conditions in homosexual men. Lancet 2:711-716 (1984)

20. Mathur-Wagh, U., Enlow, R.W., Spigland, I., et al., Longitudinal study of persistent generalized lymphadenopathy in homosexual men: Relation to acquired immunodeficiency syndrome. Lancet 1:1033-1038 (1984)

21. Abrams, D.I., Lewis, B.J., Beckstead, J.H., et al., Persistent diffuse lymphadenopathy in homosexual men: Endpoint or prodome. Ann Intern Med 100:801-808 (1984)

22. CDC., Prevention of acquired immune deficiency syndrome (AIDS): Report of inter-agency recommendations. MMWR 32:101-104 (1983)

23. Barre-Sinoussi, F., Chermann, J.C., Rey, F., et al., Isolation of a T-lymphotropic retrovirus from a patient at risk for acquired immune deficiency syndrome. Science 220:868-870 (1983)

24. Gallo, R.C., Salahuddin, S.Z., Popovic, M., Detection, isolation and continuous production of cytopathic retroviruses (HTLV-III) from patients with AIDS and pre-AIDS. Science 224:497-503 (1984)

25. Joseph, J.G., Personal communication. (1986)

26. Stevens, C., Greater New York Blood Center. Personal communication (1986)

27. New York Physicians for Human Rights. STD AIDS Risk Reduction Guidelines for Healthier Sex. Gay Men's Health Crisis. New York, NY (1984)

28. Groopman, J.E., Salahuddin, S.Z., Sarangadharan, M.G., et al., HTLV-III in saliva of people with AIDS related complex and healthy homosexual men at risk for AIDS. Science 226: 447-449 (1984)

29. Kahneman, I., ed., Behavior Under Uncertainty: Basics and Heuristics. Cambridge University Press, Cambridge (1982)

30. McKusick, L., Horstman, W., Coates, T.J., AIDS and sexual behavior reported by gay men in San Francisco. Am J Pub Health 75:493-496 (1985)

31. Puckett, S., Bart, M., Bye, L., et al., Self-reported behavioral change among gay and bisexual men - San Francisco. MMWR 34:613-614 (1985)

32. Martin, J.L., Sociomedical Research Priorities in AIDS. AIDS - the Ethical, Legal and Social Considerations. Public Responsibility in Medicine and Research Conference. Tufts University School of Medicine. (1985)

33. Siegel, K., Hirsch, D., Christ, G., Adoption of modifications in sexual behavior among asymptomatic homosexual men. International Conference on the Acquired Immune Deficiency Syndrome (AIDS). Atlanta, Georgia (1985)

34. Joseph, J.G., Emmons, C.A., Kessler, R.C., et al., Changes in sexual behavior of gay men: Relationships to perceived stress and psychological symptomatology. International Conference on the Acquired Immune Deficiency Syndrome (AIDS). Atlanta, Georgia (1985)

35. Ostrow, D., Emmons, C.A., Altman, N.L., et al., Sexual behavior change and persistence in homosexual men. International Conference on the Acquired Immunodeficiency Syndrome (AIDS). Atlanta, Georgia (1985)

36. McKusick, L., Coats, T., Stah, R., et al., Stability and change in gay sex: The case of San Francisco. International Conference on the Acquired Immunodeficiency Syndrome (AIDS), Atlanta, Georgia (1985)

37. CDC., Declining rates of rectal and pharyngeal gonorrhea among males - New York City. MMWR 33:295-297 (1984)

38. Tross, S., Holland, J., Wetzler, S., et al., Neuropsychological function in AIDS spectrum disorder patients. International Conference on Acquired Immune Deficiency Syndrome (AIDS). Atlanta, Georgia (1985)

39. Temoshok, L., Mandel, J.S., Soloman, G.F., et al., Psychosocial coping with a diagnosis of AIDS. Symposium: The Acquired Immune Deficiency Syndrome: Behavioral Medicine Research Provides a Paradigm for Understanding and Treatment. Presented at the Annual Meeting of the Society of Behavioral Medicine, San Francisco, March 5-8, 1986

40. Altman, D., AIDS in the Mind of America. Anchor Press/Doubleday, Garden City, NY (1986)

41. Feldman, D., Johnson, T., eds., The Social Dimensions of AIDS: Methods and Theory. Praeger, New York (1986)

42. Patton, C., Sex and Germs: The Politics of AIDS. South End Press, Boston (1985)

43. Gomez, M., AIDS Action Council. Personal communication (1986)

44. Hardy, A.M., Centers for Disease Control. Personal communication (1986)

45. Cohen, H., Marmor, M., Des Jarlais, D.C., et al., Risk factors for HTLV-III/LAV seropositivity among intravenous drug users. International Conference on the Acquired Immune Deficiency Syndrome (AIDS). Atlanta Georgia (1985)

46. Spira, T.J., Des Jarlais, D.C., Bokos, D., et al., HTLV-III/LAV antibodies in intravenous drug users -- comparisons of high and low risk areas of AIDS. International Conference on the Acquired Immune Deficiency Syndrome (AIDS). Atlanta, Georgia (1985)

47. Ginzburg, H., NIDA. Personal communication. (1986)

48. Friedman, S.R., Des Jarlais, D.C., Sotheran, J.L., AIDS health education for intravenous drug users. Health Education Quarterly (In Press)

49. Friedman, S.R., Des Jarlais, D.C., Sotheran, J.L., et al., AIDS and self-organization among intravenous drug users. Int J Addict (In Press)

50. Selwyn, P.A., Cox, C.P., Feiner, C., et al., Knowledge about AIDS and high-risk behavior among intravenous drug abusers in New York City. Presented at Annual Meeting of the American Public Health Association, Washington, DC, November 18 (1985)

51. French, J., New Jersey Department of Health. Personal communication (1986)

52. Chaisson, R., San Francisco General Hospital. Personal communication (1986)

53. Biernacki, P., Feldman, H., Ethnographic observations of IV drug use practices that put users at risk for AIDS. Presented at the XV International Institute on the Prevention and Treatment of Drug Dependence. Amsterdam/Noordwijkerhout, the Netherlands, April 6-11 (1986)

54. Des Jarlais, D.C., Friedman, S.r., Hopkins, W., Risk reduction for the acquired immunodeficiency syndrome among intravenous drug users. Ann Intern Med 103:755-759 (1985)

55. Des Jarlais, D.C., Hopkins, W., Free needles for intravenous drug users at risk for AIDS: Current developments in New York City. N Engl J Med 313:23 (1985)

56. Winkelstein, W., Personal communication (1985)

57. Polk, B.F., Johns Hopkins University School of Medicine. Personal communication (1986).

58. Hopkins, W., New York State Division of Substance Abuse Services. Personal communication (1986)

53
Social Barriers to the Control of HIV Infection

Peggy Clarke, David J. Sencer

Acquired immunodeficiency syndrome (AIDS) is a disease that can not occur without preceding infection by the human immunodeficiency virus (HIV). But it also is a disease predominantly of people whose life styles differ from the majority, since most persons afflicted with the disease are homosexual (gay) men or intravenous drug abusers (1)-(3).

In many parts of the United States, certain sexual activities associated with homosexuality are illegal. In all parts of the country, drug abuse is illegal and drug addicts are physically feared. Homosexuals are frequently psychologically feared. In most areas, both life styles are kept hidden. It is little wonder that AIDS is perceived as a "social disease."

Social disease used to be a euphemism for venereal disease. Today, AIDS is the euphemism that many use to express their negative social feelings toward gay men and drug addicts. AIDS is not one epidemic, but several. It is an epidemic of disease; an epidemic of fear; and epidemic of homophobia; and a media epidemic.

FEAR

A variety of events have transpired that have influenced society's response to AIDS. A national newsmagazine referred to the syndrome as the "gay plague". Public officials expressed a need to control the disease rapidly before it "spread to the rest of us!" Victims of the syndrome were referred to as the four H's: homosexuals, heroin users, hemophiliacs, and Haitians. Rock Hudson admitted he had AIDS. Much publicity was given to the isolation of the virus from tears and saliva. Claims were made that the blood test was not accurate; that HIV infection was spreading rapidly through the heterosexual community; that prostitution was a major source of transmission. All too frequently, the well documented epidemiologic data and other facts about the syndrome have not been highlighted or have been ignored. These factors led to an epidemic of proclaimed fear.

Despite the strong epidemiological evidence that the virus is limited to the well-defined risk groups and that transmission occurs either perinatally, through sexual intercourse with an infected person, or by injection of infected blood, extreme public expressions of fear have been made. This fear has been strongly vocalized by only selected segments of the population, but, nevertheless, has received much attention in the media.

Parents picketing in Queens, N.Y. in protest of a healthy child attending school, prison guards wearing masks on a ward on which there is a prisoner with AIDS, sanitation workers refusing to collect garbage at hospitals, are all images that have been pictured in the press as manifestations of this fear of AIDS. But behind these outward manifestations, were different motivating forces at work? The parents resided in a local school district that had long been battling a central Board of Education over many issues. The prison guards were involved in contract negotiations at the time of their protest against AIDS and sanitation workers are notoriously unrecognized as valued members of society. Were the actions of these groups the manifestations of their fear of AIDS alone, or was AIDS used as a manifestation of an underlying discontent? Was the media attention to these events a true reflection of the public's concerns regarding AIDS, or did it stimulate as much fear as it reported?

Yet, fear of AIDS for those who are truly at risk is clearly warranted, for the disease has taken the lives of thousands of previously healthy individuals. This fear of AIDS, along with an understanding of the mechanism of transmission, has stimulated logical behavioral changes. The incidence of sexually transmitted diseases among gay men (gonorrhea and syphilis) has decreased markedly in the last few years. This is an indication that most gay men are well aware that AIDS is associated with specific sexual practices and that risk reduction and "safer sex" have been adopted as a gay cultural norm. The stock-piling of one's own blood prior to elective surgery was also a logical indication of people's recognition that blood transfusions play a role in the transmission of the disease. However, fear was used by entrepreneurs to establish commercial operations that led to unnecessary and expensive stock-piling of blood for emergencies that might never occur. Concern among women about the possible drug use or bisexual behavior of their sexual partners (without a similar degree of concern by males), is further evidence that the public knows the basic epidemiology of AIDS, and many people are taking steps to protect themselves against its spread.

Homophobia is an emotion that is most often masked by a public outcry about AIDS, and it is prevalent throughout the United States. AIDS has provided a new avenue for expression of prejudice and hostility against the gay population. As recently as December 1985, one of the authors of this chapter was criticized by a radio commentator for allowing "perverts" to receive public assistance for the disease "that they brought upon themselves through their perverted and disgusting sexual acts."

The underlying "ultimate solution" in the minds of many has been to segregate or exclude from contact with the "general" population all people with AIDS and those who may be at risk for AIDS. While this call for quarantine may be based on a concern for public health, it is inextricably related to a misunderstanding of the disease and fear of those who are at risk.

QUARANTINE AND EXCLUSIONS

The advent of a new infectious disease always brings forth the call for quarantine: Marburg disease, Lassa fever and now AIDS. (The victims of Legionnaire's disease were spared this threat because they were either dead, recovered or thought to be suffering from a toxic exposure.)

How has the call for quarantine or exclusion been seen in the 1980's? It has been manifested during the AIDS era by the use of unnecessarily strict isolation procedures for people with AIDS in hospitals; by court attendants wearing masks and gloves during legal proceedings involving persons with AIDS; by movements to centralize treatment in a single "AIDS hospital" (but "Not in my neighborhood!"); by closure of bath-houses frequented by gays; and by the exclusion of children with AIDS from school. Public leaders have struggled to keep those who would isolate AIDS patients from practicing social ostracism in the name of public health. Appeals to reason have not, however, overcome a vocal segment of the public who wait to take action on the basis of their fear, lack of understanding of the disease or prejudice.

The State of New York ordered bath-houses closed, although their attendance was already markedly diminished. At that time, the argument made by the City of New York Department of Health to resist this, concentrated on the scientific facts: closing bath houses is a form of quarantine and quarantine has never worked.

Historically, infectiousness prior to the appearance of the signs and symptoms of a disease, or inapparent infection, has always defeated attempts to control outbreaks by isolation and quarantine. These are the factors that continue the spread of AIDS.

Quarantine may not work, but it does demonstrate some action. Public officials often believe that by doing something, they will be fulfilling their responsibilities. It is very difficult for an official to say "I don't know". It is even more difficult, but more courageous to do nothing. The data clearly show that not responding to calls for quarantine does not cause medical harm. Applied as some would have had, quarantine measures do violate the rights of individuals, and can damage society. In the case of AIDS, it may also inhibit true prevention efforts.

The prevention strategy relates to human behavior. Education can alter human behavior, governmental edicts can not. Public health is understanding, not policing. In recent decades, public health policing has been replaced by public health education. Continued transmission of the virus depends on human behavior which can and should be addressed by large educational efforts.

The Democratic National Policy Committee of Lyndon LaRouche would control AIDS with a barbed wire fence and padlock. New York City fought against the quarantine mentality. New York City officials refused to provide the names of newly reported cases to the federal government and have fought against indiscriminate testing for HIV antibody. The New York City Department of Health developed the trust of "populations at risk" (2). This trust allowed the city to work with individuals, rather than manage them.

Another type of exclusion, prevalent in many communities, is that of prohibiting children with AIDS from attending public school. This attempt has extended to children whose parents may have AIDS and to children suspected of living in the same house as a drug user or gay man.

As in the days of the struggle for equal opportunity for education, children have been the symbol of the struggle against discrimination. The public hysteria generated by children suspected of having AIDS attempting to attend school, was without scientific basis. Several studies have been conducted that show that AIDS is not transmitted between siblings in the same family. Health care workers caring for AIDS patients have not developed AIDS or even evidence of infection as manifested by the HIV antibody test. There is no evidence that air, food or the environment play a role in transmission.

Infected children are in school, some known, some unknown. In New York, after lengthy deliberation, the court ruled that the City had acted appropriately in allowing a child with AIDS to attend classes, since there was no evidence that this would endanger others. Yet in Indiana, after it was determined that a child with AIDS should go to school, there was a boycott and another law suit. The only apparent difference was that anonymity had been maintained in New York and not in Indiana. In the face of misunderstanding, hysteria and prejudice, the rights of individuals must be protected against forced exclusion.

Insurance, both life and health, have become issues in the past year (4). Treatment for AIDS is expensive, and health insurers are claiming this to be a hardship, seeking ways to either exclude from enrollment persons who may be at risk of AIDS, or adopting stringent standards for pre-existing conditions (5). Since most health insurance is written for groups rather than individuals, it is always difficult for the insurance industry to identify individuals at risk of large expenditures, but there have been highly publicized examples of denial of claims on the basis of pre-existing disease for AIDS patients if an individual has had previous care for any non-specific illness.

Life insurance, on the other hand, lends itself to screening out individuals at risk. HIV antibody testing is being used as one means of doing this. Since it is routine for some type of physical or laboratory examination to be conducted prior to insuring an individual, use of the HIV antibody test may not be unreasonable. However, with the remaining uncertainty of risk of disease after the discovery of a positive serologic test, AIDS does not lend itself to the usual rating process of the insurance industry.

In the absence of effective treatment or specific prevention, control of HIV infection is at best tenuous. Prevention of infection in the at-risk population can only be accomplished by advice, not by action (6). Those who propose to do otherwise not only will violate the rights of the individual, but will not succeed in protecting the public.

COMMUNICATION

Communication is all important in interpreting public policy. Criticism of the press and electronic media was strident in the first years of the AIDS epidemic--mostly from the gay community who felt that because the disease was predominantly affecting them, it was not considered worthy of coverage.

Whatever the reason, their criticism of lack of press attention was warranted. The New York Times Index carries only one mention of the disease in 1982. Compare that with the extended coverage given to Barney Clark, the recipient of the first artificial heart. A similar criticism could be made of lack of sensitivity by the press in the early days of reporting -- use of the term, "gay plague", exemplifies this point.

But these are usual criticisms that will be leveled against the press for any coverage or lack there of. Is this a generic communication problem that is exemplified by the current epidemic?

A recent Gallup poll revealed that over 80 percent of the public (including adolescents) knew that AIDS was not spread by casual contact, and that it was most prevalent in the gay community and among drug users; however, a majority (66%) still feared that it would spread throughout the general population.

The poll was taken just as the headlines were proclaiming that tears could "transmit" HIV infection. Press attention to preliminary findings of uncertain significance, like this, has fueled the public's fear of the unknown -- and caused undue concern and panic, at times taking attention away from the real areas of concern regarding AIDS. It is of little wonder that the public is confused (7).

Who speaks nationally for public health? The President? The Secretary of Health and Human Services? The Assistant Secretary of Health? The Public Health Service agency heads? The individual scientist in the Public Health Service? All of them rightly so. But when each interprets the public significance of critical health issues differently, it is understandable that the public becomes distrustful of national leadership.

The Public Health Service in the Fall of 1985 recommended that children be allowed to attend school if they had AIDS, but did not have manifestations of the disease that would preclude their adjusting to a school environment (8). The President of the United States publicly ignored these recommendations.

A great communicator tells the people what they want to hear. A great leader would tell the people what they need to hear. The President expressed his worry for the parents of well children. The Mayor of New York, when his panel recommended the admission of children with AIDS to school, publicly supported the recommendation.

SOCIAL ISSUES AROUND TESTING FOR HIV ANTIBODY

The test that was developed for the detection of antibody to HIV has proven a mixed blessing. It was rushed to licensure (some say to meet an over-due political time table) without the usual prelicensing testing of the system by the scientific community. It was publicly licensed in a televised press conference on a Saturday morning with the Secretary of the Department of Health and Human Services and the Commissioner of the Food and Drug Administration attempting to explain the test to the general public in highly scientific terms. The only purpose for which it was licensed was for screening of donated blood; yet immediately both the Department of Health and Human Services and the general public began demanding its expanded use.

There were and remain many misconceptions about the test. Accurate facts concerning the test include:

- The test itself does not diagnose AIDS.
- It does not measure the actual presence of the virus (antigen), as does the test used for serum hepatitis.
- The test measures the body's response to exposure (infection) with the virus.
- It does not predict disease or immunity.
- A true positive result probably equates with infectiousness.
- There is a low prevalence of false positive and false negative results.

These facts have not been easily understood by the general public unfamiliar with scientific concepts or medical terminology. All of these facts, coupled with the fear of the syndrome and its high fatality rate, make the test difficult to explain, not only to worried individuals, but also to physicians.

Initially, little was known of the results that would be obtained using the test in a non-infected population, such as would be expected at blood donation centers. Almost all of the prelicensing studies had been conducted in population groups with a high prevalence of infection--gay men and drug abusers. Yet, over-night, it was expected that the test would be applicable to all donations, and with the intention that any blood testing positive would be rejected. Ethical issues were immediately encountered.

Should individuals be told they were being tested? In New York City, it was decided that an individual not only had to be told, but that informed consent would be required before administering the test. The consent, however, was a general one and in the crush of the donation process, it is questionable whether the majority of donors realized the implications.

The blood banking community feared that many people who were in high risk groups (gay men, in particular) would use the blood banks as a means of determining their antibody status. Fearing that some of these would have a false negative test result, and thereby jeopardize the safety of the blood supply, efforts were made to discourage people in risk groups from attending blood collection facilities and to provide "alternative test sites" for people who wanted to know their serologic status.

Most gay leaders discouraged gay men from being tested believing that the test results would be of little benefit and great potential harm. It was argued that a gay man should not use his serologic status to guide his personal life. Safer sexual practices (primarily the avoidance of anal intercourse) should be practiced whether infected or not. Many gay leaders argued that beyond the psychological damage the antibody results would cause, results of testing might not remain confidential and the information could be used to discriminate against an infected individual. In fact, insurance companies are increasingly demanding the results of testing, some state health departments are developing "lists" of infected individuals, and employers are reluctant to hire antibody positive, yet well, individuals.

Because of these ramifications, the Department of Health in New York adopted stringent controls on testing. Initially, no clinical laboratory, other than blood banks and the Department of Health was licensed to perform the test. A physician who wished to have the test performed on a patient not only had to provide evidence of a signed informed consent, but also had to state that the potential liabilities of the test were discussed with the person. All tests were performed without identifying information in the Department of Health Laboratory and results provided to the physician. The Department of Health, as well as the blood banks, used a second method of testing (Western blot analysis) to add greater specificity to the test. Reports were returned to the physician who submitted the specimen to be tested, and included with the results was interpretive educational material for the doctor and the patient. The physician was encouraged to refer the patient to a Department of Health "hot-line" established for the purpose of giving information on the blood test.

Through these measures, the confidentiality of the patient was ensured, and a strenuous effort was made to make sure the individual understood the ramifications of the test. This technique also prevented the development of a list of persons with a positive blood test, which many feared could be used for discriminatory purposes.

A major problem has been to decide what information and advice to give people who test positive, since there is limited accurate information on the natural history of asymptomatic HIV infection. However, it must be assumed that a positive blood test indicates potential infectivity for others. In the absence of hard data to predict the likelihood of risk by specific sexual activity, or the probability of transmission to unborn children, prevention messages must be somewhat general and inclusive of many potential risks - resulting in a list of "don'ts" for people at risk.

With so many thorny and unanswered questions, society can be thankful that it appears that there are very few false positive reactions if ELISA positive samples are also tested by the Western blot technique. Most of the very few positive reactors identified through blood donations, have been in risk groups, and valuable experience has been gained in counseling them. Concern has been expressed over the psychological impact that notification of a positive test might have on an individual in a non-risk group. Some studies are in progress to document adverse effects and to determine modes of infection in newly discovered seropositive individuals.

An openly stated fear among gay men is that the blood test will be used as a surrogate test for homosexuality. The action of the U.S. Department of Defense in mandating HIV testing for all service-men (initially just rew recruits, but rapidly expanded to all), has made this fear real, not just theoretical. Homosexuality is a reason for discharge with less than honorable status in the US Armed Forces, as is drug abuse.

The military has offered "scientific" explanations for requiring testing such as: if a person had a depressed immune system they might respond adversely to live virus vaccines, such as smallpox; all service men are walking blood donors, and battle field conditions would preclude pretransfusion testing. It is generally believed that these reasons were less than candid, and that the test provides a mechanism by which the military may prevent gay men from entering the service or discharge them, if already members.

Following the military's implementation of the program of testing recruits, further disinformation was disseminated. Percentages of reactors have been published, but with no knowledge of the risk group status of the reactors. It is blindly assumed that the increasing percentages with age is an indication of heterosexual spread. A more tenable argument could be advanced that this pattern reflects an increasing exposure over time to drug abuse or homosexuality among military applicants or personnel. The experience of the New York City counseling service supports this hypothesis, since all the rejected military applicants who have called the hotline, have volunteered some history of risk taking behavior (exclusive of heterosexual sex).

These fears about the misuse of the antibody test were intensified by the action of some State Health Departments, and the threats from certain legislatures, to mandate the reporting of all positive reactors by name, so that lists could be maintained. As in the military, arguments for these actions have been questioned. For example, one state claims it needs the list to educate the seropositive individuals. In most areas the testing physician or health department has the responsibility for educating at the time of the test, and at the reporting of the results, thereby a third party should not be necessary.

GOVERNMENTAL RESPONSE

A basic social issue in a situation as complex as the current epidemic is the role of government in responding to the problem. Was it too little, too late, irresponsible or irresponsive? The government's response to AIDS must further be questioned to determine if the disease's emergence as a disease among gay men colored the response.

Could studies on epidemiology have been speeded or bettered? The basic facts of risk and transmission were described within a year of the recognition of the entity.

Could the etiologic agent have been isolated sooner? The putative agent was isolated within a year and a half--only the second time a retrovirus had been associated with human disease.

Could the disease have been controlled earlier? It is still not controlled but what sexually transmitted disease has been controlled without an adequate treatment? Only the small number of cases transmitted through blood transfusion has been controlled. How successful has society been in controlling or preventing narcotic addiction?

All of the above are resource dependent. Did the government make enough resources available? Resources are not just money "now", but the prior investment made in the science base.

The delineation of risk groups and modes of transmission, i.e., the epidemiology, was based on the techniques and resources pioneered by the Centers for Disease Control Epidemic Intelligence Service working with organized health departments in states and cities. The clinical and immunological descriptions of the disease were the result of work supported in the past by the National Cancer Institute, the National Institute for Allergy and Infectious Diseases, the National Institute for Alcoholism and Mental Disorders, and a host of other National Institutes. The cell lines used at the Pasteur Institute to isolate HIV were developed at the National Canter Institute prior to the advent of AIDS. ELISA technology was developed for parasitology. And so forth.

Could more money sooner have helped? Perhaps, but it could not have cloned the intellectual capacities that were brought to bear on the problem.

Many reports have recommended that the Director of the National Institutes of Health have discretionary funds available for situations such as the sudden appearance of AIDS. Would these funds have speeded research into the etiology and fundamental knowledge of the disease process, or would they have helped protect on-going research activities threatened by budget restrictions? Of course, any administrator would welcome the concept of discretionary funds, but most public administrators would prefer to have the ability to hire above an arbitrary personnel ceiling.

Perhaps a more valid criticism could be leveled at the response in public health education. This criticism can be leveled at not just the Federal government, but also most state and local authorities, except in San Francisco.

Was this discrimination against gays, or was it concern about a potential back lash if governmental monies were used to discuss explicit homosexual practices? If it were not clear that the latter was a concern, note the 400+ to 8 vote in the House of Representatives authorizing the Surgeon General to close gay bath houses, the attempts to limit Federal funds to those communities that have not closed bath houses, and the decision of the Federal government not to fund contracts that discuss explicit sexual activities, which are the basic methods of transmission of the HIV virus in the gay community.

It is not just a question of passing through governmental funds to community agencies. The issue appears to be, to what extent should tax-payer funds be used to tacitly condone practices which in many areas are illegal, and to many distasteful. A strange communication pattern has developed making it permissible for public officials to talk about anal intercourse, "fisting" and "rimming," but not all right to use public funds to support written or visual material dealing with the same activities.

On balance, scientific response has been excellent--both in terms of governmental support and actions of the scientific community. In major metropolitan areas hard hit by AIDS, scientists have demonstrated a selfless approach to AIDS that puts to shame the skeptics who believed that publish or perish is supreme. Inter-university - and even more amazing, intra-university - cooperation and sharing has been the hallmark and has shown that interdependence is sometimes preferable to independence in science.

Gay physicians speaking as the Physicians for Human Rights took the lead in pressing for adequate programs of counseling for gay men. Before the implications of the serologic test were widely known, this group took the unpopular stand of urging gay men not to be tested because of the potential misuse of the test. Their wisdom has been vindicated in the eyes of many people at risk.

"Sweet are the uses of adversity." AIDS has brought not just scientific cooperation to a higher plane than before, but has opened discussions and caused actions long over-due (9). A "Patient's Bill of Rights" includes the sexual orientation of the patient along with race, creed, national origin as forms of discrimination not condoned in the hospitals of New York City. Confidentiality is receiving public debate as the result of potential misuse of medical information by industry and the military. Homosexuality is now being discussed openly throughout the media and hopefully soon in the schools. The challenge for all, public and private persons, will be to make sure that these discussions are not misused to the detriment of those currently subjected to alienation and discrimination.

REFERENCES

1. Black, J.L., Dolan, M.P., DeFord, H.A., et al., Sharing of needles among users of intravenous drugs. N Engl J Med 314:446-447 (1986)

2. Chamberland, M.E., Allen, J.R., Monroe, J.M., Acquired immunodeficiency syndrome, New York City: Evaluation of an active surveillance system. JAMA254:383-387 (1985)

3. Curran, J.W., Morgan, W.M., Hardy, A.M., et al., The epidemiology of AIDS: Current status and future prospects. Science 229:1352-1357 (1985)

4. Lambda Legal Defense and Education Fund, Inc., AIDS Legal Guide. Lambda Legal Defense and Education Fund, Inc., New York, NY (1984)

5. City of New York Commission on Human Rights. The Gay and Lesbian Discrimination Documentation Project. Second Report Covering Nov. 1983 - Oct. 1985. City of New York Commission on Human Rights, New York, NY (1985)

6. Colorado Board of Health. Rules and Regulations Pertaining to Communicable Disease Control. Colorado Board of Health, Denver, Colorado (1985)

7. Diamond, E., Bellito, C.M., The great verbal cover-up. Washington Journalism Review 8:38-42 (1986)

8. CDC., Education on foster care of children infected with HTLV-III/LAV. MMWR 34:613-615 (1985)

9. Bayer, R., Oppenheimer, G., AIDS in the work place: The ethical ramifications. Business and Health Jan./Feb.:30-34 (1986)

54

Nursing Perspectives in the Care of Patients with AIDS: Experience from the AIDS Unit of the San Francisco General Hospital

Cliff Morrison

The first impact of what was to come with the acquired immunodeficiency syndrome (AIDS) was beginning to be felt in San Francisco in 1982. At first, there was uneasiness, anxiety and, at times, near panic among health care professionals. In many instances the new problems and issues were dealt with using an enormous amount of denial. Even today, despite the proliferation of factual information on AIDS, it is interesting to note that in many areas these reactions persist. Although the issues surrounding AIDS are complex, close examination may bring them into clearer focus for the individual health care provider. These concerns include the illness itself, factors related to contagiousness, a number of issues concerning sexuality and, most importantly, death and dying. Creation of an optimal environment for caring for persons with AIDS requires that these issues be addressed and that effective approaches for dealing with them be developed.

HEALTH CARE DELIVERY FOR AIDS PATIENTS

From the beginning, AIDS was disquieting because in part it forced examination of the inefficient delivery of health care. Issues in health care that had been suppressed for years began to emerge. AIDS has provided a perfect opportunity to begin to look at the delivery of health care and how it can be improved and made more efficient.

Institutions that are serving a significant number of persons with AIDS should have an organized plan of action to deal effectively with patients who have the disease and the pertinent psychosocial issues surrounding this illness. Each health care institution and system will have to examine its needs and resources, and more importantly, that of the community or population that it serves. Institutions caring for small numbers of persons with AIDS (a daily census of less than 10 inpatients) may be able to use their present organizational structures. Institutions and systems that are serving larger numbers, or where health care delivery issues are especially complex, may have to develop new programs or approaches to provide the level of care needed for this group of patients.

An individual designated to coordinate AIDS activities can be a tremendous asset for an institution. Such an AIDS coordinator can assist patients with educational and psychosocial issues and help to identify and interconnect with existing support systems within an institution or community. At the same time, a coordinator can provide assistance to the medical and nursing staff in areas of infection control, education, patient care, and dealing with concerns surrounding sexuality and death and dying. A Clinical Nurse Specialist is particularly suited for this assignment, based on the educational and clinical preparation for that position.

If an institution is treating larger numbers of persons with AIDS (10 to 20 inpatients at a time), it may need to develop an AIDS resource team. A resource or consult team offers major advantages when larger numbers of patients are dispersed throughout a major facility. Ideally, this team should be multidisciplinary in structure and should include a nurse, social worker, counselor and representatives from other disciplines as necessary. The team will need to coordinate with physicians, individual nursing units where the patients are located, and various hospital departments and community resources.

DEVELOPING SPECIALIZED UNITS FOR THE CARE OF AIDS PATIENTS

For institutions that are caring for even larger numbers of persons with AIDS (a daily census of more than 20 inpatients), the question of whether or not a specialized nursing care unit is needed, is raised. Some institutions have designated existing units to care for these patients. This can be successful if there is full participation of the staff already on a designated unit in planning and program development. An orientation program for members of that particular unit will be a necessity with ongoing educational programs and support groups for the staff. It will be important for the unit leadership to be very well informed and be genuinely committed for this approach to be successful. Staff that do not want to work with AIDS patients on a regular basis may have the option of transferring to another unit. However, the decision to offer this option should be examined closely because of future repercussions for the institution.

A second approach is to develop a specialized nursing care unit specifically for the treatment of persons with AIDS. In early 1983, San Francisco General Hospital designated a Clinical Nurse Specialist in the role of Clinical AIDS Coordinator for the institution. Responsibilities included: daily visits to all AIDS patients to assess their needs and to connect them to support systems in the community; education of the nursing staff in regard to issues concerning the care of individual patients; coordination with physicians; and facilitation of better communication for all the hospital staff. However, within a short period of time, the responsibilities of this position became impractical since the average daily census grew to 10 to 12 patients dispersed throughout the institution.

An inpatient unit for treatment of persons with AIDS was considered. The task of planning and setting up this unit was given to the Department of Nursing under the direction of the Clinical AIDS Coordinator. The coordinator began to discuss centralizing resources in the institution, developing clinical expertise and attempting to create a unit whose primary goal would be to "demystify" AIDS-related issues for the institution. The unit would not be an isolation unit, but instead a unit for specialized care. There was some skepticism regarding this approach. Some felt that a specialized unit would be stigmatized from the beginning. Patients would not want to be on a unit designated for AIDS. Recruitment of personnel would be difficult, if not impossible, and retention of staff would be difficult. There was fear that the community itself would not support the idea because it would be looked on as a "leper" colony. It was also believed that medical staff might shun the unit and not want to see patients located there. Plans went ahead, however, and each of the areas of concern was dealt with using proper planning, education and involvement from patients and the different agencies and organizations in the community that were attempting to provide services (1).

For an institution, or a department of nursing, that is planning to set up a specialized unit for the care of persons with AIDS, the selection of staff will be the single most important part of the process. At San Francisco General Hospital the Clinical AIDS Coordinator was the person responsible for planning and establishing the unit. The first task was to recruit qualified staff that could deal with all of the biopsychosocial issues surrounding a group of acutely ill young patients facing a life-threatening illness. Selection criteria were developed that included two years of clinical experience in an acute care setting with preference given to individuals with medical, oncology, critical care, hospice or psychiatric experience. Applicants were to be in a good general state of physical and emotional health, without unrealistic fears of contracting AIDS. Applicants were also asked if they would be willing to participate in health screening. Each person was rated on their ability to communicate and express feelings, demonstrate sensitivity to the needs of the critically ill, show acceptance of alternative lifestyles, discuss issues and feelings concerning dying, death with dignity, suicide, and discuss openly sexual issues (sexual preference or orientation was not a consideration). Each person was asked about their own support systems. Willingness to participate in staff support groups and discuss their emotional concerns openly, as well as their feelings about dealing with the media were considered. Women of child bearing age were asked to consult employee health or their personal physician. (This is no longer an issue).

Recruitment notices were posted in various areas of the hospital as well as in other institutions. Approximately 65 inquiries were received and 35 nurses were interviewed individually in information sessions. During the information session each applicant received a list of the qualifications needed for the position and a list of the issues to be discussed. Each person was asked to acknowledge in writing that they received the information. The discussion with each applicant focused on three critical concerns: comfort with one's sexuality, fears of contagion, and the ability to provide care for a person with AIDS. Applicants were told to take five days to think about the position and to discuss it with their families, roommates, significant others, etc. before making a decision. Salaries were discussed, as well as the fact that there would not be a special differential or incentive pay. The Clinical AIDS Coordinator worked closely with the union representing the nurses in establishing the unit.

After staff selection, individualized orientation programs were developed to meet the needs of each person. For example, some nurses went through orientation programs that lasted up to three months on medical units where patients with AIDS were being cared for. In addition, before the unit opened, an orientation program one week in length was conducted for the entire staff. During this orientation week classes were given on basic information on AIDS, epidemiology, immunology, infectious diseases (particularly the opportunistic infections), communication skills and group process, psychological and spiritual needs of patients, chemotherapy, infection control guidelines, death, dying and grieving, nutritional needs and primary nursing. Staff members were encouraged to examine their roles critically and to learn to recognize their own barriers to good communication with their patients (1).

The Special Care Unit for treatment of persons with AIDS at the San Francisco General Hospital (Ward 5B) opened in July of 1983. Since that time the staff have learned that they can conduct themselves in a professional manner, and at the same time be very caring and compassionate for their patients, becoming involved and sharing in their grief process (2). The support systems for the staff proved to be effective after management learned to let the staff control their own support groups. The staff of the Special Care Unit has grown professionally since the unit opened. They now take responsibility, with their head nurse and the clinical nurse specialist, in developing most of the policies and procedures relative to their area of specialty.

From a management standpoint, the Specialized Care Unit has

been a total success. In January 1986, the original 12 bed unit was closed and a new 20 bed unit was opened utilizing the same planning and orientation process. The unit has a very low attrition rate among the nursing staff, which, in itself, is a major cost savings. The nursing staff on the Special Care Unit have become the nursing experts in their clinical area. It was the responsibility of management to do the planning and to establish the unit, but it has been the nursing staff that have made it a success. It has been asked time and again why there is no "burnout" on this unit. Burnout, if it exists at all, generally occurs because staff are frustrated and feel that they are in a situation in which they have very little input or control (3). The staff of the Special Care Unit do express frustation, but they have a great deal of control over their work environment and what is happening to them and their patients. Working with this group of patients can be extremely stressful and emotionally draining for the nurse, but at the same time, both rewarding and fulfilling.

Staff members have become increasingly involved with AIDS-related issues outside of the immediate confines of the Special Care Unit. Many of the nursing staff serve on various committees throughout the hospital. Almost all are involved in some area of community work and many do public speaking. Some are writing about their experiences and others are involved in nursing research on AIDS. These experiences help in the constant process of reevaluating and upgrading the clinical program of the unit.

Creating an entirely new unit for the care of patients with AIDS has many additional positive aspects. A specialized unit for care of patients with a specific disease provides a setting where research can be done in a controlled environment. In this particular instance, working with a patient population that is very young and also willing to participate in research provides an opportunity for not only medical research, but also nursing research. Also, creative or novel programs may be piloted in a controlled setting before consideration of implementation in other areas of the hospital.

For success of such a unit, communication among all staff members has to be made a priority. Formal and informal discussions occur regularly. Nursing case conferences are presented on a regular basis. In addition, a weekly patient care conference is held where all members of the staff from the outpatient clinic and the inpatient unit are invited to discuss current treatment and patient care issues. Nurses are encouraged to participate in the physicians' rounds as well as in the daily nurse/counselor rounds. Nursing staff attend the weekly discharge planning meeting to assist in that process as well as attend regular staff meetings where all staff are encouraged to discuss current issues that are of the most importance to them. Most importantly, the staff are encouraged to attend their support groups on a regular basis.

The staff realize the importance of continuity and consistency in their approach, especially for infection control issues. The infection control coordinator and the infection control committee assist in constantly evaluating and reassessing infection control issues. Another area where communication must be ongoing is with issues concerning death and dying. Staff communicate with patients about death on a continuing basis, as well as work with families through this process.

OVERCOMING FEARS AND PREJUDICES OF HEALTH CARE PERSONNEL

One specific issue that needed to be addressed from the beginning was that of dealing with sexuality. Individuals as well as society are uncomfortable with this issue. Most health care professionals did not receive any formal instruction on this subject. To provide care effectively, it is important to view patients from a perspective above and beyond a specific disease entity (4). An individual's sexuality is often as important to the person as all other aspects of life. Consequently, it is desirable for health care providers to be able to discuss issues of sexuality, in relationship to a patient's illness, in a comfortable and non-judgemental manner. Much of the hysteria and misinformation related to sexuality have to do with the myths and stereotypes surrounding homosexuality (5). It is important to recognize that everyone in this culture has some level of homophobia, the unrealistic fear of homosexuality (1). Overcoming such prejudices requires open and frank discussions, which can be very threatening to health care personnel unless approached in a well-structured format.

Perhaps the issues surrounding AIDS causing the most hysteria to health care workers are those of death, dying and grieving, a subject that historically has been dealt with poorly (6). Our youth-oriented society uses massive denial when it comes to the issue of death. Realization that young people are dying, forces young health care professionals to come to grips with their own mortality. This in itself is probably the most threatening and difficult task for the medical community (7). Patients that have a terminal illness and are dying, in most instances, need more care than patients who are not, particularly nursing care (8). It is imperative not to abandon such patients, nor for the nursing staff, in providing care, to communicate less with the patient, or to have less hands-on contact. It is important to realize that an individual's actions convey a message to the patient. Absence of a cure is not tantamount to having nothing more to offer. In this situation care rather than cure is the issue. As health care professionals, and particularly as nurses, there is a responsibility and a commitment to provide the highest quality care possible for all patients, regardless of their race, religion, sex, sexual orientation, diagnosis and prognosis. Nurses cannot selectively decide for whom they are going to provide care. Discussions with peers or with counselors may help in dealing with biases and prejudices and permit more effective delivery of health care. It is necessary to recognize one's feelings and then attempt to deal with them.

MAINTAINING THE DIGNITY AND INDEPENDENCE OF AIDS PATIENTS

Caring for persons with AIDS means dealing with a group of patients that are young, articulate, and used to being independent. Many of these patients in San Francisco are from a middle class background, are well educated and many, despite the homosexual stereotype are assertive.

Entry into a chronic care outpatient program with the likely possibility of repeated hospitalizations places new stresses on AIDS patients. All too frequently, the hospital is a cold, sterile, and authoritarian environment. Patients are expected to adapt to a novel situation at a time when their ability to adapt has been severely impaired. It is important for all patients to be oriented to their environment, but with the chronically ill patient an orientation program from the time of entry into a treatment program will make diagnostic procedures and therapies easier to deal with later on. A simple medical and administrative booklet that explains procedures and other routine aspects of the medical care may be of great service. In addition, through conversations with the patient an attempt should be made to answer basic questions and discuss the availability of assorted services. A directed tour of the facility with introductions to staff members with whom there will be later contact is also very helpful. All these measures help to lessen the patient's level of anxiety. They can be done by nursing or counseling staff but can also be handled effectively by patient groups themselves (9).

Control is a major issue for all patients, but particularly for the young and terminally ill patient; control may be all that the individual has left. It is important to educate patients about their illness, their bodies and the aspects of care that will affect them directly. Education should be to the level that the patients can understand or wish to understand. An educated patient is able to maintain some level of control (10). Some patients will not want control and will readily relinquish it to the health care professional. If the patient chooses to do this, it is his privilege, and at the same time he is maintaining some level of control by making this decision. Also the level of anxiety for patients can be lessened through education and by involvement in their own care and in decision making processes.

One of the most important and controversial aspects in educating patients and involving them in their own care is in assisting them in setting medical and treatment parameters. It is extremely important in this process that the patients be provided adequate support in making decisions that are best for them. Psychosocial support is a major need in this situation because of the nature of the illness. Health care providers need to be objective and understanding in assisting the patient. In providing information, care must be taken not to coerce the patient, while at the same time giving support to whatever decisions that they make (11). At San Francisco General Hospital there has been an enormous amount of cooperation and compliance with treatment among the AIDS patient population. Patients appear to do better because they feel better about themselves and because they have maintained some control over their own lives. Health care providers need the cooperation of the patient to combat this disease. Epidemiologist Andrew Moss at San Francisco General Hospital's AIDS Outpatient Clinic stated recently, "The antiviral therapies that the world is waiting for are going to be tested in clinical trials on sick gay men, and the prevention trials, if we manage to get them started, will be done only with the support of seropositive gay men. And the vaccine, when it comes, like the hepatitis B vaccine, will probably be tested with the cooperation and assistance of gay men. Isn't it ironic that the cure and the prevention that the whole world is waiting for are going to come only with the support of its first and most stigmatized group of victims?" (12)

INVOLVEMENT OF THE FAMILY

A major issue in dealing with AIDS patients is how to include the family. Traditional definitions of family may not be what the patients themselves see as their family. Of course, this pertains not only to AIDS patients but to all patients. The idea of the traditional nuclear family in America is different today. Allowing patients to define family, and to designate a "significant other", gives them control over an important aspect of their life, and demonstrates that the health care profession is willing to accept them as individuals. In many instances a patient may designate a "significant other" that is a family member, for others it may be a close friend, roommate, or a lover. When a patient designates a "significant other", that individual can be included in the educational process. This not only gives the patient additional support but also gets the "family" member involved. Loved ones often feel helpless and left out, in this way the "significant other" can feel that they are making a contribution also. The feedback from patients and "significant others" to this approach has been positive. This approach helps to remove issues of guilt and fear and allows patients to concentrate on other concerns such as quality of life and the ability to maintain independence for as long as possible.

DISCHARGE PLANNING

The focus in the treatment setting should be on making the patient as independent as possible and not fostering dependence. It has been the experience at San Francisco General Hospital that this youthful patient population wants to be independent and will work with the system to stay out of the acute care setting. Therefore, from the beginning, including the patient and the family member, or "significant other", in the planning process allows the focus to be on shortening the length of stay. Discharge planning is one of the most important components of any coordinated program (13). An approach that focuses on developing a trusting relationship is a critical step for starting the discharge planning process. However, it is important to remember that the experiences of this group of patients with the health care system have generally been very negative. Therefore, it is the care providers' responsibility to initiate the basic trusting relationship.

In providing care for the patient with AIDS and in proper discharge planning, it will be important for those responsible for resource management to develop formal as well as informal relationships with outside agencies (14). Formal relationships will generally be with the more traditional agencies and organizations such as Public Health Nursing, Visiting Nurse Association, Home Health Care Agencies and Hospice. Hospice care can be an enormous asset to both the patient and the entire health care organization. Not all patients will be suitable for or be accepting of hospice care, but for those that are, hospice can coordinate their care very effectively in the community (15). The informal relationships are generally with the volunteer groups in the community, whose availability is generally dependent on the size of the community involved. These organizations can provide numerous low cost or free resources, but the referring institution has the responsibility for making the appropriate links and for networking with the different groups and organizations. In San Francisco, a large part of the success of the city wide AIDS program has been due to the fact that the organized health care system has made an effort to work directly with the community. There are enormous energies and resources to be tapped in all communities and allowing this kind of involvement enables the health care system to better educate the community concerning AIDS-related issues. Health care systems will have to learn to deal directly with the different aspects of the communities that they are serving. They can not operate separately and expect to contain costs and maintain quality care in the future (16).

Utilization of volunteers from the community can also be helpful in the institutional setting. There are many benefits to this; the most important are maintaining the trust of the community and cost containment. Since working with volunteer groups and agencies can be time consuming, it is usually appropriate to have one individual designated to coordinate volunteer services and work closely with the hospital administration to ensure that volunteers are properly oriented and closely supervised. A central AIDS coordinating office for large communities with many different services, organizations and agencies is a cost-effective means of establishing appropriate connections and eliminating duplication of services (9).

THE ROLE OF NURSING IN THE CARE OF AIDS PATIENTS

AIDS is causing the nursing profession to reexamine its role in health care. Traditionally for nurses, the primary role has been that of patient advocate which is clearly a need for the AIDS patient. AIDS is perhaps more of a nursing illness than any disease that has been seen in recent history. At this time modern medicine is limited in what it can offer persons with AIDS, yet these patients require an enormous amount of nursing care. As patient advocates, nurses and the nursing profession have to take more of a leadership role in the issues surrounding the disease. One thing that is being learned from the AIDS experience in San Francisco is how important it is for nurses to become more politically involved. Nurses need to learn to network and to communicate directly with the political systems in their various communities. AIDS is forcing all of health care, but particularly nursing, to become much more involved in political systems, legal issues and interactions with the mass media.

Nursing professionals have an enormous responsibility for staying informed and up-to-date on the most important issues for their practice. A large portion of nursing care involves education of patients, their families, and others in the community. All health care professionals are role models, but physicians and nurses have the greatest responsibility because of their visibility, both within medical institutions, and in the community. Providing education is an enormous responsibility which must not be jeopardized by nonprofessional behavior.

In the institutional setting, patient satisfaction is due in large part to nursing. It is with the nurse that the patient has the greatest contact and communication. Nursing is one discipline in health care that always attempts to care for all aspects of the patient's needs. Other disciplines tend to look at patients in terms of their diagnosis, symptoms, a specific system or in relationship to accomplishing a specific task. The concept of primary care nursing has helped to eliminate the task oriented approach and is particularly suited to the care of persons with AIDS. It is the role of the nurse in primary nursing to coordinate the patient's care and to provide all of the nursing care, not just one aspect (17). This simplifies the nurse's role and makes it much clearer for the patient, with the level of satisfaction on both sides increased significantly. The patients feel a greater sense of security because they can identify the nurse as a constant person in their care. For this approach to work, good lines of communication must be established and when jurisdictional issues do arise, it is important that they be discussed. The responsibility also rests with the primary nurse to see that the pertinent issues are dealt with. The success of the interdisciplinary approach to care will be dependent upon it.

The need for psychosocial support for all patients has been identified for some time, but with AIDS it is even more essential. The nurse will have to be particularly aware and able to assess the psychosocial needs of the patient. The nurse may be an important provider in this area but the additional expertise of counselors with specific training with AIDS patients can be extremely beneficial. At this time the issues are so complex that this additional expertise is clearly necessary. It is important for the roles to be clearly delineated and for there to be open communication between the nursing and counseling staff. All the disciplines must support each other and work in collaborative relationships in providing comprehensive care to the patient.

AIDS EDUCATION

Nursing and hospital administrators have the responsibility to provide the resources needed in the patient care setting. The most important responsibility for administration is proper planning. The planning process must include input from the different disciplines, departments and community agencies. Administration also has the responsibility to educate themselves and to provide education for the hospital staff. For success of any program, it is imperative that the managerial staff have an excellent understanding of the issues (18). It is extremely important for those in leadership positions in all areas of the hospital to be role models for their staff. One of the major reasons why care for persons with AIDS is not being delivered in a coordinated and effective manner today throughout the United States is because the leadership in health care has been unable and unwilling to deal directly and up front with the issues.

AIDS education is a responsibility that is shared by all, but it is management that must provide the resources to implement the programs. One of the problems that has been encountered with AIDS education is that the educational process itself tends to be a reactive one. Over the next few years, almost every health care institution in the country will be caring for persons with AIDS. It is important to start educational programs early. Many institutions wait until they have their first AIDS patient and there is already widespread hysteria throughout the institution. Other institutions provide educational programs to staff after sensationalistic headlines appear, or misleading information has been presented in the mass media. This approach to education is inconsistent and does not work. Educational programs for AIDS have to be well planned, coordinated and ongoing. They should be consistent and build on the knowledge that has already been gained. In educating nursing staff it is important that AIDS be presented from a nursing perspective and presented within the context of the nursing process.

AIDS is a disease of the young and it is sexually transmitted. Education has the task of shifting the focus from high risk groups to high risk behaviors, particularly sexual behavior. Failure to educate the public and to learn to deal with this disease effectively could cause this society to lose an entire generation of young talented people (19).

CONCLUSIONS

The Special Care Unit at San Francisco General Hospital is a nursing model that works and one that nurses can be proud of. Well-planned, organized and coordinated programs cost less to operate. Cost can be further contained by having a satisfied professional staff with a low attrition rate. Focusing on patient centered care, education and discharge planning, effectively reduces the length of stay. At San Francisco General Hospital the average length of stay for an AIDS patient is 11.4 days, and it costs the hospital the same to treat these patients as it does any other patient. The program at San Francisco General Hospital is not perfect, but it does offer excellent care and at the same time, cost containment.

In conclusion, there is very little that is new in dealing with AIDS. All of the issues are old issues that need to be approached in a different way. Hopefully, that approach will be from a positive point of view and health care providers will feel better about themselves and their work. Almost daily the news media carries stories concerning AIDS and the issues surrounding it. Many of these stories tell of human tragedy from a compassionate and understanding viewpoint. Others tell of prejudice, discrimination and hatreds that exist throughout society. Hopefully everyone in health care and society at large will learn valuable lessons from the AIDS experience.

REFERENCES

1. Viele, C.S, Dodd, M.J., Morrison, C., Caring for acquired immune deficiency syndrome patients. Oncology Nursing Forum 11:56-60, (1984)

2. Nelson, W.J., Maxey, L, Keith, S. Are we abandoning the AIDS patient? RN Magazine 47:18-19 (1984)

3. Blainey, C.G., Six steps to personal fulfillment in nursing. Nurs Manag 16:37-38 (1985)

4. Cross, J.R., In: Nursing Theories, (Goerge, J.B., ed), Second Edition, Prentice-Hall, Englewood Cliffs, p 258-286 (1985)

5. Dakins, D.R., Guncheon, K.F., AIDS: out of the shadows. Practitioners face psychosocial dilemmas. California Physician 1:12-19 (1985)

6. Kubler-Ross, E., On Death and Dying, Macmillan, New York, p 245-257 (1969)

7. Glaser, B., Strauss, A., Awareness of Dying, Aldine Publishing Company, Chicago, p 238-239 (1975)

8. Epstein, C., Nursing the Dying Patient, Prentice-Hall, Reston, VA, p 115, (1975)

9. Morrison, C., Establishing a therapeutic environment for the care of persons with AIDS. In: The Person with AIDS: Nursing Perspectives, (Durham, G., Cohen, F., eds), Springer, New York (In press)

10. Payne, K.W., Risch, S.J., The politics of AIDS. Science for the People, p 17-24 Sept/Oct (1984)

11. Steinbrook, R., Lo, B., Tirpack, J., et al., Ethical dilemmas in caring for patients with acquired immune deficiency syndrome. Ann Intern Med 103:787-790 (1985)

12. Staver, S., Rise in AIDS among heterosexuals seen. American Medical News, p 34 (Oct, 1985)

13. Wallace, C., Hospitals must plan for increase in number of AIDS patients. Modern Healthcare, p 52-54 (Oct, 1985)

14. Clausen, C., Staff RN: A discharge planner for every patient. Nurs Manage 15:58-61 (1984)

15. Corr, C.A., Corr, D.M., Hospice Care: Principles and Practice, Springer, New York, p 280 (1983)

16. Traska, M.R., Alternate care. No home means no home care for AIDS patients. Hospitals 60:69-70 (1986)

17. Mundinger, M., Primary Nurse. Nursing Outlook 21:642-645 (1973)

18. Burda, B., Powills, S., AIDS: A time bomb at hospitals' door. Hospitals 60:54-61 (1986)

19. Greenly, M., Chronicle, the Human Side of AIDS. Irvington, New York, p 365-369 (1986)

Index